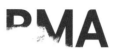

PMA

Fundamentals of Anaesthesia

Fourth Edition

Fundamentals of Anaesthesia

Fourth Edition

Edited by
Ted Lin
Department of Anaesthesia, Glenfield Hospital,
University Hospitals of Leicester NHS Trust, Leicester, UK

Tim Smith
Department of Anaesthesia, Alexandra Hospital, Worcestershire Acute Hospitals NHS Trust,
Redditch, UK

Colin Pinnock
Formerly of Department of Anaesthesia, Alexandra Hospital, Worcestershire Acute Hospitals
NHS Trust, Redditch, UK

Associate Editor
Chris Mowatt
Department of Anaesthesia, Royal Shrewsbury Hospital, Shrewsbury and Telford Hospital
NHS Trust, Shrewsbury, UK

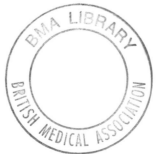

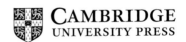
CAMBRIDGE
UNIVERSITY PRESS

CAMBRIDGE
UNIVERSITY PRESS

University Printing House, Cambridge CB2 8BS, United Kingdom

Cambridge University Press is part of the University of Cambridge.

It furthers the University's mission by disseminating knowledge in the pursuit of
education, learning and research at the highest international levels of excellence.

www.cambridge.org
Information on this title: www.cambridge.org/9781107612389

© Cambridge University Press 2017

First published by Greenwich Medical Media 1999
Second edition published 2003
Third edition published by Cambridge University Press 2009
Fourth edition published 2017

Printed in the United Kingdom by Clays, St Ives plc

A catalogue record for this publication is available from the British Library

Library of Congress Cataloging in Publication data
Names: Lin, Ted, 1945– , editor. | Smith, Tim, 1960 September 1, editor. | Pinnock,
Colin A., editor. | Mowatt, Chris, editor.
Title: Fundamentals of anaesthesia / edited by Ted Lin, Tim Smith, Colin Pinnock,
Chris Mowatt.
Description: Fourth edition. | Cambridge, United Kingdom : Cambridge University
Press, 2016. | Includes bibliographical references and index.
Identifiers: LCCN 2016000988 | ISBN 9781107612389 (pbk. : alk. paper)
Subjects: | MESH: Anesthesia | Analgesia | Analgesics–therapeutic use
Classification: LCC RD81 | NLM WO 200 | DDC 617.9/6–dc23 LC
record available at http://lccn.loc.gov/2016000988

ISBN 978-1-107-61238-9 Paperback

To our families, whose support has helped us
overcome the challenges of creating this textbook

Contents

Contributors

Rajani Annamaneni
Consultant Anaesthetist
Glenfield Hospital
Leicester, UK

Bal Appadu
Consultant Anaesthetist
Peterborough City Hospital
Peterborough, UK

Dan Bailey
Consultant Anaesthetist
Queen Elizabeth Hospital
Birmingham, UK

Gwenda Cavill
Consultant Anaesthetist
Wansbeck General Hospital
Ashington, Northumberland, UK

Mahesh Chaudhari
Consultant Anaesthetist
Worcestershire Royal Hospital
Worcester, UK

Oscar Domingo i Bosch
Consultant Anaesthetist
Alexandra Hospital
Redditch, UK

Matthew Faulds
Specialty Registrar in Anaesthetics and Intensive Care
Sheffield Teaching Hospitals NHS Foundation Trust
Sheffield, UK

Peter Featherstone
Specialty Registrar in Anaesthesia
Addenbrooke's Hospital
Cambridge, UK

Barrie Fischer
Consultant Anaesthetist
Alexandra Hospital
Redditch, UK

Smita Gohil
Consultant Anaesthetist
Warwick Hospital
Warwick, UK

Arun Gupta
Consultant in Anaesthesia and Neurointensive Care
Addenbrooke's Hospital,
Cambridge, UK

Robert Haden
Consultant Anaesthetist
Alexandra Hospital
Redditch, UK

Sue Hill
Consultant Anaesthetist
University Hospital Southampton
Southampton, UK

Jo James
Consultant Anaesthetist
Birmingham Heartlands Hospital,
Birmingham, UK

Karen Kerr
Consultant Anaesthetist
Alexandra Hospital
Redditch, UK

Ted Lin
Consultant Anaesthetist
Glenfield Hospital
Leicester, UK

Tina McLeod
Consultant Anaesthetist
Birmingham Heartlands Hospital
Birmingham, UK

Edwin Mitchell
Consultant in Anaesthesia and intensive Care
Alexandra Hospital
Redditch, UK

Nick Morgan-Hughes
Consultant Anaesthetist
Sheffield Teaching Hospitals NHS Foundation Trust
Sheffield, UK

Chris Mowatt
Consultant Anaesthetist
Royal Shrewsbury Hospital
Shrewsbury, UK

Mary Mushambi
Consultant Anaesthetist
Leicester Royal Infirmary
Leicester, UK

Jeff Neilson
Consultant in Haematology
Russells Hall Hospital
Dudley, UK

Alexander Ng
Consultant Anaesthetist and Honorary Senior Lecturer
Royal Wolverhampton Hospital NHS Trust and
University of Birmingham
West Midlands, UK

Jerry Nolan
Consultant in Anaesthesia and Intensive Care Medicine
Royal United Hospital
Bath, UK

Michael Paleologos
Staff Specialist Anaesthetist
Royal Prince Alfred Hospital
Sydney, Australia

Colin Pinnock
Formerly of Department of Anaesthesia
Alexandra Hospital
Redditch, UK

Ian Power
Professor of Anaesthesia, Critical Care and Pain Medicine
University of Edinburgh
Royal Infirmary, Edinburgh, UK

Anand Sardesai
Consultant Anaesthetist
Addenbrooke's Hospital
Cambridge, UK

Tim Smith
Consultant Anaesthetist
Alexandra Hospital,
Redditch, UK

Jim Stone
Consultant Microbiologist
Gloucestershire Royal Hospital
Gloucester, UK

Anita Stronach
Consultant Anaesthetist
Alexandra Hospital
Redditch, UK

Justiaan Swanevelder
Professor and Head of Department of Anaesthesia and
Perioperative Medicine
Groote Schuur and Red Cross War
Memorial Children's Hospitals
University of Cape Town
Cape Town, South Africa

Leon Vries
Consultant Anaesthetist
Royal Orthopaedic Hospital NHS Foundation Trust
Birmingham, UK

Andrew Wolf
Professor of Paediatric Anaesthesia and Intensive Care
University Hospitals Bristol NHS Foundation Trust,
Bristol, UK

Preface to the first edition

The advent of a syllabus for the FRCA examination, itself a requirement of the STA, seemed to me to provide an ideal opportunity for a dedicated revision textbook. It will therefore be of no surprise to readers that this volume mirrors closely the syllabus for the primary FRCA in both structure and content.

Having enlisted the willing help of my two co-editors, Tim Smith and Ted Lin, we set about recruiting authors to contribute. Chapter authors have been chosen for their ability and known prowess as teachers and a deliberate policy of not inviting 'usual' contributions from frequently seen names was taken. Having said that, several primary examiners appear as contributors and within each chapter coverage of revision topics has been kept as appropriate to the examination as possible.

To reduce the variability that is the bane of multi-author texts I have personally edited every chapter to ensure consistency of style and it is a reflection of the workload involved that it has taken three years to complete this project. I am grateful to all contributing authors for their tolerance and good humour during alteration of their golden prose.

Whilst no single book can cover the entire syllabus as a 'one stop' aid, the majority of material covered in the examination is detailed within these pages. Some items lately included in the syllabus, after completion of the manuscript, will be added in future editions (such as the anatomy pertaining to ankle block). Candidates will, however, be well served if this book is used as a general basis for revision.

I am extremely grateful to Rob Jones, who has been responsible for generating virtually all the artwork within this text, the few other diagrams being credited to their sources.

Thanks are also due to both my co-editors for their extensive work and dedication. If this volume enables any candidate to pass the primary examination, who would not have done so otherwise, then our job will have been well done.

Colin Pinnock

Preface to the second edition

I am delighted that the success of *Fundamentals* has enabled us to proceed to an early second edition. It will be apparent to the familiar reader that this edition has undergone rather more than a simple facelift. A great deal of feedback from both examiners and candidates has been used to modify and shape this current volume. New authors have been brought in to Section 1 to revise and modify the clinical chapters where necessary (incorporating several important and new areas of emerging knowledge), whilst resuscitation and trauma chapters have been updated by their original writers. Anatomy has been extended in scope to reflect subjects that are currently popular in the Primary FRCA.

In Section 2, there are new chapters on neurology and endocrinology, and an extra chapter on neonatal physiology has been incorporated to satisfy the demands of the examination syllabus.

Section 3 has been updated comprehensively with the removal of some drugs now lapsed and the incorporation of newer agents that have become available. By popular demand a new chapter on clinical trial design rounds off the pharmacology section.

It is, however, Section 4 that has undergone the most radical changes. I am very grateful to Ted Lin for the completely new physics and equipment chapters, which provide excellent core revision in these important areas. A greater number of diagrams (and many revised graphics) throughout the book and a completely new index complete the modifications over the first edition.

I thus believe that the second edition of *Fundamentals* is an even better revision aid to the Primary FRCA examination and will build on the reputation of its forerunner. Once again my thanks go to my three co-editors for their hard work and determination.

Colin Pinnock

Preface to the third edition

I am privileged to have led the creation of the third edition of this popular Primary FRCA text, ably helped by my three co-editors. Once again, feedback from users of the book has helped enormously in developing *FoA3*. The Royal College of Anaesthetists' publication of the Primary syllabus within the Competency-based Training Framework has led us to include that knowledge base, uniquely referenced to *Fundamentals*, in a new Appendix. A number of new contributors have enhanced the proportion of current and past examiners amongst our writers. The greater use of colour allows the reader to navigate more easily, and changes to technique boxes make that information easier to assimilate. This edition contains a number of new chapters in addition to widespread updates, and has been thoroughly copy-edited by Hugh Brazier to an unrivalled standard of consistency over the previous editions.

Whilst all chapters have been reviewed, there are a number of significant changes.

- Section 1 contains a significantly updated chapter in the growing field of preoperative assessment, and a brand new chapter on resuscitation. The inclusion of the DAS algorithms for airway management is a particular bonus.
- In Section 2 Ted Lin has written an additional chapter specifically covering the physiology of pain, and Colin Pinnock has edited haematology to bring it more in line with the current syllabus.
- Section 3 has a new chapter on analgesic drugs, taking account of the substantial developments in this area. The new chapter on mechanisms of drug action puts clear emphasis on the current thinking on the mechanism of anaesthesia.
- In Section 4, Ted Lin has put together a clear and concise statistics chapter, which will make preparation for this part of the exam straightforward. The inclusion of aspects of ultrasound and MRI scanning here and in the clinical section follows its incorporation into the syllabus.

Despite suggestions to expand *Fundamentals* to cover anaesthesia to higher levels and in greater depth, we have adhered to our original aim of providing a textbook specifically designed around the RCA Primary Fellowship. In so doing, we have been better able to adapt to changes in that exam as well as in anaesthetic core knowledge. The result is a much more effective exam preparation tool, which in turn is frequently used as a starting point for anaesthetists (and indeed others) of all grades including consultants, some of whom achieved exam success helped by the first edition. Finally, I am particularly grateful to Colin for his help and advice during my turn at leading the editorial process.

We were saddened to hear of the death of Dr Andy Ogilvy, author of Section 2, Chapter 11, as this edition was in preparation.

Tim Smith

Preface to the fourth edition

We are greatly pleased to be writing this introduction to our fourth edition of *Fundamentals of Anaesthesia*. Technology, clinical practice and the working environment for anaesthetists are continually changing and evolving, and we have attempted to reflect these trends in this new edition.

The curriculum for the FRCA exam is ever-expanding and presents a constant challenge for those in training. However, the basic principles for our specialty – of care for our patients, clinical skills and the application of scientific knowledge – remain constant, as they always have been.

We have taken care throughout to avoid unnecessary expansion of the material covered, and to relate material to the curriculum for the fellowship exam, as well as focusing on the basic principles of anaesthesia. One of our priorities has always been to try and make it easier for our readers to identify key facts and concepts in the mass of information that they are inevitably presented with – to gain a perspective on the topics contained in this volume.

So in this edition we introduce yellow and green boxes. Yellow boxes highlight facts or principles which we feel merit emphasis, while green boxes detail examples, calculations or techniques which are of interest but may be bypassed without interrupting the flow of the main text. The green boxes can be returned to if so desired and examined separately.

In this edition the clinical section (Section 1) has been revised and updated, taking account of the changing guidelines that influence clinical practice and focusing on the explanations behind them. The regional anaesthesia chapter now includes an introduction to ultrasound techniques.

In the physiology section (Section 2) all chapters have been revised and new chapters have been written for gastroenterology, neurophysiology, metabolism and temperature regulation, and renal physiology.

In the pharmacology section (Section 3), as well as introducing new drugs, the explanations have continued to reflect the changes in expectations for the evolving Primary FRCA examination.

The statistics chapter is now combined with the clinical trials chapter, bringing basic science and clinical research practice together, highlighting the need for basic statistical knowledge in order to interpret and design studies appropriately.

It is with great sadness that we mark the passing of our friend and colleague Colin Pinnock with this edition. He was the originator of this project and will always be remembered, not only as a prolific author but also as an uncompromising educator.

We, the editors, wish our readers an enjoyable and challenging read.

Ted Lin and Tim Smith

Acknowledgements

A number of organisations have kindly allowed us to use illustrations, tables and other material. We gratefully acknowledge the help given by the parties listed below in granting permission to use the material cited.

Alma Medical
Chapter 5
  Figure 5.27 Oxford HELP (head elevating laryngoscopy pillow) system

American College of Cardiology/American Heart Association
Chapter 1
  Figure 1.8 Clinical predictors of increased perioperative cardiovascular risk
  Figure 1.9 Surgery-specific cardiac risk for non-cardiac surgery

Association of Anaesthetists of Great Britain and Ireland
Chapter 2
  Green box Management of a patient with suspected anaphylaxis
Chapter 4
  Figure 4.1 Criteria to be met before transfer from recovery room to general ward
Chapter 5
  Figure 5.24 Indications for intubation and ventilation for transfer after brain injury
  Figure 5.25 Transfer checklist for a head-injured patient
Chapter 7
  Figure 7.5 AAGBI guidelines on the management of local anaesthetic toxicity
Chapter 46
  Figure 46.10 AAGBI checklist for anaesthetic equipment

British Journal of Anaesthesia
Chapter 46
  Figure 46.21 Mapleson classification system for breathing systems

Difficult Airway Society (UK)
Chapter 2
  Figure 2.6 Unanticipated difficult intubation during routine induction of anaesthesia
  Figure 2.7 Unanticipated difficult intubation during rapid sequence induction
  Figure 2.8 Failed intubation: rescue techniques for the 'can't intubate, can't ventilate' situation

Joint British Diabetes Societies
Chapter 5
  Figure 5.35 Suitability of patients with diabetes for day surgery

Resuscitation Council (UK)
Chapter 8
  Figure 8.2 Algorithm for in-hospital resuscitation
  Figure 8.3 Adult basic life support (BLS) algorithm
  Figure 8.4 Adult choking algorithm
  Figure 8.5 Adult advanced life support (ALS) algorithm
  Figure 8.7 Bradycardia algorithm
  Figure 8.8 Tachycardia algorithm (with pulse)
  Figure 8.9 Paediatric basic life support (BLS) algorithm
  Figure 8.10 Paediatric foreign-body airway obstruction algorithm
  Figure 8.11 Paediatric advanced life support (ALS) algorithm

The Sourcebook of Medical Illustration, ed. P. Cull. **Carnforth: Parthenon Publishing Group, 1989**

Chapter 7
  Figure 7.11 Patient positions for spinal anaesthesia
  Figure 7.26 Patient position for caudal anaesthesia
  Figure 7.27 Needle angulation for caudal anaesthesia

Chapter 18
  Figure 18.23 Structure of the eye
  Figure 18.27 Distribution of the autonomic nervous
  system

Abbreviations

2,3-DPG	2,3-diphosphoglycerate
5-HT	5-hydroxytryptamine (serotonin)
A	adenine
A&E	accident and emergency
AAGBI	Association of Anaesthetists of Great Britain and Ireland
ABC	airway, breathing, circulation
ABV	arterial blood volume
AC	alternating current
ACA	anterior cerebral artery
ACC	anterior cingulate cortex
ACE	angiotensin-converting enzyme
ACh	acetylcholine
ACT	activated clotting time
ACTH	adrenocorticotropic hormone
ACTH-RH	adrenocorticotropic hormone releasing hormone
ADCC	antibody-dependent cell-mediated cytotoxicity
ADH	antidiuretic hormone
ADP	adenosine diphosphate
ADR	adverse drug reaction
ADROIT	Adverse Drug Reactions Online Information Tracking
AED	automated external defibrillator
AER	auditory evoked response
AF	atrial fibrillation
AFE	amniotic fluid embolism
AFOI	awake fibreoptic intubation
AH	absolute humidity
AIDS	acquired immune deficiency syndrome
ALS	advanced life support
AMD	airway management device
AMP	adenosine monophosphate
AMPA	α-amino 3-hydroxy 5-methyl 4-isoxazolepropionic acid
Ang I	angiotensin I
Ang II	angiotensin II
ANOVA	analysis of variance
ANP	atrial natriuretic peptide
ANS	autonomic nervous system
ANSI	American National Standards Institute
AP	action potential
AP	anaesthetic proof
AP	anteroposterior
APC	activated protein C
APC	antigen-presenting cell
APCR	activated protein C resistance
APG	anaesthetic proof category G
APL	adjustable pressure-limiting
APTT	activated partial thromboplastin time
AQP	aquaporin
ARDS	acute respiratory distress syndrome
ARR	absolute risk reduction
ASA	American Society of Anesthesiologists
ASIC	acid-sensing ion channel
ASIS	anterior superior iliac spine
AT	anaerobic threshold
AT	angiotensin
ATLS	advanced trauma life support
ATP	adenosine triphosphate
ATPS	ambient temperature and pressure saturated
AUC	area under curve
AV	alveolar ventilation
AV	atrioventricular
AVNRT	AV nodal re-entry tachycardia
AVRT	AV re-entry tachycardia
BAER	brainstem auditory evoked response
bd	twice a day
BDNF	brain-derived neurotrophic factor
BER	basal electrical rhythm
BIS	bispectral index
BLS	basic life support
B_M	B memory cell
BMI	body mass index

BMR	basal metabolic rate	COMT	catechol-O-methyl transferase
$BMRO_2$	basal metabolic rate of oxygen consumption	COP	colloid osmotic pressure
BNF	British National Formulary	COPA	cuffed oropharyngeal airway
BNP	brain natriuretic peptide	COPD	chronic obstructive pulmonary disease
BP	blood pressure	COSHH	Control of Substances Hazardous to Health
BP	boiling point	COX	cyclo-oxygenase
BPI	Brief Pain Inventory	CP	creatine phosphate
bpm	beats per minute	CPAP	continuous positive airway pressure
BS	British Standard	CPDA	citrate phosphate dextrose adenine
BSA	body surface area	CPK MB	creatine phosphokinase (cardiac isoenzyme)
BSE	bovine spongiform encephalopathy		
C	cytosine	CPP	cerebral perfusion pressure
Ca	arterial compliance	CPP	coronary perfusion pressure
CAM	cell adhesion molecule	CPR	cardiopulmonary resuscitation
CAM	confusion assessment method	CPX	cardiopulmonary exercise
cAMP	cyclic adenosine monophosphate	C_R	respiratory system compliance
C_AO_2	alveolar oxygen content	CRP	C-reactive protein
CaO_2	arterial oxygen content	CRPS	complex regional pain syndrome
CAPD	continuous ambulatory peritoneal dialysis	CSE	combined spinal–epidural
CBF	cerebral blood flow	CSF	cerebrospinal fluid
CBG	capillary blood glucose	CSF	colony-stimulating factor
CBG	corticosteroid-binding globulin	CSM	Committee on Safety of Medicines
CBV	cerebral blood volume	CT	computerised tomography
CC	closing capacity	CTZ	chemoreceptor trigger zone
CCK	cholecystokinin	CV	controlled ventilation
CcO_2	capillary oxygen content	CvO_2	mixed venous oxygen content
CFAM	cerebral function analysing monitor	CVP	central venous pressure
cGMP	cyclic guanosine monophosphate	CVR	cerebrovascular resistance
CGRP	calcitonin gene-related peptide	CVRIII	continuous variable-rate intravenous insulin infusion
CHM	Commission on Human Medicines		
CI	cardiac index	CVS	cardiovascular system
CI	confidence interval	Cw	chest wall compliance
CJD	Creutzfeldt–Jakob disease	CYP	cytochrome P450
CK	creatine kinase	D	dopaminergic
CKD	chronic kidney disease	D&C	dilatation and curettage
CL	confidence limit	DAG	diacylglycerol
Cl	clearance	DBS	double-burst stimulation
C_L	lung compliance	DC	direct current
cmH_2O	centimetres of water (pressure)	DCR	dacryocystorhinostomy
CMR	cerebral metabolic rate	DDAVP	1-deamino-8-arginine vasopressin
$CMRO_2$	cerebral metabolic rate of oxygen consumption	DHEA	dehydroepiandrosterone
		DHFR	dihydrofolate reductase
CMV	cytomegalovirus	DHPS	deoxyhypusine synthase
CNB	central nerve block	DIC	disseminated intravascular coagulation
CNS	central nervous system	DIT	di-iodotyrosine
CO	cardiac output	DKA	diabetic ketoacidosis
CoA	co-enzyme A	DLCO	diffusing capacity of the lungs for carbon monoxide
COAD	chronic obstructive airways disease		

DNA	deoxyribonucleic acid		ESR	erythrocyte sedimentation rate
DNACPR	do not attempt cardiopulmonary resuscitation		ESV	end-systolic volume
$\dot{D}O_2$	oxygen delivery		ET	endothelium
DPP-4	dipeptidylpeptidase-4		ETC	oesophageal–tracheal combitube
DPT	dorsolateral pontine tegmentum		$ETCO_2$	end-tidal carbon dioxide
DRG	dorsal root ganglion		ETT	endotracheal tube
DVT	deep venous thrombosis		f	frequency of breaths
Ea	arterial elastance		F	gas flow
EAR	expired air respiration		F/M	feto-maternal
EBC	effective blood concentration		FA	fatty acid
EBP	epidural blood patch		F_A	alveolar tension
EC	effective concentration		FAC	fractional area change
ECA	electrical control activity		F_ACO_2	fractional alveolar carbon dioxide concentration
ECF	extracellular fluid		$FADH_2$	flavine adenine dinucleotide
ECG	electrocardiogram		FAST	focused assessment with sonography for trauma
ECMO	extracorporeal membrane oxygenation		FATE	focus assessed transthoracic echocardiography
ED_{50}	effective dose in 50% of population		FBC	full blood count
ED_{95}	effective dose in 95% of population		FDC	F-decalin
EDP	end-diastolic point		FDP	fibrin degradation product
EDPVR	end-diastolic pressure–volume relationship		Fe^{2+}	ferrous iron state
EDRF	endothelium-derived relaxing factor		$F_{\bar{E}}CO_2$	fractional mixed expired carbon dioxide concentration
EDTA	ethylenediamine tetra-acetate		FEMG	frontalis electromyogram
EDV	end-diastolic volume		FEV%	ratio of FEV_1 to FVC
EEG	electroencephalogram		FEV_1	forced expiratory volume in one second
Ees	end-systolic elastance		FFA	free fatty acid
EF	ejection fraction		FFI	fatal familial insomnia
eGFR	estimated glomerular filtration rate		FFP	fresh frozen plasma
EM	electromagnetic		FFT	fast Fourier transform
EMD	electromechanical dissociation		FG	fat group
EMF	electromotive force		FGF	fresh gas flow
EMG	electromyogram		FI	fusion inhibitor
EMLA	eutectic mixture of local anaesthetic		F_I	inspired vapour tension
EMS	emergency medical service		F_IO_2	fractional inspired oxygen concentration
ENS	enteric nervous system		FLAP	five-lipoxygenase-activating protein
ENT	ear nose and throat		FNHTR	febrile non-haemolytic transfusion reactions
EPO	erythropoietin		FRC	functional residual capacity
EPSP	excitatory postsynaptic potential		FSH	follicle-stimulating hormone
ER	endoplasmic reticulum		FSH-RH	follicle-stimulating hormone releasing hormone
ER	extraction ratio		FTPA	F-tripropylamine
ERK	extracellular signal-regulated kinase		FVC	forced vital capacity
ERPC	evacuation of retained products of conception		G	guanine
ERV	expiratory reserve volume		GABA	γ-aminobutyric acid
ESBL	extended-spectrum β-lactamase			
ESKF	end-stage kidney failure			
ESP	end-systolic point			
ESPVR	end-systolic pressure–volume relationship			

GCCR	guanylyl-cyclase-coupled receptor	HIV	human immunodeficiency virus
GCS	Glasgow coma scale	HLA	human leukocyte-associated antigen
GDNF	glial cell-line-derived neurotrophic factor	HME	heat and moisturiser exchanger
GDP	guanosine diphosphate	HMP	hexose monophosphate
GE	gradient echo	HMWK	high-molecular-weight kininogen
GFR	glomerular filtration rate	hPL	human placental lactogen
GH	growth hormone	HPV	hypoxic pulmonary vasoconstriction
GH-IH	growth hormone inhibiting hormone	HR	heart rate
GH-RH	growth hormone releasing hormone	I	current
GI	gastrointestinal	I:E	inspiratory : expiratory ratio
GIFTASUP	Guidelines on Intravenous Fluid Therapy for Adult Surgical Patients	IA	intra-arterial
		IABP	intra-aortic balloon pump
GLP-1	glucagon-like peptide 1	IASP	International Association for the Study of Pain
GLUT4	glucose transporter type 4		
GLUT5	glucose transporter type 5	IC	insular cortex
GlyR	glycine receptor	ICA	internal carotid artery
GMC	General Medical Council	ICAM	intercellular adhesion molecule
GMP	guanosine monophosphate	ICD	implantable cardioverter defibrillator
Gn-RH	gonadotropin releasing hormone	ICF	intracellular fluid
GP	general practitioner	ICP	intracranial pressure
GPCR	G-protein-coupled receptor	ICU	intensive care unit
GRK	GPCR-kinase	IDDM	insulin dependent diabetes mellitus
GSS	Gerstmann–Sträussler–Scheinker syndrome	IgA	immunoglobulin A
		IgE	immunoglobulin E
GTN	glyceryl trinitrate	IGF	insulin-like growth factor
GTP	guanosine triphosphate	IgG	immunoglobulin G
HAFOE	high airflow oxygen enrichment	iGluR	ionotropic glutamine receptor
HAS	human albumin solution	IgM	immunoglobulin M
Hb	haemoglobin	IHD	ischaemic heart disease
HbA	adult haemoglobin	IL	interleukin
HbCO	carboxyhaemoglobin	ILMA	intubating laryngeal mask airway
HbF	fetal haemoglobin	IM	intramuscular
HBF	hepatic blood flow	IML	intermediolateral
Hbmet	methaemoglobin	IMV	intermittent mandatory ventilation
HbS	sickle haemoglobin	INR	international normalised ratio
HbSul	sulphaemoglobin	INSTI	integrase strand transfer inhibitor
hCG	human chorionic gonadotrophin	IO	intraosseous
Hct	haematocrit	IOP	intra-ocular pressure
HD	haemodialysis	IP_3	inositol triphosphate
HDL	high-density lipoprotein	IPPV	intermittent positive-pressure ventilation
HDN	haemolytic disease of the newborn	IPSP	inhibitory postsynaptic potential
HDU	high dependency unit	IR	infrared
HELLP	haemolytic anaemia elevated liver enzymes low platelets	IRS	insulin receptor substrate
		IRV	inspiratory reserve volume
HELP	head elevating laryngoscopy pillow	ISI	international sensitivity index
HEMS	helicopter emergency medical services	ISO	International Organization for Standardization
HER	hepatic extraction ratio		
HFJV	high-frequency jet ventilation	I_{SPTA}	spatial-peak temporal-average intensity

IT	implant tested		MEFR	mid-expiratory flow rate
ITP	idiopathic thrombocytopenia purpura		MEPP	miniature endplate potential
IU	international unit		MET	metabolic equivalent (unit)
IUGR	intrauterine growth restriction		MEWS	modified early warning system
IV	intravenous		MFR	mannosyl–fucosyl receptor
IVC	inferior vena cava		MG	muscle group
IVIg	intravenous immunoglobulin		MGPS	medical gas pipeline service
IVRA	intravenous regional anaesthesia		MH	malignant hyperthermia
JVP	jugular venous pressure		MH	mechano-heat
KCCT	kaolin clotting time		MHC	major histocompatibility
K_F	glomerular capillary coefficient		MHRA	Medicines and Healthcare products Regulatory Agency
LAK	lymphokine-activated killer		MI	myocardial infarction
LAP	left atrial pressure		MIA	mechanically insensitive afferent
LBP	lipopolysaccharide binding protein		MIC	minimum inhibitory concentration
LBP	low back pain		MILS	manual in-line stabilisation
LC	locus coeruleus		MIR	minimum infusion rate
LD_{50}	lethal dose 50%		MIRL	membrane inhibitor of reactive lysis
LDL	low-density lipoprotein		MIT	mono-iodotyrosine
LED	light-emitting diode		MMC	migratory motor complex
LH	luteinising hormone		mmHg	millimetres of mercury (pressure)
LH-RH	luteinising hormone releasing hormone		MODS	multiple organ dysfunction syndrome
LIS	lateral intracellular space		MPAP	mean pulmonary arterial pressure
LMA	laryngeal mask airway		MR	magnetic resonance
LMW	low molecular weight		MRI	magnetic resonance imaging
LMWH	low-molecular-weight heparin		mRNA	messenger RNA
LOH	loop of Henle		MSA	mechanically sensitive afferent
LOR	loss of resistance		MRSA	meticillin-resistant *Staphyloccocus aureus*
LOS	lower oesophageal sphincter		MTC	major trauma centre
LSCS	lower-segment Caesarean section		MTD	maximum tolerated dose
LT	leukotriene		MUGA	multigated scan
LV	left ventricle		MV	minute ventilation
LVEDP	left ventricular end-diastolic pressure		MV	minute volume
LVF	left ventricular failure		MW	molecular weight
LVH	left ventricular hypertrophy		nAChR	nicotinic acetylcholine receptor
LVSWI	left ventricular stroke work index		NADH	nicotinamide adenine dinucleotide
M	muscarinic		NADPH	nicotinamide adenine dinucleotide phosphate
M3G	morphine-3-glucuronide		NAI	non-accidental injury
M6G	morphine-6-glucuronide		NANC	non-adrenergic non-cholinergic
MAC	minimum alveolar concentration		NAP3	National Audit Project 3
MAO	monoamine oxidase		NAP4	National Audit Project 4
MAOI	monoamine oxidase inhibitor		NAPQI	N-acetyl-p-benzo-quinone imine
MAP	mean arterial pressure		NBM	nil by mouth
MBL	mannan-binding lectin		NCA	nurse-controlled analgesia
MCA	middle cerebral artery		Nd-YAG	neodymium yttrium aluminium garnet
MCH	mean cell haemoglobin		NG	nasogastric
MCV	mean cell volume		NGF	nerve growth factor
MDP	maximum diastolic potential			
MEA	microwave endometrial ablation			

NHS	National Health Service	P_ACO_2	partial pressure of carbon dioxide – alveolar
NICE	National Institute for Health and Care Excellence	$PaCO_2$	partial pressure of carbon dioxide – arterial
NIOSH	National Institute for Occupational Safety and Health	PACWP	pulmonary artery capillary wedge pressure
NiPPV	nasal intermittent positive-pressure ventilation	PADP	pulmonary artery diastolic pressure
		PAF	platelet activating factor
NIST	non-interchangeable screw thread	PAFC	pulmonary artery flotation catheter
NK	natural killer	PAG	periaqueductal grey
NK	neurokinin receptor	PAH	para-aminohippuric acid
NKA	neurokinin A	PAMP	pathogen-associated molecular pattern
NMBA	neuromuscular blocking agent	P_AO_2	partial pressure of oxygen – alveolar
NMJ	neuromuscular junction	PaO_2	partial pressure of oxygen – arterial
NMDA	N-methyl-D-aspartate	PARS	patient at risk score
NMJ	neuromuscular junction	PART	patient at risk team
NNH	number needed to harm	PBP	penicillin-binding protein
NNRTI	non-nucleoside reverse transcriptase inhibitor	P_C	capillary hydrostatic pressure
		PCA	patient-controlled analgesia
NNT	number needed to treat	PCA	posterior cerebral artery
NPSA	National Patient Safety Association	PCC	prothrombinase complex concentrate
NPV	negative predictive value	PCEA	patient-controlled epidural analgesia
NRG	nucleus reticularis gigantocellularis	PCNL	percutaneous nephrolithotomy
NREM	non-rapid eye movement	PCO_2	partial pressure of carbon dioxide
NRM	nucleus raphe magnus	PCoA	posterior communicating artery
NRS	numerical rating scale	PCP	phencyclidine
NRTI	nucleoside/nucleotide reverse transcriptase inhibitor	PCP	*Pneumocystis* pneumonia
		PCWP	pulmonary capillary wedge pressure
NSAID	non-steroidal anti-inflammatory drug	PD	photodiode
NTP	normal temperature and pressure	PDE	phosphodiesterase enzyme
NTS	nucleus tractus solitarius	PDGF	platelet-derived growth factor
NV	nausea and vomiting	PDPH	post-dural puncture headache
NWC	number of words chosen	PE	potential energy
O/G	oil/gas	PE	pulmonary embolus
O/W	oil/water	PEA	pulseless electrical activity
OAA	Obstetric Anaesthetists Association	PECO2	partial pressure end-tidal carbon dioxide
OCI	oesophageal contractility index	PEEP	positive end-expiratory pressure
ODC	oxyhaemoglobin dissociation curve	PEFR	peak expiratory flow rate
OP	oxidative phosphorylation	PEP	post-exposure prophylaxis
OPAC	oximetric pulmonary artery catheter	PET	positron emission tomography
OR	odds ratio	PF4	platelet factor 4
OSA	obstructive sleep apnoea	PFC	perfluorocarbon
π	osmotic pressure	PGE	prostaglandin E
P	probability	PGG	prostaglandin G
P_{50}	PO_2 at which haemoglobin is 50% saturated	PGH	prostaglandin H
		PGI	prostaglandin I
		Pi	inorganic phosphate
PA	pulmonary artery	PI	protease inhibitor
PABA	para-aminobenzoic acid	P_{IF}	interstitial hydrostatic pressure
PAC	pulmonary artery catheter	PIH	prolactin inhibiting hormone

P_IO_2	inspired oxygen tension		RBC	red blood cell
PIP_2	phosphatidyl inositol bisphosphate		RBCV	red blood cell volume
PIS	pin index system		RBF	renal blood flow
PK	prekallikrein		RCT	randomised controlled trial
PLOC	provoked lower oesophageal contractions		RDS	respiratory distress syndrome
PMN	polymorphonuclear neutrophils		Re	Reynolds number
PNMT	phenylethanolamine N-methyl transferase		REM	rapid eye movement
PO	per os (by mouth)		RH	relative humidity
PO_2	partial pressure of oxygen		Rh	rhesus
POCD	postoperative cognitive decline		RIMA	reversible inhibitor of monoamine oxidase A
PONV	postoperative nausea and vomiting			
PPAR	peroxisome proliferator-activated receptor		RMP	resting membrane potential
PPF	plasma protein fraction		RMS	root mean square
PPI	proton pump inhibitor		RNA	ribonucleic acid
PPHN	persistent pulmonary hypertension of the newborn		RNU	regional neurosurgical unit
			ROC	receptor-operated ion channel
ppm	parts per million		ROTEM	rotational thromboelastometry
PPP	pentose phosphate pathway		RPF	renal plasma flow
PPV	positive predictive value		RQ	respiratory quotient
PPV	positive-pressure ventilation		rRNA	ribosomal RNA
PRH	prolactin releasing hormone		RR	relative risk
PRI	pain rating index		RR	respiratory rate
PRST	pressure, rate, sweating, tears		RRR	relative risk reduction
PSA	prostate-specific antigen		RRT	renal replacement therapy
psi	pounds per square inch		RS	respiratory system
PSVT	paroxysmal supraventricular tachycardia		RSI	rapid sequence induction
PT	prothrombin time		RT_3	reverse tri-iodothyronine
PTC	post-tetanic count		RV	residual volume
PTFE	polytetrafluoroethylene		RV	right ventricle
PTH	parathyroid hormone		RVM	rostral ventromedial medulla
PTT	partial thromboplastin time		RVSWI	right ventricular stroke work index
PTTK	partial thromboplastin time with kaolin		S/N	signal to noise ratio
PV	plasma volume		SA	sinoatrial
PV	pressure–volume		SAD	supraglottic airway device
PVC	poly vinyl chloride		SAGM	saline-adenine-glucose-mannitol
PVD	peripheral vascular disease		SaO_2	arterial oxygen saturation
PVG	periventricular grey		SARS	severe acute respiratory syndrome
PVR	pulmonary vascular resistance		sCJD	sporadic Creutzfeldt–Jakob disease
Q	flow		SD	standard deviation
Q	charge		SE	spin echo
$\dot{Q}$	cardiac output		SEM	standard error of the mean
QAI	quaternary ammonium ion		SFH	stroma-free haemoglobin
Qs	shunt flow		SGLT	sodium-dependent glucose co-transporter
R	resistance (electrical)		SI	stroke index
R	universal gas constant		SI	Système International d'Unités (International System of Units)
RAP	right atrial pressure			
RAS	reticular activating system		SIADH	syndrome of inappropriate ADH secretion
RAST	radioallergosorbent test		SID	strong ion difference

SIMV	synchronised intermittent mandatory ventilation		TCRE	transcervical resection of endometrium
SIRS	systemic inflammatory response syndrome		TD	transdermal
SL	semilunar		TEG	thromboelastography
SL	sublingual		TENS	transcutaneous electrical nerve stimulation
SLE	systemic lupus erythematosus		TF	tissue factor
SLOC	spontaneous lower oesophageal contractions		T_H	T helper cell
SMP	sympathetically maintained pain		THC	terahydro-cannabinol
SNGFR	single-nephron glomerular filtration rate		THR	total hip replacement
SNP	sodium nitroprusside		TIVA	total intravenous anaesthesia
SNRI	serotonin–noradrenaline reuptake inhibitor		TLC	total lung capacity
SO_2	oxygen saturation		TLV	total lung volume
SPECT	single-photon emission computed tomography		TNF	tumour necrosis factor
			TOE	transoesophageal echocardiography
SpO_2	pulse oximeter oxygen saturation		TOF	train of four
SR	sarcoplasmic reticulum		TP	threshold potential
SRS-A	slow-reacting substance of anaphylaxis		t-PA	tissue-type plasminogen activator
SSEP	somatosensory evoked potential		TPP	thiamine pyrophosphate
SSRI	selective serotonin reuptake inhibitor		TRALI	transfusion-related acute lung injury
STI	sexually transmitted infection		TRH	thyrotropin releasing hormone
STOP	suction termination of pregnancy		Trk	tyrosine kinase receptor
STT	spinothalamic tract		tRNA	transfer RNA
SV	spontaneous ventilation		TRP	transient receptor potential
SV	stroke volume		TRPV1	transient receptor potential vanilloid 1
SVC	superior vena cava		TSE	transmissible spongiform encephalopathy
SVI	systemic vascular index		TSH	thyroid-stimulating hormone
SvO_2	mixed venous oxygen saturation		TT	thrombin time
SVP	saturated vapour pressure		TTN	transient tachypnoea of the newborn
SVR	systemic vascular resistance		TUR	transurethral resection
SVWI	stroke volume work index		TURBT	transurethral resection of bladder tumour
SW	stroke work		TURP	transurethral resection of the prostate
T	absolute temperature		TV	tidal volume
T	thymine		TVT	transvaginal tension-free tape
$t_{1/2}$	half-life		TXA_2	thromboxane A_2
T_3	tri-iodothyronine		UBF	uterine blood flow
T_4	thyroxine		UOS	upper oesophageal sphincter
Tan	tangent		URT	upper respiratory tract
TBPA	thyroxine-binding prealbumin		URTI	upper respiratory tract infection
TBG	thyroxine-binding globulin		USGRA	ultrasound-guided regional anaesthesia
TBI	traumatic brain injury		UTP	uridine triphosphate
TBV	total blood volume		UV	ultraviolet
TBW	total body water		$\dot{V}$	ventilation
Tc	cytotoxic T cell		$\dot{V}/\dot{Q}$	ventilation/perfusion
TCA	tricyclic antidepressant		V_A	alveolar volume
TCI	target-controlled infusion		VAS	visual analogue scale
TCR	T-cell receptor		V_{BL}	blood volume
			VC	vital capacity
			vCJD	variant Creutzfeldt–Jakob disease
			VCO_2	carbon dioxide flux

V_D	anatomical dead space	V_{PL}	plasma volume
V_d	volume of distribution	VPN	ventral posterior nucleus of the thalamus
VER	visual evoked response		
VF	ventricular fibrillation	V_{RBC}	red blood cell volume
VIC	vaporiser inside circle	VRE	vancomycin-resistant enterococci
VIE	vacuum-insulated evaporator	VRG	vessel-rich group
V_{INT}	interstitial fluid volume	VRS	verbal rating scale
VIP	vasoactive intestinal peptide	V_T	tidal volume
VISA	vancomycin-intermediate *Staphylococcus aureus*	VT	ventricular tachycardia
		V_TCO_2	volume of carbon dioxide per breath
VLDL	very-low-density lipoprotein	VTE	venous thromboembolism
VMA	vanillylmandelic acid	vWF	von Willebrand factor
VO_2	oxygen uptake in the lungs	WBC	white blood cell
VOC	vaporiser outside circle	WHO	World Health Organization
VPC	ventricular premature contractions	WPW	Wolff–Parkinson–White

CHAPTER 1

Preoperative management

Gwenda Cavill and Karen Kerr

The safe conduct of anaesthesia requires meticulous preoperative assessment, preparation and planning. In the case of elective procedures this should occur well in advance of surgery, allowing a comprehensive review of concurrent disease, medication and social issues. This is often carried out in a dedicated preoperative assessment clinic by a multidisciplinary team comprising nursing and medical staff as well as pharmacists and specialist technicians.

While patients undergoing emergency surgery may not benefit from such a structured approach to their preoperative management, they must nevertheless undergo rigorous systematic review and preparation to ensure optimum care.

Preoperative assessment

Screening

When elective surgery is first planned, a screening questionnaire may be used to provide information regarding comorbidity that may require early preoperative review or intervention. A need for additional specialist input can be identified and acted upon at this stage.

Preoperative assessment clinic

During subsequent preoperative assessment a general medical history is taken, detailing concurrent disease and its management.

- Correspondence in the clinical notes may provide a useful outline of a disease process, giving some indication of its stability, as well as information on previous hospital admissions, current medication and recent investigation results.
- A history should be taken of previous anaesthetic experience. A family history of problems associated with anaesthesia must be noted and may require further investigation.
- The patient's general health should be assessed. In particular a history of reflux should be noted, along with smoking and alcohol habits.
- A history of recreational drug use may be appropriate.
- A list of current medication, including dosage and recent changes, is essential, along with a history of any allergic or other adverse drug reactions. The nature of the allergy or reaction should be recorded.

Fundamentals of Anaesthesia, 4th edition, ed. Ted Lin, Tim Smith and Colin Pinnock. Published by Cambridge University Press. © Cambridge University Press 2017.

- Particular attention must be paid to drugs requiring specific perioperative management, such as anti-coagulants or insulin.

A general physical examination must be carried out prior to anaesthesia and surgery.
- Of particular importance is a focused examination of the cardiorespiratory system. This aims to ensure control of conditions such as hypertension, but also to detect features such as new cardiac murmurs. The latter may require further investigation.
- A functional assessment is particularly important in patients with cardiorespiratory disease. This will be considered in more detail below.
- An assessment of the cervical spine should be made in patients with conditions likely to limit neck movement. Radiological examination is seldom necessary, but limitation of movement should be defined and recorded. The presence of neurological symptoms or signs will require further evaluation.
- The presence and location of any loose or damaged teeth should be noted, as well as dentures, crowns and orthodontic appliances.
- Airway assessment is of fundamental importance, and is generally carried out at the time of the anaesthetist's preoperative visit.

Preoperative assessment of functional capacity

Functional capacity (what a patient can physically do) not only describes exercise tolerance but gives an indication of functional reserve (the extent to which that patient can be physically challenged). This is particularly important in the preoperative assessment of surgical patients with cardiac disease.

Gross limitation or deterioration of functional capacity is of particular significance, and indicates the need for further assessment, including investigation and specialist opinion. When considered along with clinical (mainly cardiac) factors and the planned surgical procedure, an estimate of functional capacity helps us to make an assessment of perioperative risk.

We can express functional capacity in so-called *metabolic equivalent* (MET) units (Figure 1.1). A MET is expressed in terms of oxygen utilisation, and quantifies the estimated amount of energy expended at different levels of physical activity.

Figure 1.1 MET units

1 MET equates to 3.5 millilitres of oxygen per kilogram body weight per minute	
Metabolic equivalents of common daily activities	
1 MET	walk 100 metres on level ground
4 MET	climb a flight of stairs or walk up a hill
> 10 MET	strenuous exercise

A functional capacity corresponding to < 4 MET (unable to climb a flight of stairs) is associated with increased perioperative risk. A more detailed assessment can be made by referring to an activity scale such as the Duke Activity Status Index. The answers to series of questions related to daily activities provide a score related to functional capacity. Great care is needed in making such assessments, as function may be limited by factors such as arthritis or neurological disease. In such cases more specific symptoms such as orthopnoea or paroxysmal nocturnal dyspnoea are helpful in identifying cardiac disease as the factor limiting functional capacity.

A number of baseline investigations may be carried out at the time of preoperative assessment. These typically include a full blood count, electrolytes and a 12-lead electrocardiogram (ECG). Pulmonary function tests may prove helpful in some patients with respiratory disease. There are, however, comprehensive guidelines available to minimise unnecessary investigations in fit young patients. Further investigation must be guided by underlying disease and functional status. Additional blood tests, for example, might be required to assess thyroid or liver function.

In some cases there may be a need for radiological investigation, echocardiography and, occasionally, cardiopulmonary exercise testing. Such investigations should only be sought following discussion with experienced clinicians. These investigations place a heavy demand on technicians and may themselves carry risks for the patient. The likely benefits must therefore be carefully weighed up.

Some patients with serious comorbidity may be referred by the preoperative assessment clinic at this stage for further assessment by a senior anaesthetist.

Written information regarding anaesthesia and specific surgical procedures is often provided to patients at this time.

Preoperative visit

A preoperative visit by an anaesthetist is essential, and increasingly occurs on the day of surgery. Such a visit provides an opportunity for introductions, confirmation of medical conditions and an explanation of the anaesthetic role.

A general medical and surgical history is often already available, and can be discussed in further detail. Specific issues regarding previous anaesthesia and associated problems are discussed. Earlier examination findings should be available following preoperative assessment. Examination of dentition and neck movement, along with an assessment of the airway, must be made at this stage. A plan of care, including proposed anaesthetic technique, postoperative analgesia and fluid management, can be outlined to the patient.

A discussion regarding the risks and benefits of proposed procedures is usually much appreciated. This also provides an opportunity to discuss any concerns the patient may have regarding specific issues such as postoperative nausea and vomiting, and duration of immobility following regional anaesthesia.

An effective preoperative visit should do much to allay anxiety, leaving the patient well informed and confident in those caring for him or her. It may well preclude the need for premedication.

The airway

Failure to achieve adequate oxygenation and ventilation is responsible for a significant proportion of anaesthesia-related morbidity and mortality. Inadequate ventilation and difficult intubation are everyday hazards in anaesthesia and can prove catastrophic. Given the fundamental importance of adequate oxygenation, recognition of the 'difficult to ventilate' patient is essential. A number of factors are associated with difficulty in mask ventilation:

- Obesity
- Beard
- Edentulous
- Snoring
- Age > 55

Ease of intubation has been graded according to the best possible view obtained on laryngoscopy (Cormack & Lehane 1984; see Figure 2.4). Grades 3 and 4 are difficult intubations:

- Grade 1: whole of glottis visible
- Grade 2: glottis incompletely visible
- Grade 3: epiglottis but not glottis visible
- Grade 4: epiglottis not visible

The reported incidence of difficult intubation varies, but is around 1 in 65 intubations. Despite careful history and examination, 20% of difficult intubations are not predicted. The consequences may be disastrous. A history of previous difficult intubation is important, but a history of straightforward intubation several years earlier may be falsely reassuring as the patient's weight, cervical spine movement and disease process may all have changed. Some congenital conditions may predict a difficult intubation, e.g. Pierre Robin syndrome, Marfan's syndrome or cystic hygroma. Pathological conditions can make intubation difficult, e.g. tumour, infection or scarring of the upper airway tissues.

Airway assessment

As airway assessment, investigation and management becomes increasingly refined, the search for a single, reliable predictor of the difficult airway continues. A number of bedside tests are available to the anaesthetist wishing to make an assessment for features which might predict potential airway difficulties. However, unexpected airway problems can and do arise despite the ever-increasing array of assessment tools available to us. This should be borne in mind at all times.

In the modified Mallampati scoring system the patient sits opposite the anaesthetist with mouth open and tongue protruded. The structures visible at the back of the mouth are noted (Mallampati et al. 1985, Samsoon & Young 1987), as follows:

- Class 1: faucial pillars, soft palate and uvula visible
- Class 2: faucial pillars and soft palate visible, uvula masked by base of tongue
- Class 3: only soft palate visible
- Class 4: soft palate not visible

The Wilson risk factors may provide additional predictive information on the airway. The Wilson risk factors each score 0–2 points, to give a maximum of 10 points. A score greater than 2 predicts 75% of difficult intubations, although as with the Mallampati system there is a high incidence of false positives. The Wilson risk factors (Wilson et al. 1988) are:

- Obesity
- Restricted head and neck movements
- Restricted jaw movement
- Receding mandible
- Buck teeth

A number of tests of neck and jaw movement may be used to evaluate these further:

- Inability to flex the chin onto the chest indicates poor neck movement. Once the neck is fully flexed, a patient should be able to move his or her head $> 15°$ to demonstrate normal occipitoaxial movement.
- Limitation of neck (atlanto-occipital joint) extension may be predictive of difficult intubation. The normal angle of extension is $> 35°$.
- Reduced jaw movements are demonstrated by poor mouth opening (particularly if of less than two fingers' width) and by inability to protrude the lower teeth beyond the upper.
- Limited mouth opening clearly creates potential airway difficulties, and may reflect limitation of temporo-mandibular joint movement. This may be evident as a reduced inter-incisor distance (the distance between the lower and upper incisors). A distance of < 3.5 cm is predictive of a difficult airway.

The mandibular space length and its measurement have received much attention in the quest to accurately predict airway difficulties:

- The *thyromental distance*, described by Patil in 1983, is the distance between the chin and the thyroid notch with the neck fully extended. A distance of < 6.5 cm (about three finger breadths) predicts difficulty.
- The *sternomental distance* was described by Savva in 1994; it is the distance from the suprasternal notch to the chin with the neck fully extended. A distance of < 12 cm predicts difficulty.
- The *hyomental distance* is that from the chin to the hyoid bone. A distance of < 4 cm (about two finger breadths) predicts difficulty.

No one test can predict airway difficulties with a high degree of sensitivity or specificity, but a combination of tests may be helpful. Careful assessment of the airway and consideration of more than one factor is therefore recommended. The modified Mallampati classification produces a high incidence of false positives. A thyromental distance of < 6.5 cm and Mallampati class 3 or 4, however, predicts 80% of difficult intubations.

Radiological features may aid prediction of a difficult intubation, but they are not routinely performed. These include:

- Reduced distance between occiput and spine of C1 and between spines of C1 and C2
- Ratio of mandibular length to posterior mandibular depth > 3.6
- Increased depth of mandible

Other rarely used investigations include indirect laryngoscopy, ultrasonography, CT and MRI imaging.

American Society of Anesthesiologists (ASA) scoring system

The ASA scoring system describes the preoperative physical state of a patient (Saklad 1941) and is used routinely for every patient in the UK. It makes no allowances for age, smoking history, obesity or pregnancy. Anticipated difficulties in intubation are not relevant. Addition of the postscript E indicates emergency surgery. There is some correlation between ASA score and perioperative mortality, although it was never intended for use in perioperative risk prediction. Definitions applied in the ASA system are given in Figure 1.2.

Figure 1.2 ASA classification

Code	Description	Perioperative mortality
P1	A normal healthy patient	0.1%
P2	A patient with mild systemic disease	0.2%
P3	A patient with severe systemic disease	1.8%
P4	A patient with severe systemic disease that is a constant threat to life	7.8%
P5	A moribund patient who is not expected to survive without the operation	9.4%
P6	A declared brain-dead patient whose organs are being removed for donor purposes	

Preparation for anaesthesia

Premedication

As more day surgery is performed and more patients are admitted to hospital close to the scheduled time of surgery, premedication has become less common. The main indication for premedication remains anxiety, for which a benzodiazepine is usually prescribed, sometimes with metoclopramide to promote absorption. Premedication serves several purposes: anxiolysis, smoother induction of anaesthesia, reduced requirement for intravenous induction agents, and possibly reduced likelihood of awareness. Intramuscular opioids are now rarely prescribed as premedication. The prevention of aspiration pneumonitis in patients with reflux requires premedication with an H_2 antagonist, the evening before and morning of surgery, and sodium citrate administration immediately prior to induction of anaesthesia. Topical local anaesthetic cream over two potential sites for venous cannulation is usually prescribed for children. Anticholinergic agents may be prescribed to dry secretions or to prevent bradycardia, e.g. during squint surgery.

Preoperative factors

Starvation

It is routine practice to starve patients prior to surgery in an attempt to minimise the volume of stomach contents and hence decrease the incidence of their aspiration. Aspiration of solid food particles may cause asphyxiation, and aspiration of gastric acid may cause pneumonitis (Mendelson's syndrome). Guidelines for preoperative starvation are becoming less restrictive as more information becomes available. Milky drinks are not allowed because their high fat content increases gastric transit time.

Figure 1.3 Starvation guidelines

Adults
- Clear fluids and water up to 2 hours preoperatively
- Food, sweets and milky drinks up to 6 hours preoperatively
- No chewing gum on day of surgery

Children
- Clear fluids and water up to 2 hours preoperatively
- Breast milk up to 4 hours preoperatively
- Formula/cow's milk up to 6 hours preoperatively
- Food and sweets up to 6 hours preoperatively

There is evidence that chewing gum before surgery significantly increases gastric fluid volume, particularly in children.

Current recommendations for patients undergoing elective surgery are shown in Figure 1.3.

Patients undergoing emergency surgery should be treated as if they have a full stomach. Normal fasting guidance should be followed where possible.

Prolonged periods of starvation give rise to problems. Dehydration may occur, particularly in children and in patients who are pyrexial or who have received bowel preparation. Infants may become hypoglycaemic. In patients with cyanotic heart disease, sickle cell disease or polycythaemia dehydration may precipitate thrombosis. In jaundiced patients the hepatorenal syndrome may be precipitated. It is thus essential that these patients receive intravenous therapy while they are being starved.

Fluid status

Healthy patients can balance daily fluid intake and output. Adults exchange approximately 5% of body water each day, while infants exchange about 15% and so are at greater risk of dehydration. A patient's fluid status may be affected by the underlying disease process or by its treatment (Figure 1.4), and there may be associated electrolyte disturbances. In certain conditions such as trauma, infection or ileus, fluid is redistributed rather than lost from the body, but will nonetheless still require

Figure 1.4 Disturbances of fluid balance

	Increased	Decreased
Input	Excessive IV fluids	Nausea Dysphagia Nil by mouth orders Coma Severe respiratory disease
Output	Sweating Diarrhoea (including bowel preparation) Vomiting Polyuria Haemorrhage Burns	Syndrome of inappropriate ADH secretion (SIADH) Renal impairment

replacing to maintain fluid balance. If patients have been ill for longer periods, malnutrition may also be a problem.

Fluid balance should be assessed preoperatively in all patients who are at risk of disturbances, which is most likely in emergencies. A history of any of the above will direct clinical examination. Postural hypotension, tachycardia and hypotension may be found in volume depletion, while a raised jugular venous pressure (JVP) and peripheral oedema may be found in volume overload. Skin turgor, or fontanelle tension in infants, is a useful guide, and assessment of urine output is very important. Oliguria is defined as a urine output of less than 0.5 mL kg^{-1} per hour. Relevant investigations include serum electrolytes, urea and creatinine. Urea raised proportionally more than the creatinine value indicates dehydration.

Correction of fluid balance

Therapy should be guided by central venous pressure (CVP), urine output, blood pressure, heart rate and electrolyte balance. Where fluid overload is diagnosed, fluid restriction and possibly diuretic therapy are required. If fluid depletion is diagnosed, replacement of the lost fluid, plus maintenance fluids, is required. Hypovolaemia resulting from blood loss necessitates red cell transfusion. If plasma has been lost, as in burns patients, plasma protein fraction (PPF) will be required. Maintenance fluid requirements are 40 mL kg^{-1} per day in adults (greater for children). Excessive administration of 5% dextrose to correct dehydration may lead to hyperglycaemia and hyponatraemia, while excessive administration of 0.9% saline may cause hypernatraemia and peripheral and pulmonary oedema.

Electrolyte disturbances

Disturbances of electroytes may be due to the underlying disease process, to drugs, particularly diuretics, or to iatrogenic causes. It is rare for a patient to exhibit overt clinical signs, but electrolyte disturbances present several potential problems for the anaesthetist (Figure 1.5). It is particularly important to assess the volume status of the patient who has an electrolyte disturbance. Electrolyte disturbances are more likely to be acute and hence more serious in patients presenting for emergency surgery.

Preoperatively, hyponatraemia may be longstanding, commonly due to diuretics, and this situation rarely requires treatment. More acutely, preoperative hyponatraemia is often due to inappropriate intravenous therapy on the ward. Treatment should comprise the administration of intravenous normal saline and, if there are signs of fluid overload, diuretics. Severe symptomatic hyponatraemia has a high mortality, and is seen most commonly as part of the TUR (transurethral resection) syndrome (see Chapter 6). Hyponatraemia should be treated promptly with diuretics and only rarely with hypertonic saline. Too rapid correction of severe acute hyponatraemia may result in subdural haemorrhage, pontine lesions and cardiac failure. Hypernatraemia is mainly a problem when associated with volume depletion, and it should be corrected by administration of 5% dextrose intravenously, taking care not to fluid-overload the patient.

Chronic changes in plasma potassium are well tolerated, but acute changes are associated with ECG changes and cardiac dysrhythmias (Figure 1.6). It is the ratio of intracellular to extracellular potassium that is relevant to myocardial excitability. Where the disturbance is chronic, this ratio will be nearly normal. Hypokalaemia may be treated by giving potassium either orally or intravenously. Care must be taken in the presence of renal insufficiency or low cardiac output states, as hyperkalaemia may result. A flow-controlled pump should be used to control the intravenous infusion rate if the concentration of potassium exceeds 40 mmol L^{-1}, and ECG monitoring will be required, as ventricular fibrillation may occur if hypokalaemia is corrected too quickly. Hyperkalaemia should be treated over several days by the administration of calcium resonium. If ECG changes are noted, or if more rapid correction of acute changes is required preoperatively, insulin (20 units in 100 mL 20% dextrose over 30–60 minutes) may be given. This may be repeated, depending on the next serum potassium. Intravenous calcium (10 mL 10% calcium gluconate) immediately (but temporarily) improves automaticity, conduction and contractility.

Smoking

A heavy smoker is anyone who smokes 20 or more cigarettes per day. Smoking causes several perioperative problems: increased airway reactivity; increased sputum production and retention; bronchospasm; coughing and atelectasis associated with an increased risk of postoperative chest infection. Associated diseases include ischaemic heart disease and chronic obstructive pulmonary disease. Up to 15% of the haemoglobin in smokers combines with carbon monoxide to form carboxyhaemoglobin, reducing the oxygen-carrying capacity of blood. After 12–24 hours of stopping smoking the effects of carbon

Figure 1.5 Problems and causes of electrolyte disturbances

Problems	Causes
Hyponatraemia	
Confusion, fits and coma possible If water excess: hypertension, cardiac failure, anorexia and nausea	Excess water intake (particularly intravenously) Diuretics TUR syndrome Impaired water excretion (SIADH, hypothyroidism, cardiac failure, nephrotic syndrome)
Hypernatraemia	
Rarely symptoms if simple water loss If severe, there may be muscle weakness, signs of volume depletion and coma	Reduced intake (impaired consciousness, unable to swallow, no water) Increased insensible loss (fever, hot environment, hyperventilation) Impairment of urinary concentrating mechanism (diabetes insipidus, hyperosmolar non-ketotic coma or diabetic ketoacidosis)
Hypokalaemia	
Muscular weakness Potentiates non-depolarising muscle relaxants Cardiac arrhythmias Rhythm problems if on digoxin	Diuretics Gastrointestinal loss (diarrhoea, vomiting, fistula, ileus, villous adenoma of large bowel) Recovery phase of diabetic ketoacidosis and acute tubular necrosis Post relief of urinary tract obstruction Reduced intake Cushing's syndrome Hyperaldosteronism
Hyperkalaemia	
Spurious if blood sample haemolysed Cardiac arrest may occur if plasma K^+ > 7 mmol L^{-1}	Acute or chronic kidney disease Shift of K^+ out of cells (tissue damage) Acidosis (particularly diabetic ketoacidosis) Increased intake Drugs impairing secretion (K^+ retaining diuretics) Addison's disease Tissue breakdown (rhabdomyolysis)

monoxide and nicotine are significantly reduced, and after 6–8 weeks ciliary and immunological activity are restored. All smokers should be encouraged to abstain prior to theatre. Nicotine replacement therapy may prove helpful.

Concurrent medical disease

It is important to be aware of any medical condition affecting a patient and to ensure that its management prior to surgery is optimal. Emergency cases present particular problems, as nausea or vomiting may have caused the patient to omit usual medication. An understanding of the pharmacology and possible interactions of concurrent medication with anaesthetic drugs is also essential.

Respiratory disease
Viral infection

The commonest respiratory problem of relevance to anaesthesia is viral upper respiratory tract infection (URTI), which causes increased bronchial reactivity, particularly in asthmatic patients, persisting for 3–4 weeks

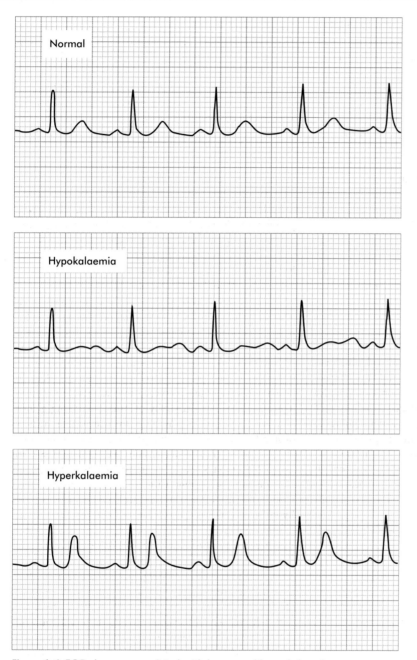

Figure 1.6 ECG changes associated with hypo- and hyperkalaemia

following resolution of the URTI. Current or recent URTI is also associated with an increased incidence of postoperative chest infection. Hence, unless surgery is urgent, such patients should be postponed for 4 weeks.

Asthma

Asthma is common, affecting 10–20% of the population. In many people the condition is mild and requires only occasional treatment, but in others there may be frequent and severe attacks requiring hospital admission and, in a few patients, ventilation on the intensive care unit. There are two main groups, although there is some overlap: **early-onset** asthma (atopic or extrinsic) and **late-onset** asthma (non-atopic or intrinsic). The symptoms of asthma are wheeze, cough, chest tightness and dyspnoea. They are caused by an inflammatory reaction within the bronchial wall which results in bronchospasm, mucosal swelling and viscid secretions. In atopic asthma exposure to allergens results in the formation of immunoglobulin E (IgE), which causes a type 1 or anaphylactic antigen–antibody hypersensitivity reaction.

The treatment of mild asthma is the occasional or regular use of inhaled selective β_2-adrenoceptor agonists such as salbutamol or terbutaline. Some patients may be using prophylactic inhaled sodium chromoglycate. In moderate cases regular inhaled corticosteroids are required. More severely affected patients may also be taking oral theophylline or regular oral steroids. Acute exacerbations of asthma may be treated with short courses of high-dose oral steroids. Regular steroids may cause adrenocortical suppression and prevent the normal stress response to surgery, and thus perioperative hydrocortisone cover may be required. Usual bronchodilator therapy should be continued preoperatively. It is common practice to prescribe a preoperative dose of inhaled β_2-adrenoceptor agonist immediately prior to the patient going to theatre, and to ensure that the patient brings his or her inhaler to theatre in case it is required postoperatively. As bronchospasm may be precipitated by anxiety, benzodiazepine premedication is often prescribed. Sedative drugs are contraindicated in anyone experiencing an acute exacerbation of asthma.

Assessment of the severity of asthma may be made from the history: frequency of attacks, whether the patient has ever been admitted to hospital with an attack or has ever required ventilation, whether oral steroids are ever necessary and if so how frequently. Nocturnal cough and frequent waking with symptoms indicate poor control of asthma. A chest radiograph in an asthmatic patient who is currently well is often normal, and is not necessary preoperatively. In longstanding cases there may be hyperinflation of the lungs. Pulmonary function tests provide a useful indication of the degree of airflow obstruction: in particular, the forced expiratory volume in 1 second (FEV_1) and the peak expiratory flow rate (PEFR) are used. If a patient's normal PEFR is known, the current state of the asthma may be ascertained from preoperative measurement of PEFR. If the patient has experienced a recent exacerbation, with an increase in symptoms, reduced PEFR and increased requirement for medication, it is appropriate to postpone elective surgery until the condition has returned to normal, which may take several weeks. Where surgery is urgent, steps should be taken to optimise the patient's condition in the time available by the use of a nebulised β_2-adrenoceptor agonist and, if it is severe, the commencement of enteral or parenteral steroids.

Chronic obstructive pulmonary disease (COPD)

Chronic bronchitis and emphysema are different pathologically but frequently coexist as chronic obstructive pulmonary disease. A patient's condition may fall anywhere in a spectrum from solely chronic bronchitis to solely emphysema, with the majority of patients possessing symptoms and signs of both. The main feature of both diseases is generalised airflow obstruction.

Chronic bronchitis is defined as daily cough with sputum production for at least three consecutive months a year for at least two consecutive years. It develops as a result of longstanding irritation of the bronchial mucosa, nearly always by tobacco smoke. The disease is more common in middle and later life, in smokers than in non-smokers, and in urban than in rural dwellers. Pathologically there is hypertrophy of mucus-secreting glands and mucosal oedema, leading to irreversible airflow obstruction. Air becomes 'trapped' in the alveoli on expiration causing alveolar distension, which may result in associated emphysema. Chronic bronchitis is a progressive disease, worsening with each acute exacerbation. Eventually respiratory failure develops, characterised by hypoxia, polycythaemia, pulmonary hypertension and cor pulmonale. Rarely, chronic hypercapnia may lead to loss of the central response to carbon dioxide, resulting in a 'blue bloater' whose hypoxia is the only stimulus to ventilation. If these patients undergo general anaesthesia they are extremely difficult to wean and to extubate. Symptoms of chronic bronchitis are cough with sputum, dyspnoea and wheeze. Clinical signs include hyperinflation of the chest, variable inspiratory and expiratory wheeze and often basal crackles, which may disappear after coughing. Peripheral oedema and raised jugular venous pressure are found with cor pulmonale, and there may be cyanosis.

Emphysema is defined as enlargement of the air spaces distal to the terminal bronchioles with destructive changes in the alveolar wall. The main cause of emphysema is smoking, although the rare genetic deficiency of α_1-antitrypsin may cause severe emphysema in young adults. The complications of emphysema include rupture of a pulmonary bulla leading to pneumothorax, and later respiratory failure and cor pulmonale may occur. Classically emphysematous patients are described as 'pink puffers'. The only symptom of emphysema is exertional dyspnoea, or dyspnoea at rest as the condition worsens. The main clinical sign of emphysema is a hyperinflated chest.

The treatment of chronic obstructive pulmonary disease is mostly symptomatic, once the patient has stopped smoking. Bronchodilators are useful if there is an element of reversible airways obstruction. Patients may be prescribed inhaled β_2-agonists, ipratropium bromide and theophylline. Diuretic therapy may be used to control right-sided heart failure. Patients who are hypoxic with pulmonary hypertension may be on domiciliary oxygen therapy, a bad prognostic indicator.

There are no characteristic radiological abnormalities due to chronic bronchitis, but coexisting emphysema may result in the appearance of hyperinflation with low flat diaphragms, loss of peripheral vascular markings and prominent hilar vessels (bat winging) and bullae. The heart is narrow until cor pulmonale develops. The presence of bullae supports the diagnosis of emphysema, and occasionally a giant emphysematous bulla will be seen, in which case surgical ablation may improve symptoms and lung function. Preoperative pulmonary function tests may help determine which of the two pathological conditions predominates. Arterial blood gas analysis is indicated to assess gas exchange if a patient has severe dyspnoea on mild or moderate exertion.

If there is a history of recent onset of green sputum production rather than white, and clinical signs support a diagnosis of chest infection, surgery should if possible be postponed and a course of antibiotics and physiotherapy commenced.

Pulmonary function tests

Peak expiratory flow rate (PEFR) is the rate of flow of exhaled air at the start of a forced expiration, and is measured using a simple flow meter. Reduced values compared to predicted values for age, height and sex indicate airflow obstruction. Serial measurements are useful for monitoring disease progress and for demonstrating a response to bronchodilator therapy.

Spirometric tests of lung function are easy to perform. If a subject exhales as hard and as long as possible from a maximal inspiration, the volume expired in the first second is the forced expiratory volume in 1 second

(FEV_1) and the total volume expired is the forced vital capacity (FVC). The measured values are compared to predicted values for age, height and sex. The ratio of FEV_1 to FVC (FEV%) is most useful (normal range 65–80%). Obstructive airways disease, e.g. asthma, reduces the FEV_1 more than the FVC, so the FEV% is low. Restrictive airways disease, e.g. pulmonary fibrosis, reduces the FVC and, to a lesser degree, the FEV_1, so the FEV% is normal or high (Figure 1.7).

Arterial blood gas analysis may be useful, and interpretation should be systematic. Look first at the pH value (acidosis or alkalosis) to determine the direction of the primary change. Although there may be partial compensation for the underlying abnormality, there is never full or over-compensation. Then look at the PCO_2, which is determined by alveolar ventilation. A low PCO_2 (hyperventilation) indicates a respiratory alkalosis or respiratory compensation for a metabolic acidosis. Conversely a raised PCO_2 (hypoventilation) indicates a respiratory acidosis. The PCO_2 does not increase above normal to compensate for a metabolic alkalosis. Next, consider the standard bicarbonate value (HCO_3^-). This is defined as the extracellular fluid (ECF) bicarbonate concentration the patient would have if the PCO_2 were normal. If standard bicarbonate is raised, there is either a metabolic alkalosis or metabolic compensation for a respiratory acidosis. If the standard bicarbonate is low, there is a metabolic acidosis or metabolic compensation for a respiratory alkalosis. The base excess is defined as the number of mmol of HCO_3^- which must be added to (or removed from) each litre of ECF to return the ECF pH to 7.4, if the PCO_2 were normal. A negative base excess (a base deficit) indicates metabolic acidosis, so is found with a low standard bicarbonate; a positive base excess, which is found with a raised standard bicarbonate, indicates metabolic alkalosis. Finally, the PO_2 should be examined. A low PO_2 indicates hypoxaemia and a raised PO_2 indicates that the patient is receiving additional oxygen.

Cardiovascular disease

Hypertension

Hypertension occurs in 15% of the UK population. Although mean systemic diastolic and systolic arterial pressure rise with increasing age, hypertension is defined by arbitrarily set levels. In 97% of these patients the cause is unknown, and they are said to have 'essential' or primary hypertension. In the remaining 3% hypertension is secondary to renal or endocrine disease, coarctation of the

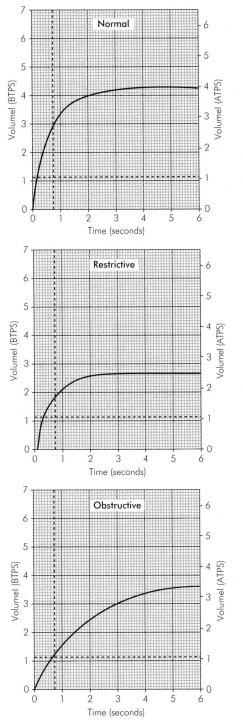

Figure 1.7 Spirometric tests in obstructive and restrictive pulmonary disease

aorta, drugs or pregnancy. It seems important that hypertension is adequately controlled preoperatively.

However, the evidence for what level of blood pressure constitutes a risk for anaesthesia and how great that risk is remains unclear. There is no evidence that patients with stage 1 (140–159 mmHg systolic and 90–99 mmHg diastolic) and stage 2 (160–179 mmHg systolic and 100–109 mmHg diastolic) hypertension in the absence of target organ damage have increased perioperative cardiovascular risk (Hartle *et al.* 2016). Patients with stage 3 (180–209 mmHg systolic and 110–119 mmHg diastolic) and 4 ($\geq$ 210 mmHg systolic and $\geq$ 120 mmHg diastolic) hypertension, who are more likely to have target organ damage, have not been rigorously tested for increased perioperative cardiovascular risk.

According to NICE (2011), in the community, clinic blood pressure should be controlled if it is above 140 mmHg systolic and 90 mmHg diastolic (150/90 in those aged 80 and over). The latest UK recommendations use documented blood pressures of below 160/90 as a cutoff for booking elective surgery and recommend that these should be provided in the referral letter from the general practitioner (Hartle *et al.* 2016). If these values are not available in the preoperative assessment clinic blood pressures, then blood pressures below 180 mmHg systolic and 110 mmHg diastolic are acceptable. It is also unclear whether or not control of hypertension prior to elective surgery will reduce perioperative complications, morbidity and mortality. The emphasis on managing the patient perioperatively is focused on the management of cardiovascular risk rather than precise blood pressure values. Isolated systolic hypertension is most prevalent in the elderly population and is a significant risk factor for stroke as well as cardiovascular morbidity in this group.

The pathogenesis of primary hypertension is not understood, but it is known that systemic vascular resistance (SVR) is increased, leading to a possible decrease in cardiac output by 15–20%. Additionally, the level of sympathetic nervous system activity is high, resulting in a greater than normal response to any stimulus. In a hypertensive patient there is a much greater fall than normal in systemic arterial pressure on induction of anaesthesia, due to a fall in cardiac output resulting from decreases in both heart rate and stroke volume. This exaggerated fall is lessened in controlled hypertension. Importantly, there is an increased risk of postoperative myocardial infarction in hypertensive patients. Hypertension is associated with other diseases of relevance to the anaesthetist such as ischaemic heart disease (IHD), peripheral vascular disease

(PVD), renal disease, cerebrovascular disease and diabetes mellitus. At preoperative assessment the anaesthetist should look for evidence of any of these conditions and for end-organ damage due to hypertension. An ECG may reveal left ventricular hypertrophy (LVH) or ischaemic heart disease. Serum urea, electrolytes and creatinine may reveal renal impairment, and serum glucose may show diabetes. Chest x-ray may reveal left ventricular enlargement, and distended upper pulmonary lobe veins indicate left ventricular failure. In advanced failure there is generalised hazy opacification spreading out from the hilum and possibly Kerley 'B' lines or pleural effusions.

Drug treatment

Usual antihypertensive therapy should be continued on the day of surgery. Antihypertensive agents tend to potentiate the hypotensive effects of general anaesthesia. Thiazide diuretics are a common first-line treatment for hypertension, particularly in the elderly. Thiazide treatment can often result in hypokalaemia or hyponatraemia. β-Adrenergic antagonists are frequently employed in conjunction with a thiazide. Despite their advantages during anaesthesia (depression of the cardiovascular response to laryngoscopy and to surgical stimulation), β-blockers may cause problems: bradycardia, atrioventricular block, decreased myocardial contractility, bronchoconstriction and altered response to inotropes. If β-blockers are stopped preoperatively, hypertension, arrhythmias and myocardial ischaemia are increased intraoperatively, as is postoperative myocardial ischaemia. Calcium channel antagonists are also prescribed for hypertension. Diltiazem and verapamil may cause bradycardia. Angiotensin-converting enzyme (ACE) inhibitors are also used for the treatment of cardiac failure, and these agents are associated with hypotension and hyperkalaemia. Angiotensin II receptor antagonists and imidazoline receptor antagonists are effective alternatives.

Sedative premedication is often prescribed for hypertensive patients to reduce endogenous catecholamine levels that may exacerbate the hypertension.

Ischaemic heart disease (IHD)

In the UK 12–20% of patients undergoing surgery have preoperative evidence of myocardial disease. This is almost always due to atheroma, although rarely other disease processes may be responsible. With increasing age atheromatous plaques form in the intima of arteries. These plaques grow and evolve with time, decreasing blood flow through a vessel and possibly occluding it.

The rate of progression of individual plaques within any patient is variable, and this explains why, although peripheral vascular and cerebrovascular disease will often coexist with coronary artery disease, the patient may be asymptomatic of these other conditions.

IHD may be diagnosed from a history of angina or myocardial infarction (MI). It may also be the underlying cause of a conduction defect or arrhythmia. A guide to the severity of angina is the exertion necessary to precipitate an attack. The distance that is regularly walked on the flat before an attack occurs should be elicited in the history. It may be that angina is only occasional, such as when climbing more than one flight of stairs or in very cold weather. If angina is precipitated by minimal exertion or is even occurring at rest (unstable angina), the patient has severe myocardial insufficiency and anaesthesia may present problems. If elective surgery is proposed, this should be cancelled and the patient investigated further with a view to cardiac intervention. It is important to establish the timing of any previous MI. Perioperative MI has a mortality of up to 70%. The risk of perioperative MI is 0.1–0.2% when there is no history of previous MI. The overall risk of reinfarction with a history of previous MI is 6–7%, this varying in relation to the time elapsed since that MI. The introduction of thrombolysis has reduced the reinfarction rate.

The progressive, episodic nature of IHD has led many workers to attempt to make predictions about the postoperative risk of cardiac complications following major non-cardiac surgery.

Perioperative assessment of cardiac risk

The Goldman cardiac risk index was one of the earlier multifactorial scoring systems designed to predict clinical risk, but despite various modifications and the introduction of alternative scoring systems, overall predictive accuracy has remained disappointingly limited.

However, much of the work supports the likelihood that certain factors consistently reduce perioperative cardiac morbidity and mortality. These include preoperative optimisation of cardiac status, aggressive invasive monitoring and prompt treatment of intraoperative haemodynamic disturbance.

The modified cardiac risk index has proved useful in the development of guidelines for the preoperative assessment of patients with documented or asymptomatic IHD, left ventricular dysfunction and valvular heart disease. In 2009 the European Society of Cardiology and the European Society of Anaesthesiology published guidelines for preoperative cardiac risk assessment and perioperative cardiac management in patients undergoing non-cardiac surgery, building on earlier guidelines from the American College of Cardiology and the American Heart Association. The guidelines integrate clinical risk factors and functional capacity with the risk for cardiac events of the planned surgical procedure when evaluating patients preoperatively. Clinical predictors of perioperative cardiac risk include cardiac and non-cardiac factors, stratified as major, intermediate and minor (Figure 1.8). A functional capacity of less than 4 MET (unable to climb a flight of stairs) is associated with increased cardiac risk.

Figure 1.8 Clinical predictors of increased perioperative cardiovascular risk

Major
- Unstable coronary syndromes
  - Acute or recent myocardial infarction with evidence of important ischaemic risk by clinical symptoms or non-invasive study
  - Unstable or severe angina (Canadian class III or IV)
- Decompensated heart failure
- Significant arrhythmias
  - High-grade atrioventricular block
  - Symptomatic ventricular arrhythmias in the presence of underlying heart disease
  - Supraventricular arrhythmias with uncontrolled ventricular rate
- Severe valvular disease

Intermediate
- Mild angina pectoris (Canadian class I or II)
- Previous myocardial infarction by history or pathological Q waves
- Compensated or prior heart failure
- Diabetes mellitus (particularly insulin-dependent)
- Renal insufficiency

Minor
- Advanced age
- Abnormal ECG (left ventricular hypertrophy, left bundle branch block, ST–T abnormalities)
- Rhythm other than sinus (e.g. atrial fibrillation)
- Low functional capacity (inability to climb one flight of stairs)
- History of stroke
- Uncontrolled systemic hypertension

ACC/AHA Guideline Update for Perioperative Cardiovascular Evaluation for Noncardiac Surgery: executive summary. *Anesth Analg* 2002; **94**: 1052–64.

Tests of functional capacity include exercise ECG, cardiopulmonary exercise testing and myocardial perfusion scans. Surgery-specific risk is considered in terms of type of non-cardiac surgery and the anticipated degree of haemodynamic stress associated with the planned procedure (Figure 1.9). Cardiovascular risk is defined in terms of myocardial infarction, heart failure and death. An algorithmic process is used to identify patients who might benefit from further investigation (such as echocardiography and radionuclide scanning) or therapeutic intervention.

These guidelines have enabled us to move away from the previously quoted intervals of 3 and 6 months' delay when considering perioperative risk following MI. Indeed, some patients would now be considered for elective surgery within 1 month of an MI. In other words, patients with cardiac disease awaiting elective surgery can be considered on a more individual basis with respect to their perioperative risk.

The electrocardiogram

As with other preoperative investigations, the indications for a 12-lead ECG have changed over time. For an ASA

Figure 1.9 Surgery-specific cardiac risk for non-cardiac surgery (combined incidence of cardiac death and non-fatal myocardial infarction)

High (cardiac risk often > 5%)
- Emergent major operations, particularly in the elderly
- Aortic and other major vascular surgery
- Peripheral vascular surgery
- Anticipated prolonged surgical procedures associated with large fluid shifts and/or blood loss

Intermediate (cardiac risk generally < 5%)
- Carotid endarterectomy
- Head and neck surgery
- Intraperitoneal and intrathoracic surgery
- Orthopaedic surgery
- Prostate surgery

Low (cardiac risk generally < 1%)
- Endoscopic procedures
- Superficial procedure
- Cataract surgery
- Breast surgery

ACC/AHA Guideline Update for Perioperative Cardiovascular Evaluation for Noncardiac Surgery: executive summary. *Anesth Analg* 2002; **94**: 1052–64.

Figure 1.10 ECG abnormalities associated with myocardial ischaemia

Conduction abnormalities	Degrees of heart block Bundle branch block
Arrhythmias	Multifocal ventricular ectopics Episodes of VT or VF
QRS	Presences of Q waves Poor R wave progression
ST segment	> 1 mm depression > 2 mm depression
T wave	Isoelectric Inverted Reverted

Figure 1.11 Diagnosis of arrhythmias

Rate	Rhythm	Diagnosis
Normal	Irregular	Multiple ectopics
Fast	Regular	Sinus tachycardia Atrial flutter Supraventricular tachycardia
Fast	Irregular	Atrial fibrillation Atrial flutter with variable block
Slow	Regular	Complete heart block
Fast and slow	Irregular	Sick sinus syndrome

1 patient undergoing minor surgery, it is only recommended if aged > 80 years. However, a 12-lead ECG is indicated if there is any evidence of cardiovascular disease, whatever the age of the patient and however minor the surgery proposed; also if the patient has severe renal disease (creatinine > 200 μmol L^{-1} or on a regular dialysis programme). For those aged > 60 years undergoing intermediate-risk surgery, an ECG is indicated. (Figure 1.10). Left axis deviation indicates IHD, while right axis deviation may be normal. Only 50% of old MIs will be seen. An exercise ECG may be indicated in patients in at-risk groups, e.g. those undergoing peripheral vascular surgery, if the resting ECG is normal, there is no LVH and no previous MI. Continuous ambulatory ECG may be useful if the patient's ability to exercise is limited. Although abnormal rhythms may be detected clinically, an ECG is needed to confirm diagnosis. Rate and rhythm should be noted (Figure 1.11), and a 24-hour ECG may be useful.

Sinus tachycardia has several common causes such as anxiety, pyrexia, cardiac failure and anaemia. Supraventricular tachycardia may be due to a congenital conduction abnormality. IHD is the main cause of the other arrhythmias, although thyroid disease should not be forgotten. Atrial tachyarrhythmias should be controlled preoperatively with digoxin or amiodarone therapy. Complete heart block, any form of bifascicular block and sick sinus syndrome require preoperative pacing. Multifocal ventricular ectopics are more significant than unifocal ectopics, indicating IHD. Atrial ectopics are not usually significant.

Other cardiac investigations

Echocardiography uses ultrasound to study blood flow, the structure of the heart and the movement of valves and cardiac muscle. Ventricular volumes, ejection fraction and gradients across valves can be estimated. The ejection fraction is particularly useful: it is normally over 60%; if it is less than 40% serious problems associated with anaesthesia should be anticipated.

Chest x-ray may show cardiomegaly, with a cardiothoracic ratio of > 0.5. Seventy per cent of patients with cardiomegaly have an ejection fraction of less than 50%.

Radionuclide scanning provides a relatively non-invasive means of accurately assessing myocardial function. In blood pool scanning [99]technetium-labelled red blood cells are injected intravenously and then both the amount of blood in the heart at each stage of the cardiac cycle and the shape of the cardiac chambers can be determined. The scanning camera may be linked to ECG and pictures collected over multiple cardiac cycles (multigated or MUGA scans). In perfusion scintigraphy, acute MI may be detected by 'hot spot' scanning. This technique also uses [99]technetium, which is taken up into the acutely infarcted myocardial tissue thus revealing the position and extent of the damage. Conversely, 'cold spot' scanning uses [201]thallium to demonstrate areas of myocardial ischaemia and scarring. [201]Thallium behaves like a potassium ion and is distributed throughout the heart muscle depending on coronary blood flow. It is taken up by normal myocardium, so areas that are not being perfused show on the scan as perfusion defects. A coronary vasodilator, such as dipyridamole, may then be given. A fixed perfusion defect indicates scar tissue while a reperfusion defect indicates ischaemia. Reperfusion defects are more significant because ischaemia may develop perioperatively, whereas a fixed perfusion defect cannot deteriorate.

Cardiopulmonary exercise testing (CPX) has been shown to identify those patients at high risk of developing cardiopulmonary complications after surgery, primarily through identification of anaerobic threshold (AT). Measurement of AT involves the patient pedaling on a static bike as the resistance is increased, while oxygen consumption (VO_2) and carbon dioxide production (VCO_2) are measured via a mouthpiece. Initially VO_2 and VCO_2 increase in parallel until, with increasing workload, anaerobic metabolism starts to occur ('the anaerobic threshold'). AT is the oxygen consumption at which lactate starts to be produced. At this point, the relationship of VO_2 to VCO_2 changes, as shown by a change in the slope of the graph of VCO_2 against VO_2. The original work on this showed patients with an oxygen consumption at AT of < 11 mL kg^{-1} min^{-1} had a higher mortality after major surgery (18%) than those with an AT > 11 (Older *et al.* 1999). Patients who had an AT < 11 and clinical IHD had a much higher mortality (42%). More recent work has confirmed the predictive value of AT (Snowden *et al.* 2010).

Implantable pacemakers and implantable cardioverter defibrillators (ICDs)

The need for cardiac pacing results from disease of the conducting system of the heart, which may or may not be associated with IHD. ICDs are used in the primary and secondary prevention of fast arrhythmias in patients who may have IHD, a familial cardiac condition, such as long QT syndrome or hypertrophic cardiomyopathy, or have undergone surgical repair of congenital heart disease. ICDs may be dual function, combining pacemaker and conventional ICD capabilities in one device.

A variety of pacemakers may be encountered, depending on the age of the unit. Modern pacemakers operate through a lead in the atrium, ventricle or both. Depolarisation arising endogenously may either inhibit or trigger a paced beat. Pacemakers are classified using a five-letter code as in Figure 1.12.

As an illustration, an AAI unit paces atrially and will be inhibited by sensing an endogenous depolarisation in the atrium. In contrast a VVT unit paces ventricularly and is triggered if an endogenous depolarisation is sensed in the ventricle.

Most modern units are dual units which work in DDD mode, providing atrial pacing in the presence of atrial bradycardia and ventricular pacing after an atrial depolarisation (endogenous or paced) if a spontaneous ventricular beat is absent.

Figure 1.12 Generic pacemaker code

1st code letter	2nd code letter	3rd code letter	4th code letter	5th code letter
Paced chamber	Sensed chamber	Response to endogenous depolarisation	Programmable functions	Antiarrhythmic function
I	II	III	IV	V
V (ventricle)	V (ventricle)	T (trigger)	P (rate)	S (scanning)
A (atrium)	A (atrium)	I (inhibited)	M (multiprogrammable)	E (externally activated)
D (double)	D (double)	D (double)	C (communicating)	
	O (none)	O (none)	R (rate responsive)	
			B (impulse burst)	
			N (normal rate competition)	
			O (none)	

The characteristics of an implanted pacemaker can sometimes be changed externally, either by application of magnets or by radiofrequency generators. The most usual indication for this is a change of demand to fixed rate. However, most modern units require a cautious approach to the use of magnets, which may expose a programmable unit to the risk of being re-set in a variable fashion. All patients who have an implanted pacemaker have a registration card with details of the device (Figure 1.13).

Preoperative assessment should be directed to determining the indication for the device, the type of unit and its characteristics. Examination of the cardiovascular system should be undertaken in detail. Chest x-ray will help identify the pulse generator siting and lead placement and number.

Surgical diathermy and pacemakers

Use of surgical diathermy in the presence of an implanted pacemaker/ICD should be avoided wherever possible, as it can give rise to electrical interference causing the device to malfunction or fail. Energy can also be induced into heart lead systems causing tissue heating at lead tips through high-frequency currents.

Where the surgical procedure is remote from the pacemaker/ICD and the device has been checked and verified in the last 3 months (especially battery condition), risk of malfunction will be minimal. However, where the procedure will be close to the implant and where the use of diathermy is likely, then risk of malfunction is increased. Support from a cardiac pacing/ICD physiologist before, during and after surgery may be required to:

- Confirm correct functioning and check condition of device before and after surgery.
- Program an ICD to 'monitor only' mode prior to surgery.
- Adjust sensing/pacing parameters if required.

Recommendations for the use of surgical diathermy in the presence of an implantable pacemaker/ICD are as follows:

- Ensure availability of temporary external/transvenous pacing and external defibrillation equipment.
- Monitor patient's ECG constantly.
- Consider using an alternative method of detecting patient's pulse, e.g. pulse oximeter or arterial line.
- Place the indifferent electrode on the same side as the operation and as far from the pacemaker/ICD as possible.

- Limit the use of diathermy as much as possible, and to short bursts.
- Use the lowest current setting possible.
- Use bipolar diathermy (but power of coagulation is less).

For emergency procedures it may not be possible to find out the details of an implantable device or involve a cardiac pacing/ICD physiologist. The recommendations above should be followed. For patients with ICDs, securing a clinical magnet over the implant site to inhibit inappropriate shock delivery for the duration of surgery can be considered. Any subsequent VT/VF will need to be treated using external defibrillation equipment. However, some ICDs may be programmed not to respond to an external magnet. With pacemakers, magnet response will vary between models and programmed settings.

Valvular heart disease

The availability of echocardiography today means that any patient with suspected valve disease should be properly investigated and a diagnosis made prior to anaesthesia. Valve angioplasty or replacement is sometimes indicated before elective surgery. Unfortunately, patients with significant valve disease may still present for emergency surgery. Any patient with a heart valve lesion, including replacement valves, requires prophylactic antibiotics for dental, genitourinary, obstetric, gynaecological and gastrointestinal procedures. The current recommended regimes are found in the British National Formulary. The main causes of valvular heart disease are shown in Figure 1.14. Note that multiple valve lesions may coexist.

Aortic stenosis

The symptoms of aortic stenosis occur late and include angina, syncope, dyspnoea and sudden death. Clinical signs are difficult to assess but generally include plateau pulse, LVH and an aortic ejection systolic murmur which is similar in character to that of aortic sclerosis. The ECG may show LVH with strain. On chest x-ray, left ventricular enlargement may not be evident and the aortic valve may be calcified. Echocardiography determines the gradient across the valve and will provide information on ventricular function. If the valve gradient is greater than 50 mmHg, angioplasty or valve replacement should be considered. The main anaesthesia-related problems are fixed cardiac output, ventricular arrhythmias and incipient cardiac failure.

Figure 1.13 Preoperative assessment of the pacemaker patient

Coded information recorded at implantation on European Pacemaker Registration Card	Symptom	01–02	unspecified
		03–04	dizziness or syncope
		05	bradycardia
		06	tachycardia
		07–09	miscellaneous conditions
	ECG rhythm	01–04	sinus or unspecified
		05–07	second-degree AV block
		08–10	complete heart block
		11–21	bundle branch or bifascicular block
	Aetiology	01–03	unspecified
		04–05	idiopathic or ischaemic
		06	post infarction
		07–11	miscellaneous conditions
ECG rhythm	(1) All beats preceded by a pacemaker spike: assume patient is pacemaker-dependent		
	(2) If native rhythm predominates: patient is unlikely to be pacemaker-dependent		
	(3) No evidence of pacemaker activity: magnet may be applied over pulse generator to switch to fixed-rate pacing		
	(4) If pacemaker spike is not followed by P or QRS wave suspect pacemaker malfunction (note: if pacemaker is activated by a magnet to pace at a fixed rate, the spike may fall in the refractory period and fail to stimulate the ventricle)		
Chest x-ray	(1) Location of pulse generator		
	(2) Location of leads in atrium, ventricle or both		
	(3) If necessary, pulse generator model can be identified		

Bloomfield & Bowler (1989)

Aortic regurgitation

Aortic regurgitation gives rise to few symptoms until the left ventricle fails, when dyspnoea occurs. Clinical signs include a collapsing pulse, left ventricular enlargement and an early diastolic murmur. The ECG shows changes of LVH, and on chest x-ray the heart will be enlarged. Echocardiography shows a dilated left ventricle and aortic root. Problems with respect to anaesthesia are poor myocardial reserve and cardiac failure.

Mitral stenosis

Symptoms of mitral stenosis are dyspnoea, tiredness and haemoptysis. Clinical signs include malar flush and a mid-diastolic murmur. Mitral stenosis may be complicated by systemic embolism or pulmonary hypertension. The ECG will often demonstrate atrial fibrillation (AF), P mitrale and right ventricular hypertrophy. On chest x-ray there may be left atrial enlargement and pulmonary venous congestion. Patients with a small valve area on

Figure 1.14 Causes of valvular disease

Valve regurgitation
- Congenital
- Rheumatic fever
- Infective endocarditis
- Syphilitic aortitis
- Valve ring dilatation, e.g. dilated cardiomyopathy
- Traumatic valve rupture
- Senile degeneration
- Damage to chordae and papillary muscles, e.g. MI

Valve stenosis
- Congenital
- Rheumatic fever
- Senile degeneration

Figure 1.15 A classification of anaemia

MCV	Cause
Microcytic	Iron deficiency (hypochromic)
	Thalassaemia (hypochromic)
	Chronic disease
Normocytic	Chronic disease (normochromic or hypochromic)
	Mixed deficiency
	Acute blood loss (normochromic)
Macrocytic	Alcohol (normochromic)
	B_{12} or folate deficiency (normochromic)
	Pregnancy
	Hypothyroidism (normochromic)
	Low-grade haemolytic anaemia with high reticulocyte count

echocardiography or moderate symptoms need surgery. Specific problems with respect to anaesthesia include fixed cardiac output, pulmonary oedema, AF and anticoagulant therapy.

Mitral regurgitation

Progressive dyspnoea and tiredness are common symptoms of mitral regurgitation. Left ventricular enlargement and a pansystolic murmur are the predominant clinical signs. The ECG shows LVH, P mitrale and atrial fibrillation. Chest x-ray demonstrates left-sided enlargement of the heart, particularly atrial enlargement, and indications of pulmonary oedema may be seen. Echocardiography is useful to assess left ventricular function. Specific problems with respect to anaesthesia include pulmonary oedema, AF and anticoagulant therapy.

Tricuspid valve lesions

Tricuspid stenosis is usually associated with mitral and aortic valve disease. Tricuspid regurgitation is usually due to right ventricular enlargement. Anaesthesia-related problems are usually due to the accompanying other valve disease rather than to the tricuspid lesion itself.

Pulmonary valve lesions

Pulmonary stenosis is usually congenital, and may be part of Fallot's tetralogy. Pulmonary regurgitation is rare, and most often secondary to pulmonary hypertension.

Haematological disease
Anaemia

A patient is considered anaemic if the haemoglobin is below the normal range and polycythaemic if it is above the normal range. For adult females this is 12–16 g dL^{-1} and for adult males 13–17 g dL^{-1}. In children the range varies: a child is considered to be anaemic if the haemoglobin value is less than 18 g dL^{-1} at birth, less than 9 g dL^{-1} at 3 months, less than 11 g dL^{-1} from 6 months to 6 years, and less than 12 g dL^{-1} from 6 to 12 years.

The causes of anaemia are blood loss, inadequate production of erythrocytes and excessive destruction of erythrocytes. Anaemia may be classified by the mean cell volume of the erythrocyte (MCV) (Figure 1.15). The mean cell haemoglobin (MCH) is also useful, and defines hypo- and normochromic types of anaemia.

Iron deficiency is the most common cause of anaemia, but the cause is often multifactorial. Those patients in whom anaemia should be suspected include all females of child-bearing age (due to menstrual loss), the elderly (due to poor diet and other diseases) and all patients who are undergoing gastrointestinal or gynaecological surgery (due to blood loss). Most patients suffering from anaemia are completely asymptomatic. If severely anaemic, symptoms may include tiredness and dyspnoea on exertion, and in the elderly angina, heart failure and confusion may be precipitated.

A full blood count also provides the platelet count (raised in acute blood loss and acute inflammation) and the white cell count (raised in infection). A differential white cell count distinguishes between neutrophilia (bacterial infection, inflammation) and lymphocytosis (viral infection). If the platelet count, white cell count and haemoglobin are all low, this indicates marrow aplasia or infiltration. Abnormalities which may be detected on examination of the blood film include a raised reticulocyte count (haemolytic anaemia, continued bleeding), sickle cells or malarial parasites. Further investigation may be indicated prior to blood transfusion, e.g. additional blood tests (ferritin, vitamin B_{12}, folate, reticulocyte count, direct Coombs test) or bone marrow aspiration.

Of most relevance to anaesthesia is a decrease in the oxygen-carrying capacity of the blood. Although anaemia decreases blood viscosity and hence improves blood flow, with a consequent increase in oxygen delivery to the tissues, once the haemoglobin is less than 10 g dL^{-1} the increase in blood flow no longer compensates for the decreased oxygen-carrying capacity. Some authorities consider a haemoglobin value of greater than 8 g dL^{-1}, rather than 10 g dL^{-1}, acceptable for anaesthesia.

A secondary anaemia-related problem is the fact that cardiac output increases in order to maintain oxygen flux. In some patients this leads to cardiac failure, and in all patients cardiac reserve is decreased, reducing the ability to compensate for the myocardial depressant effects of anaesthesia. It is important to remember that cyanosis is only evident clinically when the level of deoxyhaemoglobin equals or exceeds 5 g dL^{-1}. Hence in severely anaemic patients cyanosis is rarely seen.

In patients with chronic anaemia, there is an increase in 2,3-diphosphoglycerate (2,3-DPG) concentration in the reticulocytes, which causes the oxyhaemoglobin dissociation curve to shift to the right, improving the offloading of oxygen in the tissues. Stored blood contains decreased levels of 2,3-DPG, which take 24 hours to reach normal levels following transfusion. Hence blood transfusion in an anaemic patient immediately prior to anaesthesia confers minimal advantage and may lead to fluid overload. For elective surgery, transfusion should be completed at least 24 hours earlier.

In patients who are acutely anaemic (for example due to recent blood loss), heart rate, arterial pressure, CVP and urine output should be closely monitored during fluid replacement to ensure normovolaemia is restored prior to anaesthesia. Blood should be transfused to achieve a haemoglobin > 10 g dL^{-1} and a haematocrit > 0.3. Administration of oxygen therapy will increase oxygen delivery by ensuring maximal saturation of the available haemoglobin and an increase in the dissolved oxygen in blood. Urgent surgery may be indicated to stop the bleeding, so resuscitation may need to be continued during anaesthesia and surgery.

Sickle cell disease

Sickle cell disease is due to a haemoglobinopathy which is inherited autosomally, resulting in the formation of haemoglobin S (HbS) instead of haemoglobin A (HbA). The S variant consists of two normal α chains and two abnormal β chains in which glutamic acid has been substituted by valine in the sixth amino acid from the N-terminal. Small decreases in oxygen tension cause HbS to polymerise and form pseudo-crystalline structures which distort the red blood cell membrane to produce the characteristic sickle-shaped cells. Sickled cells increase blood viscosity and obstruct blood flow in the microvasculature, leading to thrombosis and infarction. These sickled cells are also subject to abnormal sequestration. Patients homozygous for another haemoglobinopathy, HbC, suffer minimal morbidity, but patients heterozygous for HbS and HbC (haemoglobin SC disease) suffer from a mild form of sickle cell anaemia as the presence of HbC causes the HbS to sickle more easily.

Sickle cell anaemia results from a patient being homozygous for haemoglobin S. Sickle cell trait results from a patient being heterozygous for haemoglobin S. Patients with sickle cell trait are resistant to falciparum malaria, and it is in those areas of the world where falciparum malaria is endemic that the gene is particularly common: tropical Africa, northeast Saudi Arabia, east-central India and around the Mediterranean. The prevalence of HbSS in the UK black population is around 0.25%, and the prevalence of HbAS in the same population is around 10%.

The main clinical problems for patients suffering from sickle cell anaemia are chronic haemolytic anaemia and infarction crises. Infarction crises may be precipitated by dehydration, infection, hypoxia, acidosis or cold, although they may also occur spontaneously. Crises are very painful, often involving bones or the spleen, and may also cause cerebrovascular accidents, haematuria due to renal papillary necrosis and chest pain due to pulmonary infarction. Patients with sickle cell trait have a normal haemoglobin and are clinically well. Most of their red blood cells contain less than 50% HbS, and sickling occurs only when the oxygen tension is very low.

Preoperatively all patients in the at-risk population for HbS should be screened. A Sickledex test detects the presence of HbS by precipitating sickling of the red blood cells on exposure to sodium metabisulphite. If this test is positive then electrophoresis is necessary to distinguish between the heterozygote and the homozygote. In an emergency situation, if the Sickledex test is positive but there is no history to suggest sickle cell anaemia and the haemoglobin, the reticulocyte count and the blood film are normal, then it is safe to assume that the patient has the trait only. Haematological advice should always be sought for patients with sickle cell anaemia. Evidence of renal, pulmonary or cerebrovascular complications should be assessed preoperatively. Blood transfusion prior to elective surgery may be indicated if the anaemia is particularly severe, and exchange transfusion will be necessary prior to major surgery to reduce the concentration of HbS to around 40%. An intravenous infusion should always be set up preoperatively to avoid dehydration, and heavy premedication should be avoided. Depending on the type of surgery planned, the surgeon should be sufficiently experienced to proceed without the use of a tourniquet, as its use is contraindicated in both the homozygote and the heterozygote.

Clotting abnormalities

If a patient has a history of liver disease or bleeding problems, or is taking anticoagulants, a clotting screen is indicated. Clotting may also be abnormal after massive blood transfusion or in pregnancy-induced hypertension. The activated partial thromboplastin time (APTT) measures factors VIII, IX, XI and XII in the intrinsic system. It is prolonged by warfarin therapy and liver disease. In contrast the prothrombin time (PT) measures factors I, II, VII and X in the extrinsic system and is prolonged by heparin therapy and in dilutional coagulopathy. The international normalised ratio (INR) is the ratio of the PT sample time to control time, a widely used indicator of clotting function. An INR of < 2.0 is considered safe for most surgery.

Coagulation abnormalities due to liver disease should be corrected by vitamin K administration. The effects of warfarin should be temporarily reversed by fresh frozen plasma (FFP), not by vitamin K, which will prevent the recommencement of warfarin therapy. Heparin coagulopathy is corrected by stopping the heparin or, more urgently, by protamine. FFP is required to correct a dilutional coagulopathy, as may occur with massive blood transfusion.

Disseminated intravascular coagulation (DIC) is indicated by decreased platelets, increased fibrin degradation products, decreased fibrinogen and prolonged APTT and PT. The underlying cause should be identified and treated, and clotting corrected with FFP (or cryoprecipitate) and platelet transfusion.

Thrombocytopenia may be asymptomatic, but haematological advice should be sought and platelets are usually given to ensure a platelet count above 50×10^9. For specific factor deficiencies, such as haemophilia, the purified factor or FFP should be given immediately preoperatively.

Musculoskeletal disease

Although many musculoskeletal conditions may be encountered prior to anaesthesia and surgery, by far the most common of these is rheumatoid arthritis.

Rheumatoid arthritis

Rheumatoid arthritis is an autoimmune connective tissue disease. The dominant pathological feature is a chronic destructive synovitis, which causes an inflammatory, typically symmetrical, deforming polyarthritis. Rheumatoid arthritis has many extra-articular features, which greatly influence the morbidity and mortality of the disease (Figure 1.16). Approximately 70% of patients are positive for rheumatoid factor, which is a circulating IgM antibody to the patient's own IgG. The overall prevalence is approximately 1%, with a male-to-female ratio of 1:3. Over the age of 55 years 5% of women and 2% of men are affected.

Rheumatoid arthritis is necessarily associated with a large number of drug-induced complications. Non-steroidal anti-inflammatory drugs (NSAIDs) are commonly used to treat pain and stiffness and may cause gastric erosions. The disease-modifying drugs used in the management of rheumatoid arthritis can similarly be associated with serious side effects. **Chloroquine** may cause haemolytic anaemia and ocular problems. **Sulphasalazine** rarely causes megaloblastic anaemia or hepatitis. **Oral gold** is less likely to cause marrow suppression or proteinuria than intramuscular gold.

Figure 1.16 Extra-articular features of rheumatoid arthritis

Respiratory	Fibrosing alveolitis, pleural effusion, rheumatoid nodules, bronchiolitis, Caplan's syndrome
Cardiovascular	Pericarditis, pericardial effusion, vasculitis, heart block, cardiomyopathy, aortic regurgitation
Renal	Amyloidosis (may affect other systems), drug-induced
Neurological	Cervical cord compression, peripheral neuropathy, entrapment neuropathy, mononeuritis multiplex
Haematological	Anaemia of chronic disease, iron-deficiency anaemia (NSAIDs), marrow suppression (gold), thrombocytosis, Felty's syndrome
Ocular	Keratoconjunctivitis sicca, scleritis, episcleritis, scleromalacia perforans

Methotrexate may cause marrow suppression or abnormal liver function. Although **penicillamine** may cause the nephrotic syndrome, it is also associated (rarely) with generalised marrow suppression and conditions which mimic myasthenia gravis or systemic lupus erythematosus (SLE). Some patients will be receiving systemic steroids for their disease, and others may be taking immunosuppressant drugs.

Rheumatoid arthritis most commonly affects the joints of the hands and feet, but the larger joints of the hips, knees and elbows may also be involved. Twenty-five per cent of patients with rheumatoid arthritis have cervical instability. Not all will have longstanding disease, and a quarter will have no clinical signs of cervical cord compression. The most common cervical problem is atlantoaxial subluxation, although subaxial subluxation may also occur. The atlantoaxial ligaments become lax and the odontoid peg is eroded, making neck flexion dangerous by risking cord compression. Also of interest to the anaesthetist are limited mouth opening due to temporomandibular joint involvement and, rarely,

airway obstruction due to dislocation of the cricoarytenoid joints. A hoarse voice suggests cricoarytenoid arthritis. Respiratory function may be additionally impaired by costochondrial joint disease, which can add to any restrictive defect.

It is therefore important to carefully assess the rheumatoid patient preoperatively for evidence of extra-articular involvement. A full blood count is essential and, if the patient is taking any disease-modifying drugs, serum electrolytes, urea and creatinine and liver function tests will also be necessary. Chest x-ray and pulmonary function tests may be indicated. Neck mobility and mouth opening should be assessed clinically. A lateral x-ray of the cervical spine in flexion and extension must be performed. If the gap between the odontoid peg and the posterior border of the anterior arch of the atlas is > 3 mm (or > 4 mm in those aged over 40 years), subluxation is present. Care should be taken when asking the patient to attempt maximal flexion of the cervical spine. Awake intubation may be indicated if a difficult intubation is anticipated, and if there is cervical spine involvement it will be necessary for the patient to wear a semi-rigid collar during anaesthesia to ensure perioperative cervical stability. If there is evidence of severe cervical spine instability, it is appropriate to refer the patient for surgical stabilisation.

Renal disease

Renal disease covers a wide spectrum of clinical pictures from decreased renal reserve, through varying degrees of renal impairment to end-stage kidney disease. Up to 80% of excretory function may be lost before a rise in serum urea or creatinine is seen. The creatinine value gives a useful indication of the degree of renal failure. The corresponding urea value is more readily affected by dietary protein, tissue breakdown and hydration and is therefore less useful. The cause of renal impairment or failure is very relevant to anaesthesia, because the underlying disease process may have other manifestations. Renal failure may be acute or chronic (Figure 1.17).

The majority of renal patients presenting for anaesthesia will have chronic kidney disease and most will be on a dialysis programme, involving either intermittent haemodialysis (HD) or continuous ambulatory peritoneal dialysis (CAPD). At preoperative assessment, the anaesthetist should establish the cause of renal failure and look for evidence of other systems affected by the same disease

Figure 1.17 Causes of renal failure

Chronic kidney disease
- Diabetic nephropathy
- Hypertensive nephropathy
- Chronic urinary tract obstruction
- Chronic glomerulonephritis
- Polycystic kidney disease
- Chronic bilateral pyelonephritis
- Collagen diseases
- Persisting acute renal failure

Acute kidney injury
- Pre-renal
  - Severe hypotension (hypovolaemia, cardiac failure, septic shock, drug overdose)
  - Major vessel disease (thrombosis, aortic aneurysm)
  - Intravascular haemolysis
  - Rhabdomyolysis
- Renal
  - Acute tubular necrosis (acute ischaemia, drugs, bacterial endotoxins)
  - Vasculitis
  - Acute glomerulonephritis
  - Acute interstitial nephritis
  - Coagulopathies
  - Eclampsia
- Post-renal
  - Urinary tract obstruction (prostatic hypertrophy, renal or ureteric stones, surgical mishap)

Figure 1.18 Systemic effects of renal failure

Cardiovascular
- Premature atheroma
- Hypertension
- Left ventricular failure
- Pericardial effusions

Respiratory
- Pulmonary venous congestion or oedema
- Pneumonia

Haematological
- Normochromic normocytic anaemia
- Prolonged bleeding time due to platelet dysfunction
- Increased incidence of hepatitis B carriage

Gastrointestinal
- Delayed gastric emptying
- Increased gastric acidity
- Peptic ulceration
- Impaired liver function

Neurological
- Peripheral and autonomic neuropathies
- Encephalopathy

Biochemical
- Metabolic acidosis with compensatory respiratory alkalosis
- Hyperkalaemia
- Hypocalcaemia
- Hypoalbuminaemia

process. Renal failure affects all systems of the body (Figure 1.18).

Necessary investigations include urea and electrolytes, creatinine, full blood count, clotting screen, liver function tests and hepatitis B surface antigen. Chest x-ray and ECG are also required. In evaluating the renal failure patient for anaesthesia, particular reference should be made to the fluid status. Twenty-four hours post-haemodialysis is the optimal time for elective surgery. Immediately following HD a patient may be volume-depleted. CAPD has far less effect on circulating volume and may be continued until surgery. Most patients will be chronically anaemic, but if asymptomatic and with no evidence of cardiovascular disease blood transfusion will probably not be necessary. Transfusion may precipitate fluid overload, and should be undertaken prior to or during the last HD before anaesthesia.

Hypertension should be controlled and fluid balance optimised. Acidosis and hyperkalaemia must be corrected by dialysis. The site of any arteriovenous fistula should be noted and arrangements made for it to be protected perioperatively by wrapping in gamgee. The limb with the fistula should **never** be used for intravenous access.

Endocrine disease

Patients suffering from endocrine disease should have their condition stabilised by consultation (where time allows) with the responsible physician. The most frequently encountered endocrine disease in surgical practice is diabetes mellitus, which is considered in more detail below and in Chapter 5.

Diabetes mellitus

Diabetes mellitus is characterised by a persisting state of hyperglycaemia due to lack or diminished effectiveness

Figure 1.19 Classification of diabetes mellitus

Primary

Type 1 (formerly 'insulin-dependent diabetes mellitus')

Type 2 (formerly 'non-insulin-dependent diabetes mellitus')

Secondary

Pancreatic disease, e.g. pancreatitis, pancreatectomy, neoplastic disease, cystic fibrosis

Excess production of insulin antagonists, e.g. growth hormone (acromegaly), glucocorticoids (Cushing's syndrome), thyroid hormones, catecholamines (phaeochromocytoma)

Drugs, e.g. corticosteroids, thiazides

Liver disease

of endogenous insulin. It presents problems to the anaesthetist both in respect of the need to ensure adequate perioperative control of blood glucose and in respect of the known long-term complications of the condition. Diabetes mellitus may be classified as primary or secondary (Figure 1.19). There are two types of primary diabetes mellitus: type 1 and type 2. As patients with type 2 diabetes may require insulin, the old terms of insulin-dependent diabetes mellitus for type 1 and non-insulin-dependent diabetes mellitus for type 2 are inappropriate. The prevalence in the UK is 4.2%, with approximately 15% type 1 and 85% type 2.

The aetiology of diabetes mellitus remains unclear, but it is known to be the result of environmental factors interacting with genetic factors. Type 1 usually presents before the age of 40 years and type 2 usually presents after the age of 40 years, but is increasingly presenting earlier. It is important to remember that patients with type 1 diabetes need insulin even when they are being starved. Surgery itself is a cause of stress resulting in increased secretion of the catabolic hormones (cortisol, growth hormone and glucagon), which results in increased catabolism and may lead to diabetic ketoacidosis in diabetes mellitus, both types 1 and 2. Thus type 2 patients who are undergoing major surgery will require insulin in the perioperative period, and type 1 patients will experience an increase in their insulin requirements.

Glycosuria which has been detected on routine urine testing performed preoperatively may often be the first indication that a patient has diabetes. As there is individual variation in the renal threshold for glucose, diagnosis should be confirmed by examining blood glucose. The diagnosis of diabetes mellitus may be made from a random blood glucose of > 11.1 mmol L^{-1} or a fasting blood glucose of > 7.0 mmol L^{-1}. If the patient is known to have diabetes, control may be assessed from measurement of glycosylated haemoglobin (HbA1c), as this reflects blood glucose control over the previous 6–8 weeks. Single blood glucose estimations are of little value. An elevated preoperative HbA1c is associated with adverse outcomes, but there is insufficient evidence to recommend an upper limit prior to elective surgery. The risks of proceeding when control is suboptimal should be balanced against the urgency of the procedure. An upper limit between 64 and 75 mmol mol^{-1} is acceptable, depending on individual circumstances. Postponement of surgery and referral to the local diabetes specialist team may be appropriate.

The long-term complications of diabetes are equally likely in both type 1 and type 2, and are related to the duration of the disease and the effectiveness of blood sugar control. Complications are due to disease of both large blood vessels (atheroma) and small blood vessels (microangiopathy). Atheroma causes the same pathological changes as in non-diabetic patients, but the disease occurs earlier and is both more extensive and more severe. Atheroma is the cause of the increased incidence of IHD and PVD in diabetic patients. Diabetic microangiopathy is the cause of diabetic nephropathy, retinopathy and neuropathy. Diabetes is a common cause of autonomic neuropathy, which can be detected at the bedside by demonstrating postural hypotension. Diabetic patients frequently present for surgery for the complications of their disease, and preoperative assessment must include screening for evidence of other complications. An ECG and other cardiac investigations may be indicated. Serum urea, electrolytes and creatinine should be performed to assess renal function.

While some type 2 diabetics are managed by diet alone, most will require one or more oral hypoglycaemic drugs as well as diet, and around a third will end up on insulin. The management of all type 1 diabetics is by diet and insulin. A variety of different types of oral hypoglycaemic drugs can be used, most of which depend on the presence of some endogenous insulin. **Sulphonylureas** act by augmenting insulin secretion and may also alter peripheral insulin receptor number and sensitivity. The commonly used sulphonylureas include glibenclamide, gliclazide and tolbutamide. Metformin is the only available **biguanide** and is often used in conjunction with a sulphonylurea. It enhances the peripheral action of insulin. Hypoglycaemia is very unusual with metformin, although it may cause lactic acidosis.

Acarbose inhibits intestinal α-glucosidases, delaying the digestion and absorption of starch and sucrose. The **meglitinides** nateglinide and repaglinide stimulate insulin release. Pioglitazone is a **thiazolidinedione** and reduces peripheral insulin resistance.

The **dipeptidylpeptidase-4 (DPP-4) inhibitors**, including linagliptin and saxagliptin, increase insulin secretion and lower glucagon secretion. The glucagon-like peptide 1 (GLP-1) analogues exenatide and liraglutide are given by subcutaneous injection and activate the GLP-1 receptor to increase insulin secretion.

The two main types of insulin preparation are unmodified, rapid-onset, short-acting (soluble) insulin and modified, delayed-onset, intermediate- or long-acting insulin. The insulin regime used varies from patient to patient. It may involve twice-daily or multiple injections of a combination of short- and longer-acting insulins before meals and at bedtime. Some patients use a continuous infusion of insulin via a portable infusion pump. Soluble insulin is the only form which can be given intravenously as well as subcutaneously and it is used for perioperative control of blood glucose. The management of diabetic patients presenting for surgery, including which drugs should be omitted on the day of surgery to prevent hypoglycaemia, is covered in Chapter 5.

Alcohol-related disease

As alcohol misuse increases as a social problem, so does the prevalence of alcohol-related disease.

While alcoholic liver disease may be the most obvious manifestation, there are many other potential associated conditions. These include cardiac disease such as cardiomyopathy and rhythm disturbances, haematological abnormalities, and metabolic disturbance. There may be associated neurological disease (including neuropathy).

All patients undergoing surgery should be asked about alcohol intake. Patients likely to have underlying alcohol-related disease, including dependency issues, can be sought using tools such as the CAGE questionnaire:

C Have you ever felt you should *cut down* on your drinking?

A Have you been *annoyed* by other people criticising your drinking?

G Have you ever felt *guilty* about drinking?

E Have you ever taken a drink in the morning to steady your nerves or *ease* a hangover?

A score greater than 2 prompts a more targeted history, examination and investigation pertaining to alcohol-related disease.

History and examination should focus on the possible cardiac and neurological manifestations of alcohol-related disease. In particular, evidence of cardiac failure and rhythm disturbance should be sought. Pre-existing neuropathies need to be noted and carefully documented, particularly in patients likely to be undergoing regional anaesthesia.

Investigation should include baseline blood investigations along with liver function tests and coagulation studies. Further haematological investigation may be indicated following a full blood count. A 12-lead ECG should certainly by carried out. An echocardiogram may be indicated if there are concerns regarding ventricular function.

Consideration should be given to perioperative alcohol withdrawal. Most hospitals will have local guidelines as to the management of these patients, some of whom may require a benzodiazepine, typically chlordiazepoxide.

Coagulopathy should be discussed with a haematologist preoperatively.

Obesity

Obesity continues to challenge us perioperatively and can represent a considerable anaesthetic and surgical risk.

The body mass index (BMI) is commonly used in defining obesity and is determined as weight in kilograms divided by height in metres squared ($kg\ m^{-2}$). The BMI can then be categorised as shown in Figure 1.20).

Obese patients comprise a high-risk group not just in terms of their practical anaesthesia management but also because of their associated comorbidities. Careful, targeted preoperative assessment enables us to address such comorbidities in order to guide perioperative management and evaluate risk. Obese patients are particularly at risk in terms of cardiorespiratory disease, metabolic disease and thromboembolism.

Cardiac disease

Hyperlipidaemia is common in obese patients and may underlie ischaemic heart disease. A history of

Figure 1.20 Body mass index

Body mass index (kg m^{-2})	Level of obesity*
< 25	Normal
25–27	Overweight
27–30	Mild obesity
30–35	Moderate obesity
35–40	Severe obesity
40–50	Morbid obesity
50–60	Super obesity
> 60	Super super obesity

* International Bariatric Surgery Register, USA

hypertension is common, and adequate control preoperatively must be established.

History-taking can be challenging in terms of establishing functional tolerance in these patients. Immobility due to obesity in itself can make it difficult to elicit symptoms such as angina and breathlessness which might normally alert us to cardiac ischaemia or cardiac failure. An echocardiogram may help to assess left ventricular function. Cardiopulmonary exercise testing may be helpful in assessing functional capacity but, again, obesity in itself may hamper such investigations.

Respiratory disease

Pre-existing respiratory disease in obese patients carries significant additional risk, both for anaesthesia itself and postoperatively.

A baseline assessment for patients with chronic obstructive airways disease may be indicated in the form of pulmonary function testing. This will provide information regarding reversibility and may indicate the need for a formal assessment by a respiratory physician.

It must be remembered that these patients have considerably reduced respiratory reserve and will potentially desaturate rapidly in the anaesthetic room during induction of anaesthesia, and indeed in the operating theatre when supine.

Obstructive sleep apnoea (OSA) is prevalent in obese patients. This may have been previously diagnosed and acted upon. If the patient has been using CPAP, for

instance, their equipment should be brought into hospital with them.

The Epworth Sleepiness Scale questionnaire is commonly used to identify patients who may suffer from OSA. It poses a series of questions regarding sleeping habits and determines likelihood of falling asleep during various activities in the daytime, such as while sitting reading or watching television, and reported snoring or apnoea. Thus a risk assessment may be carried out very easily in the preoperative assessment clinic using the questionnaire along with a history of snoring or sleep apnoea.

An Epworth score > 10 may indicate the need for referral and consideration of formal sleep studies, particularly if the history supports a possibility of OSA.

Metabolic disease

A history of diabetes mellitus should be sought, as this condition is common in the obese population.

Assessment can then be carried out as for any other diabetic patient. A glycosylated haemoglobin will give an indication as to adequacy of blood sugar control. Some preoperative assessment clinics are able to arrange for specialist dietary advice, although time does not always allow for this. Attempts at weight loss should be supervised and can often be facilitated by the patient's general practitioner.

Venous thromboembolism

A venous thromboembolism risk assessment is now a routine part of the preoperative preparation process. It is important that obese patients receive prophylaxis appropriate to their weight and the planned surgical procedure.

General considerations

Airway assessment is important in obese patients, as airway difficulties can be anticipated, prepared for and, hopefully, avoided.

The underlying physiology and respiratory mechanics in obese patients, e.g. reduced functional capacity, may lead to desaturation even in ideal conditions. Airway difficulties may lead to significant desaturation very quickly.

Regional anaesthesia often provides a solution regarding anaesthesia for obese patients. History and examination regarding issues which might preclude central neuraxial blockade are important, along with consideration of possible contraindications.

Morbidly obese patients sometimes require special equipment in terms of manual handling, anaesthetic room adjuncts and operating tables.

Early liaison with the anaesthetist and theatre staff will ensure that optimal, timely preparation can be put in place for such patients.

Increasingly, morbidly obese patients are presenting for surgery having already undergone bariatric surgery. Some of these patients will have devices such as a gastric band in situ. It may be necessary for intervention by the bariatric surgery team prior to the non-bariatric surgery. Some units advise elective deflation prior to general anaesthesia and surgery, although this is by no means always the case and will depend upon the nature of the surgical procedure. Most of these patients will have been provided with a contact number, and liaison with the bariatric surgery unit is generally encouraged to discuss the need for deflation.

Concurrent medication

Concurrent medication may interact with drugs administered during anaesthesia. Furthermore, the surgical procedure itself may be affected by, or indeed affect, such medication. For this reason it is important that careful consideration is given to preoperative drug management. Medication may have to be continued, stopped or modified. Alternatively, anaesthetic technique may have to be modified to minimise the risk of adverse interaction. A change in mode of administration or formulation is sometimes required.

Examples of drugs that should be continued are anticonvulsants, most cardiovascular drugs (antihypertensives, antianginals, antiarrhythmics), bronchodilators, corticosteroids and antiparkinsonian drugs. All are important in terms of providing optimal control of underlying conditions.

It is seldom necessary to stop drugs preoperatively, but a number of possible exceptions are worthy of discussion. **Warfarin** should be stopped several days preoperatively and the patient heparinised. To minimise the risk of thromboembolism **oral contraceptives** and **hormone replacement therapy** are often stopped several weeks before surgery. **Lithium therapy** should be stopped 24 hours before surgery. Most drugs that have been stopped preoperatively can be restarted when oral intake resumes. Should this be delayed, alternative routes of administration may have to be sought.

It is occasionally necessary to modify dose and formulation of a drug perioperatively, as is the case with **corticosteroid** therapy. Adrenal suppression has not been reported with prednisolone doses below 5 mg daily. Patients on higher doses undergoing major surgery will require additional corticosteroid support administered as intravenous hydrocortisone.

Monoamine oxidase inhibitors (MAOIs) irreversibly inhibit monoamine oxidase. Stopping these drugs 3 weeks prior to anaesthesia, to allow resynthesis of the enzyme, is no longer considered necessary, but anaesthetic technique may need to be modified. MAOIs interact with opioids, particularly pethidine, to cause cardiovascular and cerebrovascular excitation (hypertension, tachycardia, convulsions) or depression (hypotension, hypoventilation, coma). Hypertensive crises may be precipitated by sympathomimetic agents.

Tricyclic antidepressants competitively block noradrenaline reuptake by postganglionic sympathetic nerve endings. Patients taking these drugs are hence more sensitive to catecholamines, so sympathomimetics may cause hypertension and arrhythmias. Under the influence of anaesthesia, arrhythmias and hypotension may be seen.

Low-molecular-weight heparins (LMWH) used in thromboprophylaxis must be considered when central nerve blockade is planned during anaesthesia. To minimise the risk of vertebral canal haematoma a period of at least 12 hours should elapse between administration of an LMWH and epidural or spinal anaesthesia. Similarly, heparin administration should be delayed for a period of 6 hours following central nerve blockade.

Platelet antagonists such as NSAIDs and aspirin may be stopped in certain circumstances, usually when there is a risk of excessive bleeding. Increasingly, patients with cardiac and peripheral or cerebral vascular disease present for surgery while taking clopidogrel, a potent platelet antagonist. This must be noted at preoperative assessment, as withdrawal is frequently required prior to anaesthesia and surgery. Anaesthetic risk relates mainly to regional anaesthetic techniques and the possibility of vertebral canal haematoma following epidural or spinal anaesthesia.

While platelet antagonists should generally be stopped at least 7 days before elective surgery, the underlying reason for their use must be considered. This is particularly the case for patients taking clopidogrel following percutaneous coronary artery stenting within the last 12 months. In such a case elective surgery should ideally be postponed. When this is not possible, advice should be sought from a cardiologist.

When aspirin is prescribed for secondary prevention in cardiac and cerebrovascular disease preoperative stoppage is rarely necessary for non-neurosurgical procedures. Most hospitals have guidelines in place regarding perioperative aspirin management, and these should be sought if preoperative stoppage is being considered.

Herbal medicines have enjoyed an enormous increase in popularity recently. These drugs may not be declared by patients and should be actively sought at preoperative assessment. A number of such drugs are associated with complications such as bleeding, stroke and myocardial infarction, as well as interaction with more conventional drugs.

Garlic is a platelet inhibitor with potentially beneficial effects on blood pressure as well as serum lipid and cholesterol levels. There may be increased bleeding risk, particularly if it is taken along with more conventional platelet antagonists. Patients should be advised to discontinue garlic for 7 days preoperatively.

Ginseng may be taken to counteract stress. The active components appear to have some effects similar to steroid hormones. The drug's ability to lower blood sugar makes hypoglycaemia a potential problem perioperatively. Ginseng may also have an anticoagulant effect. It should be discontinued for 7 days preoperatively.

St John's wort may be used in the treatment of mild to moderate depression. Effects are believed to be mediated by hypericin and hyperforin and result in the inhibition of serotonin, noradrenaline and dopamine reuptake. A central serotonin syndrome can be precipitated, characterised by autonomic, neuromuscular and cognitive effects. Enzyme induction is an important feature of this drug and may affect many of the drugs used during anaesthesia. It should be discontinued for 7 days preoperatively.

Valerian is readily available as a sedative drug and is commonly found in 'herbal sleep remedies'. This drug may potentiate the sedative effects of anaesthetic drugs. This effect is believed to be GABA-mediated. Physical dependence can occur, and so abrupt discontinuation is not recommended. Postoperative withdrawal symptoms can be treated with benzodiazepines.

Concurrent surgical disease
Intestinal obstruction
Patients with intestinal obstruction often have electrolyte disturbances due to vomiting or, in the case of incomplete obstruction, diarrhoea. They may have been ill at home for several days and unable to take their usual medication for any concurrent medical condition. These patients may be dehydrated and possibly hypovolaemic due to gastrointestinal losses or to third space losses into the gut. Inappropriate intravenous fluid therapy on a surgical ward may have exacerbated the problems. Abdominal distension splints the diaphragm and decreases respiratory reserves. If longstanding, a chest infection may have developed. Fluid and electrolyte disturbances should be corrected prior to theatre, and preoperative chest physiotherapy may be useful. A nasogastric tube should be inserted before induction of anaesthesia in an attempt to empty the stomach and decrease the risk of perioperative regurgitation and aspiration.

Acute abdominal emergencies
All patients with an acute abdomen from whatever cause are at increased risk of regurgitation of stomach contents, and so a nasogastric tube should be inserted prior to theatre. Patients with testicular problems, e.g. torsion, should be included in this category because of the abdominal origin of the nerve supply of the testis.

References and further reading
Ang-Lee MK, Moss J, Yuan C. Herbal medicines and perioperative care. *JAMA* 2001; **286**: 208–16.

Association of Anaesthetists of Great Britain and Ireland. *Peri-Operative Management of the Morbidly Obese Patient.* London: AAGBI, 2007. www.aagbi.org/sites/default/files/Obesity07.pdf.

Bloomfield P, Bowler GMR. Anaesthetic management of the patient with a permanent pacemaker. *Anaesthesia* 1989; **44**: 42–6.

Chapman R, Plaat F. Alcohol and anaesthesia. *Contin Educ Anaesth Crit Care Pain* 2009; **9**: 10–13. ceaccp.oxfordjournals.org/content/9/1/10.

Cormack RS, Lehane J. Difficult tracheal intubation in obstetrics. *Anaesthesia* 1984; **39**: 1105–11.

European Society of Cardiology (ESC), European Society of Anaesthesiology (ESA). Guidelines for pre-operative cardiac risk assessment and perioperative cardiac management in non-cardiac surgery. *Eur Heart J* 2009; **30**: 2769–812.

Fleisher LA, Fleischmann KE, Auerbach AD, *et al.* 2014 ACC/AHA guideline on perioperative cardiovascular evaluation and management of patients undergoing noncardiac surgery: executive summary. *Circulation* 2014; **130**: 2215–45.

Goldman L, Caldera DL, Nussbaum SR, *et al.* Multifactorial index of cardiac risk in noncardiac surgical procedures. *N Engl J Med* 1977; **297**: 845–50.

Gupta S, Sharma R, Jain D. Airway assessment: predictors of difficult airway. *Indian J Anaesth* 2005; **49**: 257–62.

Hartle A, McCormack T, Carlisle J, *et al.* The measurement of adult blood pressure and management of hypertension before elective surgery: Joint Guidelines from the Association of Anaesthetists of Great Britain and Ireland and the British Hypertension Society. *Anaesthesia* 2016; **71**: 326–37.

Hlatky MA, Boineau RE, Higginbotham MB, *et al.* A brief-self administered questionnaire to determine functional capacity (the Duke Activity Status Index). *Am J Cardiol* 1989; **64**: 651–4.

Hopkins PM, Hunter JM (eds.). [Endocrine and metabolic disorders in anaesthesia and intensive care.] *Br J Anaesth* 2000; **85** (1): 1–153.

Johns MW. A new method for measuring daytime sleepiness: the Epworth Sleepiness Scale. *Sleep* 1991; **14**: 540–5.

Mallampati SR, Gatt SP, Gugino LD, *et al.* A clinical sign to predict difficult tracheal intubation: a prospective study. *Can Anaesth Soc J* 1985; **32**: 429–34.

Mason R. *Anaesthesia Databook: a Perioperative and Peripartum Manual*, 3rd edn. London: Greenwich Medical Media, 2001.

Medicines and Healthcare products Regulatory Agency. *Guidelines for the perioperative management of patients with implantable pacemakers or implantable cardioverter defibrillators, where use of surgical diathermy/electrocautery is anticipated.* London: MHRA, 2006. www.mhra.gov.uk.

National Institute for Health and Care Excellence. *Preoperative Tests for Elective Surgery.* NICE Guideline CG3. London: NICE, 2003. www.nice.org.uk/guidance/cg3.

National Institute for Health and Care Excellence. *Hypertension in Adults: Diagnosis and Management.* NICE Guideline CG127. London: NICE, 2011. www.nice.org.uk/guidance/cg127.

Older P, Hall A, Hader R. Cardiopulmonary exercise testing as a screening test for perioperative management of major surgery in the elderly. *Chest* 1999; **116**: 355–32.

Patil VU, Stehling LC, Zauder HL. Predicting the difficulty of intubation utilizing an intubation guide. *Anesthesiol Rev* 1983; **10**: 32–3.

Prys-Roberts C. Isolated systolic hypertension: pressure on the anaesthetist? *Anaesthesia* 2001; **56**: 505–10.

Royal College of Nursing. *Perioperative Fasting in Adults and Children: an RCN guideline for the multidisciplinary team.* London: RCN, 2005. www.rcn.org.uk.

Saklad M. Grading of patients for surgical procedures. *Anesthesiology* 1941; **2**: 281–4.

Samsoon GLT, Young JRB. Difficult tracheal intubation: a retrospective study. *Anaesthesia* 1987; **42**: 487–90.

Savva D. Prediction of difficult tracheal intubation. *Br J Anaesth* 1994; **73**: 149–53.

Snowden CP, Prentis JM, Anderson HL, *et al.* Submaximal cardiopulmonary exercise testing predicts complications and hospital length of stay in patients undergoing major elective surgery. *Ann Surg* 2010; **251**: 535–41.

Sweitzer BJ. *Handbook of Preoperative Assessment and Management.* Philadelphia, PA: Lippincott Williams & Wilkins, 2000.

Wilson ME, Spiegelhalter D, Robertson JA, Lesser P. Predicting difficult intubation. *Br J Anaesth* 1988; **61**: 211–16.

CHAPTER 2

Conduct of anaesthesia

Chris Mowatt

Preoperative preparation

The safe conduct of anaesthesia begins before the patient has arrived in the anaesthetic room. Consideration should be given to the methods of induction and maintenance of anaesthesia, airway management, positioning of the patient in theatre, necessary monitoring and the level of postoperative care required. It is important that all members of the anaesthetic and surgical team are fully informed of the planned procedure and its implications, including any foreseen difficulties that may arise.

Preoperative checks of the anaesthetic machine and all ancillary equipment are mandatory. A checklist such as that published by the Association of Anaesthetists of Great Britain and Ireland (AAGBI) is recommended.

On arrival of the patient further preoperative checks are completed. The World Health Organization surgical safety checklist improves patient safety by reducing surgical complications and mortality. Local modifications are commonplace, but the key elements are checks prior to anaesthesia induction, before skin incision, and before the patient leaves the operating room.

Induction

The aim of induction of anaesthesia is to rapidly attain a state of unconsciousness with minimal physiological disturbance. In transition from the awake to the anaesthetised state the patient passes through several stages of anaesthesia, as outlined by Guedel in 1937 using inhalational induction with diethyl ether. With modern agents and techniques transition is often too rapid to distinguish the stages and planes of anaesthesia, but inhalational induction provides the clearest development. The changes are summarised in Figure 2.1.

Various routes of delivery are available to achieve a sufficient concentration of anaesthetic agent within the central nervous system. Figures 2.2 and 2.3 show the advantages and disadvantages of methods of induction of anaesthesia.

Inhalational induction

Inhalational induction is most commonly employed in children, avoiding the distress of cannulation, and in situations where maintenance of spontaneous ventilation is desirable, e.g. upper airway obstruction or predicted difficult intubation.

Fundamentals of Anaesthesia, 4th edition, ed. Ted Lin, Tim Smith and Colin Pinnock. Published by Cambridge University Press. © Cambridge University Press 2017.

Figure 2.1 Summary of stages and planes of anaesthesia

		Breathing	Eye movement	Pupil diameter	Eye reflexes	Muscle tone
Stage 1 Analgesia		Normal	Normal	Normal	Normal	Normal
Stage 2 Excitement		Increased variability	Decreasing	Dilated	Losing lid reflex	Increased involuntary movement
Stage 3 Surgical anaesthesia	**Plane 1**		Decreasing	Decreasing	Losing corneal reflex	Decreasing response to surgical stimulation
	Plane 2		Absent	Constricted	Losing light reflex	
	Plane 3		Absent	Normal		
	Plane 4		Absent	Dilated		
Stage 4 Imminent death		Apnoea	Absent	Maximally dilated	No reflexes	

Figure 2.2 Inhalational induction of anaesthesia

Advantages
- Avoids venepuncture
- Respiration is maintained
- Slow loss of protective reflexes
- End-tidal concentration can be measured
- Rapid recovery if induction is abandoned
- Upper oesophageal sphincter tone maintained

Disadvantages
- Slow process
- Potential excitement phase
- Irritant and unpleasant, may induce coughing
- Pollution
- May cause a rise in ICP/IOP

Figure 2.3 Intravenous induction of anaesthesia

Advantages
- Rapid onset
- Dose titratable
- Depression of pharyngeal reflexes allows early insertion of LMA
- Anti-emetic and anti-convulsive properties

Disadvantages
- Venous access required
- Risk of hypotension
- Apnoea common
- Loss of airway control
- Anaphylaxis

The anaesthetic agent is introduced in increasing concentrations to the patient via a face mask, or in the case of smaller children a cupped hand. Induction is slower than with intravenous agents and there may be a prolonged stage of excitement and apnoea. More rapid induction may be achieved using a 'single breath' method with a vital capacity breath of higher concentrations of volatile agent (e.g. sevoflurane 8%).

The main factor that determines the rapidity of action of an inhalational agent is the rate at which the alveolar tension (F_A) increases to approach the inspired vapour tension (F_I): see *Uptake of inhaled anaesthetic agents in* Chapter 29. At equilibrium the partial pressure of vapour in the alveoli approximates to the effect-site tension in the brain. Several factors determine the rate at which this equilibrium is achieved:
- The blood–gas partition coefficient. Inhalational agents with low solubility in blood have a rapid onset of action.
- The inspired agent concentration.
- Pulmonary ventilation. Hyperventilation increases the rate at which the alveolar tension of an anaesthetic agent rises. A reduction in functional residual capacity

(FRC) enhances the rate at which alveolar concentration rises.
- The use of the pleasant-smelling, less irritant agents, historically halothane and most commonly sevoflurane, improves tolerability and increases the speed of induction.
- Cardiac output. Slower pulmonary transit times accelerate the rise in alveolar tension. The effect is more pronounced when agents with higher blood–gas partition coefficients are used.

The use of nitrous oxide has minor effects in accelerating the onset of anaesthesia, unless used with less soluble agents.

Intravenous induction
Intravenous induction agents are drugs that induce loss of consciousness in one arm–brain circulation time when given in an appropriate dosage. This is frequently more acceptable to the patient, with the advantage of minimising the excitement phase.

An estimated appropriate dose of intravenous agent should be given and the patient observed. The induction dose will vary according to the patient's weight, age, cardiac status, muscle and fat distribution and the use of premedicant drugs. Particular caution should be observed in circumstances where the arm–brain circulation time is likely to be prolonged, for example in hypovolaemic trauma patients and the elderly, when inadvertent overdosage with cardiovascular consequences may result. In the high-risk surgical patient or where cardiovascular instability is predicted, invasive monitoring prior to induction may be appropriate.

Alternative routes of induction
Rarely, alternative routes of induction are used. Intramuscular induction with ketamine is sometimes employed in the prehospital care setting, with agitated patients or in settings with limited resources. The rectal route is sometimes used in paediatric anaesthesia. Barbiturate agents and ketamine have been successfully used. The duration of induction is prolonged and less predictable.

Airway management
General anaesthesia inevitably results in loss of airway patency as the result of loss of pharyngeal tone and posterior displacement of the tongue. Airway management is therefore fundamental to safe anaesthetic practice.

A number of options exist for maintaining the patient's airway during anaesthesia:
- Face-mask airway
- Supraglottic airway devices, e.g. LMA
- Tracheal intubation

Face mask
The use of a face mask to maintain airway patency is an essential skill for any anaesthetist and one which may prove a considerable challenge. The face mask is employed in both spontaneous and controlled ventilation. The equipment required is simple and limits exposure to the risks of further airway instrumentation. The disadvantages are that it requires constant manipulation, which prevents the anaesthetist from attending to other tasks, and that it may prove tiring.

The successful use of a face mask relies on both a good seal around the mouth and nose and the maintenance of airway patency. Selection of the appropriate size is important in helping to maintain a gas-tight seal. Physical signs of airway obstruction should be sought constantly: noisy respiration (snoring or stridor) 'see-saw' respiration, tracheal tug and in-drawing of the soft tissues of the neck. The movement of the reservoir bag, misting of the mask and maintenance of an appropriate capnograph trace are important visual clues of airway patency. Gastric insufflation may result if face-mask ventilation is poorly applied, increasing the risk of aspiration.

Neck extension is the most effective manoeuvre in restoring airway patency, bringing the soft tissues of the neck anteriorly. Jaw thrust, applying force on the angles of the mandible to anteriorly displace the mandible and attached structures, can also be employed.

Supplementation of a face-mask airway with an airway adjunct, including oropharyngeal (Guedel) or nasopharyngeal airways, may also prove helpful in maintaining airway patency. These can be stimulating and must be inserted only at an appropriate stage of anaesthesia. Nasopharyngeal airways carry the added risk of nasal trauma and haemorrhage. Employment of the two-person technique of face-mask ventilation is potentially life-saving in the management of a difficult airway.

In current practice the face mask is most commonly applied before further airway instrumentation at induction of anaesthesia, or during short procedures such as DC cardioversion or manipulation of fractures. Nasal masks are used successfully during dental anaesthesia.

Supraglottic airway devices

Supraglottic airway devices (SADs), of which the laryngeal mask airway (LMA) is the most notable example, are the most commonly applied airway management devices in anaesthesia. Introduced in 1988, the original LMA developed by Archie Brain has been used in over 200 million anaesthetics. Supraglottic airway devices form a seal around the larynx, usually with an inflatable cuff. The LMA comes in various forms (reusable, reinforced) and sizes with guide patient weights to assist in selection.

Insertion is a blind technique which is easy to learn and requires less skill than face-mask ventilation or tracheal intubation. Appropriate positioning is confirmed by the ability to manually ventilate without significant leak, and to generate an airway pressure of 20 cmH$_2$O.

The insertion of an LMA results in less haemodynamic stimulation than laryngoscopy. During emergence coughing is less frequent than with an endotracheal tube. In some situations an endotracheal tube is exchanged for an LMA at the end of a procedure to facilitate a 'smoother' emergence. The incidence of minor laryngopharyngeal complications is similar in LMAs and endotracheal tubes. Sore throat is a frequent complication, with less common side effects including laryngeal nerve injury. Patients should be monitored closely to ameliorate the risk of displacement during surgery.

The Fourth National Audit Project of the Royal College of Anaesthetists and the Difficult Airway Society (NAP4) reported incidents of complications related to the inappropriate use of SADs, and patients who were morbidly obese featured prominently. Supraglottic airway devices do not provide reliable protection from pulmonary aspiration, and their use should be avoided in patients at risk. Modifications to the original LMA, including the ProSeal and iGel supraglottic devices, have design features to reduce the risk of pulmonary aspiration.

The LMA features at several points in the Difficult Airway Society algorithms for the management of difficult airways as a 'rescue' device. It has also been successfully employed in the prehospital setting.

Tracheal intubation

Indications

There are two major indications for tracheal intubation in the anaesthetised patient: firstly, to ensure airway patency and secondly, to protect the airway from contamination.

Indications for endotracheal intubation

• Operations where access to the airway is difficult, including
  ○ shared airway surgery
  ○ patients in the prone position
• Prolonged operations, such as
  ○ neurosurgical
  ○ cardiac
  ○ extensive abdominal surgery
• Operations involving excessive movement of the head and neck, where other forms of airway control may become dislodged
• Situations where other airway techniques have proved ineffective
• Predicted difficult airway
• Situations where a major intraoperative complication develops, such as
  ○ severe haemorrhage
  ○ anaphylaxis
  ○ malignant hyperthermia

A cuffed endotracheal tube forms an airtight seal at the level of the cuff and greatly, but not completely, reduces the risk of contamination of the lower respiratory tract. This is particularly useful in patients with an increased risk of regurgitation and during surgery when there may be extensive bleeding from the mouth, nose or oropharynx. Other indications include operations that require the isolation of one lung.

Technique

Prior to endotracheal intubation, appropriate monitoring, drugs, equipment and personnel should be available. A strategy should be devised based upon patient assessment, proposed technique and potential complications and pitfalls. This should be clearly communicated to all members of the team. Anticipated difficult airways necessitate the involvement of senior colleagues with the appropriate skills and knowledge of equipment.

Direct laryngoscopy

Positioning

The optimal position for direct laryngoscopy aligns the oral, pharyngeal and tracheal axes. Classically, the 'sniffing the morning air' position has been taught as the best way of achieving this. In this position the head is extended 15° and the neck flexed at 35°, which can be helped by elevating the head on one pillow. This serves to facilitate insertion of the laryngoscope and improves mouth opening, thereby improving the view of the larynx while limiting the risk of dental injury. In obese patients this position can be difficult to achieve. Elevation of the head so that the external auditory meatus is in alignment with the sternal notch provides optimum intubating conditions independent of age and size. Adjuncts such as the Oxford HELP (head elevating laryngoscopy pillow) system (see Figure 5.27) are useful in obese patients.

Laryngoscopy technique

Direct laryngoscopy involves moving the tongue and epiglottis anteriorly to allow visualisation of the larynx. The Macintosh laryngoscope blade has a flange on its left side to keep the tongue out of the line of sight. The blade should be inserted into the right side of the mouth and advanced centrally towards the base of the tongue. The blade is then lifted to expose the epiglottis and advanced into the vallecula with continued lifting to expose the laryngeal inlet. The views achieved were graded by Cormack and Lehane (1984) as illustrated in Figure 2.4. Inexperienced practitioners have a tendency to advance the blade insufficiently and lever the laryngoscope to achieve visualisation. This risks damage to the incisors.

Bimanual laryngoscopy, where the operator uses the free, right hand to manipulate the laryngeal cartilage to improve the view at laryngoscopy, has been advocated as a technique to improve success. A similar manoeuvre using an assistant to apply 'backwards-upwards-rightwards pressure' to the larynx has also been advocated.

Management of the difficult airway

There have been various attempts to define the 'difficult airway'. The American Society of Anesthesiologists (ASA) describes it as the situation where the trained anaesthetist has difficulty in successfully achieving adequate bag-mask

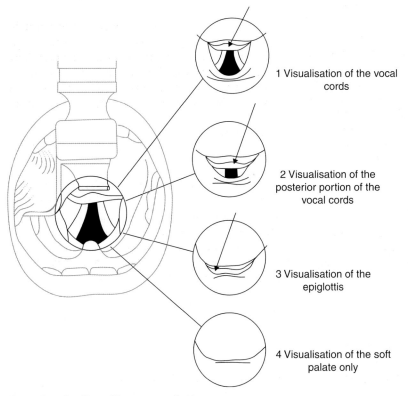

1 Visualisation of the vocal cords

2 Visualisation of the posterior portion of the vocal cords

3 Visualisation of the epiglottis

4 Visualisation of the soft palate only

Figure 2.4 Grading of laryngoscopic views

ventilation, SAD ventilation, tracheal intubation or all three. An alternative description when using direct laryngoscopy classifies a difficult airway as more than two attempts at intubation. A Cormack and Lehane view of grade 3 or 4 denotes difficult laryngoscopy (Figure 2.4).

The difficult airway may be **anticipated**, which allows for the development of a preoperative strategy, or **unanticipated**.

Airway management should be approached with a clear strategy, with the dual aims of achieving adequate gas exchange and preventing complications. All anaesthetic departments should have an explicit policy for the management of airway emergencies; the application of the techniques required in these strategies should form part of the daily practice of individuals. It is important to plan for failure, and strategies must be be outlined clearly prior to any attempts at securing the airway.

Preoperative assessment
This is described in detail under *The airway* in Chapter 1.

Preoxygenation
Adequate preoxygenation prior to induction prolongs the time between apnoea and arterial desaturation by maximising the storage of oxygen. The patient breathes 100% oxygen through a close-fitting face mask. A period of 3–5 minutes of tidal ventilation at high flows is sufficient to adequately denitrogenate the functional residual capacity (FRC) of the lungs; four vital capacity breaths may be as effective. Care should be taken to avoid leaks as indicated

by the absence of a normal capnograph trace and an empty reservoir bag. An end-tidal concentration as close to 100% as possible is the target, with a value of 90% considered acceptable. Effective preoxygenation may be difficult in some circumstances, for example the agitated, head-injured patient. Efforts should be made to actively pursue opportunities to deliver supplemental oxygen throughout the process of airway management. The rate of the arterial desaturation during apnoea is related to the FRC and oxygen consumption; as a result rapid desaturation may be seen in children, pregnancy and obesity, emphasising the importance of adequate preoxygenation in these groups.

Awake fibreoptic intubation
Awake fibreoptic intubation (AFOI) allows for an endotracheal tube to be placed through the larynx under direct vision through the oral or nasal routes without the need for the induction of general anaesthesia. AFOI is well tolerated by an awake patient and considered the safest non-invasive means of securing an airway (Figure 2.5). It has an important role in the management of **anticipated** difficult airways.

There are no absolute contraindications to the use of awake fibreoptic laryngoscopy. Care is needed in patients with potentially friable tumours or at an increased risk of bleeding. In a critically obstructed airway there is the risk of precipitating complete obstruction, and consideration should be given to other techniques.

Figure 2.5 Awake fibreoptic intubation: advantages and indications

Advantages
- Oxygenation and ventilation maintained
- Airway protective mechanisms preserved
- Muscle tone maintained, making intubation 'easier'
- Definitive check of endotracheal tube position
- High success rate

Indications
- Previous difficult intubation
- Previous AFOI
- Anticipated difficult bag-mask ventilation
- Aspiration risk
- Avoidance of iatrogenic injury (for example in the unstable cervical spine)

Awake fibreoptic intubation: technique

- Use sedative premedication cautiously, and not at all in the presence of severe airway compromise.
- Anticholinergic premedication may be given to reduce secretions.
- Prescribe aspiration prophylaxis (such as ranitidine and sodium citrate) preoperatively.
- Check all equipment in the anaesthetic room, attach monitoring and secure intravenous access.
- Prepare the airway by achieving local anaesthesia as described in Figure 7.50 (Chapter 7).
- Spray the nasal mucosa with a vasoconstrictor if this is the chosen route.
- Having loaded the chosen endotracheal tube onto the fibreoptic scope proceed via mouth or nose until the larynx is visualised.
- Pass the tube off the scope into the trachea and check for correct placement.

Inhalational induction

An inhalational technique provides another means for preserving spontaneous ventilation during attempts to secure a difficult airway. Spontaneous ventilation is preserved during a gradual induction of anaesthesia. Topical application of local anaesthetic may permit tracheal intubation in lighter planes of anaesthesia.

Difficult intubation

At times the anaesthetist may be faced with unanticipated difficulties during attempts at intubation. Figures 2.6, 2.7 and 2.8 reproduce strategies from the Difficult Airway Society to approach such situations

Maintenance of oxygenation takes priority during attempts at securing the airway. The best available help should be sought as soon as difficulty is realised.

Bougie (intubating stylet) – This simple device is a 60 cm long introducer, 5 mm in diameter, with a smooth angled tip. It is especially useful when the glottic opening cannot be visualised. Bougies are narrow and stiff and may be bent before use to aid placement. They provide tactile feedback to the operator, which facilitates blind placement. Correct placement is confirmed by the detection of 'clicks' as the tip of the bougie passes over the tracheal rings. There may also be the perception of 'hold up' as the bougie touches the carina or lodges in the smaller airways. The endotracheal tube is advanced over the bougie into the trachea; anticlockwise rotation at the laryngeal inlet facilitates passage through the vocal cords.

Alternative laryngoscope blades – The standard **Macintosh** laryngoscope blade was introduced in 1943. It has a relatively short curved blade designed to rest in the vallecula and lift the epiglottis. Several alternative laryngoscope blades are available which may be of use during the management of the difficult airway.

The **McCoy** levering laryngoscope has a 25 mm hinged blade tip controlled by a spring-loaded lever on the handle of the laryngoscope which allows elevations of the epiglottis without the use of excessive forces on the pharyngeal tissues.

The **polio** blade was originally developed to enable patients in an iron lung to be intubated. Difficulty may be encountered inserting the laryngoscope in obese patients and large-breasted women. The use of a polio blade, mounted at 135° to the handle, may be useful in these circumstances, particularly when combined with a 'stubby' handle.

Advances in digital and imaging technology have increased the availability of relatively cheap **videolaryngoscopes**, which provide a view of the glottis from a video camera or chip positioned at the tip of the laryngoscope blade. Videolaryngoscopes can offer better views of the glottis when compared with standard direct laryngoscopy and provide an option in the management of the difficult airway. They have also have some value as training tools, allowing the trainer to demonstrate airway anatomy in real time. Different models exist: those with standard Macintosh-type blades, those with a channel for tube passage, and those with angulated blades.

A different approach is required if direct laryngoscopy has failed. A secondary tracheal intubation plan (Plan B of the Difficult Airway Society guidelines) utilises techniques that allow for continuous oxygenation both during and between intubation attempts.

Supraglottic airway device – The SAD may be employed as a means of airway control in the management of difficult and failed tracheal intubation.

The **intubating LMA** (ILMA) was specifically designed to facilitate tracheal intubation while maintaining ventilation. The ILMA is a shortened version of the classic LMA with a forwardly directed metal handle. The aperture has a single wider bar which is designed to elevate the epiglottis as a narrow endotracheal tube is advanced through the lumen of the ILMA. This may be achieved either as a blind technique or guided by a fibreoptic scope.

Intubation is also possible through the classic LMA and later devices such as the iGel and Proseal SADs. Blind passage of a bougie through the lumen of the SAD into the trachea has a high failure rate. Fibreoptic guidance of intubation, using the scope as a 'directable bougie', has a higher success rate. There are potential problems with this technique. Firstly, a standard endotracheal tube may not be long enough. Secondly, a size 4 LMA will accept only a 6.5 mm internal-diameter endotracheal tube, while a size 5 LMA will accept a 7 mm endotracheal tube. This may be too small to permit adequate ventilation without excessive airway pressures. Thirdly, attempts at removing the LMA may result in accidental extubation.

The **Aintree intubation catheter** is an adaptation of the Cook airway exchange catheter. The larger internal diameter (4.8 mm) allows it to be preloaded onto a 4.0 mm fibreoptic laryngoscope. The catheter also has removable connectors which allow it to be used as a ventilatory device during airway exchange. It can be directed under video control into the airway using the LMA as a conduit. Once it is in position, the LMA can be removed and exchanged, over the catheter, for an endotracheal tube.

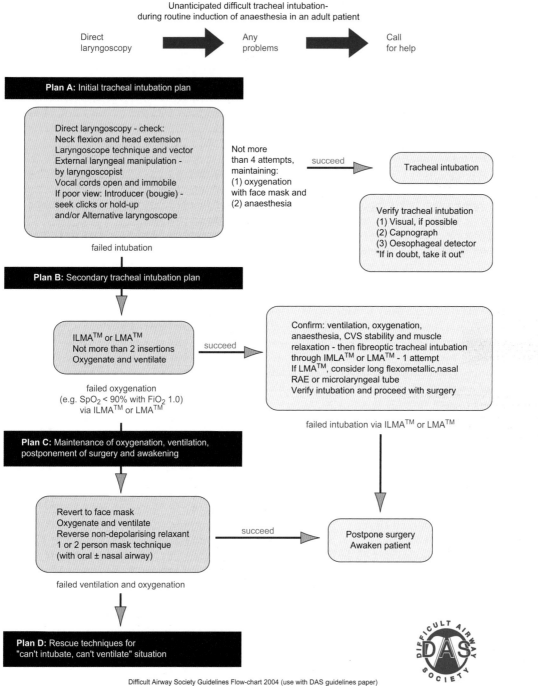

Figure 2.6 Unanticipated difficult tracheal intubation during routine induction of anaesthesia in an adult patient. Reproduced from Henderson JJ, Popat MT, Latto IP, Pearce AC. Difficult Airway Society guidelines for management of the unanticipated difficult intubation. *Anaesthesia* 2004; 59: 675–94.

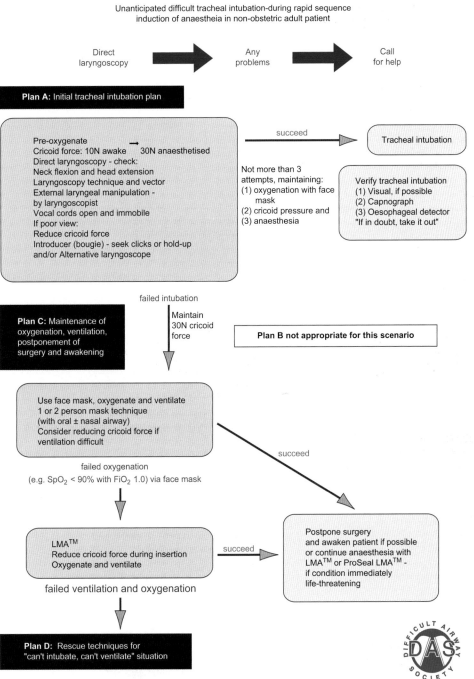

Figure 2.7 Unanticipated difficult tracheal intubation during rapid sequence induction of anaesthesia in a non-obstetric adult patient. Reproduced from Henderson JJ, Popat MT, Latto IP, Pearce AC. Difficult Airway Society guidelines for management of the unanticipated difficult intubation. *Anaesthesia* 2004; 59: 675–94.

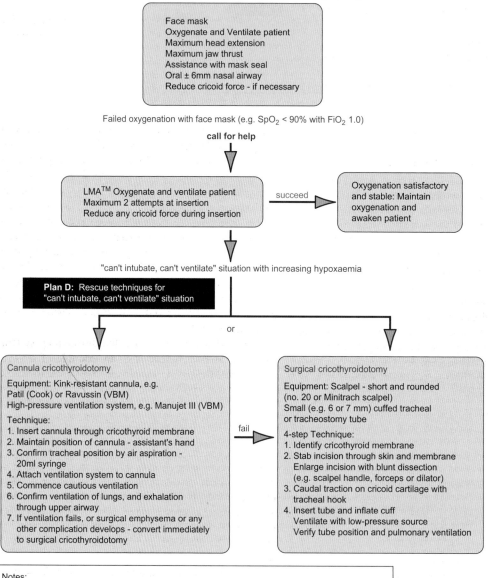

Failed intubation, increasing hypoxaemia and difficult ventilation in the paralysed anaesthetised patient: Rescue techniques for the "can't intubate, can't ventilate" situation

Failed intubation and difficult ventilation (other than laryngospasm)

Face mask
Oxygenate and Ventilate patient
Maximum head extension
Maximum jaw thrust
Assistance with mask seal
Oral ± 6mm nasal airway
Reduce cricoid force - if necessary

Failed oxygenation with face mask (e.g. SpO$_2$ < 90% with FiO$_2$ 1.0)

call for help

LMA™ Oxygenate and ventilate patient
Maximum 2 attempts at insertion
Reduce any cricoid force during insertion

succeed →

Oxygenation satisfactory and stable: Maintain oxygenation and awaken patient

"can't intubate, can't ventilate" situation with increasing hypoxaemia

Plan D: Rescue techniques for "can't intubate, can't ventilate" situation

or

Cannula cricothyroidotomy

Equipment: Kink-resistant cannula, e.g.
Patil (Cook) or Ravussin (VBM)
High-pressure ventilation system, e.g. Manujet III (VBM)

Technique:
1. Insert cannula through cricothyroid membrane
2. Maintain position of cannula - assistant's hand
3. Confirm tracheal position by air aspiration -
   20ml syringe
4. Attach ventilation system to cannula
5. Commence cautious ventilation
6. Confirm ventilation of lungs, and exhalation
   through upper airway
7. If ventilation fails, or surgical emphysema or any
   other complication develops - convert immediately
   to surgical cricothyroidotomy

fail →

Surgical cricothyroidotomy

Equipment: Scalpel - short and rounded
(no. 20 or Minitrach scalpel)
Small (e.g. 6 or 7 mm) cuffed tracheal
or tracheostomy tube

4-step Technique:
1. Identify cricothyroid membrane
2. Stab incision through skin and membrane
   Enlarge incision with blunt dissection
   (e.g. scalpel handle, forceps or dilator)
3. Caudal traction on cricoid cartilage with
   tracheal hook
4. Insert tube and inflate cuff
   Ventilate with low-pressure source
   Verify tube position and pulmonary ventilation

Notes:
1. These techniques can have serious complications - use only in life-threatening situations
2. Convert to definitive airway as soon as possible
3. Postoperative management - see other difficult airway guidelines and flow-charts
4. 4mm cannula with low-pressure ventilation may be successful in patient breathing spontaneously

Difficult Airway Society guidelines Flow-chart 2004 (use with DAS guidelines paper)

Figure 2.8 Failed intubation: rescue techniques for the 'can't intubate, can't ventilate' situation. Reproduced from Henderson JJ, Popat MT, Latto IP, Pearce AC. Difficult Airway Society guidelines for management of the unanticipated difficult intubation. *Anaesthesia* 2004; 59: 675–94.

The patient should be deeply anaesthetised with or without muscle relaxation to prevent coughing or laryngospasm during attempts to intubate through a SAD.

If two attempts at this secondary intubation technique fail, a risk–benefit assessment should be performed, balancing the risks of continuing with surgery with what may be a suboptimal airway versus postponement (Plan C of the Difficult Airway Society guidelines).

There are several factors which may influence this decision:

- Surgical factors:
  o Degree of urgency of surgery
- Patient factors:
  o Ability to maintain oxygenation
  o Risk of aspiration: is the use of cricoid pressure necessary? Does this affect airway patency?

It is important to emphasise the importance of considering alternative strategies to secure an airway in the event of difficulties. Management of difficult intubation with repeated attempts at intubation often leads to 'can't intubate, can't ventilate' situations. A change of approach is more likely to yield success than persisting with a technique which has already failed.

If ventilation is impossible and hypoxaemia is developing, then rescue techniques should be implemented (Plan D of the Difficult Airway Society Guidelines). Invasive techniques to secure the airway are not without risk, and this should be weighed against the risk of hypoxic brain injury. Rapid oxygenation is a priority in the event of severe hypoxaemia, particularly when associated with bradycardia. Immediate intervention is indicated in these circumstances.

Cannula cricothyroidotomy involves the combination of a cannula inserted through the cricothyroid membrane with high-pressure ventilation. It carries a high failure rate. This may be improved by the use of a kink-resistant cannula. It is essential to confirm correct position of the cannula before instituting high-pressure ventilation. The accumulation of air in tissue planes may preclude any further attempts at airway intervention.

Surgical 'stab' cricothyroidotomy can be performed in 30 seconds, allowing for rapid restoration of ventilation and oxygenation. This technique involves the combination of a cuffed tube in the trachea and low-pressure ventilation. The technique involves:

- Identification of the cricothyroid membrane
- Horizontal stab incision through skin and membrane with blunt dilatation

- Caudal traction on the cricothyroid membrane with a tracheal hook
- Intubation of the trachea

These are temporary steps to restore oxygenation. Definitive airway management will follow, which may mean a formal tracheostomy.

Complications at induction
Allergic reactions

During anaesthesia patients are given a large number of drugs, often in quick succession. These drugs can cause severe, life-threatening adverse reactions. Any history of known adverse reactions to drugs should be sought in the preoperative visit. This should be carefully documented and communicated to all members of the theatre team.

Adverse drug reactions may be predictable, based on knowledge of the pharmacodynamic effects of a particular drug, or unpredictable. Anaphylaxis and anaphylactoid reactions are unpredictable reactions that involve the release of histamine from mast cells. The incidence of anaphylaxis during anaesthesia has been estimated at between 1 in 10,000 and 1 in 20,000 (Fisher & Baldo 1993, Laxenaire 1999).

Anaphylaxis is a severe, life-threatening systemic hypersensitivity reaction. It is an example of a type I hypersensitivity reaction occurring in response to an antigen to which the patient has had prior exposure. Exposure to a foreign protein leads to the production of IgE which binds to and sensitises mast cells and basophils to further exposure. In the event of further exposure, antigen binds to and cross-links IgE molecules on sensitised cells resulting in degranulation and the release of pharmacologically active mediators including histamine, tryptase, platelet aggregating factor and leukotrienes. These mediators can cause smooth muscle constriction, vasodilatation and increased vascular permeability. Intravascular volume depletion is an important component of anaphylactic shock.

The commonest clinical feature of anaphylaxis is cardiovascular collapse, followed by respiratory and cutaneous manifestations (Figure 2.9). In 10% of cases cardiovascular collapse may be the only presenting feature. The severity of the reaction is graded 1–5 and ranges from mild, cutaneous reactions to death. Approximately 10% of reported anaphylactic reactions during anaesthesia prove fatal. The clinical presentation of anaphylaxis is heterogeneous and is influenced by concurrent

Figure 2.9 Presenting features of anaphylaxis

Cardiovascular • Vasodilatation • Hypotension • Bradycardia • Cardiac areest	75%
Respiratory • Bronchospasm	40%
Cutaneous • Erythema • Wheals	72%
Angio-oedema	64%

Figure 2.10 Causative agents in anaesthesia-related anaphylaxis

Neuromuscular blocking drugs	60%
Latex	20%
Antibiotics	15%
Intravenous colloids (most often gelatin)	4%
Others (chlorhexidine, NSAIDs, local anaesthetics etc.)	< 2%

medication, for example β-blockers, and comorbidity. The management of anaphylaxis-associated bronchoconstriction and respiratory failure in patients with asthma can prove very challenging.

Anaphylaxis is dose-independent and unrelated to the rate of drug delivery. It is more common when drugs are given intravenously. Neuromuscular blocking agents (NMBAs) are the most commonly implicated causative agents in anaesthesia-related anaphylaxis (Figure 2.10). Quaternary ammonium ions (QAIs) are the proposed allergenic epitope in NMBAs; it has been suggested that environmental exposure to QAIs may result in sensitisation.

Anaphylactoid reactions are not mediated by the cross-linkage of IgE. The precise mechanism is not always identifiable but may involve direct activation of mast cells and basophils and activation of the complement and coagulation cascades. Prior exposure to an agent is not a prerequisite. Agents that commonly result in histamine release include opioids and benzylisoquinolinium muscle relaxants.

Anaphylactoid reactions may be clinically indistinguishable from anaphylaxis but are typically milder.

The European Academy of Allergy and Clinical Immunology has recommended the alternative terms 'allergic anaphylaxis' in circumstances where the reaction is mediated by an immunological mechanism and 'non-allergic anaphylaxis' where it is not. These have not been universally accepted.

Management

Anaphylaxis should be considered in the differential diagnosis of any major cardiorespiratory problem. Early treatment is essential and associated with improved outcomes. Treatment is often delayed while other differential diagnoses are considered.

Every anaesthetist should be familiar with guidelines for the management of anaphylaxis under anaesthesia. Management algorithms are presented as a logical sequence of steps to take. Good teamwork and communication in emergency situations will allow for several of these steps to be taken simultaneously, for example preparing a syringe of adrenaline while assessing A, B, C (Association of Anaesthetists of Great Britain and Ireland 2009b).

Investigation

Confirmation of the diagnosis of anaphylaxis is supported by the analysis of plasma for mast cell tryptase which is highly specific (low false-negative rate) but inconsistently sensitive (true-positive rate). The first sample should be taken as soon as feasible after the onset of symptoms to capture the initial rise or peak of mast cell tryptase. A second sample is required to further characterise the pattern of tryptase release and breakdown; it is recommended that this is taken ideally 1–2 hours after the onset of symptoms but certainly within 4 hours. A further sample to exclude abnormal baseline levels of tryptase is required at 24 hours or at follow-up.

Any patient with a suspected anaphylactic reaction should be investigated fully and referred to an appropriate local allergy or immunology centre. It is important that contemporaneous records are kept, with a careful description of the sequence of events including timing and clinical findings. The patient should be kept fully informed, advised of the potential causative agents for further reference, and this information should be copied to the patient's primary care physician.

Adverse drug reactions should be reported to the appropriate agency. In the UK this is the Medicines and Healthcare products Regulatory Agency (MHRA) via the 'yellow card' scheme. The Yellow Card database (Adverse Drug Reactions Online Information Tracking, ADROIT) collates reports of adverse drug reactions experienced by patients.

Management of a patient with suspected anaphylaxis

Immediate management

- Stop administration of the suspected trigger.
- Summon assistance and inform the operating surgeon.
- Administer 100% oxygen, maintain anaesthesia. Intubate the trachea if necessary.
- Administer intravenous adrenaline. Management should be tailored to the individual patient, but there is evidence to support the early use of adrenaline. As well as α-agonist properties, the β-agonist actions – inotropy, bronchodilatation and limitation of mediator release – are valuable in anaphylaxis. An initial dose of 50 μg (0.5 mL of 1:10,000) is appropriate in adult patients. Patients may require frequent dosing, and consideration should be given to the need for a continuous infusion. Adrenaline has a short half-life.
- Start intravascular volume expansion using 0.9% sodium chloride or Hartmann's solution through a large-bore cannula. Large volumes may be required to compensate for distributive shock. Elevate the patient's legs.
- Start CPR if appropriate.

Secondary management

- Secondary management should not delay the initial resuscitation.
- Administer 10 mg IV chlorphenamine and 200 mg IV hydrocortisone.
- If bronchospasm is a significant feature administer salbutamol. This may be given intravenously, or if the appropriate equipment is available through the breathing circuit via a nebuliser or metered dose inhaler. Consider infusions of aminophylline and/or magnesium.
- The decision to continue surgery will depend on several factors including the severity of the reaction, response to immediate therapy, and the urgency and complexity of surgery.
- Arrangements should be made for postoperative care in an appropriate critical care setting.

Malplaced endotracheal tube

After intubation of the trachea, the tip of the endotracheal tube will ideally lie above the carina but below the vocal cords. The two major malplacements are accidental oesophageal and endobronchial intubation.

Endobronchial intubation is usually the result of intubation of the right main bronchus, because of its more vertical alignment. It may be the result of poor tube fixation, or it may occur due to movement of a patient's head. The smaller relative distances involved mean that this is more frequent in children. The signs of accidental endobronchial intubation are an unexplained drop in oxygen saturations, higher than expected airway pressures (and a feel of poor compliance in the reservoir bag), and asymmetrical chest movement. If auscultation confirms endobrochial intubation, deflate the cuff, withdraw until bilateral ventilation returns, then reinflate the cuff. Fibreoptic bronchoscopy will also confirm position.

Unrecognised **oesophageal intubation** is still a major cause of anaesthetic morbidity and mortality. Failure to consider oesophageal intubation as a cause of hypoxia can have serious, often fatal, consequences.

Verification of endotracheal tube position may be confirmed with clinical signs of correct endotracheal tube placement and objective measures.

Clinical signs

Direct visualisation of the tracheal tube passing through the vocal cords will confirm placement. This is not alway possible in the event of difficult laryngoscopy.

Auscultation of breath sounds should be done to ensure that the tube is correctly positioned in the trachea. This should be done repeatedly whenever there has been movement of the tube or the patient. Auscultation in both axillae to confirm symmetrical breath sounds will usually verify correct placement. There is the risk of transmitted sounds from oesophageal intubations causing confusion, particularly in smaller children. Auscultation over the epigastrium will usually reveal a characteristic gurgling sound in the event of oesophageal intubation.

Observation of chest movement should reveal symmetrical movement of the chest.

The presence of **water vapour** 'misting' the endotracheal tube and catheter mount cannot be relied upon as a clinical sign of endotracheal intubation, as it does not exclude oesophageal intubation.

Objective measures

Identification of expired carbon dioxide by **capnography** confirms correct endotracheal tube placement if the lungs are being perfused and effective alveolar ventilation is occurring. There are a number of potential causes of false-negative results which should be considered in the event of a flat capnography trace. The capnography trace may also appear normal in oesophageal intubation if exhaled gases have been forced into the stomach by vigorous bag-mask ventilation or if the patient has recently consumed a carbonated beverage. In these rare instances the trace will become flat within a few breaths.

The absence of capnography has been linked to adverse events and deaths, particularly in settings outside the normal theatre environment. The AAGBI recommends that continuous capnography should be used in all anaesthetised patients, regardless of the location.

Carbon dioxide in exhaled gases can also be detected by the use of colorimetric CO_2 detectors, which change colour reversibly on exposure to CO_2. These are often disposable devices used in prehospital settings. Continuous capnography is quickly becoming the gold standard in the UK.

Constant vigilance should be maintained after the confirmation of position; excessive movement of the head and neck, alterations in patient position, traction on the trachea or oesophagus and poor fixation may all result in tube displacement.

Confirmation of correct endotracheal tube placement

Clinical signs
- Direct visualisation of tube through the cords
- Auscultation for breath sounds
- Chest movement during positive pressure ventilation

Objective signs
- Detection of carbon dioxide

Intra-arterial injection

Unintentional intra-arterial (IA) injection can result in considerable morbidity. Inadvertent arterial cannulation can occur as the result of the normal anatomical proximity of arterial and venous vessels, or because of aberrant vascular supply, and it is more common in procedurally difficult situations. Accidental injection via known arterial cannulae for blood pressure monitoring is another potential source of risk.

Figure 2.11 Management of intra-arterial injection

Stop injecting
Leave intra-arterial cannula in place
Infuse 0.9% sodium chloride to maintain cannula patency
If not contraindicated, heparinise via intravenous cannula
Provide symptomatic relief
- Analgesia
- Elevate
- Consider nerve block
Manage arterial spasm
- Calcium channel blockers
- α-Blockers
- Antispasmodics (e.g. papaverine)
- Injection of local anaesthetics (e.g. 50 mg lidocaine)
- Consider sympathetic neural blockade (stellate ganglion or brachial plexus block)
Re-establish blood flow
- Thrombolysis
- Surgical intervention
Treat sequelae
- Surgical debridement

Historically, the most commonly associated medications with pronounced morbidity and mortality after unintentional IA injection are barbiturates and benzodiazepines.

Special patient circumstances

Traumatic brain injury

The management of patients with a significant traumatic brain injury frequently requires intubation and ventilation: to protect the airway from aspiration, to maintain adequate oxygenation and ventilation, to facilitate safe imaging, to enable inter-hospital transfer, and in the management of the agitated patient.

The goals of management are to limit primary brain injury with prompt diagnosis and treatment while preventing secondary injury.

The shocked patient

Anaesthetists are frequently faced with haemodynamically compromised patients requiring intubation and ventilation. Common scenarios include the ruptured aortic aneurysm, septic shock and trauma. Full resuscitation prior to intervention is not always possible, and in the

Management of traumatic brain injury

- The presence of cervical spine injury should be considered, and appropriate precautions taken.
- Patients should be considered to have a full stomach, and therefore require rapid sequence induction.
- The use of drugs (most frequently opioids such as fentanyl or alfentanil) to obtund the stress response and reduce the surge in intracranial pressure at induction may be desirable. This should be considered even in deeply unconscious patients.
- Care should be taken to:
  - Avoid hypoxia – single episodes of desaturation are associated with worse outcome.
  - Maintain normocarbia – hyperventilation can cause cerebral ischaemia and should be reserved for the emergency management of cerebral herniation. Continuous capnography is mandatory.
  - Maintain an adequate cerebral perfusion pressure – following correction of hypovolaemia and haemorrhage control. Vasopressors may be required to maintain an adequate MAP.
- Head-up tilt of 15–30° reduces venous congestion.
- Prevent hypoglycaemia and hypothermia.
- Treat seizures and consider prophylactic anticonvulsant therapy.
- Adequate sedation should be maintained. Coughing on the endotracheal tube causes surges in ICP and should be avoided with appropriate analgo-sedation, with neuromuscular blockade if appropriate.

example of haemorrhagic shock not desirable until haemorrhage control is possible.

Conventional anaesthetic techniques reduce cardiac output and systemic vascular resistance to varying degrees while attenuating the normal homeostatic responses to cardiovascular disturbances.

Adequate preoperative assessment is important. In the emergency situation this needs to be carefully focused on important details likely to influence anaesthetic technique.

Adequate large-bore intravenous access (two 14G cannulae or PAFC sheath) is essential prior to induction. Invasive monitoring should be considered: an arterial line will allow rapid responses to haemodynamic disturbances

during induction. Careful selection of the induction agent, its likely haemodynamic effects and the appropriate dose is important. In general, most shocked patients will exhibit a greater sensitivity to induction agents and the dose will need to be reduced. This should be balanced against the risk of awareness. In hypovolaemic shock ketamine has many favourable properties.

The patient with a full stomach

Pulmonary aspiration occurs when gastric contents enter the pulmonary tree. It is estimated to occur in 2–5 per 10,000 anaesthetics, and it is more likely in emergency surgery. The sequelae of aspiration depend on the nature of the gastric contents, the pH of the inhaled material, and its volume. The syndrome of pulmonary aspiration can vary from mild airway irritation to life-threatening acute respiratory distress syndrome (ARDS), and was originally described in obstetric patients by Mendelson in 1946. An episode of aspiration carries a mortality of around 4%.

Risk factors

Gastric contents – Larger volumes of more acidic material result in a more severe insult to the lungs. Impaired gastric emptying is seen in many situations, notably following trauma and in pregnancy after the first trimester. Pain, opioid medication and alcohol also contribute. Gastroparesis with large gastric volumes is also a common feature in many gastro-intestinal conditions; very large volumes may be seen in acute small bowel obstruction.

Integrity of lower oesophageal sphincter (LOS) – The LOS is formed at the border of the oesophagus and the stomach and prevents reflux of gastric contents into the oesophagus. The tone of the LOS is affected by conditions increasing intra-abdominal pressure, for example obesity and pregnancy, and may be affected by certain drugs including benzodiazepines. The LOS should be considered to be incompetent in patients with significant gastro-oesophageal reflux and those with a hiatus hernia. LOS incompetency contributes to the increased risk of aspiration in pregnancy.

Integrity of upper oesophageal sphincter (UOS) – The cricopharyngeus muscle acts functionally as the UOS. All anaesthetic drugs, except for ketamine, act to reduce UOS tone.

Protective reflexes – The presence of intact protective airway reflexes helps to protect the airway from aspiration. These are obtunded in patients with reduced conscious levels and in conditions affecting the

neuromuscular components of the reflex arc, for example bulbar palsy, Parkinson's disease and myotonic dystrophy.
- **Other factors** – Other factors increasing the risk of pulmonary aspiration include patient position (reverse Trendelenburg, lithotomy), metabolic disturbances, and advanced age.

Prevention of aspiration

- **Reduction of gastric volume** – The rationale for preoperative starvation is to reduce the risk and degree of regurgitation during anaesthesia. An appropriate period of starvation is considered to be 6 hours for solids (a 'light meal'), 4 hours for human breast milk and 2 hours for clear fluids. There is no evidence to support the routine use of drugs that facilitate gastric emptying, e.g. metoclopramide.
- **Increase gastric pH** – Administration of antacids, for example H_2-blockers, proton pump inhibitors (PPIs) and 0.3 M sodium citrate, acts to increase gastric pH.

The administration of preoperative H_2-blockers and PPIs significantly increases gastric pH and reduces gastric volume. There is no evidence, however, to support their routine use. Their use in high-risk patients should be considered on a case-by-case basis.

Antacid prophylaxis is recommended for routine administration in pregnant patients presenting for Caesarean section and with a high risk of operative intervention. This consists of a dose of H_2-blocker in the hours preceding surgery and 30 mL 0.3 M sodium citrate prior to anaesthesia.

- **Cricoid pressure** – Cricoid pressure has been used since the original description by Sellick in 1961. The cricoid is a complete cartilaginous ring. With direct pressure force is transmitted to the posterior lamina, occluding the oesophagus by compressing it against the vertebral bodies of the cervical spine.

Recently radiological studies have suggested that in many 'normal' subjects the oesophagus lies laterally to the cricoid ring and that the application of cricoid pressure may increase this lateral displacement in up to 90% of people. Cricoid pressure has also been shown to make bag/valve-mask ventilation more difficult and worsen the view obtained at laryngoscopy. The force required for effective cricoid pressure is also debated.

Current recommendations are that cricoid pressure should be applied during rapid sequence induction, at a force of 10 N while the patient is awake, increasing to 20–40 N as the patient loses consciousness. The force should be released if there is difficulty with laryngoscopy or passage of the endotracheal tube.

Rapid sequence induction

Patients at risk of pulmonary aspiration require a rapid sequence induction (RSI). The aim is to reduce the time between loss of consciousness, onset of neuromuscular blockade and placement of the endotracheal tube.

The essential elements are: careful preoxygenation, induction with a predetermined dose of induction agent, with the application of cricoid pressure, use of rapid-acting neuromuscular blocker, avoidance of bag/valve-mask ventilation, and intubation with confirmation of endotracheal tube placement prior to the removal of cricoid pressure.

The presence of a skilled assistant is mandatory, and a strategy should be in place for the management of difficult/failed intubation.

Classically suxamethonium is the preferred neuromuscular blocker because of its rapid onset/offset. Similar rapidity of onset can be achieved with high-dose rocuronium, and its use is now favoured by some authorities. The availability of the reversal agent sugammadex has made the use of rocuronium more widespread in RSI.

Rapid sequence induction

- Place on a tilting table.
- Check all equipment.
- Keep active suction to hand.
- Attach monitoring and secure intravenous access, connect fast-flowing fluids.
- Pre-oxygenate with a close-fitting face mask and high-flow 100% O_2 to achieve end-tidal concentrations of $O_2 > 90\%$.
- Apply cricoid pressure (10 N while patient is awake, increasing to 30 N as consciousness is lost).
- Administer sleep dose of appropriate induction agent intravenously.
- Once consciousness is lost, administer suxamethonium 1.5 mg kg^{-1} or rocuronium 1 mg kg^{-1}.
- When the patient is relaxed, intubate the trachea and confirm position before releasing cricoid pressure.

Management of pulmonary aspiration

If regurgitation or vomiting occurs during induction or surgery the upper airway should be cleared immediately by sucking out the pharynx and turning the patient head-down. Tracheal intubation limits the risk of further aspiration.

The presence of large particulate matter can cause airway obstruction and may require removal under laryngoscopic or bronchoscopic guidance. Bronchial lavage is not helpful and may result in the dissemination of aspirated material. Attempted neutralisation of gastric acid at this stage is ineffective.

Early clinical signs include a fall in oxygen saturation and the presence of bronchospasm, which may require the administration of bronchodilators. The administration of PEEP will help to maintain alveolar recruitment, and 'lung-protective' ventilation should be employed.

Of those patients that aspirate around two-thirds will have no respiratory sequelae and approximately 20% will require intubation and ventilation on ICU. The ability to maintain adequate arterial oxygen saturation with an $F_IO_2 < 0.5$ is predictive of successful extubation. A thorough clinical assessment should be made with radiography if appropriate.

Systemic corticosteroids are of no proven benefit, and antibiotics are usually reserved for the development of clear signs of secondary infection. Consideration should be given to the limitation or postponement of surgery.

References and further reading

Association of Anaesthetists of Great Britain and Ireland. *AAGBI Safety Guideline: Suspected Anaphylactic Reactions Associated with Anaesthesia*. London: AAGBI, 2009a.

Association of Anaesthetists of Great Britain and Ireland. *Management of a Patient with Suspected Anaphylaxis During Anaesthesia*. London: AAGBI, 2009b. www.aagbi.org/sites/default/files/ana_web_laminate_final.pdf.

Association of Anaesthetists of Great Britain and Ireland. Checking anaesthetic equipment 2012. *Anaesthesia* 2012; **67**: 660–8.

Cook T. Supraglottic airway devices. In Cook T, Woodall N, Frerk C, eds., *Major Complications of Airway Management in the UK. 4th National Audit Project*. London: Royal College of Anaesthetists and the Difficult Airway Society, 2011, pp. 86–95.

Cook TM, Woodall N, Frerk C; Fourth National Audit Project. Major complications of airway management in the UK: results of the Fourth National Audit Project of the Royal College of Anaesthetists and the Difficult Airway Society. Part 1: anaesthesia. *Br J Anaesth* 2011; **106**: 617–31.

Cook TM, Woodall N, Harper J, Benger J; Fourth National Audit Project. Major complications of airway management in the UK: results of the Fourth National Audit Project of the Royal College of Anaesthetists and the Difficult Airway Society. Part 2: intensive care and emergency departments. *Br J Anaesth* 2011; **106**: 632–42.

Cormack RS, Lehane J. Difficult tracheal intubation in obstetrics. *Anaesthesia* 1984; **39**: 1105–11.

Fisher MM, Baldo BA. The incidence and clinical features of anaphylactic reactions during anesthesia in Australia. *Ann Fr Anesth Reanim* 1993; **12**: 97–104.

Henderson JJ, Popat MT, Latto IP, Pearce AC. Difficult Airway Society guidelines for management of the unanticipated difficult intubation. *Anaesthesia* 2004; **59**: 675–94.

Laxenaire MC. Epidemiology of anesthetic anaphylactoid reactions. Fourth multicenter survey (July 1994–December 1996). *Ann Fr Anesth Reanim* 1999; **18**: 796–809.

Mertes PM, Lambert M, Guéant-Rodriguez RM, et al. Perioperative anaphylaxis. *Immunol Allergy Clin North Am* 2009; **29**: 429–51.

World Health Organization. *Surgical Safety Checklist*. Geneva: WHO Press, 2008.

CHAPTER 3

Intraoperative management

Chris Mowatt

The intraoperative period follows induction of anaesthesia and is terminated with the safe discharge of the patient to the recovery area. After transfer of the patient from the anaesthetic room, the anaesthetist must ensure safe positioning of the patient and the re-establishment of appropriate monitoring while maintaining an appropriate depth of anaesthesia. This represents a period of significant risk for the patient, with the anaesthetist expected to complete a series of complex tasks simultaneously.

Positioning

Patient positioning can represent a significant challenge during anaesthesia. The aim of safe positioning is to provide optimal conditions for surgical access while minimising the risk of patient harm. The main hazards are related to the physiological changes associated with a change in posture and the effects of pressure. Position-related complications remain a significant cause of patient morbidity.

Cardiovascular effects – Changes in position under general anaesthesia can have marked haemodynamic consequences. These effects are exaggerated by the loss of the normal homeostatic mechanisms which act to maintain organ perfusion during changes in position. For example reverse Trendelenburg positioning and abdominal compression in the prone position result in reduced venous return, reducing preload and cardiac output, which may result in significant hypotension.

Interruptions in monitoring should be minimised during this period, with haemodynamic compromise anticipated and treated appropriately. Patient safety should not be compromised to permit rapid positioning.

Respiratory effects – In many positions mechanical compression of the lungs results in a reduction in the functional residual capacity (FRC) and total lung volume (TLV). Ventilation/perfusion mismatches may result in significant intrapulmonary shunting. The use of mechanical ventilation and appropriate levels of positive end-expiratory pressure (PEEP) to reduce the degree of atelectasis can ameliorate some of these changes.

Nerve injury – Peripheral nerve injury, although rare, accounts for a significant number of litigation claims against anaesthetists. Commonly injured nerves include the ulnar nerve, brachial plexus, lumbosacral roots, radial, sciatic and common peroneal nerves. Injuries occur when peripheral nerves are stretched or compressed. Care must be taken to avoid excessive stretch or pressure on areas where nerves are susceptible to injury, such as the common peroneal nerve at the head of the fibula, the axillary plexus in the axilla and the ulnar nerve at the elbow. Where possible, joints should be maintained in a neutral position and pressure areas padded appropriately. Consideration should be given to individual patient risk factors,

Fundamentals of Anaesthesia, 4th edition, ed. Ted Lin, Tim Smith and Colin Pinnock. Published by Cambridge University Press. © Cambridge University Press 2017.

for example obesity, peripheral vascular disease, pre-existing neuropathy, and their influence on potential nerve injury. It may be useful to assess preoperatively whether a patient can tolerate a particular position.

Pressure areas – The development of pressure sores can result in significant morbidity. The combination of pressure-related mechanical occlusion of the vasculature and shear forces results in the development of pressure areas which can progress to necrosis and ulceration. Pressure areas should be adequately padded, skin exposure to moisture minimised, and all sheets and pads smoothed out beneath the patient. Constant vigilance is necessary, with frequent checking of the patient.

Ocular injury – Corneal abrasions are the most common type of eye injury associated with anaesthesia and are usually the result of direct trauma from foreign objects, including face masks, monitoring cables and drapes. The cornea may also be damaged if allowed to dry excessively. Particular care should be paid when the patient is placed in the prone and Trendelenburg positions, and the eyes must be protected appropriately. Frequent eye checks are recommended.

Monitoring

Continuous monitoring of the patient's physiological condition is essential for the conduct of safe anaesthesia. The uninterrupted presence of a trained, competent and appropriately experienced anaesthetist is the most important component of this. Monitoring devices should be regarded as a supplement to clinical observation of signs such as the response to surgical stimulation, movement of the chest wall and breath sounds following intubation.

The recommendations for standards of monitoring during anaesthesia and recovery are listed in Figure 3.1.

Accurate records must be kept at intervals of no more than every 5 minutes. In the clinically unstable patient measurements should be more frequent.

Maintenance of anaesthesia

The ideal for the maintenance of anaesthesia is to keep the patient safe, comfortable and appropriately relaxed to permit surgery while maintaining homeostasis. The techniques available are listed in Figure 3.2.

Figure 3.1 Standards of monitoring

A. Induction and maintenance of anaesthesia
1. Pulse oximeter
2. Non-invasive blood pressure monitor
3. Electrocardiograph
4. Airway gases: oxygen, carbon dioxide and vapour
5. Airway pressure

The following must also be available:
- A nerve stimulator whenever a muscle relaxant is used
- A means of measuring the patient's temperature

B. Recovery from anaesthesia
A high standard of monitoring should be maintained until the patient is fully recovered from anaesthesia. Clinical observations must be supplemented by the following monitoring devices:
1. Pulse oximeter
2. Non-invasive blood pressure monitor

The following must also be immediately available:
- Electrocardiograph
- Nerve stimulator
- Means of measuring temperature
- Capnograph

Figure 3.2 Maintenance of anaesthesia

Local anaesthesia
- Tissue infiltration
- Regional nerve blockade
- Central neuraxial blockade

General anaesthesia
- Inhalation of anaesthetic vapours (with or without nitrous oxide)
- Total intravenous anaesthesia (TIVA) – target-controlled infusion (TCI), intermittent injection or infusion of intravenous anaesthetic agent

Dissociative anaesthesia
- Intravenous or intramuscular injection of ketamine

Hypnosis

General anaesthesia

General anaesthesia is a pharmacologically induced reversible state of hypnosis with the components of amnesia, analgesia, muscle relaxation and to a degree amelioration of the stress response to surgical stimulation. The provision of optimal conditions, a 'balanced' anaesthetic, to permit surgery usually relies on the combination of several drugs and techniques.

Awareness

The avoidance of awareness is an absolute priority in general anaesthesia. Awareness during anaesthesia can be extremely distressing for patients with far-reaching consequences for their psychological wellbeing. The incidence of awareness is reported consistently as around 1 in 600. Up to 50% of these patients develop significant psychological sequelae. Awareness may be defined as follows:

Explicit awareness – conscious awareness with recall. This may be spontaneous or in response to postoperative questioning. Pain is not always a feature.

Implicit awareness – perception without conscious awareness or recall which may affect an individual's behaviour at a later date.

Awareness may occur at any stage during an anaesthetic from induction to emergence. The prevention of awareness requires an appreciation of the causes and risk factors.

The risk of awareness correlates directly with the depth of anaesthesia. For inhalational anaesthesia the depth of anaesthesia is related to the alveolar concentration of a volatile anaesthetic. The relative potency of inhalational agents is expressed as the minimum alveolar concentration (MAC).

In unpremedicated subjects 1 MAC is the alveolar concentration of a volatile anaesthetic which will prevent movement in response to a standard surgical stimulus in one-half of the population. MAC is thus the ED_{50} (the effective dose in 50% of patients) and shows a normally distributed variation. Thus 1 MAC may not represent a sufficient dose of anaesthetic in an individual patient. The definition of MAC does not directly encompass awareness or recall, although there is a reliable association between recall and MAC. MAC may also be influenced by other patient-related factors (Figure 3.3).

The equivalent concept can also be applied to total intravenous anaesthesia, where the term minimum inhibitory concentration (MIC) is applied. The normal distribution for MIC has a greater variability than that of MAC, and this may increase the risk of awareness. This is further compounded by the lack of ability to directly monitor, in real time, the concentration of intravenous anaesthetic agents, in contrast to inhalational agents.

Figure 3.3 Characteristics of MAC values

Normally distributed
Relate to movement and not awareness (MAC for awareness is less than MAC for movement)
Vary with age and wellbeing
Inferred from end-tidal concentration
Reduced by concurrent administration of hypnotics, sedatives and analgesics
Increased by fear and stimulant drug abuse

Figure 3.4 Risk factors for awareness under anaesthesia

1. Inadequate anaesthetic dosage
   a. accidental
   b. deliberate

2. Unrecognised equipment failure, e.g. TIVA pump failure

3. Use of muscle relaxants

4. Patient physiology
   a. age-related MAC variations
   b. metabolic state
   c. use of drugs: alcohol, cocaine and amphetamines increase MAC

Given the variability in response to anaesthesia outlined above it is important to develop a strategy for preventing awareness. This includes a thorough preoperative assessment to identify risk factors for awareness (Figure 3.4) and appropriate intraoperative monitoring. Unfortunately there are no means to directly measure level of consciousness. Clinical observation remains the mainstay of diagnosis of awareness. This may be heralded by an increase in sympathetic nervous system activity, reflected by:

- Tachycardia
- Hypertension
- Mydriasis
- Sweating
- Lacrimation

These surrogate markers for depth of anaesthesia are unreliable under certain conditions, e.g. β-blockade, presence of a pacemaker.

Modern depth of anaesthesia monitors have been developed and consist of two types: those that measure and process the electroencephalogram (EEG) to provide a measure of frontal cortical suppression, and those that measure evoked potentials. The use of depth of consciousness monitors does not prevent awareness but may reduce the risk in patients judged to be high risk.

Inhalational anaesthesia

The inhalational anaesthetics in common use produce loss of consciousness and to a variable degree muscle relaxation. With the exception of nitrous oxide they do not produce significant analgesia.

Intravenous anaesthesia

Various agents have been employed for intravenous anaesthesia. **Thiopental** was widely used in the 1950s and 1960s for continuous IV anaesthesia, but its accumulation in tissues and hence prolonged recovery phase proved disadvantageous. **Ketamine** remains a widely used agent in the prehospital field and also in developing countries. **Propofol** is the most widely used agent for total intravenous anaesthesia (TIVA). There are two popular techniques:

1. An induction dose of propofol is followed by smaller bolus doses on an empirical basis. This technique is adequate for short procedures (< 15 minutes).
2. **Target-controlled infusion (TCI)** techniques have increased in popularity with the development of sophisticated, computer-controlled devices for the administration of propofol. New concepts in pharmacokinetic modelling and computer technology have made these systems safe, reliable and user-friendly. The control of plasma levels is precise and rapid, with predictable onset and offset. A disadvantage is the lack of ability to directly monitor plasma levels of propofol in a manner similar to end-tidal gas measurement to ensure that the MIC is maintained to prevent awareness. The development of TCI software for short-acting opioids, predominantly **remifentanil**, means the two agents are frequently used together to provide a balanced anaesthetic technique. Remifentanil has a MAC/MIC sparing effect, reducing the amount of anaesthetic agent in a dose-related fashion.

Local anaesthesia

Anaesthesia may be maintained using techniques to block the transmission of nociceptive and sensory nerves with specific nerve blockade to cover the distribution of the nerves supplying the appropriate surgical field, local infiltration, or a central neuraxial blockade. A regional block in this manner may be used to supplement a general anaesthetic technique and for postoperative analgesia.

Analgesia

A balanced, multimodal approach to analgesia modified by surgical and patient factors is an important consideration for the anaesthetist. The provision of appropriate analgesia ameliorates the stress response to surgery and can help to reduce postoperative complications. Appropriate levels of analgesia also improve patient satisfaction and improve theatre productivity and patient flow.

Ventilation

Ventilation may be maintained either spontaneously or by means of artificial ventilation. The mode for maintenance of ventilation will depend on surgical factors including the site, nature, extent and (to a degree) the likely duration of the operation. Patient factors influencing the type of airway selected will also determine the mode of ventilation. For example a spontaneously breathing, inhalational technique may be more suitable for relatively less stimulating body-surface surgery than for prolonged body-cavity surgery requiring muscle relaxation.

Maintaining oxygenation to ensure adequate oxygen delivery to the tissues is essential, and consideration of the most appropriate mode to ensure this during surgery should form a part of preoperative assessment and planning.

Adequate ventilation is dependent on:

1. A patent airway. This may be provided by a face mask, supplemented with airway adjuncts if necessary or a supraglottic airway device. The depth of anaesthesia required to tolerate an endotracheal tube almost inevitably necessitates manual ventilation.
2. Central drive and the integrated response to changes in the sensors (chemoreceptors, lung receptors and influence of peripheral and 'higher' inputs) and effectors (muscles of respiration) during surgery. Central drive is reduced by opioids and both inhalational and intravenous agents, and this may necessitate mechanical ventilation. In lighter planes of anaesthesia lung receptors may be irritated, resulting in coughing, which is more pronounced in the presence of irritant agents (e.g. isoflurane).

3. Pulmonary mechanics (atelectasis, ventilation/perfusion mismatch and pre-existing pulmonary disease). Positioning has marked effects on the ability of the respiratory muscles to generate an adequate tidal volume. FRC is usually reduced and hypoxia may develop. For this reason patients under anaesthesia will require an F_IO_2 higher than preoperatively. The effects are more pronounced in certain positions, as described earlier in this chapter.

Mode of mechanical ventilation

Mechanical ventilation during anaesthesia should have the dual aims of maintaining adequate ventilation while preventing ventilator-associated harm. Mechanical ventilaton carries the risk of direct ventilator-induced lung injury (volutrauma and barotrauma). Atelectasis occurs in over 90% of patients undergoing surgical procedures, resulting in $\dot{V}/\dot{Q}$ mismatch and hypoxia and a propensity to develop pulmonary infection.

Multiple modes of ventilation are now available to the anaesthetist. Most patients who require mechanical ventilation in theatre will be paralysed and will receive a mandatory, time-cycled pressure- or volume-controlled breath.

In practice, the parameters that are set will include:

- **Minute ventilation**, as the product of tidal volume and respiratory rate. A tidal volume of 5–8 mL kg^{-1} is appropriate with a respiratory rate of 12–16 to provide sufficient CO_2 clearance as directed by the $ETCO_2$. In certain conditions the respiratory rate may need to be increased to prevent hypercapnia, most notably during laparoscopic surgery with CO_2 insufflation. Excessive tidal volumes are damaging to the lung, particularly in patients at risk of lung injury. **Plateau pressure** should be limited to less than 30 cmH_2O.
- **Inspiratory time to expiratory time ratio (I:E)**. In adult patients with healthy lungs this is 1:1.5–2. In patients with bronchospasm or lung disease which limits the rate of emptying of lung units during expiration (COPD), this may need to be prolonged.
- An appropriate F_IO_2 should be selected to maintain adequate oxygenation with SpO_2 maintained above 94% (a value at which oxyhaemoglobin is very close to the steep part of the dissociation curve). Hyperoxia should be avoided where possible, as it may result in lung injury and atelectasis.
- The use of appropriate amounts of **positive end-expiratory pressure (PEEP)** can help to maintain the recruitment of lung units, preventing atelectasis, maintaining oxygenation and keeping the lung on the mechanically advantageous steep portion of the inflation pressure–volume curve. Manipulation of PEEP can be useful in the management of hypoxia if atelectasis is felt to be responsible. The appropriate level of PEEP must be optimised to an individual patient, but a level of 5 cmH_2O is an appropriate starting point.

The development of alternative modes of ventilation including pressure support now allows for spontaneous breaths to be supported by the anaesthetic machine ventilator in theatre. These modes are comfortable for patients and mean that in certain circumstances paralysis and formal mechanical ventilation can be avoided.

Management of intraoperative fluid therapy

The aim of intraoperative fluid therapy is to maintain adequate tissue perfusion by optimising intravascular volume status and stroke volume to ensure adequate oxygen delivery to the tissues. Both hypovolaemia *and* the administration of excess amounts of fluid are harmful to the patient.

Factors affecting volume status:

- **Basal requirement**
  - Basal fluid requirements are of the order 1–1.5 mL kg^{-1} h^{-1}.
  - May be significantly increased in sepsis and hypermetabolic states.
- **Pre-existing losses**
  - Preoperative fasting should not significantly reduce intravascular volume. Patients should be encouraged to maintain hydration and limit fasting to safe, agreed limits.
  - Large-volume fluid losses can occur in conditions such as acute bowel obstruction, sepsis and pancreatitis.
  - Hypovolaemia as the result of bleeding – this may be concealed in the fit, young trauma patient.

Where possible, careful attention should be given to the preoperative assessment of fluid status and the patient delivered to theatre in a euvolaemic state.

- **Intraoperative losses**
  - Sympathetic blockade following neuraxial anaesthesia and the vasodilatation seen to a variable degree with volatile inhalational agents may result in a relative hypovolaemia necessitating fluid therapy.

o Evaporative losses from an open abdominal cavity or chest can be clinically significant if surgery is prolonged and can be in excess of $1 \text{ mL kg}^{-1} \text{ h}^{-1}$.
o Haemorrhage.

A simple formula for fluid requirement is therefore:

Input = Basal requirements + Pre-existing losses
+ Intraoperative (ongoing) losses

Clinical assessment of filling status presents a significant challenge. Assessment with 'static' measures – skin turgor, pulse, blood pressure, mucous membrane condition – is difficult under anaesthesia. Furthermore a patient can have a normal blood pressure and pulse and yet remain significantly hypovolaemic.

Studies have demonstrated that targeting an 'optimal' stroke volume for an individual patient improves operative outcomes. This has led to the development of monitors to measure dynamic indices under anaesthesia to guide adequate fluid replacement. Examples include:
• Transoesophageal Doppler
• Transcutaneous Doppler
• Pulse contour analysis with or without transpulmonary calibration
• Transthoracic impedance plethysmography

Fluid therapy can be based on the responsiveness of the circulation, measured by a change in stroke volume or stroke volume variation, to a fluid challenge (500 mL crystalloid, 200 mL colloid). In this way the patient can be maintained in an optimal position on the Frank–Starling curve, avoiding the problems of hypovolaemia and excess fluid administration.

The choice of fluid for intraoperative fluid therapy remains controversial. Hartmann's solution is the most common choice because its ionic composition is felt to most closely resemble plasma.

Critical incidents during anaesthesia
Life-threatening crises may arise during anaesthesia with limited warning. The anaesthetist must be prepared to recognise and deal with these rapidly.

Hypoxia
Hypoxia during anaesthesia is a common scenario and may occur at any point from induction to emergence. There are numerous potential causes (Figure 3.5), and anaesthetists should have a safe and systematic approach to dealing with this problem. The aim should be to ensure adequate oxygenation while attempting to identify and deal with the underlying problem. The shape of the oxyhaemoglobin dissociation curve means that at a saturation of 93% the patient is at risk of rapid desaturation and hypoxia. Desaturation should prompt immediate attention (Figure 3.6).

Figure 3.5 Causes of hypoxia

Airway
• Obstruction, including laryngospasm, occlusion of circuit
• Misplaced endotracheal tube – endobronchial intubation, accidental extubation

Breathing
• Hypoventilation
• V/Q mismatch
• Bronchospasm

Circulation
• Low cardiac output
• Embolism

Drugs
• Respiratory depressants – opioids, deep anaesthesia
• Anaphylaxis

Equipment
• Breathing circuit failure – obstruction, disconnection
• Delivery of hypoxic mixture
• Monitoring failure – incorrect trace

Figure 3.6 Desaturation algorithm

Administer high-flow oxygen, F_IO_2 1.0
Maintain anaesthesia
Consider the need for hand ventilation
Assess:
• **A**irway – confirm patency, consider intubation
• **B**reathing – manual ventilation, auscultation. Is recruitment necessary?
• **C**irculation
• Could **D**rugs be the cause?
• Consider **E**quipment failure with early use of alternative oxygen supply and breathing circuit. Exclude delivery of hypoxic mixture
Call for help early

Bronchospasm

Intraoperative bronchospasm may manifest with:

- Increased circuit pressure
- Desaturation
- Audible wheeze
- Reduction in tidal volume and hypoventilation
- Prolonged expiratory phase with upsloping of the capnography trace

Causes include:

- Allergic reaction – anaphylaxis, anaphylactoid reaction
- Airway irritation – excessive secretions, aspiration of gastric contents
- Endotracheal tube misplacement – endobronchial intubation, irritation of carina
- Pneumothorax
- Inadequate anaesthetic depth

Patients particularly at risk include smokers, patients with asthma/COPD, patients with 'reactive' airways following recent upper respiratory tract infection.

Partial occlusion of the breathing circuit may very closely mimic bronchospasm and should be excluded using an alternative breathing circuit if there are any concerns (Figure 3.7).

Figure 3.7 Bronchospasm algorithm

Administer F_IO_2 1.0
Liaise with surgeon
Deepen anaesthesia
Assess:
- **A**irway
  - if mask/supraglottic device, consider aspiration
  - if endotracheal tube, consider misplacement
- **B**reathing
  - auscultate
  - if unable to ventilate, consider alternative breathing circuit
  - is there an obstruction distal to the endoctracheal tube?
- **C**irculation
  - consider pulmonary oedema
- **D**rugs
  - consider allergic reaction
- **E**quipment
Administer salbutamol – via nebuliser or metered dose inhaler if appropriate breathing circuit connection available, or intravenously. Consider intravenous adrenaline, aminophylline or magnesium
Review and treat possible causes

Emboli

Intraoperative embolism most commonly results from thrombus, although other situations include gas, fat and rarely tumour or amniotic fluid.

Thrombus – The risk of developing intraoperative thrombosis is increased by various factors, including:

- Smoking
- Immobility
- Malignancy
- Use of the contraceptive pill
- Recent previous surgery
- Pelvic or lower limb surgery

Thrombosis usually develops in the deep veins of the lower limb and pelvis. Detachment of formed thrombus into the circulation results in venous thromboembolism, which may manifest as the clinical syndrome of pulmonary embolism.

Risk stratification should occur prior to surgery, with appropriate steps to reduce risk in some patients including: hydration, intraoperative calf compression devices and pharmacological thromboprophylaxis. The use of central neuraxial blockade may reduce the risk of venous thrombosis.

The diagnosis is usually made by a combination of signs including tachyarrhythmias, hypoxia and an acute fall in $ETCO_2$. Massive pulmonary embolism may have significant cardiovascular consequences. The increase in right ventricular wall tension caused by the rise in pulmonary artery pressure leads to impaired right ventricular function and dilatation of the right ventricle, and ultimately impaired left ventricular filling with compromised cardiac output and systemic hypoperfusion. This cycle can lead to shock, circulatory collapse and death. Management consists of increasing F_IO_2, haemodynamic support, and if indicated thrombolytic therapy or surgery. On-table echocardiography may be of value in directing therapy.

Fat embolism is rare. It is most common after bone injury, the result of either trauma or orthopaedic instrumentation with embolisation of multiple fat globules into the systemic circulation. The clinical syndrome can range from mild hypoxia to fulminant cor pulmonale with a systemic inflammatory response and disseminated intravascular coagulation (DIC). The development of a petechial rash across the chest, oral mucosa and conjunctivae is considered pathognomonic, but its appearance may be delayed. Treatment is supportive.

Significant **amniotic fluid embolism** is usually a postmortem diagnosis following the development of circulatory collapse in pregnancy and labour.

Gas embolism – Embolisation of gas results from the ingress of gas into the venous circulation. Air embolism is usually the result of subatmospheric pressure in an open large vein, as when the operative site is open and above the level of the right atrium. Examples include neurosurgery in the 'beach chair' position and shoulder surgery. Air embolism via venous catheters may also occur. Laparoscopic procedures may result in embolisation of the insufflating gas, usually CO_2.

The resulting clinical picture depends on the volume of gas entering the circulation. Embolisation of air at a rate exceeding 0.5 mL kg^{-1} min^{-1} will result in signs, usually resulting from the air reaching the cardiac chambers. The fatal amount of air is estimated at 3–5 mL kg^{-1}. Features include:

- Millwheel murmur over the chest
- Abrupt fall in end-tidal CO_2
- Hypoxia
- Tachyarrhythmias
- Raised pulmonary artery presure

With any suspicion, further entry of gas should be prevented. The surgeon should be informed, the operative site immediately flooded with saline and a wet pack. Venous pressure at the site should be increased and ventilation with 100% oxygen applied. Occasionally gas can be aspirated through an existing central venous line with the patient rotated onto the right side. Transoesophageal echocardiography can be useful in detecting air embolism in high-risk patients.

Hypotension

Hypotension during anaesthesia may be defined as a mean arterial pressure (MAP) $< 20\%$ of the preoperative value, or a reading below a MAP of 60 mmHg. If sustained, the impairment of organ perfusion may result in the ischaemic injury of end organs.

The most common causes of hypotension under anaesthesia are: (1) the result of administered drugs, (2) the reduction in SVR as the result of regional block, (3) hypovolaemia, (4) related to surgery – haemorrhage, vagal reflexes – and (5) related to cardiac arrhythmias. The presence of immediately life-threatening causes of hypotension, e.g. tension pneumothorax, cardiac

Figure 3.8 Hypotension algorithm

Confirm hypotension is real
Consider – COULD THIS BE A CARDIAC ARREST?
Liaise with surgeon
Assess:
- **A**irway
- **B**reathing
- **C**irculation
- **D**rugs
- **E**quipment

Adjust the anaesthetic dosage as appropriate
Modify posture if possible – head down, legs flat
Administer fluid – 10 mL kg^{-1} crystalloid as bolus
Give vasopressor, e.g. metaraminol 0.25–0.5 mg, ephedrine 3–6 mg, phenylephrine 25–50 µg
Review and treat possible causes
Consider invasive monitoring/further fluid or drug therapy

tamponade, massive haemorrhage, is thankfully rare. A high index of suspicion should be maintained in situations where this is more likely, for example after central venous access or during cardiac surgery (Figure 3.8).

Cardiac arrhythmias

Cardiac arrhythmias are common in the perioperative period. The aetiology is often multifactorial.

Bradycardia

A heart rate < 60 bpm is defined as bradycardia, although this may be normal in the fit or those maintained on β-blockers. A heart rate < 40 bpm is poorly tolerated and should be evaluated carefully. Cardiac output is determined by the product of heart rate and stroke volume, and therefore bradycardia may result in a significant reduction in oxygen delivery to the tissues if sustained. Treatment is recommended if signs of poor peripheral perfusion or hypotension are observed.

Bradycardia is most commonly sinus rhythm, followed in frequency by junctional bradycardia. Atrioventricular block with aberrant conduction may also present as a bradycardia.

Causes include (1) drugs (overdosage of inhalational agent, opioids, neostigmine), (2) vagal reflexes (peritoneal stretching, oculocardiac reflex), (3) hypoxia. Bradycardia may also reflect myocardial ischaemia.

Management involves treatment of the underlying cause, asking the surgeon to relieve stretch, for instance, with administration of rate-modifying drugs, most frequently atropine 0.5–1 mg or glycopyrrolate 0.2–0.6 mg. Infrequently temporary pacing, either internal or external, is required if the bradycardia is refractory to treatment.

Tachycardia

A heart rate > 100 bpm is defined as tachycardia. Sinus tachycardia is a normal response to stimulation of the sympathetic nervous system. Inadequate analgesia or depth of anaesthesia is a frequent cause.

Tachycardia is also associated with the systemic inflammatory response seen in sepsis, trauma and burns. It may also reflect an underlying metabolic disturbance (hyperthyroidism, malignant hyperthermia), or the administration of sympathomimetic drugs (ephedrine) or vagolytic drugs (atropine, pancuronium). Metabolic disturbances (acidosis, hyper/hypokalaemia and hypomagnesaemia) are related to the development of arrhythmia, and attempts should be made to correct these as far as possible before the induction of anaesthesia.

Excessive tachycardia reduces the time for diastolic filling of coronary vessels and may precipitate myocardial ischaemia, an effect more pronounced in those with underlying coronary artery disease. The development of an arrhythmia can exacerbate this and may also be precipitated by myocardial ischaemia.

Management should follow the Adult Life Support guidelines with identification of the underling rhythm, as detailed under *Management of life-threatening peri-arrest arrhythmias* in Chapter 8. The ABCDE approach to assessment of the acutely unwell patient applies when the patient is anaesthetised. Close communication with members of the surgical team is essential when planning the management of life-threatening emergencies under anaesthesia. As well as preparing surgeons for any potential disruption, plans may need to be made to abort or limit surgery in the unstable patient.

Massive haemorrhage

Massive haemorrhage may be self-evident (a traumatised patient in the emergency department), anticipated (elective cardiac, vascular or obstetric procedures), or unexpected. The definition is arbitrary, but a situation where 1–1.5 blood volumes are needed to be infused acutely or within 24 hours is sometimes cited.

The management of massive haemorrhage requires a team approach with close communication with surgeons, haematology and laboratory staff and members of the theatre team. Local procedures should be in place, and anaesthetists should familiarise themselves with the major haemorrhage protocol.

Immediate management should include:

- Haemorrhage control – haemostatic packing, tourniquet, pressure.
- Maintain adequate oxygen delivery – administer high F_IO_2.
- Fluid resuscitation – large-bore IV access with active warming of infused fluids. Consideration should be given to the use of a rapid infusion device if available.
- Blood tests should be requested to include: baseline clotting screen (near-patient ROTEM/TEG if possible), FBC and cross-match.
- Transfuse blood as appropriate. O-negative blood is usually available immediately in theatres, followed in time by type-specific and later fully cross-matched blood. Blood and blood products should be administered through a giving set with a 170–200 μm filter.
- Coagulopathy should be anticipated and ideally prevented with early administration of blood products. If present it should be managed aggressively with fresh frozen plasma (in an initial dose of 15 mL kg^{-1}) and platelets to maintain a platelet count > 75×10^9 L^{-1}. Fibrinogen should be checked and maintained above 1.5 g L^{-1} with administration of cryoprecipitate if necessary.

Haemostatic tests should be repeated regularly in the context of ongoing bleeding, with close liaison with haematology colleagues. A prothrombin time (PT) or activated partial thromboplastin time (APTT) 1.5 × normal represents etablished haemostatic failure and is associated with microvascular bleeding.

Once bleeding is controlled, aggressive attempts to normalise the metabolic disturbances associated with major haemorrhage should be made. Hypothermia and acidosis are common. Hypocalcaemia and hyperkalaemia may also feature. Disposal of the patient to a safe environment, usually critical care, is mandatory. It may not always be possible to definitively control haemorrhage, and a haemostatic pause with damage control may allow the anaesthetist to 'catch up' with resuscitation and correct abnormal physiology.

Malignant hyperthermia

Malignant hyperthermia (MH) is an inherited disorder of skeletal muscle which follows an autosomal dominant pattern, triggered by exposure to suxamethonium and *all*

Figure 3.9 Malignant hyperthermia

Clinical signs
- Hyperthermia (core temperature rising 1–2 °C per hour)
- Respiratory acidosis
- Metabolic acidosis
- Cardiac arrhythmias
- Hypoxaemia
- Cyanosis

Signs of abnormal muscle activity
- Masseter spasm following suxamethonium persisting for more than 2 minutes
- Rigidity of certain groups of muscles but not necessarily all
- Hyperkalaemia
- Myoglobinuria and acute kidney injury
- Rise in creatine kinase

Other signs
- Disseminated intravascular coagulation (DIC)
- Cerebral and pulmonary oedema

Triggering agents
- ALL the inhalational agents
- Suxamethonium
- (Avoid if possible phenothiazines, atropine)

Agents thought to be safe
- Propofol
- Thiopental
- N_2O
- Opioids
- Non-depolarising muscle relaxants

Figure 3.10 Management of malignant hyperthermia

1. Recognition
- Unexplained increase in $ETCO_2$ AND
- Unexplained tachycardia AND
- Unexplained increase in O_2 requirement

(previous uneventful anaesthesia does NOT rule out MH)

2. Immediate management
- STOP all trigger agents (anaesthetic vapours etc.)
- CALL FOR HELP. Allocate specific tasks
- Install clean breathing system and HYPERVENTILATE with high-flow 100% O_2
- Maintain anaesthesia with intravenous agent
- ABANDON/FINISH surgery as soon as possible

3. Monitoring and treatment
- Give dantrolene
  - 2.5 mg kg^{-1} immediate IV bolus. Repeat 1 mg kg^{-1} boluses to a maximum 10 mg kg^{-1}
- Initiate active cooling
- TREAT:
  - Hyperkalaemia
  - Arrhythmias
  - Metabolic acidosis
  - Myoglobinaemia – forced alkaline diuresis, consideration of RRT
  - DIC
- Check plasma CK as soon as possible

4. Follow-up
- Continue monitoring on ICU. Dantrolene may need repeat dosing for up to 24 hours
- Monitor for renal failure and compartment syndrome
- Repeat CK
- Consider alternative diagnoses (phaeochromocytoma, sepsis, thyroid storm, myopathy)
- Counsel patient and family members
- Refer to MH unit

volatile anaesthetic agents. The reported incidence varies from 1 in 40,000 to 1 in 100,000 anaesthetics. The population prevalence of the genetic susceptibility is between 1 in 5000 and 1 in 10,000. Mortality rates have fallen dramatically from 70–80% in the 1970s to 2–3% as a result of increased awareness and treatment. The metabolic disturbance produced can prove fatal if not recognised and treated promptly (Figure 3.9).

Pathophysiology
The clinical features of MH are related to disruption of skeletal muscle homeostasis. Elevated intracellular concentrations of calcium lead to:

1. Muscle rigidity due to continuous actin–mysosin interaction.
2. Hypermetabolism.
3. Rhabdomyolysis develops as the result of a generalised membrane permeability defect.

Skeletal muscle forms a large component of total body mass, and hypermetabolism quickly results in excessive heat production which outstrips the temperature-regulating capacity of the body. Oxygen delivery may not be sufficient to meet the metabolic costs of hyper-metabolism, with resulting lactic acidosis and hyper-capnia. Rhabdomyolysis results in hyperkalaemia and the leakage of myoglobin into the circulation, leading in turn to dysrhythmias and acute kidney injury.

Diagnosis and management

Diagnosis can be difficult, as the presentation may vary considerably. The onset may be insidious or a florid, rapidly life-threatening acute event. Management should follow the scheme set out in Figure 3.10.

Safe discharge

The intraoperative period is completed with the safe discharge of the patient to a designated recovery area. Transfer should only be undertaken when the patient is physiologically stable. The level of monitoring required during transfer is at the discretion of the anaesthetist and will depend on factors such as the proximity of the recovery area, level of responsiveness and stability.

The anaesthetist must formally hand over care to an appropriately trained member of staff, and the patient must be observed until he or she has regained airway control, is cardiovascularly stable, and is able to communicate.

Extubation of an endotracheal tube remains the responsibility of the anaesthetist.

The aim is to have the patient pain-free, breathing spontaneously with adequate ventilation, and cardiovascularly stable.

CHAPTER 4
Postoperative management

Tina McLeod

Care of the unconscious patient

Emergence from anaesthesia, although usually uneventful, can be associated with major morbidity. In the immediate postoperative period, patients are at risk from respiratory and cardiovascular complications, which account for approximately 70% and 20% of critical recovery room incidents respectively. The unconscious patient may develop upper airway obstruction or inadequate ventilation with subsequent hypoxaemia and hypercapnia, and is at increased risk of aspiration because of the absence of the protective airway reflexes. Ongoing blood loss and residual drug effects may compound cardiovascular compromise. The importance of observation and early intervention during this period has been recognised for many years. Hazards may be reduced by the provision of adequate postoperative recovery facilities along with fully trained staff. Guidelines for postoperative care are provided by the Royal College of Anaesthetists as part of the *Guidelines for the Provision of Anaesthetic Services*, 2014.

The recovery room

Recommendations for the situation and design of the recovery room and equipment required have been made by a working party of the Association of Anaesthetists of Great Britain and Ireland (2002).

Patient transfer from operating theatre

The design of trolleys should comply with the Association of Anaesthetists recommendations in that there is a need for oxygen cylinders, masks and tubing, airway support equipment, protective sides and a tilting mechanism. Portable monitoring equipment may be required. Transfer to the recovery room should be undertaken by suitably trained staff under the supervision of the anaesthetist, who is additionally responsible for handing over information about relevant medical conditions, the anaesthetic technique, intraoperative problems and postoperative management to the recovery staff.

Management

Until a patient can maintain his or her airway, breathing and circulation care must be provided on a one-to-one basis by a nurse trained in recovery procedures. Respiratory and cardiovascular parameters, pain severity,

Fundamentals of Anaesthesia, 4th edition, ed. Ted Lin, Tim Smith and Colin Pinnock. Published by Cambridge University Press. © Cambridge University Press 2017.

conscious level, drugs and intravenous fluids administered should be documented at appropriate intervals.

Clinical observations should be supplemented by pulse oximetry and blood pressure measurement. An ECG, peripheral nerve stimulator, temperature monitor and capnography should be immediately available.

Patient discharge

Set criteria must be met before a patient is discharged to the ward (Figure 4.1). Patients not meeting these criteria should be reviewed by an anaesthetist with a view to upgrading their level of care.

Figure 4.1 Criteria to be met before transfer from recovery room to general ward

Level of consciousness
• Fully conscious without excessive stimulation

Respiratory system	
• Upper airway	Able to maintain a clear airway Protective reflexes are present
• Respiration	Satisfactory respiratory rate (10–20 breaths min^{-1}) Satisfactory oxygenation (SpO$_2$ > 92%)

Cardiovascular system
• Haemodynamically stable
• No unexplained cardiac irregularity
• Pulse rate and blood pressure should approximate to preoperative values or be within accepted range
• No persistent bleeding
• Peripheral perfusion adequate

Pain and nausea control
• Effective pain control
• Free of nausea
• Adequate analgesic and antiemetic provisions made

Temperature
• Temperature within acceptable limits (> 36 °C)
• No evidence of developing malignant hyperthermia

Prior to discharge, recovery staff should record in the notes that the patient has met these criteria

Modified from Association of Anaesthetists of Great Britain and Ireland, 2002

Postoperative complications

Postoperative complications may be from respiratory, cardiovascular or neurological causes, and include:

- Postoperative hypoxaemia
- Hypertension
- Hypotension
- Cardiac arrhythmias
- Thromboembolism
- Hypothermia and shivering
- Failure to regain consciousness

Postoperative hypoxaemia

Hypoxaemia is defined as an oxygen saturation of less than 90%. In the postoperative period it occurs due to a combination of factors, as listed in Figure 4.2 (Mangat & Jones 1993). Prevention, early recognition and treatment are important because of the increased morbidity and mortality associated with this condition.

Clinical features

Clinical signs associated with hypoxaemia are non-specific and include central cyanosis, dyspnoea, tachycardia, arrhythmias, hyper- or hypotension and agitation. Cyanosis is a dusky, blue discoloration of the mucous membranes and skin. It is usually clinically detectable when the concentration of deoxygenated haemoglobin is greater than 5 g dL^{-1}. However, it may be absent in the hypoxaemic anaemic patient and present in the polycythaemic patient with a normal PaO$_2$, and it is therefore an unreliable indicator of hypoxaemia.

Upper airway obstruction and alveolar hypoventilation are important causes of hypoxaemia in the postoperative period.

Upper airway obstruction

> **The Fourth National Audit Project** of the Royal College of Anaesthetists and the Difficult Airway Society (NAP4) revealed that one-third of adverse events occurred during emergence or recovery, and that obstruction was the common cause. Events were twice as common in obese patients.

The causes of oropharyngeal and laryngeal obstruction are shown in Figure 4.3.

In the unconscious patient, the tongue may fall backwards and occlude the airway at the level of the oropharynx. This occurs because of a decrease in oropharyngeal

Figure 4.2 Causes of postoperative hypoxaemia

| Upper airway obstruction |
| Alveolar hypoventilation |
| Ventilation/perfusion mismatch |
| Diffusion hypoxia |
| Increased oxygen utilisation |
| Low cardiac output states |

Figure 4.3 Causes of upper airway obstruction in the postoperative period

	Oropharyngeal obstruction	Laryngeal obstruction
Common	Decreased muscle tone Secretions Sleep apnoea	Laryngospasm Secretions
Rare	Foreign body Oedema Wound haematoma Neuromuscular disease	Oedema Bilateral recurrent laryngeal nerve palsy Tracheal collapse

muscle tone, which is related to the residual effects of general anaesthesia and inadequate recovery from muscle relaxants. Patients with obstructive sleep apnoea are at particular risk in the postoperative period. Rarely, oropharyngeal obstruction results from a foreign body, e.g. failure to remove throat pack or wound haematoma after neck surgery (e.g. carotid endarterectomy, thyroidectomy, radical neck dissection). Oedema formation resulting from external compression of the venous and lymphatic drainage of the head and neck will make matters worse.

Laryngospasm is the commonest cause of laryngeal obstruction and is often associated with airway manipulation during emergence from anaesthesia, e.g. airway insertion at light levels of anaesthesia, or the presence of secretions or blood. After thyroidectomy, bilateral recurrent laryngeal nerve damage and tracheal collapse can occur, although this is rare. Laryngeal oedema secondary to prolonged or traumatic intubation can occasionally cause obstruction, although this is more likely in the paediatric than in the adult patient because of the smaller size of the airway.

Clinical features

The clinical signs of upper airway obstruction include absence of air movement, 'see-saw' motion of the chest and abdomen, and suprasternal and intercostal recession. Oxygen desaturation is a late sign. Incomplete laryngospasm typically produces stridor, an inspiratory 'crowing' noise, although this is absent if the laryngospasm is complete.

Management

Initial measures are directed at preventing the tongue from falling backwards and obstructing the airway. The unconscious patient should be recovered in the lateral position with the jaw supported. Blood and secretions should be cleared by suction and supplemental oxygen given via a face mask. If upper airway obstruction develops, a chin lift and/or jaw thrust should be used. If these measures do not rapidly clear the airway then an oropharyngeal or nasopharyngeal airway should be inserted. Care should be taken on insertion of an oral airway as this may cause laryngospasm, coughing or vomiting in the waking patient and, if in doubt, a nasal airway should be passed. If this does not immediately rectify the situation then senior help should be sought and 100% oxygen administered via a tight-fitting mask. Continuous positive airway pressure (CPAP) at this stage may help to open the airway or 'break' the laryngospasm. Deepening anaesthesia with a propofol bolus is often helpful, but in the presence of continued airway obstruction and falling oxygen saturation intravenous suxamethonium ($1–2$ mg kg^{-1}) should be given followed by manual ventilation with 100% oxygen and subsequent orotracheal intubation. In the rare event when this is not possible the failed intubation drill should be followed. Extubation of the trachea should occur when the patient has regained full muscle power and is awake. An algorithm for airway management is shown in Figure 4.4.

Upper airway obstruction secondary to wound haematoma must be immediately treated. The surgeon and an experienced anaesthetist should be called, the airway supported, 100% oxygen administered and the trachea intubated. The wound stitches should be removed and the haematoma evacuated. It is important to remember that the airway anatomy may be grossly distorted, and it may

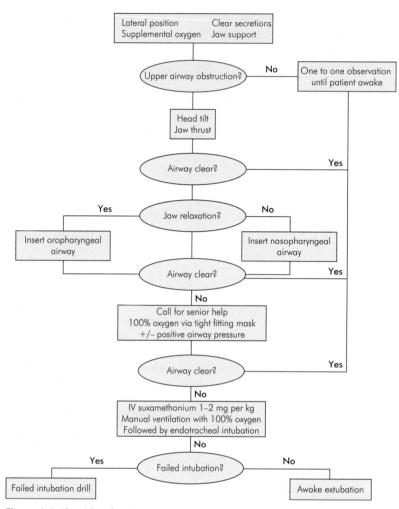

Figure 4.4 Algorithm for airway management in the unconscious patient

be impossible to intubate the trachea. In this situation, a surgical airway may be required.

Ventilation/perfusion (V̇/Q̇) mismatch

There is about a 20% reduction in functional residual capacity (FRC) after induction of anaesthesia. This may lead to airway closure in dependent parts of the lung, resulting in ventilation/perfusion (V̇/Q̇) mismatch with subsequent hypoxaemia. The very young, elderly, obese and smokers are particularly at risk, as in these groups closing capacity may equal or exceed FRC, with resultant airway closure during tidal breathing. The reduction in FRC is greatest in the supine position, and oxygen saturation may be improved by sitting the patient up, provided he or she is awake enough.

> **Causes of V̇/Q̇ mismatch** include atelectasis, bronchopneumonia, aspiration, pulmonary oedema and pneumothorax.

Atelectasis

Postoperative pulmonary collapse or atelectasis is a common cause of hypoxaemia, particularly after upper abdominal and thoracic surgery. Onset is usually within

15 minutes of induction of anaesthesia, in both spontaneously breathing and mechanically ventilated patients, and lasts up to 4 days into the postoperative period. Absorption atelectasis has been implicated in the development of postoperative pulmonary collapse. It develops when the rate of gas leaving the alveolus due to uptake into the blood exceeds the rate of inspired gas entering it. This occurs when the airway to an area of lung is closed or obstructed, usually with secretions or blood. It is also found in areas of lung with a marked reduction in $\dot{V}/\dot{Q}$ ratios. The rate of gas uptake is increased when insoluble gases such as nitrogen are replaced by soluble gases such as oxygen and nitrous oxide in an anaesthetic mixture. Effective treatment includes adequate pain control, supplemental oxygen, chest physiotherapy and promotion of deep breathing exercises and coughing.

Bronchopneumonia

Bronchopneumonia may occur after major surgery, particularly if the patient is unable to clear respiratory tract secretions because of poor cough or inability to deep breathe. Treatment follows the same pattern as for atelectasis, with the addition of appropriate antibiotic therapy.

Aspiration

There is a significant risk of aspirating gastric contents in the postoperative period, as protective airway reflexes may be absent or impaired. Patients with delayed gastric emptying (e.g. bowel obstruction, obesity, pregnancy or an incompetent gastro-oesophageal sphincter) are at increased risk. Aspiration of liquid material results in a pneumonitis of varying severity depending on the volume and acidity of the fluid. Severe pneumonitis is associated with aspiration of more than 25 mL of fluid with a pH of less than 2.5. Aspiration of solid material results in bronchial or laryngeal obstruction, and, if this is not immediately relieved, can be fatal. In the supine position, owing to the anatomy of the bronchial tree, aspiration is most likely to occur into the right lung, although, after a large aspiration, both lungs are often involved. The chance of aspiration may be reduced by recovering patients in the lateral position, and those at high risk should be extubated after full recovery of protective reflexes. The treatment of aspiration is detailed in Chapter 2.

Pulmonary oedema

This is a relatively rare cause of $\dot{V}/\dot{Q}$ mismatch in the recovery room. Causes include fluid overload or cardiac failure, and negative-pressure pulmonary oedema may occur after relief of prolonged airway obstruction.

Pneumothorax

Pneumothorax may result from direct lung or airway trauma, rib fractures, central venous cannulation, brachial plexus block, intercostal nerve and interpleural blocks and after thoracic, neck or renal surgery. A pneumothorax due to barotrauma associated with mechanical ventilation is unusual unless ventilation pressures are high. Patients with emphysematous bullae are particularly at risk.

The characteristic features are pleuritic chest pain or breathlessness, but these may not be detected if the pneumothorax is small, or may be masked by the residual effects of anaesthesia. Spontaneously breathing patients with a pneumothorax of less than 20% of the lung field may be observed and the chest x-ray repeated. Any patient with a larger pneumothorax or who is mechanically ventilated should be treated with an intercostal drain. A tension pneumothorax is associated with marked shift of the trachea and mediastinum away from the affected side, hypoxaemia, hyper-resonance to percussion and hypotension. It is a clinical diagnosis and a true medical emergency requiring immediate decompression by insertion of a chest drain at the fifth intercostal space in the anterior axillary line. A 14 gauge cannula should be inserted in the second intercostal space in the mid-clavicular line if a chest drain is not immediately available.

Diffusion hypoxia

At the end of anaesthesia nitrous oxide leaves the blood and enters the alveoli, diluting the gases already present. If the patient is breathing air, nitrogen will be absorbed into the blood at a slower rate than nitrous oxide enters the alveoli, resulting in a decrease in alveolar oxygen concentration and a potentially hypoxic gas mixture. In practice, the effect of diffusional hypoxia is transient and is simply overcome by administering supplemental oxygen for approximately 10 minutes in the immediate postoperative period.

Inadequate pulmonary ventilation

Reduced alveolar ventilation has many causes in the postoperative period (Figure 4.5). It results from a reduction in tidal volume or respiratory rate, or a combination of both, and by definition it produces a raised arterial carbon

Figure 4.5 Causes of alveolar hypoventilation in the postoperative period

Upper airway obstruction
Decreased ventilatory drive • Inhalational anaesthetics • Opioids • Benzodiazepines • Central nervous system trauma
Inadequate respiratory muscle function • Incomplete reversal of neuromuscular blockade • Neuromuscular disease • Diaphragmatic splinting (obesity, abdominal distension) • Thoracic or upper abdominal surgery • Acute or chronic lung disease

dioxide tension ($PaCO_2$). Hypoxaemia and respiratory acidosis may be associated features.

Decreased ventilatory drive

The commonest cause of central respiratory depression is the residual effect of inhalational anaesthetic agents or perioperative opioid administration. The effect of volatile anaesthetic agents is compounded, as they are predominantly excreted via the lungs.

An unconscious patient with low respiratory rate and pinpoint pupils is typical of opioid overdosage. Supportive treatment includes the administration of oxygen, maintenance of the airway and manual ventilation by mask or tracheal tube if required. Opioid-induced respiratory depression can be reversed by administration of naloxone, a competitive opioid antagonist. This agent should be given in small incremental doses of 50–100 μg intravenously in order to prevent reversal of analgesia. Tachycardia and hypertension associated with sudden development of pain increases myocardial oxygen consumption and may lead to ischaemia in susceptible patients. The onset of action of naloxone is within 1–2 minutes but the duration of action is only 20 minutes, which is shorter than that of many opioids, so a repeat dose may be required. The patient must not return to the ward until full recovery from the respiratory depressant effects of the opioid has occurred.

Benzodiazepines are often used as adjuncts to general anaesthesia. The elderly, the sick and patients with liver disease are at risk of prolonged effects from these agents. Over-sedation can be treated with flumazenil, a competitive benzodiazepine receptor antagonist. It is administered intravenously in 100 μg increments titrated against clinical response. Onset of action is within 30–60 seconds and duration of effect varies from 15 to 120 minutes.

Decreased ventilatory drive may be related to a period of intraoperative hyperventilation with a resultant marked decrease in $PaCO_2$ which may continue into the immediate postoperative phase. Neurosurgical and head-injury patients may also develop hypoventilation in the postoperative period as a direct result of central nervous system trauma.

Inadequate mechanical function of the respiratory muscles

Incomplete reversal of non-depolarising muscle blockade This is distressing and potentially dangerous to the patient. It is an important cause of both hypoventilation and upper airway obstruction. There are many factors that contribute to incomplete reversal (Figure 4.6). The use of short-acting non-depolarising muscle relaxants and neuromuscular monitoring to assess the degree of muscle blockade should help to avoid this complication.

Typically the inadequately reversed patient can initiate movements but cannot complete them, as a result of which they appear twitchy with uncoordinated actions. Adequate muscle function may be confirmed clinically if the patient can lift his or her head off the pillow for 5 seconds; strength of hand grip is also assessed, but this is more subjective. A peripheral nerve stimulator may also be used, with a train-of-four ratio of > 70%

Figure 4.6 Factors associated with prolonged neuromuscular blockade

Hypothermia	
Respiratory acidosis	
Electrolyte abnormalities	Hypokalaemia Hypocalcaemia Hyponatraemia Hypermagnesaemia
Drug interactions	Volatile agents Calcium channel blockers Aminoglycosides Diuretics
Decreased excretion	Renal failure Liver failure

and absence of fade after double burst stimulation indicating adequate recovery.

Treatment of inadequate reversal includes reassurance, along with sedation and ventilatory support if it is severe. All patients should receive supplemental oxygen, and a further dose of neostigmine 1.25–2.5 mg intravenously (maximum total dose 5 mg) may be given with the appropriate dose of anticholinergic.

Suxamethonium apnoea Recovery from the effect of suxamethonium is dependent on the enzyme plasma cholinesterase (also called butyrylcholinesterase). A prolonged neuromuscular block after suxamethonium administration is described as suxamethonium apnoea, and it can be due to both acquired and genetic factors (Davis *et al.* 1997).

Figure 4.7 Acquired causes of suxamethonium apnoea

Decreased plasma cholinesterase concentration
- Pregnancy
- Liver disease
- Chronic renal failure
- Haemodialysis
- Hypothyroidism

Decreased plasma cholinesterase activity
- Induction agents etomidate and ketamine
- Ester local anaesthetics
- Anticholinesterases

- **Acquired** (Figure 4.7) – The majority of acquired causes produce a minor prolongation of apnoea of only a few minutes. Decreased cholinesterase synthesis occurs in liver disease and to a lesser extent in pregnancy and hypothyroidism. Drugs decrease the activity of the enzyme either by competing with suxamethonium at the binding site (either reversibly or irreversibly) or by inactivating it.
- **Inherited** (Figure 4.8) – The inheritance of abnormal cholinesterase is linked to several autosomal recessive genes, which are classified by their percentage inhibition of action when exposed to different substances (for example dibucaine or fluoride).

In inherited cases, the degree of prolongation of action is related to the pattern of inheritance of the enzymes. Heterozygotes for the normal enzyme will obviously have a normal response. Two to four hours of paralysis after a 1 mg kg^{-1} dose of suxamethonium will be seen in homozygotes for the silent or atypical genes. Homozygotes for the fluoride-resistant gene will show a prolongation of effect of 1–2 hours. Most heterozygotes who have one normal and one abnormal gene will have a minor increase in duration of effect of about 20 minutes. Combinations of abnormal genes are rare, with an unpredictable result. For further details on inheritance see Chapter 32.

In cases of suxamethonium apnoea the type 1 block normally seen on using a nerve stimulator (absence of fade on train of four, no post-tetanic facilitation)

Figure 4.8 Inheritance of abnormal plasma cholinesterase

Type	Genotype		Dibucaine number	Fluoride number	Typical apnoea	Incidence
Normal	$E_1^u E_1^u$	homozygous	80	50	1–5 min	94%
Atypical	$E_1^u E_1^a$	heterozygous	60	50	10 min	1 : 25
Atypical	$E_1^a E_1^a$	homozygous	20	20	2 hours	1 : 3000
Silent	$E_1^u E_1^s$	heterozygous	80	50	10 min	1 : 25
Silent	$E_1^s E_1^s$	homozygous	minimal activity		2 hours	1 : 100,000
Fluoride-resistant	$E_1^u E_1^f$	heterozygous	75	50	10 min	1 : 300,000
Fluoride-resistant	$E_1^f E_1^f$	homozygous	65	40	2 hours	1 : 150,000

u, a, s and f are the four commonest of 25 possible gene variants for plasma cholinesterase

progresses through a transitional phase (development of tetanic fade and, later on, fade on train of four) or dual block and finally develops into a type 2 block (fade on train of four, post-tetanic facilitation).

Treatment of suxamethonium apnoea includes ongoing sedation and ventilation until there is spontaneous recovery of muscle function. Active measures such as administration of fresh frozen plasma have been used, although risk of infection and cost have limited this practice. The patient may have to be managed in the intensive care unit if recovery is prolonged.

Mivacurium apnoea The action of mivacurium is mainly terminated by plasma cholinesterase, and thus the defective forms of this enzyme will result in prolonged action of the drug. This is usually in the region of 2–4 hours from a typical dose. Other elimination pathways include liver esterase metabolism and biliary and renal excretion.

Neuromuscular disease Patients with neuromuscular disease may be particularly sensitive to the residual effects of general anaesthesia and to neuromuscular blocking agents, which, if possible, should be avoided or used at a reduced dose with monitoring of neuromuscular function.

Diaphragmatic splinting

Obese patients, those with gastric distension, and post-thoracotomy or upper abdominal surgical patients can develop diaphragmatic splinting. Good pain relief with thoracic epidural or patient-controlled analgesia, chest physiotherapy, and nasogastric tube insertion where indicated can help prevent hypoventilation in these cases.

Pre-existing lung disease

Patients with chronic obstructive pulmonary disease (COPD) are at increased risk of hypoventilation in the postoperative period. They may not be able to further increase their work of breathing to maintain an adequate $PaCO_2$, particularly if bronchospasm or excessive airway secretions are present.

Bronchospasm may occur in asthma, COPD and smokers, and in patients with acute respiratory infection. It is commonly precipitated by upper airway irritation, either during airway manipulation or if secretions are present. Other causes of wheeze include aspiration, pulmonary oedema, and bronchospasm associated with anaphylaxis. Treatment of bronchospasm will depend on the underlying cause and the severity but should include supplemental oxygen and inhaled bronchodilator therapy.

Other causes of hypoxaemia

Hypoxaemia may also occur as a result of increased oxygen consumption (e.g. shivering, pyrexia) or increased tissue oxygen extraction. These both result in a reduction in mixed venous oxygen concentration. A variable amount of mixed venous blood is shunted from the right to the left side of the heart and mixes with oxygenated blood, producing a fall in PaO_2. The extent of this fall is dependent on the mixed venous oxygen concentration and the degree of right-to-left shunt.

Hypertension

This is defined as a 20% or greater increase in preoperative systolic blood pressure, and it is often short-lived. It usually develops within 30 minutes of the end of surgery and may be precipitated by acute withdrawal of antihypertensive medication. There are multiple causes (Figure 4.9), of which pain, preoperative hypertension and blood gas abnormalities are the commonest.

Management of high blood pressure is directed at establishing and treating the underlying cause, of which pain is the most common. Other causes include hypoxia, hypercapnia and intravascular fluid overload. Further measures at this stage are determined by the degree of hypertension and associated medical or surgical factors. In general, a moderate elevation in blood pressure of 30% of the preoperative value is well tolerated.

Postoperative hypertension is usually short-lived. Agents used to treat it should therefore be short-acting, and may include the following:

- Labetalol is a β_1-adrenoceptor antagonist with some α_1-adrenoceptor antagonist activity. 5 mg bolus doses administered intravenously act within 5 minutes and last for up to an hour.
- Esmolol is a very short-acting β-adrenoceptor antagonist with a rapid onset of action. It is given as a bolus of 500 $\mu g\ kg^{-1}$ over 60 seconds followed by an infusion at a rate of 50–300 $\mu g\ kg^{-1}$ per minute depending on clinical effect. Both labetalol and esmolol are contraindicated in asthmatic patients.
- Glyceryl trinitrate, a direct-acting arterial and venous dilator, is usually used intraoperatively to control blood pressure but can be administered at a rate of 0.2–8 $\mu g\ kg^{-1}$ per minute intravenously to rapidly reduce blood pressure in the postoperative period if indicated.

Figure 4.9 Factors associated with hypertension in the immediate postoperative period

Patient factors	Agitation Preoperative hypertension Pain
Inadequate ventilation	Hypoxaemia Hypercapnia
Drug interaction	Monoamine oxidase inhibitors
Bladder distension	
Malignant hyperthermia	
Endocrine (phaeochromocytoma)	

Hypotension

Hypotension occurs frequently in the recovery room and, in the majority of cases, is transient and benign. It is usually related to the residual effects of anaesthetic and analgesic drugs (Figure 4.10).

While the causes of hypotension are many, hypovolaemia due to inadequate perioperative fluid replacement or ongoing fluid loss is the most common. Sympathetic blockade associated with spinal anaesthesia or analgesia, with a resultant fall in systemic vascular resistance (SVR), is also an important cause of hypotension in the postoperative period. The reduction in SVR related to

Figure 4.10 Causes of postoperative hypotension

Frequent causes
Hypovolaemia
 • Blood loss or third-space losses
Vasodilatation
 • Subarachnoid and extradural block
 • Residual effects of anaesthetic and analgesic agents
 • Rewarming
 • Sepsis
 • Anaphylaxis

Infrequent causes
Arrhythmias
Myocardial ischaemia / infarction
Heart failure
Tension pneumothorax
Pulmonary embolism
Pericardial tamponade
Hypothyroidism

rewarming of a hypothermic patient may also cause a decrease in blood pressure, as may rarer causes such as anaphylaxis, cardiac arrhythmias, tension pneumothorax and pulmonary embolus.

Once hypotension is evident, the cause must be sought and treatment initiated to prevent ischaemia to vital organs. The patient should be laid flat or slightly head-down and given supplemental oxygen while further assessment takes place.

The hypovolaemic patient has a tachycardia, with a low JVP, decreased urine output and poor peripheral perfusion, and there may be obvious blood loss, e.g. into drains. A rapid intravenous bolus of 250–500 mL of crystalloid or colloid should be given and the haemodynamic response assessed. Ongoing blood loss may require further surgical intervention.

Patients with marked peripheral vasodilatation can be hypotensive despite adequate volume replacement. This is commonly seen after subarachnoid or extradural anaesthesia, where administration of vasoconstrictor drugs with or without further intravenous fluid should be given. Marked vasodilatation also occurs in sepsis and anaphylaxis, where management is both supportive and aimed at treating the specific underlying abnormality.

Eighty per cent of hypotensive patients in recovery will respond to intravenous fluid therapy alone. It is potentially dangerous to use vasopressor drugs in the face of inadequate fluid replacement, as they may cause ischaemia of the visceral organs such as the liver and kidneys, but they may be useful in severe hypotension while a diagnosis is being sought, and in the presence of vasodilatation. Vasopressor agents used include the following:

 • Ephedrine, a sympathomimetic agent with α- and β-adrenoceptor agonist activity, produces peripheral vasoconstriction, and an increase in heart rate and myocardial contractility. It has a rapid onset of action when given intravenously in 3 mg boluses.
 • Metaraminol, an α-adrenoceptor agonist with some β-adrenoceptor agonist activity, can also be used in the postoperative period. It has a rapid onset of action and is given in incremental doses of 0.5 mg titrated against effect.

Cardiac arrhythmias

The majority of arrhythmias in the postoperative period are benign. They may be related to hypercapnia, hypoxaemia, electrolyte and acid–base disturbance, pain, pre-existing cardiac disease, and myocardial ischaemia or infarction.

- Sinus bradycardia (pulse < 60 beats per minute). This may be normal in the young, healthy patient, or may result from vagal stimulation, hypoxaemia or drug effects, e.g. β-adrenoceptor antagonists, neostigmine. Treatment with intravenous glycopyrrolate 0.2–0.4 mg or atropine 0.2–0.6 mg will usually increase the heart rate.

- Sinus tachycardia (pulse > 100 beats per minute). Pain, hypovolaemia, anaemia, pyrexia and an increased metabolic rate can all produce a sinus tachycardia, which is usually harmless. Treatment of the underlying cause is all that is warranted in the majority of cases. If it is associated with myocardial ischaemia, treatment with a β-blocker may be required.

- Atrial or ventricular premature contractions. No specific treatment other than correction of hypercapnia and electrolyte abnormalities is usually required.

- Non-sinus tachycardias. Hypoxaemia, hypercapnia and electrolyte imbalance should be corrected. Management of these arrhythmias depends on the degree of haemodynamic instability. Adverse signs include shock, syncope, myocardial ischaemia and heart failure. If present, synchronised DC cardioversion is indicated in the first instance. Further management and treatment of narrow or broad complex tachycardias in the absence of adverse signs is discussed in Chapter 8.

Thromboembolism

Deep venous thrombosis (DVT) and pulmonary embolus (PE) are significant causes of morbidity and mortality in the postoperative period. The incidence of DVT is difficult to assess accurately, as many cases are not clinically detected. In the postoperative period 10–80% of patients may develop DVT, depending on patient risk factors and type of surgery. The risk of subsequent PE in this group of patients is unknown, although up to 0.9% of all hospital admissions suffer fatal PE after DVT.

Deep venous thrombosis

The commonest sites for venous thrombosis are in the leg and pelvis, although any vein may be affected. The classic presentation of a painful calf which is red, swollen and warmer than the unaffected side is often not present, and many cases are asymptomatic. The investigation of choice for thrombosis is ultrasound examination.

The main aim of treatment in established venous thrombosis is to minimise the risk of subsequent PE. All patients with above-knee thrombosis must be formally anticoagulated for a period of 3 months. Treatment of below-knee thrombosis is controversial because, although a PE can occur with any DVT, it is rare in cases confined to veins situated below the knee. For this reason, observation by serial ultrasounds rather than formal anticoagulation may be carried out in this group.

Prophylaxis

Effective prevention of DVT is an important aspect of perioperative care and requires accurate identification of the at-risk patient (Figure 4.11). All surgical patients who have been identified as being at increased risk should be offered mechanical prophylaxis at admission until mobility is regained. Provided risk of bleeding is low, patients should be offered pharmacological prophylaxis according to local guidelines.

Mechanical methods available include the application of graduated compression or thromboembolic deterrent stockings and intermittent compression devices that work by preventing venous stasis. Early ambulation and leg exercises should be encouraged in the postoperative period.

Pharmacological methods include the subcutaneous administration of unfractionated and low-molecular-weight heparin (LMWH). The main advantage of LMWH is that it can be given as a once-daily dose, with a resultant improvement in patient acceptability. Oral dabigatran, a thrombin inhibitor, may also be used.

Because of the increased risk of bleeding associated with pharmacological prophylaxis, the mechanical methods are preferred in certain situations where the consequences of bleeding are severe, as in major head and neck surgery or neurosurgery.

Pulmonary embolus

This usually results from dislodgement of thrombus in the systemic veins or, rarely, from the right atrium (atrial fibrillation may promote thrombus formation) or right ventricle (postseptal/right ventricular infarction). It has a mortality of approximately 10%.

Clinical features depend on the size of the PE. A small embolus may present with exertional dyspnoea and

Figure 4.11 Thromboembolism risk assessment

Age	Risk rises exponentially with increasing age	< 40 $60–69$ > 80
Obesity		$BMI > 30 \ kg \ m^{-2}$
Varicose veins with phlebitis		
Family history of thromboembolism	First-degree relative	If relative < 50 years Or more than one first-degree relative
Thrombophilias		
Oral contraceptive medication and hormone replacement therapy (HRT)	Third-generation progestogens Oestrogens	
Pregnancy	Even higher during puerperium	
Immobility	Bed rest > 3 days Plaster cast Paralysis	
Chronic conditions	Malignancy Heart failure Inflammatory bowel disease Sickle cell disease or trait	
Surgery	Acute surgical admission	If inflammatory or intra-abdominal condition
	Critical care admission	
	Prolonged procedure (including anaesthetic time)	> 90 minutes > 60 minutes (pelvis or lower limb)
General anaesthesia $>$ epidural or spinal		
Male $>$ female		

National Institute for Health and Care Excellence. *Venous Thromboembolism: Reducing the Risk for Patients in Hospital.* NICE Guideline CG92, 2010. Scottish Intercollegiate Guidelines Network. *Prevention and Management of Venous Thromboembolism.* SIGN Publication 122, 2015.

lassitude, a moderate-sized embolus with pleuritic chest pain of sudden onset, haemoptysis and dyspnoea, and a massive embolus with severe chest pain, tachycardia, tachypnoea and syncope. Physical signs may be absent after a small PE. Larger infarcts may produce a tachycardia, gallop rhythm, right ventricular heave and a prominent 'a' wave in the jugular venous wave form. A pleural rub may be present, and signs and symptoms of DVT must be sought.

The investigation of choice is a ventilation/perfusion scan, looking for ventilated but non-perfused areas of lung. The ECG usually only shows a sinus tachycardia, although right ventricular hypertrophy, right axis deviation and right bundle branch block may be present after large emboli. The classical S wave in lead I, Q wave and inverted T wave in lead III are usually absent. The chest x-ray is also often normal. Arterial blood gas sampling usually shows hypoxaemia and hypocapnia.

Anticoagulant therapy should be initiated, after confirmation of the diagnosis, to prevent further embolisation. In cases where a delay in ventilation/perfusion scan is expected, anticoagulation should be started on clinical suspicion alone. The duration of anticoagulation depends on the risk of further venous emboli, with treatment continuing for up to 6 months. Thrombolysis with streptokinase is occasionally used after large emboli.

Hypothermia and shivering

Post-anaesthetic shivering occurs in about 1 in 4 patients (Read & White 2013). Post-anaesthetic shivering is a consequence of the body temperature being below a threshold, which in turn may be altered by anaesthetic and other drugs. Risk factors are shown in Figure 4.12. The consequences of shivering include marked increases in minute ventilation and cardiac output secondary to greater oxygen demand and carbon dioxide production. This may have a detrimental effect particularly in the patient with cardiorespiratory disease. Shivering can also interfere with postoperative haemodynamic and oxygen saturation monitoring.

The key element in most cases is the loss of body heat by peripheral vasodilatation, limited insulation from the cool operating-theatre environment and inhalation of cold gases. This is compounded by a reduction in the basal metabolic rate which is accentuated by the use of non-depolarising muscle relaxants. Anaesthesia and sedation also reset the body's thermoregulation lower.

The incidence of post-anaesthetic shivering is increased in hypothermic patients, but not all patients who shiver are hypothermic. Methods to prevent a fall in core temperature, such as raising ambient temperature in the operating theatre, warming intravenous fluids and using forced warm air blankets in the intra- and postoperative period, should be used in the at-risk patient as per NICE Clinical Guideline 65 (2008).

Treatment includes oxygen administration to prevent hypoxia, active warming and the use of specific drugs. Pethidine at a minimum dose of 0.35 mg kg^{-1} is the most effective opioid in the treatment of post-anaesthetic shivering, with a 95% success rate. Fentanyl and alfentanil have some effect, although this is less marked and shorter in duration than with pethidine. Doxapram, an agent usually used as a respiratory stimulant, is also effective at a dose of 0.2 mg kg^{-1}.

Figure 4.12 Risk factors for postoperative shivering

| Hypothermia |
| Male gender |
| Anticholinergic premedication |
| Prolonged anaesthesia |
| General as opposed to regional anaesthesia |
| Spontaneous as opposed to mechanical ventilation |
| Use of thiopental versus propofol |

Failure to regain consciousness and confusion

In most instances, failure to regain consciousness or postoperative confusion may be attributed to residual drug effects. Other causes include endocrine abnormalities such as hypoglycaemia or hypothyroidism, cerebral events including cerebrovascular accident or cerebral hypoxia, or existing physiological derangements such as hypothermia, hypoxia, hypercapnia or hypotension (Figure 4.13).

Residual drug effects may be reversed with specific antagonists if unconsciousness is particularly prolonged. These may include naloxone for opioids and flumazenil for benzodiazepines. Diabetic patients should have their blood sugar levels checked both intra- and postoperatively. Postoperative confusion is more common in elderly patients and after prolonged surgery.

If an acute confusional state is present, exclude treatable causes by appropriate history taking, physical examination and investigations. When no treatable cause is

Figure 4.13 Causes of postoperative confusion

| Sepsis |
| Drugs |
| Hypoxaemia |
| Hypoglycaemia |
| Hypercarbia |
| Biochemical abnormality, e.g. hyponatraemia |
| Urinary retention |
| Acute neurological event |
| Alcohol/nicotine/drug withdrawal |

found, management is supportive and recovery usually occurs as residual drug effects wear off and full consciousness is regained.

Oxygen therapy

Indications

Supplemental oxygen should be administered in the recovery area until the patient is fully conscious.

The indications for oxygen therapy to continue after emergence from anaesthesia are listed in Figure 4.14 (Leach & Bateman 1993). Any patient who is at risk of developing tissue hypoxia or is already hypoxaemic should be given supplemental oxygen. Research has shown that additional clinical benefits of oxygen therapy include improved wound healing, reduced nausea and vomiting and reduced hospital length of stay.

Techniques of administration

Delivery systems used in the postoperative period are listed in Figure 4.15. They may be subdivided into variable or fixed performance devices.

Variable-performance devices are so called because the inspired oxygen concentration (F_IO_2) and degree of rebreathing vary from patient to patient and during the respiratory cycle in the same patient. This depends on the respiratory rate, inspiratory flow rate and length of

Figure 4.14 Indications for oxygen therapy in the postoperative period

Patient factors
- Cardiorespiratory disease
- Obesity
- Elderly
- Shivering

Surgical factors
- Upper abdominal procedures
- Thoracic surgery

Physiological factors
- Hypovolaemia
- Hypotension
- Anaemia

Postoperative analgesic technique
- Patient-controlled analgesia
- IV opioid infusion
- Epidural infusion (both local anaesthetic agents and opioids)

expiratory pause. This type of device is most commonly used, as an accurate F_IO_2 is not required in the majority of patients. The Hudson mask is a clear plastic face mask that is placed over the nose and mouth and, at a flow rate of 4 litres per minute, provides an F_IO_2 of approximately 0.4. Addition of a reservoir bag to these masks increases the maximum obtainable F_IO_2 to approximately 98%. Patient compliance is poor due to a claustrophobic feeling and the need to remove it during eating and drinking and for routine mouth care. Nasal cannulae provide an alternative, and a flow rate of 2–4 litres per minute with these devices provides an FiO_2 comparable with the face mask.

The fixed-performance devices provide an accurate F_IO_2 and avoid rebreathing. They may be further subdivided into high airflow oxygen enrichment (HAFOE) devices, e.g. Venturi masks, or lower-flow devices such as anaesthetic breathing systems. Venturi masks use injectors of different sizes to deliver set oxygen concentrations varying from 24% to 60% by entraining air in oxygen using the Venturi principle. The appropriate oxygen flow rate for each mask is printed on the colour-coded injector. Patients who require these masks include those at risk of respiratory failure if given high oxygen concentrations, i.e. those who are reliant on a hypoxic drive for ventilation.

In patients who are taken to recovery with a laryngeal mask in situ, supplemental oxygen may be provided by a T-piece connected to it as an alternative to a Mapleson C. This may be run simply as an open-ended tube or as a fixed-performance device.

The use of anaesthetic breathing systems is reserved for the immediate postoperative period, when 100% oxygen may need to be delivered via a tight-fitting mask, for example when there is airway obstruction or laryngeal spasm.

Figure 4.15 Oxygen delivery systems in the postoperative period

Variable performance
- Hudson mask
- MC mask
- Nasal cannulae
- Nasal catheter (nasopharyngeal catheter)

Fixed performance
- Venturi masks
- Anaesthetic breathing circuits

Humidification

Humidification is only required when oxygen is delivered at high flow rates or when the upper airway humidification processes are bypassed, as occurs after tracheostomy or during prolonged tracheal intubation. It is therefore rarely required in the recovery room.

Duration

There is no consensus on how long supplemental oxygen therapy should be given. However, the incidence of hypoxaemia is greatest on the second or third postoperative night after major surgery, and the PaO_2 may not return to pre-operative levels until the fifth night. Supplemental oxygen should therefore be given, where indicated, for at least 3 days postoperatively.

Complications

Supplemental oxygen administration is a safe technique. However, problems such as barotrauma and interference with hypoxic drive in certain patients may occur when inappropriate methods are used.

Barotrauma

Barotauma occurs when oxygen is directly delivered to the lower airway without free outflow of any excess gas. A variable-performance face mask should not be placed over the open end of a tracheal tube or laryngeal mask, as there have been reports of the oxygen inlet part of the face mask impacting on the male connector of the tracheal tube. This resulted in delivery of oxygen at a flow rate of 4 litres per minute and a pressure of 400 kPa, with fatal consequences. The use of a T-piece system or Mapleson C circuit is recommended.

Loss of hypoxic ventilatory drive

Approximately 10% of patients with chronic respiratory failure depend on hypoxic ventilatory drive to maintain an adequate $PaCO_2$. In this group of patients administration of a high F_IO_2 will cause hypoventilation, with subsequent CO_2 retention and respiratory acidosis. However, the fear of causing CO_2 retention must not prevent the provision of appropriate oxygen therapy, as patients in this group do not commonly present for surgery.

Postoperative analgesia

The provision of effective pain relief during the postoperative period is dependent on anaesthetic technique, type and extent of surgery, and patient factors such as age

Figure 4.16 Adverse effects of postoperative pain

Cardiovascular
- Tachycardia
- Hypertension
- Increased myocardial oxygen demand

Respiratory
- Decreased vital capacity
- Decreased functional residual capacity
- Decreased tidal volume
- Chest infections
- Basal atelectasis

Gastrointestinal
- Nausea and vomiting
- Ileus

Other effects
- Urinary retention
- Deep venous thrombosis
- Pulmonary embolus

and personality. In practice, a combination of opioids, non-steroidal anti-inflammatory drugs (NSAIDs) and local anaesthetic techniques is often used.

Good pain control not only alleviates patient distress but also prevents or modifies many adverse effects (Figure 4.16). The increase in sympathetic activity associated with pain results in tachycardia, hypertension and increased myocardial oxygen demand, which, in patients with cardiac disease, may produce myocardial ischaemia. Postoperative chest infection and basal atelectasis are more frequent in the patient who is unable to deep breathe or cough, such as after upper abdominal or thoracic surgery. Patient immobility associated with poor pain control increases the risk of thromboembolic disease.

Treatment of pain

The 'analgesic ladder' is a widely used concept in postoperative pain management. It was originally designed by the World Health Organization (WHO) for the management of cancer pain but the principles have been widely adopted for the management of surgical pain. The ladder shown in Figure 4.17 is one such example.

Opioids

Opioids may be given via the following routes: intramuscular, subcutaneous, intravenous, oral, intrathecal or extradural.

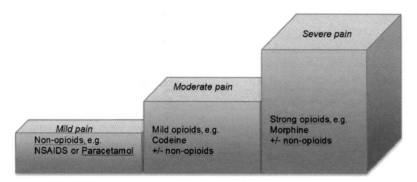

Figure 4.17 The analgesic ladder

The dose of opioid required in the postoperative period shows marked inter-patient variability. This is due to both pharmacokinetic and pharmacodynamic factors with up to a fivefold difference in plasma concentrations after identical doses of intramuscular opioid. There are also differences in opioid receptor sensitivity between patients.

On-demand intramuscular opioid often fails to provide adequate pain relief, as delays in administration, lack of patient awareness of availability and time taken for onset of action result in plasma levels falling below that required to produce analgesia. Usual dosage is 10–15 mg every 2–4 hours. There may be slow absorption in patients with poor peripheral perfusion. Subcutaneous opioid administration via indwelling cannulae is associated with similar limitations but avoids repeated needle insertion.

Intravenous opioids

Intravenous administration of opioid is generally more effective. A bolus dose can be followed by increments every few minutes until acceptable pain control is reached. This technique minimises the risk of serious side effects but is labour-intensive and is only suitable in the recovery room or high dependency unit.

Continuous intravenous administration via an infusion will ensure maintenance of adequate plasma levels but may be associated with over-sedation and respiratory depression mandating observation of the patient in a high dependency unit.

Patient-controlled analgesia (PCA) was developed to further improve opioid analgesia by accounting for the variation in opioid requirement from patient to patient and the reduction in opioid required with time. The theoretical advantage of this technique is that the patient should maintain a plasma concentration at around the minimum effective analgesic level, with resultant good pain control and reduced side effects. It is safer than intravenous infusion techniques, as the associated sedation when the patient is pain-free results in reduced usage. In practice, patients may not alleviate their pain completely with this technique because of worries about addiction and side effects. The success of PCA is dependent on patient education during the preoperative visit, adequate pain control in the recovery room and regular review by nursing and anaesthetic staff. Morphine is the most commonly used opioid, although other drugs such as alfentanil and pethidine have been used with good effect. A demand dose of morphine 1 mg is used with a lock-out period of 5 minutes. The demand dose should be large enough to provide an analgesic effect but small enough to prevent unwanted side effects, and may have to be altered depending on the clinical effect. The lock-out period must be long enough to prevent repeat administration before the initial bolus has had a maximal effect. A maximum dose per hour can also be set to prevent inadvertent overdose, although, given the large variation in opioid requirements between patients, this may prevent some patients from attaining adequate pain relief. Figure 4.18 summarises the safety requirements for PCA use.

The main side effects associated with parenteral opioid administration are nausea and vomiting, and respiratory depression. The incidence of severe respiratory depression during PCA is approximately 0.5%, which compares favourably with the intramuscular route. The risk of this is increased in patients receiving other sedative drugs. Elderly patients and those with pre-existing sleep apnoea also have an increased risk of respiratory depression.

Figure 4.18 Safety requirements for PCA use

Equipment	Lockable pump labelled for 'patient use only' Dedicated cannula or one-way valve on Y-connector Alarms to detect faults and overdose
Prescription	Standard prescription Prefilled syringe or bag Avoid concomitant use of opioids Oxygen and naloxone easily available
Monitoring	Trained staff to monitor patient and equipment Record pain score, respiratory rate, sedation score and vital signs according to local guidelines
Education	Patient instruction preoperatively Relatives and staff informed of risks of PCA by proxy

Oral opioids

Patients who are able to tolerate oral intake may benefit from opioids given by this route. It is a particularly useful technique in children as it avoids needle or cannula insertion. A dose of morphine 0.2 mg kg^{-1} is adequate in most instances. First-pass metabolism results in lower plasma concentrations after oral than after parenteral administration of the same dose.

Spinal opioids

Opioid administration via the intrathecal or extradural route can provide excellent postoperative pain control. The commonest side effects associated with this technique are nausea, pruritus, sedation and urinary retention. Respiratory depression is an infrequent complication, but it can occur up to 24 hours after administration of intrathecal opioids. Patients receiving extradural opioids are at a lower risk of developing respiratory depression, but they must also be managed on a ward where this potentially fatal complication can be recognised and treated.

The conscious level of the patient is as important as the respiratory rate, if not more so. A patient with a decreased conscious level, with or without a low respiratory rate, requires immediate treatment. Intravenous naloxone given in titrated doses is effective at reversing the opioid-induced respiratory depression without reducing the analgesic effect.

Non-steroidal anti-inflammatory drugs (NSAIDs)

This group of drugs has both analgesic and anti-inflammatory properties. They are effective for treatment of mild to moderate postoperative pain and, after the first 24–36 hours, may be used as the sole analgesic in major surgical patients. NSAIDs also have an opioid-sparing effect, with a reduction of opioid requirement after major surgery of > 20% when given regularly.

NSAIDs have several advantages over opioid analgesics. Their use is not associated with respiratory depression or gastric stasis, and as they are not controlled drugs they are readily available. However, their use is associated with potentially serious side effects, which include gastrointestinal haemorrhage, gastric ulceration, renal impairment and an increased risk of postoperative bleeding due to impairment of platelet function. NSAIDs are contraindicated in patients with a history of peptic ulcer disease, gastrointestinal bleeding, renal impairment, previous hypersensitivity reactions to aspirin or NSAIDs, asthma, and bleeding diathesis. They should be avoided in the dehydrated or hypovolaemic patient, and care should be taken when using NSAIDs in the elderly.

The salicylates are absolutely contraindicated in children under 12 years of age. Reye's syndrome, an acute encephalopathy with fatty infiltration of the liver, is associated with administration of these drugs in this age group.

Local anaesthetics

Local infiltration, peripheral nerve blocks and epidural analgesia are often used to produce postoperative pain relief, both alone and in conjunction with other analgesic methods.

The advantage of local anaesthetic techniques is that profound analgesia can be produced without respiratory depression or nausea and vomiting. However, local anaesthetic toxicity may occur as a result of inadvertent intravenous administration or after large doses. In addition, although rare, peripheral nerve damage, haemorrhage, infection, accidental arterial or subarachnoid injection and pneumothorax can all occur, depending on the site of the block.

Pain assessment

Pain, by definition, is a subjective sensation and is difficult for an observer to accurately assess. The provision of a reliable and valid means of assessing pain is important because it allows the degree of improvement, after an analgesic intervention, to be documented in a reproducible way.

There are a number of specific pain assessment scales that are used in the postoperative setting to ensure that a history of the patient's pain is recorded in a useful form so as to inform treatment decisions. These include:

- **Verbal rating scale (VRS).** This scale is simple and easy to use. The patient is asked to rate the pain as 'none', 'mild', 'moderate', or 'severe' when at rest and on movement.
- **Numerical rating scale (NRS).** This consists of a numerical scale representing the pain from 0 = 'no pain' to 10 (or 5) = 'the worst pain imaginable'.
- **Visual analogue scale (VAS).** The VAS consists of a 10 cm long line which represents a spectrum of pain intensity from 'no pain at all' on the extreme left through to 'the worst pain imaginable' on the extreme right. The patient is asked to mark the point on this line that corresponds to the severity of the pain. The VAS is primarily a research tool and, performed correctly, is arguably too complex for routine postoperative use. There is no obvious advantage of the more detailed methods in terms of practical patient management.

In very young children, physiological and behavioural indicators are used. Older children may choose from ranked facial expressions on a chart.

Acute pain service

The importance of effective postoperative pain relief, and the increased complexity of analgesic techniques such as PCA and continuous epidural infusions, has resulted in the formation of acute pain services in many hospitals. They provide a multidisciplinary approach to postoperative pain control with the involvement of anaesthetists, specialist nurses and clinical pharmacists. An acute pain service carries out regular patient assessment and provides backup for ward staff. It is also involved in 'in-house' training of medical and nursing staff to improve understanding of analgesic methods and pain assessment.

Postoperative nausea and vomiting

Postoperative nausea and vomiting (PONV) is one of the commonest complications in the postoperative period despite the use of modern-day anaesthetic techniques. It occurs in 20–40% of cases, resulting in patient discomfort and anxiety, and can produce significant morbidity in some cases. Sudden increases in intraocular and intracranial pressure associated with vomiting may be detrimental in the ophthalmic and neurosurgical patient. Fluid and electrolyte disturbances can occur if the period of vomiting is prolonged.

PONV exhibits a multifactorial aetiology and is influenced by patient, anaesthetic and surgical factors (Figure 4.19).

Females are 2.5 times more likely to develop PONV than males. The incidence also varies with age, with the lowest incidence found in infants aged less than 12 months and a peak in the 6- to 16-year-old age group, followed by a slight decrease during adult life. Increased BMI has not

Figure 4.19 Risk factors associated with PONV

Patient factors	
Female gender	
Young age	
Anxiety	
History of motion sickness	
Previous PONV	
Delayed gastric emptying	
Obesity	
Anaesthetic factors	
Drugs	Opioids
	Intravenous induction agents
	Nitrous oxide
	Neostigmine
Technique	Gastric insufflation
	Subarachnoid block
Surgical factors	
Emergency procedure	
Day-case surgery	
ENT surgery	
Strabismus correction	
Gynaecological procedures	
Gastrointestinal surgery	
Postoperative pain	
Ileus, gastric distension	

Figure 4.20 Risk management of PONV

Factor	Score
Female gender	1
Non-smoker	1
History of motion sickness or PONV	1
Use of postoperative opioids	1
Risk score 0–1	No routine prophylaxis
Risk score 2	Antiemetic prophylaxis offered, e.g. dexamethasone and 5-HT$_3$ antagonist
Risk score 3–4	Antiemetic prophylaxis offered as for risk score 2 PLUS Avoidance of volatiles and nitrous oxide, e.g. TIVA

been ratified as an independent risk factor for PONV in recent studies.

Intravenous induction agents are incriminated to varying degrees. Propofol is associated with less PONV than thiopental and may have specific antiemetic properties. Nitrous oxide is thought to be associated with PONV, possibly as a result of gut distension and raised pressure in the middle ear. Neuromuscular blocking agents are not implicated, but reversal with neostigmine has been shown to increase emesis. This is despite concurrent administration of atropine, which has antiemetic properties. The development of hypotension after spinal anaesthesia is associated with almost twice the incidence of PONV when compared with those patients where hypotension did not occur.

Prevention
Treatment of PONV is difficult, owing to its multifactorial aetiology. Risk stratification associated with appropriate therapy is the mainstay of management (Figure 4.20). The risk of PONV is 10%, 21%, 39%, 60% and 78% with 0, 1, 2, 3 and 4 risk factors respectively. Use of a single antiemetic reduces the risk by 30%, and this can be increased to 50% if two agents are used.

Treatment
Vomiting in a semiconscious patient requires immediate action. The patient should be placed in the lateral position, the pharynx cleared of any secretions and supplemental oxygen administered.

The conscious patient should be reassured and supplemental oxygen administered, although this will only have a placebo effect unless hypoxaemia is the cause. Other underlying causes such as hypercapnia, hypotension or pain should be treated. The majority of patients, however, will require a rescue antiemetic.

There are several classes of drugs used for the treatment of PONV:
- D_2 – dopaminergic antagonists
- $5\text{-}HT_3$ – serotonergic antagonists
- H_1 – histaminergic antagonists
- M_3 – muscarinic antagonists

When prophylaxis has failed a repeat dose of the drug should not be used as rescue therapy. In patients who have not received prophylaxis, treatment with a $5\text{-}HT_3$ antagonist (25% of the prophylactic dose) may be considered. There is no evidence to support the use of one rescue antiemetic over another. Selection is guided by ease of administration, cost and incidence of side effects.

Patients admitted for day-case surgery should be given instructions for its management. Those patients at high risk of developing PONV should be given rescue treatment to take home.

Postoperative fluid therapy
The aims of postoperative fluid therapy are to maintain adequate hydration, blood volume, renal function and electrolyte balance. It is indicated in patients with preoperative fluid abnormalities or ongoing fluid losses, and also in any patient undergoing a major surgical procedure.

Physiology
Total body water (TBW) for a 70 kg adult approximates to 42 L and accounts for 50–70% of body weight depending on age, sex, body habitus and fat content. TBW is distributed between three fluid compartments (see Chapter 11, Figure 11.1): the intravascular component of extracellular fluid (plasma) (8% TBW), the interstitial space (25% TBW) and the intracellular space (65% TBW). The intravascular and interstitial space together form the extracellular fluid (ECF) compartment and are separated by the endothelial cells of the capillary wall,

Figure 4.21 Causes of postoperative fluid loss in the surgical patient

Insensible losses
- Sweating
- Respiration
- Faeces
- Urine output

'Third space' losses
- Haemorrhage
- Drains
- Nasogastric
- Vomiting
- Diarrhoea

Figure 4.22 Factors influencing prescription of intravenous fluids

Fluid status – review of patient and documentation

Nature of fluid deficit if present

Type of fluid which will best treat the deficit or maintain euvolaemia

Appropriate rate of administration

Proposed clinical end point to determine volume required

Continued monitoring of fluid and electrolyte status

which are normally freely permeable to water and small ions, but not to proteins. The intracellular fluid (ICF) compartment is separated from the ECF by the cell membrane, which is selectively permeable to ions.

Surgical incision produces a neurohumoral or 'stress' response, with increasing levels of circulating catecholamines, vasopressin, aldosterone and cortisol and resultant sodium and water retention.

Postoperative fluid loss

There are many causes of fluid loss in the surgical patient (Figure 4.21). Insensible losses from the skin and lungs are approximately 0.5 mL kg^{-1} per hour. This figure increases by 12% for each degree rise in body temperature above 37 °C. 'Third space' loss is fluid lost into transcellular fluid spaces such as the bowel lumen, peritoneal and pleural cavities. It is associated with the inflammatory response to burns, trauma and surgery and varies from 1 to 15 mL kg^{-1} per hour.

Clinical assessment

Regular clinical evaluation to detect any fluid deficit should be carried out in the postoperative period. Urine output should be interpreted in the light of capillary refill time, jugulovenous pressure, trends in heart rate and blood pressure and core/peripheral temperature gradients. Trends in haemodynamic parameters are more significant than isolated measurements and can guide further fluid management. Stroke volume analysis, central venous pressure and cardiac output monitoring may be indicated in some cases.

Fluid replacement

It is difficult to predict fluid requirements in the postoperative period, particularly after major surgery. Emphasis must be placed on repeated clinical assessment. Patients undergoing minor surgery who will start drinking within a few hours of the procedure do not usually require additional intravenous fluids.

The choice of fluid replacement depends on a number of factors (Figures 4.22, 4.23). Crystalloids, which are solutions of electrolytes and sugars in water, are distributed throughout the three fluid compartments depending on their sodium concentration. Isotonic fluids such as 0.9% saline remain predominantly within the ECF compartment, whereas hypotonic solutions such as 5% dextrose are distributed throughout the ECF and ICF. Colloids, which are solutions of high-molecular-weight proteins (blood and blood products), gelatins, starches or dextrans, are mainly confined to the intravascular compartment (Figure 4.23).

Potassium should be added to maintenance fluids after the first postoperative day at 1 mmol kg^{-1} per day. Estimated 'third space' loss is replaced with a balanced salt solution such as Hartmann's solution. Blood loss is replaced with colloid on a one-to-one basis and, if the loss exceeds approximately 15% of the patient's blood volume, packed red blood cells to maintain the haemoglobin concentration at about 10 g dL^{-1}. Normal saline or Hartmann's solution can also be used to maintain intravascular volume, although a volume three times the estimated blood loss has to be infused.

A return to oral fluid administration should take place as soon as is possible once the patient is euvolaemic and haemodynamically stable.

Figure 4.23 Fluid therapy guidelines

Fluid	Indication	Associated risks
Ringer's lactate / Hartmann's solution	Crystalloid resuscitation or maintenance unless hypochloraemic For intravascular replacement use ratio of 3:1	Hypochloraemia Oedema
NaCl 0.9%	Crystalloid resuscitation or maintenance in presence of hypochloraemia, e.g. vomiting or excessive gastric drainage For intravascular replacement use ratio of 3:1	Hyperchloraemic acidosis Worsening of salt retention and oedema
4% dextrose / 0.18% saline or 5% dextrose	Water loss, e.g. diabetes insipidus	Hyponatraemia, especially in the elderly
Colloids, e.g. gelatins, starches	Blood loss < 15% of total blood volume	Allergic reaction Acute kidney injury with starch use, especially in sepsis
Blood	Blood loss >15% of total blood volume	Transmission of infection Allergic responses Promotion of antibody formation

Sequelae of anaesthesia

Complications occurring after surgery result from a combination of patient, surgical and anaesthetic factors. Morbidity directly attributable to anaesthetic practice is often relatively minor, e.g. postoperative sore throat, but can result in permanent disability, e.g. hypoxic brain damage. Increasing numbers of medico-legal claims are made against anaesthetists each year, which highlights the virtues of diligence, accurate record keeping, attention to detail and continued observation throughout the administration of anaesthesia and into the postoperative period.

The sequelae of anaesthesia are related to anaesthetic technique and patient positioning.

Eye trauma

Corneal abrasions can occur if the eyelids remain open during anaesthesia and the cornea is allowed to dry out. This is easily preventable by applying adhesive tape, which should be removed with care, to ensure that the eyelids remain closed. Corneal abrasion may also occur if the eye comes into direct contact with equipment such as catheter mounts or anaesthetic masks. Retinal ischaemia has been reported after prolonged eyeball compression, with resultant transient blindness. Eye pads should be used in addition if the prone or lateral position is adopted.

Airway trauma

Instrumentation of the oropharynx with a laryngoscope blade, a laryngeal mask or an oral airway can result in lip, tongue and gum abrasions.

Broken teeth and damaged dental work not only put the patient at risk of aspiration but are also a cause of significant inconvenience after recovery. For this reason, dental damage is a major cause of litigation. Poor dentition, loose teeth and the presence of caps, crowns and bridges should be documented at the preoperative visit. Methods employed to decrease the risk of dental trauma include the use of nasal airways, mouth guards and fibreoptic intubation.

Up to 50% of patients complain of postoperative sore throat. This may be related to tracheal intubation, although it is often associated with airway or laryngeal mask insertion, nasogastric tube placement and administration of dry gases.

Musculoskeletal trauma

Muscle pains can occur in the postoperative period and are usually related to suxamethonium administration. Suxamethonium pains are more common in the young ambulant patient with large muscle bulk. During pregnancy and childhood the muscle pains are less intense. The onset is typically delayed by 24 hours and may mimic influenza-like symptoms. Patients should be informed of the possibility of this complication.

Backache and neck pain can occur from poor patient positioning and as a result of stretched ligaments and relaxed skeletal muscle. Arms and legs can slip off operating tables or trolleys, if inadequately secured, with the potential for ligament and bony injuries.

Nerve injuries not related to regional anaesthesia have been extensively reported, and are a result of direct compression or stretching of the nerve. Correct patient positioning and extensive padding of exposed sites are mandatory. The brachial plexus can be damaged if there is excessive abduction of the arm ($> 90°$) with the humeral head impinging on the axillary neurovascular bundle. The radial nerve, as it runs down the lateral border of the arm 3–5 cm above the lateral epicondyle, is at risk of being damaged by a blood pressure cuff. The ulnar nerve is exposed at the elbow and can be damaged by direct trauma or the blood pressure cuff. The common peroneal nerve can be damaged, when the patient is placed in the lithotomy position, as it passes laterally around the neck of the fibula, resulting in foot drop and loss of sensation on the dorsum of the foot. The saphenous nerve is also at risk in the lithotomy position when there is compression of the medial aspect of the leg against the leg support, and this results in loss of sensation along the medial aspect of the calf. Facial and supraorbital nerve palsies due to direct nerve compression have also been reported.

Skin damage

Bruising and skin breakdown over pressure areas can occur after prolonged procedures and in the elderly. The occiput, elbows and heels should be padded and the undersheet smoothed out. Skin contact with metal must be prevented because of the risk of electrical burns if diathermy is used. Excessively frequent blood pressure cuff inflation is associated with localised bruising and should be avoided. In the postoperative period, patients with residual local anaesthetic blocks or epidural analgesia are at increased risk of skin breakdown due to immobility and loss of sensation.

Medico-legal issues

If a verbal or written complaint is received from a patient, a copy of all the relevant clinical information should be made. A senior member of the anaesthetic department should be informed and, if in any doubt, advice should be sought from the relevant medical defence institution. Under no account must any documented information be altered. The importance of completing an accurate and legible documentation for every patient undergoing anaesthesia cannot be stressed enough.

References and further reading

Association of Anaesthetists of Great Britain and Ireland. *Immediate Postanaesthetic Recovery*. London: AAGBI, 2002.

Carlisle JB, Stevenson CA. Drugs for preventing postoperative nausea and vomiting. *Cochrane Database Syst Rev* 2006; (3): CD004125.

Cook TM, Woodall N, Frerk C; Fourth National Audit Project. Major complications of airway management in the UK: results of the Fourth National Audit Project of the Royal College of Anaesthetists and the Difficult Airway Society. *Br J Anaesth* 2011; **106**: 617–42.

Crossley AW. Postoperative shivering. *Br J Hosp Med* 1993; **49**: 204–8.

Davis L, Britten JJ, Morgan M. Cholinesterase: its significance in anaesthetic practice. *Anaesthesia* 1997; **52**: 244–60.

Leach RM, Bateman NT. Acute oxygen therapy. *Br J Hosp Med* 1993; **49**: 637–44.

Mangat PS, Jones JG. Perioperative hypoxaemia. In Kaufman L, ed., *Anaesthesia Review* 10. Edinburgh: Churchill Livingstone, 1993, pp. 83–106.

Macintyre PE, Schug SA, Scott DA, Visser EJ, Walker SM; APM: SE Working Group of the Australian and New Zealand College of Anaesthetists and Faculty of Pain Medicine. *Acute Pain Management: Scientific Evidence*, 3rd edn. Melbourne: ANZCA & FPM, 2010.

National Institute for Health and Care Excellence. *Hypothermia: Prevention and Management in Adults Having Surgery*. NICE Guideline CG65. London: NICE, 2010. www.nice.org.uk/cg65.

National Institute for Health and Care Excellence. *Venous Thromboembolism: Reducing the Risk for Patients in Hospital*. NICE Guideline CG92. London: NICE, 2010. www.nice.org.uk/cg92.

Powell-Tuck J, Gosling P, Lobo DN, *et al. British Consensus Guidelines on Intravenous Fluid Therapy for Adult Surgical Patients (GIFTASUP)*. 2008. www.bapen.org.uk/pdfs/bapen_pubs/giftasup.pdf.

Read E, White LA. Risks associated with your anaesthetic. Section 3: shivering. London: Royal College of Anaesthetists, 2013. www.rcoa.ac.uk/system/files/PI-RISK-SERIES-2013_2.pdf.

Resuscitation Council (UK). *Resuscitation Guidelines*. London: Resuscitation Council, 2015. www.resus.org.uk/resuscitation-guidelines.

Royal College of Anaesthetists. Guidance on the provision of anaesthesia services for post-operative care. *Guidelines for the Provision of Anaesthetic Services*, Chapter 4. London: RCoA, 2014. www.rcoa.ac.uk/system/files/GPAS-2014-04-POSTOP_0.pdf.

Royal College of Surgeons of England and the College of Anaesthetists. *Pain after Surgery*. Report of a Working Party of the Commission on the Provision of Surgical Services (Chairman AA Spence), 1990.

Scottish Intercollegiate Guidelines Network. *Prevention and Management of Venous Thromboembolism: a National Clinical Guideline*. SIGN Publication 122. Edinburgh: SIGN, 2010, updated 2015.

CHAPTER 5

Special patient circumstances

Colin Pinnock, Robert Haden and Dan Bailey

The pregnant patient

Obstetric anaesthesia requires detailed knowledge of the physiological changes associated with pregnancy. While these are covered thoroughly in Chapter 23, the salient points are outlined below to aid the reader.

As pregnancy progresses, the maternal blood volume increases and, although total haemoglobin increases, the haemoglobin concentration falls by dilution. The concentration of clotting factors increases, causing a tendency to deep vein thrombosis exacerbated by pressure on the pelvic veins from the increasingly bulky uterus. Cardiac output increases throughout pregnancy due to increases in stroke volume and heart rate. Thoracic volume rises so that although tidal volume remains comparable to pre-pregnancy values, there becomes an impression of hyperinflation. At the end of pregnancy $PaCO_2$ is reduced to around 4 kPa. The hormonal changes of pregnancy cause relaxation of smooth muscle and ligaments, resulting in a reduction in lower oesophageal sphincter tone which, combined with increasing intra-abdominal pressure, leads both to functional hiatus hernia and oesophageal reflux. Gastric contents are more voluminous than usual and gastric emptying is slowed. In labour, gastric emptying virtually ceases.

Patients in the third trimester of pregnancy should not be allowed to lie in the supine position for any reason without left lateral tilt to displace the uterus, because the weight of the uterus compresses the inferior vena cava. The substantial reduction in venous return to the heart that follows may produce fainting. If compensatory

Fundamentals of Anaesthesia, 4th edition, ed. Ted Lin, Tim Smith and Colin Pinnock. Published by Cambridge University Press. © Cambridge University Press 2017.

vasoconstriction is abolished by epidural blockade, serious falls in cardiac output may result.

Analgesia in labour

Pain in labour is the result of a hollow organ, the uterus, contracting against an obstruction, the fetus, in an attempt to expel it. The pain is the result of tension in the uterine wall. The patient's response to the pain of contractions is a psychological response that depends on culture, history and preparation; therefore each patient must be taken on her own merits. The pain of labour is transmitted to the spinal cord via two routes, depending on the stage of labour. The impulses from the body and fundus of the uterus pass via the lower thoracic spinal roots, T10 to L1, while those from the cervix and birth canal pass via the sacral roots (Figure 5.1). The net result is that pain in the first stage of labour is perceived to be lower abdominal while in the second stage it changes focus to pelvis and perineum. Nociceptive impulses pass up the spinal cord and are interpreted in the brain. The various methods of providing analgesia in labour are detailed in Figure 5.2.

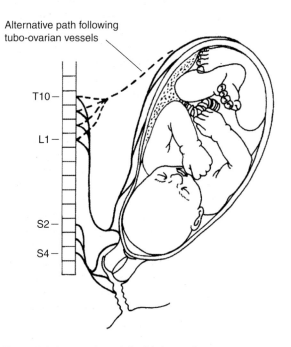

Alternative path following tubo-ovarian vessels

T10—
L1—
S2—
S4—

Figure 5.1 Innervation of the birth canal

Psychological methods

There is no doubt that adequate psychological preparation for labour significantly reduces pain. Breathing and relaxation techniques are taught routinely in antenatal classes. Attention to providing a non-clinical and stress-reducing environment is a key concern in midwifery-led units. Self-hypnosis can also be successful in the suitably motivated patient. Although still relatively uncommon, many mothers choose a water birth to aid with the pain of labour.

Complementary methods

Transcutaneous electrical nerve stimulation (TENS) can work well if introduced early enough in labour. The technique depends on the gate theory of pain transmission (as described by Melzack & Wall 1965). Stimulation must be applied to the dorsal columns of the spinal cord in the mid-thoracic region, above the level of the affected nerve roots, i.e. T10. TENS is effective early in labour but begins to lose its effect after 5 cm cervical dilatation is reached. Acupuncture has been advocated for use in labour but it is not in common use in the UK.

Systemic analgesia

Systemic administration of analgesic drugs remains popular in labour analgesia. Administration is usually by inhalation of nitrous oxide, or alternatively by intravenous or intramuscular administration of opioids.

Nitrous oxide is usually administered as a 50% mixture with oxygen (Entonox). Effective use of nitrous oxide depends on beginning the inhalation before the painful

Figure 5.2 Methods of pain relief in labour

Psychological	Antenatal education Pleasant environment
Complementary	TENS Aromatherapy Reflexology Acupuncture
Systemic analgesia	Nitrous oxide Inhalational IM opioids (pethidine) PCA (remifentanil)
Epidural	Bolus (either clinician or patient) Infusion +/- bolus

part of the contraction so that an analgesic concentration is reached by the time a contraction becomes painful, which is difficult to achieve. Subanaesthetic doses of sevoflurane (0.8%) have been shown to provide superior analgesia and patient satisfaction to nitrous oxide in the first stage of labour despite greater sedation. However, the use of volatile anaesthesia in labour has mostly been restricted to small-scale clinical trials.

Opioid analgesia may be given by either the intramuscular or the intravenous route. Local rules and preferences dictate the choice of opioid. Midwives may administer intramuscular opioids on their own responsibility, subject to local protocols relating to which drug, number of doses and accountability. Agents in widespread use include the agonists pethidine and diamorphine, while some units favour partial agonists such as meptazinol. All opioids have a reputation for causing fetal respiratory depression.

With the availability of remifentanil the intravenous route via a patient-controlled analgesia (PCA) device has witnessed a resurgence in popularity, particularly where logistical problems exclude the provision of a continuous epidural service. However, this unlicensed use of remifentanil in labour remains controversial. Although remifentanil appears to be a superior opioid it does have problems of itching and sedation with maternal desaturation and even complete apnoea. PCA devices may be simple 'elastic recoil' systems with a reservoir refilled at a fixed rate or complex computer-controlled devices with adjustable background infusions and lockout times.

Epidural analgesia

Epidural analgesia is the most effective form of labour analgesia, and remains the gold standard. However it requires the availability of a trained anaesthetist and is accompanied by rare but potentially major complications. Epidural analgesia comes into its own in long or complicated labours, malpresentations (such as occipitoposterior position or breech) and pre-eclampsia, where control of the blood pressure and improvements in placental blood flow are vital to the wellbeing of both mother and fetus. Indications for epidural analgesia are numerous, and contraindications are listed in Figure 5.3.

Contraindications to epidural analgesia

1. **Maternal refusal** is the only absolute contraindication to the technique. Anaesthetists in the UK are both morally and legally obliged to obtain informed consent for regional anaesthesia in labour. To continue, if the patient refuses after explanation of the risks and

Figure 5.3 Contraindications to epidural anaesthesia

Maternal refusal
Bleeding diathesis
Anatomical abnormality, some previous spinal surgeries
Hypovolaemia
Cardiac disease
Neurological disease
Sepsis, including local infection at injection site

benefits, constitutes assault. It is helpful if methods of labour analgesia have been discussed before the event, either as part of an antenatal class or during a pre-anaesthetic assessment. Written information improves recall of any treatment discussion, as do tools such as the Obstetric Anaesthetists Association (OAA) epidural card. Evidence suggests that the pain and distress of labour does not preclude the ability of the mother to understand, retain information and make an informed choice. Robust estimates for rarer risks were produced by the NAP3 study. The incidence of permanent harm from central nerve blockade (CNB) in obstetrics was between 1 in 80,000 and 1 in 320,000. Local estimates produced by audit may help define more common and less serious risks. Not disclosing serious risks would be unacceptable. This discussion should be documented. It is worth adding at this point that wrong-route drugs errors appear to be more common in obstetric practice, so the anaesthetist should be particularly vigilant.

2. **Bleeding diathesis**. There is controversy about the provision of epidural and spinal blockade in patients with a bleeding tendency, whether this is congenital, such as haemophilia, or acquired, such as warfarinisation. It is generally accepted that any patient whose clotting times are more than 50% extended should probably not have an epidural (in practice this means an INR > 1.5). The potential problem is the vulnerability of the epidural venous plexus and concern that if an epidural vein is punctured there will be an uncontrolled bleed from it, causing a haematoma, which could compress the spinal cord. While this sequence of events is certainly possible, it is also exceptionally rare, with an incidence between 1 in 88,000 and 1 in 140,000.

The suitability of epidural analgesia for patients taking low-dose heparin or aspirin is also controversial. Aspirin causes a permanent block of platelet thromboxane A_2, which affects any platelets in the circulation at the time the aspirin is administered. This continues for the life of any individual platelet, roughly 10 days from new. While this may appear to be a contraindication to epidural puncture, with its attendant risk of haemorrhage, the effect is quite limited because new, unaffected platelets are continually being produced. The best indicator of platelet function is the bleeding time, which suffers from poor reproducibility and a wide normal range. AAGBI have published explicit guidelines for epidural use and anticoagulation in their guide 'Regional anaesthesia and patients with abnormalities of coagulation' (2013). The risk is affected by clinical and pharmacological factors. In summary, the following limits do not increase the risk of epidural bleeding:

- 12 hours after a prophylactic dose of low-molecular-weight heparin (LMWH)
- 24 hours after a therapeutic dose of LMWH
- 4 hours after heparin (unfractionated)
- An INR < 1.5 when on warfarin
- NSAIDs without heparin
- Aspirin without heparin
- Platelet count $> 75 \times 10^9 \, L^{-1}$

In obstetric anaesthesia there are a number of other causes of acquired clotting failure, which may contraindicate epidural puncture. Pre-eclampsia is associated with deranged clotting function, particularly if severe or late in pregnancy. The platelet count will give an indication of the severity of the problem before it becomes clinically important. The HELLP syndrome (Haemolytic anaemia, Elevated Liver enzymes and Low Platelets) is a variant of pre-eclampsia. This condition is highly dangerous and causes extreme physiological upsets which can only be restored using the full facilities of an intensive care unit and haematological support. The pronounced coagulopathy that occurs in HELLP syndrome is a contraindication to epidural analgesia.

Intrauterine fetal death causes a failure of clotting as the fetus begins to macerate and breakdown products enter the maternal circulation. The process does not become significant until the fetus has been dead for more than about 5 days, but it is usual to measure clotting in this situation before an epidural is sited.

Placental abruption and other significant intrauterine bleeds may cause clotting failure secondary to the consumption of clotting factors in a vain attempt to stop bleeding from the spiral arteries. The spiral arteries pass through the myometrium to the placental bed and are usually closed off by uterine contraction after delivery. If the uterus is kept open by the presence of a fetus, blood clots or placental remnants the bleeding will continue until the uterus is emptied or the patient exsanguinates. The blood loss may not be seen as vaginal bleeding because it can remain concealed entirely within the uterus.

Amniotic fluid embolus causes a syndrome similar to major fat embolism, with clouding of consciousness, petechial haemorrhages, respiratory distress, hypotension and severe disseminated intravascular coagulation (DIC). This condition is rare but often fatal. Management consists of general supportive therapy and replacement of clotting factors and blood.

3. **Anatomical abnormalities.** Previous back surgery or spina bifida are relative contraindications to epidural analgesia because of difficulty in identifying bony landmarks or disruption of the normal anatomy of the epidural space. If the patient has had a lumbar laminectomy or spinal fusion then it is wise to check the level of surgery from previous notes or CT scans so that a level can be chosen for the puncture which has bony landmarks and avoids scar tissue or implanted metal. In spina bifida occulta, the landmarks are missing congenitally but the epidural space is relatively normal. The ligamentum flavum may, however, be absent. In the more severe forms of neural tube defect the epidural space and dural tube may be abnormal and so the situation is more complicated. None of the above situations is an absolute contraindication to epidural analgesia, but the technique may be difficult or impossible, the spread of local anaesthetic in the epidural space may be unpredictable, and the resulting pattern of block may be patchy or deficient.

4. **Hypovolaemia** must be corrected before any form of anaesthesia or analgesia, unless the situation is so dire that immediate surgery is the only way to reduce massive blood loss, in which case general anaesthesia will be indicated. In this situation, as with any hypovolaemic patient, induction must be carried out with extreme care. Sympathetic blockade caused by epidural or spinal anaesthesia in a hypovolaemic patient can have catastrophic consequences.

5. **Cardiac disease** is often taken as a contraindication to central neural blockade. In general, the effects of epidural anaesthesia are falls in both cardiac preload and afterload, which can be controlled by the cautious administration of local anaesthetic agents and by judicious use of fluids and vasoconstrictors. Pregnancy itself carries such major vascular and cardiac changes that it is difficult to reach term unless there are reasonable cardiac reserves. A growing number of patients with congenital cardiac disease, whether corrected or not, are being brought to term. In addition, the age of onset of major coronary artery disease is now falling within the childbearing years. These patients may be on the verge of major cardiac decompensation by the time they reach term. Each woman must be considered on her merits and ideally in consultation with a cardiologist. The backup of a cardiac surgical centre will be required very occasionally.

6. **Neurological disease.** Chronic neurological disease is often quoted as a contraindication to local or regional anaesthesia, without reliable evidence to confirm this view. Epidural/spinal anaesthesia is potentially dangerous in cases of raised intracranial pressure and should be discussed with a neurologist first. Spinal anaesthesia is contraindicated where there is suspicion of a tethered cord until suitable imaging is carried out. The height of the block and inclusion of opioids should be restricted if there is significant respiratory restriction due to underlying disease. Despite these caveats, most chronic neurological disorders, such as multiple sclerosis, follow a relapsing and remitting course, usually deteriorating at times of physical or mental stress and following a slow progression downward. Quality analgesia is even more important in this patient group. Childbirth is one of the stressful times likely to cause relapse, and if central nerve block is provided for analgesia or anaesthesia at this time then it is possible that any relapse will be linked to the technique, regardless of whether it is in fact to blame. Provided that this is explained and accepted by the patient, there is no reason why epidural analgesia should be withheld.

7. **Sepsis.** Systemic sepsis is a contraindication to epidural analgesia because of the cumulative detrimental affect on haemodynamic stability. Local infection at the proposed site of puncture is a relative contraindication, but there is usually a non-infected space available close by which can be used. Maternal pyrexia, however, should be taken as a contraindication because of the risk of blood-borne infection with a foreign body, the epidural catheter, in situ or a potential haematoma from epidural vein puncture providing an infective focus. Individual centres and clinicians may have different maximum maternal temperatures, above which they will not recommend epidural analgesia. Epidural analgesia limits maternal thermoregulation, and fetal death rate increases dramatically in maternal pyrexia, so it may be preferable to avoid the use of epidural anaesthesia in this situation.

Epidural technique

Detailed knowledge of the relevant anatomy is essential (Figure 5.4). For further details of epidural technique, see Chapter 7.

The epidural space is a potential space within the spinal canal. It is broadly triangular in shape with the apex posteriorly. The shape varies considerably from level to level, being more oval in the neck. Superiorly it is closed at the foramen magnum, where the spinal dura mater and the periosteum of the spinal canal fuse to form the intracranial dura mater. It is, therefore, impossible for a true epidural injection to extend intracranially. Inferiorly, the epidural space is closed at the sacrococcygeal ligament. The anterior boundary lies within the spinal canal, being formed by the posterior longitudinal ligaments of the

Figure 5.4 Anatomy of the epidural space

Boundaries	Superior	Closed at foramen magnum
	Inferior	Closed at sacrococcygeal membrane
	Anterior	Posterior longitudinal ligaments, vertebral bodies
	Posterior	Vertebral laminae, ligamenta flava
	Lateral	Open, pedicles and intervertebral foramina
Shape		Broadly triangular, apex posteriorly
Contents		Veins, arteries, fat, lymphatics, nerve roots and dural cuffs

spinal column, the vertebral bodies and the intervertebral discs. Posteriorly the space is bounded by the ligamenta flava (these may be paired at each level or one pair of continuous ligaments – opinion varies) and the vertebral laminae. There may be a plane of cleavage between the ligamenta flava that can give an impression that there is no ligament when a needle passes through it. Laterally the epidural space is bounded by the pedicles and laminae of the vertebrae and by the intervertebral foramina, and thus it is not a closed space laterally. The space contains the spinal dural sac and its contents: the spinal cord and nerve roots. The epidural space itself contains fat, arterioles, a complex of thin-walled valveless veins which drain into the azygos system, lymphatics and the spinal nerve roots after they cross the dura and before they exit through the intervertebral foramina. The nerve roots carry with them a cuff of dura that may extend out into the paravertebral space.

To reach the epidural space from the skin of the back, the tip of the needle must pass through successive layers of tissue. The bones over the lumbar area are palpated and the spaces between spinous processes identified. Once a suitable space has been identified (L2/3 or L3/4 are usually the easiest and most consistent to use) the needle is inserted through the skin, staying strictly on the midline, although a deliberate paramedian approach is acceptable. The first ligament encountered is the supraspinous ligament. This has a 'crunchy' consistency and is up to 1 cm thick. The interspinous ligament feels 'spongy' and can be up to 6 cm thick. The ligamentum flavum is very variable in thickness, up to 2 cm, but is usually tough and difficult to penetrate. The essence of the technique is that with the needle tip in the ligamentum flavum, nothing can be injected through the needle whereas after careful advancement the tip will emerge into the epidural space and there will be a sudden total loss of resistance to injection.

Ultrasound-guided epidural needle placement Ultrasound guidance is increasingly being used, both to perform epidural insertion and in the assessment of the difficult spine. It can provide information regarding position of midline structures, depth of epidural space and angle of needle entry. This may be particularly useful when planning epidural placement in the obese patient. Some evidence suggests that it may enhance learning of epidural placement, reduce the number of failed attempts and help with the management of failed catheter placement.

Combined spinal–epidural in labour Combined spinal–epidural (CSE) techniques may be used for analgesia in labour. An epidural needle is sited in the epidural space and a longer small-gauge spinal needle is typically passed through it. A small dose of a mixture of bupivacaine and fentanyl is injected into the subarachnoid space and the spinal needle is then withdrawn and an epidural catheter passed through the epidural needle. The spinal solution establishes rapid analgesia, providing good blockade of the sacral nerve roots while lessening maternal and umbilical cord concentrations of local anaesthetic. Spinal doses of 2.5 mg of local anaesthetic appear to provide satisfactory analgesia. The epidural catheter is used for further doses during the second stage of labour. The patient is allowed some mobility while the spinal solution is effective but this may be limited by the need for continuous monitoring of the fetus. Each unit must have written policies to establish the limits to mobility in labour.

Epidural test doses

It is impossible to be absolutely sure of the correct placement of an epidural catheter until a dose of local anaesthetic agent has been injected. A test dose serves two purposes, first to identify vascular placement and second to identify intrathecal placement. To achieve this, a test dose must be small enough to do no harm if in the wrong place but large enough to show an effect. Departments should have their own policies for 'testing' the epidural, and it is helpful if all practitioners follow the policy to provide consistency on what constitutes a 'failed' block. Many practitioners use a 3 mL dose of either 0.5% or 0.25% plain bupivacaine. There are advocates for both adrenaline-containing and dextrose-containing test doses but neither is in popular use.

In practice, 3 mL plain isobaric bupivacaine, placed directly into the CSF, will produce total spinal anaesthesia within 5 minutes. Hyperbaric bupivacaine (heavy Marcaine) will have a less extensive result, and if it is placed intravenously there will be no noticeable effect. Larger volumes of local anaesthetic agent injected into the lumbar epidural venous plexus tend to pass backwards up the basilar vessels and cause a short-lived loss of consciousness or at least a period of light-headedness with lingual and circumoral paraesthesia. The rationale behind using an adrenaline-containing solution is that, on intravenous injection, there will be a measurable increase in heart rate. While this may be so, the increase so caused will be within the pulse-rate variation of any woman in labour and so may not be distinguished from normal.

Having given the test dose and waited an appropriate time for an effect to appear, usually 5 minutes, the main dose may be given. Traditionally the choice was 0.25% or 0.5% plain bupivacaine by bolus top-ups of between 6 and 10 mL as necessary to relieve the pain every 30 minutes. The top-ups may be given all in one position, usually semi-reclining, or half the dose may be given in each lateral position with 5 minutes between. This method has largely been superseded by a variety of low-dose infusion and patient-controlled epidural analgesia (PCEA) techniques that have the advantage of reducing both the drug load and the unwanted effects of the traditional epidural, such as high-density motor block and an increased incidence of instrumental delivery.

The majority of infusion/PCEA epidurals begin with a single top-up to rapidly establish the analgesia before commencing the infusion. The bupivacaine/fentanyl combination appears to increase both the analgesia and the penetration of the block without any obvious drawbacks. Recent evidence suggests that there are no measurable fetal effects of the opioid at doses in current use, although addition of fentanyl clearly increases symptomatic itching in the mother. No single regime for epidural injection has gained wide acceptance. Infusion regimes vary considerably, but most are based on either 0.1–0.15% bupivacaine or 0.2% ropivacaine, each with 1–5 $\mu g\ mL^{-1}$ of fentanyl. Bolus doses in a PCEA may be 5 mL of 0.1–0.15% bupivacaine with or without 2 $\mu g\ mL^{-1}$ fentanyl followed by a lockout of 10 minutes. PCEA also allows the patient control over her analgesia, reducing breakthrough pain while waiting for a midwife/clinician-delivered bolus. Each unit should have a single standard mixture and infusion/bolus protocol with which all anaesthetists and midwives should be familiar.

Complications Epidural anaesthesia carries a risk of complications, the more major of which are listed in Figure 5.5.

Figure 5.5 Complications of epidural analgesia

| Dural tap |
| Intravascular injection |
| Intrathecal injection |
| Neurological |
| Backache |
| Pressure areas |

1. **Dural tap and post-dural puncture headache (PDPH)** occurs in about 0.5–1.5% of obstetric epidurals. The majority of these will become symptomatic. Immediate treatment involves establishing a working epidural at another lumbar interspace. The patient, midwifery and obstetric team should be notified so that a prolonged second stage can be avoided. An elective forceps or instrumental delivery may be required. The differential diagnoses for post-partum headache are shown in Figure 5.6.

   PDPH is typically postural and improves on lying down. It usually presents within 72 hours and is associated with pain in the frontal-occipital region, neck stiffness with visual and auditory symptoms. The patient should be reviewed daily by a senior member of the anaesthetic staff. The pain should initially be treated by encouraging oral fluids and by simple analgesia. If the headache becomes incapacitating, an epidural blood patch (EBP) remains the gold-standard therapy. After obtaining consent this would typically be carried out between 24 and 48 hours after the original dural puncture. Infection, pyrexia, refusal and coagulopathy will contraindicate the technique.

   Under aseptic conditions a new epidural puncture is carried out at or below the site of the original puncture and up to 20 mL of the patient's blood is injected into the epidural space. This technique should be performed with two scrubbed anaesthetists. It has been routine to send further blood for culture, although the results are usually negative. The patient is usually advised to

Figure 5.6 Postpartum headache: differential diagnoses

| Migraine |
| Meningitis |
| Post-dural puncture headache (PDPH) |
| Cortical vein thrombosis |
| Simple/tension headache |
| Subarachnoid haemorrhage |
| Pre-eclampsia/eclampsia |
| Space-occupying lesion (tumour, haemorrhage) |
| Posterior reversible leucoencephalopathy syndrome |
| Cerebral infarction/ischaemia |
| Sinusitis |

lie still for 1–2 hours afterwards before gently mobilising. Initial success rate for EBP is high, but many women (possibly up to 40%) may have a recurrence of headache requiring further treatment. Patients should be informed to immediately report pyrexia, back pain or radicular pain if it occurs after EBP. It is always worth reassessing the patient for an alternative diagnosis if she does not respond as expected to treatment.

2. **Intravascular injection.** While proper use of test doses should identify intrathecal and intravascular injections at that stage, epidural catheters can migrate into vessels or across the dura at any stage during the conduct of the technique, and the full dose of local anaesthetic may be inadvertently injected into the circulation. Clinical features and management are covered under *Local anaesthetic toxicity* in Chapter 7.

   Injection of local anaesthetic into the epidural veins may only cause paraesthesia of the tongue and lips but can also cause agitation, sudden loss of consciousness and seizures as the local anaesthetic agent affects the brain. Cardiovascular collapse may quickly follow. Advanced life support (ALS) should be delivered and an infusion of Intralipid commenced. The airway and respiration must be adequately maintained, and tracheal intubation and controlled ventilation may be necessary. Once this has been achieved the circulation must be supported by fluids, vasopressors and cardiac massage if appropriate according to standard ALS protocols.

3. **Intrathecal injection.** The effects of intrathecal injection may be slower in onset but no less of a problem than intravascular injection. Progressive rising paralysis of the whole body, including the muscles of respiration, occurs, accompanied by a significant fall in blood pressure. The feature which distinguishes intrathecal injection from massive epidural is the onset of cranial nerve effects, particularly facial paralysis, trigeminal anaesthesia and rapid loss of consciousness. As with intravenous injection, the airway and respiration must be addressed first, followed by the circulation as dictated by ALS techniques.

   These rare but major problems are the reason for direct observation of the patient for 20 minutes after an epidural injection or top-up.

4. **Neurological complications** of epidural analgesia are extremely rare and usually relate to cauda equina syndrome if there has been local neural toxicity by either too high a concentration of adrenaline in the injected drug or, more likely, the wrong drug administered. The majority of neurological complications following childbirth are related not to epidurals but to the management of labour, particularly where a large fetus has become obstructed in the second stage of labour for a prolonged time. This scenario results in compression of the roots and trunks of the lumbosacral plexus within the pelvis, especially L1 as it passes over the brim of the true pelvis. The most common defects subsequently are foot drop (lateral peroneal nerve), sciatic palsies or femoral nerve palsies. Neurological symptoms should be thoroughly documented at time of presentation and a referral made to a suitable clinician. Many symptoms will resolve slowly over time but represent a significant concern for patients. Each case should be managed with due care and appropriate follow-up.

5. **Backache.** Epidural analgesia in labour has developed a reputation for causing low-grade but persistent backache after delivery, which is probably related not to epidural analgesia itself but to the management of the back in labour. In the absence of pain sensation, proprioception and muscle tone to protect the joints and ligaments of the back, there is a possibility of musculoskeletal strain. Suitable imaging and specialist neurological input will exclude significant pathology.

6. **Pressure sores** are not usually associated with young women, but the lack of sensation and motor block provided by epidural analgesia prevent the patient moving during labour. Patients should be encouraged to move regularly to prevent pressure sores developing, particularly over the sacrum.

Operative anaesthesia

Anaesthesia for operative surgery in obstetrics falls into two main areas. First, operative delivery, for example Caesarean section and forceps procedures; second, post-delivery procedures such as retained placenta. Both are amenable to being carried out under regional or general anaesthesia. In the case of retained placenta, before considering a regional technique (such as spinal anaesthesia) which removes sympathetic tone and causes profound vasodilatation, it is essential to first accurately assess blood loss and restore circulating volume.

Regional anaesthesia

Central neural blockade for operative obstetric anaesthesia requires a different approach to the provision of analgesia in labour. In labour the only essential feature is analgesia – motor block is a distinct disadvantage. For obstetric surgery, including forceps delivery, removal of retained placenta and Caesarean section, complete anaesthesia of the relevant area is necessary. In labour the highest dermatome required is T10, whereas for Caesarean section the upper limit needs to be a minimum of T6, though there is still some debate about whether it should be even higher than this (T4) to adequately cover the variable innervation of the peritoneum. The sacral nerve roots also need to be blocked. Light touch is the modality that shows the least variability when assessing level of block. The dose of local anaesthetic agent necessary to achieve this at term is only about two-thirds of that required in the non-pregnant patient for a comparable result.

Spinal anaesthesia for obstetrics offers advantages over epidural anaesthesia because of speed of onset and intensity of block, but disadvantages because of severity and speed of onset of hypotension and the less adjustable nature of the technique, unless a combined technique is used. The major disadvantage of spinal anaesthesia in obstetric anaesthesia has always been the incidence of post-dural puncture headache (PDPH). This has been significantly reduced by the use of solid-tipped (non-cutting) needles with side holes such as the Sprotte and Whitacre point needles. The only spinal solutions with current product licences are 0.5% hyperbaric bupivacaine and 0.5% plain levobupivacaine. This latter solution is slightly hypobaric. The optimum dose for establishing an effective block (i.e. no intraoperative pain for 90–99% of parturients) remains the topic of much research.

There has been much interest in recent years in 'low-dose' spinal techniques for Caesarean section, and they have indeed become successful standard practice in some units. The definition of what constitutes a low dose varies, but the ED_{95} for 0.5% heavy Marcaine is 2.2 mL or 11 mg. The addition of an opioid (fentanyl/diamorphine) has definite advantages in extending both the duration and quality of block. Low-dose regimes have the advantage of less maternal hypotension and reduced motor blockade. However, they carry with them a slower onset and shorter duration of blockade and increased frequency of intraoperative pain and potential increased risk of conversion to general anaesthesia. They should only be used in experienced hands in obstetric units with appropriate operating conditions and the ability to supplement analgesia through an epidural catheter as part of a combined spinal–epidural

anaesthetic. This combines the speed of onset and intensity of spinal anaesthesia with the adjustability and duration of epidural anaesthesia. Spinal anaesthesia can be extended by injection of saline into the epidural catheter shortly after the spinal dose, as this increases pressure in the epidural space.

For obstetric surgery under epidural anaesthesia alone, a catheter is inserted in the usual way and, after a test dose, a main dose of local anaesthetic agent is given. This may be given as one dose or in divided doses. The local anaesthetic agent of choice should ensure rapid onset of an intense block with a duration of action in excess of 1 hour. Up to 30 mL of bupivacaine 0.5% or 20 mL of 2% lidocaine, both with 100 µg fentanyl, usually produces satisfactory blockade. The fetus should be monitored during epidural top-up and the anaesthetist should remain with the mother. If a top-up is required quickly, 20 mL lidocaine 2% with 0.1 mL of 1:000 adrenaline, 100 µg fentanyl (and 1 mL 8.4% bicarbonate) may be used.

Every patient should be assessed for the risk of venous thromboembolism, and if at risk a dose of low-molecular-weight heparin should be given 4 hours after the regional block is established or the epidural catheter removed. This should not be delayed unless there is a good reason, such as haemorrhage, coagulopathy or traumatic bloody tap. Placement or removal of an epidural catheter should occur at least 12 hours after a prophylactic dose of LMWH.

The prevention and management of hypotension as a result of central neural blockade falls into two areas: volume loading and vasopressors. Volume loading before the administration of the block requires administration of 500–1,000 mL of crystalloid solution or 500 mL of colloid solution. Traditionally ephedrine was used in small intravenous doses (3–6 mg) to correct hypotension. Ephedrine crosses the placental barrier and may thus cause a fetal tachycardia and acidosis. Prophylactic phenylephrine infusions and fluid co-hydration have made maternal hypotension much less frequent. Phenylephrine does not cross the placenta.

In the preoperative period the patient should be warned that regional anaesthesia may not give total loss of sensation. Pain during Caesarean section is a common reason for complaint and litigation. Clear honest documentation pertaining to the consent, the assessment of the block (two modalities, cold and light touch) and the management of intraoperative pain are clinical and medico-legal standards.

General anaesthesia

Obstetric general anaesthesia is usually considered to be one of the higher-risk subspecialties of anaesthesia because of the potential for urgency, uncontrolled bleeding and aspiration of gastric contents. In fact, as a cause of maternal mortality, anaesthesia ranks very low (0.31 deaths per 100,000 maternities), and deaths due to amniotic fluid embolism and obstetric haemorrhage are twice as common. This low mortality is not a reason for complacency, but a result of sustained work in eliminating the main causes of anaesthetic-related problems by intensive training in managing difficult and failed intubation, and universal antacid prophylaxis. Sadly, deaths due to failure to ventilate the lungs and postoperative aspiration still occurred in the most recent Confidential Enquiry into maternal and child health.

As a rule of thumb, there is no such thing as a pregnant woman with an empty stomach. The gastric contents also tend to be more acid than in the non-pregnant woman. Progesterone-induced relaxation of the lower oesophageal sphincter, along with the higher intra-abdominal pressure in late pregnancy, tends to encourage the regurgitation and aspiration of gastric contents into the trachea. While Mendelson actually described obstruction to respiration by solid matter, the aspiration of liquid and the resulting chemical pneumonitis are usually called Mendelson's syndrome. Acid aspiration in pregnancy causes a gross chemical pneumonitis, which distinguishes it from the aspiration pneumonia of the non-pregnant. Routine antacid prophylaxis in the delivery suite reduces both the volume and the acidity of gastric contents. Common regimes involve administration of regular oral H_2 receptor antagonists to all admissions to the delivery suite and 0.3 molar sodium citrate solution when a decision is made to proceed to surgery. Variations on this theme include the administration of intravenous ranitidine and metoclopramide, the latter to encourage gastric emptying, although this effect is difficult to show and variable. Magnesium trisilicate mixture is little used now because it is particulate and does not mix well with gastric contents.

In the second and third trimesters of pregnancy tracheal intubation is considered mandatory because of the potential for acid aspiration. For the same reasons rapid sequence induction (RSI) with cricoid pressure is also necessary. The hormonal changes of pregnancy, as pertaining to intestinal function, remain for some 48 hours post partum, and so it is wise to apply RSI for up to a week

after delivery. The standard general anaesthetic technique involves a wedge under the right buttock to displace the uterus from the inferior vena cava, RSI with thiopental and suxamethonium (propofol has no licence for use in late pregnancy, although it is increasingly used). Tracheal intubation should be followed by controlled ventilation of the lungs with 50–70% nitrous oxide and a volatile agent of choice. Suitable muscle relaxants include atracurium and vecuronium. Mivacurium should be used with care because of the reduced activity of plasma cholinesterase in late pregnancy, which may delay its offset. At the end of the procedure the tracheal tube should be removed with the patient in the lateral position, head down. The recovery period can be particularly dangerous in the postpartum patient and extubation should be considered only after the return of protective reflexes.

Tracheal intubation in the pregnant woman can be notoriously difficult. The anatomy of the chest changes in pregnancy, with an increase in functional residual capacity (FRC) giving an impression of hyperinflation. This is combined with an increase in the size of the breasts and an apparent shortening of the neck (because of the increase in FRC). Note that the majority of pregnant women have a full set of natural teeth.

Pre-eclampsia may cause laryngeal oedema, and it is now recognised that the Mallampati score may change as labour progresses, causing further difficulties. Endotracheal tube size should be reduced in expectation of difficulty. While the laryngeal mask does not provide sufficient barrier to gastric contents for routine use, in a case of failed tracheal intubation it may have a role (see Chapter 2).

Equipment for the management of difficult intubation must be available at all times and within arm's reach whenever obstetric anaesthesia is practised. Desirable equipment includes a range of laryngoscope blades and handles, including a polio blade, a variety of tube sizes down to 6.0 mm, and stylets and bougies to aid intubation. A method of transtracheal ventilation should also be readily available and staff trained in its use.

Accidental awareness is more commonly encountered in obstetric general anaesthesia than in any other specialty. The cause is usually either failure to introduce sufficiently high concentrations of vapour early enough, before the brain concentration of the induction agent begins to fall, or failure to maintain sufficiently high concentrations of vapour and nitrous oxide throughout the procedure.

> Where death has occurred after difficult or failed intubation, the cause has not been the failure to intubate but the **failure to oxygenate** the patient between attempts. **This point cannot be emphasised enough.** Regular emergency drills (possibly involving simulation) and familiarity with equipment in managing the difficult and failed airway will help to eliminate the problems of human behaviour involving fixation and denial when faced with an emergency scenario.

Non-obstetric surgery in the pregnant patient

When to consider a patient pregnant

As a general rule, the risks of acid aspiration begin to outweigh the risks of tracheal intubation at about 14–16 weeks gestation, and from this time onwards the patient should be considered as an obstetric problem. At this stage anti-acid prophylaxis is sensible. The hormonal changes of pregnancy fade rapidly after delivery, along with the effects on gastric function, and so it is probably safe to revert to non-pregnancy anaesthetic techniques at about 1 week post partum, although purely elective surgery may be delayed longer.

Non-obstetric surgery

It must be remembered that the pregnant patient may present with a variety of other surgical and medical pathologies. Common presentations include appendicitis, trauma and malignancy. Pathology or intra-abdominal surgery increases the risk of miscarriage, preterm labour and fetal demise. Timing of non-emergency surgery is important and will affect both the miscarriage rate and the chances of abnormal fetal development. The miscarriage rate after surgery in the first trimester may be as high as 10%.

The anaesthetist must take into account the health of both the mother and the developing fetus, although in an emergency the mother's life takes priority. The trimester will dictate which physiological changes are relevant to the anaesthetist. But a fundamental respect for the increased cardiac output, oxygen demand, aortocaval compression, aspiration risk and airway difficulties should always be held. Rapid sequence induction is recommended in the second trimester. MAC values are slightly reduced in pregnancy, but all volatile anaesthetics cause uterine vasodilatation and relaxation, increasing the risk of uterine bleeding.

Risks to the fetus can be minimised by early recognition of disease and consideration of placental transfer of drugs, teratogenicity and maintenance of uteroplacental perfusion, both in terms of oxygenation and flow (Figure 5.7). Maternal $PaCO_2$ should be kept normal to avoid fetal acidosis. Nitrous oxide should be avoided in the first trimester because of teratogenicity. Extubation should occur in the full lateral position with the patient fully awake.

It is worth remembering that no particular anaesthetic technique has been shown to be better than another in reducing the risk of surgery. The risk of pregnancy loss and other problems should be discussed during the consent process. Thromboprophylaxis should be considered.

The patient, an obstetrician and a midwife should be involved in discussions regards clinical management, and where possible the fetal heart should be monitored before and after the case.

Cell salvage in obstetric care

Obstetric haemorrhage is still one of the leading causes of maternal mortality in the UK. Cell salvage has the potential benefit of reducing transfusion infection risk (although salvaged blood may still be infected). It also avoids anaemia (which may occur in normovolaemic dilutional and preoperative autologous donation methods) and can be used in an emergency. It may be acceptable to those who have religious objections to receiving transfused blood products – although individual consent is still vital. It is recommended that the cell salvage machines be used whenever there is a significant risk of maternal haemorrhage (multiple previous sections, multiple pregnancies, LSCS at full dilatation, abnormal placentation etc.) or if allogenic blood is unavailable or unsuitable. Trained staff should be involved in order to reduce operator error.

Obstetric haemorrhage is unpredictable. The cell salvage machine can be set up in standby mode, consisting of simply the suction and reservoir apparatus. It can then be converted to filter blood if the need arises. The main concern in obstetric care has been the risk of alloimmunisation of RhD blood and the potential for reinfusion of amniotic fluid causing an amniotic fluid embolism (AFE). Anti-D can be used to treat reinfused rhesus-mismatched fetal erythrocytes. AFE is now considered

Figure 5.7 Anaesthetic drugs and pregnancy

Drug	Effect compared to non-pregnant state
Inhalational anaesthetic agents	
Volatile anaesthetics	Reduced MAC, decrease uterine tone, vasodilatation
Nitrous oxide	Inhibits methionine synthetase and DNA synthesis Harmful after long exposure Best avoided during first trimester
Intravenous anaesthetic agents	
Thiopental	Considered safe in appropriate doses
Propofol	Not teratogenic in animal studies
Ketamine	Avoid, increases uterine tone
Neuromuscular blockers	
Suxamethonium	Reduced plasma cholinesterases, possible increased duration of action
Non-depolarising drugs	Do not cross placenta
Local anaesthetics	Reduced protein binding, increased free concentration – increased toxicity Reduced dose needed in neuroaxial techniques
Analgesics	
NSAIDs	May increase fetal loss, causes closure of DA. Avoid
Opioids	Increased sensitivity (mother and fetus), cross placenta causing neonatal depression and dependence, possible intrauterine growth restriction (IUGR)
Anticholinergics	
Atropine	Crosses placenta causing fetal tachycardia
Glycopyrrolate	Does not cross placenta
ACh inhibitors	
Neostigmine	Crosses placenta, fetal bradycardia
Antihypertensives	
ACE inhibitors	IUGR, oligohydramnios, renal impairment
β-Blockers	IUGR, neonatal hypoglycaemia
Thiazide diuretics	Neonatal thrombocytopenia
Tocolytics	
β_2-Agonists: ritodrine, terbutaline, salbutamol	Tachycardia, pulmonary oedema, hypokalaemia, hyperglycaemia
Oxytocin antagonists – atosiban	Nausea and vomiting
Calcium channel blockers	Hypotension

Figure 5.7 (*cont.*)

Drug	Effect compared to non-pregnant state
Anticoagulants	
Warfarin	Teratogenic
Heparin	Does not cross placenta
Antiepileptics	
Phenytoin, carbamazepine, valporate	Neural tube defects
Magnesium sulphate	Muscle weakness, exacerbation of neuromuscular blockade

Based on Nejdlova & Johnson 2012.

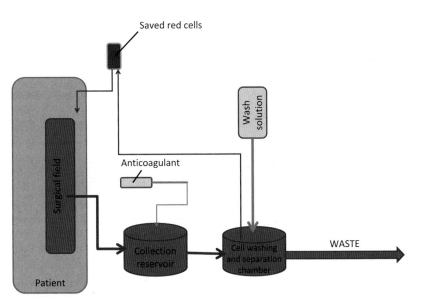

Figure 5.8 Cell saver system

Figure 5.9 Complications of cell salvage in obstetrics

Infection (bacterial, viral)
Amniotic fluid embolism (very rare)
Hypotension
Disseminated intravascular coagulation
Transfer of fetal RBCs and maternal alloimmunisation
Heparin toxicity
Red blood cell lysis
Potential sickling of transfused blood in sickle cell patients

an anaphylactoid type reaction. The incidence of AFE is reduced by having two suction systems, processing only whole bowls and using a leucodepletion filter (Figure 5.8). The second reservoir is only filled once the fetus has been delivered and the amniotic fluid removed into the waste. It has been reported that leucodepletion filters may produce hypotension due to a biochemical reaction as well as physically slowing down the rate of reinfusion. Despite the risks (Figure 5.9), no single complication that led to an adverse outcome has been exclusively attributed to cell salvage, in over 800 published cases. It is of course possible that the risk is lower than this.

The paediatric patient

This section is predominantly concerned with children of 20 kg or more in weight. In practice, this will usually equate to an age of about 5 years. A convenient formula for estimating the weight of a child is:

$$\text{Weight (kg)} = (\text{age} + 4) \times 2$$

Assessment

Preoperative assessment in children should be as rigorous as in adults, and questions should be addressed to the child even though the parents may answer for them. Most children are healthy, but chronic conditions such as asthma, multiple allergies, congenital heart disease and systemic conditions (such as muscular dystrophy) may also be encountered. The presence of one congenital abnormality should stimulate the search for others. Chromosomal abnormalities may be linked, particularly with congenital heart disease. Except for true emergency surgery, children with colds or upper respiratory tract infections should have their surgery cancelled and rescheduled to a later date. The inflamed airway is exquisitely sensitive to any kind of manipulation, resulting in laryngeal spasm. Laryngeal spasm in children is particularly dangerous because of the rapid onset of severe desaturation, made more marked by their higher metabolic rate.

There is no universally good premedicant for children. Oral midazolam (0.5 mg kg^{-1}, maximum 20 mg) usually works well. The IV dose can be given orally and its taste disguised in a small amount of clear juice. It usually takes 20–30 minutes to reach peak effect, and administration should be timed accordingly. The duration and effect of oral midazolam is sometimes unpredictable and it can cause paradoxical excitation. Day-case admission can result in insufficient time for anxiolytic premedication to take effect (and the use of sedatives in day surgery may be undesirable). All children should have topical local anaesthetic cream or gel applied to the proposed venepuncture site at least 1 hour before anaesthesia. Drug doses in children should always be calculated on a weight-related basis, a calculation which will give an approximation of the required dose. If dilution of a drug is proposed then each syringe should be labelled with the drug name and concentration. **Ambiguity must be avoided at all costs.**

Equipment

Anaesthetic equipment for patients under 20 kg body weight is quite specialised, and there is no gradation to adult equipment. For all paediatric patients the breathing system dead space and resistance should be kept to a minimum by avoiding catheter mounts, angle pieces and valves. Controlled ventilation may be preferable because of the inevitable increase in dead space after induction of anaesthesia and the increased work of breathing. The Mapleson E or F system is preferable for patients less than 20 kg, but it can also be used for heavier patients if the volume of the expiratory limb is more than the calculated tidal volume and the fresh gas flow for spontaneous ventilation is more than 2.5 times minute volume. Tidal volume approximates to 8 mL kg^{-1} in the child, and a respiratory rate of about 20 per minute is usual. If ventilation is to be controlled then a minute volume divider type of ventilator should only be used for tidal volume settings greater than 300 mL. The reason for this is that below this the ventilator becomes inaccurate in delivery because of the higher proportion of compressible volume related to total tidal volume. Many modern integrated ventilators will ventilate tidal volumes down to 50 mL, although with tidal volumes less than 300 mL either a T-piece occluder type system should be used, or a Mapleson D with a ventilator such as the Nuffield Anaesthesia Ventilator Series 200 (with Newton valve for neonates or premature babies).

If tracheal intubation is proposed then account should be taken of the increased resistance to breathing that this introduces. The resistance to flow in a tube is inversely related to the fourth power of the radius, and so halving the diameter will increase resistance by 16 times. Any tracheal tube will have a smaller internal diameter than the natural airway, particularly if the tube is cuffed. Unless there is a risk of tracheal soiling, uncuffed tubes are preferable because of the larger internal diameter that this allows. The anatomy of the child larynx is different from the adult (Figure 5.10). In consequence, the use of cuffed tubes in the under-10 age group renders the subglottic region vulnerable to oedema, particularly if an overly large tube is introduced with force. That said, there has been a recent shift to using cuffed tracheal tubes in younger children. Even small amounts of secretion in a tracheal tube will significantly increase the resistance to gas flow.

Figure 5.11 offers guidance in determining the appropriate size of endotracheal tube for use in children.

Fluid therapy

The fluid choice will depend upon the age of the child and the nature of fluid loss. Fluid requirements should take

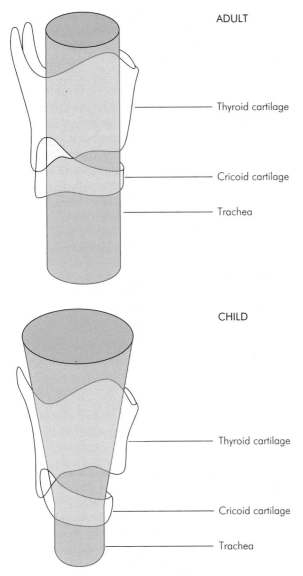

ADULT

— Thyroid cartilage

— Cricoid cartilage

— Trachea

CHILD

— Thyroid cartilage

— Cricoid cartilage

— Trachea

Figure 5.10 Anatomy of the infant larynx

Figure 5.11 ETT size in paediatric anaesthesia

ETT internal diameter (mm) = age/4 + 4 = tube diameter mm (neonate size 3–3.5)
Oral ETT length (cm) = age/2 +12
Nasal ETT length (cm) = age/2 +15

Figure 5.12 Calculation of maintenance fluid requirements in children

Weight	Rate (mL h^{-1})
0–10 kg	4 per kg of body weight
11–20 kg	40 + (2 per kg over 10 kg)
≥ 21 kg	60 + (1 per kg over 20 kg)
For example: Age 7 Weight = 7 + 4 × 2 = 22 kg Fluids = 40 + 20 + 2 = 62 mL h^{-1}	

into account maintenance fluid, deficit and ongoing losses. Resuscitation in shocked states should usually be with isotonic normal saline or Ringer's lactate (10 ml kg^{-1}). Blood sugar should be checked and glucose and potassium given as appropriate. Hypotonic solutions in particular can cause significant problems with hyponatraemia in paediatric patients.

Intravenous fluids in children should be given via a burette giving set or a volume-controlled pump and should always be calculated on a weight-related basis (Figure 5.12). A minimum of 2 mL kg^{-1} per hour should be given to those not receiving oral fluids. Blood replacement can be very difficult to calculate, and is based on replacing loss for loss when 10% blood volume has been spilt. Losses are assessed by swab weighing and accurate suction measurement. Blood volume may be estimated as 80 mL kg^{-1} in small children, falling to 70 mL kg^{-1} in adults. Blood loss of 8 mL kg^{-1} will, therefore, need replacing during surgery.

Analgesia

Much of the surgery carried out on children lends itself very well to regional anaesthesia, and this method provides very high-quality early postoperative analgesia. Caudal epidural analgesia is particularly well suited to lower abdominal and lower limb surgery and is easier to perform in children than in adults. However, it should be noted that meticulous care must be taken with indwelling epidural catheters postoperatively. Paediatric patients may not express concerns regards new symptoms, e.g. new motor block, as an adult would. Most children over 6 years of age can use a PCA machine, and a nurse-controlled version is also available (NCA). Other useful preparations involve opioid lollipops and oral

Figure 5.13 Analgesic doses in children

Drug	Paediatric dose
Paracetamol	Max 90 mg kg^{-1} day^{-1} in 4 divided doses (max 2 g day^{-1} if under 50 kg) First dose 20 mg kg^{-1} Subsequent doses 10 mg kg^{-1} at 6-hourly intervals
Ibuprofen	5 mg kg^{-1} every 8 hours (max 400 mg day^{-1})
Diclofenac	PR 1 mg kg^{-1} every 16 hours (max 150 mg day^{-1})
Codeine	1 mg kg^{-1} every 4–6 hours
Morphine	PO 0.4 mg kg^{-1} every 2–4 hours IV 0.1 mg kg^{-1} every 2–4 hours PCA (1 mg kg^{-1} in 50 mL normal saline, bolus 1 mL, 5-minute lockout, max 1 mg mL^{-1})

preparations (such as Oramorph). Rectal administration of non-steroidal agents (such as diclofenac) and paracetamol remain popular. Figure 5.13 shows paediatric doses of analgesic drugs.

Specialist surgery
General and urological surgery
Elective general and urological surgery in childhood tends to be restricted to herniotomy, orchidopexy and circumcision, all of which can be carried out on a day-case basis with a combination of general and regional anaesthesia. Appendicectomy is another frequent operation in children and is always an inpatient (emergency or urgent) procedure. Groin incisions can be covered very well by inguinal field blockade, while penile block is particularly good for circumcision. In contrast, the more widespread and bilateral anaesthesia of a caudal block may restrict mobility and be complicated by urinary retention, particularly in larger children. Oral analgesia should be given before the effect of the local anaesthetic wears off. For appendicectomy, an RSI technique should be used. Wound infiltration with local anaesthetic provides some postoperative pain relief. While some of these children are relatively well, others are pyrexial and toxic, particularly if the diagnosis is made late. These latter need to be managed very carefully and their state of hydration properly assessed and corrected in the preoperative period.

Orthopaedic surgery
Much of the orthopaedic surgery in this age group is the result of trauma. A full skeletal survey should be carried out so that other injuries are not missed, particularly head injuries and cervical spine injuries. Blood loss and analgesia requirements should receive particular attention before anaesthesia. After trauma, patients are usually assumed to have a full stomach and should be managed as such, with preoxygenation and RSI techniques. Postoperative analgesia for fractures and soft tissue injuries is best provided by regional anaesthesia, although there remains a debate about the development of compartment syndrome being masked if there are forearm or lower leg fractures. Elective orthopaedic procedures in children aged 5 years and over differ little in their anaesthesia requirements from those in adults.

Dental and ENT surgery
The core of both dental and ENT anaesthesia is the problem of the shared airway. In both types of surgery the anaesthetist and the surgeon need good access to a clear airway kept free of debris and blood. This has resulted in the development of special equipment and techniques for this situation.

Dental surgery
In the main, dental surgery in children is restricted to simple dental extraction. In some areas of the UK dental caries is still a common indication. Elsewhere, with improvements in dental hygiene and fluoridation of water, the indication has changed but the procedure has not. As a result children more often present because of crowding within the mouth or congenital dental problems. The Poswillo report (Poswillo 1990) has resulted in dental extraction under general anaesthesia being carried out almost exclusively in hospitals. They must be licensed and carry the full range of monitoring and resuscitation equipment as well as trained anaesthetic staff

Surgery is typically carried out on a 'walk in, walk out' basis, and day-case rules should be applied rigidly. Preoperative assessment is carried out as usual, with particular reference to fasting and respiratory conditions (such as asthma). There is little opportunity for preoperative investigation or correction of abnormalities. During the preoperative visit a discussion with the child and guardian is vital. This gives the opportunity to explain the induction of anaesthesia and expectations for recovery. It is useful to add at this point that the child should not be restrained by theatre staff. A frank discussion should allay most fears, help to gain trust and reduce the number of children who simply run away!

Induction of anaesthesia may be intravenous or inhalational, but venous access should be obtained in all cases. Care should be taken with intravenous drugs because of the risks of unrecognised fainting on induction, leading to hypotension and cerebrovascular insufficiency. Inhalational induction is well tolerated in children, particularly if sevoflurane is used and a good rapport is obtained between anaesthetist and patient. The standard method involves 30–40% oxygen in nitrous oxide with sevoflurane, introduced via a nasal mask. Once the mouth can be opened without resistance a pack is inserted by the surgeon which should separate the mouth from the pharynx. The teeth are then removed. The anaesthetist must maintain the airway, ensure oxygenation and anaesthesia and monitor the patient. Once the teeth have been removed and the mouth cleared of debris the inhaled anaesthetic agents are turned off and 100% oxygen administered until the child is awake. Recovery should be in the lateral 'tonsillar' position so that blood and debris are not inhaled. Debate has continued about whether the sitting or the supine position is better or safer. The supine position avoids unrecognised major falls in blood pressure but encourages regurgitation, whereas the sitting position discourages regurgitation but increases the likelihood of unrecognised fainting on induction.

Older children may accept dental extraction with local anaesthesia, but if extractions are proposed in more than two quadrants of the mouth then it is unwise to do this all at one sitting because of the inevitable risk of total anaesthesia of the tongue and palate leading to obstruction or aspiration.

General anaesthesia may be necessary for conservative dentistry in those with severe learning difficulties. This may be a prolonged procedure involving multiple restorations and should be carried out with the airway protected by either an endotracheal tube or a laryngeal mask and an absorbent pack in place. Dental drills have an incorporated water spray, which can precipitate laryngeal spasm in the unprotected airway.

ENT surgery

ENT surgery also requires a shared airway, typical procedures being tonsillectomy and adenoidectomy, where the surgeon is both operating in the airway and causing bleeding from it. Adenoidectomy in isolation requires the airway to be maintained via the mouth, either by tracheal tube or by laryngeal mask. Suction clearance of the mouth at the end of the procedure should be carried out under direct vision. Tonsillectomy in isolation may be carried out using either a nasotracheal tube or a laryngeal mask airway. The latter will require the surgeon's compliance. Suction at the end must again be carried out under direct vision, but gently, so as not to disturb the tonsillar bed. The posterior nasal space in particular should be cleared of a potential 'coroner's clot'. In both of these cases postoperative analgesia should be provided parenterally before the recovery phase. There are advocates of both spontaneous and controlled ventilation for these procedures.

Anaesthesia for myringotomy or suction clearance of the ears can be relatively simple, using intravenous or inhalational induction with face mask or laryngeal mask for airway maintenance. Most patients are best recovered in the lateral position on a tipping trolley, or alternatively with a pillow under the thorax in the 'tonsil' position (Figure 5.14). Some patients will need to return to theatre

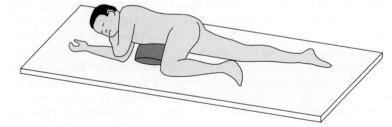

Figure 5.14 'Tonsil' position, with pillow under thorax

Figure 5.15 Return to theatre with bleeding tonsil

Clinical problem	Blood in stomach, risk of aspiration Distress (child and parents) Hypovolaemic shock Pain
Immediate management	Airway – provide supplementary oxygen Breathing – tachypnoea is a bad sign Circulation – secure IV access, send FBC, cross-match blood Resuscitate as you go Call for help Prepare theatre and surgical team
Conduct of anaesthesia	Potential difficult airway (poor view due to bleeding) Need second experienced anaesthetist RSI versus inhalational induction Keep warm Continue resuscitation Recovery, assess volume status Recovery in tonsillar position Consider NG aspiration of gastric contents before waking Keep in theatre until completely happy (the ward will thank you!)

in an emergency as a result of a post-tonsillectomy bleed (Figure 5.15).

Ophthalmic surgery

Ophthalmic surgery in the over-5s is usually for squint surgery or penetrating eye injury, probing and syringing of lachrymal ducts being confined to younger children.

Squint surgery is usually carried out as a day case, though the facility for overnight stay should always be available. Preoperative assessment should be as rigorous as for any other form of surgery. Induction of anaesthesia should include a weight-related dose of a vagolytic drug such as glycopyrrolate to prevent the severe bradycardia which results from even gentle traction on the extraocular muscles. Induction may be by the inhaled or intravenous route. Squint correction causes the same airway access

problems for the anaesthetist as other head and neck surgery. The choice of tracheal intubation or laryngeal mask airway is largely a matter of personal preference, though tracheal tubes cause much more emergence laryngospasm than do laryngeal mask airways. Ventilation may be controlled or spontaneous. Postoperative analgesia may be provided by topical local anaesthetic agents, oral paracetamol or NSAIDs.

Child protection

Abuse takes many forms: physical, neglect, sexual and psychological (Figure 5.16). It also includes fabricated or induced illness. The anaesthetist may recognise non-accidental injury (NAI) because of his or her close involvement in the care of children from admission to discharge. NAI is not uncommon (about 7% in population), but sadly too often missed. Head trauma is the commonest presentation of abuse, particularly in young children, who may present in the resuscitation department or for a CT scan. The anaesthetist must maintain a high index of suspicion when there is an unusual presentation or unexplained elements in the history of injury, including abnormal/atypical clinical signs (e.g. atypical bruising patterns). In such circumstances the anaesthetist must always act in the best interests of the child.

All anaesthetists are required to undergo training in the safeguarding of children and must be aware of the local policy for dealing with suspected cases of abuse. This normally involves gathering information and escalating the concern to a senior clinician/paediatrician or the designated clinical lead in child protection. The senior clinician/child protection lead can help decide whether there is a safeguarding issue, and if concerns are unresolved can notify the relevant child protection team. The child and his or her carers must be dealt with in an appropriate and sensitive manner throughout the process. Confidentiality still applies when you are 'considering' maltreatment, and sharing of sensitive information should be with the consent of the child/carer unless this would endanger the child. Advice should be sought from an experienced authority in the hospital, such as the Caldicott Guardian or medical director, or from a professional defence organisation. Contemporaneous, accurate, legible, written documentation of all findings, discussions and decisions is crucial.

The 2012 GMC document *Protecting Children and Young People* sets out clear principles for all doctors regarding the safety and wellbeing of children (Figure 5.17).

Figure 5.16 Clinical presentation of child abuse (NICE 2009)

Physical	Neglect	Sexual	Psychological	Fabricated
Bites	Poor hygiene and	Anogenital	Withdrawn	Symptoms and signs
Abrasions	clothing	injuries	Aggression	inconsistent with
Lacerations	Failure to provide	STIs	Eating	history
Scars	appropriate	Inappropriate	disorders	Evidence of failure of
Thermal	supervision	behaviour	Drug taking	treatment
injuries	Malnutrition	Pregnancy	Self-harm	Unexplained prolonged
Burns	Failure to care for		Domestic	illness
(cigarette)	medically		violence	Fabricated or
Scalds	Immunisation		Running away	misleading information
Cold injuries	Screening		from home	
Hypothermia	Dental caries			
Fractures				
Head injuries				
Spinal				
trauma				
Visceral				
injuries				
Oral injury				
Poisoning				

Figure 5.17 Guiding principles of child protection

All children and young people have a right to be protected from abuse and neglect

All doctors must consider the needs and wellbeing of children and young people

Children and young people are individuals with rights

Children and young people have a right to be involved in their own care

Decisions made about children and young people must be made in their best interests

Children, young people and their families have a right to receive confidential medical care and advice

Decisions about child protection are best made with others

Doctors must be competent and work within their competence to deal with child protection issues

The elderly patient

Population demographics are changing. The median age of many populations worldwide is increasing. Elderly patients more regularly need surgery than their younger counterparts, have more coexisting disease, and have greater morbidity (Figure 5.18). Health care in the next 30 years is going to be dominated by care of the elderly. As a population group there are a number of differences that require special attention by the anaesthetist. In terms of clinical evidence, the elderly in the past have been under-represented in clinical trials, being typically excluded on the basis of age or pre-existing disease.

Perioperative care of the elderly patient requires a careful preoperative assessment that attends to problems associated with the acute condition, pre-existing conditions, current functional status and those issues relating to the ageing process. It must not be forgotten that these patients require just the same risk discussions that apply to younger patients. Identical ethical principles apply in their treatment. Deliberations on what is the best course of action should always involve (where possible) the patient themselves, their family or advocates as well as the surgical team. They have an equal right to treatment with dignity and respect in a safe and caring environment as any patient, regardless of their age or illness. Intraoperative care should attend to the difficulties listed above, and postoperative care is the same as in any age group. It is a fallacy that the elderly suffer less pain from

Figure 5.18 Physiological, psychological and sociological changes associated with ageing

Gross change	Specific element	Derangement	Clinical effect
Physiological	Respiratory	Increased $\dot{V}/\dot{Q}$ mismatch Increased venous admixture Closing capacity within tidal ventilation range when supine	Reduced pulmonary reserve to hypoxaemia
		Reduced central response to hypoxaemia and hypercarbia	Increased apnoeas and respiratory depression
	Airway	Edentulous Reduction in upper airway tone Degenerative cervical spine changes	Difficulty in maintaining airway Increased OSA Limited neck movement
	Cardiovascular	Impaired autonomic nervous system Reduced baroreceptor response Reduced β-receptor sensitivity Reduced atrial pacemaker cells Poor venous access	Hypotension on induction or central neuroaxial blockade Reduced response to β-agonists and anticholinergics Atrial fibrillation, reduced maximal heart rate Bruising, extravasation, infection
	Renal	Impaired salt and water homeostasis Reduction in cortical glomeruli	Tendency to fluid overload/ dehydration and increased risk of renal impairment
	Musculoskeletal	Reduced muscle bulk Reduced soft tissue Arthritis and reduced mobility	Tendency to pressure sores Damage to fragile skin Difficulty and danger in patient positioning
	Neurological	Reduced vision Impaired hearing Autonomic disturbance Dementia (20% of those over 80) Impaired balance	Communication difficulties, impairment of cognition Impaired thermoregulation Increased mortality Increased falls
Pharmacological	Pharmacokinetic	Prolonged elimination half-life Reduction in hepatic/ renal elimination Increased volume of	Prolonged duration of action Potential increased dosing intervals

Figure 5.18 (*cont.*)

Gross change	Specific element	Derangement	Clinical effect
		distribution of lipophilic drugs	
	Pharmacodynamic	Reduced protein binding Reduced circulating volume	Increased drug effect
	Induction agents	Increased sensitivity	Reduced dose needed
		Prolonged arm–brain circulation time	Slower induction time
	Inhalational agents	MAC values reduced	Age-related MAC should be used
	Neuromuscular blockers	Reduced clearance and cardiac output Increase in extra junctional receptors	If reduced dose given, will take longer to work, but offset time similar
Sociological	Home environment	Adaptations needed to facilitate tasks of daily living	Increased dependence on external care Delays in hospital discharge due to poorly suitable home arrangements

surgical procedures. However, it may not present in the same way. A high index of suspicion is required. The requirement for good analgesia is just as great.

Postoperative cognitive deficit

Although it is not unique to an elderly population, age above 60 years is an independent risk factor for cognitive decline following anaesthesia. Pre-existing poor education, trauma and severity of surgery also contribute to the risk. Cognitive change is still underestimated in the inpatient population.

Cognition is the process whereby a person is able to process information in order to make a decision. Disorders of cognition can be categorised as delirium, postoperative cognitive decline (POCD) or dementia. The disorders vary in their presentation and time frame. Delirium commonly occurs within days of surgical/anaesthetic insult and can be either hypoactive (more common) or hyperactive in its clinical picture. A delirious patient is classically inattentive to their environment and surroundings. It is particularly common after hip fracture surgery. Emergence delirium is common at extremes of age. POCD is a more subtle condition with no consistent

definition and as such is underdiagnosed. It may occur weeks after the event and can persist indefinitely. The incidence may be up to 30% after non-cardiac surgery. It encompasses an impairment of cognitive functions, including memory, learning, concentration and speed of mental processing.

Meta-analysis has not shown a statistically proven causal link between general anaesthesia and the incidence of delirium or POCD. There is a growing body of evidence to link surgery and anaesthesia with dementia, although no causal link has yet been found. Anaesthetic agents produce long-term changes in gene and protein expression extending beyond the duration of clinical anaesthesia. They also activate numerous biochemical processes, including apoptotic pathways mediating cell death. Volatile agents have been proven to affect Alzheimer's pathogenesis both in vitro and in animal studies. This has raised concerns, particularly when anaesthetising patients in whom the brain is already damaged or is still developing.

Numerous tests exist for the diagnosis of cognition disorders, delirium (e.g. confusion assessment method, CAM) and dementia. Current therapies are lacking, antipsychotics are still indicated in acute delirium

Figure 5.19 Strategies to reduce incidence of POCD

Preoperative	Assessment of risk Assessment of pre-existing cognitive state	Normalise physiology Avoid prolonged starvation Continue normal medication as able Patient education
Intraoperative	Normalise physiology	Normothermia, normoxia, normocarbia
Postoperative	Minimise sedation	Short-acting agents – remifentanil, dexmedetomidene Avoid benzodiazepines
	Maximise sleep	Day/night cycles Melatonin
	Physical rehabilitation	Daily activity, both mental and physical Minimise invasive lines
	Prevention of pain, distress	Analgesia, avoidance of opioids
	Environment	Minimise noise Glasses Hearing aids Communication Virtual reality (creates pleasant surroundings with which patient can interact)

(haloperidol, olanzapine) and benzodiazepines should be avoided. Future treatments will rely on neuroprotection by identification of those at risk, normalisation of sleep physiology, new minimal sedation strategies and changes to the perioperative environment (Figure 5.19).

The head-injured patient

Applied physiology

The Monro–Kellie doctrine stipulates that the cranial cavity is a closed, rigid box containing brain tissue, extracellular fluid, cerebrospinal fluid (CSF) and blood. A primary brain injury causes an increase in the volume of a space-occupying lesion (e.g. tumour, blood or oedema) at the expense of the rest. The brain itself, being mostly water, is relatively incompressible. Initially any small incremental change in volume inside the cavity will be compensated for by changes in CSF or blood volume, cushioning the pressure effect of the insult. Later, if the space-occupying lesion increases in size, or causes obstruction to CSF flow, the compliance of the intracranial contents is reduced and so the pressure increase continues unbuffered. Pressure rises rapidly, directly distorting nerve tracts, producing a secondary insult by reducing cerebral blood flow (CBF) to the injured brain. Cerebral ischaemia ensues, and if untreated this will result in irreversible brain cell death.

Figure 5.20 Factors affecting cerebral blood flow

Drugs	All volatile anaesthetic agents cause dose-dependent cerebral vasodilatation and abolition of autoregulation Ketamine increases CBF All other IV induction agents reduce CBF Opioids (mediated by changes in $PaCO_2$)
Metabolic	Flow increases to metabolically active areas
Chemical	$PaCO_2$, PaO_2 (see text)
Temperature	Hypothermia reduces CBF
Pressure	Autoregulation, intracranial pressure, cerebral perfusion pressure
Neural	Sympathetic, parasympathetic control

In the normal (uninjured) brain CBF is affected by several factors (Figure 5.20). Normal cerebral blood flow is 50 mL 100 g^{-1} min^{-1}.

Arterial PCO$_2$

A relatively linear response exists at PaCO$_2$ values of 2.6–10.7 kPa. At the lower end of this range CBF will be half normal, and correspondingly double at the higher end. Reduced PaCO$_2$ decreases both cerebral blood flow and intracranial pressure (ICP), mediated by CSF pH. After a step change in PaCO$_2$, the CSF bicarbonate concentration returns to normal over the next 24 hours, and the ICP and CBF return to normal even if the change in PaCO$_2$ is maintained. Hyperventilation and artificial lowering of PaCO$_2$ creates cerebral vasoconstriction and was previously used in the short term to reduce ICP. However, there is grade II evidence that hypocapnia in the first 24 hours after injury is bad for the patient, as the accompanying cerebral vasoconstriction worsens regional ischaemia in the brain.

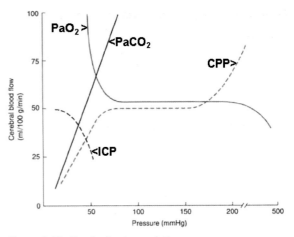

Figure 5.21 Cerebral autoregulation

Arterial PO$_2$

A small decrease in CBF occurs with the administration of 100% oxygen. Hyperbaric oxygenation in humans decreases CBF. Hypoxia, on the other hand, if severe (PaO$_2$ < 6 kPa), is a potent stimulator of arteriolar dilatation and greatly increases CBF.

Cerebral perfusion pressure

Cerebral perfusion pressure (CPP) is calculated as the mean arterial pressure (MAP) minus the sum of intracranial pressure and central venous pressure (ICP + CVP). It is the pressure that drives CBF. The normal value is around 60–70 mmHg. Regional ischaemia may occur at any pressure, but evidence suggests outcomes are poor if CPP is 30–40 mmHg or systolic blood pressure < 90 mmHg. Autoregulation maintains steady CBF between CPP values of 50 and 150 mmHg (Figure 5.21). This range is shifted upwards in the hypertensive patient. In cases of raised ICP the normal physiological response is the Cushing's reflex, which produces arterial hypertension in an attempt to maintain CPP.

Intracranial pressure

Raised ICP will obviously reduce CBF, and raised venous pressure secondarily raises ICP, with the same net result. Sudden rises in venous pressure during coughing or straining may cause serious falls in CBF, putting cerebral perfusion at risk in the compromised brain. Normal ICP is around 5–13 mmHg.

Temperature

Each degree Celsius of temperature drop reduces CBF by 5%, as well as reducing the cerebral metabolic rate for oxygen. Similarly, rises in temperature increase CBF and oxygen consumption. The therapeutic use of induced hypothermia in traumatic brain injury is still the topic of current research, but completed studies do not recommend its use outside of a well-conducted clinical trial.

Drugs

The anaesthetic induction agents, with the exception of ketamine, reduce CBF and cerebral metabolism. Ketamine and the inhalational agents cause rises in CBF via a vasodilator effect, with consequent increases in ICP. Inhalational anaesthesia is ideally avoided in cases of raised ICP. If necessary, end-tidal concentrations should be monitored and kept below 1 MAC. Optimum anaesthetic conditions for a patient with a traumatic brain injury for either surgery or transfer are produced by use of a TIVA technique using propofol and remifentanil, with keen attention to maintenance of a suitable CPP.

Management of head injury

Head injury should be considered significant if there has been certain loss of consciousness (however brief). Information on the nature and mechanism of injury, the energy involved and whether there were deaths at scene are useful factors that can be used to assess the potential severity of trauma. Blood or CSF in the ear canal/nose or bruising around both eyes may imply a base of skull fracture with the accompanying risk of meningitis due to the ingress of pathogens. In closed head injury, even of a relatively minor nature, there is a variable amount of oedema and cerebral contusion. Functional disabilities may not be seen at an early stage, particularly in extremes of age, owing to either increased compliance of the skull or additional room due to brain atrophy.

As ICP rises, so CBF falls, and the conscious level will be reduced. The standard international assessment of cerebral function is the Glasgow coma scale (GCS) (Figure 5.22). This is a very useful indicator but should not be taken in isolation. The best response in all categories gives a maximum score of 15, indicating minimal injury, while the minimum score is 3, indicating a very poor state with a very poor outcome. Trends in GCS are more valuable than single estimations. Pupil responses are a valuable additional assessment when referring the patient for definitive care. Other injuries should be sought and excluded in the primary and secondary surveys, particularly those involving the spine.

The crux of immediate management in head injury is to avoid secondary injury. The primary injury has already occurred, and any damage done will be largely irreversible. Cerebral oedema develops around the injury site, and secondary injury must be avoided by reducing ICP (especially avoiding dramatic rises in ICP) and preventing further hypoxic damage. Ensuring adequate brain tissue oxygenation requires attention to detail and maintenance of normal PaO_2, $PaCO_2$, blood sugar and core temperature. Cerebral perfusion pressure must be maintained. Systolic blood pressure should not be allowed to drop below 90 mmHg. Without invasive ICP monitoring, we can assume that in traumatic brain injury the ICP is 20 mmHg at least.

A fundamental decision to be made is whether the patient requires tracheal intubation. Tracheal intubation allows control of oxygenation and ventilation in combination with airway protection. It also facilitates surgery to other parts of the body, as well as enabling investigations such as CT scanning or allowing transport to a definitive care facility to be conducted safely. In general, a GCS < 8 indicates the need for airway intervention and intensive care management, but a downward trend in GCS of more than 2 points would also be a warning to pre-emptively take control of the airway. In addition to the GCS, the pattern of respiration, pulse and blood pressure should be taken into consideration. Spontaneous hyperventilation indicates significantly raised ICP, as does arterial hypertension accompanied by bradycardia (Cushing reflex). **Control of ICP is of the utmost importance.** Uncontrollable confusion and irritability may indicate significant brain injury, and indicates the need for intervention. Indications for intubation after head injury are listed in Figure 5.23.

Figure 5.22 Glasgow coma scale

Category	Score
Eye opening	
spontaneous	4
to voice	3
to pain	2
none	1
Verbal response	
orientated	5
confused	4
inappropriate	3
incomprehensible	2
none	1
Motor response	
obeys commands	6
localising to pain	5
withdrawing	4
flexing	3
extending	2
none	1
Total	Min = 3, max = 15

Practical technique

By and large, secondary brain injury may be minimised by good oxygenation and airway management and by avoiding rises in ICP, particularly as a result of an unmodified pressor response to intubation. Although it might appear that unconscious patients do not need to be anaesthetised before intubation, **this is not so**. In this particular situation induction agents are used not primarily for the abolition of consciousness but to reduce ICP before intubation. Intubation without previous pharmacological reduction of ICP or without modification of the

Figure 5.23 Indications for intubation and ventilation for transfer after brain injury

Coma – not obeying commands, not speaking, no eye opening, i.e. GCS $\leq$ 8
Significantly deteriorating conscious level (i.e. fall in motor score of 2 points or more)
Loss of protective laryngeal reflexes
Hypoxaemia (PaO$_2$ < 13 kPa on oxygen)
Hypercarbia (PaCO$_2$ > 6 kPa)
Spontaneous hyperventilation causing PaCO$_2$ < 4.0 kPa
Bilateral fractured mandible
Copious bleeding into the mouth (e.g. from skull base fracture)
Seizures
An intubated patient should be ventilated with muscle relaxation, and should receive appropriate sedation and analgesia. Aim for a PaO$_2$ > 13 kPa, PaCO$_2$ 4.0–4.5 kPa unless there is clinical or radiological evidence of raised ICP, when more aggressive hyperventilation is justified to a PaCO$_2$ of not less than 4 kPa. If hyperventilation is used the F$_I$O$_2$ should be increased.

Association of Anaesthetists of Great Britain and Ireland. *Recommendations for the Safe Transfer of Patients with Brain Injury.* London: AAGBI, 2006.

pressor response may cause more damage than the original injury and **should be avoided at all costs**. The sympathoadrenal response to intubation may be minimised by the administration of an adequate dose of induction agent accompanied by an opioid such as fentanyl or a target-controlled infusion (TCI) of remifentanil.

The appropriate muscle relaxant to use for intubation is potentially controversial. Rapid intubation is desirable but suxamethonium can cause a significant rise in ICP. This is certainly the case in the normal brain, but recent work suggests that it may not be the case in the injured (and therefore less compliant) brain. The rise in ICP may be an effect of the drug itself rather than the fasciculations it causes. The fasciculations of suxamethonium may be modified or abolished by pre-curarisation with a small dose of a non-depolarising relaxant (5–10 mg atracurium)

or by pretreatment with 0.1 mg kg^{-1} suxamethonium, both of which may inhibit intubating conditions.

The non-depolarising relaxants are, therefore, preferable in terms of ICP management, but the risk of aspiration must be carefully weighed against any minor advantage in ICP control. A solution lies in the administration of a large dose of a non-depolarising relaxant such as rocuronium (0.9 mg kg^{-1}), given after careful preoxygenation and the application of cricoid pressure.

Subsequently, ventilation of the lungs, if necessary, must be maintained by face mask or laryngeal mask airway until the relaxant reaches maximum clinical effect, so as to avoid coughing and movement, which will increase ICP even more than intubation itself. Once intubation has been safely achieved the pressor response to the presence of the tube must also be modified to control ICP. This can be achieved by adequate sedation or general anaesthesia with controlled ventilation. Inhalational agents (sevoflurane/isoflurane) can be used, but the dose should be restricted to less than 1 MAC because of their cerebral vasodilator effect. Anaesthesia is best maintained by a total intravenous technique (TIVA) using propofol and remifentanil. If possible, fluid loading should be restricted or avoided. Excessive crystalloid resuscitation may increase cerebral oedema. Intravenous mannitol or hypertonic saline, based on neurosurgical advice, may be used to reduce cerebral oedema and critical ICP in a crisis. They should not be given unless a urinary catheter is in situ, because the stimulation from a full bladder may increase ICP and also anaesthetic dose requirements.

Monitoring should conform to the accepted minimum monitoring standards and should include blood pressure (ideally invasive), pulse oximetry and end-tidal CO$_2$ analysis. Where possible the patient should be tilted 15° head-up to aid venous drainage of the head. The tube is better taped, to avoid ties around the neck constricting venous return. Loss from scalp wounds may be significant in itself and should not be forgotten, particularly in children.

Transfer of the head-injured patient

Head-injured patients and those with suspected intracranial haemorrhage may require transfer between hospitals, either for CT scanning or for definitive management of their injuries. This can be a difficult and dangerous enterprise and should be carried out with the greatest of care. Facilities in ambulances, helicopters and scanning rooms are limited, as is space, but nevertheless the management of the airway and ICP must take precedence over speed or convenience. The patient must be stabilised before transfer. A clear and concise discussion should occur, and should be documented, between the referring and accepting centres so that no confusion regarding optimum management occurs. The escort and their assistant must be capable of managing the predictable eventualities – reintubation, hypertension, hypotension and raised ICP – and thus must take with them sufficient equipment, drugs and fluids to maintain anaesthesia and relaxation. Ambulances should be able to travel quickly but smoothly, without the severe decelerations of fast travel. Monitoring should include invasive blood pressure, ECG, pulse oximetry and end-tidal CO_2 measurement. For CT scanning, there must be appropriate equipment in the scanning room. An anaesthetic machine with automatic ventilator, piped gases and full monitoring are essential. On arrival, the transferring team should give a thorough and accurate handover before leaving so that no crucial details are lost. The AAGBI have published specific guidelines on the transfer of the brain-injured patient, as summarised in Figure 5.24.

The day-case patient

There has been a huge push in recent years to perform more surgeries as day-case procedures, with obvious benefits to both hospital and patient. Up to 75% of elective cases could potentially be performed under this plan. The modern day-case unit is often a standalone, sometimes remote, 23-hour unit. Most patients will be admitted and discharged on the same day, even within a few hours of surgery and complete recovery from anaesthesia. For the patient, this means the shortest possible time away from the work or home environment and as little disruption as possible to their social circumstances. Some patients may stay overnight in hospital if necessary because of unresolved medical issues, for surgical reasons, or owing to lack of social support at home.

Since their inception the day-case criteria have been progressively changed, and now many patients previously deemed unsuitable are undergoing more complicated surgeries (e.g. laparoscopic abdominal surgery and minor spinal surgery) as day-case patients.

Anaesthesia and surgery remain major insults to a patient's physiology, however minor they may appear, and thus there must be rigorous policies and protocols for the day surgery unit, with patients carefully selected with regard to fitness and type of surgery.

The criteria to be applied fall into several categories:
- Social circumstances
- Surgical procedure
- Medical fitness
- Anaesthetic technique
- Admission facilities

Social circumstances

The patient's social circumstances must provide a safe environment for the postoperative care of a recently anaesthetised patient, even if the procedure has been carried out under local anaesthetic or sedation only. For the first 24 hours after anaesthesia, there must be a responsible adult present on the premises to care for the patient and to manage untoward events. The patient must be brought to, and taken from, hospital by a responsible adult. He or she must live within easy travelling distance of the hospital in case of urgent readmission (this is usually taken as within 30 minutes' to 1 hour's travelling time). Patients must not go home by public transport, and preferably not by taxi. If these criteria cannot be fulfilled then the surgery must be carried out on an inpatient basis. If the patient arrives for day surgery without these criteria being satisfied then the operation should be cancelled and admission reorganised. Part of the admission process must be to check that these criteria have been satisfied.

Specific advice should be given to each patient concerning postoperative welfare. The patient must be told to avoid alcohol for 24 hours postoperatively, because the depressant effect of alcohol acts synergistically with the residual anaesthetic drugs and, especially if barbiturate anaesthetics are used, may cause unconsciousness. Patients must be told not to drive vehicles or operate machinery, because their physical and mental reactions may not be good enough to keep them out of danger. Car insurance may be invalidated by driving under the residual influence of anaesthetics, and the police may charge the driver with driving under the influence of drugs. They should not cook or be involved in baby care. Lifetime or important decisions should not be made in the postoperative period, because patients may be residually disinhibited.

Preoperatively the day-case patient must be told these rules in front of a witness, or must sign a form to say that they have been read while not under the influence of anaesthetic drugs. The responsible escorting adult must also understand these rules.

Figure 5.24 Transfer checklist for a head-injured patient

System	Checklist
Respiration	$PaO_2 > 13$ kPa?
	$PaCO_2 < 5$ kPa?
	Airway clear?
	Airway protected adequately?
	Intubation and ventilation required?
Circulation	BP mean > 80 mmHg? (adults)
	Pulse < 100 per minute? (adults)
	Peripheral perfusion?
	Two reliable large IV cannulae in situ?
	Estimated blood loss already replaced?
	Arterial line?
	Central venous access if appropriate?
Head injury	GCS?
	GCS trend? (improving/deteriorating)
	Focal signs?
	Skull fracture?
	Seizures controlled?
	Raised ICP appropriately managed?
Other injuries	Cervical spine injury (cervical spine protection), chest injury, fractured ribs, pneumothorax excluded?
	Intrathoracic, intra-abdominal bleed?
	Pelvic, long bone fracture?
	Extracranial injuries splinted?
Escort	Doctor and escort adequately experienced?
	Instructed about this case?
	Adequate equipment and drugs?
	Can use equipment and drugs?
	Sufficient oxygen supplies?
	Case notes and x-rays?
	Transfer documentation prepared?
	Where to go in the neurosurgical unit?
	Telephone numbers programmed into mobile phone?
	Mobile phone battery fully charged?
	Name and bleep number of receiving doctor?
	Money in case of emergencies?

Association of Anaesthetists of Great Britain and Ireland. *Recommendations for the Safe Transfer of Patients with Brain Injury*. London: AAGBI, 2006.

Surgical procedure

The types of surgery suitable for day-case work include those with only minor disturbances of nutrition, which last only a short time (usually taken to be less than 1 hour of anaesthesia) and which do not typically require opioid analgesia afterwards. Surgery where significant blood loss is predicted, or where the abdomen is electively opened, is not suitable (except for laparoscopic surgery). Surgery where there will be major limitation of mobility is not suitable. Unilateral inguinal hernia repair may be suitable (especially if local anaesthesia is employed), but bilateral repair is usually not. Surgery should only be carried out by surgeons experienced in the procedure in question. Figure 5.25 indicates some procedures that may be suitable for day-case work, other factors being satisfied.

Medical fitness

Patients must be ASA 1 or 2 (see Chapter 1, Figure 1.2). Age is not necessarily a restriction subject to arrangements between the patient, the anaesthetist and the surgeon. If it is planned to carry out surgery on small children (3 years old or more in a district general hospital) organisationally it is better to arrange a full list of children with a paediatric trained nurse in attendance rather than to have children interspersed within an adult list (Department of Health 1991).

Drug-controlled diabetic patients pose a particular challenge, and guidance on their suitability is summarised later in this chapter (see *Diabetes mellitus*, under *The metabolically compromised patient*). It is recommended that these patients are done first on the morning list or early afternoon list, and that they should only miss one meal and have their medications adjusted accordingly. Essential hypertension is not necessarily a contraindication, provided control is good. Cardiovascular diseases such as angina, cardiac failure or arrhythmias are unacceptable. Controlled atrial fibrillation may be an exception to this if stable and treated.

Obesity is not acceptable (criteria differ, but body weight > 110 kg or body mass index > 35 may be taken as exclusion guidelines). These rules apply to regional anaesthesia and general anaesthesia equally.

Anaesthetic technique
Intraoperative

Anaesthesia should be restricted to simple techniques with proven good recovery characteristics, particularly in terms of postoperative nausea and vomiting and

Figure 5.25 Operations suitable for day stay

General surgery	Unilateral hernia repair
	Unilateral varicose veins (not prone)
	Sebaceous cysts
	Small benign breast lumps
	Child circumcision
Urology	Cystoscopy (± biopsy)
	Diathermy to small bladder tumours
	Hydrocoele
	Varicocoele
	Vasectomy
Gynaecology	Diagnostic laparoscopy
	Laparoscopic test of tubal patency
	Termination of pregnancy
Ophthalmology	Probing of tear ducts
	Cataract surgery (rigid application of other criteria)
	Squint surgery (single eye)
Orthopaedics	Arthroscopy (minor arthroscopic surgery)
	Joint/back manipulation
Oral surgery	Removal of third molars
ENT	Myringotomy
	Antral washout
	Nasal polypectomy
	Nasal septoplasty
	Direct laryngoscopy and pharyngoscopy
Haematology	Blood sampling and chemotherapy

analgesia. Techniques that employ regional analgesia are particularly suitable, provided that mobility is not restricted by the local block (Figure 5.26).

Figure 5.26 Regional anaesthesia and day-case surgery

Ophthalmic surgery	Peribulbar and sub-tenon blocks
	Topical anaesthesia
Orthopaedic surgery	Interscalene
	Axillary
	Individual nerve blocks
	Metacarpal/tarsal and ring blocks (fingers, toes) Ankle block
General surgery	Caudal for orchidopexy, hernias
	Penile block for circumcision
	Ilioinguinal and iliohypogastric Transverse abdominal plane (laparoscopic, hernias, gynaecology)
Dental surgery	Inferior alveolar nerve, infiltration

If ambulant patients are discharged with paralysed, insensate limbs specific printed advice regarding care of the limb should be given. Spinal anaesthesia and femoral nerve blockade are considered unsuitable because of the major inhibition of mobility that results. Caudal analgesia is acceptable in small children, but for circumcision a penile block provides good postoperative analgesia without motor effects. Spinal anaesthesia in ambulatory young people is notorious for post-dural puncture headache and for postural hypotension and should be avoided. Elective tracheal intubation should be carefully considered because of the risk of laryngeal oedema (and major nasal haemorrhage if nasal intubation is employed), but, having said that, the laryngeal mask has not yet superseded its routine use for day-stay removal of third molar teeth. Elective controlled ventilation is no longer contraindicated in day surgery because of the advent of short-acting mivacurium and sugammadex that also allows complete reversal of rocuronium-induced muscle relaxation. The use of neostigmine may reduce the likelihood of patient discharge because of its autonomic and central nervous effects. The laryngeal mask makes day-case controlled ventilation feasible where it would not otherwise be so. Thiopental is not a suitable induction agent for day-case general anaesthesia, whereas propofol is indicated because of the relatively rapid recovery without significant hangover.

Postoperative

Pain should be controlled by the use of regional anaesthetic techniques with the addition of paracetamol, non-steroidal anti-inflammatory drugs (NSAIDs) and weak opioids where suitable. Rectal diclofenac is in widespread use but should be discussed with the patient preoperatively. Account must be taken of the fact that local anaesthesia will wear off after several hours. The patient should be encouraged to take moderate analgesics before the effect of the local anaesthetic wears off, and should be discharged with a suitable supply to take home.

Admission facilities

Wherever surgery is carried out on a day-stay basis there must always be the facility to admit the patient overnight. If that facility does not exist, either because there are no inpatient beds available or because the day unit is a remote site, then surgery should not proceed.

The usual anaesthetic reasons for overnight admission following day surgery are nausea and vomiting or pain requiring opioid analgesia. Complications of surgery are a common reason for admission, as is prolonged surgery with consequent slow postoperative recovery, usually because the criteria for day surgery have been breached, either by unsuitable surgery or by an unsuitable surgeon. Audit should be performed of the reasons for refusal of day-case surgery and the incidence and reasons for unplanned postoperative admission.

The morbidly obese patient

Sadly the incidence of obesity in the general adult UK population is increasing. Morbid obesity can be defined as a body mass index (BMI) of > 35 with comorbidity, or > 40 without comorbidity. The BMI is calculated by dividing the weight (kg) by the square of the height (m^2). Obesity is associated with hypertension, ischaemic heart disease, osteoarthritis, asthma, obstructive sleep apnoea, obesity hypoventilation syndrome and diabetes mellitus. The extent of disease may be hidden by a sedentary lifestyle, and this should be sought in the preoperative assessment.

Applied physiology

Oxygen consumption and the work of breathing are increased, while chest compliance and FRC are reduced. Tidal volume and closing volume may overlap while conscious, resulting in poor aeration and a tendency to hypoxia even at rest. These factors increase shunting and the incidence of hypoxia, and shunting is further increased when FRC is reduced by anaesthesia or positional changes on the operating table. Hypoxia is commonly seen because of these changes, and because of the tendency for the diaphragm to be elevated by pressure from abdominal wall fat. Postoperative hypoxia is particularly frequently encountered and, because of the failure to adequately expand the chest, the incidence of atelectasis and hypostatic infection increases. Obesity hypoventilation syndrome results from a central problem with control of ventilation. There is a diurnal variation in breathing and an insensitivity to increased $PaCO_2$. The result is hypoxaemia, exacerbated by anaesthetic drugs, pain and the supine position.

Blood volume and cardiac output are increased, increasing cardiac work. There is also a tendency to coronary artery disease that is exacerbated by lack of exercise. The increase in both intra-abdominal and abdominal wall fat increases the intra-abdominal pressure, raising the incidence of functional and anatomical hiatus hernia. The resting volume of gastric juice is also increased, as is its acidity. The increase in intra-abdominal pressure reduces venous return from the legs, predisposing to DVT and pulmonary embolism. There is a higher incidence of wound infection and wound dehiscence. Surgical access can be difficult because of the android (apple-shaped) distribution of fat.

Anaesthesia

For the anaesthetist there are often anatomical problems in establishing venous access, and central venous access may be required, which can itself be difficult. For the uninitiated, airway maintenance may be difficult because of the tendency to a short fat neck and, in females, protruding breasts. Intubation may also be difficult, and preoxygenation is recommended. Special equipment may assist in positioning the airway optimally (Figure 5.27). Chest compliance is reduced and so the work of ventilation increases, sometimes to the extent that mechanical ventilators may be unable to generate the inflation pressure necessary to achieve adequate tidal volumes. This can also be a problem if a laryngeal mask airway is used, because the inflation pressure may exceed the LMA leak pressure. The high inflation pressures necessary will further reduce venous return, and falls in cardiac output may be significant. Periods of desaturation occur rapidly in the obese patient and respond slowly to increased F_IO_2 and increased PEEP. Hypoxaemia often persists into the postoperative period, requiring additional oxygen, chest physiotherapy and possible CPAP or NiPPV. It is sensible to admit patients with a diagnosis of obstructive sleep apnoea (Figure 5.28) overnight where they can be closely monitored. They should bring and use their own CPAP machine while in hospital.

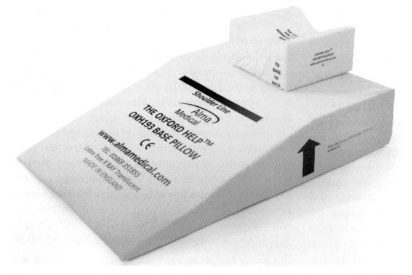

Figure 5.27 Oxford HELP (head elevating laryngoscopy pillow) system: the pillow ramps the patient up, aligning the external auditory meatus to the sternal notch, optimising the position for direct laryngoscopy. Reproduced courtesy of Alma Medical (www.almamedical.com)

Figure 5.28 Obstructive sleep apnoea (OSA)

Definition	Apnoeic episodes during sleep due to pharyngeal wall collapse
Causes	Central/mixed/obstructive
Diagnosis	Sleep studies
Features	Apnoeas (> 10 seconds) Hypopnoeas (> 5 per hour of sleep or 30 per night) Snoring Daytime somnolence Impaired concentration Morning headaches
Pathology	Hypoxaemia Hypercarbia Polycythaemia Pulmonary hypertension Right heart failure Type 2 respiratory failure

Non-invasive blood pressure measurements may give erroneous readings if the cuff size is not chosen correctly. A cuff that is too small will give falsely high readings. Regional anaesthetic techniques may be attractive but more difficult because of imprecise nerve location due to fat and loss of anatomical landmarks, and extra-long needles may be necessary. There is more fat in the epidural space and so **smaller doses of local anaesthetic agents** may produce the same effect as in the normal patient. Placing epidural and spinal needles can be particularly difficult because of the increased distance between skin and landmarks. The sitting position may help because the skin and bone midlines may come into opposition whereas in the lateral position these may be some distance apart, making the technique impossible. Finding bony landmarks with a standard hypodermic needle before inserting the epidural needle will improve the chances of success.

All induction agents and vapours are fat-soluble, and a significant proportion of the cardiac output supplies fat, so these drugs are diverted from the brain and into fat stores, increasing the requirement for induction agents and slowing the rise in brain concentration. Similarly, emergence may be slower because of the slower leaching of agents from the fat stores. This latter causes obese patients to be exposed to volatile agents for longer, thus increasing their biotransformation. Desflurane may be advantageous in these circumstances because of the low oil/gas Ostwald solubility coefficient. Some morbidly obese patients will require special equipment (such as operating tables and side extensions) to allow even simple surgeries to be conducted safely.

The metabolically compromised patient

Liver disease
Applied physiology
The liver is the largest organ in the body, receiving 30% of cardiac output. The majority of nutritional, haematological and detoxification metabolism occurs in the liver, including the breakdown or excretion of many anaesthetic drugs. Other physiological roles of the liver include the manufacture of proteins, lipoproteins and carbohydrates, including the clotting factors and the proteins to which most anaesthetic drugs are bound. Some globulins (α_1, α_2 and β) are produced in the liver, while γ-globulins are synthesised by the immune system. The liver also acts as a store for vitamins, minerals and carbohydrates. In the presence of significant liver disease, all these processes become disturbed.

Different conditions cause differing patterns of dysfunction. Excessive red cell turnover causes jaundice by overloading the pathways of haem breakdown even though other liver functions may remain relatively normal. Obstructive and cholestatic jaundice causes major disruption to metabolic pathways and to the absorption of fats and fat-soluble vitamins, causing further problems. Hepatocellular dysfunction may be toxic or infective in origin but will result in the same picture of unconjugated bilirubinaemia, fat malabsorption and metabolic disturbance. In the end stage of hepatic failure, virtually all the body's metabolic processes are disturbed. Clinical features include clotting failure, coma from ammonia toxicity because of disturbed protein metabolism, hypoglycaemia because of poor glycogen metabolism, water overload and major electrolyte imbalance. There is usually portal hypertension, which causes the formation of collateral circulation including oesophageal varices. If these bleed, then the sudden high protein meal provided by enteral haemoglobin may precipitate hepatic encephalopathy in an otherwise compensated patient, a desperate situation that may be irretrievable. Anaesthesia in liver disease is, therefore, not for the inexperienced.

Assessment of patients with liver disease
The cause of liver disease and involvement of other systems should be sought. Infectious patients should be

Figure 5.29 Risk of operative mortality: Pugh's modification to Child's criteria
(Child's A 5–6 points = < 5% risk of operative mortality, Child's B 7–9 points = 25% operative mortality, Child's C 10–15 points = > 50% risk of operative mortality)

Physiological variable	Points for worsening abnormality		
	1	2	3
Grade of encephalopathy	None	1–2	Advanced 3–4
Ascites	None	Easily managed	Poor control
Serum bilirubin (mg dL^{-1})	< 2	2–3	> 3
Serum albumin (g dL^{-1})	> 3.5	2.8–3.5	< 2.8
PT (seconds greater than control)	1–4	4–6	> 6

treated with universal precautions (see *Infective risk groups*, below). Signs of severe and decompensated disease should be documented, e.g. ascites, varices, effusions, jaundice and encephalopathy. The Pugh modification of Child's score estimates mortality in liver disease patients undergoing surgery (Figure 5.29).

Full haematological and biochemical screening results should be available to supplement clinical evaluation of the patient. Absorption of vitamin K from the gut depends entirely on the presence of bile salts, and so the synthesis of prothrombin (assessed by prothrombin time, PT) and other clotting factors, which depend on vitamin K, are sensitive barometers of liver function. Albumin has a long plasma half-life and so is an indicator of more chronic disease, when its value will be lowered. Transaminases are released from damaged hepatocytes, but as these enzymes are also present in other tissues this cannot be taken as specific to liver function (which also applies to alkaline phosphatase). Conjugated bilirubinaemia suggests obstructive jaundice whereas unconjugated bilirubinaemia suggests a prehepatic or hepatic cause. In the presence of established liver disease, anaesthetic agents and techniques must be chosen with care and with due consideration for disturbed metabolism, pharmacokinetics, and water and electrolyte balance (Figure 5.30).

Useful cardiac investigations include a 12-lead ECG and transthoracic echocardiography if physical examination reveals positive signs. A chest x-ray may reveal pleural effusions.

Fluids

Fluid and electrolyte balance must be meticulous, and blood glucose monitored frequently because of disturbed glycogen metabolism in the later stages of the disease. Large-bore IV access, a fluid warmer and a rapid infusion system are essential for any major surgery.

Anaesthetic technique

Standard general anaesthetic techniques may be used with care in liver disease. Hypoperfusion and hypoxaemia may worsen hepatocellular injury and should be avoided. Particular care should be taken if there is portal hypertension, as hepatic flow will depend mainly on hepatic artery flow. Invasive monitoring is mandatory in all major cases and should be considered in moderate/minor surgeries in patients with severe disease. Peripheral and central regional anaesthesia, including epidural and spinal techniques, are acceptable unless the INR is > 1.5 or there is significant thrombocytopenia. Specific component therapy may correct coagulation abnormalities as identified by laboratory tests or more usefully by near-patient thromboelastography. Temperature and neuromuscular monitoring are vital. Renal function is often disturbed in obstructive jaundice and is always affected in hepatic failure. Urine output must be encouraged to avoid the onset of renal failure in the postoperative period.

A note on repeat anaesthesia

In modern medicine many patients undergo repeat anaesthesia within hours and days of the original procedure without any additional complications. The dangers of a repeat halothane anaesthetic have all but completely disappeared in the UK. However, it is still used around the world and this should be considered if there is a history of recent travel to less developed countries.

Figure 5.30 Altered drug pharmacology in liver disease

Drug	Pharmacology
Benzodiazepines	Prolonged, intense effect – use with extreme caution Can precipitate encephalopathy
Opioids	Prolonged effect
Morphine	Reduced hepatic blood flow, and concurrent renal failure will delay metabolism/excretion Can precipitate encephalopathy Active metabolite (morphine-6-gluconoride)
Fentanyl	Generally safe in low doses as no active metabolites and renal excretion Will accumulate
Alfentanil	Reduced elimination, increased volume of distribution, reduced protein binding
Remifentanil	Perhaps ideal, metabolised by tissue and red cell esterases – preserved in severe liver disease
IV induction agents	Use with care
Thiopental	Reduce dose as increased free drug (reduced protein binding) and prolonged metabolism but increased distribution half-life
Propofol	Increased sensitivity to haemodynamic effects so reduce dose
Etomidate	Prolonged metabolism, little advantage over others
Muscle relaxants (NMBAs)	Monitor neuromuscular function
Suxamethonium/mivacurium	Action may be prolonged if plasma cholinesterase level reduced, clinically little difference
Non-depolarising relaxants	Apparent resistance despite decreased protein binding and excretion Increased volume of distribution
(Cis)Atracurium	Not dependent upon liver metabolism but instead upon non-specific esterases and Hoffman degradation – may have unpredictable effect particularly if significant acid/base disruption. Prolonged administration may produce toxic levels of laudanosine
Vecuronium/rocuronium	Prolonged elimination in severe disease
Pancuronium	Reduced biliary excretion will prolong effect
Volatile agents	Little effect
Halothane	Not specifically contraindicated (unless for other reasons) but usually avoided now because there are better alternatives
Local anaesthetics	Delayed excretion, coagulation abnormalities may limit regional anaesthesia

The main considerations at preoperative assessment for repeat anaesthesia are to identify, if possible, the anaesthetic technique used, the drugs involved and any related problems. Problems of particular interest are nausea and vomiting, difficult airway management, difficult intubation, drug reactions and the use of halothane.

Derangement of liver function following halothane exposure shows two clinical pictures. In type I hepatotoxicity, a mild and transient disturbance in liver function is seen, and this may be accompanied by mild pyrexia. Resolution is seen within a few days without permanent sequelae. It is suggested that the mechanism underlying this mild picture is the result of the phase 1 transformation products of halothane reacting directly with hepatic macromolecules to cause tissue necrosis. Other volatile agents are metabolised to a much lesser extent than halothane and do not cause type I hepatotoxicity. In type II hepatotoxicity, massive and fulminant hepatic necrosis occurs. Although it is rare, mortality is in the region of 40–70%. Type II hepatotoxicity appears to be immune-mediated. Halothane is oxidatively metabolised to produce trifluoroacetyl metabolites to an intermediate compound. These metabolites bind liver proteins and, in genetically susceptible patients, antibodies are formed to this metabolite (hapten)–protein complex. The antibodies in turn mediate subsequent cellular toxicity. Inactivation of cytochrome P450 (CYP) and neutrophil involvement are currently under investigation as other possible causes. The other volatile agents can also cause type II hepatotoxicity.

The Committee on Safety of Medicines (CSM), now replaced by the Commission on Human Medicines (CHM), issued a recommendation for the repeated use of halothane which stated that it should not be used within 3 months of a previous administration unless there is an overwhelming clinical reason for the second use, and that it should not be used if there was unexplained pyrexia or jaundice within 1 week after a previous exposure.

Even though a patient may be a regular patient, it is important to go through a full preoperative assessment each time because there is always the possibility of new intercurrent disease, particularly in the elderly.

Renal disease
Applied physiology

The kidneys excrete water, electrolytes, water-soluble drugs and water-soluble products of metabolism. Plasma electrolytes, urea, creatinine and estimated glomerular filtration rate (eGFR) provide an indication of renal function. While the plasma urea also depends on liver function, the creatinine concentration also depends on the level of protein metabolism in the body. Renal dysfunction causes multiple problems for the anaesthetist (Figure 5.31). For the plasma creatinine to rise, renal function must be < 30% of normal. As renal function is reduced below this the creatinine and urea will rise. Electrolyte abnormalities typically include sodium and water retention, hyperkalaemia (> 6 mmol L^{-1}), hypocalcaemia, hypermagnesaemia and hyperphosphataemia.

A failure to excrete organic acids and make bicarbonate produces a metabolic acidosis which worsens hyperkalaemia. The production of new red cells is depressed by reductions in erythropoietin secretion. There is accompanying platelet dysfunction despite normal laboratory tests of coagulation.

A failure to metabolise or excrete protein and amino acid by-products creates uraemia. Uraemia has widespread metabolic effects that when combined with the failure of the endocrine functions of the kidney ultimately lead to death. Therapies for end-stage kidney failure (ESKF) include renal transplant, ambulatory peritoneal dialysis and haemodialysis.

Renal failure can be acute or chronic in onset. The cause of renal impairment can be usefully divided into pre-renal, renal and post-renal pathologies (Figure 5.32). In established chronic kidney disease (CKD) the GFR will be less than 10% of normal (20 mL min^{-1}) and in ESKF < 5% (10 mL min^{-1}).

Figure 5.31 Pathophysiological abnormalities encountered in chronic kidney disease

Biochemical	Clinical	Endocrine/metabolic
Hyper/ hyponatraemia	Ischaemic heart disease	Secondary hyperparathyroidism
Hyperkalaemia	Hypertension	Disruption of renin/angiotensin mechanism
Hypocalcaemia	Autonomic neuropathy	Normochromic, normocytic anaemia
Hyperphosphataemia	Nausea	Inhibition of cell-mediated immunity and humoral
Hypermagnesaemia	Poor wound healing	defence mechanisms
Water overload	Gastric paresis	Impairment of vitamin D metabolism
Hypoalbuminaemia	Peptic ulcer disease	
	Peripheral neuropathy	

Figure 5.32 Causes of renal failure

Pre-renal	Hypovolaemia Renal vascular disease Diabetes Hypertension Infection (sepsis) Hepatorenal syndrome
Renal	Drugs/toxins Glomerular disease Tubular disease Trauma Polycystic kidney disease Tumour Infection (pyelonephritis)
Post-renal	Obstruction (stones, tumour, prostate)

Figure 5.33 Drugs to be used with extreme caution in renal failure

β-Blockers
ACE inhibitors
Potassium-sparing diuretics
NSAIDs
Angiotensin antagonists
Antimicrobials (aminoglycosides, ciclosporin)

Anaesthetic technique and drugs

All patients should be assessed for biochemical abnormality, acid–base status and fluid status. Patients presenting with renal failure can be hypervolaemic pre-dialysis and significantly hypovolaemic immediately post-dialysis. A period of stability should be allowed to occur after dialysis before operating, if the urgency of the surgery will allow it. Emergency renal replacement therapy may be required perioperatively, to treat uraemic encephalopathy, severe acidosis, and cardiac failure due to fluid overload and significant/symptomatic hyperkalaemia.

Patients in renal failure (even if mild) should not be transfused to correct their anaemia unless there is a situation of acute blood loss. To do so will precipitate cardiac failure by volume overload and will suppress the production of normal red cells. Owing to changes in 2,3-DPG concentration, stored red cells do not carry oxygen at their full capacity for some 24 hours after transfusion, and so the effect of transfusion can be a reduction of oxygen delivery to the tissues.

Care should be taken to avoid those drugs that are excreted solely through the kidney or those that cause direct renal impairment (Figure 5.33). Fortunately, all of the induction agents undergo redistribution and biotransformation to inactive products before excretion. Renal impairment may delay the excretion of the opioids and prolong their action. Suxamethonium should be avoided, as it causes the release of potassium from muscle cells and may precipitate cardiac arrhythmias in an already

hyperkalaemic patient. The volume of distribution of the non-depolarising relaxants may be increased, reducing their effect while their breakdown and excretion are reduced. Mivacurium, atracurium and *cis*-atracurium may have a relatively normal duration of action, altered only by acidosis. Pancuronium and vecuronium should be used with great care, because they are largely excreted unchanged in the urine.

Doses of highly protein-bound drugs (thiopental, benzodiazepines) should be reduced because of reduced protein binding in renal disease. Lipid-soluble analgesic drugs may be metabolised by the liver but often their active metabolites (e.g. morphine-6-gluconoride) are renally excreted, so caution must be exercised in the timing of repeat doses.

Renal impairment has little bearing on the choice of anaesthetic vapours, though there is a theoretical risk of additional renal toxicity if enflurane or isoflurane is used in high concentration for prolonged periods, as fluoride ions are released during their metabolism and high concentrations of fluoride are known to be nephrotoxic. Exposure of sevoflurane to soda lime produces the renally toxic metabolite 'compound A', although this is not thought to represent a real clinical problem.

Aminoglycoside antibiotics should be used with extreme care in renal impairment, as they are renally excreted and both nephrotoxic and ototoxic at the high and sustained levels which are found if normal doses are given to patients with impaired excretion. Attention to fluid and electrolyte balance must be rigorous, replacing only that which has been lost and avoiding potassium-containing fluids. Occasionally a patient may present who maintains renal function only if he or she has a high urine output, or with a high-output type of renal failure. These patients must not be fluid-restricted in the preoperative period.

Venous access must be considered very carefully in patients likely to need dialysis, as chronic fistula or shunt formation may be necessary. It is better to preserve the vessels in one arm if possible. If a fistula is already present, then this limb should be avoided at all costs and the limb protected from pressure during surgery. Regional anaesthesia is useful in the renally impaired patient provided that there are no other contraindications or coagulopathy. Doses of local anaesthetics should be reduced because of reduced protein binding and a lower seizure threshold in the uraemic patient.

Diabetes mellitus

Diabetes mellitus is the most common endocrine disorder, and one of the more common coexisting conditions in patients presenting for surgery.

Complications

The complications of diabetes are listed in Figure 5.34.

Patients with diabetes may present for incidental surgery or for surgery related to their diabetes,

Figure 5.34 Complications of diabetes

Nephropathy
Peripheral neuropathy
Autonomic neuropathy
Cerebrovascular disease
Coronary artery disease
Peripheral vascular disease
Retinopathy
Lipoatrophy
Fetal macrosomia
Hypoglycaemia
Hyperglycaemia
Ketoacidosis
Lactic acidosis
Obesity
Infection
Wound infection
Delayed healing

particularly abscesses, wound debridement, amputations and cataract surgery – although diabetic patients do not have a higher incidence of cataracts, simply an earlier presentation of the condition. Whether the surgery is incidental or not, and whether the diabetes is insulin- or non-insulin-dependent, there is an interaction between the surgical insult and the diabetes that needs to be properly managed to maintain stability and avoid further complications of both the diabetes and the surgery. Inadequately managed diabetes can result in hyper- or hypoglycaemia, ketoacidosis, wound infection and delayed healing. Occasionally the surgical condition can result in instability and toxic confusion, which will, of course, make the diabetes more unstable and worsen the surgical condition.

Patients should not be presented for anaesthesia unless their diabetes is under reasonable control with blood glucose between 4 and 12 mmol L^{-1} during the preoperative fasting period. Any patient whose blood glucose is outside this range should have the surgery postponed until the situation has been corrected, unless the surgical condition is a true emergency. Similarly, any tendency to acidosis or ketosis and any coexisting electrolyte disturbance must be corrected before anaesthesia. Unfortunately, there are many patients with gangrene or infection of ischaemic tissue whose diabetes will not come into adequate control until debridement has been carried out. This should not prevent the attempt being made. Patients presented for elective surgery should be seen by their GP before the day of operation so that their diabetes is under optimal control. If control is difficult in the community (e.g. recurrent hypoglycaemic episodes or HbA1c > 69 mmol mol^{-1} (8.5%)) they should be referred to a secondary care team specialising in diabetes. Those admitted acutely should be referred to a diabetic specialist team.

Effect of complications on anaesthesia

Nephropathy causes hypertension and electrolyte disturbances, particularly of potassium and creatinine. These disturbances are a reflection of renal function and give some indication of the adequacy of fluid and electrolyte homeostasis and drug excretion.

Neuropathy. Diabetic peripheral neuropathy is unpredictable in both distribution and effect. This may make the testing of peripheral nerve blocks more difficult. Autonomic neuropathy is not usually formally sought, the test being a formal Valsalva manoeuvre, but it is probably present in a large number of diabetic patients. The heart may be partly denervated, and so physiological variations in heart rate may not follow the expected patterns. Similarly the peripheral autonomic responses may not be adequate to prevent variations in blood pressure. Gastrointestinal autonomic neuropathy may delay gastric emptying, increasing the likelihood of regurgitation.

Vascular disease. Diabetic vascular disease tends to involve small rather than large vessels, and though there may be no obvious major coronary or cerebral vessel disease, as a general rule it should be assumed that anyone who has peripheral vascular disease also has central and coronary vascular disease. As it is mostly small vessels that are affected, the fall in blood pressure associated with regional or central nerve blockade tends not to be so manifest.

Pregnancy. Diabetic management in pregnancy can be very difficult, with significant increases in insulin requirement during the pregnancy and major, sudden falls in requirement in the puerperium. Diabetic women tend to have large premature babies that may need forceps delivery or Caesarean section. All pregnant diabetic women should be managed by a specialist diabetologist in addition to their obstetrician. Gestational diabetes will also need careful management to prevent complications.

Elective surgery and the diabetic patient

Diabetes may be controlled by diet, oral therapy or insulin. Management of the diabetic patient is influenced by the severity of the disease, current treatment and the planned surgical intervention. Perioperative metabolic disturbances of diabetes may take the form of hypo- or hyperglycaemia, ketoacidosis or lactic acidosis. The starvation and trauma that accompanies surgery creates a catabolic state with a reduction in production of endogenous insulin and an initial insulin resistance. In a diabetic patient this typically produces a slight hyperglycaemia. The demand for insulin is increased in prolonged surgeries, and in those patients who are obese, or who have concomitant glucocorticoid use or a concurrent infection. Patients should be supported to help manage their condition themselves if able. Oral carbohydrate loading like that seen in enhanced recovery programmes is not suitable for diabetic patients.

Guidelines for the management of diabetic patients undergoing elective surgery

The NHS has commissioned guidance on the management of adults with diabetes undergoing surgery and elective procedures (Joint British Diabetes Societies 2015). A summary of the recommendations relating to day surgery is shown in Figure 5.35.

Preoperative

- Ensure the patient is in the best possible condition for surgery, optimised by GP.
- Ensure that the patient is well informed, understands the treatment options and has realistic expectations about the risks and benefits of surgery and the processes involved.
- HbA1c monitored (< 69 mmol mol^{-1} or $< 8.5\%$); if unable or recurrent hypoglycaemias then secondary care referral.
- Recognise and optimise comorbidities prior to surgery.
- Take all diabetic drugs and normal diet on day before surgery.
- Minimise starvation period.
- Management plan agreed by patient and diabetic team – written instructions given to patient regarding any treatment modifications.
- Identify high-risk patients (poor control, multiple comorbidities, concurrent infections).

Perioperative

- Prioritise patient on operating list if possible (avoid evening lists).
- Written guidance to hospital staff regards modification of normal hypoglycaemic agents (see drugs section below).
- Determine treatment pathway, depending on usual control (diet, tablets, insulin) and number of missed meals (see drugs section below).
- Assess venous thromboembolism risk (avoid stockings if contraindicated).
- Fluids: 0.45% saline and 4% dextrose for continuous variable-rate intravenous insulin infusions (CVRIII): see Figure 5.38.
- Aim for capillary glucose 6–10 mmol L^{-1} (4–12 acceptable); avoid swings and exceptionally tight control.
- Prescribe and administer insulin according to National Patient Safety Association (NPSA) guidelines.

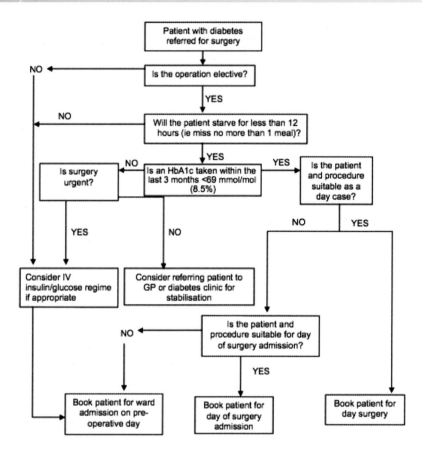

Figure 5.35 Suitability of patients with diabetes for day surgery. Reproduced with permission from Joint British Diabetes Societies for inpatient care (JBDS-IP). *Management of Adults with Diabetes Undergoing Surgery and Elective Procedures: Improving Standards*. 2011, updated 2015

- Some long-acting insulins may be continued (see drugs section below).
- Plan postoperative location (i.e. HDU).

Postoperative
- Involve diabetic team if therapeutic targets are not met.
- Thromboembolic prophylaxis if appropriate.
- Discharge planning.
- Return to normal diabetic control.
- Written instructions given to the patient.

Day-case surgery
Patients with diet-controlled diabetes are all suitable for day-case surgery if the procedure itself is suitable for day surgery and all other criteria are fulfilled.

People with diabetes controlled by oral or injected medication are suitable for day-case surgery if:
- They fulfil all day-case criteria.
- They can be first, or early, on a morning or afternoon list.

See Figure 5.35 for guidance.

Emergency surgery
By definition there will be no opportunity for pre-admission planning. The blood glucose should be closely monitored hourly, and if it rises above 10 mmol L^{-1} a CVRIII should be commenced and continued until the patient is eating and drinking. The HbA1c should be measured to assess the level of pre-admission blood

glucose control as this may influence subsequent diabetes management. Early involvement of the critical care and diabetes specialist teams is recommended in the management of any high-risk surgical patient.

The management of fluids for diabetics during surgery

- Provide intravenous fluid as required according to individual need until the patient has recommenced normal oral intake.
- Maintain serum electrolytes within the normal ranges.
- Avoid hyperchloraemic metabolic acidosis.
- Hartmann's solution should be used in preference to 0.9% saline.
- Glucose-containing solutions should be avoided unless the blood glucose is low.

Further detailed recommendations can be found in the 2008 *British Consensus Guidelines on Intravenous Fluid Therapy for Adult Surgical Patients* (GIFTASUP).

The management of diabetic drugs during surgery

Oral hypoglycaemics

For diabetic patients controlled on oral hypoglycaemics recommendations are given in Figure 5.36.

Insulin

For diabetic patients using insulin recommendations are given in Figure 5.37.

Continuous variable rate intravenous insulin infusion (CCVRIII)

Under certain circumstances some diabetic patients may require a variable rate intravenous insulin infusion during their admission. In such cases the rate of infusion will be adjusted according to bedside capillary glucose measurements. See Figure 5.38.

Administration of CVRIII

- Make up a solution in a 50 mL syringe with 49.5 mL of 0.9% sodium chloride.
- The initial crystalloid solution to be co-administered with the CVRIII is 0.45% NaCl with 5% glucose and 0.15% KCl. This should be given by a volumetric pump.
- Subsequently, the substrate solution used alongside the CVRIII should be either:
  - 0.45% saline with 5% glucose and 0.15% KCl
  - 0.45% saline with 5% glucose and 0.3% KCl
- Selection should be based upon daily electrolytes.
- Very occasionally the patient may develop hyponatraemia without overt signs of fluid or salt overload. In these rare circumstances it is acceptable to prescribe one of the following solutions as the substrate solution:

Figure 5.36 Recommendations for diabetic patients taking oral hypoglycaemics

Tablets	Day prior to admission	Day of surgery	
		am surgery	pm surgery
Acarbose	Take as normal	Omit morning dose if NBM	Give morning dose if eating
Meglitinide (e.g. repaglinide)	Take as normal	Omit morning dose if NBM	Give morning dose if eating
Metformin* (not requiring contrast media)	Take as normal	Take as normal	Take as normal
Sulphonylurea (e.g. gliclazide)	Take as normal	Once daily, am: omit Twice daily: omit am	Once daily, am: omit Twice daily: omit am and pm
Pioglitazone	Take as normal	Take as normal	Take as normal
DPP-4 inhibitor (e.g. sitagliptin) GLP-1 analogue (e.g. exenatide)	Take as normal Take as normal	Omit on day of surgery	Omit on day of surgery

*If contrast medium is to be used and eGFR < 50 mL min^{-1} 1.73 m^{-2}, then metformin should be omitted on day of procedure and for 48 hours afterwards.

Figure 5.37 Recommendations for diabetic patients using insulin

Insulins	Day prior to admission	Day of surgery	
		am surgery	**pm surgery**
Once daily (evening) (e.g. long-acting insulins – Lantus or Levemir, Insulatard, Humulin I, Insuman)	No dose change*	Check glucose on admission	Check glucose on admission
Once daily (morning) (e.g. long-acting insulins)	No dose change	No dose change* Check glucose on admission	No dose change* Check glucose on admission
Twice daily (e.g. Novomix 30, Humulin M3, Humalog Mix 25, Humalog Mix 50, Insuman Comb 25, Insuman Comb 50, twice-daily Levemir or lantus)	No dose change	Halve morning dose. Check glucose on admission. Leave evening meal dose unchanged	Halve morning dose. Check glucose on admission. Leave evening meal dose unchanged
Twice daily – separate injections of short-acting (e.g. animal neutral Novorapid, Humulin, Apidra) **and intermediate-acting** (e.g. animal isophane, Insulatard, Humulin I, Insuman)	No dose change	Calculate the total dose of both morning insulins and give half as intermediate acting only in the morning. Check glucose on admission. Leave evening meal dose unchanged.	Calculate the total dose of both morning insulins and give half as intermediate acting only in the morning. Check glucose on admission. Leave evening meal dose unchanged.
3, 4 or 5 injections	No dose change	**Basal bolus regimes:** omit morning and lunchtime short acting insulins. Keep basal unchanged* **Premixed am insulin:** halve morning dose and omit lunchtime dose. Check glucose on admission.	Take usual morning insulin dose(s). Omit lunchtime dose. Check glucose on admission

*Consider reducing the long-acting dose by 1/3 if patient grazes during the day.

- o 0.9% saline with 5% glucose and 0.15% KCl
- o 0.9% saline with 5% glucose and 0.3% KCl
- The rate of fluid replacement must be set to deliver the hourly fluid requirements of the individual patient and should not be altered thereafter without senior advice.
- Some patients will require additional concurrent crystalloid via a second infusion line.
- Insulin should not be infused without substrate unless in an HDU/ICU setting.
- If increased doses of insulin are consistently being required (blood glucose > 15 mmol L^{-1} and

Figure 5.38 Continuous variable-rate intravenous insulin infusion (CCVRIII)

Bedside capillary blood glucose (mmol L^{-1})	Initial rate of insulin infusion (units per hour)
< 4.0	0.5 (0.0 if background long-acting insulin has been continued)
4.1–7.0	1
7.1–9.0	2
9.1–11.0	3
11.1–14.0	4
14.1–17.0	5
17.1–20	6
> 20	Seek expert advice

not falling), advice should be sought from the specialist diabetes team.
- Continue the substrate solution and CVRIII intra-operatively and postoperatively until the patient is eating and drinking and back on their usual glucose lowering medication.
- Ideally the postoperative sodium intake should not exceed 200 mmol per day.

Diabetic management under specific conditions
Patients undergoing surgery with a short starvation period (one missed meal)
- Monitor blood glucose on admission and hourly during the stay.
- Aim for glucose 6–10 mmol L^{-1} (4–12 mmol L^{-1} acceptable).
- Adjust normal drugs as shown in Figures 5.37 and 5.38.

Patients anticipated to have a long starvation period (two or more missed meals) or decompensated diabetes
These patients will normally need a variable-rate intravenous insulin infusion (CVRIII: see Figure 5.38). The aim is to achieve and maintain normoglycaemia, CBG 6–10 mmol L^{-1} (4–12 mmol L^{-1} is acceptable).
- There is no one-plan-fits-all.

- Although controversial, if already on a long-acting insulin analogue, these should be continued.
- Heavier patients often need more insulin per hour.
- Initial insulin infusion rate should be determined by CBG measurement.
- Hourly bedside CBG should guide infusion rate.
- If the CBG remains over 12 mmol L^{-1} for three consecutive readings and is not dropping by 3 mmol L^{-1} h^{-1} then the rate of insulin infusion should be increased.
- If the CBG is less than 4 mmol L^{-1} then the insulin infusion rate should be reduced to 0.5 U h^{-1} and the low blood glucose treated according to the protocol below (*Management of hypoglycaemia*). If the patient has continued on their background insulin then the CVRIII can be switched off but regular CBG measurements need to continue.

Management of hyperglycaemia
- Hyperglycaemia with ketoacidosis (glucose > 12 mmol L^{-1} either before or after surgery):
  - Check capillary blood ketone levels if possible.
  - If capillary ketones are > 3 mmol L^{-1} or urinary ketones > +++ cancel surgery. Follow diabetic ketoacidosis (DKA) protocol. Contact diabetic team.
- Preoperative hyperglycaemia without ketoacidosis (glucose > 12 mmol L^{-1} and blood ketones < 3 mmol or urinary ketones < +++):
  - Type 1 diabetes: Give SC rapid-acting analogue insulin. 1 unit will drop blood glucose by 3 mmol L^{-1}, but be guided by the patient if possible. Recheck after 1 hour. If surgery cannot be delayed then commence CVRIII (see Figure 5.38).
  - Type 2 diabetes: Give 0.1 units kg^{-1} of rapid-acting insulin. Recheck after 1 hour. Commence CVRIII if surgery cannot be delayed.
- Postoperative hyperglycaemia (without ketoacidosis):
  - Type 1 diabetes: Give SC rapid-acting analogue insulin. 1 unit will drop blood glucose by 3 mmol L^{-1} but be guided by the patient if possible. Recheck after 1 hour. Repeat after 2 hours if still above 12 mmol L^{-1} guided by response to original dose. If still uncontrolled commence CVRIII.
  - Type 2 diabetes: Give 0.1 units/kg of rapid acting insulin. Recheck after 1 hour. Recheck after 1 hour. Repeat after 2 hours if still above 12 mmol L^{-1} guided by response to original dose. If still uncontrolled commence VRII.

Management of hypoglycaemia

- To avoid perioperative hypoglycaemia, consider the risk if the admission glucose is less than 6 mmol L^{-1}. Patients on diet control alone are not usually at risk of hypoglycaemia.
- If capillary blood glucose (CBG) is 4–6 mmol L^{-1} and the patient is symptomatic, consider giving 50–100 mL of 10% dextrose as a stat IV bolus and repeat CBG after 15 minutes.
- If CBG is < 4 mmol L^{-1}, give 80–100 mL of 20% glucose and repeat the blood glucose after 15 minutes.
- Try to avoid stopping the CVRIII in patients with type 1 diabetes. If stopped, then recommence as soon as CBG rises above 5 mmol L^{-1}.
- Persistent hypoglycaemia should be referred to the on-call specialist team.
- Increase frequency of monitoring until normoglycaemia is achieved and then revert to hourly monitoring until eating and drinking.

Infective risk groups

The major risk to healthcare workers is represented by the blood-borne viruses, a group which contains hepatitis A, B and C as well as human immunodeficiency virus (HIV), though the prion diseases have stimulated considerable interest.

Prion diseases

The prion diseases are a group of transmissible neurodegenerative diseases also known as the transmissible spongiform encephalopathies (TSE). While their clinical pictures vary, their common feature is the deposition of an abnormal prion protein in the brain, causing neuronal dysfunction and cell death. All of these diseases are inevitably fatal. Their incubation periods may be very prolonged. Currently there are two animal and seven human prion diseases recognised (Figure 5.39). There are no serological tests which can identify this infection during the incubation period, and there is no identifiable immune response.

These diseases have stimulated much scientific interest because the transmissible agent is non-bacterial and non-viral. It appears that the transmissible agent is the protein itself. Despite species differences in the protein, cross-species transmission has been recognised both in the laboratory and in the food chain.

Prion protein is a membrane-associated glycoprotein normally present in the animal brain. Its function is not

Figure 5.39 Types of prion disease

Human	Animal
Sporadic Creutzfeldt–Jakob disease Familial Creutzfeldt–Jakob disease Iatrogenic Creutzfeldt–Jakob disease Variant Creutzfeldt–Jakob disease Kuru Familial fatal insomnia Gerstmann–Sträussler–Scheinker syndrome	Scrapie (sheep) Bovine spongiform encephalopathy (cattle)

known. The disease process is triggered by a replication of this protein leading to deposition of an abnormal form of the protein. The difference between the normal and abnormal forms is in the tertiary structure rather than the amino acid sequence. How the disease is triggered is not known.

Different routes of inoculation vary in their efficiency of transmission. The intracerebral route is the most efficient, with intravenous, intraperitoneal and oral each less efficient. The National Blood Service undertakes measures including leucodepletion, obtaining plasma for fractionation from countries other than the UK and exclusion of donors who themselves received transfusions before 1980 in order to reduce the risk of transmission in transfused blood.

Because of the differences between prion proteins of different species, there is also a species barrier of variable efficiency. Transmission by any route between species is unpredictable but does occur, both in the laboratory and in nature.

After ingestion, the agent replicates in the lymphoreticular system before entering the spinal cord and brain, possibly via the autonomic nerves. Before the onset of clinical disease, the neural and lymphoreticular tissues may contain high concentrations of the infective agent. This is a major concern both in the food industry and in medicine, because of the possibilities of transmission from food animals to humans by ingestion and between humans by surgical instruments, grafts, blood transfusion and organ transplants.

The human prion protein gene is situated on chromosome 20. There is a polymorphic region at codon 129 that expresses either methionine or valine. Homozygosity for methionine at this codon increases susceptibility to sporadic Creutzfeldt–Jakob disease (CJD). Variations in other codons within this area also seem to increase susceptibility to other prion diseases.

Sporadic CJD (sCJD) has a worldwide distribution at an incidence of about 1 in 1,000,000. It tends to be a disease of late middle age, presenting with a rapidly progressing dementia with cerebellar ataxia, myoclonus and rigidity. Mean survival is about 4 months from onset. As it is sporadic, it is suggested that this is the result of a spontaneous mutation in the prion protein which then becomes a template for self-replication.

Iatrogenic CJD follows medical interventions where infected material from one patient is implanted into another. Transmission has occurred following corneal grafts, dura mater grafts and use of human-derived pituitary growth hormone. It has also occurred where surgical instruments used on the brain of a CJD-affected patient have subsequently been used on another patient. The high density of abnormal prion protein in the tonsils and appendix of affected patients has caused concern about the possibility of transmission unless disposable instruments (both surgical and anaesthetic) are used. Unfortunately, when disposable instruments were substituted for reusable instruments in tonsillectomy, the postoperative mortality increased because of an increase in the occurrence of secondary haemorrhage. Tonsillectomy is carried out with reusable instruments, but only if the surgeon believes that the surgery is strictly necessary.

Familial CJD. The concept of a familial transmissible disease may seem paradoxical. There is a higher than normal incidence of CJD in Slovakia and in Libyan-born Israelis. These populations are highly inbred and may have an excessive dietary exposure to scrapie-affected sheep, these factors acting as multipliers of the abnormal protein genes.

Gerstmann–Sträussler–Scheinker syndrome (GSS) and **fatal familial insomnia** (FFI) are also familial but very rare prion diseases. There seem to be more than 20 mutations of the prion protein gene in GSS, and a mutation at codon 178 in FFI. This is believed to lead to an instability of the protein structure.

Variant CJD (vCJD) was first described in 1996 following a cluster of cases whose neuropathology was dissimilar to sCJD. The mean age at onset in vCJD is 29 years, in contrast to 66 years in sCJD. Variant CJD tends to present with psychiatric disorders which then progress to ataxia, dementia and choreiform movements. The duration of decline is considerably longer than for sCJD: up to 18 months. There are also histological differences. The suggestion that vCJD is a variety of bovine spongiform encephalopathy (BSE) that has crossed species is supported by the consistent clinical and pathological picture, the time relationship between the appearance of vCJD as a new disease and the epidemic of BSE in the late twentieth century. The number of infected but non-clinical cases is unknown, but person-to-person infection remains an ongoing risk.

Kuru was first shown to be a prion disease in 1966. Before that time kuru was endemic in the Fore region of Papua New Guinea and was a major cause of death in the affected population. This population practised ritual cannibalism. The women and children tended to consume internal organs and brain, and were the most likely to be affected. Ritual cannibalism ceased in 1960 and the incidence of kuru has declined since.

The appearance of vCJD has highlighted deficiencies in the cleaning, disinfection and sterilisation procedures used for reusable surgical instruments. Washing by hand (as previously used) does not remove protein deposits from the micropits found in metal surgical instruments. The prion protein is also resistant to the usual chemicals used in the disinfection process, even those that disrupt nucleic acids, and so every hospital sterilisation unit has been upgraded to new standards. Autoclaving at > 121–132 °C for at least 1 hour is considered to provide an acceptable level of safety. Cycles less than this are recognised as only being partially effective. Despite the risk of lymphocyte contamination being unquantified, an inevitable move to disposable laryngoscope blades has occurred. The use of disposable laryngoscope handles is now recommended by recent coroner's advice following the likely transmission of a fatal strain of *Streptococcus* A via a shared laryngoscope handle.

Hepatitis A

The hepatitis A virus is a common infection acquired by close contact with infected persons or by food contamination, particularly sewage-contaminated water and shellfish. The incubation period is 2–7 weeks. Carriers have not been reported.

There is a prodromal 'flu-like' illness with marked myalgia proceeding to hepatocellular jaundice, which resolves spontaneously without chronic damage. Serum transaminases can take many months to return to normal levels after the clinical picture has improved.

Hepatitis B

Infection with the hepatitis B virus is much more serious than hepatitis A in that hepatic failure is more common, chronic damage is frequent, the disease is endemic in many parts of the world and some 10% of all those infected will become chronic carriers with B surface antigen (HBsAg) present. The infection may be acquired by vertical transmission from mother to child in utero, or in childhood, or by heterosexual or homosexual contact or direct inoculation of body fluids. The virus is highly infective in small inoculates, unlike HIV. In countries with adequate blood transfusion services this route of transmission is now rare.

The prodromal illness may be severe, with arthralgia and urticaria followed by hepatocellular jaundice. The illness is not usually severe, and the majority of patients clear the virus within a few weeks. All healthcare workers should be immunised against this condition, though occasionally the immunisation may have to be repeated several times.

Hepatitis C

Hepatitis C is indistinguishable from the other viral hepatitides except on serological testing. The usual route of transmission is parenteral inoculation. Infectivity depends upon the presence and quantity of hepatitis C viral RNA in the blood. The risk of developing hepatitis C after occupational exposure is around 2%. Some may be offered post-exposure immunoglobulin. Exposure can confer partial immunity against future infection, but reinfection is possible. There is no vaccine against hepatitis C infection. Until recently, transfusion of blood and blood products was the major route of infection, which suggests that there must be a pool of chronic carriers in the community. Blood products can now be screened for this infection, but there must be a large number of previously transfused patients who carry the disease.

A high proportion of those infected will develop progressive chronic hepatitis, 20% progressing to cirrhosis and 3% to hepatocellular carcinoma.

HIV/AIDS

Infection with the human immunodeficiency virus (HIV) was only recognised in 1983, but there must have been numerous unrecognised cases before that. The virus is delicate, easily destroyed and has low infectivity. The primary route of transmission is by sexual activity (both heterosexual and homosexual). Other less common routes of transmission include mother to fetus, intravenous drug use (sharing needles) and blood transfusion. Many haemophiliacs were infected by pooled blood transfusion products, which came from an infected community before the problem was recognised. New transfusion safety guidelines were introduced in 1995 to prevent this happening again. The risk of developing the disease after percutaneous inoculation/needlestick from a positive person is around 0.3%. The risk of contracting the disease depends upon type of exposure and the patient's viral load. The risk is greater in the case of a large inoculate or frequent small inoculation from an infected population, such as when performing surgery in sub-Saharan Africa. HIV and hepatitis B frequently occur together, particularly in prostitutes and in the homosexual and drug-abusing communities.

In 2014 there were > 100,000 people living with HIV in the UK, of whom probably 25% were unaware of the diagnosis.

The Centers for Disease Control classification of HIV infection recognises four stages of disease, which may overlap:

1. Acute seroconversion illness, a flu-like illness that usually occurs within 3 months of infection. There is a high viral load but patients tend to remain asymptomatic.
2. Asymptomatic infection. 10% progress to AIDS within 2–3 years, while the remainder progress to AIDS later, with a median of 10 years.
3. Persistent generalised lymphadenopathy.
4. Symptomatic HIV infection.

HIV is one of a family of retroviruses, which have reverse transcriptase as part of their make-up. This enzyme allows the viral RNA to be transcribed into DNA, which is then incorporated into the host cell genome. This virus preferentially infects T-helper lymphocytes, destroying them progressively and leading to a susceptibility to opportunistic infections and malignancies.

Diagnosis is dependent on detection of anti-HIV IgG. But antibodies may not develop until many weeks after inoculation.

In the US there are now six different classes of drug available to treat HIV. These include the nucleoside/

nucleotide reverse transcriptase inhibitors (NRTI, e.g. zidovudine), non-nucleoside reverse transcriptase inhibitors (NNRTI, e.g. nevaripine), protease inhibitors (PI, e.g. saquinavir), fusion inhibitors (FI, e.g. enfuvirtide), CCR5 antagonists (e.g. maraviroc) and integrase strand transfer inhibitors (INSTI, e.g. raltegravir). Over 20 individual drugs can be used in combination to tailor a suitable regimen for each patient. A typical regimen may involve three drugs with the aim of reducing viral load, and improving quality and duration of life. Complex patterns of administration and the high incidence of side effects tend to reduce compliance.

Preoperative assessment of HIV-infected patients should be as thorough as for any other patient. In particular, HIV-infected patients may have respiratory infections with *Pneumocystis*, *Aspergillus*, herpes, and cytomegalovirus, *Mycobacterium* or *Candida*. They may have cardiac valvular infections and vegetations, particularly if they are also intravenous drug users. Chronic diarrhoea may be caused by CMV, *Cryptosporidium* or *Candida*. The neurological complications of HIV include aseptic meningitis, herpes encephalitis, polyneuropathy or HIV-related dementia. Kaposi's sarcoma, a skin malignancy, is diagnostic of HIV infection.

The depression of cellular immunity that occurs after general anaesthesia appears to be transient in these patients and causes no obvious deterioration in their condition. Regional anaesthesia is not contraindicated by HIV alone.

HIV-infected patients may require periods of intensive care, often because of respiratory failure as a consequence of *Pneumocystis jirovecii* (*P. carinii*) infection. Aggressive antibiotic and antiretroviral therapy during mechanical ventilation brings surprisingly good results.

Universal precautions

Hepatitis B and C may cause chronic liver damage, and due account should be taken of liver function in those patients known to be carriers or known to have had hepatitis B or C. Hepatitis A does not produce chronic sequelae but patients may present for surgery during the active or prodromal phases of the disease, and again liver function should be tested and the anaesthetic managed accordingly. The AIDS-related conditions may be of interest to the anaesthetist when the patient presents for surgery, but the possibilities are so broad that each must be taken on its merits. Patients may present for lymph node biopsy.

Unfortunately, the majority of people infected with hepatitis B, hepatitis C and HIV are asymptomatic and not known to the medical community. While precautions against cross-infection are usually taken in those patients known to be infected, it is more logical to take precautions in all patients and assume that every patient is potentially infectious. It is thus wise for anaesthetists to develop the habit of wearing gloves and eye protection in all cases where there will be exposure to bodily fluids. Contaminated needles should **never** be re-sheathed, but disposed of immediately in sharps disposal containers. Safety cannulae are now readily available and may reduce the risk of needlestick injury. Syringes, ampoules and saline flush bags should not be shared between patients. The person using sharps should dispose of them to reduce the number of staff potentially exposed. All cuts and abrasions on both staff and patients should be covered with waterproof dressings, and all spillages of body fluids should be cleaned immediately with a viricidal solution.

In anaesthetising patients known to have one of the HIV-related syndromes, extreme care should be taken to avoid introducing infections into the patient, who has a life-threatening immune deficiency akin to immunosuppressed leukaemics or transplant recipients. This involves effective skin disinfection before venepuncture and full aseptic technique for other invasive procedures. All other equipment used should be either disposable single-use or have been autoclaved and be re-autoclaved as soon as possible after the event. Figure 5.40 details recommended precautions to prevent occupational transmission of HIV from patients to healthcare workers.

Needlestick injury

Although great care is taken to avoid needlestick injury, inevitably occasional accidental inoculation can occur. Following injury the puncture site should be encouraged to bleed vigorously and thoroughly washed with soap and water. Eye splashes should be rinsed with sterile eye-wash or water.

Occupational exposure must be reported and recorded as a critical incident. Each unit should have a stringent protocol for this. Advice should be sought from the occupational health department in hours but most require attendance at A&E. Blood should be taken from the victim, and in high-risk scenarios from the patient (only after informed consent). If, after consideration of the relative risk (taking into account HIV and hepatitis status), post-exposure prophylaxis (PEP) is considered desirable, this should be instituted. Triple therapy is usual:

Figure 5.40 Risk of occupational exposure to HIV and precautions to minimise risk

Exposure with a significant potential to transmit HIV	Precautions to minimise risk of transmission
Percutaneous injury from needles, instruments, bony fragments and bites which break the skin	Wear gloves Dispose of sharps yourself immediately Do NOT resheath needles Post-exposure prophylaxis (PEP)
Exposure of broken skin (eczema, cuts, abrasions) to contaminated blood	Cover with waterproof dressings Wear gloves PEP
Exposure of mucous membranes including the conjunctivae	Wear goggles Wear mask Minimise handling of airway equipment PEP
Deep injury	Universal precautions PEP
Visible blood on the device which caused the injury	Gloves, apron, goggles, mask Minimise handling Decontaminate and sterilise after use PEP
Injury with a needle or device which had been placed directly into a source patient's artery, vein, body cavity	Decontamination and sterilisation policy Single-use items PEP
Terminal HIV-related illness in the source patient	Universal precautions WHO checklist
Exposure to larger volumes of blood, particularly if viral load is high	Universal precautions WHO checklist PEP

this comprises three antiviral drugs, a combination of protease inhibitors and nucleoside analogue reverse transcriptase inhibitors. PEP is most effective if given within 1 hour of injury but may be beneficial up to 2 weeks after the injury. Counselling should be made available through the occupational health department.

Latex allergy

Allergy to natural rubber latex is an increasing problem for healthcare workers, who may have to carry out procedures on patients who react to latex or who may themselves develop reactions to latex. The reactions tend to fall into two groups, irritant contact dermatitis (a delayed type IV reaction mediated by T cells) and IgE-mediated anaphylactic shock. Both are serious problems, and no distinction should be made between them. Natural latex

contains a variety of highly allergenic proteins, which cause reaction by repeated exposure and hypersensitivity. Continued exposure increases the severity of the reaction. It is interesting that there are reports of cross-reactions to similar proteins in fruits such as banana, avocado and kiwifruit as well as nuts.

If a patient reports possible latex allergy, skin testing by dermatologists is possible, but it is time-consuming and potentially dangerous – so it may be wise to accept the report at face value and treat such patients as if they are positive.

Perioperative care

For planned surgery the patient should be first on a morning operating list, to avoid the possibility of latex particles being in the operating theatre atmosphere. All staff should be familiar with the local latex allergy policy and aware of their responsibilities. Traffic in the room should be kept to a minimum; signs on the entrances and exits to the theatre will facilitate this.

All staff should wear non-latex gloves.

It should now be possible to ensure that all anaesthetic breathing system tubing is made of plastics or man-made rubbers such as neoprene. In some countries this may still not be possible – in which case circuits should be covered with stockinet gauze to prevent transfer of particles from the rubber to the patient by staff handling the exposed rubber. Similarly, blood pressure cuff bladders and tubing should be covered so that there is no contact with the patient. All breathing systems should have a bacterial filter at the patient end to prevent latex particles entering the patient's airway. For airway maintenance PVC tracheal tubes and laryngeal mask airways are acceptable, as they do not contain latex. Face masks should be made of plastic. Intravenous cannulae are usually latex-free, though it is always wise to check beforehand.

Syringes should be checked for latex, though most modern syringes are latex-free and labelled as such. Standard blood-giving sets may contain latex in the injection port at the cannula connection. These should be avoided. Even supposedly latex-free fluid-giving sets may contain latex in injection ports. These should be removed, but if this is not possible they should not be used as injection ports because of the possibility of coring and embolising particles of latex. A three-way tap is preferable.

Equipment for local and regional anaesthesia does not usually contain latex, but each anaesthetic department should identify which products are latex-free and keep a stock of these products.

Note that the rubber seals on drug ampoules do not usually contain latex.

An anaphylaxis pack should be available in every operating theatre while a latex-allergic patient is present. The patient should be anaesthetised in the operating theatre and recover in the same room rather than being transferred to a recovery room where the atmosphere is less well controlled.

Each anaesthetic and operating theatre department should develop a policy on the management of latex allergy and a box containing latex-free equipment. All staff should familiarise themselves with both of these.

Jehovah's Witnesses

In general, a patient's religious beliefs have little impact on the conduct of anaesthesia, though there may be dignity and dietary issues, and issues around the care of the dying and the newly dead.

In the case of Jehovah's Witnesses there are a number of issues around consent for administration of blood and blood products and transplantation. This becomes more complex where children are involved. The Association of Anaesthetists of Great Britain and Ireland (2005b) has produced a booklet which gives a very good summary of the situation and is recommended reading for all anaesthetists. In general it may be safer to ask the patient and their religious advisors about specific issues rather than making assumptions that may be in error. Interviews are best conducted on a one-to-one basis rather than having the advisors in the room. This may avoid any suggestion of coercion by the advisor.

Infusion or reinfusion of blood is not usually acceptable once that blood has left the circulation, even if it is the patient's own blood. For some patients the cell-saver systems used as a continuous circuit may be acceptable. Reinfusion from cardiopulmonary bypass machines may be acceptable provided the blood does not come to a standstill. In general, stored blood or blood products/fractions are not acceptable, though if the patient will die without, they may be acceptable. A special consent form may be available that lists specific blood-derived products and therapies to be used as part of the informed consent process.

Preoperative iron therapy is acceptable, though in the presence of a normal haemoglobin concentration it will make little difference. Erythropoietin may be acceptable if it is the recombinant rather than the human-derived form.

In children there are complex legal issues concerning the child's autonomy. This has been complicated rather than clarified by the Children Act. Children who are able to understand the need for surgery and the possible risks and outcomes are autonomous and capable of making their own decisions regarding blood and blood products, regardless of the views of the parents. Remember, the physician has a legal duty of care to act in the patient's best interests while also respecting the patient's wishes. In the situation where the child will die without transfusion it would be wise to garner a second senior consultant opinion *and* to consult the hospital's legal department. These situations are relatively uncommon but present a real ethical and legal challenge. It is prudent to document all discussions and the thinking behind any clinical decision taken in these circumstances.

In general, Jehovah's Witnesses are willing to donate or receive almost any other type of transplant, though there should always be discussion on an individual case basis, especially if blood or blood products may be involved.

Magnetic resonance imaging

Magnetic resonance imaging (MRI) has specific requirements for anaesthesia. The need for anaesthetic input arises from the need for a patient to remain motionless during the scan, while maintaining patient comfort and safety. The traditional cylindrical bore design could cause significant claustrophobia, but new open scanners are now coming on stream. Nonetheless, deep sedation or general anaesthesia may be necessary, particularly with children and some adults. Except in purpose-built environments, radiology departments are typically remote from the rest of anaesthetic activity, equipment and expert assistance, while space is often confined. In a few specialist centres MRI may be used in the operating theatre itself, which demands exemplary safety protocols to be followed by a fully trained team.

The problems with the powerful magnetic field (0.5–3 tesla) are summarised in Figure 5.41.

The long-term effects of very strong magnetic field exposure remain unknown. The patient would usually be stabilised on sedation or anaesthesia, ideally in a designated adjacent anaesthetic room outside the 5G line and then transferred into the scanner on a non-ferrous trolley. The patient is then monitored at a distance. A secure airway is strongly recommended, as a poorly functioning LMA will be difficult to identify and adjust due to inaccessibility of the head once scanning has begun. Pilot balloons on cuffed endotracheal tubes should be taped down to avoid interference with the scan. Breathing circuits may be very long, resulting in increased resistance to breathing and increased compliance of the tubing. Elective ventilation may therefore be worthwhile, and it has the additional advantage of giving controlled apnoea for the purpose of improved scan quality. Gas-sampling tubes of a similar length lead to some mixing within the tube and a significant delay to the signal. Specially constructed monitoring devices, anaesthetic machines and infusion pumps

Figure 5.41 Problems with MRI

	Problem	Solution
Static magnetic field	Attraction of ferrous magnetic materials towards magnet Generates dangerous projectiles Interferes with function and position of cardiac pacemakers, defibrillators and other implanted devices Will damage eye if metal fragments within globe	Clearly marked 5 Gauss line MRI safety check for all persons
Time-varying magnetic gradient fields	Induced currents may cause damage or involuntary movements	Limited field strength
Noise	Volume > 85 dB	Ear protection
Radiofrequency heating	Local heating within/on patient can cause burns	Avoid patient contact with metal, leads, Rf coils, other conductive materials Case reports of burns with conventional pulse oximetry – fibreoptic cables are safer
Helium escape	Helium is used in the superconductor. Will rapidly vaporise if MRI undergoes an unexpected shutdown Will drop room oxygen and prevent door opening	Emergency vent to outside of building – must be patent Rapid evacuation of room in event of a 'quench'

that are shielded against the effects of magnetic interference and are MR safe are now readily available – but may not exist in every department. The anaesthetist should be aware of the safety of any equipment used in the local centre. Some equipment is safe to use under a specific set of conditions (MR conditional), while some is known to be MR unsafe. The AAGBI states that all monitoring equipment should be placed in the control room. The physics of MRI is covered in Chapter 44.

References and further reading

Association of Anaesthetists of Great Britain and Ireland. *HIV and Other Blood Borne Viruses: Guidance for Anaesthetists.* London: AAGBI, 1992.

Association of Anaesthetists of Great Britain and Ireland. *Day Surgery*, 2nd edn. London: AAGBI, 2005a.

Association of Anaesthetists of Great Britain and Ireland. *Management of Anaesthesia for Jehovah's Witnesses*, 2nd edn. London: AAGBI, 2005b.

Association of Anaesthetists of Great Britain and Ireland. *Recommendations for the Safe Transfer of Patients with Brain Injury.* London: AAGBI, 2006.

Association of Anaesthetists of Great Britain and Ireland, Obstetric Anaesthetists' Association and Regional Anaesthesia UK. Regional anaesthesia and patients with abnormalities of coagulation. *Anaesthesia* 2013; **68**: 966–72.

Centre for Maternal and Child Enquiries (CMACE). Saving Mothers' Lives: reviewing maternal deaths to make motherhood safer: 2006–2008. The Eighth Report on Confidential Enquiries into Maternal Deaths in the United Kingdom. *BJOG* 2011; **118** (Suppl 1): 1–203.

Department of Health. *Welfare of Children and Young People in Hospital.* London: HMSO, 1991.

El-Orbany M, Woehlck H, Salem MR. Head and neck position for direct laryngoscopy. *Anesth Analg* 2011; **133**: 103–9.

General Medical Council. *Protecting Children and Young People: the Responsibilities of All Doctors.* Manchester: GMC, 2012.

Joint British Diabetes Societies for inpatient care (JBDS-IP). *Management of Adults with Diabetes Undergoing Surgery and Elective Procedures: Improving Standards.* 2011, updated 2015.

Lloyd DG, Ma D, Vizcaychipi MP. Cognitive decline after anaesthesia and critical care. *Contin Educ Anaesth Crit Care Pain* 2012; **12**: 105–9.

Liumbruno GM, Liumbruno C, Rafanelli D. Autologous blood in obstetrics: where are we going now? *Blood Transfus* 2012; **10**: 125–47.

Mason SE, Noel-Storr A, Ritchie CW. The impact of general and regional anesthesia on the incidence of post-operative cognitive dysfunction and post-operative delirium: a systematic review with meta-analysis. *J Alzheimers Dis* 2010; **22** (Suppl 3): 67–79.

Michenfelder JD. *Anaesthesia and the Brain.* Edinburgh: Churchill Livingstone, 1988.

Nejdlova M, Johnson T. Anaesthesia for non-obstetric procedures during pregnancy. *Contin Educ Anaesth Crit Care Pain* 2012; **12**: 203–6.

National Institute for Health and Care Excellence. *Child Maltreatment: When to Suspect Maltreatment in Under 18s.* NICE Guideline CG89. London: NICE, 2009. www.nice.org.uk/guidance/cg89.

Poswillo DE (chairman). *General Anaesthesia, Sedation and Resuscitation in Dentistry.* Report of an Expert Working Party. Standing Dental Advisory Committee, 1990.

Rucklidge MW, Paech MJ. Limiting the dose of local anaesthetic for caesarean section under spinal anaesthesia: has the limbo bar been set too low? *Anaesthesia* 2012; **67**: 347–51.

Reddy U, White MJ, Wilson SR. Anaesthesia for magnetic resonance imaging. *Contin Educ Anaesth Crit Care Pain* 2012; **12**: 140–4.

Rutala WA, Weber DJ. Creutzfeldt–Jakob disease: recommendations for disinfection and sterilization. *Clin Infect Dis* 2001; **32**: 1348–56.

Steward DJ, Lerman J. *Manual of Paediatric Anaesthesia*, 5th edn. Edinburgh: Churchill Livingstone, 2001.

Yeo ST, Holdcroft A, Yentis SM, Stewart A, Bassett P. Analgesia with sevoflurane during labour: ii. Sevoflurane compared with Entonox for labour analgesia. *Br J Anaesth* 2007; **98**: 110–15.

CHAPTER 6

The surgical insult

Colin Pinnock and Robert Haden

Surgery of any kind represents a traumatic insult to the body and is accompanied by a verifiable stress response dependent on the magnitude of the insult. While the general principles of broad-based anaesthesia have been covered in Chapters 2, 3 and 4, the purpose of this chapter is to alert the reader to operative procedures that have specific problems or caveats associated with them. For reasons of space, only the more frequently encountered operations have been included.

General surgery

Laparotomy

The majority of patients requiring laparotomy will present an aspiration risk, and therefore require rapid sequence induction (RSI) and subsequent muscular relaxation with controlled ventilation. In the case of a perforated viscus (duodenal ulcer, for example), electrolyte imbalance, dehydration and cardiovascular instability make for a high-risk procedure. The presence of faecal soiling of the peritoneum is a particularly bad prognostic indicator. Anastomosis of the bowel requires special consideration. Survival of anastomoses is maximised if the blood supply to the joined section is not compromised in any way. In practice, this requires the avoidance of reversal drugs (and therefore a careful choice of relaxant and its dose) and the use of epidural anaesthesia, usually combined with general anaesthesia if there are no contraindicating factors to the technique (such as poor haemodynamic resuscitation). Epidural anaesthesia provides better postoperative pain relief than patient-controlled analgesia (PCA), which is important in the avoidance of pneumonia after upper abdominal incisions. Extubation of patients following a surgical procedure that has involved handling of the

Fundamentals of Anaesthesia, 4th edition, ed. Ted Lin, Tim Smith and Colin Pinnock. Published by Cambridge University Press. © Cambridge University Press 2017.

bowel should be left until the protective reflexes have returned, as the risk of regurgitation is ever-present. In cases of intestinal obstruction, the use of nitrous oxide may cause the bowel to enlarge dramatically, making it difficult for the surgeon to close the abdomen.

Head and neck surgery

Surgery to the head and neck, whether thyroid, parathyroid or salivary glands are the target, encompasses the same basic principles. Airway security is of paramount importance, and the likely situation is one of obscuration of the patient and breathing circuitry with head towels, making intubation and subsequent controlled ventilation preferable to the use of the laryngeal mask airway, although this device is in use. Avoidance of coughing is important and adequate muscular relaxation and depth of anaesthesia will ensure that this complication does not arise. Spontaneous respiration is not recommended. In the case of thyroid surgery, adequate assessment of the airway is necessary if there is any degree of goitre. Parathyroidectomy can be a prolonged procedure, in which case warming precautions (mattress and fluids) should be used. Patients covered with head towels require suitable eye protection to avoid corneal damage.

Rectum and anus

Surgery to the rectum and anus (e.g. manual dilatation of the anus and haemorrhoidectomy) is highly stimulating and requires adequate depth of anaesthesia to prevent the development of hypertension, tachycardia and laryngeal spasm. Caudal anaesthesia is appropriate in this situation but may be technically difficult in adults. Pilonidal sinus deserves special mention. Many of these patients are obese and for reasons of surgical access require placing in the prone position. Airway security is best achieved by endotracheal intubation followed by controlled ventilation, and eye protection should be employed. Caudal anaesthesia is contraindicated in the presence of active infection close to the site of injection.

Laparoscopic cholecystectomy

While recovery from laparoscopic cholecystectomy is both quicker and less problematic than from the traditional open operation, the procedure itself carries a considerably greater physiological insult and greater morbidity. Patients who are fit for the open procedure may not be fit for a laparoscopic procedure. The abdomen is filled to high pressure with carbon dioxide and the patient

is required to be positioned in a steep head-up position with left rotation. The diaphragm therefore becomes splinted and the lungs compressed, widening the carina and moving it to a higher position in the chest. A properly placed tracheal tube may enter a main bronchus once the abdomen is inflated. The heart may be rotated from its usual position, distorting the great vessels. The venous return from the lower half of the body is compromised by the intra-abdominal pressure and position. Hypertension is induced by the absorption of carbon dioxide. These factors combine to produce a patient with poor venous return, low cardiac output and high systemic resistance, a recipe for significant cardiac strain even in the absence of coronary artery disease. The increased intragastric pressure encourages regurgitation. Peritoneal stretching can also induce severe vagal bradycardia. The standard anaesthetic technique for this procedure is a controlled ventilation technique via a tracheal tube. A dose of a vagolytic drug may be given before the start of surgery in order to avoid the vagal bradycardia of peritoneal stretching. Postoperative analgesia with systemic opioids and nonsteroidal anti-inflammatory drugs (NSAIDs) is usually sufficient, though the pneumoperitoneum causes shoulder pain which may be resistant to opioids until the carbon dioxide has been absorbed. There is a risk that laparoscopic procedures may be converted to open procedures if the anatomy is difficult or if bleeding becomes a problem.

Laparoscopic techniques are increasingly being used to assist in major surgery, to reduce the size of the surgical incision. While this may be carried out by traditional laparoscopy, in some techniques an artificial cavity is created within the preperitoneal or retroperitoneal space. These procedures may be more prolonged than traditional open surgery, and carry a risk of significant surgical emphysema or gas embolism. They may be accompanied by significant postoperative pain, although this is usually short-lived.

Urological surgery

Transurethral resection of the prostate (TURP)

Open prostatectomy has become a very infrequent procedure, the majority being undertaken as transurethral resection of the prostate (TURP). Prostatic hypertrophy, whether benign or malignant, tends to coincide with comorbidities such as ischaemic heart disease, hypertension, diabetes and respiratory disease. These must all be taken into account when planning anaesthesia. Patients requiring prostatectomy may have disturbed plasma electrolytes because of chronic back pressure on the kidneys. This situation may improve with good preoperative drainage by urethral or suprapubic catheterisation, but the electrolyte results rarely return to normal, and thus mild elevations of urea or creatinine values are common. Urethral instrumentation is notorious for causing Gram-negative septicaemia, and so patients with indwelling catheters or those known to have pre-existing infection should have their operations covered by a suitable antibiotic (such as gentamicin) with a dose related to renal function.

Blood loss in prostatectomy is related to resection time rather than size of the prostate, and is generally accepted to be less if spinal anaesthesia is used rather than general anaesthesia. This also has the advantage that any catheter manipulations or bladder washouts necessary in the immediate postoperative period will be covered by the residual effects of the anaesthetic. Spinal anaesthesia has advantages in those with pre-existing respiratory disease, though its use in the presence of ischaemic heart disease is more contentious. Prolonged surgery with continuous irrigation can cause dramatic falls in the patient's temperature, which can only be partly corrected by warming the irrigation and intravenous fluids. Blankets covering the upper body may also help, but the majority of rewarming must be done in the postoperative period. Blood loss at prostatectomy can be difficult to assess, though a variety of methods are available. The lithotomy position tends to increase peripheral resistance until the patient is returned to the supine position, when there is a major fall in peripheral resistance often accompanied by a fall in arterial pressure – which should, therefore, be measured and corrected before transfer from the operating theatre into recovery.

A possible complication of this procedure is the TUR syndrome (Figure 6.1).

Radical prostatectomy

Radical prostatectomy has become common for younger, fitter men with prostate-confined cancer. This is a major undertaking and is not the same operation as a retropubic prostatectomy.

This operation involves a laparotomy-type incision, often a head-down or 'arched back' position, and a potential for major blood loss. It may be a prolonged procedure. General anaesthesia with epidural analgesia would be the norm. Airway maintenance is usually with a tracheal tube,

Figure 6.1 TUR syndrome

Endoscopic surgery requires continuous irrigation with a solution of glycine (1.5% in water). At 200 mOsm L^{-1} this is the minimum non-haemolysing concentration. This solution is deliberately non-electrolytic so that the diathermy current is applied to the tissue rather than being dissipated in the fluid.

If significant volumes of this solution get into either the general circulation or the tissues, from where it is absorbed, then there may be serious fluid and electrolyte disturbances.

The most obvious are water excess and hyponatraemia. Cerebral oedema develops, leading to confusion, hypertension and bradycardia, though loss of consciousness or convulsions is not uncommon. Respiratory distress accompanied by hypoxia (because of interstitial pulmonary oedema) and cardiac effects such as rhythm and contractility changes may also be seen.

Glycine is an inhibitory neurotransmitter and can lead to temporary blindness. It has an intravascular half-life of 85 minutes, and breakdown products include oxalate and ammonia. The plasma sodium concentration may fall to extreme levels: below 100 mmol L^{-1} is not unknown.

If the irrigation fluid is in the tissues or free in the peritoneal cavity then laparotomy for drainage may be the only possible method of treatment. Emergency anaesthesia in this situation is fraught with difficulties, but it is one of those occasions when the patient must be accepted as they are, without any attempt to improve the situation in the preoperative period. General anaesthesia employing intubation and controlled ventilation is the first choice.

A glycine solution containing 1% ethanol enables the use of breath alcohol estimations, which can give an estimate of fluid absorption during the procedure. This technique is increasingly being used for resectoscopic surgery.

and invasive monitoring is common. Management of the circulation can be difficult if the patient is placed in the 'arched back' position because of venous pooling in the legs and in the upper body, with reduced cardiac output as a consequence. Postoperative admission to a high dependency unit is usual.

Cystectomy

Urinary cystectomy is a major procedure involving removal of the bladder and prostate (in men) and formation of a urinary diversion by implantation of the ureters into an isolated loop of small bowel. Anaesthesia for this would normally involve general anaesthesia with tracheal intubation, epidural analgesia and invasive monitoring, followed by admission to an intensive care bed. There is a potential for significant blood loss. Once the ureters have been disconnected from the bladder, blood loss and urine output may be difficult to assess because the urine drains into the abdominal cavity and is removed by suction along with any blood loss. Again, this procedure is often carried out in the 'arched back' position. The surgery may be prolonged, with its attendant problems.

Transurethral resection of bladder tumour (TURBT)

Bladder tumours are not usually large and rarely result in major blood loss. Occasionally patients will be anaemic at presentation from frank blood loss over a period of time. Anaemia should be corrected. Use of diathermy in the bladder can stimulate the obturator nerve, which is close by in the pelvis, lateral to the bladder. This causes mass movement of the patient's legs, which can result in perforation of the bladder and vascular or bowel damage by the resectoscope. This situation can only be prevented by using muscular relaxation and controlled ventilation. Good relaxation is also necessary for adequate bimanual surgical assessment of the tumour and the bladder, and anaesthesia should not be terminated until this is complete. Patients with bladder tumours become regular attenders, and so at each attendance the anaesthetist must establish the time since the last general anaesthetic, which agents were used and the patient's response to them. As time passes, new medical conditions may appear or pre-existing conditions deteriorate, so a full preoperative assessment should be carried out at each admission.

A possible complication of this procedure is the TUR syndrome (Figure 6.1).

Nephrectomy

Nephrectomy for benign disease is usually carried out through a loin incision, whereas if malignancy is involved (including ureteric disease) the operation is generally performed through a laparotomy. The essential difference is the position of the patient, supine for laparotomy but in the lateral position for the loin approach. When in the lateral position the operating table may be arched to increase the distance between the rib cage and the pelvis to improve surgical access. This may cause kinking of the great vessels in the abdomen. In both positions there may be significant blood loss because of damage to renal vessels close to the aorta or inferior vena cava. In left-sided operations the diaphragm and pleura are in danger, and the anaesthetist should be prepared to deal with pneumothorax.

The vessels of the dependent arm may be partly occluded in this position, and therefore all monitoring and infusions should be on the upper arm. Loin incisions are particularly painful postoperatively because of their proximity to the ribcage. Continuous epidural analgesia is particularly effective for both types of incision. Pyeloplasty is usually carried out in the lateral position through a loin incision, and the above comments apply.

Percutaneous nephrolithotomy (PCNL)

Percutaneous nephrolithotomy is an endoscopic procedure to remove stones from the kidney without open surgery. The patient is placed prone. A large needle is passed under x-ray control into the relevant renal calyx and a large-bore cannula passed along the track. The endoscope is then passed through this cannula accompanied by continuous irrigation with glycine or saline, depending upon the method used to extract the stones. Saline is used with electrohydraulic lithotripsy, whereas glycine or saline may be used with the lithoclast.

PCNL can take several hours, and it therefore becomes difficult to maintain patient temperature throughout, particularly when large volumes of irrigant are used. There can be considerable blood loss and significant absorption of irrigating solution causing facial and cerebral oedema. If glycine is used there may be features of the TUR syndrome (Figure 6.1). Severe pain is common in the immediate postoperative period. Standard anaesthetic techniques for this involve tracheal intubation, controlled ventilation and epidural analgesia for postoperative pain relief. The epidural dressing must be waterproof, and it must be placed away from the operative puncture site. The usual precautions are necessary for the prone position, particularly eye protection and padding of pressure points. Care should be exercised in the tension of any bandage used to tie in the tracheal tube, as the facial oedema may cause this to cut into the patient, increasing the possibility of a restricted cerebrovascular supply.

This procedure can be a major physiological strain on patients with ischaemic heart disease. It carries a significant mortality. The patients should be admitted to a high dependency unit for the immediate postoperative period, though less healthy patients may require the full facilities of an intensive care unit on a planned basis.

Transvaginal tension-free tape (TVT)

Transvaginal tension-free tape support of the bladder neck is a relatively new procedure for stress incontinence. It is often performed using spinal anaesthesia because of the surgeon's need to adjust the tension of the buttressing tape to the minimum (which prevents leakage). This involves the patient either coughing or straining part way through the procedure, and thus it is necessary to limit the level of block to no higher than the T10 dermatome so that some power remains in the abdominal musculature. This is difficult to achieve in a predictable way. Some practitioners are using propofol and remifentanil infusion techniques, awakening the patient when required. Obviously this requires acceptable analgesia, for which local anaesthetic infiltration is used.

Orthopaedic surgery

Joint replacement surgery

The most frequently performed operations in this category are hip and knee arthroplasty. Total hip replacement may be carried out under epidural, spinal or general anaesthesia. Peripheral nerve blockade may be useful for postoperative analgesia (e.g. paravascular '3 in 1', iliac crest and lumbar plexus block) but the hip joint is not easy to denervate in this manner because of its multiple nerve supply. Hip replacement may be carried out in the supine or lateral positions, and it is essential, especially in this relatively older patient group, that great care is taken in positioning the patient and protecting any potential pressure areas (see Chapter 3 for other positioning guidance). Revision surgery and bone grafting to the acetabulum complicate the procedure greatly and add to the likelihood of extensive blood loss and the need for close haemodynamic monitoring.

The most major incident to anticipate is cement reaction, which generally occurs with cementing of the femoral, rather than the acetabular, prosthesis. Various mechanisms have been suggested as implicated in cement reactions, and these are listed in Figure 6.2. The clinical picture is one of hypotension accompanied by falling oxygen saturation which usually reverts over a 10–20 minute time course. Increase of inspired oxygen and circulatory support may become necessary. It is important

Figure 6.2 Mechanisms of cement reaction

Pulmonary embolisation	Marrow Fat Cement Air
Methylmethacrylate absorption	
Pressurisation of femoral cavity	
Heat from cement reaction within femoral cavity	

that fluid balance is adequate before the cementing of the femoral component. Measures which have been used to reduce the likelihood of cement reaction include a distal bone plug in the shaft to limit the spread of cement, venting of the shaft to reduce pressure and air trapping, and waiting for the mixture to be relatively non-viscous before insertion to reduce the likelihood of monomer absorption. Although less common, a similar reaction may be seen after cemented humeral prostheses.

Anaesthesia for total knee arthroplasty is broadly similar but does not show the same picture of cement reaction unless extra-long femoral components are used after extensive reaming. Femoral and sciatic blockade may be used for analgesia or operation, and in general techniques of anaesthesia are as for hip arthroplasty. The use of a tourniquet restricts blood loss intraoperatively, but postoperative losses may be brisk. After release of the tourniquet metabolic products are released into the circulation, representing an acid load which may cause temporary acidosis and a rise in end-tidal carbon dioxide. Bilateral joint replacements are severe surgical insults that should not be undertaken lightly.

Laminectomy

The primary requirement of back surgery is the prone or knee–chest position. Adequate eye care is important, and there is no substitute for endotracheal intubation (possibly with an armoured tube) and controlled ventilation using individual drugs of choice. The patient's arms must be carefully and symmetrically moved when turning into the prone position to avoid shoulder dislocation, and pressure points should be padded. A suitable support should be employed to avoid abdominal compression, which will both embarrass ventilation and cause venous congestion in the epidural plexus. The Montreal mattress and Toronto frame are frequently used.

Fractured neck of femur

There are several operations for the treatment of fractured neck of femur (e.g. dynamic hip screw, cannulated screws), depending on the precise site of the break. The majority of patients presenting for this procedure are elderly and frail, and they may be the victims of severe polypharmacy. A picture of dehydration and cardiac decompensation is frequently seen. As the operation is urgent rather than emergency, attention should be paid to the correction of reversible comorbidities such as uncontrolled atrial fibrillation and electrolyte imbalance.

Spinal anaesthesia is the most commonly employed technique for this procedure, although care must be taken to ensure adequate fluid resuscitation, otherwise severe hypotension may result from sympathetic blockade of the lower limbs. Turning the patient for spinal insertion may necessitate analgesia (particularly in the case of heavy solutions when the injured leg will be underneath) and small incremental doses of IV ketamine with or without midazolam are frequently used. Epidural and general anaesthesia may also be used, and although the mortality from general anaesthesia is higher in the short term, there is very little difference after 3 months or so have elapsed, when death rates from all techniques approximate. Mortality is lowest where surgery is carried out within 24–48 hours of admission.

Gynaecological surgery

Hysterectomy

Hysterectomy may be undertaken by an abdominal or a vaginal route. Abdominal hysterectomy equates to a laparotomy in its anaesthesia requirements, although the use of a low transverse incision has encouraged the use of the laryngeal mask airway instead of endotracheal intubation (assuming no other contraindications, such as morbid obesity). Muscular relaxation and controlled ventilation are usually required, with volatile agent and opioid of choice. Postoperative pain relief may be delivered by the use of epidural infusions or PCA. The combination of PCA with a rectally administered NSAID (such as diclofenac 100 mg) is widespread. Rectal administration of NSAIDs in gynaecological surgery is especially indicated, as the high concentrations of the drug which are found in the pelvic venous plexus after absorption ensure delivery to the surgical field. Vaginal hysterectomy is less of an insult than abdominal hysterectomy but has broadly similar anaesthesia requirements. Caudal injection of local anaesthetic agents provides a degree of postoperative analgesia, although it is unlikely that the level of block from this technique will reach sufficient height to be fully effective (T10); therefore, additional analgesia should be provided. If rectal drug administration after pelvic floor repair is desired, this is best administered by the operating surgeon after completion, when the suppository can be gently inserted without damage to the suture line.

Transcervical resection of endometrium (TCRE) and microwave endometrial ablation (MEA) are replacing hysterectomy as a treatment for uncomplicated menorrhagia. In TCRE a resectoscope is inserted through the cervix, after which endometrium is resected by laser or diathermy under direct vision. Fluid irrigation of the uterus is necessary in this procedure. The irrigating solution is isotonic glycine, and the problems of absorption are identical to those occurring during transurethral resection of the prostate (Figure 6.1). The use of irrigating solutions containing 1% alcohol is recommended, as absorption can be monitored by the measurement of breath alcohol using a suitable meter and normogram tables. TCRE is not accompanied by significant postoperative discomfort. In terms of anaesthetic requirement, MEA varies little from dilatation and curettage (D&C). General anaesthesia with spontaneous ventilation via a face mask or laryngeal mask is therefore adequate.

Laparoscopy

Laparoscopy involves the inflation of the abdomen with carbon dioxide before the insertion of an endoscope to examine the abdominal contents. The degree of inflation of the abdomen varies greatly between surgeons. Although the procedure is possible with the patient breathing spontaneously, this is not recommended, and controlled ventilation with muscular relaxation is the norm (suitable agents being mivacurium and atracurium). Use of the laryngeal mask airway is common but not universal. The procedure is usually of short duration and not accompanied by great postoperative discomfort except in the case of sterilisation or other tubal surgery, where the presence of occluding clips on the Fallopian tubes may precipitate spasm. In this situation opioid drugs may be needed postoperatively, although NSAIDs are a preferred first-line treatment (especially for a day-case patient).

The most alarming problem during laparoscopy is a severe bradycardia which may be precipitated on inflating the abdomen. Vagolytic drugs should be always at hand, and if necessary the abdomen should be deflated until the heart rate stabilises. Asystolic arrest has been reported.

Laparoscopy may be used to confirm the diagnosis of ectopic pregnancy. The patient must be carefully assessed to ensure that there is no great degree of concealed blood loss. The onset of muscle relaxation under anaesthesia in a patient with a bleeding ectopic pregnancy can result in sudden massive haemorrhage, in which case aggressive fluid replacement and urgent laparotomy are required. Large-scale blood replacement should always be followed by haematological assessment of coagulation and appropriate remedial therapy.

Evacuation and termination (ERPC/STOP)

Evacuation of retained products of conception (ERPC) and suction termination of pregnancy (STOP) are similar in their anaesthesia requirements. As the volatile anaesthetic agents have a relaxant effect on the uterus, their use is associated with increased blood loss, although this may not reach clinical significance. For this reason a technique of intermittent (or infused) induction agent is usual. Propofol with or without supplemental opioid is popular for what is a short, minimally disruptive procedure. Patients requiring ERPC should be assessed for preoperative blood loss and resuscitated as necessary. The use of oxytocic agents during anaesthesia for STOP is occasionally accompanied by untoward effects (peripheral vasoconstriction, for example).

Ear, nose and throat surgery

Laryngoscopy

Direct laryngoscopy and its variants (which may include the use of lasers in the airway) demand special techniques of airway management because the surgeon works directly in the airway and needs access to the larynx. Specially designed small tracheal tubes, tubes with a cuff and an insufflation port, or special laser-proof tubes are available, and all have their uses. Because of the difficulties of maintaining spontaneous or controlled ventilation under these circumstances, the usual techniques involve a total intravenous technique with controlled ventilation using an insufflation device such as the Sanders injector or high-frequency jet ventilator. If lasers are to be used in the airway then great care must be taken to isolate the trachea below the tube cuff from the airway above the cuff, because any backwash of gas containing oxygen might result in an explosion or fire when the laser is next fired. Nitrous oxide is flammable.

Tonsillectomy

Anaesthesia for tonsillectomy with or without adenoidectomy requires defence of the shared airway from blood and debris. This necessarily involves endotracheal intubation after induction, which may be inhalational or intravenous. If an uncuffed tube is used in the child patient, a suitable pack (ribbon gauze, for example) should be placed around the laryngeal additus to protect the larynx from contamination of blood and saliva. Use of a Boyle–Davis gag will prevent compression of the tube during surgical positioning. Having decided upon intubation, controlled ventilation should be used, and commonly a non-depolarising relaxant, opioid, vapour combination is used for the maintenance of anaesthesia. Extubation should be undertaken in the head-down lateral position after adequate pharyngeal suction. There are two choices for timing of this event: while the patient is still deep, or after protective reflexes have returned. The latter is more common today. Blood loss should be particularly carefully assessed in young children. The potential for transmission of prion disease by surgical and anaesthetic instruments is discussed in Chapter 5.

Post-tonsillectomy haemorrhage is a specific problem that requires mention. Following post-tonsillectomy haemorrhage, the patient will usually be pale, tachycardic and sweaty. Intravenous resuscitation is essential before induction, and two different techniques of anaesthesia have been recommended. In both situations the patient should be placed head-down, in left lateral position, with suction to hand. Following preparation of all equipment a choice may be made between intravenous or gaseous induction. In the first instance after the usual RSI precautions (pre-oxygenation, cricoid pressure) a cautious dose of induction agent is given, followed by suxamethonium and securing the airway by endotracheal intubation. Alternatively, a gaseous induction of vapour and oxygen may be employed, using suction as necessary and enough time to achieve a plane of anaesthesia deep enough to permit laryngoscopy and intubation. Maintenance and extubation are as described above. Some authorities recommend the emptying of swallowed blood from the stomach with a nasogastric tube before extubation, which would appear wise.

Middle ear surgery

Middle ear surgery has one main requirement which differentiates it from other surgical procedures. This is the need to control blood loss in order to provide the surgeon with the best possible view down the microscope. In practice, 'smooth' anaesthesia is desirable (for example no coughing or straining) and a relaxant, opioid, vapour technique is usually employed after intubation with an armoured endotracheal tube. Lidocaine spray to the larynx has been advocated before intubation to reduce the response to the presence of the tube, as has the use of alfentanil with induction. Arterial hypotension is often requested, and provided there are no contraindications this may be achieved by the use of sodium nitroprusside by controlled infusion or β-blockade (esmolol is a suitable choice). Inspired oxygen concentration should be increased and a slight head-up tilt will reduce bleeding by aiding venous drainage. It has been suggested that avoidance of nitrous oxide is beneficial to avoid pressure rises in the middle ear as it diffuses in. Oxygen–air mixtures are therefore recommended in this situation. An antiemetic drug should be administered during the procedure, as nausea from disturbance of labyrinthine function is frequent and postoperative vomiting is particularly undesirable.

Tracheostomy

The majority of elective tracheostomies are performed on intensive care patients following long-term oral intubation. In this instance anaesthesia is usually maintained by the use of opioid agents with or without volatile supplementation and muscle relaxants as required to facilitate controlled ventilation. The critical element of the procedure is to avoid completely withdrawing the existing endotracheal tube before the surgeon has gained control of the airway with the tracheostomy tube and secured it in place. If this is not achievable, the original tube can be re-advanced and oxygenation maintained. If the endotracheal tube has been removed without securing the tracheostomy tube correctly, a potentially dangerous situation develops which may be fatal. Transfer of connecting tubing from old to new tube should be as quick as possible to avoid desaturation.

Emergency tracheostomy is a difficult and hazardous procedure best performed under local anaesthesia.

Ophthalmic surgery

Cataract surgery

Cataracts may be congenital, traumatic, steroid- or radiation-induced, or degenerative. In degenerative cataracts there will also be other medical conditions associated with ageing. While people with diabetes have no more cataracts than the general population, they tend to present earlier and so there seems to be a preponderance of diabetic patients presenting for cataract surgery. Steroid-induced cataracts present in patients taking long-term steroids for other conditions, particularly eczema or asthma, which should be taken into account.

Cataract surgery demands a still eye with low intra-ocular pressure. This can usually be achieved by smooth anaesthesia with muscle relaxation and controlled ventilation to achieve mild hypocapnia, whether via a tracheal tube or a laryngeal mask. The latter is preferable, because of the lack of intubation pressor response or laryngeal spasm and coughing on extubation. Local anaesthesia is also an alternative for cataract surgery, but has a higher failure rate, more complications and less predictable reduction of intraocular pressure. Patients who cannot lie flat without coughing or distress, or who cannot communicate because of language, deafness or dementia, cannot safely have their cataract surgery under local anaesthesia. They may or may not be fit for general anaesthesia.

Squint surgery

The majority of patients for squint surgery are children, though occasional adults may present for cosmetic corrections. This operation is difficult to carry out with local anaesthesia because of the age of the patient and the manipulations necessary in the orbit. General anaesthesia should be carried out with the airway maintained by either a laryngeal mask or a tracheal tube. There is little to choose between spontaneous and controlled ventilation. All patients having squint surgery should receive a weight-related dose of a vagolytic such as glycopyrrolate to obtund the oculocardiac reflex, which can cause severe bradycardia on traction of the extraocular muscles. This is much easier to prevent than treat. Tracheal tubes in small children restrict the cross-sectional area of the airway with a consequent increase in resistance to gas flow (resistance is inversely proportional to the 4th power of the radius). After extubation, the smallest amount of laryngeal or tracheal oedema can cause major falls in oxygen saturation. Laryngeal spasm at extubation causes sudden dramatic falls in saturation, and the facilities for reintubation with a muscle relaxant should be immediately to hand. Waiting for the spasm to break is a recipe for disaster. The tracheal tube used during the surgery should not be disposed of until the patient leaves the recovery room.

Retinal surgery

Retinal detachments present sporadically, but are not usually so urgent that they have to be done immediately on presentation. The patients are often hypertensive, though whether this is cause or effect is debatable. The surgery may be prolonged and is often carried out in semi-darkness. In this situation too soft an eye may be a disadvantage in that the low intraocular pressure may cause further tearing of the retina. Controlled ventilation is advantageous, given the duration of the surgery. A vagolytic agent should be used to prevent the oculocardiac reflex during surgical manipulation of the globe. The oculocardiac reflex also occurs during exenteration or enucleation. Occasionally the surgeon may wish to introduce a gas bubble between the vitreous and retina to tamponade the retina. If this is planned then nitrous oxide should be avoided or turned off as soon as the decision is made. Nitrous oxide diffuses into closed gas-filled spaces and increases the volume of the bubble or, if the area has low compliance, the pressure will rise. While this may be acceptable during the procedure, it will diffuse out in the postoperative period and the pressure or volume will reduce, reducing the tamponade effect.

Penetrating eye injury

Penetrating eye injuries may require induction of anaesthesia in the presence of a potentially full stomach. Unfortunately, suxamethonium causes a significant rise in intraocular pressure, which may cause further damage, especially if there is already vitreous loss or the lens is disrupted. An alternative is a rapid sequence induction using a generous dose of a rapid-onset non-depolarising relaxant instead of suxamethonium. Vecuronium or rocuronium are suitable choices. Rocuronium at 1.5 mg kg^{-1} gives equivalent intubating conditions to suxamethonium. It should be noted, however, that this dose ($3 \times ED_{95}$) may last up to 1 hour. If the penetration of the globe has been with metallic fragments then the search for these may involve magnets or repeated x-rays, which can require multiple changes of position or prolonged surgery.

Dacryocystorhinostomy (DCR)

Dacryocystorhinostomy is a potentially bloody procedure usually requiring an anaesthetic technique designed to reduce blood loss. The patient is usually placed with the table head up to improve venous drainage. A vasoconstrictor is introduced inside the nose to reduce mucosal bleeding. The blood pressure is often lowered to further reduce bleeding. Hypotension may be achieved by increasing the inspired concentration of anaesthetic vapour, or by introducing agents which cause peripheral vasodilatation such as trimetaphan or sodium nitroprusside. Trimetaphan is a ganglion-blocking drug, and its use causes the pupils to become fixed and dilated. These agents must be used with extreme caution. Mild hyperventilation will also help to reduce the blood pressure. The airway is usually maintained with a tracheal tube, though the laryngeal mask will avoid the pressor response to the presence of the tube and so may avoid the need for active reduction of blood pressure. A pharyngeal pack is essential to absorb blood that trickles down from the nasopharynx.

Oral and maxillofacial surgery

Dental extraction

Simple dental extraction demands good control of a shared airway and a degree of understanding between anaesthetist and dentist. Dental extraction should be carried out with the same standard of equipment and monitoring as in the best hospital operating theatres, including ECG, oximetry, non-invasive blood pressure monitoring and expired gas analysis. The majority of dental extractions are carried out on a day-case basis unless there is significant coexisting disease. There is still some debate as to whether the traditional sitting position or the supine position is better. The latter provides some protection against fainting on induction of anaesthesia, but encourages regurgitation of stomach contents.

Induction of anaesthesia may be by inhalation or intravenous injection, but in both cases venous access should be obtained first. The sudden falls in blood pressure associated with propofol tend to limit its use in the dental chair, particularly in the sitting position.

There is no need for intravenous opioids, and simple analgesics are adequate in the postoperative period. Many children prefer inhalational induction, which should be with halothane or sevoflurane in a nitrous oxide/oxygen mixture. Isoflurane has too pungent a smell and enflurane causes too much coughing and salivation to be useful. Desflurane also carries a significant incidence of airway irritation. Inhalational induction and maintenance are carried out using a nasal mask. Once adequate anaesthesia has been established, the mouth is opened and a pack inserted between the mouth cavity and the pharynx, separating the nasal airway from the oral airway. In this way, the extraction can be carried out without dilution of the anaesthetic gases by mouth breathing, and the airway can be maintained without contamination by blood and debris. Recovery should be in the lateral position, preferably head down.

Removal of wisdom teeth

Surgical removal of wisdom teeth demands that the surgeon has good access to the mouth cavity while the airway is protected from debris, water and blood. This is usually achieved by nasal intubation and use of a pharyngeal pack. The reinforced laryngeal mask is also used by experienced anaesthetists. Nasal intubation can cause significant bleeding and pharyngeal tears. An accidental pharyngeal mucosal tear must be recognised and treated with a broad-spectrum antibiotic to avoid major infective complications (including potential mediastinitis).

The anaesthetist must choose between spontaneous and controlled ventilation. If spontaneous ventilation is used then there is a high incidence of cardiac arrhythmia, particularly with halothane. Most of the disturbances resolve with emergence from anaesthesia and require no intervention. Care must be taken to remove the pharyngeal pack at the end of the procedure. Recovery should be in the lateral position with observation of blood loss, and postoperative pain relief provided by NSAIDs.

Fractured mandible

Surgical treatment of a fractured mandible involves stabilisation of the fracture against the mandible itself or against the maxilla via the upper teeth. The fracture may be plated, in which case the airway at the end of the procedure is clear, or the mandible may be wired to the upper teeth, in which case the mouth is closed at the end. It can be difficult to establish at the beginning of the procedure which situation will pertain at the end.

Provided that the mouth can be opened before anaesthesia is induced, an IV induction may be used, followed by nasal intubation and a pharyngeal pack. Ventilation may be controlled or spontaneous but with due consideration for the duration of surgery and the recovery phase. An antiemetic should be given before the end of the procedure, because vomiting in a semiconscious patient with a closed mouth is disastrous. The pack must be removed before the end of the surgery. Spontaneous respiration must be re-established in the operating theatre, following which the tube must not be removed until the patient is conscious and can maintain his or her own airway. The tracheal tube used must be retained until the patient leaves the recovery room. If the mouth is wired closed then a pair of wire cutters must go with the patient everywhere while in hospital in case the wires need to be cut in an emergency. NSAIDs are suitable for postoperative analgesia. The opioids are less suitable because of their sedative effects. There is a case to be made for patients with wired jaws to be nursed on an HDU or ICU overnight for airway observation.

Fractured zygoma

Fracture of the zygoma indicates that severe trauma has taken place, and the preoperative assessment should take into account the possibility of closed head injury. The fracture is usually reduced via an incision above the temporal hair line, so the anaesthetist must be remote from the head. Intravenous induction should be used, followed by controlled or spontaneous ventilation via an oral tracheal tube or a reinforced laryngeal mask airway. Whichever airway device is used, it must be securely fixed, because there may be significant head movement during the reduction. There is always the possibility of further open surgery if the initial manipulation fails.

Fractured maxilla

Anaesthesia for fractured maxilla is not for the inexperienced. The fracture indicates severe trauma, and preoperative assessment should take into account the possibility of closed head injury. The combination of significant head injury and maxillary fracture is an indication for tracheostomy as part of the surgical procedure, as is fracture of both maxilla and mandible together. The surgical procedure may involve stabilisation of the maxilla against the mandible or the skull, either of which will cause airway management problems. A compromised airway is an indication for inhalation induction followed by an 'exploratory' laryngoscopy before a muscle relaxant is given. An oral tracheal tube may be used unless the mouth is to be wired closed, in which case an oral tube will suffice while a tracheostomy is performed. Nasal tubes should not be used, because displacement of the maxilla is usually backward. Ventilation should be controlled and the anaesthetic machine placed remotely. Access to the head is difficult, particularly at the end of the procedure if a halo device is used to fix the maxilla to the skull. The patient should be nursed on an ICU/HDU after surgery.

Trismus

Fractures of the mandible and infection or haematoma in the mouth can cause significant swelling, inflammation of the tissues and spasm of the muscles of mastication, resulting in an inability to open the mouth adequately. The spasm may or may not relax after induction of anaesthesia. In this situation, intravenous induction can prove rapidly fatal because the patency of the airway is only maintained by muscle power, which is lost on induction of anaesthesia. If at this point it proves impossible to open the mouth or maintain the airway then the patient will die of hypoxia unless a cricothyrotomy is performed immediately. The presence of trismus, for whatever reason, demands inhalational induction. If, during the induction, the airway becomes compromised, then the anaesthetic may be terminated without risk to the patient and consciousness restored. Alternatives must then be considered with the patient awake. Tracheostomy under local anaesthesia is one option. If the inhalational anaesthetic proceeds without difficulty then the degree of trismus can be assessed while the patient is unconscious, with a view to tracheal intubation or laryngeal mask airway placement. Muscle relaxants should not be used unless a good view of the glottis has been obtained under anaesthesia. Blind nasal intubation has no place in this scenario, because of the risk of torrential haemorrhage in an uncontrollable airway and because success is not guaranteed.

References and further reading

Williamson KM, Mushambi MC. Complications of hysteroscopic treatment of menorrhagia. *Br J Anaesth* 1996; **77**: 305–8.

Yentis SM, Hirsch NP, Smith GB. *Anaesthesia and Intensive Care A–Z*, 3rd edn. Oxford: Butterworth-Heinemann, 2004.

CHAPTER 7

Regional anaesthesia

Barrie Fischer and Oscar Domingo i Bosch

Regional anaesthesia has its origins in 1884, 38 years after the discovery of general anaesthesia, when Carl Koller instilled a solution of cocaine into a patient's eye and performed glaucoma surgery 'under local'. This landmark discovery led to an explosion of interest in blocking nerve conduction as surgeons looked for less dangerous alternatives to the general anaesthetic techniques then available.

General principles of management

Several important factors, common to all major regional anaesthesia techniques, require consideration to minimise risks and promote high standards of patient care.

Patient preparation

Preoperative preparation of the patient for regional anaesthesia should fulfil the same standards of care as for general anaesthesia, because regional anaesthesia should not be regarded as a shortcut for high-risk patients. A full explanation of the intended block should cover the conduct of the injection, patient management during surgery and recovery from the effects of the block. The advantages to patient, surgeon and anaesthetist may be discussed. The more common side effects that may be experienced should be outlined and the patient offered the choice of

Figure 7.1 Contraindications to regional anaesthesia

Patient refusal despite adequate explanation
Uncooperative patient (e.g. obtunded conscious)
Anticoagulation or coagulopathy
Untreated hypovolaemia (particularly applies to spinal anaesthesia)
Major infection
Trauma or burns over injection site
Raised intracranial pressure (particularly central blockade)

whether to remain fully conscious during surgery, have a sedative premedication or intravenous sedation during the procedure. Major complications of regional anaesthesia are rare (less than 1%).

Contraindications to regional anaesthesia are also relatively uncommon, and are shown in Figure 7.1.

Local anaesthetic toxicity

Local anaesthetic toxicity may be **local**, **systemic** or related to **hypersensitivity reactions**. Local reactions are

Fundamentals of Anaesthesia, 4th edition, ed. Ted Lin, Tim Smith and Colin Pinnock. Published by Cambridge University Press. © Cambridge University Press 2017.

Figure 7.2 Maximum recommended doses of local anaesthetics

	Adult dose (mg)		mg kg^{-1} equivalent	
	Plain	With adrenaline	Plain	With adrenaline
Ester				
Cocaine	100	a	1.5	a
Amides				
Bupivacaine	150	150	2	2
Levobupivacaine	150	150	2	2
Lidocaine	200	500	3	7
Prilocaine	400	600 (felypressin)	6	8.5 (felypressin)
Ropivacaine^{b}	250	N/A	3.5	N/A

^{a} Unnecessary and contraindicated
^{b} 150 mg (2 mg kg^{-1}) for epidural Caesarean section

usually related to direct neural or muscle injury. Hypersensitivity reactions are more frequent with ester-type local anaesthetics which are metabolised via a degradation process to a para-aminobenzoic acid (PABA) metabolite which is highly allergenic. Allergy to amides is extremely rare, and the reaction can range from local hypersensitivity to anaphylaxis.

The incidence of severe systemic toxicity to local anaesthetics is around 7.5 per 10,000 procedures. The development of toxicity depends on the build-up of harmful plasma levels either by direct intravascular injection or by absorption from the injection site. This in turn is dependent on the physicochemical properties of the agent used (lipid solubility, intrinsic vasoactivity), site of injection (vascularity) and cumulative dose. Thus toxicity may develop immediately or be delayed, especially in the case of catheter placement. Recognition can be challenging. The anaesthetist must maintain a high level of vigilance and assess risk on a case-by-case basis. The maximum recommended doses for some local anaesthetics are shown in Figure 7.2.

Clinical effects of local anaesthetic toxicity
Systemic effects
Central nervous system
Central toxicity results from high levels of local anaesthetic agent within the brain. This may be due to direct spread from subarachnoid injection or by excessive systemic absorption. Transfer across the blood–brain barrier is influenced by lipid solubility and ionisation. At a neuronal level, initial suppression of inhibitory pathways results in early excitatory phenomena, superseded by later depressant effects.

CNS effects of local anaesthetic toxicity

- Numbness and paraesthesiae of tongue, mouth and lips
- Metallic taste
- Light-headedness
- Tinnitus
- Slurred speech
- Muscle twitching
- Shivering
- Tremors
- Grand mal convulsions
- Coma
- Apnoea

Apnoea and convulsions result in hypoxia, hypercapnia and metabolic acidosis. The acidosis increases the proportion of ionised local anaesthetic agent. Toxicity results from the presence of ionised drug within the cell blocking the ion channel. Acidosis effectively reduces the proportion of diffusible drug within the cells, and slows clearance.

Cardiovascular system

Most local anaesthetic agents (except cocaine) relax vascular smooth muscle, causing vasodilatation. In addition, centrally administered drugs cause vasodilatation by sympathetic blockade. Direct cardiovascular toxicity is caused by the membrane-stabilising activity of the drugs on myocardial muscle, which is a feature of blockade of voltage-gated fast sodium channels. This reduces the maximum rate of rise of the cardiac action potential and reduces the duration of the action potential. Conduction of the action potential through the myocardium is slowed. Other voltage-gated and ligand-gated ion channels are also affected. Bupivacaine blocks transient outward potassium flux, decreasing baseline cardiac membrane potential and interfering with myocardial repolarisation. Calcium ion release from the sarcoplasmic reticulum is impaired. Bupivacaine may bind to the enzyme protein carnitine-acylcarnitine translocase of the mitochondria, preventing entry of the fatty acids which serve as energy substrates to power myocardial contraction.

Cardiovascular effects of local anaesthetic toxicity

- Prolongation of PR interval
- Supraventricular tachycardia
- Decreased automaticity
- Widening of QRS complex
- Ventricular ectopic beats
- Prolongation of ST interval
- T-wave changes

Respiratory system

The respiratory effects of local anaesthetic agents are due to a combination of peripheral neuronal blockade and systemic toxicity.

Respiratory effects of local anaesthetic toxicity

- Apnoea with systemic toxicity affecting the respiratory centre
- Bronchodilatation secondary to relaxation of bronchial smooth muscle

---

Other effects

Local anaesthetic drugs have a weak neuromuscular blocking action. Amides block plasma cholinesterase. A direct antiplatelet effect (probably due to membrane stabilisation) reduces platelet aggregation and blood viscosity. These effects are of minor clinical significance.

Anaphylactoid reactions

Anaphylactoid reactions are very rare with amide local anaesthetics, and some of those reported have been due to preservatives (such as metabisulphite and methylparaben). Effects range from local erythema and swelling to systemic hypotension and bronchospasm. More commonly, the reactions are due to co-administration of adrenaline, intravascular injection or psychological effects (vasovagal episodes). Reactions are relatively common with esters, and cross-sensitivity may occur. The metabolism of procaine produces para-aminobenzoic acid (PABA), which may be allergenic.

Factors affecting toxicity of local anaesthetics

The toxic effects resulting from systemic absorption of local anaesthetic agent are dependent on various factors.

Factors affecting toxicity of local anaesthetics

- Fraction of unbound drug within the plasma
- Peak plasma concentration
- Rate of rise of plasma concentration
- Plasma clearance
- Plasma pH

Following an accidental IV bolus the plasma concentration will fall as redistribution and elimination occur, exactly as with other intravenously administered drugs. Slow absorption from a tissue plane (correctly administered drug) will result in much slower rise and lower peak of plasma concentration. The speed of absorption and the elimination rate will determine the maximum plasma concentration that occurs. The maximum recommended doses for various local anaesthetic agents are shown in Figure 7.2.

The pattern of toxicity is broadly similar for all local anaesthetic agents, but variations exist in the relative severity of the cardiovascular and neurological effects.

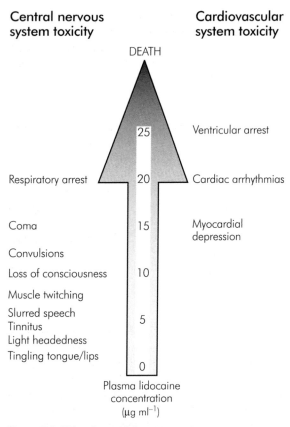

Figure 7.3 Lidocaine toxicity

Figure 7.3 shows the dose-dependent effects of lidocaine on CNS and CVS. Bupivacaine has a narrower safety margin between CNS and cardiovascular toxicity and is particularly dangerous if cardiac effects do occur, as dissociation from the myocardium is slow, and successful resuscitation following cardiac arrest is unlikely unless prolonged CPR is instituted. Bupivacaine should not be used for intravenous regional anaesthesia (Bier's block).

Cardiovascular and central nervous system toxicity depend on the mass of drug reaching the systemic circulation. The transfer of drug (by diffusion) from the circulation to organs is determined by the Fick principle (see Chapter 14). The mass of drug reaching the circulation after peripheral administration is influenced by the following factors:

- Mass of drug administered
- Site of injection
- Tissue protein binding and metabolism
- Vascularity of the injection site

Dose

The volume and concentration of local anaesthetic agents, considered individually, have little influence on systemic spread. Systemically the mass of drug rather than its administered concentration is more important.

Absorption

Absorption from different sites is influenced by the blood flow to the tissue and the uptake of the drug into the vascular compartment, which is a function of solubility. Absorption occurs in the following order of magnitude:

intercostal > epidural > plexus > peripheral
> subcutaneous

Absorption is particularly high when agents are applied topically to mucosa (such as lidocaine spray in the oropharynx). A vasoconstrictor may be added to reduce absorption. Cocaine produces vasoconstriction in its own right and is used on the nasal mucosa to reduce vascularity before some ENT procedures.

Accidental IV injection bypasses the absorption process and subjects the patient to potentially toxic levels of drug. Intravenous regional anaesthesia (IVRA) involves the deliberate introduction of local anaesthetic into the venous system of a limb isolated by tourniquet. The safety of this procedure is dependent on the drug becoming predominantly tissue-bound by the time the tourniquet is released, which should not be for at least 20 minutes. Further improvements in safety can be achieved by using relatively non-cardiotoxic drugs, typically prilocaine.

Distribution

Absorbed drug passes through the lungs, where a large amount of the local anaesthetic agent may become tissue-bound and in some cases metabolised. However, this ability is soon saturated by direct IV injection. After passing through the lungs, local anaesthetic drugs reach vessel-rich tissues which have a high affinity. Some is distributed to muscle and fat, and later gradually released for subsequent metabolism.

Metabolism

Ester local anaesthetics are rapidly metabolised by plasma cholinesterase, and systemic toxicity is rarely a problem. Amide local anaesthetics are metabolised by the liver, but hepatic failure must be very severe before local anaesthetic breakdown is compromised. Lidocaine has a high extraction ratio, and metabolism is therefore dependent on

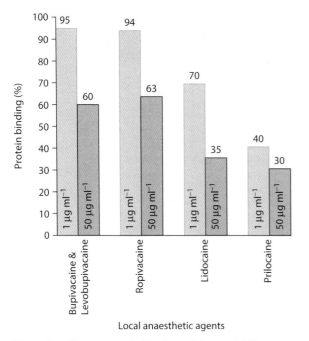

Figure 7.4 Plasma protein binding of drugs at different plasma concentrations

Plasma protein binding

α_1-Acid glycoprotein and albumin are the main sites for local anaesthetic binding within the plasma. α_1-Acid glycoprotein has a high affinity but a low capacity, while albumin has a low affinity but a high capacity for local anaesthetics. Figure 7.4 shows the plasma protein binding of drugs at different plasma concentrations.

Protein binding acts as a buffer to changes in plasma concentration. The chemical bonds are weak and the protein readily releases the local anaesthetic as concentration falls. Toxicity is therefore not directly linked to plasma protein binding, and tissue binding is the more important factor.

Pregnancy

Fetal blood rapidly equilibrates with maternal blood levels of free local anaesthetic agent, but as there is more α_1-acid glycoprotein in fetal blood the overall concentration will be higher. Metabolism is less well developed in the fetus,

but the drug rapidly passes back to the mother as maternal levels decline; therefore this does not present a problem. The pH of the fetal fluids is lower than maternal, which acts to increase the proportion of ionised local anaesthetic agent.

Management of local anaesthetic toxicity

Guidelines are available from the Association of Anaesthetists of Great Britain and Ireland (2010) (Figure 7.5).

Prevention

Careful observation of patients receiving local anaesthetic agents, and a high degree of suspicion both during and after administration, is essential. Make use of the maximum recommended doses as a guide, and combine that with careful technique and an appreciation of the anatomy. If any suspicion of central toxicity arises then stop the injection and re-evaluate.

Treatment

If toxicity does occur, then first stop injecting the local anaesthetic. Call for help. Supportive measures for airway and circulation are the mainstay of successful treatment. Seizures should be controlled with incremental midazolam, thiopental or propofol. Sodium channel blocking agents should not be used, as they will only worsen the situation. If cardiac arrest occurs then inotropes, vasopressors and vagolytics may help. Lidocaine, of course, must be avoided. Bupivacaine is particularly tissue-bound, and cardiac massage for an hour or more may be required.

Lipid emulsion

The use of lipid emulsion is primarily based on animal studies, although case reports have appeared for bupivacaine, levobupivacaine and ropivacaine. Although the exact mechanism of action is unknown, the following have been postulated:

- Intravascular bupivacaine is absorbed into the lipid (very slow for removing myocardial bupivacaine).
- The lipid delivers a significant concentration of fatty acids to the energy-starved myocardium, allowing replenishment of the ATP as cardiac resuscitation continues.

Picard & Meek (2006) provide a useful discussion of the potential benefits. Uptake into the lipid phase is dependent on the lipid/aqueous plasma partition coefficient,

---

hepatic blood flow, which may be particularly relevant when IV lidocaine is used to stabilise ventricular myocardium in low-cardiac-output states.

AAGBI Safety Guideline

Management of Severe Local Anaesthetic Toxicity

1 Recognition

Signs of severe toxicity:
- Sudden alteration in mental status, severe agitation or loss of consciousness, with or without tonic-clonic convulsions
- Cardiovascular collapse: sinus bradycardia, conduction blocks, asystole and ventricular tachyarrhythmias may all occur
- Local anaesthetic (LA) toxicity may occur some time after an initial injection

2 Immediate management

- Stop injecting the LA
- Call for help
- Maintain the airway and, if necessary, secure it with a tracheal tube
- Give 100% oxygen and ensure adequate lung ventilation (hyperventilation may help by increasing plasma pH in the presence of metabolic acidosis)
- Confirm or establish intravenous access
- Control seizures: give a benzodiazepine, thiopental or propofol in small incremental doses
- Assess cardiovascular status throughout
- Consider drawing blood for analysis, but do not delay definitive treatment to do this

3 Treatment

IN CIRCULATORY ARREST
- Start cardiopulmonary resuscitation (CPR) using standard protocols
- Manage arrhythmias using the same protocols, recognising that arrhythmias may be very refractory to treatment
- Consider the use of cardiopulmonary bypass if available

GIVE INTRAVENOUS LIPID EMULSION
(following the regimen overleaf)

- Continue CPR throughout treatment with lipid emulsion
- Recovery from LA-induced cardiac arrest may take >1 h
- Propofol is not a suitable substitute for lipid emulsion
- Lidocaine should not be used as an anti-arrhythmic therapy

WITHOUT CIRCULATORY ARREST
Use conventional therapies to treat:
- hypotension,
- bradycardia,
- tachyarrhythmia

CONSIDER INTRAVENOUS LIPID EMULSION
(following the regimen overleaf)

- Propofol is not a suitable substitute for lipid emulsion
- Lidocaine should not be used as an anti-arrhythmic therapy

4 Follow-up

- Arrange safe transfer to a clinical area with appropriate equipment and suitable staff until sustained recovery is achieved
- Exclude pancreatitis by regular clinical review, including daily amylase or lipase assays for two days
- Report cases as follows:
    in the United Kingdom to the National Patient Safety Agency
    (via **www.npsa.nhs.uk**)
    in the Republic of Ireland to the Irish Medicines Board (via **www.imb.ie**)
If Lipid has been given, please also report its use to the international registry at **www.lipidregistry.org**. Details may also be posted at **www.lipidrescue.org**

Your nearest bag of Lipid Emulsion is kept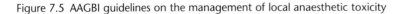

Figure 7.5 AAGBI guidelines on the management of local anaesthetic toxicity

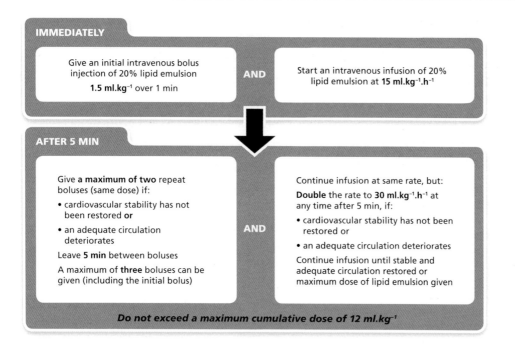

IMMEDIATELY

Give an initial intravenous bolus injection of 20% lipid emulsion
1.5 ml.kg⁻¹ over 1 min

AND

Start an intravenous infusion of 20% lipid emulsion at **15 ml.kg⁻¹.h⁻¹**

AFTER 5 MIN

Give **a maximum of two** repeat boluses (same dose) if:
- cardiovascular stability has not been restored **or**
- an adequate circulation deteriorates

Leave **5 min** between boluses

A maximum of **three** boluses can be given (including the initial bolus)

AND

Continue infusion at same rate, but:
Double the rate to **30 ml.kg⁻¹.h⁻¹** at any time after 5 min, if:
- cardiovascular stability has not been restored or
- an adequate circulation deteriorates

Continue infusion until stable and adequate circulation restored or maximum dose of lipid emulsion given

Do not exceed a maximum cumulative dose of 12 ml.kg⁻¹

An approximate dose regimen for a 70-kg patient would be as follows:

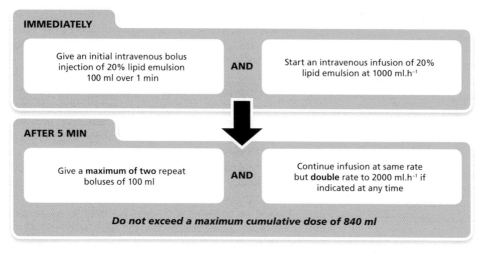

IMMEDIATELY

Give an initial intravenous bolus injection of 20% lipid emulsion 100 ml over 1 min

AND

Start an intravenous infusion of 20% lipid emulsion at 1000 ml.h⁻¹

AFTER 5 MIN

Give a **maximum of two** repeat boluses of 100 ml

AND

Continue infusion at same rate but **double** rate to 2000 ml.h⁻¹ if indicated at any time

Do not exceed a maximum cumulative dose of 840 ml

This AAGBI Safety Guideline was produced by a Working Party that comprised:
Grant Cave, Will Harrop-Griffiths (Chair), Martyn Harvey, Tim Meek, John Picard, Tim Short and Guy Weinberg.

This Safety Guideline is endorsed by the Australian and New Zealand College of Anaesthetists (ANZCA).

© The Association of Anaesthetists of Great Britain & Ireland 2010

Figure 7.5 (*cont.*)

which varies with Intralipid mixture and species. It is important to appreciate that propofol, while useful to treat convulsions, in the volumes that could be given has too little lipid to make any impact on treating toxicity. Intralipid 20%, by comparison, would be given in a bolus of the order of 100 mL followed by an infusion.

Insulin/glucose/potassium infusions

This method has not become part of the management of local anaesthetic toxicity, but the underlying mechanism may be of relevance. Kim *et al.* (2004) induced cardiovascular collapse without arrest in dogs using a bupivacaine infusion. They then stopped the bupivacaine and gave one group a bolus of insulin. Potassium and glucose were then infused. All the dogs in the insulin group gradually improved and survived while the entire control group died. It is postulated that the successful resuscitation using insulin was due to a reversal of bupivacaine-induced changes to potassium ion flux, calcium ion transport in the sarcoplasmic reticulum and maybe improved mitochondrial glucose and pyruvate levels as well.

Performing the block

Major regional anaesthetic techniques require formal sterile precautions, especially central nerve blocks, where meningitis and epidural abscess are rare but definite risks. Direct contact of chlorhexidine skin preparation with neural tissue has been implicated in cases of permanent neurological harm following neuraxial block. Scrupulous attention should be paid to avoiding contact of chlorhexidine with equipment and gloves, and it should be given time to dry before beginning the procedure. Chlorhexidine 0.5% is as effective as a 2% preparation in achieving asepsis and is theoretically less toxic.

In addition to the potentially toxic properties of local anaesthetic drugs discussed above, all regional anaesthesia techniques have associated complications. Airway and resuscitation skills are essential to the practice of regional anaesthesia. Figure 7.6 describes the general requirements for successful practice.

Perioperative management

During performance of the block verbal contact with the patient should be maintained to offer reassurance and explanation of the unfolding events. Staff within the operating theatre must be aware of the impact of their noise and activity on the patient. Patients who have received premedication or intravenous sedation often sleep during surgery once the block is fully established and the initial surge

Figure 7.6 Requirements for performing major regional anaesthesia techniques

Secure intravenous access
Full resuscitation apparatus
Adequate patient monitoring equipment
Ability to administer general anaesthesia rapidly
Fully trained anaesthetic assistance
Suitable sterile packs (reusable or disposable)
A full range of sterile needles and other necessary equipment
Adequate space to maintain sterility
Surroundings that offer privacy, good lighting and warmth

of activity during preparation for surgery has subsided. Occasional verbal contact should still be maintained as part of the routine monitoring of the patient. Central neural blocks have the potential to cause hypotension due to peripheral vasodilatation and reduced venous return. Hypotension responds to changes in posture. Slight head-down tilt with elevation of the legs will restore venous return, and intravenous fluids may be required. Bradycardia should be treated with appropriate vagolytic therapy (e.g. glycopyrrolate 200–400 μg IV), and vasopressors (e.g. ephedrine 3–6 mg IV or metaraminol 0.25–0.5 mg IV) may be necessary if hypotension does not respond to the above measures.

The patient will be unable to protect anaesthetised limbs from pressure or extremes of posture and, if the procedure is prolonged, may become distressed by being unable to change position. It is therefore important to protect the anaesthetised parts of the body and to maintain a comfortable posture for the patient. Postoperatively, the affected limbs need protection from injury and pressure, and patients should be mobilised with care to guard against postural hypotension until the effects of the block have worn off.

Central neural blockade

There are three neuraxial techniques in common use, and their terminology can confuse because terms are used interchangeably. **Spinal** (synonym: intrathecal or subarachnoid), **epidural** (synonym: extradural or peridural) and **caudal** (synonym: sacral epidural) are the preferred terms for anaesthesia and analgesia within the boundaries of the spinal column.

Spinal anaesthesia

Indications for spinal anaesthesia

Spinal anaesthesia is used for a wide variety of both elective and emergency surgical procedures below the level of the umbilicus. For surgery above the umbilicus, high spinals are now rarely used because of associated difficulties of maintaining spontaneous ventilation and abolishing the painful stimuli from traction on the peritoneum and pressure on the diaphragm.

Anatomy

Spinal anaesthesia requires the injection of a small volume of local anaesthetic agent directly into the cerebrospinal fluid (CSF) in the lumbar region, below the level of L1/2, where the spinal cord ends. Figure 7.7 shows the typical anatomy of the lumbar spine in cross-section.

The meninges surround the spinal cord from the foramen magnum as far down as the second sacral segment (S2). The dura mater is a tough fibroelastic membrane, beneath which lies the delicate arachnoid mater. The dura mater invests the spinal cord and the spinal nerve roots, forming the dural cuffs which extend laterally as far as the intervertebral foramina. Although the arachnoid is attached to the dura there is a potential space between the layers (the subdural space), and inadvertent injection into this space is a recognised complication of both spinal and epidural injections. The pia mater is a delicate vascular layer closely adherent to the spinal cord. Lateral projections of the pia form the dentate ligaments, which attach to the dura and stabilise the spinal cord. The filum terminale is the caudal extension of the pia that anchors the spinal cord and dura to the periosteum of the coccyx. There are 31 pairs of spinal nerves (8 cervical, 12 thoracic, 5 lumbar, 5 sacral, 1 coccygeal) arising from the spinal cord, which extends from the foramen magnum to the L1/2 vertebral level. Below this level, the lumbar and sacral nerves form the cauda equina, which offers a large surface area of nerve roots covered only by the pia mater and accounts for the sensitivity of these nerves to local anaesthetic agents administered centrally.

Physiology

Cerebrospinal fluid (CSF) is a clear fluid with a mean specific gravity of 1.006 at 37 °C, which is actively secreted by the choroid plexi in the lateral and fourth ventricles at a rate of up to 500 mL per day. With a CSF volume of 150 mL that means that the total volume changes 3–4 times a day. There is no active flow, movement occurring by diffusion and changes in posture. Absorption occurs (at equilibrium with production) via the arachnoid villi of the major cerebral sinuses. The typical composition of CSF is shown in Figure 7.8. A number of factors affect the spread of local anaesthetic within the CSF, and these are listed in Figure 7.9.

The maximal spread, duration and quality of the block is mostly influenced by the posture of the patient during and immediately after the injection, and the density of the solution. The ratio of the density of the solution to that of CSF is expressed as baricity (where isobaricity = 1.0). If the injection is made at the L3/4 interspace with the patient in the left lateral position and the patient is then immediately turned supine, hypo- and

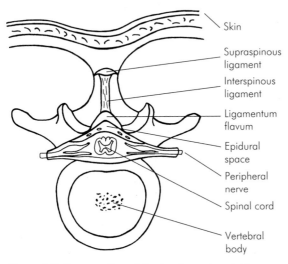

Figure 7.7 Cross-section of the lumbar spine at L1

Skin

Supraspinous ligament

Interspinous ligament

Ligamentum flavum

Epidural space

Peripheral nerve

Spinal cord

Vertebral body

Figure 7.8 Composition of CSF

Total volume (brain and spinal cord) approximately 130 mL	
Volume around spinal cord approximately 35 mL	
CSF pressure in lumbar region	6–10 cmH$_2$O (lateral position)
	20–25 cmH$_2$O (sitting)
Hydrogen ion concentration 40–45 nmol L^{-1}	
Protein content 20–40 mg L^{-1}	

Figure 7.9 Factors influencing intrathecal spread of solutions

Major influence

- Baricity of solution
- Posture of patient
- Volume of solution
- Mass of drug injected
- Volume of CSF

Minor influence

- Intervertebral level of injection
- Height of patient
- Age of patient
- Weight of patient
- Speed of injection
- Induced turbulence (barbotage)
- Posture

hyperbaric solutions produce different effects due to their distribution patterns. Hypobaric solutions are not commonly available in the UK now but have been used in the past for lower abdominal and lower extremity surgery, as they tend to be restricted to the top of the lumbar lordosis when the patient lies supine. With the use of head-up tilt, the height of the block can be encouraged in a cephalad direction but at the expense of a patchy quality of anaesthesia and an unpredictable height. Head-down tilt will restrict the caudad limit of the block. Commercially produced bupivacaine (normally described as isobaric) is slightly hypobaric (0.999) at body temperature and can produce unpredictable results with changing posture. Hyperbaric bupivacaine is commonly used for spinal anaesthesia in the UK at present. As hyperbaric solutions are hypertonic they remain affected by posture for up to 30 minutes after injection, and so sensory levels may change within that time. This explains why so-called saddle blocks and unilateral spinals can rarely, if ever, be achieved with hyperbaric solutions. Isobaric solutions (chirocaine) are also being increasingly used. The block in this case is not influenced by posture, but mainly determined by level of injection and volume.

The effects of a spinal anaesthetic on the physiology of the major organ systems are related primarily to the height of the block. Specific organ systems affected are detailed below.

Nervous system

As a rule there is total neural blockade caudad to the injection site while cephalad to it the concentration of local anaesthetic decreases, producing a differential nerve block of the sensory, motor and autonomic fibres. Sympathetic fibres are most sensitive and may be blocked two to six segments higher than sensory fibres, which in turn may be blocked a few segments higher than the associated motor block.

Respiratory system

Below the thoracic nerves, spinal anaesthesia has no clinical effect on respiratory function but as the intercostal nerves become progressively blocked, active expiratory mechanics are impaired, producing a reduction in vital capacity and expiratory reserve volume. Tidal volume and other inspiratory mechanics remain normal due to increased diaphragm movement. Patients may complain of dyspnoea and may lose the ability to cough effectively. If there is exceptional cephalad spread and the cervical nerves become affected, apnoea due to phrenic nerve blockade can occur.

Cardiovascular system

Progressive blockade of the thoracolumbar sympathetic outflow produces increasing vasodilatation of the resistance and capacitance vessels and a reduction of 15–18% in systemic vascular resistance. If the cardiac output is maintained, there will be a similar fall in mean arterial pressure. If, however, the cardiac output falls due to a reduction in preload (for example due to hypovolaemia or a reduction in venous return due to postural changes) then hypotension may develop rapidly, especially if the block reaches the cardioaccelerator fibres above the level of T4/5, when a reflex bradycardia may occur. Above the level of the block there is usually compensatory vasoconstriction, but this is not sufficient to prevent significant falls in arterial pressure if the block is extensive.

Gastrointestinal system

Sympathetic blockade allows vagal parasympathetic activity to predominate. Gastric emptying and peristalsis continue, sphincters relax and the bowel is generally contracted. This may preclude the use of central blockade in patients with obstructed bowel, at least until the obstruction has been relieved. However, the incidence of postoperative ileus is reduced by spinal and epidural blockade, and this is one of their main benefits. Nausea

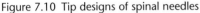
Quinke

Whitacre

Sprotte

Figure 7.10 Tip designs of spinal needles

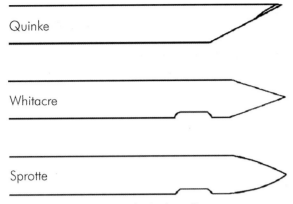

Spinous
process
L4

Tuffier's
line

Figure 7.11 Patient positions for spinal anaesthesia

and vomiting can occur as a result of the unopposed vagal activity, if the peritoneal contents are stimulated in the awake patient.

Equipment

Spinal anaesthesia requires specialised needles and introducers in addition to the general equipment necessary for central nerve blocks (Figure 7.10). There is an inevitable incidence of post-dural puncture headache (PDPH) with spinal anaesthesia, ranging from 0.2% to 24%, and many designs of needle have been introduced to try and reduce this problem. Currently the lowest incidence of PDPH is associated with narrow-gauge, short-bevel needles (26–29 G) and 24 G pencil-point Whitacre tip designs, or the more specialised Sprotte designs with a large side-opening hole. The narrow gauge and relatively blunt tips of these needles necessitate insertion through a properly designed introducer, which should be closely matched to the type of spinal needle being used, to avoid tip damage.

Technique

Successful spinal anaesthesia depends on a reliable lumbar puncture technique. First establish venous access with a wide-bore cannula and then position the patient either in the lateral position with the spine flexed maximally to open up the gaps between the vertebral spines or in the sitting position with the feet placed on a low stool at the side of the bed and the elbows resting on the thighs (Figure 7.11). Each position has drawbacks and advantages, and the choice is usually made on personal preference. In either case, a skilled assistant is necessary to position the patient correctly, maintain and support the

posture and establish a rapport with the patient during the conduct of the block.

A line joining both iliac crests (Tuffier's line) passes across the spine of L4 and is a useful topographical landmark for locating the L3/4 interspace, which is usually easily defined and is the one most often used. Ultrasound can be used to assist identification of the midline and lumbar interspaces in patients with poorly recognizable landmarks.

The technique for spinal anaesthesia is described in Figure 7.12.

Note that 22 G needles are robust enough to be used in patients with calcified ligaments or other anatomical difficulties, and they are recommended for elderly patients, where these problems are more common and the risk of PDPH is very low. If an introducer is required, it should be inserted into the deep layers of the interspinous ligament, so that the needle has only a short distance to travel. Narrow-gauge needles may deviate or be damaged by the ligamentum flavum, calcified ligaments or osteophytes and also will give little feedback. After performing the block the blood pressure, pulse rate and ECG should be monitored, as the onset of sympathetic nerve blockade is quite rapid. When using 3 mL bupivacaine 0.5% in 8% glucose (so-called hyperbaric solution), motor and

Figure 7.12 Technique for spinal anaesthesia

Sterilise the skin over the lumbar spine with a spirit-based antiseptic and raise a skin weal with lidocaine 1% over the appropriate interspace. Inject 2–3 mL more lidocaine into the subcutaneous tissue. Anchor the skin over the interspace by pressing the non-dominant index finger on the spine of the cephalad vertebra and insert the needle or introducer in the midline at 90° to the skin. Feedback from the needle tip will monitor the progress of the needle through the supraspinous and interspinous ligaments, the ligamentum flavum and sometimes the dura mater. If bone is contacted, withdraw the needle to the subcutaneous tissue and redirect slightly cephalad in the first instance. Puncture of the dura is usually obvious, and when the stylet is removed CSF should flow freely.

Figure 7.13 The Bromage motor block scale (1965)

Degree of motor block	Bromage criterion	% score
(1) No block	Full flexion of knees and feet	0
(2) Partial block	Just able to flex knees plus full flexion of feet	33
(3) Almost complete	Unable to flex knees, some foot flexion still	66
(4) Complete	Unable to move legs or feet	100

sensory loss will be apparent within a few minutes but the block may not be fully complete for up to 25 minutes. Sensory block can be tested using a blunt pinprick or loss of temperature sensation with an alcohol swab. Dermatomes should be tested bilaterally starting in the dermatome nearest to the level of injection. Motor loss is usually estimated using the Bromage scale (Figure 7.13).

Normally, the whole procedure is conducted with the patient conscious or lightly premedicated, so as to maintain verbal contact and cooperation. If turning the patient is likely to be painful (for example in those with fractured neck of femur) then intravenous ketamine 0.5 mg kg^{-1} may be administered to provide analgesia during insertion of the spinal.

Figure 7.14 Drug doses in spinal anaesthesia

Operation site	Block level	Drug volume (hyperbaric bupivacaine 0.5%)
Perianal	L 4/5	2.5 mL
Urogenital	T 10	2.75–3.0 mL
Lower abdominal	T 6/7	3.0–3.25 mL

Drugs, doses and volumes

Figure 7.14 gives a guide to drug administration for various operative sites, based on a fit adult of normal stature (70 kg); smaller volumes may be necessary for higher-risk patients. Hyperbaric bupivacaine 0.5% gives a reliable surgical block for 2–3 hours. Plain 'isobaric' bupivacaine 0.5% 3–4 mL is also commonly used but is less reliable above T10.

Complications

Some complications (hypotension, urinary retention, bradycardia) are actually physiological consequences of central neural blockade and should not represent a clinical problem if correctly managed. If management is inappropriate, secondary effects such as nausea and vomiting, faintness or vasovagal loss of consciousness may follow. Total spinal blockade requires urgent supportive management, which may include leg elevation, ventilatory support including intubation, IV fluids and vasopressors. The Third National Audit Project, *Major Complications of Central Neuraxial Block in the United Kingdom* (NAP3) examined the incidence of complications. The main findings are outlined in Figure 7.15.

Headache

Loss of CSF through the dural puncture site will produce a low-pressure headache due to traction on the cranial meninges. The main characteristics of a spinal headache are that it is minimal when lying flat, is severe when sitting up or standing, occurs in the occipital and bifrontal distribution, and may be worsened by coughing or straining. In severe cases the traction may produce cranial nerve symptoms with alterations in vision and hearing. Onset is usually within 24 hours of the injection, and the majority of PDPH diminishes rapidly with rest, oral analgesia and adequate hydration and should resolve

Figure 7.15 Main findings of NAP3 report

The NAP3 report (published in 2009) covered injuries reported in 700,000 CNB cases
46% spinals, 41% epidurals
45% obstetric, 44% perioperative

Results
84 'major' incidents out of 700,000 cases reported
67% resolved completely
Injuries were judged either 'optimistically' or 'pessimistically' according to the census reports submitted

Permanent injuries
Between 14 (optimistic) and 30 (pessimistic) permanent injuries
2.0–4.2 per 100,000 cases (between 1 in 54,000 and 1 in 24,000)
60% after epidurals, 23% after spinals, 13% after CSE

Deaths or paraplegias
Between 5 (optimistic) and 13 (pessimistic)
0.7–1.8 per 100,000 cases (between 1 in 140,000 and 1 in 50,000)

within 7 days. Occasionally more invasive treatment is required in high-risk groups such as pregnant women and after puncture with large-bore needles. An epidural blood patch, in which up to 20 mL of the patient's blood is withdrawn from a vein under the strictest sterile precautions and injected through an epidural needle placed as close to the level of the dural puncture as possible, is very effective at relieving a PDPH, with > 90% success with the first injection. Other causes of headache should be considered before ascribing the cause to the spinal and a careful history of events should be elicited, as headaches are a very frequent complaint after surgery or labour.

Neurological sequelae

Temporary symptoms of paraesthesia, hypoaesthesia and motor weakness may follow spinal anaesthesia but are not necessarily the result of trauma to a spinal nerve root. These symptoms occur from pressure, surgical trauma or stretching of the root or peripheral nerve, and the great majority resolve spontaneously within a few weeks. Serious, permanent neurological damage is extremely rare, but in view of the serious consequences of such an event, any neurological sequelae should be formally examined by a neurologist with experience of this type of damage as

soon as the problem arises. Other rare causes of neurological damage include brain damage and anterior spinal artery syndrome due to excessive and prolonged hypotension, infection (meningitis and epidural abscess), arachnoiditis and cauda equina syndrome (both associated with the injection of incorrect solutions), and are usually the result of a failure of technique.

Epidural anaesthesia
Indications

Surgery can be undertaken within the abdomen and the lower limbs using an epidural as the sole anaesthetic technique, but it is more usual to combine epidural anaesthesia and a general anaesthetic. Epidural infusions are extensively used for postoperative analgesia following thoracic and major abdominal surgery, as well as in the management of some acute and chronic pain conditions (Figure 7.16).

The salient significant differences between spinal and epidural approaches are summarised in Figure 7.17. These differences apply to single-shot, local anaesthetic blocks; the addition of adjuvant drugs (such as opioids or α_2-agonists) can alter the characteristics of each technique. For epidural administration it is customary to insert a catheter to allow top-up doses or prolonged infusions, whereas spinal catheters are not commonplace. Combined spinal and epidural (CSE) anaesthesia is used, especially for obstetric surgery, to utilise the benefits of both techniques. Surgical block can be rapidly established with a small dose of spinal bupivacaine (2–2.5 mL hyperbaric solution) followed by the slower onset of a low-dose epidural, which can be used to extend operating time and postoperative analgesia. However, the NAP3 study demonstrated an increased relative risk with this combined technique, compared to when spinal and epidural techniques are used alone, and a careful evaluation of individual risk should be discussed with the patient.

In summary, spinals provide rapid-onset, short-duration surgical anaesthesia below the umbilicus with small doses of drug. Epidurals have a slower onset time, require large doses of drug and produce less dense surgical anaesthesia but can be used more flexibly in the lumbar and thoracic regions, and their duration may be extended to days or weeks for analgesia by the insertion of a catheter.

Anatomy

The anatomy of the epidural space is described in Chapter 5. Refer also to Figure 7.7.

Figure 7.16 Indications for epidural anaesthesia and analgesia

Surgery

- Thoracic
- Pulmonary
- Cardiac
- Vascular
- Abdominal
- Gastrointestinal
- Gynaecological
- Urological
- Orthopaedic and trauma

Acute pain relief

- Postoperative analgesia
- Trauma
- Miscellaneous (pancreatitis, ischaemic pain)

Chronic pain states

- Chronic benign pain
- Cancer pain

Figure 7.17 Differences between spinal and epidural techniques

	Spinal	Epidural
Onset	2–5 minutes	20–30 minutes
Duration	2–3 hours (single shot)	3–5 hours
Drug volume	2.5–4 mL	20–30 mL
Quality of block	Rapid surgical anaesthesia	May be inadequate in some dermatomes

Figure 7.18 Factors affecting spread of epidural solutions

Factors	Comment
Drug mass	Drug mass is critical, and more important than either volume or concentration
Drug volume	For a given drug mass, larger volume gives more spread than a small volume
Site of injection	The epidural space increases in volume in a caudal direction. Thus a given volume will spread further in the cervical > thoracic > lumbar > sacral Onset is fastest and the block most intense in the dermatomes nearest the site of injection
Age	A given volume spreads further with increasing age over 40 years
Raised abdominal pressure	Smaller volumes may be needed in pregnancy and morbid obesity
Patient position	Prolonged sitting position may reduce upward spread. Earlier onset of block in dependent side
Injection technique	Slow 'unfractionated' injection of dose through needle gives fewer incomplete blocks than 'fractionated' or incremental doses

Physiology

The effects of epidural anaesthesia on the major organ systems are similar to those of spinal anaesthesia, with the height of the block being the major determinant. In a patient with compromised cardiovascular or respiratory reserve, the slower onset of epidural blockade gives more time to manage the onset of hypotension and other side effects, although against this advantage must be weighed the risks of the need for a much larger dose of local anaesthetic drug. The spread of local anaesthetic solution within the epidural space and thus the ultimate height of block is determined by a number of factors (Figure 7.18).

Equipment

In addition to the equipment necessary for spinal anaesthesia (see above) a suitable epidural pack will be required. There are several commercial packs readily available, and these will contain a loss-of-resistance syringe, Tuohy needle, catheter and bacterial filter as a basic set.

Figure 7.19 Technique for epidural insertion

The Tuohy needle, the loss-of-resistance syringe, the catheter and filter must be examined and prepared for use. Connect the filter and catheter and fill with saline to ensure free passage of solution. Position the patient in either the lateral or sitting position as for a spinal injection and identify the appropriate vertebral interspace. Sterilise and drape the area, raise a skin weal with lidocaine 1% and anchor the skin over the cephalad spine of the interspace with the non-dominant index finger. Insert a 21 G hypodermic needle at right angles to the skin exactly in the midline of the interspace to inject more local anaesthetic into the interspinous ligaments and identify the route of the Tuohy needle. Insert the Tuohy needle in the direction indicated by the hypodermic needle. The needle will pass easily through the superficial layers, but as it passes through the supraspinous and interspinous ligaments resistance will become more obvious. If the needle strikes bone, withdraw it slightly and re-angle slightly cephalad but still in the midline. At this point remove the trochar and attach the loss-of-resistance syringe filled with air or saline as required. Carefully advance the needle and syringe combination through the deep layers of the interspinous ligament and into the ligamentum flavum. Constantly check for loss of resistance as the needle is advanced through the ligament, which is 3–5 mm thick in the midline. As the tip of the needle enters the epidural space, there will be a simultaneous loss of resistance in the syringe, an audible 'click' and a tactile feeling of the needle advancing more easily, which requires great control to prevent sudden advancement within the epidural space. Immobilise the Tuohy needle once the loss of resistance occurs, carefully remove the syringe and check that no blood or CSF drains from the needle. CSF will normally emerge from a Tuohy needle with sufficient volume and velocity to leave no doubt as to its identity.

Technique

The practical technique of lumbar midline approach to the epidural space is described in Figure 7.19.

The description in Figure 7.19 relates to loss of resistance to air (LORA), although many clinicians use a continuous-pressure loss of resistance to saline (LORS). Each technique has its own benefits and drawbacks. These are summarised in Figure 7.20.

Figure 7.20 Loss of resistance to air (LORA) or saline (LORS)

Air	Saline
Requires LOR syringe	Ordinary syringe
Intermittent testing and movement of needle	Continuous pressure on plunger and movement of needle
Easy to learn	More difficult to learn
Air bubbles may form space and expand with N_2O	Saline may be confused with CSF

If air is used, only 3 mL (or less) should be injected in order to minimise bubble formation; similarly the volume of saline injected should be minimised to avoid dilution of the local anaesthetic and confusion with CSF. In distinguishing saline from CSF, saline should be cold on the skin compared with CSF, and CSF will show positive for glucose on proprietary stick testing. The use of ultrasound can identify the midline, bony structures and intervertebral spaces. Ultrasound can also measure the depth to the epidural space.

Drugs, doses and volumes
Injection of the local anaesthetic agent

Single-shot technique. A test dose through the needle of 3 mL lidocaine 2% plus adrenaline 1:200,000 may detect inadvertent spinal or intravascular injection, denoted by the rapid onset of a spinal block or a sudden tachycardia (although there is an incidence of false-negative test doses). The local anaesthetic agent may be injected slowly over 2 minutes in 5 mL aliquots to allow for detection of signs of impending toxicity.

Catheter techniques. The initial dose of local anaesthetic agent may be administered via the needle followed by insertion of a catheter for subsequent top-up doses. This method dilates the epidural space, allows easier insertion of the catheter, and produces a more rapid onset of anaesthesia and fewer missed segments. Alternatively, the catheter is inserted immediately loss of resistance is confirmed, the test dose administered and the main dose given in incremental doses via the catheter. Figure 7.21 shows some indicative dosing requirements for a fit adult male with the injection made at L3/4. Lidocaine is usually

Figure 7.21 Drug doses in epidural anaesthesia

Block height	Drug and volume			Duration
Lumbosacral (L1–S5 approx)	Lidocaine	2.0%	20–25 mL	2–3 h
	Bupivacaine	0.5%	18–20 mL	4–6 h
	Bupivacaine (racemic or levo)	0.75%	10–15 mL	4–6 h
	Ropivacaine	7.5 mg mL^{-1}	20–25 mL	4–6 h
Thoracolumbar (T5–L4/5 approx)	Lidocaine	2.0%	25–30 mL	2–3 h
	Bupivacaine	0.5%	20–25 mL	4–6 h
	Bupivacaine (racemic or levo)	0.75%	15–20 mL	4–6 h
	Ropivacaine	7.5 mg mL^{-1}	15–25 mL	4–6 h

used with 1:200,000 adrenaline to reduce absorption and prolong duration. Bupivacaine 0.75% offers the same duration as 0.5% solution but gives a better-quality sensory and motor block.

Whichever method of epidural injection is used, the ECG, heart rate, oxygen saturation and blood pressure must be monitored frequently as the block develops over 15–20 minutes. The development of segmental sensory loss should be followed by testing of dermatomal levels as for a spinal block.

Complications

Complications of epidural block are similar to those of a spinal block, but there is a difference of severity and incidence for each of the following complications.

Post-dural puncture headache

This complication of accidental dural puncture carries a higher risk of headache developing and the headache is more severe, because of the larger hole made in the dura. In non-obstetric patients about half of those who have a dural puncture will develop a headache severe enough to require a blood patch, but in the obstetric population over 90% of sufferers will require one.

Back pain

Back pain is sometimes reported after epidural (and spinal) anaesthesia, and it may be related to several causes (Figure 7.22).

Figure 7.22 Causes of back pain after epidural or spinal block

Cause	Notes
Needle track pain	Localised and temporary
Postural	Extremes of posture during surgery or labour
Drug or additive	2-Chloroprocaine and EDTA
Epidural abscess or haematoma	Rare but important to treat
Recurrence of previous low back pain	

Vertebral canal haematoma

Although reported after diagnostic lumbar puncture, haematoma formation is rare after spinal and epidural anaesthesia. The risk factors for spinal haematoma occurrence are summarised in Figure 7.23. The majority of reported cases occur in patients with a coagulopathy or anticoagulant treatment. The NAP3 study recorded 5 cases of vertebral canal haematoma out of 293,050 epidurals. Permanent harm of any form in epidurals alone occurred in less than 1 in 20,000 cases. Current knowledge suggests that it is safe to use spinal and epidural techniques in patients receiving prophylactic heparinisation for surgery. In cases of doubt the AAGBI guidelines (2013) can be used.

Figure 7.23 Risk factors for spinal haematoma after CNB

Patient factors	Technique factors
Spinal abnormalities	Technical difficulty
Age over 70 years	Repeated attempts
Female	Traumatic puncture
Anticoagulant therapy	Catheter placement
Coagulopathy	Catheter removal

Figure 7.24 Indications for caudal anaesthesia

Adult
Surgery • anorectal • gynaecology • orthopaedic surgery
Obstetric • episiotomy • removal of placenta
Chronic pain • coccydynia • spinal manipulation
Paediatric
Major abdominal and orthopaedic surgery
Inguinal hernia repair
Surgery to genitalia

Caudal anaesthesia

Indications

The caudal route for injection of local anaesthetic agents provides a way of administering a sacral epidural. There are multiple indications for the use of caudal anaesthesia, listed in Figure 7.24.

Anatomy

The normal anatomy of the sacrum is subject to great variation in the extent to which the laminae of the five sacral vertebrae fuse in the midline to form the sacral canal. The sacral hiatus normally results from the failure of the laminae of S4 and S5 to fuse, but it can vary in size from complete absence (approximately 5% of the population) to complete bifida of the sacrum. The dural sac ends

at the S2 level in adults, a level which approximates to a line drawn between the posterior superior iliac spines. In pre-adolescent children there is a predictable relationship between age, volume of injection and height of block, but pubertal growth changes the volume and shape of the sacral canal and this relationship is lost in adults.

Physiology

The effect of caudal anaesthesia is limited to the lumbar and sacral nerves, and therefore there will be less effect on cardiovascular, respiratory and gastro-intestinal performance than with other epidural techniques. Motor weakness is limited to the legs, and sensory loss is usually subumbilical. Autonomic disturbance is limited to bladder and anorectal dysfunction as both sympathetic and pelvic parasympathetic outflow is blocked.

Equipment

A 22 G short-bevel needle should be used for adults and larger children, and a 23 G hypodermic needle for smaller children and babies. For prolonged anaesthesia and postoperative analgesia in children, continuous caudal epidurals, employing a 20 G epidural catheter inserted through an 18 G Tuohy needle, are becoming popular.

Technique

It is most common to administer a caudal after inducing general anaesthesia. The practical technique is described in Figure 7.25.

Drugs, doses and volumes

Paediatric. The linear relationship between age, volume and segmental spread is utilised in a number of formulae. The best known is that of Armitage (1979), and this is shown in Figure 7.28. If the volume of bupivacaine used exceeds 20 mL, motor blockade can be minimised by using bupivacaine 0.19% (dilute 3 parts bupivacaine 0.25% with 1 part normal saline) and use the calculated volume as in Figure 7.28. Lidocaine 1% in the same volumes gives analgesia for 3–4 hours, compared with 6–8 hours for bupivacaine.

Adults. 25–30 mL bupivacaine 0.5% provides 6–8 hours of subumbilical analgesia with a variable degree of segmental spread and motor blockade. If analgesia is necessary only within the sacral nerves, 20 mL is sufficient.

Complications

Incorrect needle placement is the commonest problem of the technique, and is usually a matter of difficulty palpating landmarks. If the needle is too superficial, then the only adverse effect is a subcutaneous injection and a failed block. If the needle is inserted too deeply, it can pass through the sacrococcygeal joint into the pelvic cavity and thus the viscera, risking contamination of the epidural space. Intravascular injection is a risk, due to the rich plexus of veins within the sacral canal. If the marrow of the sacral vertebra is cannulated and the dose injected, rapid systemic absorption can occur. Infection from a dirty technique in a potentially unsterile area is a constant

Figure 7.25 Technique of caudal anaesthesia

Place the patient in the lateral position as for a spinal or lumbar epidural. Note that the posterior superior iliac spines and the sacral hiatus form an equilateral triangle (Figure 7.26). Use the index finger of the non-dominant hand to palpate the sacral cornua either side of the hiatus, which normally feels like a small depression between the bony landmarks. With the hiatus located, sterilise and prepare the area and insert the needle at an angle of about 60° to the skin through the subcutaneous tissues. The sacrococcygeal membrane is tough and offers obvious resistance to the needle; once through the membrane, re-angle the needle to 20–30° (Figure 7.27) and carefully advance the needle a few millimetres, ensuring that it remains in free space. If it strikes bone or will not advance freely, withdraw slightly and reposition the needle or begin the whole procedure again. Do not advance the needle more than a few millimetres within the sacral canal, especially in children, because the dural sac extends beyond S2 in some individuals. Aspirate to check for blood and CSF and then slowly inject 3 mL of the chosen solution to test for low resistance to injection. If this feels normal and there is no subcutaneous swelling denoting needle misplacement in the superficial tissues, slowly inject the main dose, with frequent aspiration checks.

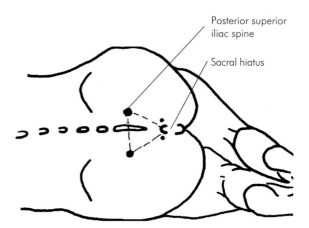

Figure 7.26 Patient position for caudal anaesthesia

Figure 7.28 Drug doses for paediatric caudal block (bupivacaine 0.25%)

Block height	Volume (mL kg^{-1})
Lumbosacral	0.5
Thoracolumbar	1.0
Mid-thoracic	1.25

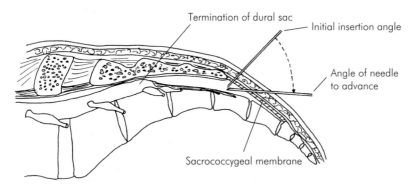

Figure 7.27 Needle angulation for caudal anaesthesia

risk. Dural puncture is an uncommon but important complication because of the potentially large volume of local anaesthetic solution that can be inadvertently injected intrathecally.

Ultrasound-guided regional anaesthesia (USGRA)

The use of utrasound-guided techniques in regional anaesthesia (USGRA) when performing peripheral nerve blocks was first described by Ting and Sivagnanaratnam in 1989. Over recent years, with improvements in technology and equipment, USGRA has developed to the point where it is now the standard of care in regional anaesthesia.

Advantages and disadvantages of USGRA

Advantages
- Visualisation in real time of anatomical structures
- Easier recognition of unexpected pathological structures
- Easier recognition of simple anatomical variations
- Decreased risk of accidental intravascular, intraneural, visceral or pleural puncture
- Application of lower-intensity electrical neurostimulation, meaning the experience is usually well tolerated by the awake patient
- Reduction in the volume of local anaesthetics
- Visualisation of local anaesthetic distribution and increased efficacy of block
- Safe to use in patients with a cardiac pacemaker

Disadvantages

- Results depend on the skill of the anaesthetist
- Equipment is expensive
- Sonographic artefacts can affect the quality of the scan image (Figure 7.29)

Performing a block with ultrasound guidance

Using ultrasound guidance to perform a peripheral nerve block should ideally be used against a background knowledge of the corresponding landmark technique, together with knowledge of the appropriate surface and regional anatomy. In this way ultrasound guidance can only enhance block results, and it can also lead to the development of new approaches to regional anaesthesia.

Figure 7.29 Some examples of sonographic artefacts

Shadowing – blocking of ultrasound by target due to high reflectivity or attenuation, leaving a 'shadow' distal to it
Acoustic enhancement – increased reflection from an area distal to a fluid-containing cyst or vessel due to low acoustic impedance in the fluid
Anisotropy – echogenicity varying with the angle of incidence of the ultrasound beam
Reverberation – where ultrasound bounces between two interfaces, resulting in a 'stripe' pattern which may obscure the target

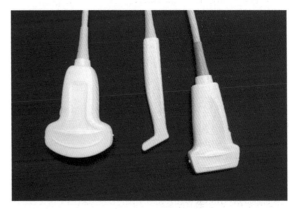

Figure 7.30 Types of ultrasound probes
From left to right:
Curved array transducer (2–5 MHz, 60 mm) – Compromises resolution in favour of penetration. Ideal for deep structures
Hockey-stick transducer (6–18 MHz, 25 mm) – Good resolution with reduced penetration. This probe has a small area of contact, which is ideal for paediatric cases
Linear array transducer (6–18 MHz, 38 mm) – High frequency with good resolution and less penetration

Interpretation of ultrasound scans in USGRA (sonoanatomy) and detailed description of USGRA blocks are provided in more specialised texts.

Selection of ultrasound probe

Probe selection is a compromise between the resolution obtained and the depth of penetration required. Low ultrasound frequencies penetrate the tissues further, but the lower the frequency used the worse the resolution obtained (Figure 7.30).

Obtaining the best scan

Adjustment of depth and gain settings. A compromise has to be decided to adjust the settings to achieve the best resolution for the depth of the target. Depth should be adjusted to visualise the target in the lower half of the screen. Gain should be optimised to obtain the best view of targets but avoid unwanted reflections that can obscure them. The gain is a feature in the ultrasound machine that amplifies the return signal and increases the 'brightness' of the scan. Time gain compensation may be used to improve the view of deeper areas.

Ergonomics and operator positioning. These factors are important not only for the success of a block but also to prevent musculoskeletal injuries in the sonographer. Optimum alignment of operator's eyes, hands and screen are achieved using:

- Correct screen tilt and height
- Comfortable sitting conditions
- Relaxed shoulders and arms position
- Stable probe and needle-holding technique

Scanning technique. The transducer should be orientated to obtain a 'left and right' orientation on the scanner screen corresponding to the sonographer's view of the patient. In this way the adjustment of the probe when performing the block becomes intuitive. Probe stabilisation is a basic competency, and the hands of the operator, the probe, the needle and the area of scanning must be maintained in a stable configuration. The use of phantoms is extremely helpful in developing these skills.

A coupling medium should be used and evenly applied to optimise ultrasound transmission from the probe to the tissues.

Sterile conditions should be maintained, especially when indwelling catheters are inserted.

Selection of needle and trajectory

When performing a block, it is important to ensure delivery of the local anaesthetic to the correct location and to avoid unwanted trauma to neighbouring structures. In particular it is important to identify the tip of the needle. Visualisation of the needle is dependent on the amount of ultrasound reflected back to the probe from the shaft and tip of the needle.

Needle selection. The ideal needle should have good visibility at all angles of insonation with very low artefact formation. Needles with a short bevel ($15°$) are recommended. By facing the bevel toward the ultrasound probe a 'double step' image will appear, which will facilitate tip identification. Avoid air in the needle by flushing prior to injection. Some manufacturers have improved needle visibility by etching the surface of the needle shaft to improve reflection of ultrasound back to the probe.

The path or trajectory chosen for the needle. Maximum reflection and visibility will occur when the angle between the needle and the face of the probe is $0–30°$. Thus, where possible, pass the needle at a shallow angle with respect to the face of the probe. The trajectory of the needle may also be chosen to lie 'in plane' or 'out of plane' (Figure 7.31). In plane, the shaft and tip of the needle will be visible. Out of plane, only a single point where the needle crosses the plane of the ultrasound beam will be visible.

Probe manoeuvres to optimise ultrasound images (P.A.R.T.)

Pressure – vary pressure applied with the probe to distinguish compressible vessels (veins) from incompressible vessels (arteries).

Alignment – use accurate alignment to maintain visualisation of the needle and longitudinal views (axial) of vessels or nerves. Useful in tracking the course of and passing catheters into or next to these structures.

Rotation – rotate the probe through $90°$ to obtain longitudinal and transverse views of a structure. This can help to verify the identity of nerves and vessels as well as obtaining a 3D impression of the local sonoanatomy.

Tilt – tilt the probe to reduce the effect of anisotropy. The view of certain structures can be optimised using tilt. Both nerves and tendons show anisotropic properties.

Wrong-sided blocks

Inadvertent wrong-sided peripheral nerve block is thankfully uncommon, but may carry significant consequences. The identification of contributory factors (Figure 7.32) has led to the development of a National Patient Safety initiative, the 'Stop Before You Block' campaign.

Injection of local anaesthetic

Injection should occur under continuous view of the tip of the needle. High injection pressures should be

RA31 'In plane' and 'out of plane' needle trajectories

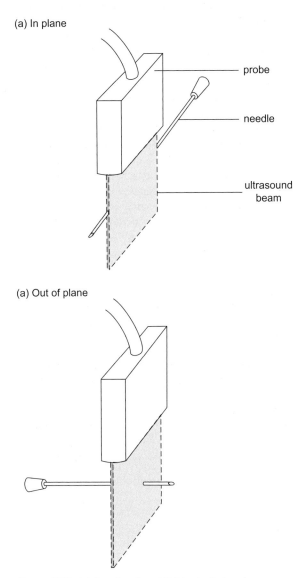

Figure 7.31 (a) 'In plane' and (b) 'out of plane' needle trajectory

Figure 7.32 Factors increasing the risk of wrong-sided block

Distraction in anaesthetic room (e.g. noisy room, too many people, continuous interruptions)
Time delay between sign-in and performance of the nerve block
Concealment of surgical mark
Positional changes relative to the anaesthetist
Temporary staff unfamiliar with local guidelines assisting or performing the block (e.g. locums, trainees)

Peripheral nerve blockade

There are several peripheral nerve blocks that have an important role in providing anaesthesia and postoperative analgesia for surgery of the upper and lower extremities and the body surface (Pinnock *et al.* 1996). A select few are detailed below. This section of the book focuses on the general principles of peripheral nerve blocks rather than offering a detailed explanation of every specific nerve block. This is best achieved by illustrating the traditional landmark techniques for blocks. We encourage the reader to refer to specialised texts for a more comprehensive description of the different blocks, and for the use of USGRA.

The traditional method of performing blocks is based on the clinician's knowledge of surface and regional anatomy, and is referred to as **landmark technique**. However, the efficacy and safety of peripheral nerve block procedures has been greatly enhanced by the introduction of **ultrasound guidance** into the performance of peripheral nerve blocks. Ultrasound-guided regional anaesthesia requires not only a sound knowledge of surface and regional anatomy (as for landmark techniques), but also a knowledge of the anatomical features of regional ultrasound scans (sonoanatomy).

Brachial plexus block
Indications
Brachial plexus anaesthesia is indicated for a wide variety of surgical procedures and for the management of acute and chronic pain (Figure 7.33).

Anatomy
The important practical feature is the fascia that invests the plexus from its origins at the cervical roots between the middle and anterior scalene muscles to the five

avoided by injecting the local anaesthetic slowly and in small increments. The tip should be placed tangentially to the nerve and not aiming directly at it. The aim should be to obtain an image where the nerve is surrounded by a hypoechoic (dark) area ('doughnut' or 'isle in the ocean' sign).

Figure 7.33 Indications for brachial plexus blockade

Indication	Notes
Trauma and orthopaedic surgery • fracture manipulation or fixation • joint replacement • soft tissue trauma	Possibility of compartment syndrome with closed trauma
Vascular and reconstructive surgery • shunt formation • plastic reconstruction • microvascular surgery	Prolonged sympathetic blockade improves blood flow to critical perfusion areas
Acute pain • postoperative analgesia • continuous passive movement (after joint surgery)	Up to 24 h analgesia with bupivacaine 0.75%
Chronic pain • reflex sympathetic dystrophy • terminal cancer pain	Catheter insertion into sheath allows prolonged infusions

terminal nerves at the mid-humeral level. Blockade of the brachial plexus is theoretically possible with entry into this fascia at any level, although the resulting block will vary according to the volume and subsequent spread of solution. There are several techniques described in the literature, but the three most common are the **interscalene** (which blocks at the level of the five cervical roots), the **supraclavicular** (which blocks at the level of the three trunks) and the **axillary** (which blocks at the level of the five terminal nerves). Only the supraclavicular and the axillary are described below, as the interscalene is technically more demanding.

Equipment

For single-shot injections, a short-bevel 22 G, 3.5 cm regional block needle is ideal as it relays considerable information to the user about the tissue layers, particularly the sheath itself. The tactile response from the needle plus the frequent paraesthesiae when the needle is correctly placed should ensure a high success rate (> 85%). In the UK, most clinicians use a peripheral nerve stimulator to confirm accurate needle placement, and this is a useful adjunct to teaching blocks or performing them in sedated or anaesthetised patients. Care should be taken to ensure that the needle is not displaced by manipulating or changing the syringes during injection. A short extension set from the needle to the syringe allows the operator to carefully control the needle while an assistant makes the injection or changes the syringes.

The use of ultrasound-guided regional anaesthesia (USGRA) has increased in popularity since Ting & Sivagnanaratnam first described the use of ultrasound in axillary block. USGRA allows visualisation of the anatomical structures (sonoanatomy), location of the needle tip and the pattern of local anaesthetic spread.

Techniques

The axillary approach is the easiest technique to learn, and carries the lowest risk of serious complications. The landmark technique in the absence of ultrasound facilities is described in Figure 7.34, and patient position is shown in Figure 7.35.

Note: the needle may enter the axillary artery, in which case apply gentle aspiration and continue to slowly advance the needle through the posterior wall of the artery until blood can no longer be aspirated. At this point the patient may experience parasthesiae within the distribution of the radial nerve, and after careful negative aspiration the injection can be completed – the transarterial approach. Firm digital pressure must be maintained for several minutes if the artery is punctured. Direct visualisation of the artery with ultrasound should minimise this risk.

In a fit adult, 40 mL local anaesthetic will usually produce an effective brachial plexus block, but it may not uniformly block all five terminal nerves because of variable spread within the sheath. Thus a partial block may occur with a nerve territory being missed (usually the musculocutaneous) rather than a dermatomal pattern of failure as would be the case with an interscalene block, where the injection is made at the level of the roots. With a supraclavicular block, partial failure is manifested as both a dermatomal (C8/T1) and nerve territory (median or ulnar) failure, because the inferior trunk is the most likely to be missed. USGRA can help to identify the different terminal branches individually. The ultrasound scan in Figure 7.36 illustrates the sonoanatomy of the axillary brachial plexus. It is clear that a thorough

Figure 7.34 Landmark technique for brachial plexus block, axillary approach

Position the patient supine with the shoulder abducted to 90° and the elbow flexed to 90° (Figure 7.35). Identify the lateral border of the pectoralis major and palpate the axillary arterial pulse at this level on the medial surface of the arm. Follow the pulsation proximal into the axilla to identify where the pulse is most obvious, and raise a skin weal with a 25 G needle and 1–2 mL of local anaesthetic over this point. Fix the artery with the non-dominant index finger and insert a 22 G short-bevel, 3.5 cm needle either above or below the index finger, aiming towards the pulse, at a depth of 1–2 cm. In a normal adult arm there will be resistance from the fascial sheath followed by a distinct 'pop', and the patient may experience parasthesiae in the distribution of the ulnar nerve. The needle should be immobilised at this stage and the injection made after negative aspiration. Digital pressure applied distal to the needle during the injection and maintained while the needle is removed and the arm adducted after injection will encourage proximal spread of solution.

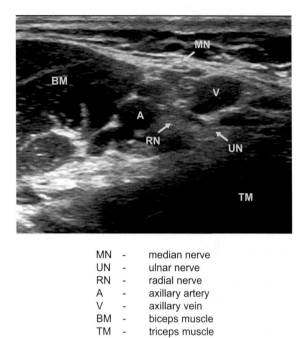

MN	-	median nerve
UN	-	ulnar nerve
RN	-	radial nerve
A	-	axillary artery
V	-	axillary vein
BM	-	biceps muscle
TM	-	triceps muscle

Figure 7.36 Sonoanatomy of the axillary brachial plexus

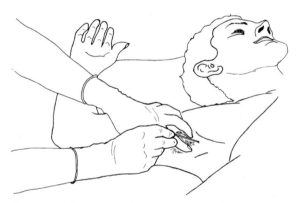

Figure 7.35 Patient position for axillary brachial plexus block

knowledge of the regional anatomy is still required in order to interpret the scan.

The supraclavicular approach. Identification of the interscalene groove is essential in order to perform this block effectively and safely. A line drawn from the cricoid cartilage laterally across the sternocleidomastoid muscle meets its posterior border at the point where the interscalene groove emerges. The interscalene groove runs caudally and laterally between the anterior and middle scalenus muscles, towards the midpoint of the clavicle. Injection is commonly performed at this point under ultrasound guidance, by placing a linear probe across this point aligned parallel to the clavicle. USGRA has become a standard approach for this block as it visualises the vessels and pleura as well as the brachial plexus. This significantly reduces the risk of complications. See Figure 7.39 for the sonoanatomy of the supraclavicular brachial plexus block.

This block may also be performed by landmark technique in the absence of ultrasound facilities. The landmark technique is described in Figure 7.37, and patient position is shown in Figure 7.38.

Drugs, doses and volumes

Figure 7.40 illustrates the drugs, volumes and average duration of block for surgical anaesthesia with respect to axillary and supraclavicular approaches to brachial plexus block. Although the relatively large volumes indicated may be above data-sheet maxima, they are more effective than smaller volumes, widely used, and known to be safe because of the low rates of systemic absorption from the

Figure 7.37 Landmark technique for brachial plexus block, supraclavicular approach

Position the patient supine with the head supported by a single pillow and turned slightly away from the side to be blocked and the arm extended downwards, beside the thigh, to depress the clavicle (Figure 7.38). If the muscular landmarks are difficult to identify, ask the patient to lift his or her head slightly off the pillow to throw the muscle into relief; the interscalene groove can be highlighted by vigorous sniffing. Trace the interscalene groove distally with the non-dominant index finger until the pulsation of the subclavian artery is palpable – usually about 1 cm behind the midpoint of the clavicle. Raise a skin weal of local anaesthetic at this point and then insert a 22 G short-bevel 3.5 cm needle parallel to the neck in the horizontal plane towards the pulse of the subclavian artery. It is not crucial to feel the arterial pulse, if the groove can be identified accurately. Advance the needle until the sheath is detected at a depth of about 1–2 cm as an increased resistance with a distinct 'pop' when the needle penetrates. The patient may experience parasthesiae in the distribution of the superior trunk (C5/6, median, musculocutaneous or radial nerves). Aspirate to ensure that the needle has not entered the subclavian artery and slowly make the injection. If arterial blood is aspirated, carefully withdraw the needle a few millimetres until aspiration is negative; the needle will still be within the fascial sheath and the injection can be made as normal. Digital pressure proximal to the needle insertion will encourage distal spread as the large volume is injected.

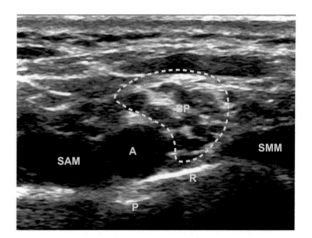

BP	-	brachial plexus
SAM	-	scalenus anterior muscle
SMM	-	scalenus medius muscle
A	-	subclavian artery
R	-	first rib
P	-	pleura

Figure 7.39 Sonoanatomy of the supraclavicular brachial plexus block

Figure 7.40 Drug doses and duration for brachial plexus block

Drug	Volume	Duration
Lidocaine 1.5% + adrenaline	40–50 mL	3–4 h
Bupivacaine 0.5% (racemic or levo)	35–40 mL	9–11 h
Ropivacaine 0.5%	35–40 mL	9–11 h

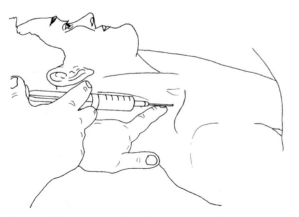

Figure 7.38 Patient position for supraclavicular brachial plexus block

brachial plexus sheath. Attention should always be paid to maximum doses of local anaesthetic agent when calculated on a body-weight basis. For axillary block the technique will be most effective in the medial aspect of the upper arm, forearm and hand, whereas for supraclavicular block distribution is fairly uniform below the shoulder but may be less dense in the ulnar aspect of the hand. A reduction in the total volume of local anaesthetic agent can be achieved by using USGRA, which also allows targeting of the individual components of the plexus and visualisation of the spread of the local anaesthetic.

Figure 7.41 Complications of brachial plexus block

Axillary
- Haematoma
- Vascular damage

Supraclavicular
- Phrenic nerve block
- Horner's syndrome
- Recurrent laryngeal nerve block

Pneumothorax

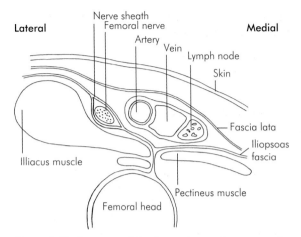

Figure 7.42 Anatomy of the femoral nerve in cross-section

Complications

Some complications may be considered as inevitable side effects of a successful block, whereas others are potentially dangerous (Figure 7.41).

Femoral nerve block
Indications
The femoral nerve may be used in combination with sciatic, obturator and lateral cutaneous nerve blocks, as appropriate, to ensure an adequate block for the proposed site of surgery. The main indication is for major orthopaedic procedures of the lower limb, especially surgery to the femur and knee joint. Postoperative analgesia following a total knee replacement or cruciate ligament reconstruction can be impressive, as a single-shot femoral nerve block may last up to 24 hours if bupivacaine 0.375% is used.

Anatomy
The femoral nerve is the largest branch of the lumbar plexus and enters the thigh lateral to the femoral artery in its own fascial sheath (Figure 7.42). It can be discretely blocked as a single nerve using 10–15 mL solution. Larger volumes (20–30 mL) have been used to produce, in effect, a distal approach to the lumbar plexus which also blocks the obturator nerve and lateral cutaneous nerve of the thigh. This was traditionally known as the '3-in-1 block', but it is unlikely that all three nerves are reliably blocked with this approach.

Technique
USGRA is commonly used to obtain a femoral nerve block, but this block can also readily be performed by the traditional landmark technique without ultrasound. The landmark technique of femoral nerve blockade is given in Figure 7.43.

Figure 7.43 Landmark technique for femoral nerve block

Position the patient supine and identify the inguinal ligament and the femoral arterial pulse immediately distal to it. The point of injection should be 1 cm lateral to the pulsation and 1–2 cm distal to the inguinal ligament. Having raised a skin weal of lidocaine, insert a 22 G short-bevel regional block needle at about 45°, aiming cephalad. A distinct pop as the needle pierces the fascia lata may be felt, followed by a secondary pop as it enters the nerve sheath. Parasthesiae in the distribution of the femoral or saphenous nerves indicates close proximity to the nerve. After aspiration, slowly inject the chosen volume. In anaesthetised patients, a peripheral nerve stimulator will aid accurate location.

Drugs, doses and volumes
Figure 7.44 shows the duration of a single-shot femoral nerve block using a long-acting local anaesthetic solution. Duration can be extended by the insertion of a catheter into the femoral nerve sheath for continuous infusion.

Complications
The only significant complication of femoral nerve block is the accidental injection of local anaesthetic into the femoral vessels, which are immediately adjacent to the nerve. Attention to detail when performing the block, careful aspiration prior to injection, and use of USGRA will prevent this avoidable complication. The limb will be

Figure 7.44 Drug doses for femoral nerve block

Drug	Volume	Duration
Bupivacaine 0.5% (racemic or levo)	15 mL	12–18 h
Bupivacaine 0.75%	12 mL	18–24 h
Bupivacaine 0.5% (racemic or levo) (for 3-in-1)	20–30 mL	8–12 h

anaesthetised for many hours, and it must therefore be protected from pressure sores and prolonged immobility.

Ankle block
Indications
The nerve supply to the foot can be blocked at the ankle to provide surgical anaesthesia and postoperative pain relief for any operation performed distal to the malleoli. The main indications are orthopaedic and trauma surgery to the forefoot and digits. Surgery such as correction of hallux valgus is very painful, and ankle blocks, using bupivacaine 0.5%, can provide 18–24 hours analgesia. Although it is usual to perform a combination of blocks at the ankle under general anaesthesia, it is possible to use the technique in conscious patients.

Anatomy
The five nerves which supply the foot and the ankle are the terminal branches of the femoral and sciatic nerves. The saphenous nerve is the terminal branch of the femoral nerve and supplies the skin over the medial malleolus and a variable amount of the medial border of the foot. It passes anterior to the medial malleolus, accompanied by the saphenous vein. The other nerves are branches of the sciatic nerve, which divides into the common peroneal and tibial nerves within the popliteal fossa. The deep and superficial peroneal nerves emerge onto the dorsum of the foot at the level of the extensor skin crease between the pulse of the dorsalis pedis and the tendon of extensor hallucis longus. The deep peroneal nerve supplies the deep structures of the dorsum of the foot and the skin of the first webspace only; the superficial peroneal nerve supplies the skin of the dorsum of the foot and the lateral three webspaces. The tibial nerve runs in a sulcus behind the medial malleolus, deep to the medial collateral ligament of the ankle, accompanied by the corresponding tibial

vessels, and divides into medial and lateral plantar nerves which supply the sole of the foot and the deep plantar structures. The sural nerve runs subcutaneously between the lateral malleolus and the calcaneus to supply the lateral border of the foot.

Technique
The landmark technique of ankle block is described in Figure 7.45.

Drugs, doses and volumes
Bupivacaine 0.5% will provide surgical anaesthesia for 3–4 hours and 12–18 hours analgesia, although up to 24 hours is possible. For minor surgery, especially in ambulant patients, lidocaine 2% will provide 1–2 hours surgical anaesthesia and 4–6 hours analgesia. Each nerve requires approximately 5–6 mL; thus the total volume used depends on the number of nerves blocked, although a maximum of 20 mL is recommended.

Complications
The main complications of these nerve blocks are the potential for intravascular injection or vascular trauma, as all the injections are made into neurovascular bundles (except the sural nerve). However, the volumes of local anaesthetic are small, the needle used should be no larger than 23 gauge, and aspirating the needle before each injection will minimise the risk. USGRA reduces the risk of vascular damage and increases the efficacy of these blocks, allowing a reduction in volumes of local anaesthetic required.

Many patients will be mobilised soon after surgery, and they must be supervised and non-weight bearing while the blocks are still working because they will have no sensory or proprioceptive awareness in the sole of the foot if the tibial nerve has been blocked.

Abdominal wall blocks
Inguinal field block
Indications
Inguinal field block in combination with light general anaesthesia is ideally suited to day-case repair of a hernia. The technique offers rapid recovery from anaesthesia and postoperative analgesia lasting for 6–8 hours. If the surgery is to be performed using local anaesthesia as a sole technique, a larger volume of more dilute local anaesthetic is preferable, and the surgeon may need to reinforce the anaesthesia by direct infiltration of the deeper structures within the inguinal canal.

Figure 7.45 Landmark technique for ankle block

Tibial nerve
Palpate the lower border of the medial malleolus and the medial surface of the calcaneal tuberosity. At the midpoint of a line between these two bony landmarks insert a 23 G needle at 90° to the skin until it just touches the periosteum of the calcaneus just below the sustentaculum tali, which can be felt as a crescent-shaped protuberance on the calcaneus. Withdraw the needle 1–2 mm, aspirate and slowly inject 5–6 mL. If the injection is in the correct plane, deep to the medical collateral ligament, the local anaesthetic will spread proximally and distally along the course of the tibial nerve.

Deep peroneal nerve
Position the foot at right angles to the tibia and palpate the pulse of dorsalis pedis. Identify the tendon of extensor hallucis longus by moving the great toe and insert a 23 G needle between these two landmarks at 45° to the skin until contact is made with the distal end of the tibia. Withdraw the needle 1–2 mm, aspirate and slowly inject 4–5 mL of local anaesthetic.

Superficial peroneal nerve
Withdraw the needle into the subcutaneous tissue having completed the deep peroneal injection, and realign it, aiming towards the lateral border of the foot. Advance the needle slowly and inject 4–5 mL of local anaesthetic subcutaneously to produce a weal of local anaesthetic extending laterally across the dorsum of the foot. This weal can be gently massaged to spread it further laterally.

Sural nerve
Palpate the lower border of the lateral malleolus and the lateral aspect of the calcaneal tuberosity and make a subcutaneous injection of 5 mL of local anaesthetic between these two points.

Saphenous nerve
Identify the saphenous vein, if possible, anterior and proximal to the medial malleolus, and inject a subcutaneous weal of 3–4 mL of local anaesthetic around the vein, using a 23 G needle. Take care to avoid intravenous injection and trauma to the vein.

Anatomy

The inguinal area is supplied by the ilioinguinal and iliohypogastric nerves, which are terminal branches of spinal nerve L1. In addition a small area of the medial

Figure 7.46 Landmark technique for inguinal field block

Lie the patient in the supine position and identify the anterior superior iliac spine (ASIS) and the pubic tubercle – the bony landmarks which define the two injection points. The top injection point will be 1 cm medial and 2 cm caudal to the ASIS. Make a skin weal of lidocaine at this point and insert a 22 G short-bevel regional block needle, at right angles to the skin, directly downwards through the skin and subcutaneous tissue. At a depth of 1–2 cm (more in obese patients), the needle will encounter the external oblique aponeurosis, which will offer marked resistance to penetration. Move the needle from side to side in a horizontal plane and a distinct scratching over the surface of the aponeurosis will be felt. The iliohypogastric nerve (T12/L1) lies just deep to the aponeurosis, so once the needle penetrates it, immobilise the needle and inject 5 mL of local anaesthetic. Carefully advance the needle another 0.5–1 cm to penetrate the internal oblique muscle (there is often a slight loss of resistance as the needle leaves the inner surface of the muscle) and inject a further 5 mL of solution to block the ilioinguinal nerve (T12/L1), immediately deep to the muscle. Withdraw the needle to the subcutaneous tissues and infiltrate a subcutaneous, fan-shaped area, using 10 mL of solution to block the terminal fibres of the subcostal nerve (T12).

The second part of the injection should be made over the pubic tubercle. Insert the needle directly down to the tubercle and inject 5 mL of solution around the external inguinal ring to anaesthetise the genitofemoral nerve (L1/2). Make a second fan-shaped subcutaneous infiltration to block any fibres that may cross the midline.

thigh and lateral aspect of the scrotum or labia majora are covered by the genitofemoral nerve (L1,2). The ilioinguinal and iliohypogastric nerves run in the plane between the internal oblique and transversus abdominis muscles. The genitofemoral nerve enters the inguinal canal and runs in the spermatic cord or with the round ligament of the uterus, to exit and become subcutaneous at the pubic tubercle.

Technique

The landmark technique of inguinal field block is detailed in Figure 7.46.

Drugs, doses and volumes

Bupivacaine 0.5% with adrenaline 1:200,000 to a total of 30 mL for supplementation of light general anaesthesia will provide up to 8 hours postoperative analgesia. For local anaesthesia as a sole technique, 50 mL prilocaine 1% is suitable, but only 2–3 hours postoperative analgesia will result.

Complications

There are few important complications, as the technique is mainly one of infiltration together with the discrete blockade of three small peripheral nerves. From the first point of injection, puncture of the peritoneum and viscera is possible if a long needle is used. Inadvertent intravascular injection is always a possibility with the second point of injection, especially the femoral vessels. It is also possible to block the femoral nerve from the same point, and the patient may complain of pain in the hernia site and a numb, heavy leg.

Transversus abdominal plane (TAP) block
Indications

The TAP block is a more recently developed technique, which targets the somatic nerves innervating the muscles and skin of the anterior abdominal wall. It provides effective supplementary analgesia after lower abdominal surgery, with a reduction in pain scores and opioid requirements.

Anatomy

The myocutaneous nerves which supply the anterior abdominal wall (T6–L1) lie within the muscular plane between internal oblique and transversus abdominis, referred to as the transversus abdominal plane (TAP). The point of needle insertion is identified by palpating the triangle of Petit, an area posterior to the mid-axillary line circumscribed by the iliac crest, latissimus dorsi and external oblique muscles. For an extensive incision extending into the epigastrium a subcostal TAP block may be added to ensure complete coverage of the upper and lower anterior abdominal wall.

Technique

This block has particularly evolved with the advent of USGRA, since ultrasound guidance is required to identify the transversus abdominis plane. See Figures 7.47 and 7.48 for the technique and sonoanatomy of the TAP block.

Figure 7.47 USGRA technique for TAP block

Lie the patient in the supine position. The point of needle insertion is identified by palpating the triangle of Petit, an area posterior to the mid-axillary line circumscribed by the iliac crest, latissimus dorsi and external oblique muscles. The needle is inserted perpendicular to the skin and advanced until the space between internal oblique and transversus abdominis is identified by a loss-of-resistance technique similar to the one described for the inguinal field block ('pop technique'). In many patients the identification of the triangle can be challenging, generally due to excessive adipose tissue but also to the anatomical variation in its location on the lateral abdominal wall.

This block is particularly suited for USGRA. Ultrasound demonstrates the three muscular layers (see Figure 7.48 for sonoanatomy of the TAP block). An in-plane technique enables the advance of the needle in an anteromedial direction to be made under direct observation, to the plane between internal oblique and transversus abdominis muscles. Hydrodissection is generally well visualised as the local anaesthetic is injected and a hypoechoic (dark) lens shape develops between two distinctive 'tramlines'.

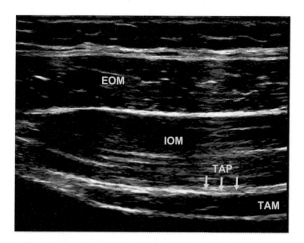

EOM -	external oblique muscle
IOM -	internal oblique muscle
TAM -	transversus abdominis muscle
TAP -	transversus abdominis plane

Figure 7.48 Sonoanatomy of the TAP block

Drugs, doses and volumes

Usually a volume of 20 mL of local anaesthetic agent is adequate. The concentration has to be adjusted accordingly to minimise toxicity. This will be especially relevant in the case of performing a bilateral block.

Complications

Intraperitoneal penetration and visceral perforation has been reported with the landmark technique. Using USGRA reduces this risk.

Penile block
Indications

The main indication for penile block is for postoperative analgesia for adult and paediatric male circumcision, although any surgery on the shaft of the penis will benefit. Analgesia is comparable with that produced by a caudal block and avoids the motor and sensory effects on the legs and the autonomic dysfunction of bladder and bowel control. There are no major complications provided that adrenaline or other vasoconstrictors are not used and intravascular injection is avoided.

Anatomy

The shaft and glans of the penis are supplied by a pair of nerves (the dorsal penile nerves) which are terminal branches of the pudendal nerve (S2, 3, 4). The paired nerves emerge beneath the inferior surface of the pubic symphysis separated by the suspensory ligament and deep to Buck's fascia (the fascial sheath surrounding the corpora cavernosa). The perineal nerves (from the other branch of the pudendal nerve) which innervate the anterior part of the scrotum and the midline ventral surface of the penis need to be blocked for complete penile analgesia.

Technique

See Figure 7.49 for a description of the technique of penile nerve block.

Drugs, doses and volumes

Avoid local anaesthetic solutions that contain adrenaline. Bupivacaine 0.5% will provide 6–8 hours postoperative analgesia following circumcision. 10 mL is sufficient for an adult; children need 3–6 mL according to body weight and size. Limit total dose of bupivacaine to 2 mg kg^{-1} body weight.

Figure 7.49 Technique for penile nerve block

Palpate the inferior edge of the pubic symphysis with the non-dominant index finger and insert a 21 G (adult) or 23 G (paediatric) needle at about 45° until it contacts the pubis or passes just caudad to it. If the needle contacts the pubis, re-angle it to walk it off the inferior edge and through Buck's fascia, which may be detectable as a slight resistance to the needle. After careful aspiration, make a single injection in the midline (both dorsal nerves may be reliably blocked by a single injection). In an adult, inject 7 mL and then inject a further 3 mL as a subcutaneous weal across the midline of the ventral surface of the penis at its junction with the scrotum, starting approximately 1 cm lateral to the midline raphe and finishing 1 cm lateral on the other side. It is important to keep the needle subcutaneous while making this injection as the urethra is superficial at this point. In children the volume needs to be reduced pro rata according to body weight and penile size.

Local anaesthesia of the upper airway

The mucosal surfaces of the mouth, oropharynx, glottis and larynx may be anaesthetised by a combination of topical anaesthesia and discrete nerve blocks.

Indications

Intubation of the trachea in patients with difficult airway due to trauma or disease.

Anatomy

The nerve supply of the airway comes from three sources. The trigeminal nerve supplies the nasopharynx, palate (V2) and anterior aspect of tongue (V3). The glossopharyngeal nerve supplies the oropharynx, posterior aspect of tongue and soft palate. The vagus nerve gives off two nerves – the superior laryngeal and recurrent laryngeal nerves – which supply motor and sensory fibres to the airway below the epiglottis. The superior laryngeal nerve emerges beneath the inferior edge of the greater cornu of the hyoid before it divides into the internal and external branches.

Technique

The technique of local anaesthesia of the upper airway comprises three parts, topical anaesthesia, superior

Figure 7.50 Technique for local anaesthesia of the airway

To topically anaesthetise the mouth and oropharynx, sit the patient up with the mouth open maximally and spray four metered puffs of lidocaine (10 mg per spray) onto the tongue and wait a few minutes for it to take effect. Depress the tongue and spray a further four puffs onto the posterior part of the tongue and pharynx.

Although the superior laryngeal nerve can be topically anaesthetised by placing a pledget soaked in lidocaine 2% into each pyriform fossa with Krause forceps, once the mouth and tongue are blocked, it is more usually blocked discretely as follows. Place the patient supine with the head extended and palpate the hyoid bone just cephalad to the thyroid cartilage. Displace the hyoid slightly towards the side to be blocked and insert a 25 G, 2.5 cm needle just under the inferior border of the hyoid and inject 2–3 mL of lidocaine 1%, moving the needle gently in and out through the thyrohyoid membrane (Figure 7.51). Repeat on the other side.

To complete the airway anaesthesia, with the patient in the same position as above, palpate the inferior border of the thyroid cartilage and, having first anaesthetised the skin, insert a 21 G, 2.5 cm needle through the cricothyroid membrane into the lumen of the trachea. Ensure that air is freely aspirable and then rapidly inject 3–4 mL of lidocaine 2%. This will precipitate brisk coughing, which spreads the local anaesthetic throughout the trachea and up into the larynx and vocal cords (Figure 7.52). Total dose of lidocaine in an average 70 kg adult should not exceed 200 mg.

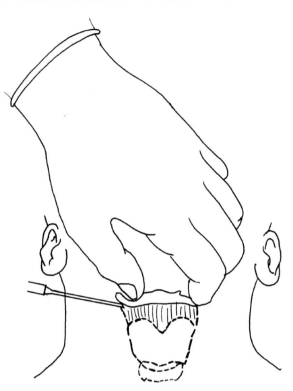

Figure 7.51 Superior laryngeal nerve block

laryngeal nerve block and transtracheal anaesthesia. Practical details are given in Figure 7.50.

Intravenous regional anaesthesia (IVRA)

The technique in current use differs from the original description of August Bier in 1908, although it is often called 'Bier's block'. Bier placed two tourniquets on the forearm and injected procaine directly into a vein isolated by surgical cut-down. Although a two-tourniquet technique has been re-evaluated recently, one tourniquet is used in modern practice.

Indications

Any surgery lasting less than 1 hour below the level of the elbow in the arm or the ankle in the leg.

Equipment

The tourniquet used must be properly maintained with regular calibration of the pressure gauge and must be of an approved design. Sphygmomanometer cuffs should never be used. Specially designed double-cuff tourniquets are available: these allow the proximal cuff to be blown up while the block is established, and then the distal cuff is inflated over anaesthetised skin for use during surgery and the proximal one deflated. This improves comfort during prolonged procedures, but the patient may still experience deep pain from ischaemic muscle.

Technique

The practical technique for performing IVRA is shown in Figure 7.53.

Analgesia will be complete within 15 minutes using prilocaine 0.5%. The cuff should remain inflated for at

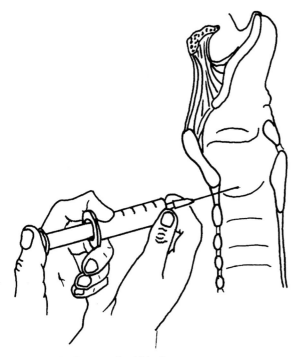

Figure 7.52 Transtracheal block

Figure 7.53 Technique for performing IVRA

Place an intravenous cannula in the dorsum of both hands, one for injection of the local anaesthetic and the other to allow for drug and fluid requirements during surgery. Wrap a layer of wool padding around the upper arm and place the tourniquet over the padding, ensuring that it is of the correct dimensions for the limb and properly secured. Elevate the limb and use a compression bandage to exsanguinate it or simply compress the axillary artery and keep the arm elevated for three minutes. Inflate the tourniquet to 100 mmHg above the patient's systolic blood pressure, remove the compression bandage and observe the arm for one minute to ensure that the veins remain empty. If blood begins to flow under the tourniquet the procedure should be repeated, using a pressure 150 mmHg above systolic, or an alternative anaesthetic technique considered. Inject the local anaesthetic solution slowly (20 mL per minute) to avoid high intravenous pressures which could force it under the tourniquet.

least 20 minutes, after which time deflation of the cuff and systemic release of the local anaesthetic drug should not cause untoward reactions, although occasionally some transient minor systemic symptoms such as light-headedness or tinnitus are reported. IVRA in the leg is not practical if the cuff has to be placed around the thigh, as inflation pressures of 300–400 mmHg above systolic and very large volumes of local anaesthetic are required. If the surgery is limited to below the ankle, however, then a cuff around the calf is possible, using pressures and drug volumes similar to those in the arm, although exsanguination may not be ideal as the lower leg has a two-bone compartment and vessels between the tibia and fibula will not be compressed. There is also a risk of damage to the peroneal nerve in the region of the head of the fibula if a high tourniquet is applied.

Drugs, doses and volumes

The local anaesthetic agent currently licensed for IVRA is prilocaine 0.5%. For an adult male, 60 mL 0.5% (300 mg) produces good sensory and motor block and is well within the maximum recommended dose of 600 mg.

References and further reading

Armitage EN. Caudal block in children. *Anaesthesia* 1979; **34**: 396.

Association of Anaesthetists of Great Britain and Ireland, Obstetric Anaesthetists' Association and Regional Anaesthesia UK. Regional anaesthesia and patients with abnormalities of coagulation. *Anaesthesia* 2013; **68**: 966–72.

Bromage PR. A comparison of the hydrochloride and carbon dioxide salts of lidocaine and prilocaine in epidural analgesia. *Acta Anaesthsiol Scand Suppl* 1965; **16**: 55–69.

Brown DL. *Regional Anesthesia and Analgesia*. Philadelphia, PA: Saunders, 1996.

Greene NM. Distribution of local anaesthetic solutions within the subarachnoid space. *Anesth Analg* 1985; **64**: 715–30.

Kim JT, Jung CW, Lee KH. The effect of insulin on the resuscitation of bupivacaine-induced severe cardiovascular toxicity in dogs. *Anesth Analg* 2004; **99**: 728–33.

Lin E, Gaur A, Jones M, Ahmed A. *Sonoanatomy for Anaesthetists*. Cambridge: Cambridge University Press 2012.

Picard J, Meek T, Weinberg G, Hertz P. Lipid emulsion for local anaesthetic toxicity. *Anaesthesia* 2006; **61**: 1116–17.

Pinnock CA, Fischer HBJ, Jones RP. *Peripheral Nerve Blockade*. Edinburgh: Churchill Livingstone, 1996.

Royal College of Anaesthetists. *Major Complications of Central Neuraxial Block in the United Kingdom*. The 3rd National Audit Project of The Royal College of Anaesthetists (NAP3). London: RCoA, 2009.

CHAPTER 8

Principles of resuscitation

Anita Stronach

Cardiorespiratory arrest

The contents of this chapter have been updated in accordance with scientific evidence and audit data accrued since the year 2005 (Nolan *et al.* 2010), and are firmly linked to the teaching and algorithms of the Resuscitation Council (UK) (2015) and the European Resuscitation Council (2015).

Causes

A person suffers a cardiorespiratory arrest either because of a primary cardiac problem or secondary to non-cardiac causes. The majority of cardiac arrests occurring in adults outside hospital are from ventricular fibrillation (VF) due to myocardial ischaemia arising from pre-existing ischaemic heart disease (IHD). Other cardiac conditions which may lead to cardiorespiratory arrest include valvular heart disease, cardiomyopathy, myocarditis, endocarditis and conduction defects, e.g. Wolff–Parkinson–White syndrome or prolonged atrioventricular (AV) block.

An important secondary cause of cardiorespiratory arrest is uncorrected hypoxia resulting from airway obstruction. Hypoxia leads to myocardial failure, which is compounded by the resulting hypercarbia and acidosis. A bradycardia will

develop, and this will be followed by an asystolic cardiac arrest unless the airway obstruction is cleared. Some causes of airway obstruction are listed in Figure 8.1.

Non-cardiac causes of cardiac arrest

- Electrocution
- Electrolyte abnormalities
- Hypothermia
- Intracerebral haemorrhage
- Mechanical
  - massive pulmonary thromboembolism or air embolism
  - tension pneumothorax
  - pneumopericardium
  - cardiac tamponade
  - hypovolaemia
- Muscular disorders
- Neurological disorders
- Poisoning

Despite trained cardiac arrest teams being present in hospitals and readily available to manage cardiac arrests,

Fundamentals of Anaesthesia, 4th edition, ed. Ted Lin, Tim Smith and Colin Pinnock. Published by Cambridge University Press. © Cambridge University Press 2017.

Figure 8.1 Causes of airway obstruction

Cause	Nature of obstruction
Coma	Tongue displacement
Anaphylaxis	Tongue, oropharyngeal and laryngeal oedema, bronchospasm, pulmonary oedema
Foreign body	Oropharyngeal, laryngeal, tracheal and bronchial obstruction, bronchospasm
Trauma	Oropharyngeal and laryngeal damage
Infection	Oropharyngeal, laryngeal and pulmonary oedema
Asthma	Bronchospasm
Irritants/poisons/ burns/smoke inhalation	Tongue/oropharyngeal/ laryngeal oedema, laryngeal/bronchospasm, pulmonary oedema
Near-drowning	Pulmonary oedema
Neurogenic shock	Pulmonary oedema
Aspiration	Pulmonary oedema

Adapted from European Resuscitation Council Guidelines for Resuscitation 2005. *Resuscitation* 2005; **67** (Suppl. 1): S1–190.

fewer than 20% of patients who suffer an in-hospital cardiac arrest will survive to go home. Most of those who do survive are in cardiac monitored beds and are rapidly resuscitated from VF secondary to myocardial ischaemia.

Unmonitored patients who suffer cardiac arrest have often shown evidence of hypoxia and hypotension for several hours prior to their arrest, which either goes unnoticed or is poorly treated. The presenting rhythm at these cardiac arrests is usually pulseless electrical activity (PEA) or asystole, and the outcome is poor. It is therefore imperative that, as well as being able to recognise a patient who is having a cardiorespiratory arrest, systems are put in place to allow early identification and management of those patients who if left untreated will deteriorate and suffer a cardiorespiratory arrest.

Recognition

Previously, guidelines have recommended palpating for the presence of a pulse to diagnose a cardiorespiratory arrest. However, checking for a carotid pulse, whether by trained healthcare professionals or by lay rescuers, has been shown to be not only time-consuming but also an inaccurate method of confirming either the presence or absence of circulation. The guidelines now advise that an unconscious, unresponsive patient who is not moving and not breathing normally should be diagnosed as having a cardiorespiratory arrest. Agonal breathing, which is seen as occasional gasps, slow, laboured or noisy breathing, is a common sign in the early stages of cardiac arrest and should be recognised as a sign of cardiac arrest and not mistaken for normal breathing.

As well as being able to recognise patients who have suffered a cardiorespiratory arrest, it is important to identify acutely ill patients whose condition is deteriorating, since cardiac arrest in this group of patients is often predictable and may be preventable. Early-warning scoring systems such as MEWS (modified early warning system) and PARS (patient at risk score) have been established in hospitals for several years. These scoring systems use data obtained from regular monitoring of vital signs, so that appropriate help is called at an early stage. Effective treatment can then be started to prevent further deterioration. Such systems, however, rely on the accuracy of recorded physiological parameters, which are not always recorded either regularly or accurately on general wards.

The most important determinant of survival at a cardiac arrest is the presence of someone who is trained, willing, able and equipped to act in an emergency. In many hospitals, medical emergency teams, made up of medical and nursing staff from critical care and medical backgrounds, have replaced cardiac arrest teams. These have been established to respond not only to cardiac arrests but also to patients with acute physiological deterioration. It is now recognised that medical emergencies, and not only cardiorespiratory arrests, need the presence of appropriately trained personnel (Figure 8.2).

Cardiopulmonary resuscitation

Although cardiopulmonary resuscitation (CPR) is traditionally divided into basic life support (BLS) and advanced life support (ALS), this division is arbitrary when cardiac arrests occur in hospital. The immediate response will depend both on the skills of the initial rescuer and on the equipment available. The aim of

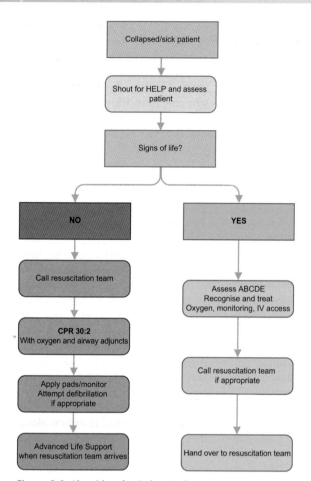

Figure 8.2 Algorithm for in-hospital resuscitation. Reproduced with the kind permission of the Resuscitation Council (UK). © Resuscitation Council (UK) (2015)

quality chest compressions with minimal interruptions, as there is evidence that this is associated with improved survival.

The recommendation of a specific cardiac compression: ventilation ratio is a compromise between the need to generate forward blood flow and the need to supply oxygen to the lungs to optimise oxygen delivery to the brain and other vital organs. A 30:2 ratio is recommended, taking into account evidence available to optimise outcomes during CPR. The guidelines have been kept simple to aid learning and retention of BLS skills.

The adult BLS algorithm is as shown in Figure 8.3. Before approaching a collapsed person, a priority is to ensure both personal safety and that of bystanders. Although this is more important outside hospital, there are still safety issues to be considered within the hospital environment. Check for a response by shaking the person's shoulders gently and asking loudly 'are you alright?' If there is no response, shout for help and turn the patient onto his or her back, except in pregnancy (see *Resuscitation of the pregnant patient*), and commence BLS.

Airway

The maintenance of a patent airway during the management of a cardiorespiratory arrest is imperative. In an unconscious patient the tongue falls backwards and the airway is obstructed at the oropharyngeal level. Three simple airway manoeuvres, head tilt, chin lift and jaw thrust, can all be used to open the airway. In a patient who is still making respiratory effort, this may prevent the patient from deteriorating and suffering a cardiorespiratory arrest. The **head tilt**, which flexes the lower cervical spine while extending the head at the atlanto-occipital joint, and the **chin lift** may be sufficient to open an obstructed airway. If not, a **jaw thrust** may be added to further displace the tongue forwards.

In trauma cases where there is a suspected cervical spine injury, manual in-line traction must be applied and jaw-thrust/chin-lift techniques used to open the airway. If still unable to adequately clear the airway, a gentle head tilt may be added. Although all these airway manoeuvres are associated with some cervical spine movement, the maintenance of an open airway is the overriding priority and damage to spinal cord from excessive head tilt has never been reported in cases where cervical spine injury has been suspected.

Look in the mouth to check for any obvious obstruction and use a finger sweep to clear any visible foreign body present within the oropharynx. Then, taking no

effective CPR is to restore a spontaneous circulation to the patient as soon as possible. Although in most circumstances it is possible to support ventilation for prolonged periods effectively, there is no equivalent method of providing circulatory support without a heart beating in an effective rhythm producing cardiac output.

Basic life support

Basic life support (BLS), strictly defined, is the maintenance of a clear airway while supporting ventilation and circulation without the use of specialist equipment other than a protective airway device, e.g. a pocket mask. Current guidelines place a greater emphasis on good-

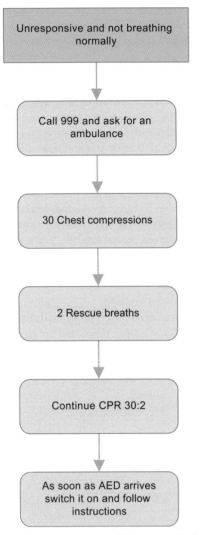

Figure 8.3 Adult basic life support (BLS) algorithm. Reproduced with the kind permission of the Resuscitation Council (UK). © Resuscitation Council (UK) (2015)

correct hand position for cardiac compressions is found by placing the heel of the dominant hand in the centre of the chest between the nipples. The heel of other hand is then placed on top and the fingers interlocked, ensuring that pressure is applied over the sternum and not the ribs or abdomen. The rescuer assumes a position vertically above the patient's chest and with straight arms applies compressions to a depth of 5–6 centimetres and at a rate of 100–120 compressions per minute.

The time taken for compression and release should be equal. After each compression all pressure on the chest must be released without losing contact between hands and sternum. If chest recoil is not complete it may lead to significantly increased intrathoracic pressure, decreased venous return and decreased coronary and cerebral perfusion.

Properly executed cardiac compressions are tiring, and there is evidence that the quality of chest compressions deteriorates as the rescuer tires. If there is more than one rescuer present, change the person performing cardiac compressions every 2 minutes.

Cardiac compressions generate forward blood flow by increasing intrathoracic pressure and directly compressing the heart. Although the mean carotid arterial pressure, even with good-quality cardiac compressions, seldom exceeds 40 mmHg, it provides a small but critical blood flow to the brain and myocardium.

During a VF arrest, blood continues to flow into and dilate the right ventricle. Early CPR prevents the right ventricle dilating and thereby increases the likelihood that a defibrillatory shock will terminate VF and enable the heart to resume an effective rhythm. It may also prevent an initial rhythm of VF deteriorating to asystole. With evidence that a patient stands the best chance of survival if rapidly resuscitated from VF, automated external defibrillators (AED) are being introduced widely in public places as well as becoming standard equipment on many hospital wards. For in-hospital cardiac arrests the use of an AED is an integral part of BLS.

Allowance has now been made in the guidelines for the rescuer who is unable or unwilling to perform mouth-to-mouth ventilation. Chest compressions alone are recommended in this situation. This will only be effective for the first few minutes, and then only in cases of non-hypoxic cardiac arrests, as within 4–6 minutes all oxygen stores are depleted. It is not recommended as standard management.

longer than 10 seconds, **look** for chest moments, **listen** for breath sounds, and **feel** for air movement. If the respiratory pattern is not normal and the patient is unresponsive, call for help and start cardiac compressions.

Circulation

Chest compressions must be started with the patient placed in a supine position on a firm surface. The

Rescue breathing

Expired air ventilation is the standard method used for rescue breathing in BLS, and produces an inspired oxygen content of 16–17%. Using chin-lift/head-tilt and/or jaw-thrust manoeuvres, the airway is opened while the rescuer takes a normal breath. If a pocket mask is not readily available, the soft part of the nose is closed by pinching between the index finger and thumb and the rescuer's lips are placed round the patient's mouth, making sure that a good seal is achieved before expiration. As well as mouth-to-mouth and mouth-to-nose ventilation, if the mouth is clenched shut or is badly injured, mouth-to-tracheal stoma ventilation is effective. The chest must be observed to rise and fall during each rescue breath.

Each rescue breath is given over 1 second, at a rate of 10–12 breaths per minute, to produce tidal volumes of about 500 mL. This limits interruptions to cardiac compressions and minimises gastric distension. Gastric distension splints the diaphragm and interferes with ventilation as well as increasing the risk of aspiration. Large tidal volumes increase intrathoracic pressure, decreasing coronary and cerebral perfusion, and in animals have been shown to reduce the chance of successful return of spontaneous circulation. Oxygenation is not impaired by the use of small tidal volumes, and the resulting hypercarbia and acidosis has not been shown to adversely affect outcome. The time taken to give two rescue breaths should be less than 5 seconds, which limits interruptions to cardiac compressions.

Only stop resuscitation if there are signs of regaining consciousness such as coughing, opening eyes, speaking or moving purposefully and there is resumption of normal respiration. Once cardiac output and normal respiration have been re-established, the patient should be turned into the recovery position. This is a stable lateral position, with the head dependent and no pressure on the chest to impair breathing. With increasing levels of obesity, the risks of injury to the rescuer when turning the patient must be balanced against the risks associated with leaving the patient supine.

Special situations
Foreign-body airway obstruction

Choking in adults tends to occur when eating, and should be promptly recognised and treated. If not, and the airway is severely compromised, the victim's condition will

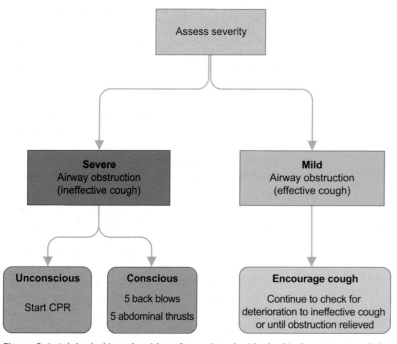

Figure 8.4 Adult choking algorithm. Reproduced with the kind permission of the Resuscitation Council (UK). © Resuscitation Council (UK) (2015)

rapidly deteriorate to a cardiorespiratory arrest. If there is mild respiratory distress, characterised by the ability to speak, breathe and cough, the victim should be encouraged to cough to clear the obstruction.

If there is severe airway obstruction, the victim will be unable to speak, breathe or cough. If the victim remains conscious, stand to one side slightly behind them and, while supporting the chest with one hand, lean the victim forwards so that the obstructing object when dislodged comes out of the mouth. Immediately give up to five back blows between the shoulder blades with the heel of your hand. The aim is to dislodge the foreign body with each blow, rather than to give all five.

If this fails to relieve the airway obstruction, give up to five abdominal thrusts. Stand behind the victim, with both arms around the upper part of the abdomen, between the umbilicus and xiphisternum. Clench your fist and, while holding this with your other hand, pull sharply inwards and upwards. Repeat the abdominal thrust manoeuvre up to five times. There is no evidence to suggest which method should be used first. If the obstruction is still not relieved, continue alternating five back blows with five abdominal thrusts.

If the patient is initially unconscious or loses consciousness at any time, call for help and start BLS (Figure 8.3).

Cardiorespiratory arrest secondary to hypoxia

In cases of identifiable asphyxia, e.g. drowning, trauma and intoxication, the victim should receive 1 minute of CPR before a single rescuer calls for help. Five initial rescue breaths are given before starting chest compressions.

Advanced life support

Advanced life support (ALS) is a continuum of BLS and involves the use of extra equipment to aid resuscitation attempts. The adult ALS algorithm (Figure 8.5) provides a standardised approach to the treatment of all adult patients presenting in cardiac arrest.

Arrhythmias associated with a cardiac arrest are divided into two groups: shockable rhythms (ventricular fibrillation (VF) and ventricular tachycardia (VT)) and non-shockable rhythms (asystole and pulseless electrical activity (PEA)). The main difference in the management of these arrhythmias is the need for early defibrillation in patients with VF/VT. Subsequent actions, including advanced airway management, ventilation, good-quality chest compressions, venous access and administration of adrenaline, are common to both groups.

During CPR it is imperative that repeated attempts are made to identify and treat potentially reversible causes (Figure 8.5).

Airway

Even when correctly performed by experienced personnel, the simple airway manoeuvres as taught in BLS do not always allow maintenance of a clear airway. The use of mechanical aids should help, but if these are used by inadequately trained personnel there may be increased complications without any improvement in airway management.

Forceps or suction are used to remove any foreign material visible in the oropharynx.

Pharyngeal airways, inserted by either the oral or the nasal route, overcome the backward displacement of the soft palate and tongue. The oropharyngeal airway can only be used in unconscious patients and must be removed if there is gagging or retching. The nasopharyngeal airway is useful in situations where the mouth cannot be opened, but must be inserted gently as there is a risk of haemorrhage. In most cases the benefit of improved airway patency outweighs this risk.

A laryngeal mask airway (LMA) or iGel is relatively easy to insert and provides more efficient ventilation than standard bag-mask ventilation. Cardiac compressions may still need to be interrupted to enable adequate ventilation without an excessive air leak. The LMA only offers partial airway protection during CPR, but there have been few case reports of aspiration in this situation.

Endotracheal intubation remains the gold standard in airway management during CPR. Its use protects the airway from aspiration, prevents gastric distension, allows suction of airway secretions, provides a route for drug administration and allows cardiac compressions to continue uninterrupted during ventilation. Disadvantages include a comparatively high failure rate when performed by non-anaesthetists, the risk of a misplaced tube, and prolonged periods of time without cardiac compressions while attempts are made to intubate. Endotracheal intubation should therefore only be attempted by trained personnel, taking no longer than 10 seconds to complete the process, in order to minimise interruptions to cardiac compressions. Correct placement of the endotracheal tube

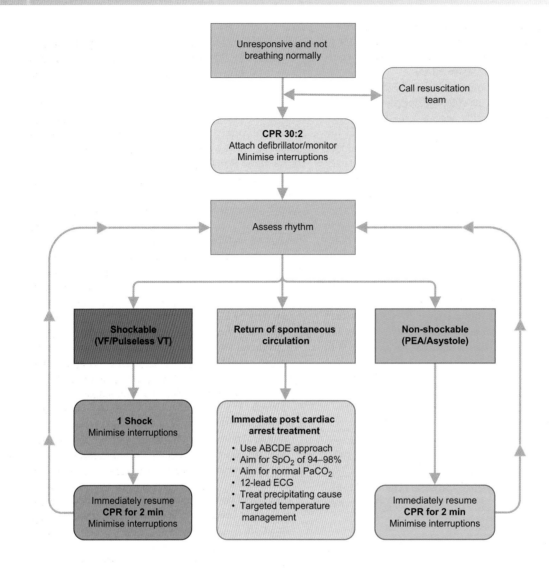

Figure 8.5 Adult advanced life support (ALS) algorithm. Reproduced with the kind permission of the Resuscitation Council (UK). © Resuscitation Council (UK) (2015)

must be confirmed, as with intubation in theatre. The 2015 guidelines for ALS recommend the use of capnography to both confirm and continually monitor tube placement. An increase in end-tidal carbon dioxide concentrations may provide an early indication of the return of a spontaneous circulation.

A needle or surgical cricothyroidotomy can be life-saving in the 'can't intubate, can't ventilate' scenario when there is extensive facial trauma or laryngeal obstruction secondary to oedema or foreign-body ingestion. Percutaneous or surgical tracheostomies are not recommended in this emergency situation, as they take too long to perform.

Ventilation

As in BLS, inspiratory time for ventilation should be limited to 1 second, producing a tidal volume of about 500 mL at a rate of 10–12 breaths per minute. This allows adequate ventilation without excessive interruptions to cardiac compressions. Although expired air ventilation provides effective ventilation, an inspired oxygen concentration of only 16–17% can be achieved. A self-inflating bag will deliver 21% oxygen, and this can be increased to 45% if oxygen is attached directly to the bag. With the addition of a reservoir system and oxygen at 15 L per minute, an inspired oxygen concentration exceeding 85% can be achieved.

To effectively ventilate a patient with a bag-mask technique is difficult, and meticulous attention must be paid to maintaining an open airway while observing the rise and fall of the chest. Even when skilled in airway management, bag-mask ventilation is often a two-person technique. Endotracheal intubation will in most cases, and the use of a LMA may, allow ventilation at a rate of 10 breaths per minute, without interruptions of cardiac compressions.

Circulation

When an unmonitored patient suffers a cardiac arrest, initial attention should be focused on providing good-quality minimally interrupted chest compressions as described for BLS (cardiac compressions : ventilation ratio 30:2). Chest compressions should only be briefly paused to allow a specific intervention to take place. As soon as a defibrillator arrives the cardiac rhythm must be monitored and the appropriate limb of the ALS algorithm (Figure 8.5) followed, depending on the diagnosis.

Shockable rhythms (VF/VT)

The most common presenting rhythm at a cardiac arrest is VF, and if VF is present for more than a few minutes the myocardium is depleted of oxygen and metabolic substrates. A brief period of chest compressions before defibrillation will deliver small amounts of oxygen and energy substrates, which will increase the probability of restoring a perfusing rhythm after shock delivery. Early defibrillation has been shown to improve the chances of survival in VF/VT arrests.

Once VF or pulseless VT has been diagnosed, defibrillation should be attempted as soon as possible. Shock energies should start at 150 J and may be repeated or increase with subsequent shocks to a maximum of 360 J. Chest compressions should continue while the defibrillator is charged to minimise the pre-shock pause. CPR should resume immediately after the first shock and continue for 2 minutes before reassessing the rhythm. If VT/VF persists, give a second shock and restart CPR immediately. Continue for a further 2 minutes before pausing to reassess the rhythm and, if still in VT/VF, give a third shock, resume CPR, and give adrenaline, 1 mg IV, and amiodarone, 300 mg IV. Continue the 2-minute CPR, rhythm/pulse check, defibrillation sequence, and if VF/VT persists, on alternate cycles give adrenaline 1 mg IV immediately following shocks (approximately every 3–5 minutes).

If at any time organised electrical activity is seen when checking the rhythm, and there are no clinical signs of spontaneous circulation (i.e. signs of regaining consciousness such as coughing, opening eyes, speaking or moving purposefully, normal respiration, or increasing end-tidal carbon dioxide concentrations on capnography), change to the non-shockable limb of the algorithm; similarly if the rhythm deteriorates to asystole.

Fine VF is very difficult to distinguish from asystole, and is unlikely to be shocked into a perfusing rhythm. Repeated attempts at defibrillation not only cause myocardial damage but also repeatedly interrupt chest compressions. If fine VF is suspected start CPR, which may increase the amplitude and frequency of VF and the chances of successful defibrillation.

A precordial thump is now recommended only in the case of a witnessed cardiac arrest when a defibrillator is not immediately available. Although a precordial thump may convert VT to sinus rhythm, and has been reported to convert VF into sinus rhythm if given within 10 seconds of a VF arrest, rare adverse effects have also been reported. These include rate acceleration of VT, conversion of VT to VF, complete heart block and asystole.

A precordial thump is performed by using the ulnar edge of a tightly clenched fist to deliver a sharp impact to the lower half of the sternum from a height of about 20 cm. The fist should immediately be retracted to create an impulse-like stimulus. The mechanical energy of the thump is converted to electrical energy, which may be sufficient to achieve defibrillation.

Electrical defibrillation

Electrical defibrillation is the passage of an electrical current across the myocardium that is of sufficient magnitude to depolarise a critical mass of myocardium. If the heart is still viable, normal pacemakers will take over and produce coordinated electrical activity, which will restore spontaneous circulation. The optimum energy to use is that which achieves defibrillation of a critical mass of myocardium while causing minimal myocardial damage. Transthoracic impedance, typically 70–80 Ω in adults, is at its lowest at the end of expiration, and defibrillation should be attempted at this point of the respiratory cycle. Shaving a hairy chest may also further reduce impedance by improving contact between pad/paddle and skin.

Self-adhesive pads are preferred to manual paddles as they not only allow delivery of shocks more rapidly and defibrillation from a safe distance, but also facilitate continuation of chest compressions during charging of the defibrillator. Pads or paddles can be placed in the antero-apical position, with the right sternal pad to the right of the sternum below the clavicle and the apical pad in the mid-axillary line in the V6 ECG electrode position. An alternative position is to place pads/paddles anteroposteriorly, which may provide more effective defibrillation. However, this must be balanced against the difficulty in applying the posterior pad/paddle to an unconscious patient. If there is a pacemaker or implantable cardioverter defibrillator (ICD) present, it is safer to place the pads away from the device if possible.

ALS guidelines advise a single-shock protocol (Figure 8.5), and not three stacked shocks as previously recommended. The stacked-shock protocol led to significant periods of time without cardiac compressions, which has been shown to be detrimental to a patient's chance of survival. Defibrillator technology has also advanced, producing biphasic waveforms, which are more efficient than the monophasic waveforms produced by older defibrillators. The success of the first shock from a biphasic defibrillator now exceeds 90%, and failure to terminate VF/VT indicates the need for further CPR to improve myocardial oxygenation rather than the need for further shocks. Biphasic devices produce either truncated exponential waveforms or rectilinear biphasic waveforms, and these require different energy levels for defibrillation. Manufacturers should display an effective waveform energy range on the biphasic device, but if unsure use 200 J for the first shock.

Even if defibrillation is successful, it is very rare for a pulse to become palpable immediately after defibrillation, and CPR must therefore be restarted immediately after delivery of a shock. If a perfusing rhythm has not been restored, this avoids a further interruption of CPR. If a perfusing rhythm has been restored, CPR is not detrimental and will not precipitate further episodes of VF/VT. If the shock has converted VF/VT into asystole, then a further period of CPR may induce VF, which has a better prognosis.

Non-shockable rhythms (pulseless electrical activity and asystole)

Pulseless electrical activity (PEA) is when cardiac electrical activity is present but there are no palpable pulses. A PEA arrest resulting from primary myocardial pump failure carries a very poor prognosis; however, it is often secondary to potentially reversible causes listed in Figure 8.5, and if these are rapidly identified and appropriately treated, PEA is often survivable.

When **PEA** is diagnosed CPR must be started immediately according to the ALS algorithm, and when IV access is achieved 1 mg of adrenaline (IV) should be given. Continue CPR at a ratio of 30:2 until the airway is secured with an endotracheal tube, and then continue cardiac compressions uninterrupted with a ventilation rate of 10–12 breaths per minute. After 2 minutes of CPR recheck the rhythm, and if an organised rhythm is present also check for a pulse. If PEA persists, continue with 2-minute cycles of CPR, giving further adrenaline 1 mg IV on alternate cycles (every 3–5 minutes). Repeated attempts should be made to identify and treat any potentially reversible causes.

As soon as **asystole** is diagnosed start CPR immediately. While continuing CPR, check that all monitoring devices are correctly attached and that there is not a disconnection producing an apparent asystolic trace. Establish IV access, give 1 mg of adrenaline (IV), and continue with CPR for 2 minutes, before rechecking the rhythm. If asystole persists, the airway should be secured and CPR continued in accordance with the ALS algorithm

(Figure 8.5). Adrenaline (1 mg IV boluses) should be given every 3–5 minutes. During rhythm checks the ECG should be carefully scrutinised for the presence of P waves: if present, pacing may restore a perfusing rhythm.

If at any time the rhythm changes to VF/VT then the shockable limb of the ALS algorithm should be followed.

Drug usage

The most common route for drug administration during a cardiorespiratory arrest is via a peripheral IV cannula. It is relatively quick and easy to establish, when compared with central venous access, and is safer. When drugs are given peripherally each dose should be flushed with 10–20 mL of saline and the limb elevated for 10–20 seconds to facilitate drug delivery. If a central venous line is present it should be used in preference to peripheral lines, as higher peak drug concentrations are achieved and drug circulation times are shorter. However, to insert a central venous line at the time of a cardiac arrest is time-consuming, which necessitates time without chest compressions, and is associated with a high risk of complications.

It is now recommended that if intravenous access has not been established within 2 minutes, the intraosseous (IO) route should be considered in adults as well as in children. With the ease of gaining IO access using semi-automated devices and the knowledge that plasma concentrations achieved from tracheal administration of drugs are variable and unpredictable, giving drugs via the endotracheal tube is no longer recommended.

Adrenaline

Adrenaline 1 mg IV remains the vasopressor of choice in all forms of cardiac arrest. It has potent α effects, causing widespread vasoconstriction, which increases coronary and cerebral perfusion pressure, and β-adrenergic effects, which increase coronary and cerebral blood flow through inotropic and chronotropic actions. However, some of these beneficial β-effects may be offset by increased myocardial oxygen consumption and increased ventricular arrhythmogenicity. Although its use is still recommended, there remains no good evidence which shows that the use of any vasopressor at any stage during CPR increases neurologically intact survival.

Vasopressin

A meta-analysis demonstrated no statistical difference, in terms of return of spontaneous circulation, between the use of vasopressin and adrenaline (Aung & Htay 2005). Vasopressin is a naturally occurring antidiuretic hormone (ADH) and has powerful vasoconstrictor effects through its action on smooth muscle V_1 receptors. There is insufficient evidence to recommend a change to the use of vasopressin as a first-line vasopressor in cases of cardiac arrest.

Atropine

The routine use of atropine during the management of a cardiac arrest is no longer recommended. Asystole is mainly caused by primary myocardial pathology, rather than excessive vagal tone, and studies have failed to provide evidence to support its routine use.

Amiodarone

Amiodarone is a membrane-stabilising antiarrhythmic drug that increases the duration of both the action potential and the refractory period in atrial and ventricular myocardium, as well as slowing atrioventricular conduction. It has mild negative inotropic actions and causes peripheral vasodilatation.

Amiodarone is used in shock-refractory VF/VT, and if VF/VT persists after three shocks, amiodarone, 300 mg IV, should be given. A further dose of 150 mg followed by an infusion of 900 mg over 24 hours is then recommended. Its use is also indicated in haemodynamically stable VT.

Lidocaine

Lidocaine has been superseded by amiodarone as the first-line antiarrhythmic drug. Lidocaine has a membrane-stabilising action and increases the refractory period. It can be used in a dose of 1 mg kg^{-1} in shock-refractory VF/VT if amiodarone is not readily available. It should not be used if amiodarone has already been given.

Sodium bicarbonate

The routine use of sodium bicarbonate during a cardiac arrest is not recommended. The best treatment for an acidosis resulting from cardiorespiratory arrest is good-quality CPR and a rapid return of spontaneous circulation. Bicarbonate has a number of adverse effects, including the exacerbation of intracellular acidosis, negative inotropic effects on an ischaemic myocardium, a large sodium load, and the shift of the oxyhaemoglobin dissociation curve to the left, which further inhibits release of oxygen to tissues.

The use of 50 mmol of sodium bicarbonate is indicated if a cardiac arrest is associated with hyperkalaemia or tricyclic antidepressant overdose, or in patients with pre-existing metabolic acidosis. The use of bicarbonate when the arterial pH is < 7.1 remains controversial. A repeat dose of bicarbonate may be given, depending on the patient's clinical condition and repeated blood gas analysis.

Arterial blood gases do not accurately reflect acid–base status of tissues during a cardiorespiratory arrest. There is a rapid accumulation of carbon dioxide and lactic acid due to poor tissue perfusion and a marked arteriovenous difference in pH. Theoretically a mixed venous gas, or venous gas taken from a central line, will provide a closer estimate of tissue acid–base status.

Calcium

The routine use of calcium during a cardiac arrest is not recommended. Calcium must not be given simultaneously with bicarbonate through the same IV/IO access.

Calcium has a vital role in cellular mechanisms underlying myocardial contraction. It is indicated in PEA secondary to hyperkalaemia, hypocalcaemia, overdose of calcium blocking drugs and overdose of magnesium. The initial dose is 10 mL of 10% calcium chloride (6.8 mmol Ca^{2+}).

Calcium should be used cautiously, as high levels are harmful to ischaemic myocardium and may impair cerebral recovery. It may also slow the heart and cause arrhythmias.

Intralipid

Intravenous intralipid 20% is a sterile fat emulsion, which has been successfully used to treat tachyarrhythmias associated with local anaesthetic toxicity. An initial bolus of 1.5 mL kg^{-1} of 20% lipid emulsion, given over 1 minute, is followed by an infusion of 15 mL kg^{-1} h^{-1}.

Magnesium

Magnesium (4 mL of 50% solution; 8 mmol) should be given for refractory VF when there is any suspicion of hypomagnesaemia, e.g. patients on potassium-losing diuretics. It should also be considered in other ventricular tachyarrhythmias as well as torsades de pointes and digoxin toxicity.

Aminophylline

Aminophylline is a phosphodiesterase inhibitor which has chronotropic and inotropic actions. It may be used in

asystolic cardiac arrest or peri-arrest bradycardia which is refractory to atropine.

Fibrinolytics

Fibrinolytics should be considered in patients with proven or suspected pulmonary embolism. There is insufficient evidence to recommend its use in cardiac arrest from other causes.

Complications of CPR

Iatrogenic complications of CPR are relatively common, and some of these may lead to problems in the post-resuscitation period. However, since the alternative to CPR is death, CPR can be justified in most circumstances providing that care is taken to minimise the risks both to the patient and to the rescuer.

Frequent complications of chest compressions include rib and sternal fractures, and less commonly visceral and cardiac trauma. Poor airway management may lead to aspiration of gastric contents or unrecognised oesophageal intubation.

Other post-resuscitation problems, not necessarily resulting from substandard CPR, include pulmonary oedema, recurrent cardiac arrest, cardiogenic shock, multiple organ dysfunction and adverse neurological outcome (see below). Evidence is emerging that the use of protocol-driven post-cardiac arrest care may improve outcome.

Complications associated with defibrillator use

A clear 'stand back' command should be given prior to defibrillation to avoid accidental defibrillation of a member of the resuscitation team.

There have been several reports of burns to patients through the incorrect use of defibrillator paddles. Poor contact between defibrillator paddles/pads and the patient's chest increases transthoracic impedance, which causes arcing of current and burns to the patient. The use of self-adhesive pads reduces this risk, but if manual metal paddles are still used they must always be used with conduction gel or gel pads. Excessively hairy patients may need to be shaved to ensure good paddle/pad contact prior to defibrillation, but this should not excessively delay defibrillation. Glyceryl trinitrate (GTN) patches must also be removed prior to defibrillation.

Sparks from poorly applied defibrillator paddles/pads may cause a fire in an oxygen-rich environment. Risks of fire from oxygen during defibrillation may be minimised by the following strategies. If using bag-mask ventilation the oxygen mask should be moved to a distance of at least

1 metre from the patient's chest during defibrillation. A ventilation bag should remain attached to an endotracheal tube provided the oxygen source is more than 1 metre away. In the critical care/theatre setting the ventilator should be left connected to the patient.

Transmission of infection

There have been isolated reports of rescuers becoming infected with tuberculosis and severe acute respiratory syndrome (SARS) from patients during CPR. The transmission of HIV through CPR has never been reported. Universal safety precautions should be taken when dealing with patients known to have serious infections, e.g. tuberculosis, HIV, hepatitis B virus or SARS.

Neurological injury

Although not entirely preventable, poor neurological outcome may be minimised by meticulous care in the immediate post-resuscitation period. Ideally the patient should be transferred to a critical care setting, where they may require a period of intubation, sedation and controlled ventilation to optimise oxygenation and maintain normocarbia. Invasive monitoring, inotropes, vasodilators and diuretics may be required to optimise the patient haemodynamically. Insulin should be given to ensure tight glycaemic control, and hyperthermia should be treated aggressively with antipyretics. A period of active cooling to induce therapeutic hypothermia, 32–34 °C for 12–24 hours after the arrest, may improve neurological outcome, particularly when the presenting rhythm is VF. Seizures should be controlled by the use of anticonvulsants, e.g. benzodiazepines, phenytoin, sodium valproate and/or barbiturates.

Management of life-threatening peri-arrest arrhythmias

Life-threatening peri-arrest arrhythmias can be divided into two broad groups, those that are stable and can be treated with antiarrhythmic drugs, and those that are unstable and need immediate cardioversion or pacing. In general the action of drugs is slower and less reliable than electricity. All antiarrhythmic treatments – physical manoeuvres, drugs and electrical cardioversion – can also be pro-arrhythmogenic, and antiarrhythmic drugs may also cause myocardial depression and hypotension. Initial management is to assess the patient, give oxygen, gain IV access, record a 12-lead ECG (Figure 8.6) and correct any electrolyte abnormalities, particularly potassium, magnesium and calcium.

Signs of an unstable arrhythmia include pallor, sweating, impaired conscious level and hypotension, which all reflect an inadequate cardiac output. Chest pain, secondary to myocardial ischaemia, is often precipitated by excessive heart rates. Similarly, low heart rates may not be tolerated in patients with poor cardiac reserve. Signs of heart failure – pulmonary oedema, raised jugular venous pressure and hepatic engorgement – may also be present.

Bradycardias

A bradycardia is defined in an adult as a heart rate of less than 60 bpm; however a slow heart rate does not always need treating as it may be physiological, as in athletes, or drug-induced by β-blockers, diltiazem, digoxin or amiodarone.

In a symptomatic patient give atropine 500 µg IV, and if the patient remains symptomatic, repeat this dose every 3–5 minutes up to a maximum of 3 g (Figure 8.7). If there has been a calcium antagonist or β-blocker overdose consider using glucagon.

If the patient is at risk of developing asystole, transvenous pacing may be required. Risk factors for a bradycardia deteriorating to asystole include a recent episode of asystole, Mobitz type II AV block, third-degree (complete) heart block (Figure 8.6), or ventricular standstill of more than 3 seconds. Complete heart block with narrow complexes may not require immediate pacing, as AV junctional ectopic pacemakers can provide a stable cardiac output.

Transvenous pacing is the definitive treatment, but if expertise is not readily available, patients may be managed temporarily with either transcutaneous pacing or an adrenaline infusion in the range of 2–10 µg per minute. If there is no pacing equipment immediately available, fist pacing may be attempted. Apply serial rhythmic blows with a closed fist over the left sternal edge to pace the heart at physiological rate of 50–70 times a minute.

Tachycardias

Guidelines for the management of tachycardias are now contained in a single algorithm that includes treatment of narrow complex tachycardias, broad complex tachycardias and atrial fibrillation (Figure 8.8).

In an unstable patient, electrical cardioversion should be attempted immediately. The shock must be synchronised to occur with the R wave of the electrocardiogram. If not, and it is delivered during a relatively refractory

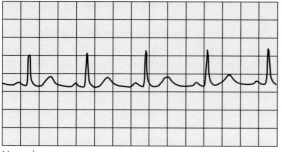

Normal

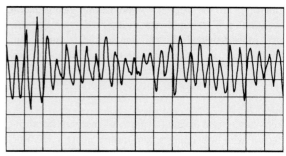

Ventricular fibrillation

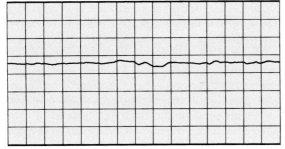

Asystole

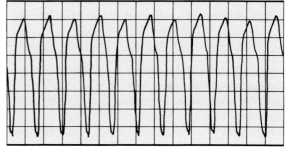

Broad complex tachycardia

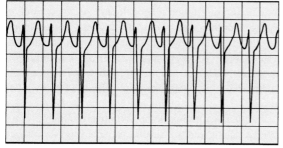

Narrow complex tachycardia

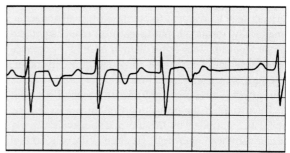

Atrioventricular block, second degree, Mobitz type I
(Wenkebach)

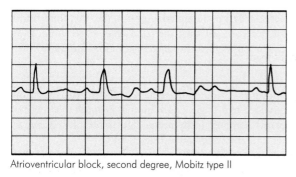

Atrioventricular block, second degree, Mobitz type II

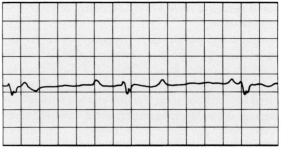

Atrioventricular block, third degree, complete heart block

Figure 8.6 Examples of electrocardiogram tracings

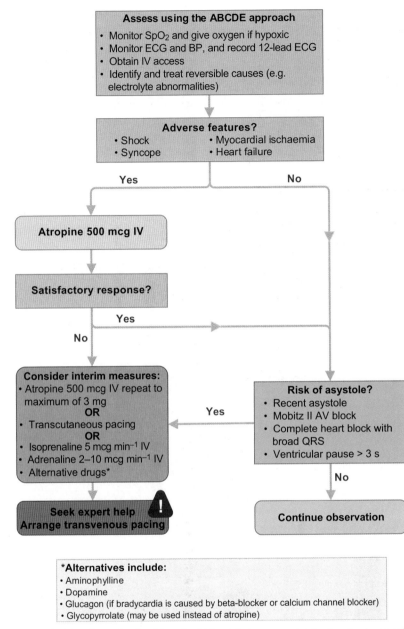

Assess using the ABCDE approach
- Monitor SpO$_2$ and give oxygen if hypoxic
- Monitor ECG and BP, and record 12-lead ECG
- Obtain IV access
- Identify and treat reversible causes (e.g. electrolyte abnormalities)

Adverse features?
- Shock
- Syncope
- Myocardial ischaemia
- Heart failure

Yes   No

Atropine 500 mcg IV

Satisfactory response?

Yes

No

Consider interim measures:
- Atropine 500 mcg IV repeat to maximum of 3 mg
  OR
- Transcutaneous pacing
  OR
- Isoprenaline 5 mcg min^{-1} IV
- Adrenaline 2–10 mcg min^{-1} IV
- Alternative drugs*

Yes

Risk of asystole?
- Recent asystole
- Mobitz II AV block
- Complete heart block with broad QRS
- Ventricular pause > 3 s

No

**Seek expert help
Arrange transvenous pacing**

Continue observation

***Alternatives include:**
- Aminophylline
- Dopamine
- Glucagon (if bradycardia is caused by beta-blocker or calcium channel blocker)
- Glycopyrrolate (may be used instead of atropine)

Figure 8.7 Bradycardia algorithm (includes rate inappropriately slow for haemodynamic state). Reproduced with the kind permission of the Resuscitation Council (UK). © Resuscitation Council (UK) (2015)

portion of the cardiac cycle, VF may be induced. A starting energy level of 120–150 J biphasic (200 J monophasic) should be used, except in atrial flutter and other narrow complex tachycardias, which will often cardiovert at lower energy levels (70–120 J biphasic, 100 J monophasic). Although electrical cardioversion is effective it does not prevent the occurrence of subsequent arrhythmias, which should be treated with drugs, e.g. an

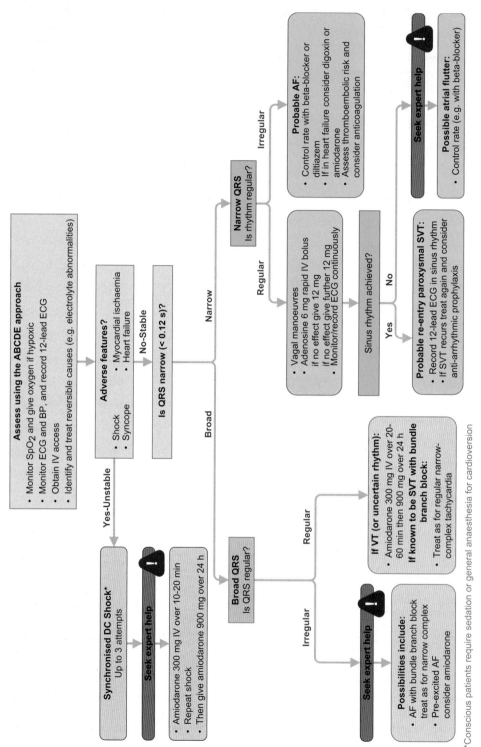

Assess using the ABCDE approach
- Monitor SpO₂ and give oxygen if hypoxic
- Monitor ECG and BP, and record 12-lead ECG
- Obtain IV access
- Identify and treat reversible causes (e.g. electrolyte abnormalities)

Adverse features?
- Shock
- Syncope
- Myocardial ischaemia
- Heart failure

Yes-Unstable

No-Stable

Is QRS narrow (< 0.12 s)?

Broad

Narrow

Synchronised DC Shock*
Up to 3 attempts

Seek expert help

- Amiodarone 300 mg IV over 10-20 min
- Repeat shock
- Then give amiodarone 900 mg over 24 h

Broad QRS
Is QRS regular?

Regular

Irregular

If VT (or uncertain rhythm):
- Amiodarone 300 mg IV over 20-60 min then 900 mg over 24 h
If known to be SVT with bundle branch block:
- Treat as for regular narrow-complex tachycardia

Seek expert help

Possibilities include:
- AF with bundle branch block treat as for narrow complex
- Pre-excited AF consider amiodarone

Narrow QRS
Is rhythm regular?

Regular

Irregular

- Vagal manoeuvres
- Adenosine 6 mg rapid IV bolus if no effect give 12 mg if no effect give further 12 mg
- Monitor/record ECG continuously

Sinus rhythm achieved?

Yes

No

Probable re-entry paroxysmal SVT:
- Record 12-lead ECG in sinus rhythm
- If SVT recurs treat again and consider anti-arrhythmic prophylaxis

Probable AF:
- Control rate with beta-blocker or diltiazem
- If in heart failure consider digoxin or amiodarone
- Assess thromboembolic risk and consider anticoagulation

Seek expert help

Possible atrial flutter:
- Control rate (e.g. with beta-blocker)

*Conscious patients require sedation or general anaesthesia for cardioversion

Figure 8.8 Tachycardia algorithm (with pulse). Reproduced with the kind permission of the Resuscitation Council (UK). © Resuscitation Council (UK) (2015)

infusion of amiodarone. If initial electrical cardioversion fails to re-establish sinus rhythm and the patient remains unstable, give amiodarone 300 mg IV over 15–20 minutes before re-attempting electrical cardioversion.

Tachycardias are relatively common in the critically ill patient. As well as treating the arrhythmia, if the patient is clinically compromised, the underlying cause (e.g. sepsis, electrolyte disturbances) must also be treated. In patients with normal hearts, adverse signs are unlikely to occur with heart rates of less than 150 bpm.

Broad complex tachycardia

A broad complex tachycardia has a QRS complex > 0.12 seconds. They are usually ventricular in origin, but can also be supraventricular with aberrant conduction. If the patient is unstable, treat with electrical cardioversion.

Broad complex tachycardia

If stable, determine whether the arrhythmia is regular or irregular.

- A regular broad complex tachycardia is likely to be VT or a supraventricular rhythm with bundle branch block. Treat with amiodarone 300 mg IV followed by 900 mg over 24 hours. If the arrhythmia is known to be supraventricular with bundle branch block, treat as a narrow complex tachycardia.
- An irregular broad complex tachycardia is most likely to be atrial fibrillation with bundle branch block, and should be treated as narrow complex atrial fibrillation.

Other possible causes for broad complex tachycardias include atrial fibrillation with ventricular pre-excitation, i.e. patients with Wolff–Parkinson–White (WPW) syndrome, or torsades de pointes (polymorphic VT). In a stable patient who is known to have WPW, the use of amiodarone is probably safe. Adenosine, digoxin, verapamil and diltiazem must be avoided, as these drugs block the AV node and will cause a relative increase in pre-excitation. If possible, expert cardiological advice should be sought in the assessment and management of these patients. Electrical cardioversion remains the safest option for the treatment of the unstable patient.

Torsades de pointes is treated by stopping all drugs known to prolong the QT interval and correcting electrolyte abnormalities. Magnesium sulphate (2 g IV over 10

minutes) should also be given. Expert help is often required to manage these patients, who may require ventricular pacing. If the patient's condition deteriorates, proceed to synchronised electrical cardioversion or, if the patient is pulseless, commence the ALS algorithm (Figure 8.5).

Narrow complex tachycardia

A narrow complex tachycardia has a QRS interval < 0.12 seconds. Sinus tachycardia is a common physiological response to exercise or anxiety and is also seen in patients who are anaemic, in pain, pyrexial or shocked. The management of the tachycardia in these cases is by treating the cause.

Narrow complex tachycardia

Other causes of a regular narrow complex tachycardia include:

- AV nodal re-entry tachycardia (AVNRT). This is the commonest type of paroxysmal supraventricular tachycardia (PSVT). It is often seen in people without any heart disease, and is usually benign. It is a regular narrow complex tachycardia with P waves often not visible.
- AV re-entry tachycardia (AVRT). This occurs in patients with WPW, and is usually benign unless there is coexisting structural heart disease. Again it is a regular narrow complex tachycardia, with P waves often not visible.
- Atrial flutter with regular AV conduction. This usually presents as a 2:1 block and produces a tachycardia with a rate of 150 bpm. Flutter waves may be difficult to see.

An unstable patient presenting with a **regular** narrow complex tachycardia should be treated with electrical cardioversion. If this is not immediately available, adenosine should be given as a first-line treatment.

A stable patient presenting with a regular narrow complex tachycardia should initially be treated by vagal manoeuvres such as carotid sinus massage or the Valsalva manoeuvre, as these will terminate up to a quarter of episodes of PSVT. Carotid sinus massage should be avoided in the elderly, especially if a carotid bruit is present, as it may dislodge an atheromatous plaque and cause a stroke.

If the tachycardia persists and is not atrial flutter, 6 mg of adenosine should be given as an IV bolus, followed by a 12 mg bolus if no response. A further 12 mg bolus of adenosine may be given if the tachycardia persists. Vagal manoeuvres or adenosine will terminate almost all AVNRTs or AVRTs within seconds, and therefore failure to convert suggests an atrial tachycardia such as atrial flutter. If adenosine is contraindicated, or fails to terminate a narrow complex tachycardia, without first demonstrating it as atrial flutter, give a calcium channel blocker, e.g. verapamil 2.5–5 mg IV over 2 minutes. Atrial flutter should be treated by rate control with a β-blocker.

An **irregular** narrow complex tachycardia is most likely to be atrial fibrillation (AF) with an uncontrolled ventricular response, but may also be atrial flutter with variable block. If the patient is unstable, synchronised electrical cardioversion should be used to treat the arrhythmia.

Treatment options for a stable patient with AF include:

- Rate control by drug therapy. Drugs used to control the heart rate include β-blockers, digoxin, magnesium, calcium antagonists or a combination of these.
- Rhythm control by amiodarone to encourage cardioversion. Amiodarone is given as a 300 mg IV bolus, followed by 900 mg IV over 24 hours.
- Rhythm control by electrical cardioversion. This is more likely to restore sinus rhythm than chemical cardioversion.
- Treatment to prevent complications. Patients who are in AF are at risk of atrial thrombus formation and should be anticoagulated.

Resuscitation of the pregnant patient

Although there are two potential patients, the best chance of fetal survival is the prompt management of the critically ill mother. It is essential, therefore, that when dealing with a cardiorespiratory arrest in a pregnant patient there is early involvement of a senior obstetrician and neonatologist. A decision to perform a perimortem Caesarean section must be taken early during the resuscitation attempt. If the gestational age of the fetus is more than 24–25 weeks a Caesarean section must be performed, as it may save the life of both mother and baby. If the gestational age is 20–23 weeks a Caesarean section will improve the chances of survival of the mother and should

therefore be performed, even though the baby is highly unlikely to survive.

Prompt delivery of the fetus of more than 20 weeks gestation, ideally within 5 minutes of the cardiac arrest, relieves aortocaval compression and improves thoracic compliance. This increases the efficiency of both chest compressions and ventilation, and improves the chances of survival of both baby and mother.

There are a number of factors that tip the balance of resuscitating the pregnant patient towards non-survival when compared with a non-pregnant patient of similar age. Airway management is made more difficult by the presence of laryngeal oedema and obesity. Other physiological changes of pregnancy predispose a pregnant patient to a greater risk of aspiration owing to the incompetence of the gastroesophageal sphincter and increased intragastric pressure. In addition, the maintenance of adequate oxygenation through ventilation is made more difficult by increased oxygen demand, decreased chest compliance and a reduced functional residual capacity.

Causes

The incidence of cardiac arrests occurring during late pregnancy is 1 in 30,000. Indirect deaths from medical conditions exacerbated by pregnancy are much more frequent than deaths from conditions that arise as a result of pregnancy itself. Causes of cardiorespiratory arrest that also occur in non-pregnant women of a similar age group include acute coronary syndromes, often in patients with pre-existing IHD, congenital heart disease, anaphylaxis, trauma and drug overdose.

Additional causes of cardiac arrest relating to pregnancy

- Haemorrhage
- Hypertensive disease of pregnancy
- Peripartum cardiomyopathy
- Amniotic fluid embolism
- Pulmonary embolism

As in the non-pregnant patient, common and reversible causes of cardiorespiratory arrest should be promptly recognised and treated during CPR.

Basic life support

BLS should be performed in accordance with the standard adult algorithm (Figure 8.3). However, there are a number of issues which make the resuscitation attempt more difficult in the pregnant patient.

- The **airway** will need to be managed with the patient in the semi-lateral position in order to avoid aortocaval syndrome. Pregnant patients are at an increased risk of aspiration, and cricoid pressure should be applied as soon as expertise is available. The patient should be intubated as soon as possible.
- Rescue **breathing** is more difficult as there is reduced chest compliance secondary to flaring of the ribs, splinting of the diaphragm by abdominal contents and the presence of hypertrophied breasts.
- The hand position for **cardiac compressions** should be moved up the sternum, as the diaphragm is displaced upwards by the abdominal contents. Aortocaval compression, a risk from about 20 weeks gestation, must be avoided by lateral displacement of the uterus. To achieve this, the patient can be tilted onto the rescuer's knees, or purpose-made wedges or pillows may be used. Effective forces for chest compression can still be generated up to a 30-degree tilt. Manual displacement of the uterus may also be performed.

Advanced life support

ALS is performed in accordance with the standard adult algorithm (Figure 8.5).

Factors which make airway management more difficult in the pregnant patient include the presence of full dentition, hypertrophied breasts, obesity and laryngeal oedema. Tracheal intubation should be carried out as soon as possible. A smaller size of endotracheal tube may be needed and a polio blade required to facilitate access.

It is more difficult to apply paddles/pads for defibrillation owing to the presence of hypertrophied breasts and obesity. There is no evidence of adverse effects of defibrillation to the fetus, and standard energy levels for adults should be used.

Tachyarrhythmias secondary to bupivacaine toxicity are likely to be refractory to management in line with standard protocols. Cardiac massage may have to be sustained for long periods of time, up to an hour, as bupivacaine is highly tissue-bound and sinus rhythm may not be successfully re-established until some recovery of the myocardium has occurred. Animal studies and case reports suggest that tachyarrhythmias secondary to local anaesthetic toxicity may respond to treatment with IV lipid emulsion.

Drug usage

Drugs should be given in accordance with ALS recommendations.

Magnesium sulphate is increasingly used in the management of pre-eclampsia and eclampsia, and if high magnesium concentrations are thought to have contributed to the cardiac arrest then calcium chloride or calcium gluconate should be given intravenously.

Resuscitation of infants and children

There is little scientific evidence looking specifically at resuscitation in infants and children, and much of the evidence used in producing the following guidelines has been extrapolated from adult studies. The guidelines have been simplified so that there is now a single cardiac compression : ventilation ratio (15:2) for all infants and children regardless of age. When a child reaches puberty the adult resuscitation guidelines should be used.

In the following guidelines an infant is a child of less than 1 year, and a child is from the age of 1 year until puberty.

Causes

Cardiac arrests tend to occur less commonly in children than in adults, and the aetiology is usually different. They are usually secondary to either respiratory or circulatory failure, rather than originating from a primary cardiac problem. The presenting rhythm is either a severe bradycardia or asystole resulting from hypoxia. Causes of secondary cardiac arrest in children include trauma, drowning and poisoning.

Primary cardiac arrests resulting in VF are relatively rare, comprising 7–15% of all paediatric arrests. VF tends not to be seen in children unless they are known to have heart disease, and more often occurs in hospitals on critical care units and cardiac wards. In a previously normal child who presents with VF/VT, hypothermia, drug effects and electrolyte disturbances must be considered.

Basic life support

If only the adult BLS algorithm is known, it can be used in children, but the paediatric BLS algorithm has certain modifications which make it more suitable for this age group (Figure 8.9).

Confirm that a cardiac arrest has occurred, by gently stimulating the child and asking loudly 'are you alright?' Do not shake the child if a cervical spine injury is

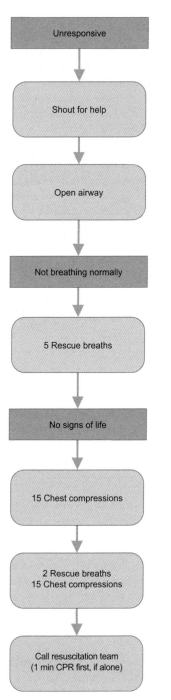

Figure 8.9 Paediatric basic life support (BLS) algorithm. Reproduced with the kind permission of the Resuscitation Council (UK).© Resuscitation Council (UK) (2015)

suspected. For the single rescuer, 1 minute of CPR is recommended before calling for help, because the cardiac arrest is more likely to be secondary to hypoxia, which may rapidly respond to rescue breathing. Five initial rescue breaths should be given before starting cardiac compressions. However, if a sudden collapse is witnessed, it is more likely to be due to a primary cardiac arrhythmia, and defibrillation takes priority.

Airway

Simple manoeuvres should be used to open the airway. Place a hand on the child's forehead and gently tilt the head back while performing a chin lift. An infant's airway should be managed in the neutral position, although a gentle head-tilt manoeuvre may be required to achieve this as the occiput is relatively large. Care must be taken when positioning fingers so as not to compress the soft tissues, as this may cause airway obstruction. If unable to clear the airway by these manoeuvres alone, the jaw thrust can also be used in children.

Breathing

Assess whether the child or infant is breathing normally by looking for chest movements, listening at the nose and mouth for breath sounds, and feeling for air movement. This assessment should last no longer than 10 seconds.

If the child or infant is not breathing normally, or is only taking infrequent irregular breaths, then rescue breathing should be commenced immediately, and five breaths should be given consecutively. For a child, mouth-to-mouth or mouth-to-nose rescue breathing may be used. In infants, a technique of mouth to mouth-and-nose rescue breathing may be required. Inflation should last for 1–1.5 seconds and the chest observed to rise and fall.

If, despite optimal positioning, having cleared the mouth of any obvious obstructions, adequate rescue breathing is not achieved, move straight on to cardiac compressions.

Circulation

As in adults, signs of circulation include movement, coughing or normal breathing. If confident to do so, check for a pulse, but take no longer than 10 seconds. In a child the carotid or femoral pulse should be used for assessment, and in infants the brachial or femoral pulse. If circulation is present continue rescue breathing only. If there are no signs of circulation or the pulse rate is less than 60 bpm with poor perfusion, rescue breathing should be combined with cardiac compressions.

Cardiac compressions should compress the chest by at least one-third of its depth at a rate of 100 compressions per minute. The correct ratio of cardiac compressions to rescue breaths is 15:2 for two rescuers, but if alone use the adult ratio of 30:2, which will allow a single rescuer to perform the recommended 100 compressions per minute. The advice is to push hard, push fast, minimise interruptions and allow for full chest recoil.

To locate the correct position for hand placement in children, identify the xiphisternum and place the hands one finger's breadth above this. Depending on the size of the child one or two hands may be used. It is important that the pressure is applied over the lower third of the sternum and not the ribs.

In infants either two fingertips may be used to apply cardiac compressions or, when two or more rescuers are present, the two-thumb encircling technique. The two-thumb encircling technique has been shown to produce higher coronary perfusion pressures, as the correct depth and force of compressions are more consistently achieved. However, for the single rescuer it is difficult to swap from cardiac compressions to rescue breathing, so the two-finger technique is preferable.

Once spontaneous circulation and ventilation is established the child must be placed in the recovery position.

Foreign-body airway obstruction

The majority of choking episodes in children and infants are witnessed and occur during play or eating. The child or infant is usually conscious in the initial stages, but if the obstruction is not rapidly cleared, cardiac arrest secondary to hypoxia will ensue. Choking, which occurs suddenly, must be differentiated from other causes of upper airway obstruction in children and infants, such as laryngitis, epiglottitis and croup, in which they are systemically ill and require different management.

The management of choking in children is very similar to that in adults (Figure 8.10). If the victim is conscious

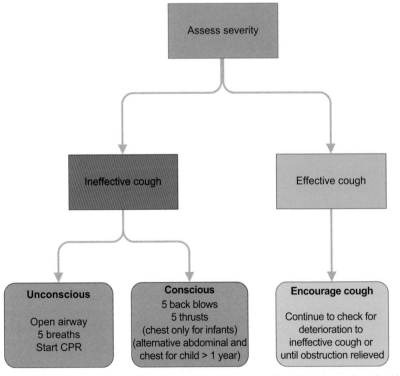

Figure 8.10 Paediatric foreign-body airway obstruction algorithm. Reproduced with the kind permission of the Resuscitation Council (UK). © Resuscitation Council (UK) (2015)

and coughing then further coughing should be encouraged. If there is an inadequate cough, and the child remains conscious, then back blows followed by abdominal thrusts should be used to attempt to dislodge the foreign body. In infants, chest thrusts should be used in place of abdominal thrusts. These are similar to chest compressions, but sharper in nature and delivered at a slower rate. Abdominal thrusts should not be used to treat choking in infants, because the more horizontal position of their ribs leaves the upper abdominal viscera more exposed to trauma.

All these manoeuvres create an 'artificial cough' with the aim of increasing intrathoracic pressure and dislodging the foreign body. The head of the patient should be kept dependent. Obviously the position used will depend on the size of both the child and the rescuer.

If at any time the child becomes unconscious, commence the paediatric BLS algorithm (Figure 8.9).

Advanced life support

As in the adult ALS guidelines, the emphasis for paediatric ALS is continuous cardiac compressions, minimising the 'time off chest' for assessment of cardiac rhythm, defibrillation and endotracheal intubation. The paediatric ALS algorithm (Figure 8.11) provides a standardised approach for the treatment of a cardiac arrest in infants and children. During resuscitation attempts reversible causes should be identified and treated as soon as possible.

Airway

Simple oropharyngeal or nasopharyngeal airways, or LMAs, may be used in children, and although they help provide a clear airway for ventilation, they do not protect against aspiration or inadvertent gastric distension. Endotracheal intubation remains the airway of choice as it ensures a secure protected airway and, once the patient is intubated, cardiac compressions can be performed continuously.

Traditionally uncuffed endotracheal tubes have been used in children below the age of puberty. There is some evidence that there is no greater risk of complications when cuffed tubes are used in preference to uncuffed tubes even in young children (Cox 2005). A smaller size of cuffed tube may need to be used, and meticulous care must be taken when inflating cuffs, since excessive pressures will lead to ischaemic necrosis of surrounding laryngeal tissues and stenosis.

Ventilation

100% oxygen should be used for ventilation during resuscitation. Ventilation should be performed at a rate of 12–20 breaths per minute, and the ideal tidal volume should achieve a modest chest wall rise. The increasing use of capnography during resuscitation attempts not only provides a monitor of the effectiveness of chest compressions but may also give an early indication of return of spontaneous circulation.

Circulation

Assess the patient for signs of spontaneous circulation, and monitor the cardiac rhythm using either cardiac electrodes in the standard positions or paediatric defibrillator pads/paddles placed just below the right clavicle and at the left anterior axillary line. In small children and infants, placing the pads/paddles front and back may be more appropriate. The cardiac rhythm will determine which limb of the ALS algorithm to follow.

Cardiac compressions should be performed as described for BLS. The person performing cardiac compressions should be changed after every 2-minute cycle, to avoid the quality of compressions decreasing with fatigue.

Non-shockable rhythms (asystole or PEA)

Asystole and PEA should be managed according to the non-shockable limb of the paediatric ALS algorithm (Figure 8.11) with repeated doses of adrenaline (10 μg kg^{-1} IV or IO) once IV/IO access has been established and then every 3–5 minutes.

Shockable rhythms (VF/VT)

VF and VT should be managed according to the shockable limb of the paediatric ALS algorithm (Figure 8.11). The recommendation for the use of a single-shock protocol is based on extrapolated evidence from adult studies. The optimum energy for safe and effective defibrillation in children is unknown, but relatively high energies are known to cause less myocardial damage in children than in adults. The use of biphasic defibrillation is more effective and causes less post-shock myocardial dysfunction. The recommended energy level for defibrillation in children is a non-escalating level of 4 J kg^{-1} (for both monophasic and biphasic defibrillators).

If using an AED device, purpose-made paediatric pads are available which attenuate the output of the machine to 50–75 J. These should be used in children aged 1–8 years.

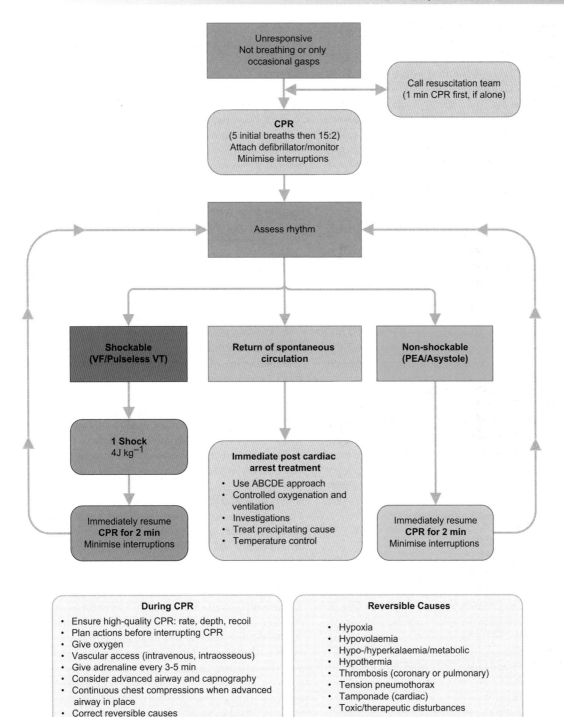

Figure 8.11 Paediatric advanced life support (ALS) algorithm. Reproduced with the kind permission of the Resuscitation Council (UK). © Resuscitation Council (UK) (2015)

Above the age of 8 use the adult energy levels. AEDs are not recommended for use in infants.

Once VF or VT is identified, attempt defibrillation as soon as possible and then continue with CPR for 2 minutes before rechecking the rhythm. If VF/VT persists give a further shock at the same energy level. Again resume CPR for a further 2 minutes, prior to reassessing the rhythm. If VF/VT continues, adrenaline (10 µg kg^{-1} IV or IO) and amiodarone (5 mg kg^{-1} IV or IO) should be given immediately after the third shock.

If VF/VT persists, 2-minute cycles of CPR should be performed, pausing only briefly to assess the rhythm. Adrenaline should be given on alternate cycles and a dose of amiodarone should be repeated after the fifth cycle.

Drug usage

IV access for fluid and drug administration can be very difficult to establish in small children. If not rapidly achieved, insert an IO needle into the proximal tibia to provide vascular access. When using the IO route for drug administration each dose of drug should be followed by a bolus of normal saline to disperse the drug beyond the marrow cavity into the central circulation.

Since hypovolaemia is a potentially reversible cause of cardiac arrest, unless there are obvious signs of volume overload volume expansion is always indicated. A 20 mL kg^{-1} bolus of an isotonic saline solution should be given, and repeated as necessary. The use of dextrose-based solutions should be avoided, unless there is hypoglycaemia, since it leads to hyponatraemia and hyperglycaemia, both of which are associated with poor neurological outcomes after cardiac arrest.

Adrenaline

The use of adrenaline in paediatric cardiac arrest improves coronary and cerebral perfusion due to its potent α- and β-adrenergic actions. The recommended dose in children and infants is 10 µg kg^{-1} (IV/IO). The use of higher doses of adrenaline has not been shown to improve either survival or neurological outcome in children and is not recommended. The exception to this is if the cardiac arrest is secondary to β-blocker overdose.

Amiodarone

Amiodarone is now the antiarrhythmic drug of choice in the management of persistent VT/VF. An initial 5 µg kg^{-1} IV/IO bolus should be used. When given via a peripheral vein, amiodarone causes thrombophlebitis and should therefore be flushed through with either dextrose or saline. As in adults, lidocaine is only recommended when amiodarone is unavailable.

Atropine

There is no evidence for the use of atropine in asphyxia bradycardias or asystole. It may still be of use if bradycardia/asystole is known to be secondary to high vagal tone.

Calcium

The routine use of calcium should be avoided, as it is known to be harmful to the ischaemic myocardium and may impair cerebral recovery. Indications for its use are hyperkalaemia, hypocalcaemia and overdose of calcium blocking drugs.

Magnesium

Magnesium is a major intracellular cation and cofactor in many enzyme reactions. Its use is indicated in hypomagnesemia or polymorphic VT regardless of cause.

Sodium bicarbonate

The routine use of sodium bicarbonate during a cardiac arrest is not recommended (see *Drug usage* in adult guidelines). The best treatment of acidosis developing during a cardiac arrest is good-quality cardiac compressions and ventilation. A dose of 1–2 mL kg^{-1} of 8.4% solution (IV or IO) is recommended if there is hyperkalaemia or if arrhythmias are secondary to tricyclic antidepressant overdose.

Ethical considerations in CPR

The issues that surround ethical decision making during cardiorespiratory resuscitation all relate to life-and-death decisions and the appropriateness of either starting or continuing resuscitation attempts. These decisions are often emotive and distressing, but this does not mean that they ought not to be made. It should be remembered that 70–90% of resuscitation attempts are unsuccessful, and therefore death is inevitable in the majority of cases.

The concept of CPR was originally introduced in the 1960s as a treatment for sudden unexpected deaths, but over the next two decades it evolved to be used for the majority of patients who suffered a cardiorespiratory arrest in hospital. Over the last 30 years guidelines have been developed to enable decisions to be made to stop or withhold resuscitation when inappropriate (BMA 2007). There continues to be a lot of misunderstanding surrounding do-not-attempt-cardiopulmonary-resuscitation

(DNACPR) orders. A DNACPR order simply means that if a patient suffers a cardiorespiratory arrest, cardiac compressions, ventilation or defibrillation should not be attempted. DNACPR does not mean 'for no treatment', and all other supportive care should be continued until it is decided that active treatment is inappropriate. At this point there should be a move from aggressive active care towards palliative care. Good communication and documentation of discussions is paramount when making DNACPR and limitation of treatment decisions.

Justification of resuscitation

In order to justify resuscitation attempts, CPR must provide an overall benefit to the patient. This is the prolongation of life with a quality that is of value to the patient. For most people, as a minimum, this will be considered to be a life with awareness of their surroundings as well as the ability to interact with others and experience relationships. DNACPR decisions are influenced by individual, cultural and religious factors.

There are a number of situations in which CPR will offer no benefit to the patient and should be considered futile. Examples include patients with metastatic malignant disease, those who are already showing signs of irreversible death, and patients who are in a critical care setting with deteriorating vital organ function despite being on maximal therapy, e.g. progressive septic or cardiogenic shock.

Whose decision?

As with any other medical decision, a patient with capacity who is fully informed has the right to refuse an attempt at resuscitation. Similarly, an advance decision ('living will') should be considered legally binding.

Ultimately a decision to withhold or stop resuscitation is a medical decision. DNACPR orders should be written by a senior doctor, but this should only be done after wide consultation with other healthcare professionals involved in the patient's care. In most cases the patient should also be involved in the decision-making process. If the patient lacks capacity the DNACPR decision must be made in accordance with the guidance in the Mental Capacity Act (2005). The decision will be made in the patient's best interests, and relatives should be approached to gain information about the patient's values and what the patient would have wanted to happen in this situation; however, they must not be made to feel that they have made the decision. It must also be remembered that not all families will have the patient's best interests at heart,

and they may well have a vested interest in the patient's death or continued existence.

Although a patient with capacity may refuse resuscitation, they cannot demand an inappropriate treatment, and this includes a resuscitation attempt which is deemed to be futile. Where a patient is demanding an inappropriate resuscitation attempt, a second opinion or consultation with a clinical ethics forum should be sought. Application to the courts should be a last resort. There is no ethical imperative requiring a doctor to perform medical procedures in the absence of any medical benefit.

Withholding and withdrawing resuscitation

If there is any uncertainty as to the appropriateness of a resuscitation attempt, then CPR should be started immediately. There is no ethical difference between stopping a resuscitation attempt that has started and withholding resuscitation in the first place. Starting resuscitation allows for information to be gathered to aid decision making.

There are many factors to consider when deciding whether to abandon a resuscitation attempt. These include the medical history of the patient as well as the progress of the resuscitation attempt, e.g. the likely time gap between the cardiac arrest and the start of CPR and the duration of the resuscitation attempt. The longer the resuscitation attempt continues, the smaller the chance of the patient surviving either neurologically intact or to discharge from hospital. The duration of any individual resuscitation attempt is a matter of clinical judgement by the doctors present at the time. If VF persists and it was considered appropriate to start resuscitation, then it is probably worth continuing all the time the patient remains in VF/VT. For a non-VF/VT arrest, if at 20 minutes there continues to be asystole, and no reversible causes have been identified, then to continue CPR is probably futile.

When all the relevant information has been gathered, if it is found there is no justification to continue with resuscitation, CPR should be stopped.

DNACPR orders in patients presenting for surgery

A DNACPR order in a patient presenting for surgery is not a contraindication to proceeding with surgery. However, discussion needs to take place between the anaesthetist, the surgeon and the patient before surgery in order to clarify the goals and limitations of the proposed treatment. During anaesthesia and surgery there are often periods of increased cardiorespiratory instability, and there needs to be clear documentation regarding which interventions are appropriate. Clearly tracheal intubation, ventilation and the use of vasopressors may be needed, but it may still be felt that electrical cardioversion and cardiac compressions are inappropriate. In some cases, it may be appropriate to suspend the DNACPR order, but this should only be taken after full discussion with the patient and surgeon regarding prognosis. General assumptions cannot be made in this situation, and decisions will need to be made on an individual patient basis.

Presence of relatives during resuscitation attempts

The concept of relatives being present during resuscitation attempts was first introduced during the 1980s, mainly in the case of paediatric resuscitation. Subsequent surveys showed that the majority of relatives found the experience of great value, and were the circumstances to be repeated they would wish to be present again. They found it gave them a realistic view of resuscitation, and they could see that everything was being done for their child. It also helped them come to terms with the reality of death and eased the bereavement period.

However, for this to work there must be a dedicated member of staff with the sole responsibility of looking after the relatives and explaining the events of the resuscitation attempt. The relatives must not be allowed to impede resuscitation, and may have to be removed if they do. The attempt must be well run, under good leadership, and the resuscitation team must be comfortable with the concept of family members being present.

The doctor in charge decides when to stop the resuscitation effort, not the patient's family, and this must be expressed with sensitivity and understanding.

References and further reading

Aung K, Htay T. Vasopressin for cardiac arrest: a systematic review and meta-analysis. *Arch Intern Med* 2005; **165**: 17–24.

British Medical Association, Resuscitation Council (UK), Royal College of Nursing. *Decisions Relating to Cardiopulmonary Resuscitation*. London: BMA, 2007.

Cox RG. Should cuffed endotracheal tubes be used routinely in children? *Can J Anaesth* 2005; **52**: 669–74.

European Resuscitation Council. European Resuscitation Council Guidelines for Resuscitation 2015. *Resuscitation* 2015; **95**: 1–312.

Nolan JP, Hazinski MF, Billi JE, *et al.* 2010 International consensus on cardiopulmonary resuscitation and emergency care science with treatment recommendations. *Resuscitation* 2010; **81**: e1–e330.

Resuscitation Council (UK). *Resuscitation Guidelines 2015*. London: Resuscitation Council, 2015.

CHAPTER 9
Major trauma

Jerry Nolan

National Audit Office data indicate that major trauma kills 5400 people in England annually, and it is the commonest cause of death in those under 40 years. The advanced trauma life support (ATLS) course (American College of Surgeons 2008) provides a basic framework onto which hospital specialists can build their individual skills. The ATLS course focuses on the initial management of patients with major injuries during the so-called 'golden hour'. The golden hour reflects the importance of timely treatment. A severely injured patient who is hypoxic, in haemorrhagic shock, or who has an expanding intracranial haematoma, for example, will need rapid, effective resuscitation. The aim is to restore cellular oxygenation before the onset of irreversible shock.

Pathophysiology of trauma and hypovolaemia

Several mechanisms are involved in the development of cellular injury after severe trauma. The commonest is haemorrhage, causing circulatory failure with poor tissue perfusion and generalised hypoxia (hypovolaemic shock). Myocardial trauma may cause cardiogenic shock, while spinal cord trauma may cause neurogenic shock. Severe trauma is a potent cause of the systemic inflammatory response syndrome (SIRS), and this may progress to the multiple organ dysfunction syndrome (MODS) and multiple organ failure (Xiao *et al.* 2011).

Physiological responses to haemorrhage

Trauma compromises tissue oxygenation because haemorrhage reduces oxygen delivery while at the same time tissue injury and inflammation increase oxygen consumption.

Compensatory responses to haemorrhage are categorised into immediate, early and late. The loss of blood volume is detected by low-pressure stretch receptors in the atria and arterial baroreceptors in the aorta and carotid artery. Efferents from the vasomotor centre trigger an increase in catecholamines, which causes arteriolar constriction, venoconstriction and tachycardia. Early compensatory mechanisms (5–60 minutes) include movement of fluid from the interstitium to the intravascular space and mobilisation of intracellular fluid. Long-term compensation to haemorrhage is by several mechanisms: reduced glomerular filtration rate, salt and water reabsorption (aldosterone and vasopressin), thirst, and increased erythropoiesis.

Hypovolaemic shock can be conveniently divided into four classes according to the percentage of the total blood volume lost and the associated symptoms and signs (Figure 9.1). Blood loss of 15–30% of the total blood volume will typically be associated with a tachycardia > 100 bpm and reduced pulse pressure; the increase in diastolic pressure reflects peripheral vasoconstriction. A decrease in systolic pressure suggests a loss of > 30%

Fundamentals of Anaesthesia, 4th edition, ed. Ted Lin, Tim Smith and Colin Pinnock. Published by Cambridge University Press. © Cambridge University Press 2017.

Figure 9.1 A classification of haemorrhage (adapted from the Advanced Trauma Life Support manual)

	Class 1	Class 2	Class 3	Class 4
Blood loss (% of TBV)	< 15%	15–30%	30–40%	> 40%
Blood loss/70 kg (mL)	750	750–1500	1500–2000	> 2000
Systolic BP	Normal	Normal	Reduced	Very low
Diastolic BP	Normal	Raised	Reduced	Very low
Heart rate	< 100	> 100	> 120	> 140
Respiratory rate	14–20	20–30	30–40	30–40
Urine output (mL h^{-1})	> 30	20–30	10–20	0
Mental state	Alert	Anxious or aggressive	Confused	Drowsy or unconscious

of total blood volume (approximately 1500 mL in a 70 kg adult). Pure haemorrhage without the presence of significant tissue injury may not cause this typical pattern of a stepwise increase in heart rate. Occasionally, the heart rate may remain relatively low until the onset of cardiovascular collapse.

Haemorrhagic shock causes a significant lactic acidosis: once the mitochondrial PO_2 is less than 2 mmHg oxidative phosphorylation is inhibited and pyruvate is unable to enter the Krebs cycle. Instead, pyruvate undergoes anaerobic metabolism in the cytoplasm, a process that is relatively inefficient for adenosine triphosphate (ATP) generation. ATP depletion causes cell membrane pump failure and cell death. Resuscitation must restore oxygen delivery rapidly if irreversible haemorrhagic shock and death is to be prevented.

Systemic inflammatory response syndrome

Crushed and wounded tissues activate complement, which in turn triggers a cascade of inflammatory mediators (C3a, C5a, tumour necrosis factor α (TNF-α), interleukin 1 (IL-1), IL-6 and IL-8). Thus, severe trauma is a potent cause of SIRS. The diagnostic features of SIRS are summarised in Figure 9.2.

In response to trauma, large numbers of polymorphonuclear neutrophils (PMNs) are released from human bone marrow. Depending on the presence of various modulators, the PMNs adhere tightly to endothelium and migrate into the surrounding parenchyma, where they are activated to release superoxide anion (O_2^-) and elastase. This inflammatory response plays a key role in the development of acute respiratory distress syndrome (ARDS) and MODS. The metabolic response to severe

Figure 9.2 The systemic inflammatory response syndrome (SIRS)

Manifested by two or more of the following conditions:
- Temperature > 38 °C or < 36 °C
- Heart rate > 90 beats min^{-1}
- Respiratory rate > 20 breaths min^{-1} or $PaCO_2$ < 4.3 kPa
- WBC > 12,000 cells mm^{-3}, < 4000 cells mm^{-3}, or > 10% immature (band) forms

trauma is biphasic. SIRS occurs during the initial 3–5 days; during this phase, a second insult (or hit), such as surgery, may provoke an exaggerated inflammatory response. Up to 50% of the patients developing organ failure early after trauma do so in the absence of bacterial infection. The initial phase is followed by a period (perhaps 10–14 days) of immunosuppression, when the patient is prone to infection. Multiple organ failure can occur during either of these phases.

Assessment and management of the trauma patient

Prehospital phase

In the UK, prehospital management of severely injured patients is performed mainly by paramedics, although doctors are increased involved, particularly with helicopter emergency medical services (HEMS). Paramedics are trained to minimise on-scene time; a prolonged time to definitive care will increase mortality. Unless the patient is trapped, on-scene interventions should be restricted to control of the airway and ventilation, and stabilisation of the spine. The prehospital presence of a doctor will enable rapid sequence induction (RSI) and intubation to be undertaken in patients with severe traumatic brain injury (TBI) and others in whom control of the airway and ventilation is considered important before transfer to hospital. The receiving hospital should be given advanced warning of the impending admission of a severely injured patient. Ambulance personnel should be able to communicate directly with emergency department staff via a talk-through link. Concise and essential information on the patient's condition and estimated time of arrival must be given. Emergency department staff can then decide whether to alert the trauma team.

Trauma networks

There is evidence from the United States that severely injured patients who are treated in specialised trauma centres have better outcomes than those treated in smaller hospitals that treat relatively few such patients. In the UK, trauma networks were implemented widely in 2012 and severely injured patients are transferred directly to a major trauma centre (MTC) unless they have immediately life-threatening injuries that require initial stabilisation at the nearest trauma unit (usually a district general hospital) before secondary transfer to the MTC.

Preparation for resuscitation

With advance warning, medical and nursing staff can prepare a resuscitation bay in readiness for the patient's arrival. This will include running through drip sets, turning on fluid warmers, and drawing up anaesthetic drugs. Members of the resuscitation team put on protective clothing comprising gloves, plastic aprons and eye protection. The relevant nurses and doctors are assigned tasks before the patient arrives. In hospitals with formal trauma teams, the roles of individual team members are usually well established (Figure 9.3). The team leader should be a suitably experienced doctor from one of the relevant specialties, e.g. emergency medicine, anaesthesia, general surgery or orthopaedic surgery.

Primary survey and resuscitation

The initial management of the trauma patient is considered in four phases:

- Primary survey
- Resuscitation
- Secondary survey
- Definitive care

Figure 9.3 Composition and role of a typical trauma team

Team leader	Primary and secondary surveys, coordination of team, overall responsibility for the patient while in the emergency department
Doctor 1 & Nurse 1	Airway, ventilation, central venous access, difficult peripheral access, fluid balance, analgesia
Doctor 2 & Nurse 2	All other procedures, chest drain, fracture splintage, urethral catheter
Nurse 3	Measure vital signs, record data, remove clothes, assist other team members
Radiographer	Chest and pelvis x-rays; other x-rays as requested by team leader
Porter	To take samples to pathology labs, to retrieve urgent blood from blood bank

Although the first two phases are listed consecutively, they are performed simultaneously. The secondary survey, or head-to-toe examination of the patient, is not started until the patient has been adequately resuscitated. The aim of the primary survey is to look sequentially for immediately life-threatening injuries, in the order that they are most likely to kill the patient. The correct sequence is:

A. Airway with cervical spine control
B. Breathing
C. Circulation and haemorrhage control
D. Disability – a rapid assessment of neurological function
E. Exposure – while considering the environment, and preventing hypothermia

If life-threatening problems are detected, treat them immediately (resuscitate) before proceeding to the next step of the primary survey. In the presence of exsanguinating external haemorrhage it may be more appropriate to apply a CABC sequence, in which external bleeding is first controlled with external pressure or, if a limb is involved, by the application of a tourniquet. Use of the CABC sequence is particularly common in military settings.

Airway and cervical spine

Unless there is catastrophic external haemorrhage (when CABC applies), the first priority during the resuscitation of any severely injured patient is to ensure a clear airway and maintain adequate oxygenation (Crewdson & Nolan 2011). Place a pulse oximeter probe on the patient's finger. Knowing the patient's arterial blood oxygen saturation is very valuable, although sometimes peripheral vasoconstriction will make it impossible to obtain a reliable reading. If the airway is obstructed, immediate basic manoeuvres such as suction, chin lift and jaw thrust may clear it temporarily. A soft nasopharyngeal airway (size 6.0–7.0 mm) may be particularly useful in the semiconscious patient who will not tolerate an oropharyngeal airway. Give high-concentration oxygen to every patient with multiple injuries. In the unintubated, spontaneously breathing patient this is provided with a mask and reservoir bag ($F_IO_2 = 0.85$).

Care of the cervical spine

Every patient sustaining significant blunt trauma, particularly above the clavicles, should be assumed to have a cervical spine injury until proven otherwise. Such patients should have their cervical spines immobilised at the accident scene. The most effective method comprises a combination of an appropriately sized semi-rigid cervical collar, lateral supports and straps (Figure 9.4). Undertake all airway manoeuvres carefully without moving the neck. Significant subluxation of the cervical spine can occur during aggressive chin lift or jaw thrust despite the presence of an appropriate collar. Mask ventilation can

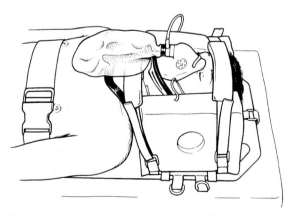

Figure 9.4 Cervical spine immobilisation with semi-rigid collar, lateral blocks and spine board

displace the cervical spine as much as oral intubation. Manual in-line stabilisation of the neck will minimise movement of the cervical spine during oral intubation, but avoid excessive traction, which may distract a cervical fracture. In the resuscitation room, the cervical spine cannot be deemed undamaged until the patient has been examined by an experienced clinician and/or appropriate radiological procedures have been completed. A reliable clinical examination cannot be obtained if the patient has sustained a significant closed head injury, is intoxicated, or has a reduced conscious level from any other cause.

Advanced airway management

In the unconscious patient, or in the presence of haemorrhage from maxillofacial injuries, for example, the airway must be secured by placing a cuffed tube in the trachea. Other reasons for intubating the trauma patient during the resuscitation phase are to optimise oxygen delivery and to enable appropriate procedures to be performed on uncooperative patients. The choice of technique for intubating a patient with a suspected or confirmed cervical spine injury will depend on the indication and on the skill and experience of the individual clinician. If performed with care, tracheal intubation of a patient with a cervical spine injury carries relatively little risk (Crosby 2006). Occasionally, awake fibreoptic intubation may be appropriate, but this will take much longer to achieve and is rarely applicable in the resuscitation phase. Do not attempt blind nasal intubation.

The technique of choice for emergency intubation of a patient with a potential cervical spine injury is direct laryngoscopy and oral intubation with manual in-line stabilisation (MILS) of the cervical spine, following a period of preoxygenation, intravenous induction of anaesthesia, paralysis with suxamethonium and application of cricoid pressure. Manual in-line stabilisation reduces neck movement during intubation, but excessive axial traction must be avoided. An assistant kneels at the head of the patient and to one side to leave room for the intubator. The assistant holds the patient's head firmly down on the trolley by grasping the mastoid processes. The tape or straps, lateral blocks and front of the collar are removed. The front of a single-piece collar can be folded under the patient's shoulder, leaving the posterior portion of the collar in situ behind the head. Do not attempt laryngoscopy and intubation with the collar in place – it will make it very difficult to get an adequate view of the larynx. Placing the patient's head and neck in neutral alignment will make the view at laryngoscopy worse: in this position the view of the larynx will be grade 3 or worse in approximately 20% of patients. Intubation will be aided greatly by the use of a gum-elastic bougie – it enables less force to be applied to the laryngoscope because intubation can be achieved despite a relatively poor view. The McCoy levering laryngoscope may also be useful: it reduces the incidence of grade 3 or worse views to 5%. A variety of videolaryngoscopes are now available, and use of these devices in the trauma setting is likely to become the standard of care.

If intubation of the patient proves impossible the airway should be secured by surgical cricothyroidotomy. A supraglottic airway device (SAD) may provide a temporary airway, but does not guarantee protection against aspiration (Timmermann 2011). A second-generation SAD, such as the ProSeal LMA, is probably better under these circumstances. The laryngeal tube and iGel are reasonable alternatives.

Needle cricothyroidotomy and jet insufflation of oxygen from a high-pressure source (400 kPa) is an alternative method of providing temporary oxygenation, but it seemed less successful than surgical cricothyroidotomy in the Fourth National Audit Project (NAP4) study (Cook *et al.* 2011). Standard cannulae may kink and become obstructed, so use a device manufactured specifically for needle cricothyroidotomy.

Breathing

Look and listen to the chest to confirm that both sides are being ventilated adequately, and measure the respiratory rate. The following chest injuries are immediately life-threatening and must be diagnosed and treated in the primary survey:

- Tension pneumothorax
- Open pneumothorax
- Flail chest
- Massive haemothorax
- Cardiac tamponade

Tension pneumothorax

Reduced chest movement, reduced breath sounds and a resonant percussion note on the affected side, along with respiratory distress, hypotension and tachycardia, indicate a tension pneumothorax. Deviation of the trachea to the opposite side is a late sign, and neck veins may not be distended in the presence of hypovolaemia. Treatment is immediate decompression with either a large cannula placed in the 2nd intercostal space, in the mid-clavicular line on the affected side, or a rapid thoracostomy (small incision into the pleural space) in the 5th intercostal space in the anterior axillary line. Once intravenous access has been obtained, insert a large chest drain (32 F) in the 5th intercostal space in the anterior axillary line, and connect to an underwater seal drain.

Open pneumothorax

Cover an open pneumothorax with an occlusive dressing and seal on three sides: the unsealed side should act as a flutter valve. Insert a chest drain away from the wound in the same hemithorax.

Flail chest

Multiple fractures in adjacent ribs will cause a segment of the chest wall to lose bony continuity with the thoracic cage. This flail segment will move paradoxically with inspiration. The immediately life-threatening problem is the underlying lung contusion, which can cause severe hypoxia. The patient must be given effective analgesia – in the cardiovascularly stable patient a thoracic epidural is ideal (see below). Assisted ventilation, via a tracheal tube or by a non-invasive technique, is required if hypoxia persists despite supplemental oxygen.

Massive haemothorax

A massive haemothorax is defined as more than 1500 mL blood in a hemithorax, and it will cause reduced chest movement, a dull percussion note and hypoxaemia. Start fluid resuscitation and insert a chest drain. The patient is likely to require a thoracotomy if blood loss from the chest drain exceeds 200 mL per hour, but this decision will depend also on the patient's general physiological state.

Cardiac tamponade

While not a disorder of breathing, it is logical to consider the possibility of cardiac tamponade while examining the chest, particularly if the patient has sustained a penetrating injury to the chest or upper abdomen. Distended neck veins in the presence of hypotension are suggestive of cardiac tamponade although, after rapid volume resuscitation, myocardial contusion will also present in this way. Ultrasound examination in the resuscitation room is the best way to make the diagnosis, and now that focused assessment with sonography for trauma (FAST) scanning is included in the emergency medicine curriculum there is usually someone immediately available to undertake this examination. If cardiac tamponade is diagnosed and the

Figure 9.5 Insertion of chest drain

- Place the patient supine with the ipsilateral arm at right angles to the chest
- The insertion point is in the 5th intercostal space (nipple level) in the anterior axillary line
- Infiltrate down to the upper border of the rib with 1% lidocaine
- Make a 3 cm incision along the upper border of the 5th rib. Using forceps, bluntly dissect down into the pleural cavity
- Insert a finger into the pleural cavity and sweep around to ensure that the lung is clear of the chest wall
- Select a large chest drain (32 F), remove the trochar, and insert the forceps through the distal side hole. Insert the chest drain into the pleural cavity using the forceps as a guide
- Suture the chest drain securely to the skin and connect it to an underwater drainage system
- Obtain a chest x-ray to check for lung expansion and tube position. Leave the drain in situ until the lung is re-expanded and drainage of fluid and/or air has stopped
- Do not clamp chest drains in a patient receiving positive-pressure ventilation – the intrapleural pressure is always positive and the patient can be transported safely as long the drains are not moved above the level of the chest

patient is deteriorating, a resuscitative thoracotomy and pericardiotomy is indicated. Needle pericardiocentesis is often unsuccessful because, contrary to traditional teaching, the pericardial blood is often clotted or re-accumulates rapidly once aspirated.

Chest drainage

Indications for chest drainage in the trauma patient are a tension pneumothorax (after decompression), simple pneumothorax, haemothorax, and multiple rib fractures in a patient requiring positive-pressure ventilation. Do not use a trochar for chest drain insertion: it can cause serious lacerations of the lung and pulmonary vessels. The practical technique is given in Figure 9.5. It is reasonable to observe carefully (but not insert a chest drain initially) in cases where there is a small pneumothorax that is seen on CT scan but not a chest x-ray ('occult pneumothorax') or when positive-pressure ventilation is used in the presence of relatively undisplaced rib fractures. In both these

cases, ensure that there is immediate access to the chest in case a chest drain is required.

Circulation

Control any major external haemorrhage with direct pressure. Severe haemorrhage from open limb injuries may be controlled with a properly applied tourniquet. In the past, use of tourniquets in this way was discouraged, but recent military experience with blast injuries, in particular, has shown them to be very effective. Rapidly assess the patient's haemodynamic state and attach ECG leads. Until proven otherwise, hypotension should be assumed to be caused by hypovolaemia. Less likely causes include myocardial contusion, cardiac tamponade, tension pneumothorax, neurogenic shock and sepsis.

Intravenous access

Insert two short large-bore intravenous cannulae (14 gauge or larger) into a peripheral vein. Most anaesthetists are confident in inserting central lines but this may not be easy in the hypovolaemic patient and there is a risk of creating a pneumothorax. The femoral vein provides a good route for a large-bore cannula. In the severely injured patient, central venous access is valuable because it enables delivery of multiple drug infusions as well as central venous pressure (CVP) monitoring. The intraosseous (IO) route (usually via the proximal tibia) is useful and modern devices enable infusion of fluids at up to 200 mL min^{-1}, which makes this route useful for fluid resuscitation of adults as well as children. Insert an arterial cannula for continuous direct blood pressure monitoring and send a sample for arterial blood gas analysis – severely injured patients will have a marked base deficit, and its correction will help to confirm adequate resuscitation.

Fluids

An initial fluid challenge is made with crystalloid. There is no evidence for use of colloids in the resuscitation phase except, of course, for early use of blood in the exsanguinating patient. Failure to improve the vital signs after 1–2 litres of crystalloid suggests exsanguinating haemorrhage, and the need for immediate surgical intervention and transfusion of blood (a full cross-match will take 45 minutes, group-confirmed blood can be issued in 10 minutes, and group O blood can be obtained immediately). A transient response to this fluid challenge suggests that the patient may have lost 20–40% of circulating blood volume and has ongoing bleeding; he or she will require immediate surgical assessment and is likely to need blood. A sustained reduction in heart rate and increase in blood pressure implies only moderate blood loss (< 20% blood volume).

Recently, there has been a trend away from giving large-volume crystalloid fluid challenges in hypovolaemic trauma patients and instead giving blood and blood products much earlier. Observational data from both military and civilian settings have documented increased survival rates associated with earlier use of platelets and FFP particularly when given with blood in ratios approximating 1:1:1. There are significant methodological weaknesses associated with these non-randomised studies – the most important being that patients dying early are inevitably less likely to have received blood products (survivor bias). More recently, it has been suggested that a blood-to-FFP ratio of 2:1 to 1.5:1 may be optimal. There is good evidence that tranexamic acid (1 g over 10 minutes given within 3 hours of injury and then an infusion of 1 g over 8 hours) reduces mortality from bleeding in trauma patients. A multicentre randomised placebo-controlled phase III trial failed to show benefit for activated recombinant factor VII in severely injured trauma patients with bleeding refractory to standard treatment. The use of recombinant factor VII may still be considered if coagulopathy persists despite adequate treatment with other blood products, but the initial enthusiasm for this expensive product is waning.

In the absence of obvious external haemorrhage, the likely sources of severe haemorrhage are the chest, abdomen or pelvis. Explore these possibilities and treat them during the primary survey. Careful examination of the chest should exclude massive haemothorax. Obvious abdominal distension mandates a laparotomy, while an equivocal abdominal examination is an indication for computerised tomograpy (CT) or ultrasound (see under *Secondary survey*, below). If significant pelvic injury is suspected, apply a pelvic binder. Springing the iliac crests to detect a pelvic disruption is no longer recommended, because it aggravates bleeding. All patients with major injuries should be CT scanned (head, spine, chest and pelvis), ideally within 30 minutes of arrival, unless there is an indication to go directly to the operating room. If the patient is going directly to the operating room, rapidly obtain chest and pelvic x-rays.

Fluid warming

Warm all intravenous fluids, especially blood products. A high-capacity fluid warmer will be required to cope with the rapid infusion rates used during trauma patient resuscitation. Hypothermia (core temperature < 35 °C) is a serious complication of severe trauma and haemorrhage and is an independent predictor of mortality.

Hypothermia has several adverse effects

- It causes a gradual decline in heart rate and cardiac output while increasing the propensity for myocardial dysrhythmias. One study has shown an increase in the incidence of morbid cardiac events in mildly hypothermic patients undergoing a variety of surgical procedures.
- The oxyhaemoglobin dissociation curve is shifted to the left by a decrease in temperature, thus impairing peripheral oxygen delivery in the hypovolaemic patient at a time when it is needed most.
- Shivering may compound the lactic acidosis that typically accompanies hypovolaemia, and this may be further aggravated by a decreased metabolic clearance of lactic acid by the liver.
- Hypothermia contributes to the coagulopathy accompanying massive transfusion. The likely mechanisms involved include retarding the function of enzymes in the clotting cascade, enhanced plasma fibrinolytic activity, and reduced platelet aggregation.
- Mild hypothermia in the perioperative period increases the incidence of wound infection.

Resuscitation end points

Simply returning the heart rate, blood pressure and urine output to normal does not represent a suitable resuscitation end point for the trauma patient. Plasma lactate and base deficit are better end points to use.

Hypotensive resuscitation

Aggressive fluid resuscitation before surgical control of the bleeding is likely to be harmful: in the presence of active bleeding, increasing the blood pressure with fluid accelerates the loss of red blood cells and may hamper clotting mechanisms. However, older patients and those with a significant head injury will require fluid resuscitation to restore vital organ perfusion. The balance is between the risk of inducing organ ischaemia and the risk of accelerating haemorrhage.

Disability

Record the size of the pupils and their reaction to light, and rapidly assess the Glasgow coma scale (GCS) score, which is described in Chapter 5 (Figure 5.22). If the patient requires urgent induction of anaesthesia and intubation, a quick neurological assessment should be performed first.

Exposure and environmental control

It is likely that the patient's clothes will have been removed by this stage. If not, undress them completely and apply a forced-air warming blanket to keep the patient warm.

Tubes

Insert a urinary catheter: urine output is an excellent indicator of the adequacy of resuscitation. Before inserting the catheter, check for indications of a ruptured urethra such as scrotal haematoma, blood at the meatus or a high prostate. If any of these signs are present, ask a urologist to assess the patient – the specialist may make one attempt to gently insert a urethral catheter before using the suprapubic route. Insert a gastric tube to drain the stomach contents and reduce the risk of aspiration. If there is any suspicion of a basal skull fracture, use the orogastric route, which eliminates the possibility of passing a nasogastric tube through a basal skull fracture and into the brain.

Radiology

Technological advances in computed tomography (image quality and speed) combined with increasing recognition of the limitations of plain radiographs has led to a much greater reliance on whole-body CT as the primary radiological investigation in severely injured patients. The modern standard is to obtain a CT scan within 30 minutes of patient arrival in the emergency department. Chest and pelvic x-rays should be considered if the patient is going directly to the operating room or if they are haemodynamically very unstable (e.g. systolic blood pressure < 90 mmHg or heart rate > 120 despite 2 units of Group O negative blood). Any x-rays must be taken without interrupting the resuscitation process – this is achievable if members of the trauma team are wearing lead coats. There is no indication for a lateral x-ray of the cervical spine in the severely injured patient – it will not change the patient's management, and a cervical spine injury is assumed until ruled out with a CT scan with or without clinical examination.

Secondary survey

Do not undertake the detailed head-to-toe survey until resuscitation is well under way and the patient's vital signs are stable. Re-evaluate the patient continually, so that ongoing bleeding is detected early. Patients with exsanguinating haemorrhage may need a laparotomy as part of the resuscitation phase. They should be transferred directly to the operating theatre (within 30 minutes of arrival in the emergency department); the secondary survey is postponed until the completion of life-saving surgery. Alert staff in the operating theatre and ICU as soon as any severely injured patient is admitted to the resuscitation room. The objectives of the secondary survey are: to examine the patient from head to toe and front to back; to take a complete medical history; to gather all clinical, laboratory and radiological information; and to devise a management plan.

Head

Inspect and feel the scalp for lacerations, haematomas or depressed fractures. Look for evidence of a basal skull fracture:

- Panda (raccoon) eyes
- Battle's sign (bruising over the mastoid process)
- Subhyaloid haemorrhage
- Scleral haemorrhage without a posterior margin
- Haemotympanum
- CSF rhinorrhoea and otorrhoea

Brain injury can be divided into primary and secondary groups. Primary injury (concussion, contusion and laceration) occurs at the moment of impact and, other than preventive strategies, there is nothing that can be done about it. Secondary brain injury is compounded by hypoxia, hypercarbia and hypotension. These factors can be prevented or rapidly treated. Guidelines for the management of severe head injury are published by the Brain Trauma Foundation (last updated in 2007). Goals include a mean blood pressure of at least 90 mmHg, $SaO_2 > 95\%$ and, if mechanically ventilated, a $PaCO_2$ of approximately 4.5–5.0 kPa.

The conscious level is assessed using the GCS, which is reliable and reproducible. As the GCS is a dynamic measurement, the trend of conscious level change is more important than one static reading. Record the pupillary response and the presence of any lateralising signs. A dilated pupil in a patient in coma can be caused by pressure on the occulomotor nerve from a displaced medial temporal lobe, and is a sign of ipsilateral

Figure 9.6 Indications for urgent CT brain scan in adult trauma patients (NICE 2014).

Within 1 hour of identifying risk factor
- GCS < 13 on initial assessment in the emergency department
- GCS < 15 two hours after the injury on assessment in the emergency department
- Suspected open or depressed skull fracture
- Any sign of basal skull fracture
- Post-traumatic seizure
- Focal neurological deficit
- One or more episodes of vomiting

Within 8 hours of injury
- Age > 65 y
- History of bleeding or clotting disorder
- Amnesia of > 30 minutes events before injury
- Dangerous mechanism of injury (e.g. struck by vehicle or fall from > 1 metre)

haematoma or brain injury. A haematoma pressing on the motor cortex usually causes contralateral motor weakness. However, it may be of such a size that the whole hemisphere is shifted, pressing the opposite cerebral peduncle against the edge of tentorium. This will cause ipsilateral weakness, although its clinical detection is masked because the patient will be deeply comatose. If there is right/left asymmetry, use the best motor response for documenting the GCS. A GCS score of less than 9 defines a severe head injury, a score of 9–12 is a moderate head injury, and head injuries associated with a score of 13–15 are minor.

Indications for urgent CT scan after head injury have been defined by the National Institute for Health and Care Excellence (2014) and are shown in Figure 9.6.

A GCS < 9 is generally cited as the primary indication for intubating the head-injured, but in practice virtually all patients with a moderate head injury are normally intubated and ventilated for at least the duration of the CT scan. Depending on the results of the CT scan, these patients are often sedated and mechanically ventilated for at least 24 hours even if their pre-induction GCS was > 9.

Major trauma networks will have their own criteria for transfer of the head-injured patients to the MTC but, traditionally, referral to the regional neurosurgical unit is indicated for:
- All patients with an intracranial mass
- Primary brain injury requiring ventilation
- Compound depressed skull fracture

- Persistent CSF leak
- Penetrating skull injury
- Patients deteriorating rapidly with signs of an intracranial mass lesion

Mannitol 0.5–1.0 g kg^{-1} may be considered after discussion with the neurosurgeon; it can reduce intracranial pressure and will buy time before surgery.

Face and neck

Palpate the face and look for steps around the orbital margins and along the zygoma. Check for mobile segments in the mid-face or mandible. While an assistant maintains the head and neck in neutral alignment, inspect the neck for swelling or lacerations. Carefully palpate the cervical spinous processes for tenderness or deformities. In the patient who is awake, alert, sober, neurologically normal and without distracting injuries, the cervical spine may be cleared if there is no pain at rest and, subsequently, on flexion and extension. All other patients who have head injuries or multisystem trauma will require a CT scan of their cervical spine (occiput to T1) (Como et al. 2009). Most of these patients will also have scans of their chest, abdomen and pelvis, which will include the entire spine. Obtunded patients will have their spines cleared (and spinal immobilisation removed) using the CT images alone; however, if a reliable clinical examination is considered possible within 24 hours, some clinicians will continue spinal immobilisation until this examination is completed (there is a very small possibility of clinically significant ligamentous injury that is not detected by CT scan).

Thorax

There are six potentially life-threatening injuries (two contusions and four 'ruptures') that can be identified by careful examination of the chest during the secondary survey:
- Pulmonary contusion
- Cardiac contusion
- Aortic rupture (blunt aortic injury)
- Ruptured diaphragm
- Oesophageal rupture
- Rupture of the tracheobronchial tree

Pulmonary contusion

Inspect the chest for signs of considerable decelerating forces, such as seatbelt bruising. Even in the absence of rib fractures, pulmonary contusion is the commonest potentially lethal chest injury. Young adults and children have compliant ribs and considerable energy can be transmitted to the lungs in the absence of rib fractures. The earliest indication of pulmonary contusion is hypoxaemia (reduced PaO_2/F_IO_2 ratio). The chest radiograph will show patchy infiltrates over the affected area, but it may be normal initially. Increasing the F_IO_2 alone may provide sufficient oxygenation but, failing that, the patient may require continuous positive airway pressure (CPAP) by face mask, or tracheal intubation and positive-pressure ventilation. Check the ventilator settings continually. Use a small tidal volume (5–7 mL kg^{-1}) and keep the peak inspiratory pressure below 35 cmH$_2$O to minimise volutrauma and barotrauma. The patient with chest trauma requires appropriate fluid resuscitation, but fluid overload will worsen lung contusion.

Cardiac contusion

Consider cardiac contusion in any patient with severe blunt chest trauma, particularly those with sternal fractures. Cardiac arrhythmias and ST changes on the ECG may indicate contusion, but these signs are very non-specific; elevated plasma troponin may be slightly better. An elevated CVP in the presence of hypotension will be the earliest indication of myocardial dysfunction secondary to severe cardiac contusion, but cardiac tamponade must be excluded. Echocardiography may confirm the diagnosis of cardiac contusion. The right ventricle is most frequently injured, as it is predominantly an anterior structure. Patients with severe cardiac contusion tend to have other serious injuries that will mandate their admission to an intensive care unit. Thus the decision to admit a patient to ICU rarely depends on the diagnosis of cardiac contusion alone. The severely contused myocardium is likely to require inotropic support.

Blunt aortic injury

The thoracic aorta is at risk in any patient subjected to a significant decelerating force, e.g., a fall from a height or a high-speed road traffic crash. Only 10–15% of these patients will reach hospital alive. The commonest site for aortic injury is at the aortic isthmus, just distal to the origin of the left subclavian artery at the level of the ligamentum arteriosum. Deceleration produces huge shear forces at this site because the relatively mobile aortic arch travels forward relative to the fixed descending aorta. The tear in the intima and media may involve either part or all of the circumference of the aorta, and in survivors

the haematoma is contained by an intact aortic adventitia and mediastinal pleura. Patients sustaining traumatic aortic rupture usually have multiple injuries and may be hypotensive at presentation. However, upper extremity hypertension is present in 40% of cases as the haematoma compresses the true lumen, causing a 'pseudo-coarctation'. The supine chest radiograph will show a widened mediastinum in the vast majority of cases, but these days diagnosis is achieved with urgent CT angiography. If a rupture of the thoracic aorta is suspected, maintain the blood pressure at 80–100 mmHg systolic (using a β-blocker such as esmolol) to reduce the risk of further dissection or rupture. Pure vasodilators, such as sodium nitroprusside (SNP), increase the pulse pressure and will not reduce the shear forces on the aortic wall. When bleeding from other injuries has been controlled, transfer the patient to the nearest cardiothoracic unit. The majority of these blunt aortic injuries are now treated with endovascular stents instead of the more traditional open operative repair.

Rupture of the diaphragm

Rupture of the diaphragm occurs in about 5% of patients sustaining severe blunt trauma to the trunk. It can be difficult to diagnose initially, particularly when other severe injuries dominate the patient's management, and consequently the diagnosis may be made late. Early detection has been improved by the routine use of high-quality CT in virtually all severely injured patients. Approximately 75% of ruptures occur on the left side. The stomach or colon commonly herniates into the chest, and strangulation of these organs is a significant complication. Signs and symptoms detected during the secondary survey may include diminished breath sounds on the ipsilateral side, pain in the chest and abdomen, and respiratory distress. Diagnosis can be made on a plain radiograph (elevated hemidiaphragm, gas bubbles above the diaphragm, shift of the mediastinum to the opposite side, nasogastric tube in the chest). Multislice CT will usually provide the definite answer. Once the patient has been stabilised, the diaphragm will require surgical repair.

Oesophageal rupture

A severe blow to the upper abdomen may result in a torn lower oesophagus, as gastric contents are forcefully ejected. The conscious patient will complain of severe chest and abdominal pain, and mediastinal air may be visible on the chest x-ray. Gastric contents may appear in the chest drain. The diagnosis is confirmed by contrast study of the oesophagus, CT and, if necessary, endoscopy. Urgent surgery is essential, since accompanying mediastinitis carries a high mortality.

Tracheobronchial injury

Laryngeal fractures are, fortunately, rare. Signs of laryngeal injury include hoarseness, subcutaneous emphysema and palpable fracture crepitus. Total airway obstruction or severe respiratory distress will have been managed by intubation or surgical airway during the primary survey and resuscitation phases. This is the one situation where tracheostomy, rather than cricothyroidotomy, is indicated. Less severe laryngeal injuries are assessed by CT before any appropriate surgery. Transections of the trachea or bronchi proximal to the pleural reflection cause massive mediastinal and cervical emphysema. Injuries distal to the pleural sheath lead to pneumothoraces. Typically, these will not resolve after chest drainage, since the bronchopleural fistula causes a large air leak. Most bronchial injuries occur within 2.5 cm of the carina and the diagnosis is confirmed by bronchoscopy. Tracheobronchial injuries require urgent repair through a thoracotomy.

Abdomen

A thorough examination of the whole abdomen is required. The priority is to determine quickly the need for laparotomy and not to spend considerable time trying to define precisely which viscus is injured. Inspect the abdomen for bruising, lacerations and distension. Careful palpation may reveal tenderness. A rectal examination is performed to assess sphincter tone and to exclude the presence of pelvic fracture or a high prostate. If abdominal examination is unreliable, exclusion of intra-abdominal injury will require CT scan, often preceded by ultrasound. Focused assessment with sonography for trauma (FAST) scanning will detect significant free fluid in the regions defined by the four Ps: pericardial, perihepatic, perisplenic and pelvic. While ultrasound is good for detecting blood, CT will provide information on specific organ injury; however, CT may miss some gastrointestinal, diaphragmatic and pancreatic injuries.

In patients with multiple injuries, 'damage control' surgery is often undertaken. This emphasises rapid but definitive haemostasis, closure of all hollow-viscus injuries or performing only essential bowel resections, and delaying the more standard reconstruction until after the patient has been stabilised and all physiological parameters have been corrected.

Major pelvic trauma resulting in exsanguinating haemorrhage should be dealt with during the resuscitative phase.

Extremities

Inspect all limbs for bruising, wounds and deformities, and examine for vascular and neurological defects. Correct any neurovascular impairment by realignment of any deformity and splintage of the limb.

Spinal column

A detailed neurological examination at this stage should detect any motor or sensory deficits. The patient will need to be log-rolled to enable a thorough inspection and palpation of the whole length of the spine. A safe log roll requires a total of five people: three to control and turn the patient's body, one to maintain the cervical spine in neutral alignment with the rest of the body, and one to examine the spine. The person controlling the cervical spine should command the team.

Reconstruction in the sagittal plane of the images obtained from the CT scan of the chest, abdomen and pelvis will provide 'scanograms' of the thoracolumbar spine, and these can be used to clear the thoracolumbar spine. Lateral and AP x-rays are no longer used for this purpose.

Medical history

Obtain a medical history from the patient, relatives and/or the ambulance crew. A useful mnemonic is AMPLE:

A Allergies
M Medications
P Past medical history
L Last meal
E Event leading to the injury and the environment

It is possible that a patient's pre-existing medical problem contributed to or precipitated an accident, e.g. myocardial infarction while driving a car.

The paramedics will be able to give invaluable information about the mechanism of injury. The speed of a road traffic crash and the direction of impact will dictate the likely injury patterns.

Analgesia

Systemic analgesia

Give effective analgesia as soon as practically possible. If the patient needs surgery imminently, then immediate induction of general anaesthesia is a logical and very effective solution to the patient's pain. If not, titrate intravenous opioid (e.g. fentanyl or morphine) to the desired effect. Head-injured patients will require adequate pain relief for any other injuries. Careful titration of intravenous morphine or fentanyl will provide effective pain relief without serious respiratory depression.

Non-steroidal anti-inflammatory drugs (NSAIDs) provide moderate analgesia but are relatively contraindicated in patients with hypovolaemia; these patients depend on renal prostaglandins to maintain renal blood flow. In normovolaemic trauma patients, use of NSAIDs may reduce the need for opioids.

Local and regional analgesia

Local anaesthetic blocks are ideal in the acute trauma patient. Unfortunately, there are relatively few blocks that are both simple and effective. One of these is the femoral nerve block for a fracture of the femoral shaft.

Regional analgesia has a useful role in some acute trauma patients. Exclude hypovolaemia and coagulopathy before attempting epidural or spinal analgesia in the acute trauma patient. In patients with multiple rib fractures, including flail segments, a thoracic epidural will provide excellent analgesia. This will help the patient to tolerate physiotherapy and to maintain adequate ventilation. All these factors help to reduce the requirement for intubation and mechanical ventilation. A lumbar epidural will benefit patients with lower limb injuries and, assuming there are no contraindications, this can be placed intraoperatively.

Management of burns

The standard ABC principles apply to treating patients with severe burns. Patients with severe burns should be stabilised and transferred to the nearest burns centre. The patient with a thermal injury to the respiratory tract may develop airway obstruction rapidly from the oedema. Give humidified high-concentration oxygen to all patients suspected of having thermal or smoke injury to the respiratory tract. Undertake arterial blood gas analysis and measure the carboxyhaemoglobin concentration. Consider the need for early intubation in the presence of any of the following:

- Altered consciousness
- Direct burns to the face or oropharynx
- Hoarseness or stridor
- Soot in the nostrils or sputum
- Expiratory rhonchi
- Dysphagia
- Drooling and dribbling saliva

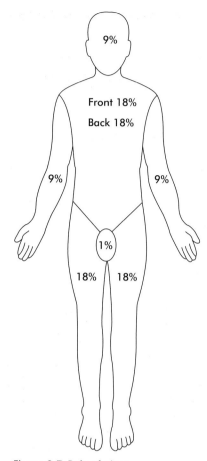

Figure 9.7 Rule of nines

Having established intravenous access, start fluid resuscitation and cover burnt areas with cling film. The simple 'rule of nines' (Figure 9.7) enables an approximate calculation of the surface area of the burn, which is determined more precisely later using a Lund and Browder chart (Figure 9.8). Most burns centres use crystalloid for initial fluid resuscitation. Give 2–4 mL of crystalloid per kilogram body weight per percent burn area in the first 24 hours. Give one-half of this fluid in the first 8 hours, and the remainder over the next 16 hours. The exact volume of fluid given depends on vital signs, central venous pressure and urine output. Recent data suggest that this formula tends to overestimate fluid requirement in many of these patients. Patients with full-thickness burns of > 10% of the body surface area

CHART FOR ESTIMATING SEVERITY OF BURN WOUND

NAME _____ WARD _____ NUMBER _____ DATE _____

AGE _____ ADMISSION WEIGHT _____

LUND AND BROWDER CHARTS

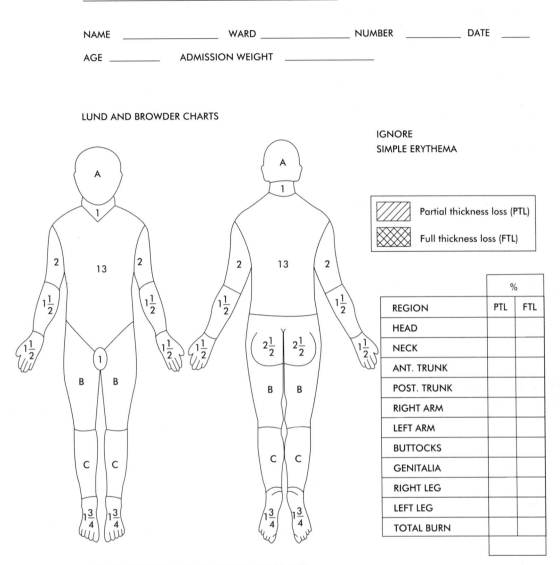

IGNORE
SIMPLE ERYTHEMA

Partial thickness loss (PTL)

Full thickness loss (FTL)

REGION	%	
	PTL	FTL
HEAD		
NECK		
ANT. TRUNK		
POST. TRUNK		
RIGHT ARM		
LEFT ARM		
BUTTOCKS		
GENITALIA		
RIGHT LEG		
LEFT LEG		
TOTAL BURN		

RELATIVE PERCENTAGE OF BODY SURFACE AREA
AFFECTED BY GROWTH

AREA	AGE 0	1	5	10	15	ADULT
A = $\frac{1}{2}$ OF HEAD	$9\frac{1}{2}$	$8\frac{1}{2}$	$6\frac{1}{2}$	$5\frac{1}{2}$	$4\frac{1}{2}$	$3\frac{1}{2}$
B = $\frac{1}{2}$ OF ONE THIGH	$2\frac{3}{4}$	$3\frac{1}{4}$	4	$4\frac{1}{2}$	$4\frac{1}{2}$	$4\frac{3}{4}$
C = $\frac{1}{2}$ OF ONE LEG	$2\frac{1}{2}$	$2\frac{1}{2}$	$2\frac{3}{4}$	3	$3\frac{1}{4}$	$3\frac{1}{2}$

Figure 9.8 Lund and Browder chart

will probably require blood. Patients with severe burns need potent analgesia, which is best given by carefully titrating intravenous opioids.

Anaesthesia for patients with severe trauma

Induction of anaesthesia

A smooth induction of anaesthesia and neuromuscular blockade provides optimal conditions for intubating high-risk trauma patients. All anaesthetic induction drugs are vasodilators and respiratory depressants and have the potential to produce or worsen hypotension. There is no evidence that the choice of induction drug alters survival in major trauma patients. Their appropriate use during resuscitation involves a careful assessment of the clinical situation and a thorough knowledge of their clinical pharmacology. The safest strategy is for the anaesthetist to use drugs with which he or she is familiar: the trauma resuscitation room is not the place for experimentation. Anaesthetic requirement is assessed individually, and the risk of awareness kept to a minimum. Severely injured patients requiring intubation fall generally into one of three groups:

1. Stable and adequately resuscitated. These patients should receive a standard or slightly reduced dose of induction drug.
2. Unstable or inadequately resuscitated but require immediate intubation. These patients should receive a reduced, titrated dose of induction drug.
3. In extremis – severely obtunded and hypotensive. Induction drugs would be inappropriate, but muscle relaxants may be used to facilitate intubation. Give anaesthetic and analgesic drugs as soon as adequate cerebral perfusion is achieved.

Suxamethonium retains its status as the neuromuscular blocker with the fastest onset of action, and remains the most popular relaxant for intubation of the acute trauma patient. In the presence of adequate anaesthesia, suxamethonium does not increase intracranial pressure in severely head-injured patients. Rocuronium is almost as fast in onset and is favoured by some trauma anaesthetists, particularly as rapid reversal with sugammadex is now possible. In practice, if airway management is difficult, waking the patient up is often not feasible because these patients need urgent resuscitation, assessment, and definitive surgery,

Intraoperative management

The following considerations are of relevance to the anaesthetist during surgery for the severely injured patient:

- **Prolonged surgery.** The patient will be at risk from pressure areas and from heat loss. Anaesthetists (and surgeons) should rotate to avoid exhaustion.
- **Fluid loss.** Be prepared for heavy blood and 'third space' losses. The combination of tissue injury, hypothermia and massive transfusion will cause profound coagulopathy. Expect to see a significant metabolic acidosis in patients with major injuries. This needs frequent monitoring (arterial blood gases) and correction with fluids and inotropes, as appropriate. Massive haemorrhage is treated with blood, FFP, platelets and cryoprecipitate guided by coagulation tests and clinical evidence of coagulopathy (Rossaint et al. 2010). Give tranexamic acid as early as possible and certainly within 3 hours of injury. Consider the use of recombinant factor VIIa if coagulopathy persists despite adequate treatment with other blood products.
- **Multiple surgical teams.** It is more efficient if surgical teams from different specialties are able to work simultaneously; however, this may severely restrict the space available to the anaesthetist!
- **Acute lung injury.** Trauma patients are at significant risk of hypoxia from acute lung injury. This may be secondary to direct pulmonary contusion or to fat embolism from orthopaedic injuries. Advanced ventilatory modes may be required to maintain appropriate oxygenation.

References and further reading

American College of Surgeons Committee on Trauma. *Advanced Trauma Life Support for Doctors. Student Course Manual.* Chicago, IL: American College of Surgeons, 2008.

Brain Trauma Foundation. Guidelines for the management of severe traumatic brain injury. 3rd Edition. *J Neurotrauma* 2007; **24**: S1–106.

Como JJ, Diaz JJ, Dunham CM, *et al.* Practice management guidelines for identification of cervical spine injuries following trauma: update from the Eastern Association for the Surgery of Trauma Practice Management Guidelines Committee. *J Trauma* 2009; **67**: 651–9.

Cook TM, Woodall N, Harper J, Benger J; Fourth National Audit Project. Major complications of airway management in the UK: results of the Fourth National Audit Project of the Royal College of Anaesthetists and the Difficult

Airway Society. Part 2: intensive care and emergency departments. *Br J Anaesth* 2011; **106**: 632–42.

Crewdson K, Nolan JP. Management of the trauma airway. *Trauma* 2011; **13**: 221–232.

Crosby ET. Airway management in adults after cervical spine trauma. *Anesthesiology* 2006; **104**: 1293–318.

National Institute for Health and Care Excellence. *Head Injury: Assessment and Early Management*. NICE Guideline CG176. London: NICE, 2014. www.nice.org.uk/guidance/cg176.

Rossaint R, Bouillon B, Cerny V, *et al.* Management of bleeding following major trauma: an updated European guideline. *Crit Care* 2010; **14**: R52.

Timmermann A. Supraglottic airways in difficult airway management: successes, failures, use and misuse. *Anaesthesia* 2011; **66** (Suppl 2): 45–56.

Xiao W, Mindrinos MN, Seok J, *et al.* A genomic storm in critically injured humans. *J Exp Med* 2011; **208**: 2581–90.

CHAPTER 10
Cellular physiology

Ted Lin

Organisation and control

The physiology of the body divides itself into different levels of functional organisation. Natural boundaries define three major levels, those of metabolism, cellular function and organ systems.

Control mechanisms direct physiological function towards the ultimate goal of homeostasis, using both negative and positive feedback mediated by the endocrine and nervous systems.

Homeostasis can be defined as maintenance of the composition and properties of both intracellular and extracellular fluid.

Cell functions

Cell functions can be divided into those which are intracellular and those which are extracellular.

Intracellular functions

Intracellular functions are highly dependent on the intracellular milieu, which is in turn determined by the composition and properties of the extracellular fluid.

> **Intracellular functions include:**
> - Maintaining the internal milieu
> - Reproducing DNA
> - Production of RNA
> - Repairing cell structures
> - Synthesis of substances for export
> - Metabolism of imported substances
> - Production of chemical energy
> - Cell motility

Extracellular functions

Extracellular functions involve interaction and communication with other cells. This interaction may occur via mechanical, chemical or electrical mechanisms.

> **Chemical messengers**
>
> The most common form of intercellular communication is via chemical messenger. Common groups of messengers are neurotransmitters, neurohormones, endocrine hormones and paracrine secretions.

Fundamentals of Anaesthesia, 4th edition, ed. Ted Lin, Tim Smith and Colin Pinnock. Published by Cambridge University Press. © Cambridge University Press 2017.

Cell interactions can result in different types of response. Cells interacting with other cells in the immediate vicinity can produce local homeostatic responses such as an inflammatory response triggered by tissue injury. Coordinated functioning of masses of similar cells can result in specialised tissue or visceral activity such as myocardial contraction or gut peristalsis. Finally, interaction may occur with remote cells, as occurs in the systemic effects of hormones or systemic responses of the immune system. Intercellular communication mechanisms are discussed in more detail below.

Local homeostatic responses

> **Local homeostatic responses** involve the secretion of chemical messengers by cells in the immediate vicinity of the target cell (paracrine secretion). Alternatively, messengers may be secreted by a cell to act on itself (autocrine secretion).

An example of such a local response is the inflammatory response in the case of injury, when local metabolites are released to increase blood flow to the injured tissues.

A group of paracrine agents commonly encountered is the eicosanoids, which are derivatives of arachidonic acid. These include prostaglandins, prostacyclin, leukotrienes and thromboxanes. These agents exert a wide spectrum of effects in many physiological processes including blood coagulation, smooth muscle contraction, pain mechanisms and local inflammatory responses.

Intracellular control

Control of intracellular processes is achieved by various molecular mechanisms. All of the above cellular functions are influenced by chemical messengers produced by the endocrine system (Figure 10.1), or produced locally as paracrine or autocrine secretions. Chemical messengers are received at the extracellular membrane surface by receptors and often activate secondary chemical messengers at the inner surface of the cell membrane, which mediate intracellular changes.

Organ systems and homeostatic control

Organ systems and their control mechanisms provide the macroscopic means of controlling homeostasis and interfacing the body with its external environment.

> ## Intracellular control mechanisms
>
> - Activation or inhibition of enzymes
> - Regulation of gene expression
> - Changes in membrane permeability
> - Regulation of membrane receptor activity
> - Changes in membrane potential

The traditionally described systems, such as the cardiovascular, respiratory and neurological systems, all exert their control over the body's physiology by well-recognised mechanisms.

Negative feedback systems

The most common homeostatic control mechanism is the negative feedback system. A negative feedback system operates to maintain a constant output parameter or steady state, even if the output parameter is disturbed by an applied stimulus. When the steady state is disturbed the system first detects the change in the output parameter. It then produces an opposite polarity signal (negative feedback signal) proportional to the output deviation, and feeds this signal back to the input of the system. This feedback signal changes the input, and thus acts to correct the output deviation (Figure 10.2).

The physiological parameter may be a variable such as mean arterial blood pressure, which rests normally at its operating point. When a change occurs in the blood pressure, the change is detected by a baroreceptor that relays a signal to an integrating centre (vasomotor centre of the medulla). The integrating centre then transmits a signal to an effector (vascular smooth muscle), which exerts a response to oppose the original change.

Positive feedback systems

Positive feedback systems are also used for physiological control, although in these cases the system is not used to control a specific physiological parameter, but rather to produce a systemic response directed towards maintaining homeostasis. In such a system there is no polarity change in the feedback signal, and thus, instead of opposing the detected physiological change, the feedback signal acts to increase the deviation. This produces a cascade effect that can be identified in certain physiological responses, such as the coagulation cascade during blood clot formation.

Figure 10.1 Hormone effects on cell metabolism

Hormone	Gland	Metabolic effects
Insulin	Beta cells in the islets of Langerhans	↑ glycolysis ↑ glycogen synthesis ↑ protein synthesis ↑ triacylglycerol synthesis ↑ fatty acid synthesis ↓ glycogenolysis ↓ ketone formation ↓ breakdown of triglycerides
Glucagon	Alpha cells in the islets of Langerhans	↑ glycogenolysis ↑ ketone formation ↑ gluconeogenesis
Adrenaline	Adrenal medulla	↑ glycogenolysis ↑ gluconeogenesis ↑ lipolysis
Cortisol	Adrenal cortex	↑ gluconeogenesis ↑ lipolysis ↑ protein catabolism ↓ DNA synthesis
Growth hormone	Anterior pituitary	↑ gluconeogenesis ↑ lipolysis
Thyroid hormone	Thyroid	*Normal concentrations* ↑ RNA synthesis ↑ protein synthesis *High concentrations* ↑ basal metabolic rate ↓ protein synthesis uncouples oxidative phosphorylation

Cell structure

Cellular function is reflected by cell structure. In broad terms, a cell consists of the cell plasma membrane, the cytosol, intracellular organelles and the nucleus.

Basic cell morphology

A basic cell is illustrated in Figure 10.3. The outer cell membrane surrounds various functional structures or organelles, the largest of which is the nucleus. The medium surrounding the nucleus is the cytoplasm.

Cytoplasm

'Cytoplasm' is used to describe all intracellular contents outside the nucleus. It consists of the cytosol and the organelles.

Cytosol

Cytosol refers to the intracelluar fluid containing proteins and electrolytes. Intracellular fluid forms 40% of body weight and possesses an electrolyte composition, which is discussed in Chapter 11.

Organelles

A summary of the organelles and their functions is shown in Figure 10.4.

Cytoskeleton

This system of microscopic fibres maintains the cell structure and enables cell movement to occur. Its main components are:

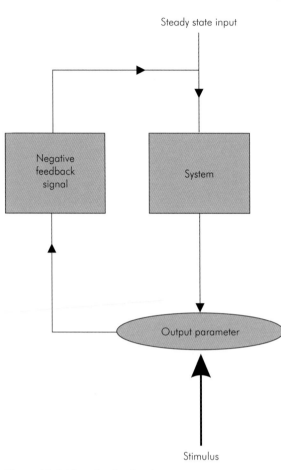

Figure 10.2 Negative feedback system

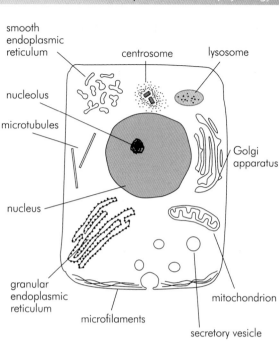

Figure 10.3 A basic cell

- Microtubules – 25 nm diameter structures with 5 nm thick walls. Tubule length is a dynamic balance between assembly (at the positive end) and disassembly (at the negative end) of protein subunits
- Muscle thick filaments – composed of myosin 15 nm in diameter
- Intermediate filaments – solid fibres about 10 nm in diameter
- Microfilaments – solid fibres about 5 nm in diameter made of polymerised actin

Cellular motion, shape changes and ciliary or flagellar movement all involve molecular motor mechanisms based on the action of ATPases. These form moving flexible cross-bridges between cytoskeletal components and membranes or organelles. The actin–myosin mechanism responsible for muscle contraction is a molecular motor mechanism that occurs universally in other cells. Other examples of molecular motors include dynamin and kinesin, which act on microtubules.

Mitochondria

These are sausage-shaped structures with outer and inner membranes. Their main function is to produce chemical energy in the form of ATP by oxidative phosphorylation. The inner membrane is folded to form cristae, which are studded with units containing the oxidative phosphorylating and ATP-synthesising enzymes (Figure 10.5). The matrix contains enzymes required to drive the citric acid cycle, which in turn provides the substrate for oxidative phosphorylation. Mitochondria also contain a small amount of DNA, which is solely of maternal origin.

Endoplasmic reticulum (ER)

This membranous structure is composed of complex folds and tubules. In its granular form, ribosomes are attached to the cytoplasmic surfaces and are the primary site for protein synthesis in the cell. Agranular ER is free from ribosomes and is the site of steroid synthesis and detoxification.

Figure 10.4 Intracellular organelles and their functions

Cytoskeleton	Maintains the structure of the cell
Membrane	Container for cell, nucleus and other organelles Structural support and control of environment on either side
Mitochondria	Energy source for the cell, generating ATP via oxidative phosphorylation
Nucleus	Contains the genetic material in the form of chromosomes The central site of cell division or mitosis Nucleolus synthesises ribosomes
Centrosome	Formation of mitotic spindle in cell division
Endoplasmic reticulum (ER)	Rough (granular) ER has ribosomes attached and is responsible for protein synthesis Smooth (agranular) ER is the site of steroid synthesis and detoxification
Ribosome	The actual site of protein synthesis in the ER, or may occur free in cytoplasm
Golgi apparatus	Processes proteins for secretion from cell
Lysosomes	Breakdown and elimination of intracellular debris or exogenous substances
Peroxisomes	Catalyse various anabolic and catabolic reactions, e.g. breakdown of long chain fatty acids
Cilia	Used by the cell to propel mucus or other substances over exposed mucosal surfaces

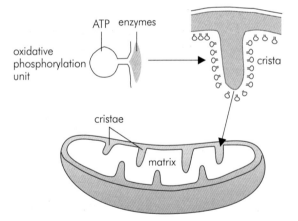

Figure 10.5 Mitochondrion structure

Ribosomes

Ribosomes are about 32 nm in diameter, with large and small subunits. They are composed of 65% RNA and 35% protein, and are the sites of protein synthesis. Free ribosomes exist in the cytoplasm and synthesise haemoglobin, peroxisomal and mitochondrial proteins.

Centrosome

This is composed of two centrioles at right angles to each other. The centrioles are cylindrical structures in which nine triplets of microtubules form the walls. A cylinder of pericentriolar material surrounds these structures. The whole structure is situated near the nucleus and is activated at the start of mitosis. Initially the centrioles replicate, and then the centriole pairs separate to form the mitotic spindle.

Golgi apparatus

This consists of flattened membranous sacs or cisterns that are stacked together to form a polarised structure with *cis* and *trans* ends, separated by a middle region. The Golgi apparatus prepares proteins for secretion (via exocytosis) by receiving the proteins from the ER at the *cis* side, coding them for destination and finally producing

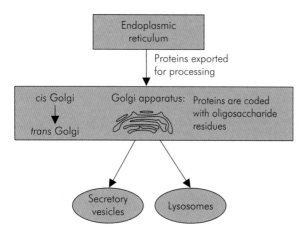

Figure 10.6 Golgi apparatus and protein processing

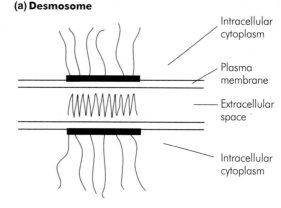

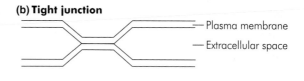

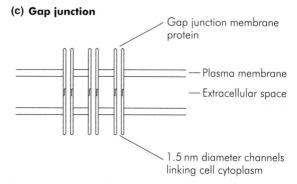

Figure 10.7 Intercellular junctions

secretory granules or vesicles at the *trans* side (Figure 10.6).

Intercellular junctions

The organisation of cells into tissues involves the formation of specialised junctions between the cells and the formation of an extracellular matrix surrounding the cells. Connective tissues such as bone and tendon are predominantly extracellular matrix with the cells anchored to the matrix rather than forming intercellular junctions. Epithelial tissues consist of layers of cells anchored to a basement membrane with little extracellular matrix, but dense specialised intercellular junctions determining the functions of the epithelium.

Some basic types of junction (Figure 10.7) are:

- Anchoring junctions – forming cell–cell adhesions and cell matrix adhesions, and providing anchorage for the cytoskeleton. These give the tissue mechanical stability.
- Occluding junctions – circumferential junctions that seal the extracellular space between epithelial cells, preventing the passage of molecules between cells.
- Channel-forming junctions – small channels (diameter 1.5 nm) that allow transfer of small ions and molecules between cells.
- Signal relaying junctions – allowing communication between cells.

Cilia

These projections on the luminal surface of epithelial cells are motile processes that move secretions and other substances across the surface of the cell. They are composed of nine pairs of microtubules arranged circumferentially around a central pair of microtubules. Each cilium is attached to a basal granule that has a structure similar to that of a centriole. Ciliary movement is produced by molecular motor mechanisms that cause the microtubules to slide relative to each other.

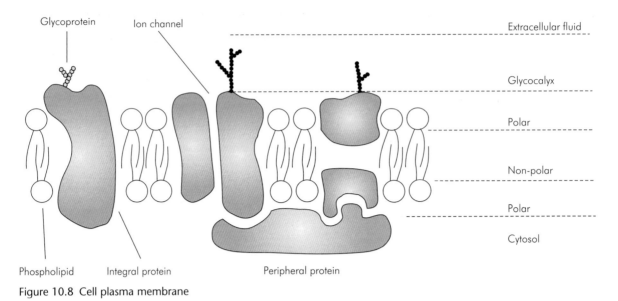

Figure 10.8 Cell plasma membrane

The cell membrane

> **Membranes** surround all cells and the majority of intracellular organelles. The cell membrane has a primary function of controlling the passage of substances across it to maintain the intracellular environment, which is an essential requirement for cellular metabolism. Controlling the movement of ions across the membrane also establishes ion concentration gradients and electrical potential differences (membrane potential) across the membrane, which enable cells to generate action potentials in excitable tissues.

Membrane functions

A summary of cell membrane functions is as follows:
- Regulation of the passage of substances across it for intracellular homeostasis
- Establishment of ion concentration gradients (K^+ and Na^+) and membrane potential
- Generation of action potentials
- Container for cell contents
- Anchorage for cytoskeleton
- Structural function for tissues acting as a site for intercellular connections
- Communication via chemical messengers
- Communication via action potentials

Membrane structure

Cell membranes are based on a double phospholipid layer structure. The phospholipid molecules are amphipathic, with one end charged and the other non-polar. The membrane is formed by a double layer of these amphipathic molecules with the polar ends orientated outwards. The double layer is interrupted by integral membrane protein molecules, which often span the membrane completely and are referred to as transmembrane proteins. Membrane proteins and lipids may possess polysaccharide chains attached to their extracellular surface, which appears as a fuzzy coat visible on electron microscopy, known as the glycocalyx (Figure 10.8).

Integral membrane proteins

Integral membrane proteins have various functions. Some form controllable channels for the passage of ions or water. Another group transmits chemical signals across the cell membrane by acting as active carriers. Cell adhesion molecules determine the cell's ability to attach to the extracellular matrix, basal membranes and other cells. Types of integral membrane proteins include:
- Ion channels
- Transport carriers
- Cell adhesion molecules
- G proteins
- Second messenger enzymes

Peripheral membrane proteins are located on the cytoplasmic membrane surface, where they are attached to polar regions of the integral membrane proteins. These peripheral proteins are associated with cell motility and shape.

Cell adhesion molecules (CAMs)

Cell adhesion molecules form a large group of membrane proteins with several subdivisions and a wide range of functions. Some of the processes cell adhesion molecules are involved in include:

- Transduction of signals controlling differentiation, gene expression and motility
- Programmed assembly of cells to form the complex architecture of individual tissues
- Morphogenesis of embryological tissues and organs
- Formation of intercellular connections in epithelial tissues
- Adhesion of leukocytes to vascular endothelium
- Enablement of leukocyte motility
- Directing of leukocyte migration in inflammation
- Platelet adhesion in blood coagulation
- Pathogenesis of airway inflammation in asthma
- Epithelial cell adhesion to basement membranes and the pathogenesis of bullous diseases

An outline of the different CAMs is summarised in Figure 10.9.

Cell adhesion molecules (CAMs) form the basis for cells to adhere either to other cells (cadherins) or to the extracellular matrix (integrins). CAM properties also include signal transduction and transmission. The scope of CAM function thus extends well beyond a simple structural role, and involves both normal and pathological processes.

G proteins

This group of membrane proteins has a high affinity for guanine nucleotides. Over 16 G proteins have been identified, composed of α, β and γ subunits, suggesting the existence of many more. Activation of the G protein enables it to bind guanosine triphosphate (GTP) and interact with an effector protein. The activated G protein then deactivates itself by intrinsic GTPase activity (Figure 10.10). This reduces the GTP to GDP, thus deactivating the G protein.

Activation of the G protein system can result in various effects. It can control the release of second messengers via Gs- and Gi-type proteins that have stimulatory or inhibitory effects on enzymes such as adenylyl cyclase. Some

Figure 10.9 Families of CAMs and their properties

Integrins	Platelet adhesion Expressed on leukocytes and bind to IgSF (endothelium) Leukocyte motility Cell-matrix adhesion
Selectins	Expressed on circulating leukocytes Stored in endothelial cells and allow rolling of leukocytes Stored in platelets Leukocyte–endothelial adhesion
Cadherins	Morphogenesis of tissues Metastasis of tumours Embryological development
Immunoglobulin superfamily (IgSF)	Expressed on endothelium and bind to integrins (leukocytes) Expressed on gut mucosa and bind integrins and selectins (lymphocytes)

G proteins are directly coupled to ion channels, and thus control membrane permeability to ions. Others can increase intracellular calcium concentrations and activate intracellular kinases.

G protein function

The heterogeneous nature of G proteins means that a first messenger common to several tissues can produce a spectrum of different cellular responses according to the tissue targeted. This variability is further increased by the fact that more than one G protein may be activated by a single receptor, and several effector proteins can be coupled to a single G protein.

Second messenger enzymes

The production of second messengers – cyclic adenosine monophosphate (cAMP), cyclic guanosine monophosphate (cGMP), inositol triphosphate and diacylglycerol – takes place at the cell membrane. The enzymes responsible for their production are adenylyl cyclase, guanylyl cyclase and tyrosine kinase. The activities of these enzymes are

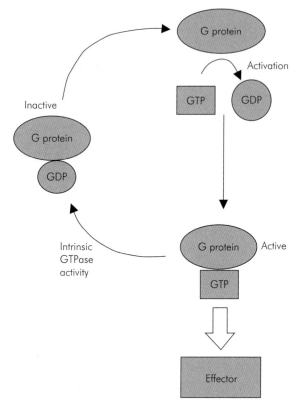

Figure 10.10 G protein activation and deactivation

and osmosis are passive and do not require the expenditure of energy. Active transport is mediated by integral membrane proteins and uses energy often in the form of ATP. Membrane transport mechanisms include:

- Diffusion
- Osmosis
- Ion channel diffusion
- Facilitated diffusion
- Primary active transport
- Secondary active transport
- Exo- and endocytosis

Diffusion

This describes the movement of solute molecules due to their random thermal motion. It is a passive process, and net movement of the solute occurs when a concentration gradient is present (from a high to a low concentration). Certain molecules can diffuse across the phospholipid bilayer areas of a cell membrane.

The rate of diffusion across the cell membrane:

- Increases with concentration gradient
- Increases with surface area
- Decreases with membrane thickness
- Increases with temperature
- Increases with lipid solubility
- Decreases with molecular weight
- Decreases with electrical charge of particle

A cell membrane acts as a diffusion barrier to solute molecules and can reduce their rates of diffusion by a factor of between 10^3 and 10^6, compared with free diffusion rates in water.

Osmosis

This term describes the net movement of water molecules due to diffusion between areas of different concentration. Pure water has a molar concentration of 55.5 M. In a solution, the addition of solute reduces the water concentration by replacing some water molecules with a solute molecule (or ion). Thus, a 1 M solution of glucose will have a reduced water concentration of 55.5 – 1 = 54.5 M.

Osmolarity

The concentration of a solution can be expressed in terms of its osmolarity, reflecting the osmotic effect of the solute particles. The osmolarity of the 1 M glucose solution is thus 1 osmole per litre (1 Osm L^{-1}).L^{-1}.

controlled by various pathways, which involve both activation and inhibition. Second messenger effects are multiple and widespread intracellularly.

Membrane transport of substances

Cell membranes control the movement of a wide range of particles and substances between the intra- and extracellular spaces. These include gases, ions, water, proteins and intracellular granules or debris. Different components of the membrane are associated with different mechanisms of transport. The phospholipid bilayer areas of the membrane allow diffusion of water, small molecules and lipid-soluble substances. Transmembrane proteins provide active mechanisms for transport and allow ion diffusion via channels. Examples of substances transported across membranes are shown in Figure 10.11.

Membrane transport mechanisms

Various mechanisms exist for the transport of substances across the cell membrane. Mechanisms such as diffusion

Figure 10.11 Examples of substances transported across membranes

Substance	Size (nm)	Site	Mechanism
Water	0.13	Lipid bilayer	Osmosis
Oxygen	0.12	Lipid bilayer	Diffusion
Nitrogen	0.12	Lipid bilayer	Diffusion
Carbon dioxide	0.12	Lipid bilayer	Diffusion
Sodium ions	0.19	Lipid bilayer	Ion diffusion
		ATPase pump	Active transport
Potassium ions	0.23	Ion channel	Ion diffusion
		ATPase pump	Active transport
Calcium ions	0.17	Ion channel	Ion diffusion
		ATPase pump	Active transport
Urea	0.23	Lipid bilayer	Diffusion
Steroids	< 1.0	Lipid bilayer	Diffusion
Fatty acid	< 1.0	Lipid bilayer	Diffusion
Glucose	0.38	Transport proteins	Facilitated diffusion
Proteins	> 7.5	Vesicles	Exocytosis Endocytosis

Osmotic pressure

A concentration gradient of water can be produced between two compartments separated by a semipermeable membrane, such as a cell membrane, which is permeable to water but impermeable to solute. In this case, net diffusion of water molecules will occur from the compartment with the lower concentration of solute (higher concentration of water) across the membrane into the higher solute concentration (lower concentration of water). The movement of water into a compartment due to osmosis will have the physical effects of increasing the volume of the compartment and/or increasing the pressure in the compartment. This movement of water can be opposed by an increase in pressure in the compartment.

> The **osmotic pressure of a solution** contained by a semipermeable partition is the pressure required to oppose the net movement of water into that solution. This is a property of the solution dependent on its osmolarity (Figure 10.12).

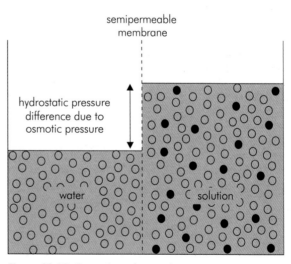

Figure 10.12 Osmosis and osmotic pressure

Tonicity

In a cell, changes in volume can be produced according to the osmolarity of the intra- and extracellular fluids. Net movement of water into the cell occurs when the cell is placed in a solution of lower osmolarity (hypotonic), giving rise to swelling and ultimately cell disruption or haemolysis. Placing a cell in a solution of higher osmolarity than the intracellular contents (hypertonic) causes shrinking. Normal extracellular fluid has an osmolarity of 300 mOsm L^{-1}, which is equal to that of the intracellular fluid (isotonic). Since intra- and extracellular solute concentrations are maintained by the cell membrane permeability properties, no net movement of water occurs into or out of cells and they remain in equilibrium. Hyperosmotic, hypo-osmotic and iso-osmotic describe solution osmolarity irrespective of the membrane permeability to the solute contained. Thus, the tonicity of such a solution may not correspond to its osmolarity.

Tonicity refers to the ability of the solution to cause swelling or shrinkage of cells placed in it. It will depend on the solution osmolarity and the cell membrane permeability to solute particles in the solution.

Ion diffusion

Although the phospholipid bilayer portions of the cell membrane are impermeable to ions, ion channels formed by transmembrane proteins render the cell membrane selectively permeable to Na^+, K^+, Ca^{2+} and Cl^-. The walls of these channels are formed by polypeptide subunits, which may number up to 12 per channel (Figure 10.13). Rapid changes in ion concentrations (such as in the production of action potentials) are produced by opening and closing the channels (gating) and consequently producing dramatic changes in permeability to a given ion. The gating of ion channels may be controlled by chemical messengers binding to the subunits (ligand gating, e.g. acetylcholine receptors), changes in membrane potential (voltage gating, e.g. Na^+ channel) and stretching of the membrane (mechanical gating).

Factors determining permeability of a cell membrane to a given ion are:

- Chemical messenger concentration
- Membrane potential
- Membrane conformation
- Density of specific ion channels

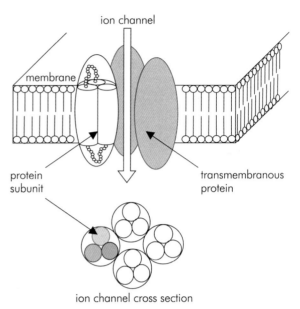

Figure 10.13 Ion channel

Active transport

Active transport is mediated by integral membrane proteins or carriers that bind a substance on one side of the membrane, undergo a conformational change, and then release the substance on the opposite side of the membrane. Carriers may be specific for a given substance (uniport), or they may transport a combination of substances (symport), or finally they may exchange one substance for another (antiport). Factors affecting rate of active transport include:

- Degree of carrier saturation
- Density of carriers on membrane
- The speed of carrier conformational change

Primary active transport

Active transport requires the expenditure of energy, since it usually moves substances against a concentration or electrical potential gradient (i.e. against an electrochemical gradient). In primary active transport, energy is obtained directly from the hydrolysis of ATP and then catalysed by the carrier, which binds the released phosphate (Figure 10.14). Phosphorylation of the carrier produces covalent modulation of its structure. $Na^+K^+ATPase$ is an antiport carrier responsible for maintaining transmembrane ion gradients of Na^+ and K^+. This carrier

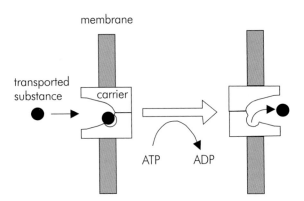

Figure 10.14 Primary active transport

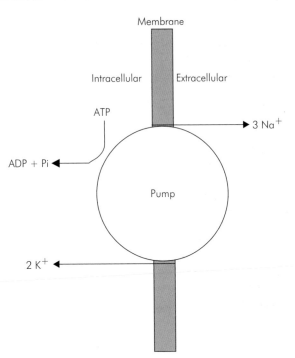

Figure 10.15 Na⁺K⁺ pump

'pumps' three Na^+ ions out of the cell in exchange for two potassium ions (Figure 10.15), both against their respective concentration gradients. Other ion pumps (uniport systems) move calcium (Ca^{2+}ATPase) and hydrogen ions (H^+ATPase) across cell and organelle membranes against electrochemical gradients.

Secondary active transport

In this process a symport carrier transports a substance and an ion (usually Na^+) together. The carrier possesses two binding sites, one for the substance and one for the ion. The substance binds to the first carrier site. The change in carrier conformation required to release the substance on the opposite side of the membrane is then powered by the ion binding to the second site, which produces allosteric modulation of the carrier structure. Since the ion always passes from high to low concentrations, there is no direct energy input required, and the energy for this secondary transport process is ultimately derived from the energy required to maintain the ion concentration gradient. The transported substance can travel in the same direction as the ion (co-transport) or in the opposite direction (counter-transport). An example of such a system is the transport of glucose and Na^+ in the gut (Figure 10.16).

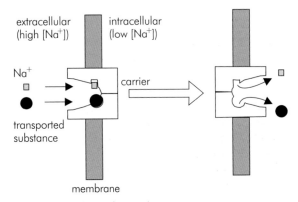

Figure 10.16 Secondary active transport

Facilitated diffusion

This is a misnomer, since no diffusive process is involved. Facilitated diffusion describes the transport of a substance from a high to low concentration via a carrier. No energy coupling is required for this process, since movement occurs down the concentration gradient. However, diffusion is not involved, and thus the transport kinetics are characteristic of carrier-mediated transport (Figure 10.17) and carrier saturation occurs. An example of this process is the transport of glucose into the cell, which occurs via a set of four different carriers.

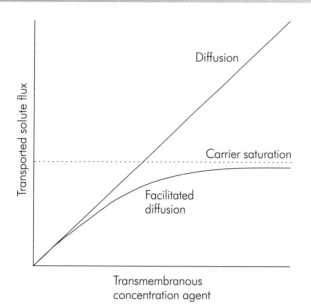

Figure 10.17 Facilitated diffusion and carrier kinetics

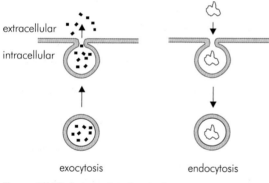

Figure 10.18 Exo- and endocytosis

Exo- and endocytosis

This mode of transport does not require substances to pass through the membrane structure, but transports substances contained in membrane-covered vesicles. In endocytosis, extracellular material is absorbed by being packaged into vesicles at the cell membrane. The vesicles are formed by invagination of the membrane. An equivalent process in reverse is exocytosis, which allows the cell to export intracellular substances or debris (Figure 10.18).

Cell nucleus

Nucleus and nucleolus

Most cells in the body carry a single nucleus (exceptions are skeletal muscle cells, which are multinucleate, and red blood cells, which are anucleate). The nucleus is surrounded by a double membrane – the nuclear envelope. This envelope is interrupted at intervals by openings – the nuclear pores – that allow the passage of specific proteins into and out of the nucleus.

Genetic material is contained as a DNA–protein complex and forms the bulk of the nuclear contents. In addition, there is a dense patch of granules visible under light microscopy known as the nucleolus. The nucleolus is rich in RNA; it synthesises the ribosomal subunits for export to the cytoplasm, where the complete ribosomes are assembled and act as sites for protein synthesis.

Nucleic acids

Nucleic acids are nucleotide polymers. Each nucleotide consists of a purine or pyrimidine base, a sugar (deoxyribose or ribose) and a phosphate group. The DNA molecule is a double helix, each component helix being a chain of nucleotides. DNA nucleotides contain deoxyribose sugar combined with one of the following bases: adenine (A), guanine (G), cytosine (C) and thymine (T). The deoxyribose molecules are linked by phosphate bonds to form the backbone of each spiral, and the spirals are linked via the protruding bases to form the DNA double helix (Figure 10.19).

Genetic information is coded linearly along the double helix structure by the sequence of the base pairs. The alphabet for this genetic code is formed by triplets of bases, each triplet coding for an amino acid, e.g. the triplet sequence cytosine–guanine–thymine (CGT) codes for the amino acid alanine. Figure 10.20 shows the DNA coding for a small polypeptide.

RNA is a single-stranded nucleotide polymer that differs from DNA in function and structure (Figure 10.21). Three types of RNA are recognised: messenger (mRNA), transfer (tRNA) and ribosomal (rRNA). They are all synthesised in the nucleus using DNA as a template, but differ from each other in molecular size and function. The bulk of cellular RNA is rRNA, which together with specific proteins forms the ribosomal subunits. The large and small ribosomal subunits are two thirds rRNA and a third ribosomal proteins.

Nucleic acids

The most important substances in the nucleus are the nucleic acids deoxyribonucleic acid (DNA) and ribonucleic acid (RNA).

- The DNA acts as a store of coded information for the synthesis of proteins.
- RNA acts as a mobile template to transcribe specific sequences from the DNA and transport these to the cytoplasm for protein synthesis.

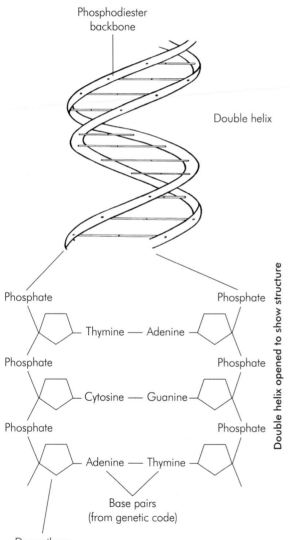

Phosphodiester backbone

Double helix

Phosphate

Phosphate

Thymine —— Adenine

Phosphate

Phosphate

Cytosine —— Guanine

Phosphate

Phosphate

Adenine —— Thymine

Double helix opened to show structure

Base pairs
(from genetic code)

Deoxyribose

Figure 10.19 Double helix of DNA

The human genome

The total genetic material in the nucleus forms a blueprint for the individual and is referred to as the genome. The genetic information is coded into giant molecules of DNA. These DNA molecules form large complexes with proteins, which appear as clumps of stained material, chromatin, under light microscopy. During cell division the chromatin forms paired bodies in the nucleus known as chromosomes. The human genome is contained in 46 chromosomes (23 pairs), each chromosome consisting of a single DNA molecule–protein complex. The genetic coding responsible for producing a single polypeptide is known as a gene, which represents a unit of hereditary information. There are between 50,000 and 100,000 genes in the human genome, containing 3×10^9 base pairs.

Cell division

Two forms of cell division occur in the body, mitosis and meiosis.

Mitosis is the division of the parent cell to produce two daughter cells which are identical with the parent cell. Each daughter cell possesses the same number of chromosomes ($n = 46$). The mitotic process starts with nuclear division and ends with cytokinesis or splitting of the nucleated daughter cells from each other. The sequence of events in nuclear division is described in the following stages:

Prophase – separation of centrioles and chromosome formation

Prometaphase – nuclear membrane and nucleolus disintegrate

Metaphase – chromosomes line up on cell equator

Anaphase – chromatids separate

Telophase – chromosomes, nuclear membranes and nucleoli reform. Cytokinesis begins

Meiosis is the division of a parent cell to produce four daughter gametes each of which is haploid, possessing half the number of chromosomes of the parent ($n = 23$). In many ways meiosis is similar to mitosis, but it is more complicated due to the extra replication of chromosomes and division of cells required to produce four gametes from a single parent cell

Protein synthesis

The process of synthesising proteins from the genetic information coded on DNA in the nucleus is outlined in Figure 10.22. Transcription describes the first stage, in which mRNA is synthesised by RNA polymerase bound

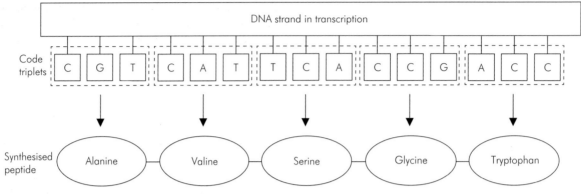

Figure 10.20 DNA coding for a peptide

Figure 10.21 Properties of DNA and RNA

	DNA	**mRNA**	**tRNA**	**rRNA**
Structure	Double helix	Single strand	Single strand	Single strand
Nucleotide sugar	Deoxyribose	Ribose	Ribose	Ribose
Purines	Adenine	Adenine	Adenine	Adenine
	Guanine	Guanine	Guanine	Guanine
Pyrimidines	Cytosine	Cytosine	Cytosine	Cytosine
	Thymine	Uracil	Uracil	Uracil
Number of bases in a molecule	$< 10^5$	$< 10^3$	80	
Function	Stores amino acid sequences for protein synthesis	Transfers amino acid sequence as codons from DNA to ribosomes	Links amino acids to mRNA codons	Forms structure of ribosomes and catalyses peptide bond formation

to the gene for the protein being synthesised. The mRNA then undergoes post-transcriptional processing. The processed RNA passes from the nucleus into the cytoplasm, where one end binds to the surface of a ribosome. Free amino acids are concentrated around the ribosomal surface, where they are loaded onto tRNA by aminoacyl-tRNA synthetase.

The surface-bound region of the mRNA is the site where the polypeptide is gradually elongated by the addition of amino acids in sequence. It provides two adjacent codons that recognise and bind tRNA by the corresponding anticodon. The first codon binds tRNA carrying the incomplete peptide chain. The adjacent site binds tRNA carrying the next amino acid in the sequence, which is then added to the chain. The addition of each new amino acid is then completed by a shift of the active region along the mRNA strand by one codon. The cycle can then be repeated to add the next amino acid to the peptide.

Control of protein synthesis

Genes possess different regions, of which only the exons are transcribed to produce mRNA for protein synthesis (Figure 10.23). At any given time, only a fraction of the genes in a cell are being transcribed. Control of the transcription process in each gene is exerted via a promoter region to which RNA polymerase binds before commencing transcription. Control of protein synthesis is exerted via transcription factors that allow RNA polymerase to bind to the promoter site and to commence transcription. These controlling factors may originate from within the same cell, or originate from other cells via the extracellular fluid. A single transcription factor may control transcription for several genes.

Control of the rate of protein synthesis may also be exerted at the translation stage and by controlling the breakdown of mRNA in the cytoplasm.

Cell communication

Intercellular communication is the basic machinery through which homeostatic control is applied. Cells almost always use a chemical messenger to communicate with target cells, which may be local or remote in location. One group of chemical messengers is formed by the neurotransmitters, which are secreted by one neurone to target a neighbouring neurone just a synapse away. On the other hand, a hormone travels in the circulation

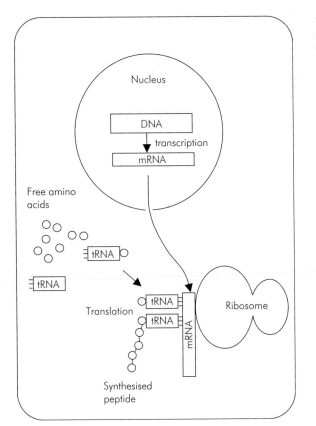

Figure 10.22 Protein synthesis

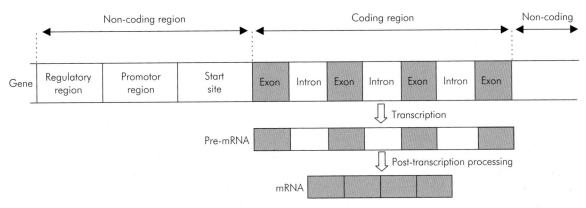

Figure 10.23 Gene regions

to target multiple tissues remote from the secreting cells. In general terms, chemical messengers (ligands) are usually received by cell-membrane proteins (receptors), and this interaction triggers the required cellular response by various mechanisms.

Chemical messengers

> **First chemical messengers** reach target cells in the extracellular fluid, whether via the circulation or through the interstitium. The action of a first chemical messenger often results in the intracellular release of an active ligand, which is termed a **second messenger**.

Various groups of first messengers are recognised, such as neurotransmitters, neuromuscular transmitters, hormones, paracrine agents and autocrine agents. These are differentiated by their origin, the route travelled by the messengers and the cells targeted. Some examples are shown in Figure 10.24.

All chemical messengers or ligands interact with their target cells by binding to receptors, and they therefore have common properties that determine their performance.

Properties of a ligand

Ligands show the following properties:

- Affinity – strength of binding with the receptor
- Competition – ability of different ligands to bind to the same receptor
- Agonist activity – ability of a ligand to trigger the cell response
- Antagonist activity – ability of a ligand to bind to a receptor without triggering the cell response, i.e. to block the receptor
- Half-life – time taken for ligand to be metabolised to half its concentration
- Lipid solubility – lipid-insoluble ligands activate receptors at the membrane surface; lipid-soluble ligands activate intracellular or intranuclear receptors

Receptors

'Receptor' refers to the region of a protein molecule that provides a binding site for a ligand. Receptors are usually situated on integral membrane proteins, and are activated

Figure 10.24 Types of first chemical messenger and their target cells

Messenger	Origin	Route	Target cell
Neurotransmitters • noradrenaline • acetylcholine serotonin	Neurone	Synapse	Adjacent neurone
Hormones • thyroxine • insulin • cortisol	Gland	Circulation	Multiple tissues
Neurohormones • vasopressin • oxytocin • ACTH • TSH	Neurone	Circulation	Multiple tissues Endocrine glands
Neuromuscular transmitter • acetylcholine	Neurone	Circulation	Muscle cell
Paracrine agents • eicosanoids • cytokines	Local cell	Extracellular fluid	Neighbouring cells
Autocrine agent • eicosanoids • cytokines	Local cell	Extracellular fluid	Cell of origin

by lipid-insoluble messengers at the membrane surface. Lipid-soluble messengers may cross the membrane to activate intracellular receptors. Receptors are not fixed components of the membrane, but are free to change position and to alter in population density.

Receptor properties
The properties of receptors are:
- Specificity – selectivity of a receptor, determining how specifically it binds to a single ligand
- Saturation – percentage of receptors already occupied by a ligand
- Down-regulation – a decrease in the number of receptors available for a given ligand
- Up-regulation – an increase in the number of available receptors for a given ligand
- Sensitivity – responsiveness of a target cell to a given ligand, dependent on the density of receptors
- Supersensitivity – increased sensitivity of a cell as a result of up-regulation

Binding site modulation
The first stage in transduction is the production of a change in shape or modulation of the binding site, when the ligand binds to the receptor. There are two main mechanisms by which this occurs, allosteric modulation and covalent modulation (Figure 10.25).

Allosteric modulation
In this case the receptor possesses two binding sites, one (the functional site) for the ligand and the other (the regulatory site) for a modulator molecule. Binding of the modulator molecule enables ligand binding to occur at the functional site.

Covalent modulation
This form of modulation requires the attachment of a phosphate group to the receptor (phosphorylation) to enable the functional site to bind the ligand.

Membrane signal transduction
When a ligand binds to a receptor, modulation sets off a sequence of events which can be thought of as transduction of a chemical signal received by the cell. Signal transduction ultimately results in alterations in cell function. These changes can affect:
- Membrane permeability
- Membrane potential
- Membrane transport
- Contractile activity
- Secretory activity
- Protein synthesis

Different mechanisms are activated following modulation of the receptor protein.

Membrane signal transduction mechanisms
- Receptors act as ion channels that are opened or closed by ligand binding (Figure 10.26).

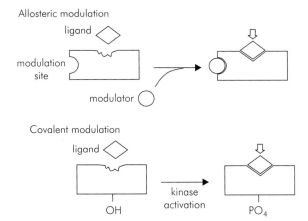

Figure 10.25 Allosteric and covalent modulation

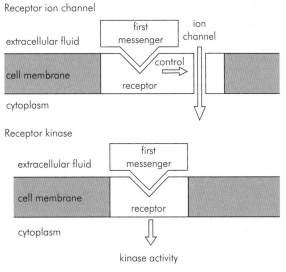

Figure 10.26 Signal transduction mechanisms

G protein ion channel

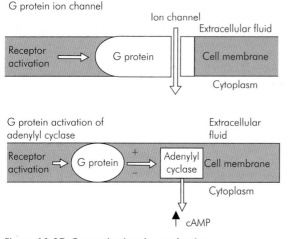

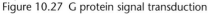

G protein activation of adenylyl cyclase

Figure 10.27 G protein signal transduction

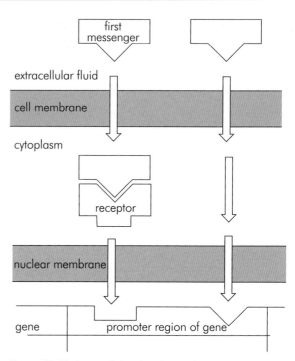

Figure 10.28 Intracellular signal transduction

- Receptors function as protein kinases that are activated on ligand binding (Figure 10.26).
- Receptors activate G proteins, which then mediate further actions. These include gating ion channels or releasing second messengers intracellularly (Figure 10.27).

Intracellular transduction

Lipophilic first messengers, such as steroids, can cross the phospholipid bilayer and activate intracellular receptors in the following ways (Figure 10.28):

- Ligand crosses cell membrane to form complex with cytosol receptor. This complex moves into nucleus and binds to promoter region of gene.
- Ligand moves across cell and nuclear membranes to form complex with nuclear receptor. This complex binds to promoter region of gene.

Second chemical messengers

This term refers to substances released intracellularly, following G protein activation of effector proteins (enzymes such as adenylyl cyclase and guanylyl cyclase). The second messengers released diffuse through the cytosol and exert wide-ranging effects, usually by activation of a protein kinase (Figure 10.29). The kinase in turn activates or inhibits a range of cellular functions by enzyme phosphorylation. This sequence of events can be thought of as a cascade triggered by a single messenger. The cascade effectively amplifies and processes the effect of

low concentrations of a ligand to produce widespread cellular changes, tailored to the needs of different tissues.

The second messengers cAMP and cGMP are metabolised by phosphodiesterase, which can be inhibited by methylxanthines (caffeine, theophylline). These compounds thus augment the second messenger effects.

Intracellular calcium

The extracellular-to-cytosol concentration gradient of calcium is $> 10^4$. Thus calcium enters the cytosol readily via calcium channels that are controlled by ligand or voltage gating. Alternatively, calcium can be released internally from the endoplasmic reticulum, which acts as a store. Active decrease of intracellular calcium levels is mediated by a $Ca^{2+}H^+ATPase$, a Na^+Ca^{2+} antiport system and reuptake into the endoplasmic reticulum.

Calcium exerts wide-ranging effects intracellularly by binding to a group of proteins including calmodulin, troponin and calbindin.

Calmodulin is one of the most prominent of these proteins, with wide-ranging activation of protein kinases involved in many aspects of cellular function (Figure 10.30).

Figure 10.29 Second messengers and their functions

Second messenger	Precursor or origin	Mediator	Examples of cell functions influenced
Cyclic AMP (cAMP)	ATP	Adenylyl cyclase	Protein synthesis Calcium ion transport DNA synthesis RNA synthesis Lipid breakdown Glycogen breakdown Glycogen synthesis Ion channels Active transport
Cyclic GMP (cGMP)	GTP	Guanylyl cyclase	Physiology of vision
Inositol triphosphate (IP$_3$)	Phosphotidyl inositol diphosphate (PIP$_2$)	Phospholipase C	Release of calcium from endoplasmic reticulum
Diacylglycerol (DAG)	Phosphatidyl inositol diphosphate (PIP$_2$)	Phospholipase C	Activation of protein kinase C used in membrane protein regulation
Calcium	Entry via calcium channels	G proteins	Activation of protein kinases via calmodulin or directly
	Release from endoplasmic reticulum	G proteins	Skeletal, smooth and cardiac muscle contraction
			Synaptic function
			Protein synthesis

Ageing

> **Ageing** is a physiological process that involves general changes in the body systems that are distinct from the pathological changes associated with disease. The changes usually reflect a decline in function.

The changes occurring in ageing are illustrated in Figure 10.31, which shows parameters in relation to those of an equivalent young adult. Functional deterioration occurs in all of the physiological systems, including those shown in Figure 10.32.

Ageing and dyshomeostasis

The deterioration normally associated with the ageing process leads to a reduction in the effectiveness of homeostatic control mechanisms, or dyshomeostasis. This contributes to an increased prevalence of certain conditions with age. These include:

- Dehydration
- Hypokalaemia
- Hyponatraemia
- Ankle oedema
- Diabetes mellitus
- Hypothyroidism
- Hypothermia

Theories of ageing

> Three theories on the origins of ageing have been put forward: wear and tear, adaptive evolution and non-adaptive evolution.

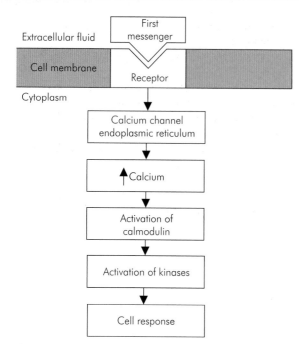

Figure 10.30 Calcium as a second messenger

Figure 10.31 Changes in physiological parameters due to ageing

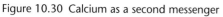

Parameter for a 70-year-old male	% of young adult value
Muscle mass	74
Total body water	87
Cardiac output at rest	64
Cardiac reserve	50
PaO$_2$	90
Oxygen consumption at rest	74
Maximal oxygen consumption	65
Renal blood flow	60
Max urine concentration	64
Cerebral blood flow	80

Figure 10.32 Effects of ageing on physiological systems

System	Change due to ageing
Cardiovascular	↓ cardiac output and reserve ↓ heart rate ↓ stroke volume ↓ LV compliance
Respiratory	↓ PaO$_2$ ↓ lung elasticity ↓ chest wall compliance ↓ vital capacity ↑ residual volume
Gastrointestinal	↓ sense of smell and taste ↓ coordination of swallowing and peristaltic reflexes ↓ gastric and pancreatic secretion ↓ large bowel motility
Endocrine	↑ noradrenaline levels ↓ renin and aldosterone levels ↓ carbohydrate tolerance ↑ vasopressin levels ↓ oestrogen in female ↓ testosterone in male
Renal	↓ kidney mass ↓ ability to concentrate urine ↓ renal response to vasopressin ↑ prostate mass
CNS	↓ brain mass ↓ acetylcholine activity ↓ cerebral blood flow ↓ short-term memory and learning ability ↑ reaction time
Musculoskeletal	↓ bone and muscle mass ↓ muscle effectiveness
Immunity	↓ cellular and humoral immunity

Wear and tear

This states that the ageing process is a natural deterioration as a result of the continuous functioning of a highly complex organism.

Adaptive evolution

Adaptive evolution suggests that ageing is a genetically programmed termination of life in the interests of evolutionary selection.

Non-adaptive evolution

Non-adaptive evolution suggests that the ageing process has evolved as an optimum balance between the limited energy sources available to the organism and the demands of normal function and repair.

Several cellular mechanisms are associated with ageing. It is unclear at present whether any of these predominate in determining the rate and extent of the process. The more important processes are:

- Accumulation of cells with random DNA mutations
- Increased cross-linking of collagens and proteins by glycosylation
- Accumulation of cytoplasmic lipofuscin granules
- Accumulation of oxidant radicals
- Genetic clock determining the number of cell reduplications
- Pleiotropic genes with 'good' effects early in life and 'bad' effects later in life

In general, it remains fair to say that the ageing process is incompletely understood at present.

CHAPTER 11
Body fluids

Mahesh Chaudhari

Fluid compartment volumes

Total body water (TBW)

In a young adult male, water accounts for about 60% of body weight. This percentage varies with build, sex and age in the following manner:

- TBW in the adult can range from 45% to 75% of body weight. This large variation is the result of individual differences in adipose tissue, which contains relatively little water.
- In the young adult female TBW only forms about 50% of body weight. This difference between the sexes develops during puberty and is due to the higher proportion of adipose tissue in females.
- TBW as a proportion of body weight may be as high as 80% in the neonate.

TBW is divided into several fluid compartments (Figure 11.1), the main division being between intracellular fluid (ICF) and extracellular fluid (ECF).

The variations of TBW (% body weight) and ECF (% body weight) with age are shown in Figure 11.2.

- In the young adult male **total body water** (TBW) forms approximately 60% of body weight.
- In the young adult female TBW forms approximately 50% of body weight.
- In the elderly TBW may decrease to 45% of body weight.
- In the neonate TBW may be 80% of body weight.

Intracellular fluid (ICF)

The ICF compartment contains approximately 66% of TBW, equivalent to 40% of body weight. The water content and composition of ICF varies according to the function of the tissue. Water moves freely across, but the cell membrane is only selectively permeable to the ions. Water movement across the cell membrane helps to maintain osmolalities of ICF and ECF at equilibrium.

Fundamentals of Anaesthesia, 4th edition, ed. Ted Lin, Tim Smith and Colin Pinnock. Published by Cambridge University Press. © Cambridge University Press 2017.

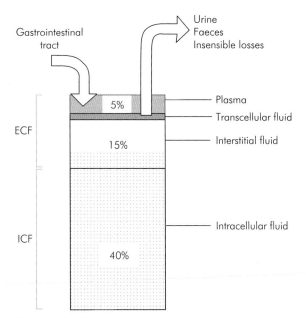

Figure 11.1 Body fluid compartments as percentage of body weight

Figure 11.2 Variation of TBW and ECF with age

Age	TBW (% body weight)	ECF (% body weight)
Neonate	80	45
6 months	70	35
1 year	60	28
5 years	65	25
Young adult	60	22
Elderly	50	20

Extracellular fluid (ECF)

Extracellular fluid is about one-third of total body water (or 20% of body weight). Approximately 25% of ECF is in the vascular system and the remainder (75%) is interstitial fluid. Although ECF as a percentage of body weight varies with age (Figure 11.2), when expressed as an index of body surface area it remains relatively constant throughout life. ECF is composed of several components (Figure 11.3).

Figure 11.3 Components of ECF in a 70 kg adult

Fluid	% body weight	Volume (litres)
Interstitial fluid	15	10.5
Plasma	5	3.5
Transcellular fluid	1	0.7
Total ECF	21	14.7

Capillary endothelium is permeable to water, ions, and soluble substances such as urea and glucose, but impermeable to proteins. Therefore, the solute composition of plasma and interstitial fluid is similar except for the protein content. Because of the higher concentration of protein in the plasma, electrical neutrality across the two compartments is maintained by a slightly higher concentration of Cl^- in interstitial fluid.

> ### ICF and ECF
>
> - ICF forms approximately two-thirds of TBW.
> - ECF forms approximately one-third of TBW.
> - 25% of ECF is intravascular.

Plasma

Plasma volume equates to the intravascular component of ECF and amounts to about 5% body weight. The total blood volume is composed of plasma and the red blood cell volume. Plasma volume (V_{PL}) can be measured using a dilution technique. The fractional red blood cell volume is readily available as the haematocrit (%). Given these values, the total blood volume (V_{BL}) can be calculated:

$$V_{PL} = 3.5 \text{ litres}$$
$$\text{Haematocrit (Hct)} = 45\%$$
$$\text{Total blood volume } (V_{BL}) = \frac{V_{PL} \times 100}{(100 - \text{Hct})}$$
$$= 6.4 \text{ litres}$$

Transcellular fluid

The transcellular fluid compartment is composed of fluids that have been secreted but are separated from the plasma by an epithelial layer. These include:

- Cerebrospinal fluid
- Intraocular fluid
- Gastrointestinal fluid
- Bile
- Pleural, peritoneal and pericardial fluid
- Sweat

The composition of transcellular fluid differs from both plasma and interstitial fluid, since it is controlled by the secretory cells.

Measurement of fluid compartment volumes

Compartment volumes are estimated by radioactive dilutional techniques. In these methods, an indicator dye that is freely distributed (but contained) within the compartment being estimated is injected into the compartment. The mass of indicator used and the concentration in the fluid are measured. Then the size of the compartment can be determined using the formula:

$$\text{Volume of compartment} = \frac{\text{Mass of indicator}}{\text{Concentration in compartment}}$$

Indicator methods used to estimate the volume of various compartments are summarised in Figure 11.4.

Solutions and semipermeable membranes

Concentration of a solution

The concentration of a solution is usually expressed in terms of the amount of solute present in a given amount of solvent. In the body, concentrations can be varied in fluid compartments by the movement of solute or solvent (water) into a compartment. The concentrations of various substances can be critical for normal function (e.g. extracellular potassium). Several units are used to express concentration, and the following definitions should be noted.

Amount of solute

A given amount of any substance can simply be measured by its mass. In chemical reactions, activity of a substance is related to the number of molecules present, and it is more useful to use a unit of mass that relates to the number of molecules present, the **mole** (symbol = mol), rather than a unit of absolute mass such as the kilogram.

> **One mole** of a substance is defined as the mass of substance containing 6.022×10^{23} (Avogadro constant) molecules.

Figure 11.4 Measurement of fluid compartment volumes

Compartment	Indicator	Comments
Total body water (TBW)	Antipyrine D_2O	Tendency to underestimate uniform distribution
Extracellular fluid (ECF)	Radioisotopes of Na^+, Br^-, Cl^-	These enter cells and so overestimate
	Saccharides (mannitol, inulin)	Incomplete distribution and so underestimate
Plasma volume (V_{PL})	Radioisotope ^{131}I albumin	Total blood volume (V_{BL}) may be derived from V_{PL} and haematocrit (Hct)
Red cell volume (V_{RBC})	Red cells tagged with radioisotope ^{51}Cr	Measures fraction of red blood cells tagged to determine V_{RBC}
		Measures concentration of tagged cells to determine V_{BL}
Intracellular fluid (ICF)		Derived from: ICF = TBW − ECF
Interstitial fluid volume (V_{INT})		Derived from: V_{INT} = ECF − V_{PL}

> The **Avogadro constant** is defined as the number of atoms in 12 grams of pure carbon-12 (^{12}C). It has a value of $6.02214129 \times 10^{23}$.

Chemical and electrochemical activity of a solution

The effects exerted by a solution are related to concentration. This is most commonly expressed as mass per unit volume (mg mL^{-1}, g L^{-1}, kg m^{-3}). However, the chemical and electrochemical activity of a solution is more closely related to the number of molecules present in a given amount of solution. Concentration of a solution is thus better expressed in terms of its molarity or its molality.

> - **Molarity** – moles of solute per litre of solution (solute plus water) (mol L^{-1})
> - **Molality** – moles of solute per kilogram of solvent (water) (mol kg^{-1} H$_2$O)

Equivalent weight

Chemical reactions between elements occur with fixed proportions of different elements by weight.

> - A **gram equivalent weight** can be defined for each element. This is the weight of an element that reacts with 8.000 g O$_2$.
> - An **electrical equivalent weight** can also be defined for an ion, which is equal to the atomic weight divided by its valency.

Thus, the electrical equivalent weight of Na$^+$ (atomic weight = 23) is 23/1 = 23, while the electrical equivalent weight of Ca^{2+} (atomic weight = 40) is 40/2 = 20.

> ### Normal solution
>
> The concentration of a solution may be measured in terms of its **normality**, where a normal solution (1 N solution) contains 1 g equivalent solute per litre solution.

Movement of water across a membrane

The membranes separating the fluid compartments generally allow the free passage of water, but not solutes, across them. Such membranes are known as semipermeable membranes. If a semipermeable membrane separates two aqueous solutions of different concentrations, water molecules will diffuse across the membrane to equalise the concentrations. **Osmosis** describes this diffusion process. The osmotic activity of the solutes is dependent on the number and not the type of free particles in solution.

Osmotic pressure

The osmotic activity of solute particles in an aqueous solution can be visualised as exerting an **osmotic pressure**, which would potentially draw water into the solution. This can be demonstrated as a hydrostatic pressure difference between two compartments separated by a semipermeable membrane, one containing solution and the other containing water alone.

> **Osmotic pressure** is defined as the pressure required to prevent osmosis when the solution is separated from pure solvent by a semipermeable membrane (Figure 11.5).

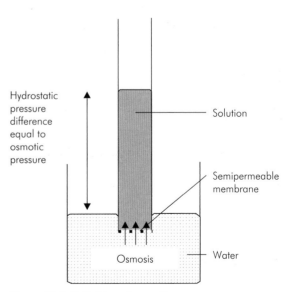

Figure 11.5 Definition of osmotic pressure

Calculation of osmotic pressure from molality of a solution

The osmotic pressure of a solution can be calculated from the solution molality. In a dilute solution, with a solute which does not dissociate or associate, osmotic pressure (π) is dependent on temperature and molal concentration. This can be expressed as:

$\pi \propto$ absolute temperature (T) at a given concentration

Also:

$\pi \propto$ absolute concentration (C) at a given temperature

---

van't Hoff equation for osmotic pressure

In 1877, van't Hoff noted the similarity of behaviour between dilute solutions and gases. Combining the two relations above gives the van't Hoff equation for the osmotic pressure exerted by a dilute solution as:

osmotic pressure (π) = RTC (pascals)
where: R = universal gas constant (= 8.32 J K^{-1})
$\quad$ T = absolute temperature (K)
$\quad$ C = osmolality (mOsm kg^{-1} H$_2$O)

This can be applied to find the osmotic pressure of plasma at body temperature (T = 307 K, C = 290 mOsm kg^{-1} H$_2$O), thus:

Osmotic pressure of plasma $= 8.32 \times 307 \times 290$ Pa
$\qquad\qquad\qquad\qquad = 740729.6$ Pa
$\qquad\qquad\qquad\qquad = 740.7$ kPa

The osmole

The concentration of solute particles in solution can be expressed in osmoles (Osm), to reflect the osmotic activity of the solution, where:

1 osmole = amount of solute that exerts an osmotic
$\qquad\qquad$ pressure of 1 atm when placed in 22.4 litres
$\qquad\qquad$ of solution at 0 °C

For a substance that does not associate or dissociate in solution (e.g. glucose),

1 osmole = 1 mole

For a substance which dissociates into two osmotically active particles (e.g. NaCl → Na$^+$ + Cl$^-$),

1 osmole = 1 mole/2

Osmolality and osmolarity of a solution

Osmolarity is the concentration of a solution expressed in osmoles of solute per litre of solution (solute plus water). The units of osmolarity are thus osmoles per litre (Osm L^{-1}) or milliosmoles per litre (mOsm L^{-1}).

Osmolality is the concentration of a solution expressed as osmoles of solute per kilogram of solvent (water alone). The units of osmolality are thus osmoles per kg water (Osm kg^{-1} H$_2$O) or milliosmoles per kg water (mOsm kg^{-1} H$_2$O). Osmolality is thus independent of temperature and the volume occupied by the solute.

As **osmolality** is independent of temperature, and independent of the volume taken up by the solutes within the solution, it is the preferred term in most physiological applications.

Osmolality of body fluids

The osmolality of a body fluid is usually higher than its osmolarity because of protein and lipid content, which occupy a small but finite volume. In practice this difference is insignificant except in cases of gross hyperproteinaemia or hyperlipidaemia.

Plasma osmolality ranges from 280 to 295 mOsm kg^{-1} H$_2$O, and is maintained constant at about 290 mOsm kg^{-1} H$_2$O throughout the body. The similar osmolality of all major body fluids is due to the free permeability to water of the endothelium and plasma membranes, which separate the various fluid compartments. The distribution and number of osmotically active particles contained by each primarily determine the size of these compartments.

Regulation of body fluid osmolality

The regulation of body fluid osmolality is inextricably linked to the control of total body water (TBW). It involves the secretion of vasopressin (antidiuretic hormone, ADH) in response to an increase in osmolality or a decrease in TBW. Although osmoreceptors appear sensitive enough to respond to small changes in osmolality, their response can be overridden by the haemodynamic response to changes in effective circulating volume. An outline of these responses is shown in Figure 11.6.

Measurement of osmolality

The osmolality of a solution can be estimated in practice by measuring depression of freezing point of the solution, when compared with the pure solvent. Plasma osmolality

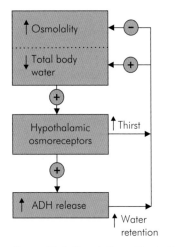

Figure 11.6 Regulation of body fluid osmolality

proteins raise the plasma osmotic pressure above that of the interstitial fluid by an amount referred to as the colloid osmotic pressure (or oncotic pressure). Quantitatively, the most important protein contributing to the colloid osmotic pressure is albumin, which is responsible for up to 75% of the total 25 mmHg colloid osmotic pressure.

Distribution of a solute across a membrane

> **Solute particles** are distributed between fluid compartments according to the permeability of the separating membrane to each type of particle.

can also be estimated from the molality of the major solutes: sodium, chloride, urea and glucose:

$$
\begin{aligned}
\text{Plasma osmolality} &= 2 \times [\text{Na}^+] + [\text{glucose}] + [\text{urea}] \\
&= 2 \times 140 + 5.0 + 5.0 \\
&= 290 \text{ mOsm kg}^{-1}\text{H}_2\text{O}
\end{aligned}
$$

Tonicity of a solution

> **Tonicity** describes the relative osmolality between two fluid compartments. All solutes in ECF contribute to osmolality; however, only solutes which do not cross the cell membrane contribute to the tonicity.

Tonicity determines movement of water between two compartments. If one compartment contains a solution of lower osmolality, it is hypotonic compared with the higher-osmolality compartment. Usually this term is used to describe the effective osmotic pressure of a solution relative to that of plasma.

In an isotonic solution cells can be suspended without a change in cell volume. Cells placed in a hypertonic solution will shrink in volume, and in a hypotonic solution they will increase in volume.

A 0.9% solution of NaCl is approximately isotonic (308 mOsm kg^{-1} H$_2$O).

Plasma colloid osmotic pressure

The capillary endothelium is impermeable to the plasma proteins, albumin and globulins. The retained plasma

Both passive and active mechanisms determine the movement of solutes across a membrane. Active processes such as carrier proteins or ion channels selectively transport or allow the diffusion of substances across a membrane. Passive movement of particles can occur through *pores* or *fenestrations*, or even through the membrane, depending on lipid solubility.

Movement of solute across a capillary wall generally occurs in the filtrate as it passes from the capillary lumen into the interstitium. Large protein molecules remain in the capillary plasma unable to be filtered out because of their size. This capillary filtration process, and the balance of forces (Starling forces) driving it, is described in Chapter 15.

> The main transport mechanisms involved across capillary endothelium are:
> - **Filtration**, which describes the action of hydrostatic pressure forcing fluid out of the capillaries. It is opposed by the plasma colloid osmotic pressure.
> - **Diffusion**, which is the passive movement of substances under the influence of concentration gradients, and occurs through fenestrations and intercellular junctions. The main diffusion barrier is the basement membrane.
> - **Transcytosis**, which is the active transfer of a substance by endocytosis from the capillary lumen, followed by exocytosis out of the endothelial cells. It represents only a small fraction of the total transport across capillary endothelium.

The structure of capillaries and the composition of fluids passing across the capillary walls differ between tissues. These differences reflect the variation in function between vessels, such as between glomerular capillaries in the kidneys, and capillaries found in skeletal muscle.

Gibbs–Donnan effect

Passive movement of solute particles usually occurs under the influence of a chemical concentration or electrical gradient. Consider the case of two compartments (A and B) each containing NaCl but separated by a semipermeable membrane. The diffusion of Na^+ and Cl^- occurs between the compartments to equalise chemical concentration gradients and to maintain electrical neutrality on either side of the membrane (Figure 11.7a).

If protein is trapped in one of the compartments it can affect the distribution of the diffusible ions by the Gibbs–Donnan effect. This occurs due to the negative charge on protein molecules, which acts by holding Na^+ back on one side of the membrane to preserve electroneutrality in the compartment (Figure 11.7b). The chemical gradient of Na^+ across the membrane will then redistribute Na^+ (followed by Cl^- to preserve electroneutrality) between the compartments until equilibrium is reached (Figure 11.7c), when:

$$[cation]_A \times [anion]_A = [cation]_B \times [anion]_B$$
$$[Na^+]_A \times [Cl^-]_A = [Na^+]_B \times [Cl^-]_B$$
$$9 \times 4 = 6 \times 6$$

This mechanism is referred to as the Gibbs–Donnan effect and, in vivo, it affects the distributions of Na^+ and Cl^- between the intravascular and interstitial compartments in the body.

In vivo the Gibbs–Donnan effect gives rise to:

- Unequal distributions of diffusible ions, Na^+ and Cl^-, between intravascular and interstitial compartments
- Higher Na^+ concentration in the protein-containing plasma compartment and higher Cl^- concentration in the interstitial compartment
- A small electrical potential difference across the membrane

---

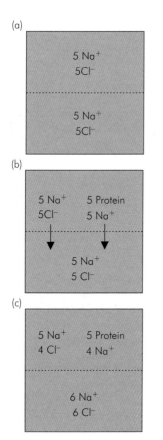

Figure 11.7 Gibbs–Donnan equilibrium

Calculation of potential difference across capillary wall

The magnitude of this potential difference can be calculated using the Nernst equation, and it is dependent on the ratio of the diffusible ion concentrations on either side of the membrane at equilibrium. Thus, applying the Nernst equation to a capillary wall:

$$\text{Potential difference} = \frac{RT}{FZ_{Na}} \times \ln\frac{[Na^+]_{INT}}{[Na^+]_C}$$
$$= 62 \times (145/153)$$
$$= -3.24\text{mV}$$

Thus there is a potential difference across the capillary wall of about 3 mV, the endothelial surface being negative with respect to the interstitium.

The Gibbs–Donnan effect is significant in the distribution of diffusible ions across a largely passive semipermeable membrane such as capillary endothelium separating intravascular and interstitial compartments.

The Gibbs–Donnan equilibrium described above results when the diffusion of the ions down their chemical concentration gradients is balanced by the electrostatic attraction of the protein molecules trapped in one compartment of the model. This balance between chemical and electrostatic forces produces an electrical potential difference across the membrane of about 3 mV.

Composition of body fluids

The compositions of the major body fluids – plasma, interstitial and intracellular – are shown in Figure 11.8.

Intracellular fluid

ICF composition varies according to cell function. There are general differences between ICF and interstitial fluid. These include low intracellular Na^+, Cl^- and HCO_3^- concentrations compared with the extracellular values. The predominant cation is K^+, and the organic phosphates and proteins are the principal intracellular anions.

Figure 11.8 Compositions of major body fluids (mmol L^{-1})

Substance	Plasma	Interstitial fluid	Intracellular fluid
Cations			
Na^+	153	145	10
K^+	4.3	4.1	159
Ca^{2+}	2.7	2.4	< 1
Mg^{2+}	1.1	1	40
Total	161.1	152.5	209
Anions			
Cl^-	112	117	3
HCO_3^-	25.8	27.1	7
Proteins	15.1	< 0.1	45
Others	8.2	8.4	154
Total	161.1	152.5	209

The composition of ICF is maintained largely by the cell plasma membrane in a stable but dynamic state of flux.

Interstitial fluid

The composition of interstitial fluid is dependent on the filtration of plasma through the capillary wall. This is largely a passive process driven by the balance of hydrostatic and colloid osmotic pressures. The diffusible ions are therefore of approximately equal concentrations in plasma and interstitial fluid. The retention of protein in the capillaries, however, results in a small discrepancy due to the Gibbs–Donnan effect.

Plasma

The distinguishing component in plasma is the retained plasma protein. There is a total protein content in plasma of about 7 g per 100 mL. The various plasma proteins are outlined in Figure 11.9.

Albumin

Albumin accounts for 60% of plasma protein. One of its main functions is to act as a transport protein binding free fatty acids and bilirubin. It is also the principal component responsible for plasma colloid osmotic pressure. Of plasma albumin, 5% circulates through the interstitial fluid compartment each hour, while 60% of the total mass

Figure 11.9 Plasma proteins

Plasma protein group	Name
Proteolytic systems	Kinins
Carrier proteins	Albumin Haptoglobulin Transferrin Ceruloplasmin Pre-albumin Transcortin Transcobalamin
Protease inhibitors	α_1-Antitrypsin α_2-Macroglobulin Antithrombin III
Acute phase proteins	Interleukin 1 Tumour necrosis factor C-reactive protein
Immunoglobulins	IgG, IgA, IgM, IgD, IgE

of albumin is actually extravascular. The intravascular half-life of albumin is 19 days.

Immunoglobulins

Immunoglobulins form about 20% of plasma proteins and are split into five groups, each with differing functions and structures. IgG, IgD and IgE are monomers with molecular weights between 150,000 and 190,000 daltons; IgA is secreted as a dimer with a molecular weight of 400,000; IgM is a pentamer with a molecular weight of 900,000. IgM immunoglobulin is completely confined to the intravascular space.

Transcellular fluids

Some of the transcellular fluids differ considerably from plasma in composition. Excessive losses of different transcellular fluids can give rise to significant water and electrolyte disturbances, when disease is present. Some examples of transcellular fluid composition are given in Figure 11.10.

Intravenous fluids

Composition of IV fluids

The electrolyte content of commonly used IV fluids is shown in Figure 11.11.

Figure 11.10 Composition of transcellular fluids (mmol L^{-1})

Substance	Saliva	Gastric juice	Bile	Sweat
Na^+	33	60	149	45
K^+	20	9	5	5
Cl^-	34	84	101	58
HCO_3^-	0	0	45	0
pH	6.6	3	8	5.2

Distribution of IV fluids in fluid compartments

On intravenous administration of a litre of 0.9% solution, which is an isotonic fluid, all of it remains in ECF. However, infusion of a litre of 0.45% saline (osmolality 154 mOsm kg^{-1}) causes a decrease in the osmolality of ECF leading to a shift (of about a third of a litre) in water from ECF to ICF.

If 5% glucose solution is administered intravenously, initially it will stay in the ECF compartment. Once glucose is metabolised, water distributes into both ECF and ICF compartments according to their proportional volumes.

Maintenance fluid requirements

- In normal circumstances, in adults, daily water requirement is about 30–35 mL kg^{-1} for maintenance.
- Daily requirement for sodium and potassium is 1 mmol kg^{-1} of each.
- This fluid and electrolyte need can be met by 2500 mL of glucose 4%/saline 0.18% or 2000 mL of glucose 5% with 500 mL of 0.9% saline, plus potassium as KCl 5 g (65 mmol).

Fluid requirements in the perioperative period

In certain circumstances abnormal fluid loss, sensible or insensible, occurs. This is common in the perioperative period. In the presence of fever or tachypnoea, insensible loss of water can be significant. 'Third space' fluid loss (loss of fluid that does not take part in normal metabolic processes) is frequent at the site of tissue injury or from bowel (e.g. in intestinal obstruction). Often it is difficult to

Figure 11.11 Electrolyte content of commonly used intravenous fluids

Solution	Electrolyte (cations)	Level (mmol L^{-1})	Electrolyte (anions)	Level (mmol L^{-1})	Osmolality (mOsm kg^{-1})
Hartmann's solution	Na, K, Ca	131, 5, 4	Cl, HCO_3	112, 29	281
Normal saline	Na	154	Cl	154	308
5% glucose	Nil	–	Nil	–	278
Glucose-saline (glucose 4%, saline 0.18%)	Na	31	Cl	31	284

correctly estimate fluid loss in the gut. If it is isotonic fluid loss, only ECF volume is affected, but loss of hypotonic fluid or water leads to a shift of water from ICF to ECF to equalise osmolality. Such fluid losses should be corrected using water and appropriate electrolytes.

The infusion of inappropriate fluid can cause significant electrolyte and acid–base imbalance. For example, replacement of significant 'third space' fluid loss by intravenous 0.9% saline only (instead of appropriate electrolytes and water replacement) can cause hyperchloraemic acidosis. This occurs because excessive infusion of chloride ions leads to renal elimination of bicarbonate ions to maintain electrolyte neutrality.

Disorders of water and electrolyte balance

Sodium and water

> The regulation of total body sodium is inextricably linked to the loss or retention of water, and disturbances in total body sodium content will thus be compensated for by changes in total body water. Similarly, compensation for a disturbance of TBW will include readjustment of body sodium levels.

Disturbances of total body water

Some examples of body water disturbances are outlined in Figure 11.12.

Abnormalities of plasma sodium

Although total body sodium and total body water are different physiological entities, they are interdependent, so that a disturbance in one quantity will activate compensatory mechanisms which affect both. In practice, they are not readily measured, and the clinical management of sodium/water disturbances often relies on the measurement of plasma sodium levels and osmolalities.

Hypernatraemia

Hypernatraemia occurs when plasma sodium is > 150 mmol L^{-1}. It often presents with an altered sensorium, this being dependent on the speed of plasma sodium change and plasma osmolality. Coma ensues at plasma osmolalities > 350 mOsm kg^{-1} H_2O. Acute hypernatraemia is associated with osmotic shift of water from the intracellular compartment, causing reduction in cell volume and water content of the brain. Hypernatraemia may occur with decreased or increased ECF volume and increased or decreased total body sodium, depending on the cause of the original disturbance (Figure 11.13). Intracellular dehydration due to ECF hyperosmolality is an abnormality common to all hypernatraemic states. The clinical signs and symptoms accompanying hypernatraemia may reflect hypervolaemia or hypovolaemia (diabetes

Figure 11.13 Features of hypernatraemia

Cause	ECF volume	Total body free water	Total body sodium
Diuresis, vomiting, pyrexia	Low	↓↓	↓
Over-transfusion with hypertonic sodium solutions	High	↑	↑↑

Figure 11.12 Body water disturbances

Condition	Definition	Causes
Dehydration	A decrease in TBW with or without a loss of sodium	↓ intake, e.g. nil by mouth, dysphagia ↑ insensible loss, e.g. pyrexia, hyperhidrosis, hyperventilation
Water deficiency	A decrease in TBW without a comparable decrease in body sodium	↑ urinary loss, e.g. diabetes insipidus, diabetes mellitus ↑ gastrointestinal losses, e.g. vomiting, diarrhoea
Water intoxication	An increase in TBW without a comparable increase in body sodium	Renal failure, inappropriate vasopressin secretion, hepatic failure, IV infusion of dextrose

insipidus, fever, severe exercise in hot climate). Where hypovolaemia is present, sodium deficit can be replaced relatively rapidly compared with the replacement of free water. Free water deficits should be replaced gradually (over 48–72 hours) to avoid an increased risk of cerebral oedema.

Pathophysiology of hypernatraemia

Assessment of urine output and the measurement of urine and plasma osmolality are helpful in the diagnosis of hypernatraemia.
- High urine osmolality (≥ 750 mOsm kg^{-1}) and low urine output indicates normal ADH function, and most likely cause is extrarenal water loss (diarrhoea, vomiting) or inadequate intake.
- High urine output with high urine osmolality suggests osmotic diuresis.

Treatment of hypernatraemia

Iatrogenic hypernatraemia can occur due to administration of excessive hypertonic sodium bicarbonate during resuscitation, or when insensible losses (which should be replaced only by water or 5% glucose) are replaced by 0.9% saline. Management of hypernatraemia in such conditions includes loop diuretics or haemofiltration.

Hypernatraemia without volume depletion is corrected by 5% glucose. However, commonly volume depletion is present in hypernatraemic patients, and in such patients isotonic saline is the initial treatment of choice. Once volume depletion is corrected, further water deficit can be replaced by hypotonic fluids.

In hypernatraemic patients, water deficit is estimated from:

$$\text{Water deficit} = (\text{measured Na concentration}/140 \times \text{TBW}) - \text{TBW}$$

Hyponatraemia

Hyponatraemia occurs when plasma sodium is < 135 mmol L^{-1}. There are different clinical syndromes associated with hyponatraemia, depending on the underlying cause (Figure 11.14).

Pathophysiology of hyponatraemia

- Hyponatraemia will be associated with water intoxication, which is described above, and is due to excessive water intake or excessive water retention due to inappropriate vasopressin secretion.
- Hypervolaemia will accompany hyponatraemia when the primary disturbance is an increase in TBW, and regulatory mechanisms attempt to maintain plasma osmolality by sodium retention.
- Hypovolaemia and hyponatraemia occur when the primary disturbance is an excessive loss of water and sodium with inappropriate (hypotonic fluids) and inadequate resuscitation.

Clinical signs and symptoms of hyponatraemia are those of hypovolaemia or hypervolaemia, depending on the underlying disturbance. The decrease in plasma osmolality results in movement of water into the ICF, causing expansion of brain cells. Central signs range from mild lethargy to seizures and respiratory arrest.

Figure 11.14 Features of hyponatraemia

Cause	ECF volume	Total body free water	Total body sodium	Urinary sodium
Cardiac failure, renal failure, hepatic failure, TUR syndrome	High	↑↑↑	↑	< 20 mmol L^{-1}
Inappropriate vasopressin secretion	Normal ECF volume, plasma osmolality $<$ 290 mOsm kg^{-1} H$_2$O	↑	→	< 20 mmol L^{-1}, urine osmolality $>$ 100 mOsm kg^{-1} H$_2$O
Adrenal failure	Low	↓	↓↓↓	> 20 mmol L^{-1}

Figure 11.15 Features of potassium, calcium and magnesium imbalance

Disorder	Cause	Symptoms and signs
Hypokalaemia	Acute – administration of insulin and glucose, familial periodic paralysis, vomiting, diarrhoea	Tachycardia, extrasystoles, cardiac dilatation
	Chronic – dietary insufficiency, malabsorption, diuretics, hyperaldosteronism, Cushing's syndrome	Weakness, hypotonia and paralysis of muscle, metabolic alkalosis
Hyperkalaemia	Renal failure, Addison's disease, iatrogenic (spironolactone, administration of potassium supplements)	Cardiac arrhythmias, heart block, cardiac arrest in diastole. Weakness, numbness, paraesthesiae, listlessness, confusion
Hypocalcaemia	Hypoparathyroidism, post-thyroidectomy, vitamin D deficiency, renal failure, hyperventilation	Tetany, convulsions, cataracts, ectopic calcification in CNS
Hypercalcaemia	Hyperparathyroidism, malignancy, sarcoidosis, multiple myeloma, vitamin D toxicity, milk-alkali syndrome	Nephrolithiasis, personality changes, muscle weakness and atrophy, abdominal discomfort, corneal calcification
Hypomagnesaemia	Diarrhoea, malabsorption, hyperaldosteronism	'Calcium-resistant' tetany, muscular weakness, depression, irritability, convulsions
Hypermagnesaemia	Renal failure, iatrogenic administration	Prolonged AV and intraventricular conduction rates

Treatment of hyponatraemia

Acute symptomatic hyponatraemia is a medical emergency, but rapid correction can lead to central pontine myelinolysis, a disorder characterised by coma, paralysis and death. Hypertonic saline is administered to raise the plasma sodium concentration to 125 mmol L^{-1} only over a period of at least 12 hours. The amount of sodium required to achieve the desired concentration is calculated as follows:

$$Na\,required\,(mmol\,L^{-1}) = [(desired\,Na - measured\,Na)\,concentration] \times TBW$$

Potassium

Potassium is the main intracellular cation and plays an important role intracellularly in protein synthesis, acid–base balance and maintaining osmolality.

Although extracellular concentrations are comparatively low, extracellular levels are also important because they affect membrane potentials and plasma acid–base balance. Potassium level is primarily regulated by the kidney. Some details of potassium excess (hyperkalaemia) and potassium deficit (hypokalaemia) are outlined in Figure 11.15.

Hypokalaemia is more common than hyperkalaemia. Generally, a reduction in K^+ level of 1 mmol L^{-1} reflects a total body potassium deficit of about 100 mmol. The potassium infusion rate should not exceed 0.5 mmol $kg^{-1}\,h^{-1}$, to allow equilibration with the intracellular compartment.

In a hyperkalaemic patient, a plasma potassium concentration in excess of 7 mmol L^{-1}, or ECG changes, warrants immediate treatment.

Calcium

Calcium is quantitatively the most common mineral in the body, with a total body content of about 1200 g. More than 99% of this calcium is in bone, the remainder being in body fluids, partially ionised and partially protein-bound. Ionised calcium is important as a cofactor, particularly in the coagulation cascade. Calcium is central in maintaining excitability of the myocardium, skeletal muscle, smooth muscle and nerves. It also has a significant role in the regulation of membrane permeability. See Figure 11.15 for some details of calcium imbalance.

Magnesium

The total body content of magnesium is about 25 g, of which half is contained in bone and teeth. The normal plasma level is about 1.1 mmol L^{-1}. The most important function of magnesium systemically is its role as a cofactor, since it is essential for the activity of all kinases. These enzymes catalyse phosphorylation reactions by ATP. Since this is the main mechanism for the transfer of chemical energy in intermediate metabolism, magnesium plays a key role in functions such as muscle contraction as well as pathways such as glycolysis. Regulation of magnesium levels in the body is not clear, but it may involve parathyroid hormone and aldosterone. Figure 11.15 details the effects of magnesium imbalance.

Acid–base imbalance and electrolyte replacement

Metabolic acidosis

> **Metabolic acidosis** is characterised by low pH, decreased HCO_3^-, and low $PaCO_2$.

For the purposes of treatment, it is useful to classify the metabolic acidosis in relation to the anion gap.

Anion gap is the difference between measured cations and anions in the plasma. Because of unmeasured anions (proteins, phosphates, lactates, organic anions) in the plasma, a discrepancy exists in the number of measured anions and cations. The normal anion gap is 12–18 mmol L^{-1}.

Metabolic acidosis with normal anion gap is caused by loss of bicarbonate ions and replacement with chloride. Metabolic acidosis with increased anion gap occurs due to overproduction of acids (e.g. lactates, diabetic ketoacidosis) or ingestion of exogenous acids (e.g. salicylates).

Treatment involves correction of the cause of metabolic acidosis. Sodium bicarbonate (1.4%, isotonic, or 8.4%, hypertonic) can be used to restore pH to near normal value, but this must only be done in cases of life-threatening acidaemia. Use of sodium bicarbonate solution can cause respiratory acidosis, as carbon dioxide is generated during the buffering process; this is particularly significant in patients with tissue hypoxia (e.g. septic shock, cardiac arrest).

Metabolic alkalosis

> **Metabolic alkalosis** is characterised by high pH, an increased HCO_3^-, and raised $PaCO_2$.

For the purposes of diagnosis and treatment, the metabolic alkalosis can be classified as chloride-resistant or chloride-responsive. The urinary chloride level is measured to differentiate two groups of patients.

In chloride-resistant metabolic alkalosis (urinary chloride > 20 mmol L^{-1}), HCO_3^- loss is increased by using acetazolamide or acid loss is minimised/replaced (e.g. by use of proton pump inhibitors to minimise hydrogen ion loss). Hypokalaemia causes this type of metabolic alkalosis.

In chloride-responsive metabolic alkalosis (urinary chloride < 20 mmol L^{-1}), 0.9% saline infusion results in loss of bicarbonate due to increase in chloride ion availability.

Strong ions

The compounds which dissociate completely in a solution form strong ions. The strong ions are always present in a fully dissociated state. In blood, commonly occurring strong ions (measurable ions) include Na^+, K^+, Ca^{2+} and Mg^{2+}. Generally strong acids or strong bases dissociate completely in a solution.

The difference between the strong positive ions (cations) and the strong negative ions (anions) is called a strong ion difference (SID). In plasma, the difference between the strong positive ions and the strong negative ions is commonly labelled as the anion gap.

Special fluids

Lymph and the lymphatic system

The lymphatics are a system of blind-ending tubules with endothelium similar to blood capillaries. There is neither basement membrane nor intercellular gaps, and pinocytosis makes the vessels permeable to proteins. Lymph nodes are encapsulated collections of specialised tissue situated along the course of the lymphatic vessels. They are populated by phagocytic cells lining medullary and cortical sinuses. These engulf bacteria so that under normal conditions the lymph exiting the nodes is sterile.

Ultimately two main vessels, the right lymphatic and thoracic duct, drain into the subclavian veins. The 24-hour production of lymph is 2–4 litres. The low resistance of the lymphatic branching system, the presence of valves and positive intrathoracic pressures promote forward flow. There is also a high resistance to returning to the interstitial space.

The lymphatic capillaries supplement the venous capillaries in the drainage of tissue fluid. Lymph pumps augment fluid removal. These take the form of adjacent arteriolar pulsations compressing and dilating the lymph vessels, as is found in skeletal muscle. Excessive accumulation of tissue fluid is oedema. Other functions of the lymphatics include the return and absorption of nutrients. Plasma lipids are transported as lipoproteins and neutral fat as chylomicrons, and concentrations vary with dietary intake. Chylomicrons are small fat globules comprising lipid and protein that are created by the intestinal mucosa.

Features of lymph and the lymphatic system

- The lymphatic system aids drainage of tissue fluid and helps in the transport and delivery of nutrients.
- Protein content is lower than plasma and depends on the drained organ.
- Contains all coagulation factors, especially hepatic lymph.
- Antibodies are found in high concentrations.
- Electrolyte composition is similar to plasma.
- Lymphocytes are common, red cells and platelets are rare.

Cerebrospinal fluid (CSF)

About 150 mL cerebrospinal fluid surrounds the structures of the CNS and fills the cerebral ventricles. This fluid is continually produced at 600 mL per 24 hours, it circulates and is reabsorbed into the cerebrovenous system. The majority of CSF (70%) is produced by the choroid plexuses within the cerebral ventricles; the remaining 30% is produced in the endothelium of cerebral capillaries. The choroid plexuses are networks of cerebral blood vessels exposed to the CSF in the third and lateral ventricles. They produce the CSF by modified ultrafiltration from the plexus capillaries into the ventricles. The filtration

barrier consists of capillary endothelium, basement membrane and choroid epithelium, which also actively modifies the composition of the CSF produced.

Circulation of CSF

The CSF flows through the lateral ventricles to the brainstem, where it passes via the third and fourth ventricles, aided by ciliated ependymal cells, which line the ventricles. From the fourth ventricle the CSF exits to the subarachnoid space via the lateral foramina of Luschka and the median foramen of Magendie. It then circulates around the brainstem, brain and spinal cord in the subarachnoid space, finally to be reabsorbed by arachnoid villi in the venous sinuses of the skull. The rate of reabsorption is proportional to CSF outflow pressure. This is normally 11.2 cmH$_2$O. Reabsorption ceases if it is < 7 cmH$_2$O.

Composition of CSF

As noted, the filtration process producing the CSF in the choroid plexuses is ultrafiltration, which is modified (by active secretion) by the ependymal cells. The concentrations of the major constituents in CSF are given in Figure 11.16.

Ionic homeostasis

The ionic composition of interstitial fluid in the CNS is tightly controlled. Both the CSF and the cerebral capillaries contribute to the formation of interstitial fluid. CSF is in free communication with the interstitial fluid in the

Figure 11.16 Concentrations of major substances in CSF and plasma

Substance	CSF	Plasma
Protein (g L^{-1})	0.3	70
HCO$_3^-$ (mmol L^{-1})	23	25
Glucose (mmol L^{-1})	4.8	8
Na$^+$ (mmol L^{-1})	147	150
K$^+$ (mmol L^{-1})	2.9	4.6
Cl$^-$ (mmol L^{-1})	112	100
pH	7.32	7.4
Osmolality (mOsm kg^{-1} H$_2$O)	290	290
PCO$_2$ (kPa)	6.6	5.3

brain and has the same composition, but there can be a significant time lag in the equilibration of changes between CSF and interstitial fluid. The formation of interstitial fluid and the CSF occurs across a blood–brain barrier located in the cerebral capillaries and the choroid plexuses respectively. This barrier separates the cerebral circulation from the cerebral tissue and serves several functions, which are to:

- Provide tight control over ion concentrations in the CNS
- Protect the brain from transient changes in plasma glucose
- Protect the brain from endogenous and exogenous toxins
- Prevent the release of central neurotransmitters into the systemic circulation

CNS chemoreceptor respiratory control

The central chemoreceptors involved in respiratory control are situated on the ventral surface of the medulla and the floor of the fourth ventricle. The chemoreceptors are bathed in interstitial fluid, which as noted is in communication with the CSF, as well as being formed by cerebral capillaries. The blood–brain barrier is freely permeable to CO_2 but relatively impermeable to H^+ and HCO_3^-. Thus, CO_2 diffuses across into the CSF and interstitial fluid in proportion to arterial PCO_2. The low protein concentration in CSF and interstitial fluid limits its buffering capacity, and pH changes are greater than those in plasma for a given change in PCO_2.

The initial response to increasing plasma PCO_2 is formation of H^+ and HCO_3^- in the epithelial cells, catalysed by carbonic anhydrase. Compensation then takes place through the secretion of HCO_3^- buffering CSF and interstitial pH. The concentration of HCO_3^- in CSF and cerebral interstitial fluid is always lower than in plasma, because of the lack of protein buffering in these fluids. The chemoreceptor response to H^+ is to stimulate hyperventilation.

Functions of CSF

- 150 mL of CSF surrounds the spinal cord and brain, and fills the ventricles.
- CSF provides buoyancy and protection.
- CSF aids ionic homeostasis in the CNS.
- CSF participates in respiratory control.

Intraocular fluid

Aqueous and vitreous humour are formed from plasma. Aqueous is a plasma dialysate with a continuous hourly turnover, and it provides the metabolic and respiratory substrate for the anterior chamber. Specialised cells in the ciliary body actively secrete aqueous humour. The principal route of drainage is via the canal of Schlemm. Production and drainage maintains intraocular pressure at 15–18 mmHg. Vitreous humour in the posterior chamber contains the gelatine-like protein vitrein.

Pleural fluid

Capillaries on the surface of highly vascular visceral and parietal pleurae form a thin lubricating layer of fluid. The forces of ultrafiltration and reabsorption apply as in the formation of any transcellular fluid discussed above. The hydrostatic pressure in pulmonary capillaries is low compared with a high plasma colloid pressure. The Starling shifts are in favour of reabsorption, leaving a thin intrapleural layer of fluid.

CHAPTER 12

Haematology and immunology

Jeff Neilson and Ted Lin

Red blood cells

The main function of red blood cells (erythrocytes) is the carriage of oxygen. They are specialised cells which lack organelles and a nucleus. Over 95% of the protein content is the oxygen transport protein haemoglobin, the remainder being enzymes required to maintain haemoglobin in a functional, reduced state and enzymes for glycolysis.

The biconcave shape of erythrocytes increases their surface-area-to-volume ratio, making gas exchange more efficient, and also makes the cell more deformable in order to navigate the microvasculature.

Erythropoiesis

Erythropoiesis (production of erythrocytes) occurs predominantly in the bone marrow from the seventh month of gestation. Under normal circumstances the average survival of erythrocytes is 120 days, and the rate of production of erythrocytes equals their rate of destruction. However, production can respond to unusual demands as in hypoxia, haemorrhage, haemolysis or anaemia. Erythropoiesis is stimulated by erythropoietin (EPO), which is a glycoprotein produced mainly in the kidney but also in the liver. Hormones such as corticosteroids, androgens, thyroxine and growth hormone also increase EPO production due to their effect in increasing metabolic rate. The bone marrow is one of the most proliferative tissues in the body, with a high requirement for iron (for haem), vitamin B_{12}, folate and pyridoxine (for DNA synthesis), riboflavin, vitamin E and copper.

Haemoglobin

Haemoglobin is the main oxygen-carrying molecule, increasing the oxygen-carrying capacity of blood more than 50 times since oxygen is relatively insoluble in aqueous solution. Haemoglobin is also involved in the transport of CO_2 and hydrogen ions (H^+). Myoglobin is also an oxygen-carrying molecule; it is present in skeletal muscle and acts as an oxygen store, releasing oxygen when needed.

Fundamentals of Anaesthesia, 4th edition, ed. Ted Lin, Tim Smith and Colin Pinnock. Published by Cambridge University Press. © Cambridge University Press 2017.

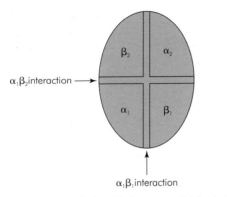

Figure 12.1 Relationship between globin chains in haemoglobin

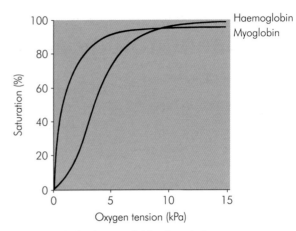

Figure 12.2 Oxyhaemoglobin dissociation curve

Structure and function of haemoglobin

The haemoglobin A molecule has four polypeptide chains (two α and two β chains), each of which has a covalently bound haem group consisting of a porphyrin ring with a central iron atom in the ferrous (Fe^{2+}) state. A single oxygen molecule can bind to the central iron atom of each haem group. The cross-links between the polypeptide chains consist of non-covalent electrostatic salt links. There are two distinct types of salt link in the haemoglobin molecule (Figure 12.1).

The haemoglobin molecule changes configuration during oxygen uptake and release. Deoxyhaemoglobin is in the taut (T) configuration, while the binding of oxygen produces a more relaxed (R) configuration by breaking salt links in the $\alpha_1\beta_2$ and $\alpha_2\beta_1$ interactions. The first oxygen molecule binds relatively weakly to haemoglobin, since more salt links must be broken (and therefore more energy is required) compared with the subsequent two oxygen molecules, and less energy still is required for the binding of the fourth oxygen molecule. This sequential increase in oxygen affinity explains the sigmoid shape of the oxyhaemoglobin dissociation curve of haemoglobin (Figure 12.2). Myoglobin, being a single-chain molecule, has a hyperbolic-shaped oxyhaemoglobin dissociation curve.

Regulation of oxygen carriage in haemoglobin

Haemoglobin is a good example of an allosteric molecule in that its oxygen binding properties are regulated by the binding of other substances at sites remote from the oxygen binding sites. These regulator substances are CO_2, H^+ and 2,3-diphosphoglycerate (2,3-DPG).

Effect of CO_2, H^+

CO_2 binds to the terminal amino groups of haemoglobin as bicarbonate, which is formed in the red cell by the action of carbonic anhydrase:

$$CO_2 + H_2O \leftrightharpoons HCO_3^- + H^+$$

This lowers the oxygen affinity of haemoglobin, shifting the oxyhaemoglobin dissociation curve to the right. Much of the hydrogen ion generated by this reaction is taken up by deoxyhaemoglobin, which has a higher affinity for H^+ than oxyhaemoglobin:

$$HbO_2 + H^+ \leftrightharpoons HbH^+ + O_2$$

Hence, under acid conditions the equilibrium between deoxy- and oxyhaemoglobin shifts in favour of deoxyhaemoglobin – this is called the 'Bohr effect'. Acidic conditions, therefore, reduce the oxygen affinity of haemoglobin and shift the oxyhaemoglobin dissociation curve to the right. In the highly oxygenated environment of the alveolar capillaries of the lungs the above reactions are reversed.

Effect of 2,3-DPG

Metabolism in the erythrocyte is mainly via anaerobic glycolysis, following the Embden–Meyerhof pathway. 2,3-Diphosphoglycerate (2,3-DPG) is a product of glycolysis binding to haemoglobin in the ratio of one molecule of 2,3-DPG per tetramer.

2,3-DPG reduces the oxygen affinity of haemoglobin 26-fold (oxyhaemoglobin dissociation curve moves to the right). In the absence of 2,3-DPG, haemoglobin would unload little oxygen in the capillaries.

Part of the 'storage lesion' of blood for transfusion is a fall in 2,3-DPG levels to about 30% of normal after 3 weeks storage of whole blood in CPDA medium (citrate-phosphate-dextrose-adenine). This is improved with storage of plasma-reduced blood in SAGM (saline-adenine-glucose-mannitol). The clinical significance of the low 2,3-DPG is only likely to be of importance in recipients with severe anaemia or cardiac ischaemia. 2,3-DPG levels are restored to at least 50% of normal in 24 hours and 95% of normal at 72 hours after transfusion.

An increase in body temperature is capable of shifting the oxyhaemoglobin dissociation curve to the right and is an appropriate response to exercise. The converse is also true, but in hypothermic individuals the oxygen requirement also falls.

Genetic control of haemoglobin and haemoglobinopathies

The genes for the α-globins are located on the short arm of chromosome 16, while the β-globin gene cluster is located on the short arm of chromosome 11. Alteration of the coding regions (exons) of the globin genes is likely to alter the amino acid sequence of the corresponding globin chain, and the end result is a haemoglobinopathy (e.g. sickle cell disease). On the other hand, if there is lack of expression of a globin chain as a result of deletion or mutation at critical control regions (e.g. RNA splice sites) then a thalassaemia results. Although sickle cell and thalassaemia are the two most common anomalies of haemoglobin, there are other abnormal forms.

Sickle cell disease
Pathophysiology

> **Sickle cell disease** is a result of a single DNA base change (adenine to thymine) which results in the substitution of valine for glutamic acid at position 6 of the β-globin chain.

Sickle haemoglobin (HbS) polymerises into microfibrils (crystals) in the deoxygenated state. It is thought that the formation of parallel HbS microfibrils causes red cell membrane damage, which results in the classical sickle cell deformity. The effect of this is to shorten the survival of sickle red cells (to 5–15 days in homozygous sickle cell disease), causing haemolytic anaemia. In addition, the deformed red cells are more rigid and less capable of passing through the microcirculation. The result is obstruction, clinically manifest as 'crises', e.g. bone pain, pulmonary syndrome and stroke.

The rate of polymerisation of HbS is related to the 50th power of its concentration. Polymerisation is also affected by the presence of other haemoglobin types, which may inhibit this process to varying degrees. Haemoglobin C and D are not sickling haemoglobins, but inhibit the sickling of HbS much less than HbA and HbF. Hence, persons with double heterozygosity for HbS and HbC or HbD have a sickling disorder, whereas heterozygotes for HbS do not.

Sickle cell disease exists widely throughout Africa and in parts of Asia, the Arabian peninsula and southern Europe. The high prevalence of this debilitating disease is a result of balanced polymorphism driven by the relative resistance of heterozygotes to malaria. The majority of sickle cell disease seen in the UK is found in African-Caribbean populations in large cities, where up to 10% of individuals carry the β^S gene. In Africa this may be as high as 45%.

Clinical features: sickle trait

Sufferers of sickle trait have normal growth, development, exercise tolerance and life expectancy. There are rare reports of high-altitude splenic infarction, though it must be stressed that most persons with sickle trait tolerate high altitude with impunity.

Clinical features: sickle cell disease

The clinical features of sickle cell disease can be summarised as follows:

- **Anaemia** – universal. Most patients have a haemoglobin level between 5 and 10 g dL^{-1}. It is generally well tolerated and does not require therapy.
- **Vaso-occlusive (painful) crises** – the most common manifestation that brings the patient into hospital contact. There is sudden onset of severe pain, usually in bones and joints, which reflects bone marrow ischaemia due to sickling in the bone marrow sinusoids. It may be precipitated by infection or exposure to cold, although often no precipitant can be identified. Abdominal crises may present as an acute abdomen and can be difficult to distinguish from biliary colic. The absence of bowel sounds, however, should alert the physician to a disorder requiring surgical intervention.
- **Acute chest syndrome** – features include pleuritic chest pain, fever, tachypnoea, pulmonary infiltrates

and leucocytosis. It is difficult to distinguish infection, infarction due to sickling, and pulmonary embolism. Hypoxia is common and ventilatory support is sometimes needed.

- **Stroke** – perhaps the most important complication, with the majority occurring in children. Infarction is the usual pathology.
- **In children** – aplastic crises (parvovirus), splenic sequestration (major cause of death in children under 2 years old), dactylitis, delayed growth and development.
- **Long-term complications in adults** – include cholelithiasis, sickle retinopathy, leg ulcers (more common in the tropics), renal impairment and chronic bone damage from recurrent crises.

Diagnosis

Some other haemoglobin types may mimic sickle cell disease. To obtain an exact diagnosis, haemoglobin electrophoresis should be performed.

Medical management

Ideally all patients should be managed in centres with experience in managing haemoglobinopathies. Management of specific problems is as follows:

- Vaso-occlusive crises – adequate and prompt pain relief is essential. Opioids are often required. Adequate hydration is essential. Broad-spectrum antibiotics should be given if infection is suspected. Hypoxia is the only proven indication for oxygen therapy.
- Pregnancy – transfusion therapy during pregnancy reduces the incidence of painful crises but has not been shown to alter pregnancy outcome.
- Prophylaxis – penicillin V 250–500 mg bd (important in hyposplenic status). Vaccination against pneumococcus, *Haemophilus influenzae* and meningococcus is recommended.

Perioperative management

- Consult with haematologist preoperatively, to confirm diagnosis and possible antibodies due to previous transfusion.
- Consider transfusion preoperatively to reduce the HbS level to < 30% and correct anaemia.
- Special attention to be paid to hydration, oxygenation, hypothermia, acidosis preoperatively and postoperatively, as well as during surgery.

- Increased infection risk requires antibiotic prophylaxis.
- Monitor the use of tourniquets carefully and ensure effective exsanguination before inflation.

Thalassaemias

> The **thalassaemias** are genetic disorders of globin chain synthesis (α or β). The genetic lesion results in failure of expression of the globin chain gene involved.

In the α-thalassaemias gene deletion is the usual mechanism, and in the β-thalassaemias gene mutation, resulting in abnormal processing, occurs most often. Heterozygotes are said to have thalassaemia trait; they are asymptomatic but may have characteristic blood count abnormalities.

Alpha-thalassaemia

In α-thalassaemias there is reduced or absent α-chain synthesis. It is critical in the understanding of these disorders to recall that there are two α-chain genes on each chromosome and therefore four genes in any diploid cell. Either one gene is deleted on the same chromosome (α^+) or both are (α^0). The homozygous condition in which no α chains are produced (—/— or $\alpha^0\alpha^0$) is not compatible with life, the fetus being stillborn at 28–40 weeks or surviving a few hours after birth. It is termed the Hb Barts–Hydrops syndrome.

> **Alpha-thalassaemia trait** may be suspected in persons having thalassaemic indices (MCH < 27 pg, low MCV, raised RBC) with normal HbA_2 level and who are iron-replete.

Beta-thalassaemia

In β-thalassaemia there is reduced or absent β-chain synthesis. Each diploid cell has two β-chain genes. Mutation is the usual abnormality at the DNA level, which results in transcriptional dysfunction, RNA processing error or non-functional mRNA. This can result in either reduced β-chain production from that gene (β^+) or absent production (β^0). Each racial group affected has its own repertoire of mutations. Affected populations originate from the Mediterranean, Indian subcontinent or Southeast Asia.

Homozygous β-thalassaemia – thalassaemia major (Cooley's anaemia)

There is absent or greatly reduced β-chain synthesis. This becomes apparent with the natural fall in fetal haemoglobin ($\alpha_2\gamma_2$) levels due to the switch from γ- to β-chain production. The infant presents with anaemia during the first 6 months of life. If transfusion therapy is not instituted then the infant may demonstrate the typical thalassaemic facies (frontal bossing, maxillary hyperplasia). With transfusion therapy there is normal development for the first decade, but iron overload then becomes clinically apparent in the absence of chelation therapy (desferrioxamine) and death occurs in the second or third decade. Chelation is usually started in infancy, and with good compliance patients can expect to live well into their 30s and perhaps longer. In a select group of children bone marrow transplantation is an option, but not without risk of transplant-related death.

Beta-thalassaemia trait

This is asymptomatic with a thalassaemic blood picture. The HbA_2 ($\alpha_2\delta_2$) level is elevated due to a relative reduction in β-chain synthesis with normal δ-chain synthesis. Iron deficiency can reduce HbA_2 levels into the normal range, and therefore HbA_2 should be measured for diagnostic purposes when the individual is iron-replete.

Transfusion medicine

Transfusion medicine involves the procurement, processing, testing and administration of blood and its components. It is also concerned with the prevention, investigation and treatment of transfusion-related complications.

> **ABO incompatibility** remains an important cause of life-threatening transfusion reaction, and most often as a result of clerical error.

The blood group systems were recognised following a reaction between the recipient's serum and donor red cells. Historically, this occurred in vitro and/or in vivo as a transfusion reaction or haemolytic disease of the newborn (HDN), such reactions being simple antibody–antigen reactions. If the particular antibody is able to fix complement (IgM, IgG), then lysis occurs. If this occurs in vivo, an immediate (intravascular) haemolytic transfusion reaction occurs.

Figure 12.3 Relative frequencies of ABO groups

Blood group	Naturally occurring antibodies (IgM)	UK (%)
O	Anti-A, anti-B	47
A	Anti-B	42
B	Anti-A	8
AB	None	3

ABO system

> The **ABO system** is the most important blood antigen system, because of the presence of naturally occurring IgM antibodies to groups A and B in subjects lacking these antigens.

The IgM antibodies are active at 37 °C and readily cause immediate haemolytic transfusion reactions in ABO incompatibility. They are not present at birth, and are thought to arise after exposure to foreign antigens in infancy. Figure 12.3 gives the frequencies of the ABO groups in the UK. Among blood group A and AB individuals approximately one-quarter have a lower density of A antigen on the surface of the red cells, and such subjects are referred to as A_2 and A_2B (the rest are A_1/A_1B). Some A_2 and A_2B people have low levels of anti-A_1 in their serum, though this is rarely of clinical significance as it is not active at 37 °C.

The majority (80%) of individuals can secrete ABO substances in their saliva and other bodily secretions. Persons who are group O and are secretors secrete a precursor substance (H) in the saliva, group A secretors secrete A and H, and so on.

Rhesus system

> The **rhesus sytem** is the second most important system, not because of naturally occurring antibodies as in the ABO system, but because rhesus D (RhD) antibodies are readily formed when blood from a RhD-positive donor is infused into a RhD-negative recipient or when a RhD-negative mother bears a RhD-positive infant. Rhesus antibodies are IgG, and can therefore cross the placenta to cause haemolytic disease of the newborn (HDN).

Alongside the D antigen there are four other Rh antigens of importance – C, c, E, e – although a total of at least 50 Rh antigens have been described. The antigens C and c are allelic, as are E and e. There is no d antigen; the letter is used to indicate a lack of D antigen. D is the most important of the Rh antigens as it is more than 20 times more immunogenic than c, the next most important antigen. Because of the RhD testing of all donors and recipients, and immunoprophylaxis with anti-D during pregnancy and at delivery, the relative frequency of anti-D compared with other Rh antibodies has declined significantly in recent years. Red cell units are still labelled RhD-positive or negative, but a proportion will also have a Rh genotype label. The reason for this is to indicate a lack of certain antigens (c and e in the examples given); these units are, therefore, suitable for patients whose serum contains the corresponding antibodies. Numerous other red cell antigens also exist.

Group and screen

It is of critical importance that blood samples for compatibility testing are correctly identified. The ABO and RhD groups are established by using monoclonal typing reagents (anti-A, anti-B, anti-A+B and anti-D). In ABO grouping, the reverse group is also performed by mixing the patient's serum with A_1 and B red cells. Then an antibody screen is performed. The patient's serum is tested against red cells that between them carry the antigens listed above. If there is a positive reaction in the antibody screen, then the antibody is identified by testing the patient's serum against a panel of red cells. This is done either in the hospital blood bank or at the regional transfusion centre. Once an alloantibody is identified, appropriate red cell units, lacking the red cell antigen, are selected.

Red cell selection and cross-matching

If a red cell alloantibody is detected, then blood should be selected that is known to be negative for that antigen and is ABO- and Rh-compatible. A cross-match follows, where the patient's serum is tested against red cells from the units to be transfused. If the cross-match is negative, then a compatibility label, giving patient details, is attached to the unit and the blood and a compatibility report issued.

Emergency situations

If the situation is life-threatening then group O blood is issued. If the patient is a premenopausal female,

O RhD-negative must be issued. There is generally a shortage of O RhD-negative blood due to high demand for universal usage in emergency situations. Usually, there is sufficient time to perform ABO and RhD groups on the patient sample by rapid techniques and to do an immediate spin cross-match before issue. This may take 10–15 minutes. An antibody screen is then performed by the laboratory retrospectively. A label stating that standard pre-transfusion testing has not been performed is attached to the blood bag. In massive transfusion, where one blood volume has been given within 24 hours, ABO- and RhD-compatible blood can be issued without further serological testing, provided no alloantibodies were present by earlier testing.

Transfusion reactions
Immediate life-threatening reactions
Immediate haemolytic transfusion reactions

These are most often due to ABO incompatibility arising from clerical error. Less commonly, they may be due to antibodies against RhD, Duffy, Kidd and Kell antigens. The antibodies (IgM, IgG1 and IgG3) fix complement and this causes intravascular haemolysis. Features include pain at infusion site, chest and back pain, hypotension, DIC, haemoglobinuria. The mortality rate is 10%.

Anaphylaxis

Anaphylaxis is rare but may be fatal. It is most often related to IgA deficiency in the recipient associated with complement-fixing anti-IgA.

Delayed life-threatening reactions
Bacterial contamination

This is rare but is usually fatal if red cells are contaminated. One of the most frequent organisms responsible is *Yersinia enterocolitica*. There is rapid development of septic shock and collapse. The contaminated blood may be clotted or have a purple discoloration. Platelets can sometimes be contaminated with bacteria, most often Gram-positive organisms such as *Staphylococcus epidermidis*. This relates to storage of platelets at 22 °C.

Transfusion-related acute lung injury (TRALI)

This is rare. It is due to antileukocyte antibodies in donor plasma, and most often seen associated with fresh frozen plasma (FFP). Hypoxia develops during or in the hours following transfusion. There are associated bilateral lung infiltrates radiographically. This syndrome is easily confused with ARDS, and in the critical care setting TRALI may be overlooked as a cause of this clinical picture. Respiratory support is often required, and IV methylprednisolone should be given. In contrast with ARDS, recovery is usual within 48 hours. Recurrence is not a problem, as the antibodies existed in the *donor* plasma.

Congestive cardiac failure (usually LVF)

This is a common adverse effect of transfusion in the elderly, and can be late in onset. Patients with ischaemic heart disease are most at risk. It can be avoided by prophylactic diuretics and transfusion of only two units a day by slow infusion – one unit in 3 hours.

Non-life-threatening reactions
Febrile non-haemolytic transfusion reactions (FNHTR)

This is the most common type of transfusion reaction. It is due to recipient antileukocyte antibodies. These may be acquired following pregnancy or after transfusion of cellular blood components. The patient may experience a rigor, but temperature may rise without one. There are no signs or symptoms to suggest a haemolytic reaction, but severe FNHTRs may be associated with moderate hypotension, nausea, vomiting, cyanosis and collapse. If FNHTRs have already been experienced, further reactions can be prevented by paracetamol before transfusion. Leucodepletion of blood components may be indicated if reactions persist despite this measure. Primary prevention of FNHTR by leucodepletion is appropriate in some situations, e.g. aplastic anaemia, renal transplant candidates, transfusion-dependent patients.

Urticarial reactions

Urticarial reactions to donor plasma proteins may be treated with antihistamines. If there are repeated reactions unresponsive to antihistamines, washed red cells should be given.

Delayed haemolytic transfusion reactions

These reactions occur in patients who have been previously sensitised by transfusion or pregnancy. Red cell antibody titres in such patients may fall to undetectable levels over time, and subsequent re-exposure to the corresponding antigen in a later transfusion can result in a secondary immune response and haemolysis of the transfused cells. IgG antibodies are generally responsible, and haemolysis is generally extravascular, though occasionally it can be intravascular.

Clinical features include fever and a fall in haemoglobin level associated with jaundice between 4 and 14 days after transfusion. If the haemolysis is intravascular, then there may be haemoglobinuria. The clinical severity is related to the volume of incompatible blood transfused. Diagnosis requires a positive direct antiglobulin test and the demonstration of an alloantibody either in the serum or in a red cell eluate, which is antibody eluted from the red blood cells.

Use of blood components

Guidelines are available for the use of platelets, fresh frozen plasma (FFP) and cryoprecipitate. Figures 12.4, 12.5 and 12.6 give indications for the use of these components.

Figure 12.4 Indications for the use of platelet concentrates

Bone marrow failure – if this is reversible (e.g. after chemotherapy), prophylaxis to maintain platelets $> 10 \times 10^9 \, L^{-1}$ is appropriate. In chronic bone marrow failure platelets are generally given if the patient is haemorrhagic
Platelet function disorders – very occasionally required prior to surgery
Massive blood transfusion – clinically significant dilutional thrombocytopenia occurs after the transfusion of about 1.5 blood volumes. The platelet count should be maintained $> 50 \times 10^9 \, L^{-1}$
Cardiopulmonary bypass surgery – platelet functional abnormalities and thrombocytopenia are common in this situation. Platelet transfusion should be reserved for patients with non-surgical bleeding. Prophylaxis is not indicated
Disseminated intravascular coagulation (DIC) – in acute DIC with haemorrhage and thrombocytopenia. Fibrin degradation products (FDPs) impair platelet function. In the absence of bleeding and in chronic DIC platelet transfusion is not indicated
Prior to surgery and invasive procedures – platelet count should be raised to $50 \times 10^9 \, L^{-1}$. For operations on critical sites (e.g. brain and eye) the platelet count should be raised to $100 \times 10^9 \, L^{-1}$

Note that a 'standard dose' of platelets in an adult may be considered as 4 units m^{-2}.

Figure 12.5 Indications for the use of fresh frozen plasma

Replacement of single coagulation factor deficiencies where a specific concentrate is not available

Immediate reversal of warfarin effect – but in life-threatening bleeding due to warfarin prothrombinase complex concentrates (PCC = intermediate purity factor IX) and factor VII concentrates are indicated, together with vitamin K (5 mg IV)

DIC if there is haemorrhage and coagulation abnormality – if there is no haemorrhage or the condition is chronic, FFP is not indicated

Thrombotic thrombocytopenic purpura – a rare disorder which is treated with plasmapheresis using cryoprecipitate-poor FFP

Massive transfusion if there are abnormal coagulation tests (PT and/or APTT ratio ≥ 1.5) and fibrinogen > 1.5 g L^{-1} (if < 1.5 g L^{-1} cryoprecipitate indicated). Coagulation tests need to be repeated frequently to assess the need for further components

Liver disease – if there is bleeding, or prior to surgery/procedures if the PT ratio is prolonged ≥ 1.5

Cardiopulmonary bypass – if there is non-surgical bleeding and a coagulation abnormality with normal platelet count and function

Note that a 'standard' dose of FFP in an adult may be considered as 4 units.

Figure 12.6 Indications for the use of cryoprecipitate

Emergency treatment of haemophilia and von Willebrand disease when specific concentrates are not available and on the advice of a haematologist

Dysfibrinogenaemia associated with bleeding

Massive transfusion if the fibrinogen level is < 1.5 g L^{-1}

DIC if there is bleeding and the fibrinogen level is < 1.5 g L^{-1}

Bleeding associated with renal failure

Bleeding following thrombolytic therapy. Inhibitors of fibrinolysis (e.g. tranexamic acid) may also be required if the situation is life-threatening, but may result in the formation of large clots at the site of bleeding

Note that a single unit of cryoprecipitate contains 400–460 mg of fibrinogen. A 'standard' dose of cryoprecipitate is 2 pools of 5 units each, which will raise the plasma fibrinogen level by 1 g L^{-1}.

Haemostasis

The arrest of bleeding following an injury is a rapid and complex process that involves changes in the involved vessel (smooth muscle constricts and the endothelium becomes procoagulant), platelets (become activated and aggregate) and plasma (fibrin formation). Simultaneous inhibitory mechanisms ensure these processes are confined to the site of injury. Subsequently, the removal of the clot (fibrinolysis) occurs as part of tissue remodelling. Although there are newer theories of the mechanism of clot formation, the classical division into intrinsic and extrinsic systems still has validity and aids understanding.

Abnormal coagulation tests are among the commonest reasons for seeking haematological advice. In many cases, the underlying coagulation abnormality and its treatment can be deduced from a basic knowledge of the coagulation mechanism. The classical theory of blood coagulation describing intrinsic and extrinsic systems is useful for understanding in vitro coagulation tests. However, apparent paradoxes exist with the classical theory, such as the fact that haemophiliacs bleed, while patients with factor XII deficiency do not. These may be explained by more recent theories.

The classical coagulation cascade is shown in Figure 12.7. Such cascade reactions allow for considerable amplification as well as many opportunities for control of the process.

Extrinsic pathway

The extrinsic pathway is so called because to activate coagulation via this pathway a substance (i.e. tissue factor) which is normally present outside the vascular system is required. Tissue factor is a ubiquitous lipoprotein found in particularly high concentrations in placenta, brain and lung. It is also found in monocytes and endothelial cells but is only expressed when these cells are activated, e.g. by endotoxin. Tissue factor is not an enzyme, but a cofactor serving to increase the catalytic activity of factors VII and VIIa in the cleavage of factors X–Xa.

Prothrombin time (PT)

This tests the integrity of the extrinsic pathway. A source of tissue factor (thromboplastin) is added to a citrated

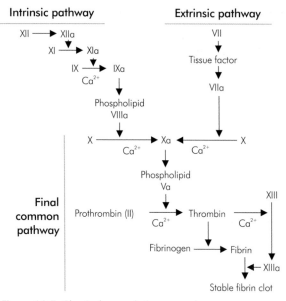

Figure 12.7 Classical coagulation cascade

Figure 12.8 Causes of a prolonged prothrombin time

Oral anticoagulant drug administration
Liver disease, hepatocellular (decreased production of factors II and VII), obstructive (decreased absorption of vitamin K)
Vitamin K deficiency
Disseminated intravascular coagulation
Hypofibrinogenaemia
Massive transfusion
Inherited deficiency of factor VII, X or V
Heparin

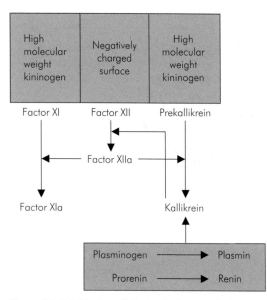

Figure 12.9 Initiation of the intrinsic coagulation pathway

plasma sample, which is followed by calcium chloride to overcome the anticoagulant effect of citrate. The time taken for a clot to form is then measured. In some laboratories the PT is expressed as an INR (international normalised ratio), in order to standardise the PT between laboratories for the purpose of monitoring anticoagulation with coumarins. The INR is the ratio of the PT to mean normal PT, raised to the power of the ISI (international sensitivity index) of the thromboplastin used in the system. Since sensitive thromboplastins (ISI close to 1.0) are usually used in the UK, the INR often approximates to the PT ratio. The commonest causes of a prolonged PT are given in Figure 12.8.

Intrinsic pathway

The intrinsic pathway was thought to activate blood coagulation by involving only substances present in the plasma. Initiation of coagulation via this pathway requires 'contact activation'. This occurs when prekallikrein (PK) and factors XII and XI are activated in the presence of high-molecular-weight kininogen (HMWK) on exposure to certain surfaces: in vivo to negatively charged surfaces such as collagen, in vitro to glass or kaolin (Figure 12.9). The sequential activation of factors XI and IX then occurs, culminating in the activation of factor X by factor IX with factor VIII as a cofactor.

Activated partial thromboplastin time (APTT)

APTT tests the intrinsic pathway and is also known as the PTTK (partial thromboplastin time with kaolin) and the KCCT (kaolin cephalin clotting time). The plasma is preincubated with kaolin and phospholipid to activate the contact factors, calcium chloride is then added, and the time for a clot to form is recorded. The sensitivities of different phospholipid reagents to deficiencies of the clinically important factors (VIII and IX) in the intrinsic pathway vary. APTT is used to monitor heparin therapy;

Figure 12.10 Causes of a prolonged APTT

Heparin therapy
Sample contamination by heparin, e.g. by taking sample from a line through which heparin has been administered (including 'Hepflush')
Liver disease
Disseminated intravascular coagulation
Hypofibrinogenaemia
Massive transfusion
Coagulation inhibitor, e.g. lupus anticoagulant, acquired factor VIII inhibitor
Inherited deficiency of factors XI, VIII, IX, X, PK or HMWK

Figure 12.11 Causes of a prolonged TT

Hypofibrinogenaemia • Disseminated intravascular coagulation • Fibrinolytic therapy • Massive transfusion • Inherited deficiency (rare)
Dysfibrinogenaemia (abnormal fibrinogen molecule) • Inherited (rare) • Acquired (liver disease most common cause)
Raised FDP levels – DIC or liver disease
Heparin

unfortunately, it has not yet been possible to standardise these reagents for the monitoring of heparins in the same way that thromboplastins have been for oral anticoagulant control, making local derivation of therapeutic ranges for heparin necessary. The most frequent causes of a prolonged APTT are shown in Figure 12.10.

Final common pathway

The final common pathway sees the conversion of prothrombin to thrombin by factor Xa, with factor Va as a cofactor. Thrombin is central in coagulation, with multiple roles:

- It cleaves fibrinogen to form fibrin monomers. These then aggregate to form fibrin strands which are subsequently cross-linked by factor XIIa, resulting in a stable clot.
- It activates factor XII.
- It activates the cofactors V and VIII.
- It induces platelet aggregation.
- It combines with thrombomodulin to activate protein C, an anticoagulant protein, which deactivates factors V and VIII.

Deficiency of factors X, V, II and fibrinogen causes prolongation of both the PT and the APTT. Hence the function of the final common pathway can be monitored by using both tests. In reality, since isolated deficiency of factors X or V is rare, the commonest reason for prolongation of both tests in a patient not receiving oral anticoagulants is hypofibrinogenaemia.

Thrombin time (TT)

The TT tests the key reaction in the coagulation cascade: the conversion of fibrinogen to fibrin. Conceptually it is the simplest of all the coagulation tests as it consists of simply adding a solution of thrombin to platelet-poor plasma and measuring the time taken for a clot to form; the addition of calcium is not necessary. TT is very sensitive to low levels of heparin, this probably being the most common reason for a prolonged TT; other reasons are shown in Figure 12.11. In many laboratories the TT is not performed as part of a routine coagulation screen, and instead the fibrinogen is measured.

Coagulation tests summary

- Prothrombin time (PT) – tests the extrinsic pathway and is used to monitor coumarin therapy
- Activated partial thromboplastin time (APTT) – tests the intrinsic pathway and is used to monitor heparin therapy
- APTT and PT – tests the final common pathway
- Thrombin time (TT) – tests fibrinogen levels

'In vivo' coagulation

The classical cascade is important in understanding what occurs in the screening coagulation tests, but it does introduces some anomalies. For example, while patients deficient in factors VIII and IX (haemophiliacs) bleed spontaneously, those with factor XII, PK or HMWK deficiency do not have a bleeding diathesis, in spite of considerably prolonged APTTs. Thus an alternative view of in vivo coagulation is required in order to

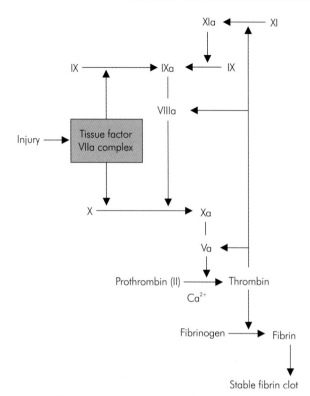

Figure 12.12 A revised coagulation hypothesis

then occurs via two highly efficient reactions, resulting in thrombin formation.

Natural inhibitors of coagulation

The cascade structure of the coagulation system ensures very rapid activation of coagulation: for example, it has been estimated that 10 mL plasma can generate sufficient thrombin to clot all the body's fibrinogen in 30 seconds; clearly this may be deleterious, so powerful inhibitors of coagulation in the plasma ensure that the haemostatic response is confined to the vicinity of the platelet plug and vascular injury.

Natural coagulation inhibitors

- Tissue factor pathway inhibitor.
- Serine protease inhibitors, the most important of which is antithrombin.
- Coagulation cofactor inhibitors (VIIIa and Va). These are protein C and protein S.

Tissue factor pathway inhibitor

Factor VIIa–TF complex is rapidly inhibited by tissue factor pathway inhibitor, so factor Xa generation must occur via the intrinsic pathway factors VIIIa/IXa. This is augmented by factor XIa, which is activated by thrombin, this being a late step in the pathway. The critical roles of factors XIa and VIIIa in this scheme are demonstrated by the severity of the bleeding when these factors are deficient. Contact activation has no place in coagulation in vivo.

Antithrombin

Antithrombin (previously called antithrombin III) complexes with the serine protease coagulation factors (thrombin, Xa, XIIa, XIa and IXa, but not VIIa) and inactivates them. The resulting inhibitor–protease complex is rapidly removed by the liver. The affinity for thrombin is highest, followed by factor Xa. Heparin binds to antithrombin and induces a 2300-fold increase in thrombin inactivation. Endothelial glycosaminoglycans act in a similar fashion. Reduction in plasma antithrombin levels results in a tendency to venous thrombosis.

Other serine protease inhibitors include heparin cofactor II, α_1-antitrypsin, C_1-esterase inhibitor, α_2-antiplasmin and α_2-macroglobulin. Deficiency of these inhibitors has not been clearly associated with thrombosis.

take into account the paradoxes offered by the classical cascade (Figure 12.12).

It is important to realise that coagulation reactions occur on surfaces, e.g. platelets, activated endothelium and subendothelial collagen. When coagulation is initiated thrombin is formed in the absence of activated factors V and VIII, and trace amounts of thrombin then activate factors V and VIII. These are large molecules that act as cofactors in their respective reactions and localise reactions to surfaces. The overall result is an increase by many thousand-fold in the efficiency of the coagulation mechanism.

Tissue factor (TF) initiates coagulation in vivo by forming a complex with factor VIIa and then activating factor X (it is not clear how factor VII is activated). This complex also activates factor IX, which is a significant departure from the classical hypothesis. The importance of this is only realised upon activation of factors V and VIII: the predominant action of the VIIa–TF complex becomes activation of factor IX, and massive amplification of the coagulation mechanism

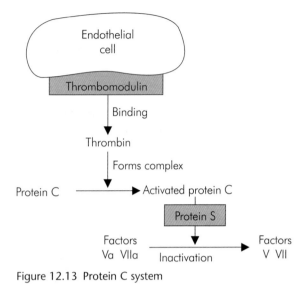

Figure 12.13 Protein C system

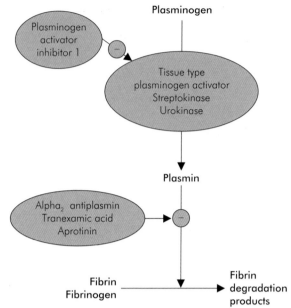

Figure 12.14 Fibrinolytic system

Protein C system

The protein C system is responsible for the inactivation of the activated cofactors Va and VIIIa. Proteins C and S are vitamin K-dependent factors. The system is represented in Figure 12.13.

Thrombin behaves as an anticoagulant when it binds to thrombomodulin, which is present on the endothelial surface. The resulting complex activates protein C, which in the presence of protein S inactivates factors Va and VIIIa by cleavage. Thus thrombosis is prevented from propagating along normal vessels close to a point of injury.

Reduced plasma levels of protein C and S are associated with thrombosis and can be inherited in an autosomal dominant fashion. Deficiency of thrombomodulin has not been described, and probably results in nonviability. The most common inherited cause of a thrombotic tendency is a mutation of factor V (factor V Leiden) which alters the activated protein C (APC) cleavage site. This is an autosomal dominant trait that results in reduced APC-induced cleavage and is demonstrated in vitro by the APC resistance (APCR) test.

Fibrinolysis

Tissue-type plasminogen activators (t-PA) are synthesised by endothelial cells and their release stimulated by venous occlusion, thrombin, adrenaline, vasopressin and strenuous exercise. t-PA activity increases dramatically when it is bound to fibrin. Intrinsic activation of fibrinolysis, via kallikrein, is also possible, but the physiological relevance is uncertain.

In vivo activity of the fibrinolytic system is assessed clinically by measuring fibrin degradation products (FDPs), which do not rely on the presence of fibrin. D-dimers, on the other hand, are only produced by digestion of crosslinked fibrin and are therefore a more specific indicator of fibrinolysis that can be used as an indicator of suspected pulmonary embolism (Figure 12.14).

Platelets

Platelets are responsible for forming the primary haemostatic plug following injury. They are produced in the bone marrow by the cytoplasmic budding of megakaryocytes. They are biconvex discs with a diameter of 2–4 μm and a volume of 5–8 fl (fl is the abbreviation for the SI unit femtolitre, L^{-15}). The normal lifespan of a platelet is between 8 and 14 days. They contain granules of which the most numerous are α granules (the contents of which are listed in Figure 12.15). Dense bodies are less numerous but are of importance as their deficiency (storage pool disease) can result in significant haemorrhage. Dense bodies contain platelet nucleotides (ADP, ATP, 5-HT).

Figure 12.15 Contents of platelet α granules

Coagulation factors – V, X, protein S
Adhesive proteins – von Willebrand factor, fibrinogen, fibronectin, vitronectin
Growth factors • platelet-derived growth factor (PDGF) • platelet factor 4 (PF4) • β-thromboglobulin

Platelets function by:

- Adhesion to the site of injury
- Aggregation to form a platelet plug at the site of injury
- Providing the surfaces to enhance the coagulation reaction
- Changing shape and releasing α granules containing growth factors which stimulate tissue repair

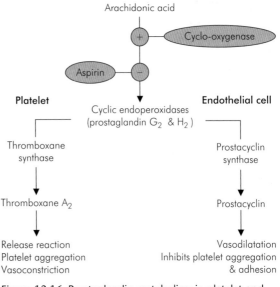

Figure 12.16 Prostaglandin metabolism in platelet and endothelial cell

Global platelet function can be tested by measuring the bleeding time, which is best performed by experienced laboratory staff using the template method (normal < 9 minutes). It should be remembered that thrombocytopenia results in prolongation of the bleeding time. Qualitative platelet defects can be assessed by platelet aggregometry to various stimuli.

Platelet aggregation

At the site of injury ADP is released from damaged cells and, following platelet release reaction, this binds to platelets and exposes the glycoprotein IIb–IIIa complex. Fibrinogen binds to this receptor, and as it is a dimeric molecule is capable of forming bridges between platelets. The other main physiological inducer of platelet aggregation is thromboxane A_2, which is a product of arachidonic acid metabolism in the platelet.

Prostaglandin metabolism in platelets

This is a critical part of platelet activation, because blocking it (with aspirin) prevents the release reaction. Arachidonic acid is released from membrane phospholipid by phospholipase A_2. Prostaglandin metabolism in the platelet and endothelial cell is shown in Figure 12.16.

Platelet adhesion

Blood vessel injury results in exposure of subendothelial collagen and microfibrils. Larger von Willebrand factor (vWF) molecules bind to the microfibrils and platelets adhere to the vWF via platelet glycoprotein Ib. Following this, the glycoprotein IIb–IIIa complex becomes exposed, which increases adhesion and is also involved in aggregation.

Platelet shape change

This occurs within seconds of adhesion. The platelet becomes more spherical and spiky, which enhances interaction between platelets. The platelet granules migrate towards the surface.

Platelet release reaction

This follows immediately and involves the release of the contents of platelet granules. It is sustained for several minutes. Thus coagulation factors, adhesive proteins, growth factors and nucleotides are delivered to the site of injury.

von Willebrand factor

von Willebrand factor consists of large molecules (multimers) made up of a variable number of subunits. It is produced in endothelial cells and megakaryocytes, then stored in Weibel–Palade bodies of endothelial cells and α granules of platelets. The main function of vWF is in platelet adhesion; however, it also acts as a carrier of factor VIII. vWF deficiency results in the most common inherited bleeding tendency – von Willebrand disease, which is estimated to occur in up to 1% of the population. It is most commonly a mild quantitative (type 1) deficiency, but type 2 (qualitative) and type 3 (severe quantitative) also occur. Deficiency of vWF produces two haemostatic defects – a prolonged bleeding time due to failure of platelet adhesion and a coagulation defect due to reduced levels of factor VIII.

The immune system

The immune system provides the body with a number of complex responses which defend it against invasion by pathogens. Defences which evolved early on in more primitive species still form part of the immune system in vertebrates. These are the 'innate' defence mechanisms, which are non-specific and are triggered at the site of infection by pathogens. Pathogens include organisms such as viruses, bacteria and protozoa as well as reproductive molecules like prions.

'Adaptive' defences have developed more recently in the evolutionary process and are part of the immune defences in vertebrates. They are highly specific, with an immunological memory enabling a more rapid and powerful response to be mounted in the event of repeated exposure to the same pathogen, thus providing long-term protection.

Both 'innate' and 'adaptive' responses integrate in the common immunological pathways of the inflammatory response and the complement cascade.

Innate and adaptive immune defences

- First-line physical barriers (innate) – skin, mucous membranes, mucociliary function
- First-line chemical barriers (innate) – tears, saliva, gastric acid, lysozyme
- Second-line cellular response (innate) – phagocytosis by neutrophils and macrophages
- Second-line chemical response (innate) – complement system, interferons
- Third-line defence (adaptive) – specific responses depending on 'immunological memory' and the production of antibodies to specific antigens, mediated by B cells and T cells

---

Innate defences

These form the first- and second-line defences in the body. Simple physical barriers such as the epidermis, mucosa and ciliary action obstruct the ingress of pathogens. These barriers are enhanced by secretions which contain chemically active substances (gastric acid, lysozyme).

Many bacteria have common surface molecules (pathogen-associated molecular patterns, PAMPs), which act as immunostimulants to the innate system, triggering phagocytosis by neutrophils and dendritic cells or activating the complement system. Mannan-binding lectin (MBL) is a serum protein which binds to the mannose and fucose residues common to many bacterial walls, and activates the MBL complement pathway.

The innate system may also activate the more powerful and selective adaptive defences in peripheral lymphoid tissue.

Phagocytosis

Phagocytosis is the ingestion of pathogens by cells of the immune system which migrate to sites of infection stimulated by chemotactic components released by microorganisms. They can then bind, engulf and kill pathogens, utilising oxidant free radicals and peroxides. Phagocytic cells include:

- **Macrophages** – which have the ability to recognise pathogens by their surface immunostimulant molecules (PAMPs). They reside in tissues or circulate as monocytes.
- **Granulocytes** – short-lived cells which provide a rapid response in large numbers at a site of infection and do not usually survive the acute encounter.
- **Dendritic cells** – which ingest pathogens but have the special function of transporting the products of ingestion to peripheral lymphoid tissue in order to activate the adaptive defence system. These cells are antigen-presenting cells (APCs).

Macrophages have specific receptors on their surface that allow them to bind to microorganisms. These include the mannosyl–fucosyl receptors (MFRs) which bind to microbial saccharides and a lipopolysaccharide binding protein (LBP) which binds Gram-negative bacteria. Once bound, the microbes are ingested to form a phagosome.

Lysosomes then merge with the phagosome, and the microorganism is killed and digested. The lysosome contents include proteolytic enzymes, peroxidase, elastase and collagenase. The presence of complement receptors on macrophages and neutrophils improves phagocytic efficiency if microorganisms are opsonised (coated) with complement. Fcγ receptors are present on the surface of monocytes/macrophages and bind the Fc portion of IgG, which also serves as an opsonin.

Cytokines

Cytokines are small peptides or glycopeptides, released by T cells, B cells and other cells of the immune system, in order to signal other cells. They play an important role in both cellular and humoral immunity responses and the inflammation pathway. These defences are central in a host reaction to infection, sepsis, cancer or trauma.

Examples of cytokines include the interleukins (lymphokines), interferons, colony-stimulating factors (CSFs) and tumour necrosis factor (TNF). Macrophages release TNF in response to invasion by microorganisms, an important part of the inflammatory response. TNF also enhances granulocyte and macrophage microbicidal capacity.

The complement cascade

'Complement', coined by Ehrlich, refers to the activity in serum which when combined with antibody results in the lysis of bacteria. Activation occurs via three main pathways.

> ### Pathways activating the complement system
>
> - The classical pathway – mediated by antigen–antibody complexes
> - The mannan-binding lectin (MBL) pathway – activation by serum protein MBL which binds to mannose and fucose residues in bacterial walls
> - The alternative pathway – direct activation by surface molecules on bacterial walls

The complement system consists of a cascade reaction involving about 20 serum proteins synthesised in the liver. Activation of the cascade results in the following. The central event of the complement pathway is the cleavage of C3 to form C3b and C3a (Figure 12.17). C3b attaches to microorganisms or immune complexes and acts as a site of membrane attack complex formation. It also acts as an opsonin. The small peptide cleaved from C3, C3a, stimulates mast cell degranulation and smooth muscle contraction.

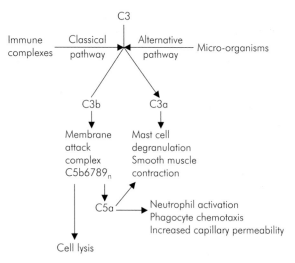

Figure 12.17 Central role of C3 in the complement pathway

> ### Functions of the complement system
>
> - Opsonisation (coating) of bacteria and immune complexes
> - Activation and attraction (chemotaxis) of phagocytes
> - Lysis of target cells by the membrane attack complex
> - Activation of phagocytosis
> - Activation of adaptive defence responses

Formation of the membrane attack complex

This is the final common pathway of complement activation. The first step is cleavage of C5 to C5a (a mediator of inflammation) and C5b. C5b can then aggregate with C6 and C7 to produce C5b67 which, being hydrophobic, attaches to plasma membranes. C8 then binds to a site on C5b and penetrates the membrane. The resulting C5b678 complex polymerises a number of C9 molecules to form the membrane attack complex (C5b6789n), which is essentially a pore in the cell membrane; lysis is thus produced.

Once the C5b67 complex is formed it can attach to any nearby membrane and produce lysis – this is sometimes called the 'innocent bystander' effect. This is prevented in the fluid phase by proteins such as vitronectin inactivating this complex. On cell membranes a protein

(MIRL, membrane inhibitor of reactive lysis) performs a similar function against membrane attack complex.

Adaptive defences

The adaptive defence system is formed by the thymus, spleen, peripheral lymphoid tissue and lymphatics. The active cells are millions of lymphocyte clones, each clone being identified by a unique cell surface receptor which recognises a specific antigen. The lymphocytes originate from haemopoietic stem cells in the bone marrow. Two types of lymphocyte mature from these stem cells: T cells, which develop in the thymus, and B cells, developing in the bone marrow. The lymphocytes circulate continuously between the blood and lymphatic system. The adaptive system is responsible for two powerful responses. Firstly, a humoral reponse using circulating antibodies and mediated through the B cells. Secondly, a cellular response involving the T cells.

Antigen presentation

Antigens are presented to T cells in order to activate them and convert the T cells to their active form, known as effector T cells. The main antigen-presenting cells (APCs) are the dendritic cells which present antigen to T cells in peripheral lymphoid tissue. Ingested pathogens are digested by the APCs into small peptides that are processed and expressed on the cell surface as complexes with class II major histocompatibility complex (MHC) proteins. Dendritic cells have many fine, long projections which maximise the surface area over which interaction with T cells can occur. They are found in the T-cell-rich areas of lymphoid tissue.

Other cell types, when stimulated, can also function as antigen-presenting cells, and these include endothelial and epithelial cells.

MHC proteins

This group of histocompatibility proteins exists on the surface of all nucleated cells, and they act as markers to distinguish 'self' tissue from 'non-self' tissue. They were originally discovered as the main antigens initiating allograft or xenograft transplant rejection. These proteins are encoded by a group of genes known as the major histocompatibility complex (MHC). There are more than 12 MHC genes with over 400 alleles, making it rare for any two individuals to have identical MHC proteins (i.e. to be tissue-matched for transplantation). Human MHC proteins are known as human lymphocyte-associated antigens (HLAs), since they were first identified in human lymphocytes.

Class I and class II MHC proteins are distinguished by structural differences. They are both transmembrane proteins with an exposed protein binding site, which enables them to form a complex with antigenic protein fragments. The peptide binding site is a groove facing outwards from the cell membrane and normally binds peptide fragments produced by normal protein degradation from within the cell.

Virtually all tissue cells express such class I MHC protein–peptide complexes, which enable the cell to be recognised as 'self' by T cells. If a cell is infected, pathogenic MHC protein–peptide complexes are formed on its surface, which marks it for T-cell destruction.

Class II MHC proteins are confined to antigen-presenting cells which ingest pathogens and form pathogenic MHC complexes on their surface to be presented to T cells and B cells in the activation of adaptive responses.

Antibody-mediated response

The antibody response recruits the complement system to kill bacteria and invading organisms; it also inactivates bacterial viruses and microbial toxins. Antigen binds to the surface immunoglobulin of specific B lymphocytes. It is processed and expressed in association with MHC molecules. The B cell is now capable of interacting with specific helper T cells (T_H cells), which will have been activated by interaction with APCs. This B–T interaction results in delivery of stimulatory cytokines by the T_H cells, and the result is the proliferation and then differentiation of B cells to produce plasma cells and then antibody (Figure 12.18).

When activated, **B cells** produce a systemic response by releasing antibodies into the circulation which:

- Inactivate bacterial toxins
- Activate the complement system which kills pathogens
- Inactivate viruses

A proportion of B cells, rather than differentiating to form plasma cells, enter a resting phase to become memory B cells (B_M). Similarly a subpopulation of the stimulated T_H population will become memory T_H cells.

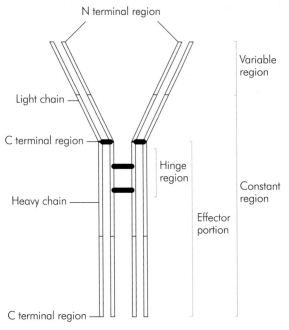

Figure 12.19 Antibody structure

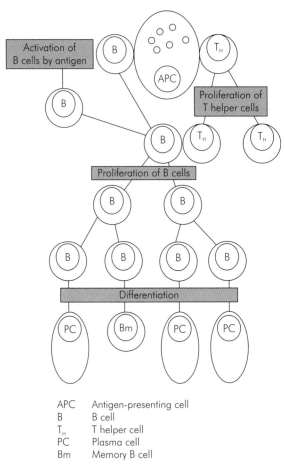

APC	Antigen-presenting cell
B	B cell
T$_H$	T helper cell
PC	Plasma cell
Bm	Memory B cell

Figure 12.18 B-cell activation and interaction with T cells

Antibody structure, subtypes and diversity

Immunoglobulins are composed of four peptide chains – two heavy chains (IgH) and two light chains (Figure 12.19). There are five structural heavy chain variants to produce IgG, IgM, IgA, IgD and IgE. IgM is pentameric and IgA dimeric. There are two structural light chain variants – κ and λ. Most of the molecule consists of framework on which the highly variable antigen binding site is located. Diversity of antigen binding sites is achieved by immunoglobulin gene rearrangement at the DNA level where a variable gene (V, one of several hundred), joining gene (J, one of six) and diversity gene (D, one of 30) are combined to produce a unique gene in each developing B cell, which then produces the unique antigen binding site. More refinement is achieved with point mutation of the VDJ recombination, and this may occur during B-cell activation and proliferation. Subsequently the best antigen–antibody matches selectively proliferate, enhancing the overall response. The relatively frequent occurrence of recombinational inaccuracy of the VDJ adds a further mechanism of diversity generation.

Primary and secondary antibody responses

Following an initial antigen challenge there is a lag phase where no antibody is detectable. Then there is a logarithmic increase in antibody levels to a plateau, and there follows a decline to low or undetectable levels. Such a primary response consists predominantly of IgM, with IgG present but appearing slightly later. If the individual is challenged again, then there is a shorter lag phase before antibody is detected, the rise in antibody titre is up to 10 times greater than in the primary response, the plateau is more prolonged and the decline is slow. The secondary response consists almost entirely of IgG, and the affinity of the antibodies is greater, a process called antibody maturation.

A typical example of primary and secondary antibody responses occurs with a delayed haemolytic transfusion reaction. Initial exposure to the foreign red cell antigen results in no clinical effects, but low-level antibody is produced and subsequently declines. Antibody screening after the decline may miss a low-level antibody, but should the individual be exposed to the antigen again, a brisk secondary response occurs which results in the destruction of the antibody-coated transfused red cells by the mononuclear phagocyte system. Clinically this is apparent after 4–14 days when the patient presents with anaemia, fever and jaundice.

Cell-mediated immunity

Cell-mediated immunity in the adaptive system is mediated via T cells which have been activated. These activated T cells are known as effector T cells. Effector T cells come in three types: cytotoxic T cells, helper T cells and regulatory T cells.

> **Effector T cells** migrate to infection sites to produce a cellular response. Three different types of effector T cells are formed:
>
> - Cytotoxic T cells – which kill infected cells by inducing apoptosis
> - Helper T (T_H) cells – which activate B cells, macrophages, dendritic cells and cytotoxic T cells by displaying proteins and secreting cytokines
> - Regulatory T cells – which inhibit the function of cytotoxic T cells, helper T cells and dendritic cells

T-cell receptors (TCRs)

Effector T cells express a diverse set of receptors on their surface (TCRs) which enable them to bind to MHC–peptide complexes presented to them. TCRs are dimers which are transmembrane bound, and consist of two chains, an α and a β chain. The antigen binding site is provided by the ends of these chains, which protrude away from the cell membrane. T cells use similar mechanisms to generate TCR diversity as employed by B cells in generating antibody diversity. The genes for α and β chains are located on two different chromosomes with V, D and J segments.

Interaction between antigen-presenting cells (APCs) and T lymphocytes

When a pathogen is ingested by an APC, peptide fragments from the ingested pathogen bind to the peptide groove of MHC forming MHC–peptide complexes, in the rough endoplasmic reticulum of APCs. These MHC

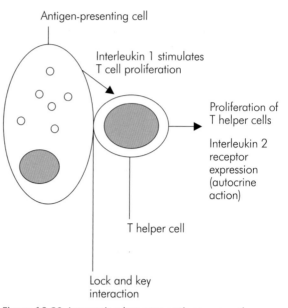

Figure 12.20 Interaction between antigen-presenting cell and T_H cell

complexes are then expressed on the cell surface as pathogenic complexes which can be recognised by T-cell receptors (TCRs), resulting in the activation of cytotoxic T cells and helper T cells. APC antigen presentation can also render T cells tolerant to a presented antigen, enabling effector T cells to recognise 'self' tissue.

Further molecular interactions occur once the cells are brought into close proximity by this interaction (Figure 12.20). The result is an exchange of cytokines including interleukin 1 (IL-1), produced by macrophages, which stimulates T_H proliferation and expression of interleukin 2 (IL-2) receptors on T_H cells. Activation of T cells also results in the production of interferon γ, which stimulates the expression of MHC molecules on macrophages, producing positive feedback.

These processes are the first events following challenge by a new antigen, and the development of an effective immune response depends on the production, by proliferation, of adequate numbers of T_H cells. An immune response follows, and this can be antibody-mediated (a B-cell function) or cell-mediated (a T-cell and macrophage function).

Similar expression of pathogenic MHC complexes occurs in cells which have been infected by viruses. These complexes label the damaged cells for destruction by cytotoxic T cells, which activate apoptosis.

CD4 and CD8 co-receptors

The affinity between MHC–peptide complexes and TCRs alone is not strong enough to produce a functional interaction between an APC and a cytotoxic or helper T cell. An accessory or co-receptor is needed to increase the adhesion between APC and T cell before activation of the T cells can occur. CD4 and CD8 proteins are the best recognised co-receptors on T cells. The co-receptors recognise MHC class II and MHC class I proteins respectively, and provide the enhanced adhesion required for APC and T-cell interaction to take place.

T-cell mechanisms

Cytotoxic T cells (Tc)

A subpopulation of peripheral blood lymphocytes forms cytotoxic T cells (Tc). These recognise antigen when presented in association with the relevant MHC molecules. Tc cells are important in recognising and destroying virus-infected cells.

The antigen associated with an MHC molecule is recognised by the T-cell receptor (TCR) in the same way that T_H cells recognise antigen presented by APCs. The TCR is analogous to the immunoglobulin molecule expressed on the surface of B cells in that diversity is generated by similar mechanisms.

Other cytotoxic cells

- Natural killer cells (NK cells) do not have rearranged TCR genes. It is thought that they recognise tumour-associated antigens. They also have Fc receptors on their surface and can destroy antibody-coated cells.
- Lymphokine-activated killer cells (LAK cells) are formed by the culture of peripheral lymphocytes in IL-2. Enhanced tumour killing results. It is thought that LAK cells are activated NK cells.
- Antibody-dependent cell-mediated cytotoxicity (ADCC) requires effector cells to have an Fc receptor. Antibody-coated cells are thus recognised and destroyed. Cells capable of such killing are Tc cells, NK cells, mononuclear phagocytes and granulocytes.

The role of T_H cells in cell-mediated immunity is very important, as T_H cells provide cytokines necessary for activation and proliferation.

The inflammatory response

The clinical signs of inflammation are heat, redness, swelling, pain and reduced function. Inflammation is a response to injury or invasion by pathogens. Three fundamental events are involved:

- **Hyperaemia** – there is an increase in blood supply to the affected area. This is a result of arteriolar relaxation.
- **Exudation** – there is an increase in capillary permeability resulting from retraction of endothelial cells. Larger molecules are allowed to pass across the endothelium, and thus plasma enzyme systems reach the site of inflammation.
- **Emigration of leucocytes** – initially phagocytes and then lymphocytes migrate between endothelial cells into the surrounding tissues along chemotactic gradients.

Pathologically, inflammation is diagnosed when there are increased numbers of granulocytes, macrophages and lymphocytes in a tissue section.

Mediators of inflammation

The kinin system

The products of this system mediate the immediate vasoactive response (Figure 12.21).

Histamine and leukotrienes (B_4 and D_4)

These are released by basophils and their tissue equivalent, mast cells, after stimulation by microbes, and result in increased vascular permeability. Leukotrienes together with neutrophil chemotactic factor (also produced by mast cells) stimulate the migration of granulocytes to sites of invasion or injury. Leukotrienes are products of arachidonic acid metabolism via the lipoxygenase pathway.

Neutrophil adhesion and migration across the endothelium

Under normal, steady-state conditions, while leucocytes flow in close proximity to the endothelium they do not adhere to it. At sites of inflammation, endothelial cells become activated by mediators such as TNF-α, and one of the effects of this is adhesion molecule synthesis and expression on the surface of endothelial cells. One of the first to be expressed is E-selectin (4–12 hours); later, intercellular adhesion molecule 1 (ICAM-1) is produced.

Neutrophils, upon stimulation by inflammatory mediators, express preformed adhesion molecules such as LFA-1 and CR3. The result is neutrophil adhesion. The neutrophil then, attracted by chemotactic agents, migrates between endothelial cells and along the subendothelial matrix of collagen, laminin, etc., using different adhesion

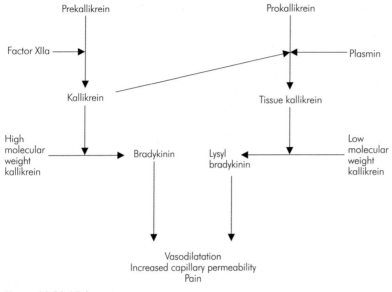

Figure 12.21 Kinin system

molecules, to sites of injury. Lymphocytes and macrophages migrate in a similar way, but later than neutrophils.

Once present at the site of injury, neutrophils release mediators including platelet activating factor (PAF), which stimulates mediator release from platelets and increases vascular permeability and smooth muscle contraction. PAF also activates other neutrophils. Macrophages and monocytes also migrate along the same chemotactic gradients and engulf microbes, as well as presenting antigens to T and B lymphocytes as described above. Mononuclear cells and lymphocytes release cytokines.

Tumour necrosis factor

TNF is a mediator of inflammation released by macrophages and lymphocytes in the presence of bacterial pathogens. It activates endothelial cells and enhances phagocytic function. Activated endothelium becomes procoagulant, adhesive and more permeable, and produces increased nitric oxide, resulting in smooth muscle relaxation and vasodilatation. TNF and nitric oxide are important mediators of septic shock.

Complement

Complement components C3a and C5a are inflammatory mediators, and their production is described below. Both stimulate mast cell degranulation and smooth

muscle contraction. C5a also increases capillary permeability, activates neutrophils and stimulates phagocyte chemotaxis.

Other plasma enzyme systems are also involved in inflammation, namely the coagulation cascade and the fibrinolytic system. FDPs are capable of increasing vascular permeability and stimulating neutrophil and macrophage chemotaxis.

Hypersensitivity

Hypersensitivity occurs when an otherwise beneficial immune response is inappropriate or exaggerated, resulting in tissue damage. It occurs on re-exposure to the antigen concerned, and the damage may be due to one or more of four mechanisms – referred to as types I, II, III and IV hypersensitivity.

Type I

Type I hypersensitivity, also referred to as immediate hypersensitivity, is an IgE-mediated response. IgE is released by B cells and binds to tissue mast cells via their Fc receptors. If the antigen is subsequently encountered it binds to the mast-cell-bound IgE, and stimulates mast cell degranulation and release of preformed mediators (Figure 12.22). The clinical effects depend on the site where the antigen is encountered. In the skin eczema or urticaria will result; if the antigen is

Figure 12.22 Mediators released by tissue mast cells and their actions

Mediator	Action
Histamine	Vasodilatation Increases vascular permeability, smooth muscle contraction
Platelet activating factor (PAF)	Platelet degranulation and aggregation leading to microthrombi formation & neutrophil chemotaxis
Tryptase	Protease acting to cleave C3 to C3a and C3b
Kininogenase	Activates kinin system
Cytokines, e.g. IL-5, TNF-α, IL-8	Granulocyte chemotaxis including eosinophils and basophils
Leukotriene B$_4$	Basophil chemotaxis
Leukotriene C$_4$ & D$_4$	Smooth muscle contraction Mucosal oedema Increased mucus secretion

inhaled asthma occurs; in the nasal passages allergic rhinitis (hay fever) develops.

In severe cases the reaction can be generalised, producing anaphylactic shock. The mechanism is the same but there is widespread mediator release. This response should be distinguished from the anaphylactoid reaction that can be induced by certain drugs (e.g. codeine and morphine) which act on mast cells directly and not via IgE.

Mast cell tryptase testing in anaphylaxis

Beta-tryptase is an abundant protease stored in mast cell granules, and it is released in anaphylactic and anaphylactoid reactions. Testing for peak mast cell tryptase levels following a suspected anaphylactic reaction can be performed to help in the diagnosis of the cause of cardiovascular collapse during anaesthesia. An initial blood sample should be taken as soon as possible, following the commencement of resuscitation (as long as this does not delay treatment in any way), and following this a further sample between 1 and 2 hours after onset.

Figure 12.23 Examples of immune-complex-related diseases

Infections
- Bacterial endocarditis
- Hepatitis B
- Dengue fever

Autoimmune diseases
- Rheumatoid arthritis
- Systemic lupus erythematosus (SLE)
- Polyarteritis nodosa and microscopic polyarteritis
- Polymyositis
- Cutaneous vasculitis
- Fibrosing alveolitis
- Cryoglobulinaemia

Type II

This occurs when IgG and/or IgM molecules interact with complement to produce target cell damage. An example of this is Goodpasture's syndrome, where an antibasement membrane immunoglobulin is produced. This together with complement is deposited on the glomerular and pulmonary basement membranes, resulting in renal failure and pulmonary haemorrhage.

Type III

This is a result of the production of large quantities of immune complex that cannot be adequately cleared by the mononuclear phagocyte system. There is often widespread deposition of these immune complexes that activate complement via the classical pathway. There are numerous diseases that are immune-complex-related (Figure 12.23), and their clinical features reflect the sites of deposition.

Type IV

Type IV hypersensitivity reactions are produced by cell-mediated mechanisms and generally take > 12 hours to develop. Previously called delayed hypersensitivity, three types are described:
- Contact hypersensitivity, which is a cutaneous reaction, maximal at 48–72 hours. Most commonly this is in response to a hapten, which is a molecule too small to induce an immune response.
- Tuberculin-type hypersensitivity, which is maximal at 48–72 hours, is the reaction that occurs after intradermal injection of tuberculin.

- Granulomatous hypersensitivity is most important clinically because it is responsible for diseases such as tuberculosis, leprosy, schistosomiasis, leishmaniasis and sarcoidosis. Again, T_H cells are critical in the production of these reactions, which result from a continuous antigen stimulus or where macrophages are unable to destroy the antigen. The result is granuloma formation in the presence of antigen.

Immunodeficiency

Immune-deficient states may result from congenital conditions such as Down's syndrome, oroticaciduria or hereditary asplenia. Immune deficiency may be acquired following infection (e.g. with HIV) or associated with leukaemias or lymphomas. Iatrogenic immunodeficiency may also occur following the administration of steroids or immunosuppressants.

HIV and AIDS

The human immunodeficiency virus (HIV) is responsible for the aquired immunodeficiency syndrome (AIDS). HIV is a member of the retroviruses, which are characterised by their ability to synthesise their own DNA from the host cell RNA (using reverse transcriptase) and incorporate this DNA into the host cell genome.

The incorporated HIV genome down-regulates the CD4 co-receptor protein in T-cell lymphocytes, stimulates a release of virions from infected cells and produces a fall in the CD4 T-lymphocyte count, which may fall to < 200 per microlitre.

HIV infection can result in a spectrum of clinical conditions:

- Category A states – which may be largely asymptomatic with lymphadenopathy
- Category B states – with conditions such as candidiasis, cervical dysplasia and herpes zoster
- Category C states – which include the category B conditions as well as a range of more severe conditions such as sarcomas, lymphomas, herpes simplex and *Pneumocystis* infections

---

Occupational transmission of HIV

HIV infection can be transmitted via needlestick injury from a person with known HIV infection. The risk of this occurring has been estimated at 0.3%. The incidence of seroconversion following mucous membrane or unbroken skin exposure is thought to be considerably lower than this. It is thought that the larger the volume of infected blood involved in an exposure through broken skin the greater the risk of seroconversion. Following exposure, the use of an antiretroviral agent such as zidovudine can reduce the risk of seroconversion.

Muscle physiology

Edwin Mitchell

Muscle is a specialised type of excitable tissue that provides several functions:

- Physical support of body tissues
- Mechanical response to environmental and endogenous stimuli
- Metabolic stores of glycogen and glucose
- Metabolic stores of protein for gluconeogenesis
- Thermoregulation (shivering)

There are three main types of muscle fibre in the body:

1. Skeletal (striated)
2. Smooth
3. Cardiac

Although all three types share some common characteristics, there are also important differences which will be individually discussed below. Cardiac muscle will be more fully described in Chapter 14. A summary table is provided in Figure 13.1 highlighting the differences between the muscle types and should be referred to in concert with the fuller descriptions.

Skeletal muscle

Skeletal muscles function to maintain posture and enable movement. They are under voluntary control and consist

Figure 13.1 Comparison of muscle types

Property	Skeletal muscle	Smooth muscle	Cardiac muscle
Structure			
Motor endplate	Yes	No	No
Mitochondria	Plentiful	Few	Plentiful
Sarcomere	Yes	No	Yes
Sarcoplasmic reticulum	Well developed	Poorly developed	Well developed
Syncytium	No	Yes	Yes
Function			
Pacemaker	No	Sometimes	Yes
Response	All or none	Graded	All or none
Actin:myosin ratio	6:1	10:1	4:1
Tetanic contraction	Yes	Yes	No

Fundamentals of Anaesthesia, 4th edition, ed. Ted Lin, Tim Smith and Colin Pinnock. Published by Cambridge University Press. © Cambridge University Press 2017.

of a muscle belly attached by tendons at either end to bony structures.

Anatomy of skeletal muscle
Macroscopic structure
The muscle belly contains several fasciculi and is enclosed within the epimysium. The individual fascicles are made up of bundles of muscle cells, or muscle fibres, which are surrounded by a perimysium. Individual fibres are surrounded by an endomysium made up of connective tissue, and containing capillaries and lymphatics (Figure 13.2).

Microscopic structure
Each muscle cell runs the length of the muscle belly and is polynucleate. The vast majority of muscle cells are innervated by a single nerve ending, located at the centre of the muscle belly. The cell wall of the muscle cell is called the sarcolemma, which contains both the lipid bilayer membrane and an outer layer of polysaccharide and collagen which fuse together at the ends of the fibre with the tendons. Within the sarcolemma, each muscle fibre contains hundreds of myofibrils suspended in the specialised cytoplasm called sarcoplasm. The sarcoplasm is notable for containing the large numbers of mitochondria needed to power muscle contraction, and the sarcoplasmic reticulum. The sarcoplasmic reticulum is a specialised organelle and provides an intracellular store of calcium ions. It is wound tightly around the myofibrils. Long invaginations of the sarcolemma called T tubules penetrate deep into the cell and provide a mechanism for surface depolarisation to reach all parts of the mechanical apparatus contained within the myofibrils.

Myofibrils are compsed of adjacent blocks of actin and myosin, called sarcomeres, giving a characteristic 'light' and 'dark' pattern on polarised light microscopy (Figure 13.3). The light band is referred to as the 'I' band and contains only thin myofilaments containing actin, whereas the dark or 'A' bands contain both thick myofilaments made of myosin and the overlapping ends of some actin filaments. A and I refer to the anisotropic and isotropic appearance of the bands on polarised light microscopy. Each block of actin and myosin is separated by a Z line, and an H line is seen running through the middle of the I band. The side-by-side arrangement of actin and myosin is maintained by titin, a large protein.

There are two T tubules for each sarcomere, positioned at each end of the myosin filaments (Figure 13.4).

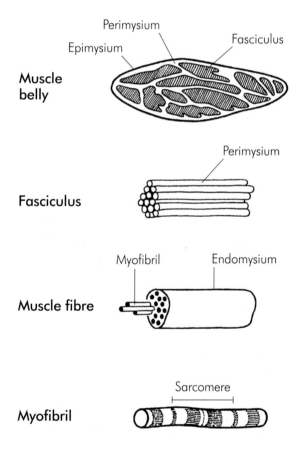

Figure 13.2 Macroscopic structure of skeletal muscle

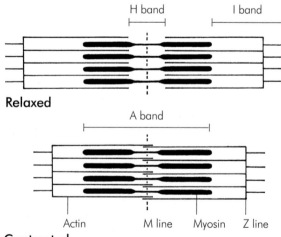

Figure 13.3 Structure of a sarcomere

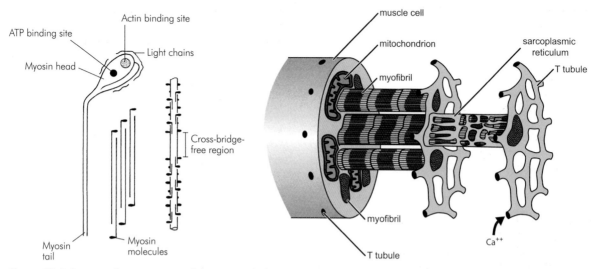

Figure 13.4 Separated components of the sarcotubular system

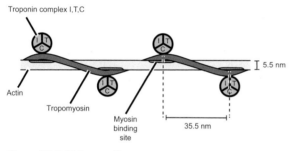

Figure 13.5 Thin myofilament

Thin myofilament

The thin myofilament comprises a complex of two molecules of actin and a molecule of tropomyosin bound up in a helical arrangement (Figure 13.5). At each half-turn of the helix, another protein complex called troponin is bound to the actin/tropomyosin structure. Troponin is made up from three complexes, troponin I, troponin T and troponin C.

Thick myofilament

The thick myofilament is made of myosin molecules. Each myosin molecule consists of a long 'tail' and two shorter 'head' regions (Figure 13.6). Each head region contains an ATP and an actin binding site. The myosin molecules are packed together in a helical bundle, with the heads

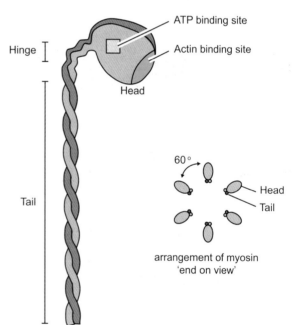

Figure 13.6 Thick myofilament

sticking outwards, between the thin myofilaments. The 'headless' region between adjacent myosin chains corresponds to the H line seen on light microscopy.

Actin and myosin bind strongly to each other, forming links between the head of the myosin molecules and active sites on the actin molecules. In the presence of tropomyosin and troponin, this binding does not occur. It is thought that the inhibitory action of tropomyosin and troponin itself has to be inhibited to allow muscle contraction to occur.

The sequential steps in muscle contraction

1. Action potential depolarises nerve ending attached to muscle cell, releasing small amounts of acetylcholine.
2. Acetylcholine acts as a neurotransmitter and on binding with acetylcholine receptors on the muscle cell membrane causes depolarisation of the sarcolemma, identically to a nerve membrane.
3. Depolarisation spreads rapidly across the sarcolemma, including the portions deep within the cell, via the T tubules.
4. Depolarisation of the cell causes release of calcium from the sarcoplasmic reticulum.
5. Calcium ions bind to troponin C, releasing the inhibition of tropomyosin on actin and allowing actin to bind to myosin.
6. Repeated binding of actin and myosin causes the molecules to slide alongside one another, causing muscular shortening.
7. The calcium is pumped back into the sarcoplasmic reticulum, troponin/tropomyosin inhibits actin and myosin binding once again, and contraction stops.

Muscle contraction

Muscle contraction occurs as a sequence of events beginning with depolarisation of the motor nerve cell endings and resulting in shortening of the myofibrils. The process linking nerve cell depolarisation to muscle cell contraction is known as **excitation–contraction coupling**.

Excitation–contraction coupling

Nerve endings attached to muscles form specialised neuromuscular junctions (NMJs). The end of the nerve is flattened into an unmyelinated terminal button and the muscle cell wall opposite is thickened and convoluted into junctional folds. Between the two cells there is a space, the junctional gap (Figure 13.7).

When the nerve ending is depolarised, vesicles containing acetylcholine (ACh) fuse with the cell membrane, releasing the ACh into the junctional gap. Approximately 60 vesicles fuse, each containing around 4000 molecules of ACh. The ACh diffuses across the gap, and binds to nicotinic acetylcholine receptors on the muscle wall. Each muscle end plate contains around 50 million acetylcholine receptors, but activation of as few as 25,000 is sufficient to cause muscle depolarisation. With approximately 240,000 molecules of ACh being released with each nerve ending depolarisation, there is a 10:1 excess of neurotransmitter above the necessary threshold, ensuring reliable neurotransmission.

The nicotinic acetylcholine receptor is made of five protein subunits and spans the lipid bilayer of the muscle

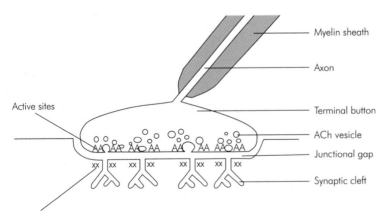

Figure 13.7 Structure of the NMJ

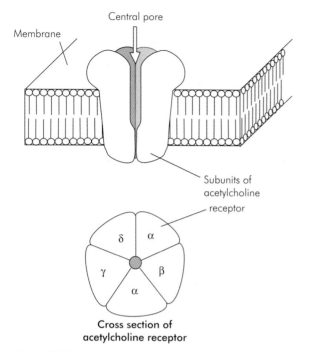

Figure 13.8 Acetylcholine receptor structure

Ryanodine receptors

These receptors function as calcium channels when activated, and calcium moves down its concentration gradient out of the sarcoplasmic reticulum and into the sarcoplasm where the calcium concentration increases 100- to 1000-fold (10^{-8} to 10^{-5} mol L^{-1}).

Ryanodine receptor mutations are important in anaesthesia because they are responsible for malignant hyperthermia and central core disease, and dantrolene is an inhibitor of the ryanodine receptor.

cell. Binding of acetylcholine on the α subunit causes a conformational change and opens a pore in the receptor, allowing the rapid passage of sodium down its concentration gradient into the cell and causing muscle cell membrane depolarisation (Figure 13.8).

Myofibril depolarisation is analogous to nerve cell depolarisation, but with some differences. The resting membrane potential of muscle is around –90 mV and the action potential lasts 2–4 ms. Conduction of the action potential travels at around 5 m s^{-1}. Initiation of myofibril contraction involves the interaction of three components of the sarcotubular system, the T-tubule, the sarcoplasmic reticulum and the sarcolemma. These form the 'sarcotubular triad' (Figure 13.9).

Depolarisation of the sarcolemma is sensed by dihydropyridine receptors in the T tubules. Dihydropyridine receptors are voltage-sensitive calcium channels and are attached to ryanodine receptors. Ryanodine receptors span both the sarcoplasmic reticulum membrane and connect to sarcolemma. The signal received from the dihydropyridine receptors induces a conformational change in the ryanodine receptor.

The released calcium binds to troponin C, causing it to change the physical shape of the other troponin (I and T) molecules. The whole troponin complex then displaces tropomyosin on the actin molecule, exposing myosin binding sites. Myosin binding to actin causes a further displacement of the tropomyosin molecule, exposing more myosin binding sites on the actin molecule and encouraging further cross-bridges to be made.

Myosin binding to actin triggers a conformational change in the myosin molecule, causing the head to move backwards, and as a result the two molecules start to move. This is the so-called 'power stroke' (Figure 13.10). Once the myosin head has changed position, it is released by the actin, is reset and is free to bind to the actin once again. This process, repeated thousands of times, causes the molecules to 'walk' past each other, resulting in macroscopic muscle contraction. This process continues in each sarcomere until the myosin molecules reach the Z plate. Each sarcomere may shorten from around 3.5 to 1.5 μm in length.

Evidence for these conformational changes comes from electron microscopy and x-ray interference studies.

Approximately 50 ms after a single depolarisation, the calcium ions are pumped back into the sarcoplasmic reticulum, actinomyosin slides back over the actin active sites and relaxation occurs (Figure 13.11). The calcium pump in the sarcoplasmic reticulum is continually active throughout this muscle contraction, and calcium concentration in the sarcoplasm starts to fall before maximum power is generated by the sarcomere. Although muscle cells exhibit a refractory period (like nerves), repeated depolarisation allows the concentration of calcium in the sarcoplasm to increase faster than the calcium pump can return it to the sarcoplamic reticulum, and maximum power may then be generated.

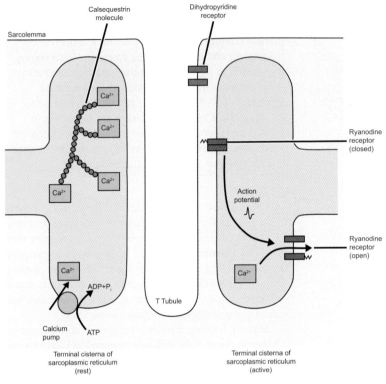

Figure 13.9 Sarcotubular triad

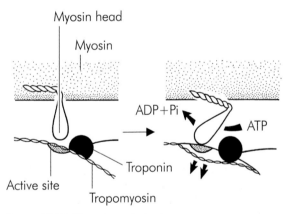

Figure 13.10 The power stroke

Mechanics of skeletal muscle contraction
Single fibre

A single fibre responds to a single nerve impulse by generating a single contraction, known as a 'twitch' (Figure 13.12). The strength of the twitch is dependent on the muscle type and the applied load.

Motor unit

The nerve supplying a muscle will have multiple branches, each branch innervating a number of muscle cells. The muscle cells innervated by a single nerve branch are called a 'motor unit', since all the muscle cells contract together as one. Muscles requiring a fine amount of control have small motor units, muscles where less control is required have larger motor units. For example, in the eye, a motor unit may consist of 20 muscle cells, in the calf muscles a motor unit may be 2000 muscle cells. The muscle cells within a motor unit may be distributed throughout the muscle evenly or concentrated within a particular part of the muscle.

Motor unit summation

The motor signal from the central nervous system producing a muscular movement consists of a sequence of impulses, which continues as the muscle contracts. The α motor nerve cells are activated in a particular order, so that motor units are recruited sequentially. Smaller motor units are activated first, followed by larger more powerful motor units.

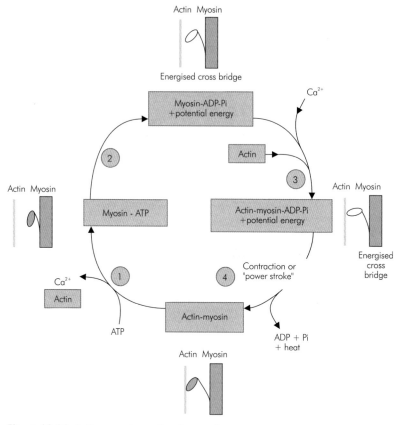

Figure 13.11 Actin–myosin contraction cycle:

1. ATP binds to myosin, releasing the actin and Ca^{2+}.
2. ATP is hydrolysed, energising the myosin but retaining the ADP and Pi produced.
3. In the presence of Ca^{2+} and actin reattachment of the energised myosin occurs.
4. The power stroke occurs with release of the ADP and Pi.

Henneman's size principle

This decribes the order in which motor units are recruited when a muscle movement is initiated. Small motor units contract first, followed by larger units. This allows a graduated response, preserving fine control at the beginning of a movement, and is energy-efficient. Small motor units typically have fatigue-resistant muscle fibres, permitting low-power movements to be made for prolonged periods. Recruitment of the larger muscle units allows more powerful work to be done, but only for short periods of time.

Frequency summation

To maintain a contraction within a muscle, multiple nerve impulses are sent to the motor units. At low frequencies of nerve impulses, single twitches are generated within the motor units, but as the frequency increases, there is insufficient time for calcium ions to be pumped back into the sarcoplasmic reticulum and the muscle cell stays in a state of tetanic contraction (Figure 13.13). Another feature of this is that the strength of the individual muscle cell contraction increases as the actin and myosin contractile apparatus becomes flooded with calcium ions.

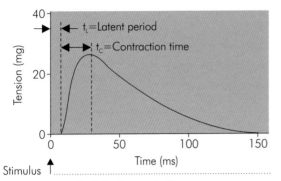

(a) Isometric twitch of single muscle fibre

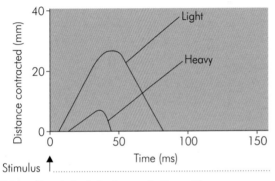

(b) Isotonic twitch of single muscle fibre with light load and heavy load

Figure 13.12 Single fibre twitch response

The duration of continuous whole muscle contraction

This is limited by:

- Exhausting glycogen stores within the muscle
- Decreased firing rate of the motor nerve cells
- Reduction of the blood supply through the contracted muscle
- Diminishing oxygen supply as the blood supply decreases

Muscle tone

Skeletal muscle movements do not occur without motor nerve stimulation. However, most muscles are partially contracted at all times, a state known as tone. This helps to maintain posture via a low-frequency discharge of motor nerve cells controlled by the central nervous system using feedback from muscle spindles (see below).

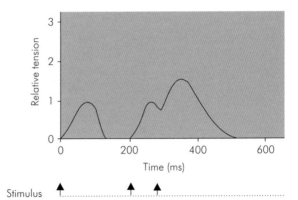

(a) Repeated isometric twitches of single muscle fibre

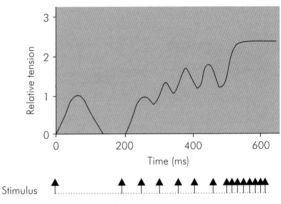

(b) High-frequency twitches of single muscle fibre giving tetany

Figure 13.13 Single fibre repeated twitch response

Rigor mortis

Rigor mortis is a state of muscle contraction that occurs after death. The calcium pump in the sarcoplasmic reticulum stops and calcium ions are available in the sarcoplasm to remove the inhibitory effect of tropomyosin. Actin binds to myosin, and muscle contraction occurs. There is no ATP available to release the myosin from the actin, however, and the muscles remain contracted. The muscles remain in rigor mortis until autolysis physically destroys the muscle proteins.

Skeletal muscle fibre types

It has long been recognised that different muscles have different speeds of contraction in response to a stimulus, and that this correlates to a degree with the macroscopic

Figure 13.14 Characteristics of different striated muscle fibre types

Characteristic	Type Ia	Type IIa	Type IIx (also known as IIb)
Colour	Red	Red	White
Capillary network	Dense	Dense	Sparse
Myoglobin content	High	High	Low
Mitochondria content	High	High	Lower
Contraction speed	Slow	Moderate	Fast
Size of motor neurone	Small	Medium	Large
Metabolism	Fast oxidative	Slow oxidative	Fast glycolytic
Fatigue rate	Slow	Slow	Fast
Glycogen content	Low	Medium	High
Needed for (e.g.)	Long-distance running	Middle-distance running	Sprinting
Myosin heavy chain gene	MYH7	MYH2	MYH1

colour of the muscle, with red muscles contracting more slowly than white muscles. Further investigations have shown that the red muscles contain a higher amount of myoglobin and a denser capillary network than white muscles, and although they contract more slowly they are more adapted for performing work over a prolonged period. Although most muscles contain a mixture of 'white' and 'red' muscle cells, all the cells belonging to a particular motor unit are the same colour. Red muscle motor units are activated first in any particular muscle contraction.

Histochemical staining for ATPase (on the myosin heads) and the predominant type of muscle metabolism allows classification of muscle cells into three groups (Figure 13.14).

Classically, a sprinter's muscles contain large amounts of white cells, and an endurance runner's muscles large amounts of red cells. Muscular training can affect the relative proportions of red and white fibres. With ageing and inactivity, the relative proportion of white fibres increases as the red fibres appear to atrophy preferentially.

Modulation of the motor response
Muscle spindles
Sequential activation of motor units provides the basic control for strength response. The muscle spindle system provides backgound tone and modulation for accurate movements. Muscle spindles are fusifom structures located within each muscle belly (Figure 13.15). They are innervated by both sensory (Ia and IIa afferents) and γ motor nerves.

Static and dynamic muscle spindle signals

Muscle spindles provide both a static signal, to report their current length, and a dynamic signal as they are stretched by muscle movement. The static signal helps to maintain current muscle length, and hence functions such as posture. The dynamic signal helps modulate the rate of contraction and helps smooth out muscle contraction.

When muscle spindles are stretched, stretch-sensitive ion channels in the sensory nerves open, causing depolarisation and generation of action potentials in the Ia and IIa nerves. Ia nerve cells synapse monosynaptically with α motor neurones within the spinal cord to increase the rate of α motor nerve cell firing to the muscle generating the signal and thus oppose the stretch. They also interact polysynaptically (via Renshaw cells) with inhibitory motor neurones of antagonistic muscles. IIa nerves have

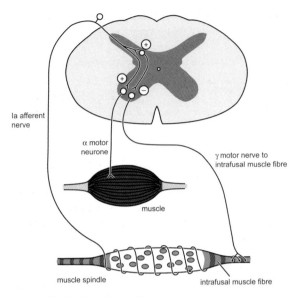

Figure 13.15 Muscle spindle

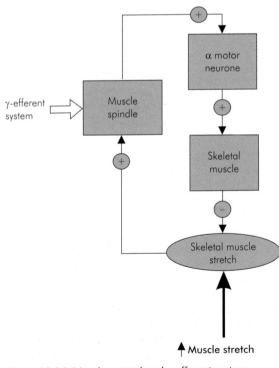

Figure 13.16 Muscle control and γ-efferent system

a smaller velocity-sensitive response than Ia nerves, and may be more important in proprioception.

The γ fibres cause contraction of the muscle fibres within the muscle spindles (Figure 13.16). This effectively pre-tensions the spindles and sets their sensitivity. When γ tone is low, muscles become flaccid and have low tone. When γ tone is high, the muscles become hypertonic and respond to stretch vigorously. γ-Efferent system tone is controlled by the central nervous system.

Golgi tendon organs

Golgi tendon organs are encapsulated specialised nerve endings that are wrapped around small bundles of tendon fibres, just distal to where the muscle cells fuse with the tendon (Figure 13.17). Each tendon organ encapsulates around 10–20 muscle fibres, and signals from them are passed via Ib nerves to the spinal cord.

Tendon organs sense tension developing in the muscle, and their discharge is inhibitory in nature, i.e. it is a (poly-synaptic) negative feedback mechanism (Figure 13.18). This mechanism prevents too much tension developing in the muscle and potentially damaging the muscle itself. However, the organ is active at all muscle tensions, not just at the extremes of power generation as had previously been thought. It has also been suggested that the tendon organ has a role in equalising the tension developed by different parts of the muscle.

Muscle metabolism

Hydrolysis of ATP to ADP and Pi provides the energy to drive the power stroke of the muscle.

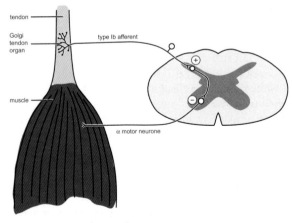

Figure 13.17 Golgi tendon organ

muscle contraction may be sustained for up to a minute anaerobically as a result of glycolysis.

Oxidative phosphorylation in mitochondria

This process supplies most energy during moderate exercise and requires oxygen. Myocytes are packed full of the mitochondria required to produce large amounts of ATP.

Metabolic fuel

Breakdown of muscle glycogen provides the glucose needed for glycolysis and oxidative phosphorylation. The intracellular stores are sufficient for around 10 minutes of moderate exercise. After glycogen is exhausted, blood glucose and fatty acids provide the energy, with a slow switch towards burning fatty acids almost exclusively after around 40 minutes of sustained exercise.

Even under ideal circumstances, muscle is only around 25% efficient. Most of the chemical energy stored in the foodstuffs is dissipated as heat rather than converted into

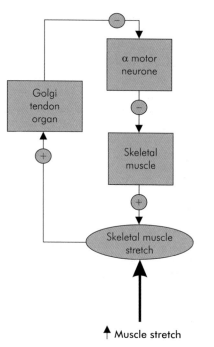

↑ Muscle stretch

Figure 13.18 Golgi tendon organ reflex

ATP is generated in three ways

- Phosphorylation of ADP by creatine phosphate
- Glycolytic phosphorylation
- Oxidative phosphorylation in mitochondria

Phosphorylation of ADP by creatine phosphate

Creatine phosphate provides a limited but immediate supply of high-energy inorganic phosphate. The creatine system is depleted within a few (2–7) seconds of muscle contraction, but is important for providing energy for explosive movements before oxidative phosphorylation and glycolytic phosphorylation take over. This pathway produces the waste product creatinine. During periods of relative rest, excess ATP may be used to regenerate creatine phosphate via several creatine kinases

Glycolytic phosphorylation

Glycolytic phosphorylation occurs in the cytoplasm. The substrate is pyruvate derived from the glycolysis of glycogen. It is a relatively inefficient, anaerobic process and produces only small amounts of ATP under normal circumstances. The waste product is lactic acid. Maximal

---

Energy for muscle contraction

This is provided in the form of ATP. The ATP releases the myosin from the actin and restores the myosin head to the 'cocked' or 'energised' position, i.e. the position in which it is ready to bind to actin. This conformational change causes the ATP to be hydrolysed to ADP and inorganic phosphate (Pi), which are released as the myosin binds to the actin and undergoes the backwards movement of the head. The myosin head acts as an ATPase enzyme.

---

mechanical work, during the multiple chemical reactions required to form ATP.

Smooth muscle

Smooth muscle is involuntary muscle under the control of the autonomic nervous system. It is found in viscera and blood vessel walls, providing the motility patterns required in visceral function. Smooth muscle may be divided into single-unit or multi-unit types. In single-unit smooth muscle the whole muscle contracts as one, whereas in multi-unit smooth muscle individual cells may contract alone. Most smooth muscle is single unit in nature, leading to coordinated contractions in organs such as the uterus and the bowel. Multi-unit smooth muscle occurs in the iris of the eye and in large arteries.

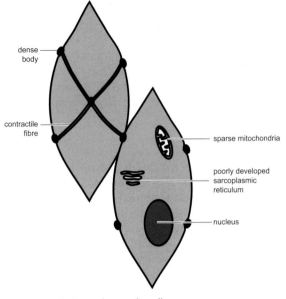

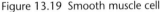

Figure 13.19 Smooth muscle cell

Anatomy of smooth muscle

Smooth muscle is considered smooth, or non-striated, from its appearance under light microscopy. There are many similarities but several important differences between smooth and striated muscle (Figure 13.1). Smooth muscle cells are much smaller than their striated muscle counterparts, and rather than being arranged in parallel bundles, may be found in clusters or sheets.

The basic contractile apparatus consists of actin and myosin, but the arrangement of the molecules is different from that of striated muscle. Likewise, the contraction mechanism is calcium-dependent, but the method of activation is somewhat different.

The actin molecules in smooth muscle are attached to so-called dense bodies, rather than Z plates, some of which are attached to the cell wall, and others of which are found within the cell cytoplasm (Figure 13.19). Myosin filaments are found in bundles in association with the actin molecules, but are arranged differently, with the heads of the myosin pointing in opposing directions. This allows smooth muscles to contract to much shorter lengths than striated muscle, by as much as 80% of the resting length compared with the 30% or so of skeletal muscle. Compared to striated muscle, smooth muscle contains proportionately more actin and less myosin. The actin and myosin molecules are

distinctly separate isoforms in skeletal and smooth muscle, and coded for by different genes.

Speed and force of contraction in smooth muscle

Depolarisation of the cell opens voltage-sensitive calcium channels in the cell membrane. The action potential relies largely on a calcium gradient, rather than the sodium gradient typical of skeletal muscle. Release of calcium into the cytoplasm also occurs from the sarcoplasmic reticulum, but rather than an interaction with troponin, calcium binds to calmodulin in the cytoplasm. Calmodulin activates the myosin light chain kinase and induces cross-bridge formation and cycling. Troponin is absent from smooth muscle cells. Tropomyosin is present in smooth muscles, but its relationship to the actin molecule is different to that in skeletal muscle and its function is unknown.

Smooth muscle contracts much more slowly than striated muscle, but the force generated per cell may be much greater. Both of these phenomena may be due to the poorer ATPase of the smooth muscle myosin, so that the actin and myosin units bind together for longer, reducing the cycling rate and hence speed of contraction, but providing more cross-links at any one time, increasing strength.

Many smooth muscle cells have an unstable resting membrane potential. In isolated single units of smooth muscle this may lead to irregular contractions, but where there is lots of smooth muscle together, particular cells may depolarise more frequently than others, and then spread a wave of depolarisation throughout the smooth muscle sheet. This 'pacemaker potential' is the basis for regular organised contractions of smooth muscle such as gut peristalsis. Although not observed in skeletal muscle, regular rhythmic depolarisation of muscle cells also occurs in cardiac muscle.

Smooth muscle cells are physically joined together by adherens junctions, and electrically linked together by gap junctions in the cell membrane. Single-unit smooth muscle typically contains lots of gap junctions, allowing waves of depolarisation to pass through the muscle.

Smooth muscle may also be induced to contract by physical stretch. Mechanical force induces the opening of ion channels in the cell membrane, causing depolarisation and subsequent contraction. As smooth muscle cells are tethered together by adherens junctions, contraction in one cell may trigger contraction in neighbouring cells. The stretch response of smooth muscle is important for the autoregulation seen in blood vessels. If smooth muscle is tensioned and then it is maintained at the longer length after stretching, the tension developed within the muscle gradually decreases. This is known as the plasticity of smooth muscle.

Smooth muscle control

Smooth muscle may come under extrinsic controls to a greater extent than skeletal muscle, in which activity is largely modulated by the nervous system alone. Smooth muscle contraction may be modified by:

- Autonomic nervous system – e.g. vagal tone affects gut motility.
- Hormones – e.g. progesterone typically causes smooth muscle contraction.
- Local humoral factors – e.g. calcium concentration in the extracellular fluid.

The relative degree of extrinsic control that smooth muscle is under depends on the exact type and location of the muscle.

CHAPTER 14

Cardiac physiology

Justiaan Swanevelder

The heart

The cardiovascular system acts as a transport system for the tissues and functions by:

- Supplying oxygen and removing carbon dioxide
- Delivering nutrients and removing metabolic waste products
- Delivering hormones and vasoactive substances to target cells

The heart is the driving force behind this system. It consists of a right-sided low-pressure pump and a left-sided high-pressure pump. Each of these pumps is composed of an atrium and a ventricle. The atria prime the ventricles which in turn eject the cardiac output into either the pulmonary or the systemic circulation. This chapter examines the heart and its functions.

Structure of cardiac muscle

Cardiac muscle is striated, the striations being due to the structure of the contractile intracellular myofibrils. The myofibrils are composed of sarcomere units which are identical to those of skeletal muscle, and are composed of thick and thin filaments which are arranged to give the characteristic Z line, A band and I band striations.

The thick filaments are composed of myosin molecules, whose tails are linked to form the filament leaving the 'heads' of the myosin molecules free. Each thick filament is surrounded by six thin filaments composed of a double spiral of actin molecules in combination with tropomyosin and troponin. These thin filaments form a hexagonal tube around the thick myosin filament. Contraction of the sarcomere is produced by a coupling and decoupling reaction between the myosin heads and actin

Fundamentals of Anaesthesia, 4th edition, ed. Ted Lin, Tim Smith and Colin Pinnock. Published by Cambridge University Press. © Cambridge University Press 2017.

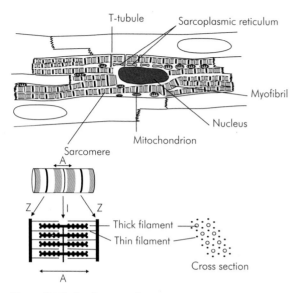

Figure 14.1 Cardiac muscle structure

fibres, which offer a low resistance to the propagation of action potentials along the axis of muscle cells, owing to the intercalated discs. The intercalated discs allow rapid transmission of action potentials between cells via gap junctions which are composed of connexons or open channels connecting the cytosol of adjacent cells.

Finally, cardiac muscle cells contain much greater numbers of packed mitochondria and are more richly supplied with capillaries than skeletal muscle, since the myocardium cannot afford to incur an oxygen debt by using anaerobic metabolism.

- The actin–myosin coupling and decoupling reaction lies at the heart of the contractile process and is fuelled by ATP and calcium.
- The sarcoplasmic reticulum acts as a reversible intracellular store for calcium ions.
- Cardiac muscle is a functional syncytium with an all-or-nothing contractile response

filaments which results in a 'walking' action of the myosin heads along the thin filaments. This causes the thick filaments to slide along the axis of the actin tubes.

Sarcoplasmic reticulum

Each cardiac muscle cell is surrounded by a cell membrane, the sarcolemma. This forms invaginations penetrating deeply into the cell which are called transverse or T tubules. These tubules are located at the Z lines and spread the action potential into the interior of the muscle cell. A system of closed cisterns and tubules, the sarcoplasmic reticulum (SR), surrounds each myofibril, the cisterns being closely related to the T tubules.

Differences between cardiac muscle and skeletal muscle

Cardiac muscle differs from skeletal muscle in that the individual cells or fibres are tightly coupled, mechanically and electrically, to form a functional syncytium. This is achieved by branching and interdigitation of the cells and specialised end-to-end membrane junctions called intercalated discs. Intercalated discs are located at positions corresponding to the Z lines (Figure 14.1). The result functionally is an all-or-nothing contractile response of the myocardium when stimulated. Cardiac muscle is not a true syncytium, as each cardiac muscle cell has a single nucleus and is surrounded by the sarcolemma.

A further difference from skeletal muscle lies in the electrical conductive characteristics of the cardiac muscle

Excitation–contraction coupling

This term describes the events which are initially triggered by an action potential and which culminate in contraction of a myofibril. Propagation of an action potential along the sarcolemma and into the muscle cell through the T-tubule system causes calcium ions (Ca^{2+}) to enter the cell through voltage-dependent and receptor-dependent channels, and also by passive diffusion across the sarcolemma. This initial rise in Ca^{2+} triggers further release of Ca^{2+} from the sarcoplasmic reticulum. As a result intracellular Ca^{2+} levels increase from resting values of 10^{-7} mmol L^{-1} to concentrations of 10^{-4} mmol L^{-1} (Figure 14.2). The released calcium acts on the thin filaments, binding to troponin C and causing tropomyosin to move and reveal the actin binding sites for the myosin heads. This enables the myosin heads to attach themselves to the actin filaments, and contraction commences. Contraction proceeds by a 'walk-along' or 'ratchet' process, in which ATP is hydrolysed to ADP by ATPase in the myosin head. The energy released produces the 'power stroke' that slides the myosin on the actin.

The strength of cardiac muscle contraction is highly dependent on the calcium concentration in the extracellular fluid. At the end of the action potential plateau the calcium flow into the cell decreases, and the intracellular Ca^{2+} is actively pumped back into the sarcoplasmic reticulum and T tubules by a calcium–magnesium ATPase pump.

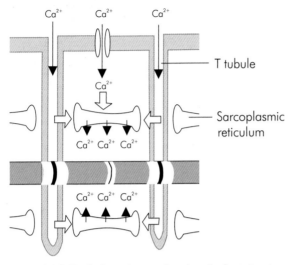

Figure 14.2 T tubule and sarcoplasmic reticulum structure

The chemical interaction between actin and myosin ceases and the muscle relaxes until the next action potential.

Cardiac action potentials

An action potential (AP) is a spontaneous depolarisation of an excitable cell's membrane, usually in response to a stimulus.

> Two different types of **action potential** are found in the heart, the fast-response and the slow-response. In the myocardium two cell types produce fast-response action potentials. These are the contractile myocardial cells and the conduction system cells. Slow-response APs are normally produced by the pacemaker cells in the sinoatrial (SA) node and the atrioventricular (AV) node. These pacemaker cells spontaneously depolarise to produce slow-response APs, exhibiting a property called automaticity.

Fast-response action potential

The fast-response AP of the cardiac muscle cell can be divided into five distinct phases (Figure 14.3):

Phase 0 – initial rapid depolarisation/upstroke
Phase 1 – early rapid repolarisation
Phase 2 – prolonged plateau phase
Phase 3 – final rapid repolarisation
Phase 4 – resting membrane potential

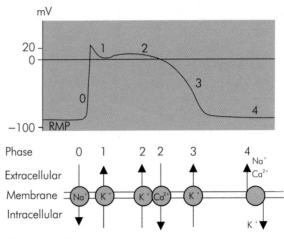

Figure 14.3 Fast-response action potential

Resting membrane potential (RMP)

The RMP is the electrical potential across the cell membrane during diastole and is approximately –90 mV, the intracellular membrane surface being negative with respect to the extracellular surface. The RMP is maintained by the permeability properties of the cell membrane, which retains negative ions (anions) in the cell but allows positive ions (cations) to diffuse out of the cell. The cell membrane is impermeable to negatively charged ions such as proteins, sulphates and phosphates, which therefore remain intracellular. In contrast membrane permeability to potassium is higher, allowing it to diffuse out of the cell under its concentration gradient of approximately 30:1. Potassium diffuses out of the cell until an equilibrium is reached at which the electrostatic attraction of the retained anions balances the chemical force moving the potassium down its concentration gradient out of the cell. This equilibrium is expressed mathematically by the Nernst equation.

The intracellular–extracellular concentration gradient of potassium must be maintained if the RMP is to stay constant. This is achieved by the active transport of potassium from the extracellular fluid to the intracellular space by a sodium–potassium pump.

Other ions also contribute to the RMP by producing transmembranous potentials due to the balance between chemical and electrostatic forces acting on them. For instance, sodium will diffuse across the cell membrane in the opposite direction to potassium (i.e. extracellular to intracellular) because of the normal resting sodium concentration gradient. Accordingly

Application of the Nernst equation to calculate RMP

Electrostatic force $=$ Chemical force

$$\text{Equilibrium potential} = \frac{RT}{FZ_K} \times \log_e \frac{[K_o^+]}{[K_I^+]}$$

where
$[K_I^+]$ = potassium concentration inside cell membrane
$[K_o^+]$ = potassium concentration outside cell membrane
R = the gas constant
T = absolute temperature
F = Faraday's constant
Z_K = the valency of potassium
Thus:

$$\text{Membrane potential due to } k^+ = 62 \times \log \frac{[K_I^+]}{[K_O^+]}$$

But resting membrane potential (RMP) is due mainly to the distribution and diffusion of potassium ions (see below), therefore:

$$\begin{aligned} \text{RMP} &= 62 \times \log_{10} \frac{[5]}{[150]} \\ &= -94 \, \text{mV} \end{aligned}$$

RMP is maintained by three mechanisms

- The retention of many intracellular anions (proteins, phosphates and sulphates) to which the cell membrane is not permeable.
- The selective permeability of the cell membrane, which is almost 100 times more permeable to potassium than to sodium, allowing potassium to flow down its concentration gradient out of the cell while keeping sodium extracellular.
- The maintenance of an intracellular–extracellular concentration gradient for potassium ions by a sodium–potassium ATPase pump. This transports potassium actively into the cell and sodium out of the cell (three Na^+ ions for every two K^+ ions) and is dependent on energy supplied by the hydrolysis of ATP.

this movement of sodium into the cell will reduce the membrane potential set up by potassium. However, because membrane permeability to sodium under resting conditions is relatively low, this effect is small, only reducing the membrane potential by approximately 4 mV. Similarly the cell membrane is relatively impermeable to other ions in the resting state, and therefore the RMP is primarily determined by the intracellular/extracellular distribution of potassium ions.

Phase 0 – rapid depolarisation
An action potential is produced when an electrical stimulus increases the RMP (causes it to become less negative) to a threshold potential (TP). At this value, fast sodium channels open for a very short period of time and potassium channels close. Sodium rapidly enters the cell under the influence of its concentration gradient and the electrostatic attraction of the intracellular anions, to make the inside positive in comparison to the outside by +20 mV. At the end of this stage the sodium channels close. This phase coincides with the 'all-or-nothing' depolarisation of the myocardium and the QRS complex of the ECG.

Phase 1 – early rapid repolarisation
This describes a brief fall in membrane potential towards zero following the rapid rise in phase 0. This occurs due to the start of potassium flow out of the cell under the positive intracellular electrical gradient and chemical gradients. At the same time slow, L-type Ca^{2+} channels open, providing a prolonged influx of calcium ions which maintains the positive intracellular charge. There is also movement intracellularly of chloride following sodium into the cell along the electrical gradient. All of this leads to an initial rapid repolarisation of the cell membrane to just above 0 mV.

Phase 2 – plateau phase
During this phase the continued influx of calcium via the slow L-type Ca^{2+} channels is balanced by the continued efflux of potassium commenced in phase 1. This maintains the zero or slightly positive membrane potential and corresponds in time with the ST segment of the ECG.

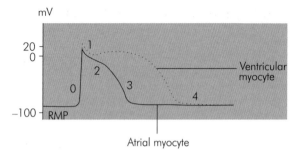

Figure 14.4 Atrial and ventricular myocyte action potentials

Phase 3 – final rapid repolarisation

Potassium permeability rapidly increases at this stage and potassium flows out to restore the transmembrane potential to –90 mV. Although repolarisation of the membrane is complete by the end of phase 3, the normal ionic gradients have not yet been re-established across the membrane

Phase 4 – restoration of ionic concentrations and resting state

During this phase ATPase-dependent ion pumps exchange intracellular sodium and calcium ions for extracellular potassium, thus restoring the resting ionic gradients. When an equilibrium state is reached electrostatic forces equal the chemical forces acting on the different ions and RMP is re-established. This phase corresponds to diastole.

Atrial cell action potentials

Atrial myocyte action potentials are also of the rapid-response type but vary from the ventricular action potentials in having a shorter-duration plateau (phase 2). This effect is due to a much greater early repolarisation current (phase 1) in the atrial AP than in the ventricular case (Figure 14.4).

Excitability of cardiac cells

Excitability describes the ability of cardiac tissue to depolarise to a given electrical stimulus. It is dependent on the difference between RMP and TP, and thus changes in RMP will alter myocardial excitability. When RMP decreases (becomes more negative), this difference becomes greater and the heart becomes less excitable. Similarly, excitability is increased as the difference

between RMP and TP decreases. Various factors affect excitability, including:

- Catecholamines
- β-Blockers
- Local anaesthetics
- Plasma electrolyte levels

Refractoriness

During rapid depolarisation (phase 0) and the early part of repolarisation (phases 1, 2 and the initial part of 3), the cell cannot be depolarised to produce another AP regardless of stimulus strength. The sodium and calcium channels are inactivated and repolarisation must occur before they can open again. This is called the absolute refractory period. During the latter part of phase 3 and early phase 4 a stronger than normal impulse can lead to an AP. This is called the relative refractory period. During this period the heart is particularly vulnerable because an impulse at this time might produce repetitive, dyssynchronous depolarisation (e.g. ventricular fibrillation or tachycardia). The absolute and relative refractory periods together form the effective refractory period.

Pacemaker cells

The heart continues to beat even after all nerves to it are sectioned. This happens because of the specialised pacemaker tissue (P-cell) that makes up the conduction system of the heart. These cells are found in the SA and AV nodes and also in the His–Purkinje system. Pacemaker cells exhibit automaticity (the ability to depolarise spontaneously) and rhythmicity (the ability to maintain a regular discharge rate). Normally atrial and ventricular myocardial cells do not have pacemaker ability, and they only discharge spontaneously when injured. There are however latent pacemakers in other parts of the conduction system that can take over when conduction from the SA and AV nodes is blocked.

Slow-response action potential

The action potential produced when a pacemaker cell depolarises spontaneously is called a slow-response action potential (Figure 14.5). The most negative potential reached just before depolarisation is called the maximum diastolic potential (MDP), which is only –60 mV compared to the RMP of –90 mV for a myocardial muscle cell. The reason for this is that the pacemaker cell membranes are more permeable to sodium ions in their resting state.

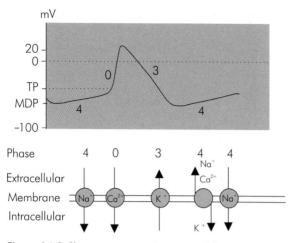

Figure 14.5 Slow-response action potential

Effectively phase 1 is absent and phase 2 is very brief, resulting in the absence of a plateau effect.

> **Differences between pacemaker and myocardial cell action potentials**
>
> Pacemaker action potentials have the following features which differ from those of the myocardial cells:
> - Less negative phase 4 membrane potential
> - Less negative threshold potential
> - Spontaneous depolarisation in phase 4
> - Less steep slope in phase 0 (dependence on T-type Ca^{2+} channels)
> - Absence of phase 2 (plateau)

Phases can be identified in the slow-response action potential which correspond superficially to some phases of the rapid-response AP, although the underlying events differ.

Phase 4 – restoration of ionic gradients and resting state

These cells do not maintain a stable RMP, but instead depolarise spontaneously because of increased membrane permeability to cations during this phase. Sodium and calcium slowly 'leak' into the cell. Although potassium diffuses out simultaneously during this phase, the inward 'leak' of sodium predominates to cause the membrane potential to gradually increase until a threshold potential (TP) is reached at approximately –40 mV. This property is called spontaneous diastolic depolarisation or pacemaker automaticity, and is directly related to the positive slope of phase 4.

Phase 0 – rapid depolarisation

Rapid depolarisation occurs at TP and is mainly due to calcium influx through transient or T-type Ca^{2+} channels, which are slower than the rapid sodium channels responsible for phase 0 in the myocardial cell APs. The slope of phase 0 is therefore less steep than in the rapid AP case. The phase 0 slope in these cells is also reduced because of onset at a less negative transmembrane potential.

Phase 3 – repolarisation

In the slow response, repolarisation is effectively a single phase equivalent to phase 3 in the rapid response.

Ion channels and action potentials

Action potentials owe their basic characteristics to voltage-controlled changes in membrane permeability to different ions. The main ions concerned are potassium, sodium and calcium, whose membrane permeabilities are dependent on various types of ion diffusion channel. The basic ion diffusion channel is described in Chapter 10. These ion channels have been described in vitro by controlling and varying membrane potentials in different ion solutions, using a technique called 'patch clamping'. Different channels can then be identified by the changes in current produced as the channels open and close according to their control potentials. Some of these channels are outlined in Figure 14.6.

Automaticity of pacemaker cells

Automaticity is the ability of pacemaker cells to maintain a spontaneous rhythm, and it depends mainly on the leakage of sodium into the cell in phase 4 of the AP. This occurs via specific sodium channels which are activated when the membrane potential has become hyperpolarised, i.e. reached a value of approximately –50 mV during repolarisation. These channels then allow an inward hyperpolarisation current (I_f), which commences the spontaneous depolarisation of phase 4. The sodium current (I_f) is aided to a small extent by overlap of the decaying rapid depolarisation calcium current and opposed by extracellular diffusion of potassium. Automaticity is dependent on the slope of phase 4 of the AP, which is influenced by the autonomic system and various drugs.

Figure 14.6 Voltage-controlled ion channels in action potentials

Action potential	Phase	Ion	Channel/gating mechanism
Rapid response (ventricular)	0	Na$^+$	Fast channels with 'm' activation and 'h' inactivation gates
	1,2,3	K$^+$	Transient outward current (i_{to}) channel
	2,3,4	K$^+$	Inward rectifier K$^+$ current (i_{K1}) channel
	2,3,4	K$^+$	Delayed rectifier K$^+$ current (i_K) channel
	2	Ca^{2+}	Slow (long-lasting, L-type) Ca^{2+} channel blocked by calcium antagonists
Slow response (pacemaker)	0	Ca^{2+}	Transient (T-type) Ca^{2+} channel
	4	Na$^+$	Specific channels 'leaking' sodium current (I_f) into pacemaker cells

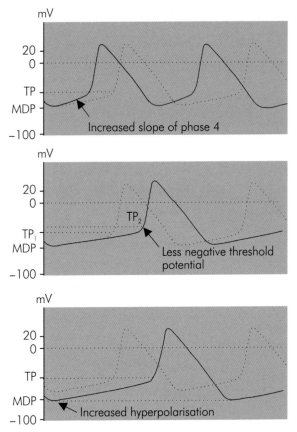

Figure 14.7 Changes in pacemaker action potential causing variation of discharge rate

Pacemaker discharge rate

Pacemaker discharge rate is controlled primarily by the autonomic system. This is discussed in further detail later (see *Heart rate*, below). This control is mediated by changes in action potential characteristics. The following characteristics are associated with variation of the discharge rate (Figure 14.7):

- Slope of phase 4 in AP – An increase in the slope of phase 4 reduces the time to reach TP during spontaneous depolarisation and thus increases pacemaker rate. Similarly a decrease in the phase 4 slope results in a slower pacemaker rate. Phase 4 slope can be varied by the autonomic nervous system.
- Threshold potential – If this becomes less negative the pacemaker rate will decrease. Drugs such as quinidine and procainamide have this effect.
- Hyperpolarisation potential – If hyperpolarisation is increased, i.e. the membrane potential becomes more

negative, spontaneous discharge will take longer to reach TP during phase 4 and the pacemaker rate will decrease. This occurs with increases in acetylcholine levels.

Conduction system anatomy

The conduction system of the heart is composed of specialised cardiac tissues which form the following structures (Figure 14.8):

- Sinoatrial node
- Atrial conduction pathways
- Atrioventricular node
- Bundle of His
- Bundle branches
- Purkinje fibres

The sinoatrial (SA) node is the normal cardiac pacemaker, with a resting rate of between 60 and 100 per minute. It is

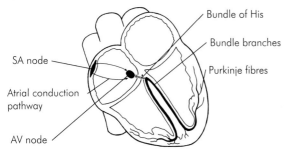

Figure 14.8 Anatomy of the conduction system

Figure 14.9 Arrhythmias due to conduction system defects

Site	Arrhythmia	Features
Sinoatrial node	Sick sinus syndrome	Sinus arrest, sinus bradycardia, tachycardias
Atrial conduction pathways	Wolff–Parkinson–White syndrome	Supraventricular tachycardia
Atrioventricular node	AV junctional rhythm	Bradycardia with abnormal P waves
Bundle of His	Complete (third-degree) AV block	Bradycardia with dissociated P waves
Bundle branches	Bundle branch block	Abnormal broad QRS complexes (> 0.12 s)

a group of modified myocardial cells located close to the junction of the superior vena cava with the right atrium. Its blood supply is usually from a branch of the right coronary artery. Depolarisation spreads from the SA node through the atria and converges on the AV node.

The two atria are electrically separated from the two ventricles except for three internodal communication pathways. The anterior (Bachmann), middle (Wenckebach) and posterior (Thorel) bundles connect the SA node to the AV node, which is located in the right posterior part of the right atrium close to the tricuspid valve and the coronary sinus opening. Anomalous accessory pathways (like the bundle of Kent) can sometimes connect the atria directly to the ventricle or other areas of the conducting system and cause a pre-excitation syndrome with arrhythmias. Blood supply to the AV node is also from a branch off the right coronary artery. The AV node is connected to the bundle of His, which distributes the impulse to the ventricles via the left and right bundle branches in the interventricular septum. There is a slight delay (about 0.13 seconds) of the impulse before it enters the AV node, inside the AV node and in the bundle of His. This delay permits completion of both atrial electrical activation and conduction before ventricular activation is started. The left bundle branch divides into the anterior and posterior fascicles. These bundles and fascicles run subendocardially down the septum and into the Purkinje system, which spreads the impulse to all parts of the ventricular muscle. Conduction velocity through the bundle branches and the Purkinje system is the most rapid of the conduction system. The AP as well as contraction begins endocardially and spreads out to the outside of the heart. However, repolarisation occurs from the outside to the inside. Ventricular activation is earliest at the apex and latest at the base of the heart, giving it an apical-to-basal contraction pattern.

Conduction system defects

Defects can arise in any part of the conduction system. Some examples of arrhythmias occurring due to lesions in different parts of the conduction system are shown in Figure 14.9.

The electrocardiogram

In an electrophysiological sense the heart consists of two chambers. The two atria function as a single electrophysiological unit and are separated from the biventricular unit by the fibrous atrioventricular ring. Electrical communication between these two units is only possible through the specialised conduction system. The main electrical events of the cardiac cycle are the mass depolarisation and repolarisation of the atria and ventricles. These can be thought of as waves of depolarisation (or repolarisation) which propagate through the cardiac tissues. As they propagate they generate potentials which can be sensed by electrodes on the skin surface. The electrocardiogram (ECG) is a recording of the signals picked up by a standard pattern of skin electrodes over the chest. When an electrode detects depolarisation moving towards it a positive deflection on the ECG is

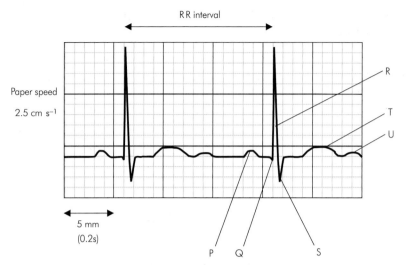

Figure 14.10 Sample electrocardiogram trace

produced. Alternatively, if depolarisation is moving away from the electrode, it produces a negative deflection.

ECG waves and the cardiac cycle

The normal ECG consists of P, QRS, T and U deflections (Figure 14.10). Electrical activity precedes corresponding mechanical events during the cardiac cycle as follows:

- The P wave is associated with atrial depolarisation and contraction. The atria repolarise at the same time as ventricular depolarisation, so the atrial repolarisation wave is usually obscured by the prominent QRS complex.
- The PR interval is between the beginning of the P wave and the start of the QRS complex. This represents the time from onset of atrial contraction to the beginning of ventricular contraction. The normal PR interval is approximately 0.16 seconds, but it varies with heart rate.
- The QRS complex reflects ventricular depolarisation and precedes ventricular contraction. A normal QRS complex has smooth peaks with no notches or slurs and has a duration of less than 0.12 seconds. The amplitude is dependent on multiple factors including myocardial mass, the cardiac axis, the distance of the sensing electrode from the ventricles and the anatomical orientation of the heart.
- The QT interval lies between the beginning of the Q wave and the end of the T wave. This is approximately 0.35 seconds at a normal resting heart rate. The QT interval shortens with tachycardia and lengthens with bradycardia and can be normalised to a heart rate of 60 beats per minute, by using Bazett's formula:

$$QTc = \frac{QT}{\sqrt{R-R}}$$

where R–R is the interval measured between two R waves.

- The ST segment and T wave are associated with ventricular repolarisation. The ventricles remain contracted until a few milliseconds after repolarisation ends.
- The U wave remains controversial in its origin. It may represent the slow repolarisation of the papillary muscles.

Electrical axis of the heart

Electrical activity in the heart can be represented by a vector, since it possesses both amplitude and direction. A single or resultant vector can be drawn showing the magnitude and direction of the electrical activity in the heart at any instant. This will change continuously throughout the cardiac cycle. Thus a vector can be drawn to represent maximum electrical activity for any wave of the ECG. During the QRS complex, a maximum vector is normally produced pointing downwards and to the left.

This vector reflects peak electrical activity during mass depolarisation of the ventricles, and its direction is referred to as the electrical axis of the heart or the cardiac axis. Various factors may vary the direction of this axis, including the anatomical position of the heart and different pathological conditions (e.g. left ventricular hypertrophy).

ECG leads

An electrical signal is a potential difference detected between two points. In the ECG, signals are recorded between two active surface electrodes, or an active electrode and a common or indifferent point. Each signal recorded is called a lead and may have an amplitude of several millivolts. There are 12 conventional ECG leads. They may be divided into two groups:

- Frontal-plane leads:
  - Standard leads I, II and III
  - Unipolar limb leads aVR, aVL and aVF
- Horizontal-plane leads:
  - Precordial/chest leads V_1–V_6

Standard limb leads I, II, III

These leads are recorded with a combination of two active electrodes at a time and are therefore bipolar leads. Each signal is recorded in the direction of the sides of an equilateral triangle with an apex on each shoulder and the pubic region, and the heart at its centre. This is called Einthoven's triangle (Figure 14.11).

- Lead I – The negative electrode is placed on the right arm and the positive electrode on the left arm.
- Lead II – The negative electrode is placed on the right arm and the positive electrode on the left foot.
- Lead III – The negative electrode is placed on the left arm and the positive electrode on the left foot.

The ECGs of these three leads are very similar to each other. They all record positive P waves, positive T waves and positive QRS complexes.

Unipolar limb leads aVR, aVL, aVF

These unipolar leads record the difference between an active limb electrode and an indifferent (zero potential) electrode at the centre of Einthoven's triangle (Figure 14.11). These signals are of lower amplitude than other leads and require increased amplification (hence referred to as augmented leads):

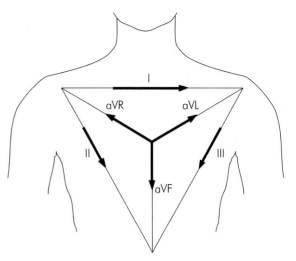

Figure 14.11 Einthoven's triangle

- aVR – The augmented unipolar right arm lead faces the heart from the right side and is usually orientated to the cavity of the heart. Therefore all the deflections P, QRS and T are normally negative in this lead.
- aVL – The augmented unipolar left arm lead faces the heart from the left side and is orientated to the anterolateral surface of the left ventricle.
- aVF – The augmented unipolar left leg lead, orientated to the inferior surface of the heart.

Precordial chest leads

These horizontal-plane unipolar leads are placed as follows:

- V_1 – Fourth intercostal space immediately right of the sternum
- V_2 – Fourth intercostal space immediately left of the sternum
- V_3 – Exactly halfway between the positions of V_2 and V_4
- V_4 – Fifth intercostal space in the midclavicular line
- V_5 – Same horizontal level as V_4 but on the anterior axillary line
- V_6 – Same horizontal level as V_4 and V_5 on the midaxillary line

Anatomical orientation of ECG electrodes

Although there is considerable variation in the position of the normal heart, the atria are usually positioned posteriorly in the chest while the ventricles form the base and anterior surface. The right ventricle is anterolateral to the left ventricle. The ventricles consist of three muscle masses. These are the free walls of the left and right ventricles and the interventricular septum. Electrical activity in the left ventricle and the interventricular septum is predominant. ECG electrodes will pick up signals from the closest structures and those producing the greatest electrical signals. Therefore ECG signals recorded from the anterior aspect of the heart are mainly due to activity in the interventricular septum, with only a small contribution from the right ventricular wall. Since ECG lead signals reflect activity in different parts of the heart because of their position, they are said to 'look' at different aspects of the heart:

- sII, sIII and aVF look at the inferior surface of the heart.
- sI and aVL are orientated towards the superior left lateral wall.
- aVR and V_1 face the cavity of the heart, and the deflections are mainly negative in these leads.
- Leads V_1 to V_6 are orientated towards the anterior wall. V_1 and V_2 are anterior leads, V_3 and V_4 are septal leads, and V_5 and V_6 are lateral leads.
- V_1 and V_2 examine the right ventricle, while V_4 to V_6 are orientated towards the septum and left ventricle.
- There is no lead which is orientated directly to the posterior wall of the heart.

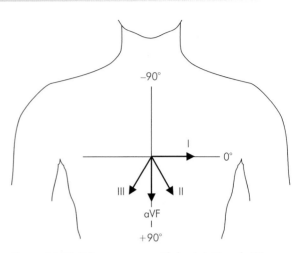

Figure 14.12 Reference axes with leads I–III and aVF

Calculation of heart rate from ECG

The heart rate in beats per minute can be determined from the ECG by measuring the time interval (in seconds) between two successive beats (R–R interval), and dividing this into 60 seconds.

Thus if R–R interval = 0.6 seconds:

Heart rate = 60/0.6
           = 100 beats/min

The time scale of the ECG depends on the recording paper speed. Normal paper speed is 2.5 cm s^{-1}, meaning that each large square (5 mm) of the ECG trace represents 0.2 seconds (Figure 14.10). In the above example the R–R interval is 3 large squares (15 mm) which is equal to 0.6 seconds. If the R–R interval were to become 5 large squares (1 second) this would give a heart rate of 60 bpm.

Calculation of cardiac axis

The direction of the electrical axis of the heart is usually calculated in the frontal plane only, and can be done using two of the frontal ECG leads (these are the standard limb and unipolar limb leads). It is determined as an angle referred to the axes shown in Figure 14.12, the normal range lying between 0° and +90°.

The cardiac vector, like any vector, can be resolved to give an effect or 'component' in any given direction. The amplitudes of the QRS complexes in the frontal leads represent components of the cardiac vector in the direction of the leads. The cardiac axis can therefore be found by the vector summation of any two of these components to find their resultant (here sI and aVF are taken for convenience since they lie at angles of 0° and 90° respectively). The direction of the cardiac axis is then given by the angle, θ, of the resultant. A simple algorithm to determine the cardiac axis from sI and aVF is presented in the green box and in Figure 14.13.

Monitoring in the operating room

During routine non-cardiac surgery sII and V_5 are usually used as continuous monitoring leads. The P wave is best detected in sII, which facilitates detection of junctional or ventricular dysrhythmias. Chest lead V_5 is most sensitive to ST segment changes and can warn the anaesthetist about possible ischaemia.

Calculation of the cardiac axis from ECG leads sI and aVF

(shown in Figure 14.13)

- Determine the amplitudes of the QRS complexes in sI and aVF by subtracting the height of the S wave from the height of the R wave in each lead.
- Construct a rectangle with the sides in proportion to the amplitudes of sI and aVF. The diagonal then represents the resultant of sI and aVF (i.e. the cardiac vector).
- Determine the direction of the cardiac axis from the angle θ by taking the tangent of θ as the ratio of [amplitude of aVF] / [amplitude of sI].

Cardiac axis estimation by inspection of standard limb leads

In practice a rapid estimation of the cardiac axis can be made simply by inspection of the frontal ECG leads. Convenient leads to use are the standard limb leads sI, sII, sIII and aVF, which lie at 0°, 60°, 120° and 90° respectively (Figure 14.12).

Initially some basic facts about the relationship between a vector and its components should be noted. The QRS amplitudes in these leads are components of the cardiac vector. The amplitude of a component depends on the angle between the component and the vector it is derived from. As this angle increases the amplitude of the component decreases.

- For angles less than 90° the component is positive.
- When the angle between vector and component is zero, i.e. the component is acting in the direction of the vector, the component is maximum and equal to the vector.
- At 60° the amplitude of the component is half of the vector.
- At 90° the amplitude of the component becomes zero.
- For angles greater than 90° the component becomes negative.

Applying these simple principles confirm the following estimations:

sII = 0, the cardiac axis is at − 30° (left axis deviation)

aVF = 0, the cardiac axis is at 0°

sI = sII, then the cardiac axis is at + 30°, bisecting the angle between them

sI and sIII are each half of sII, the cardiac axis is at + 60°

sI = 0, the cardiac axis is at + 90°

sIII > sII, the cardiac axis is at > 90° (right axis deviation)

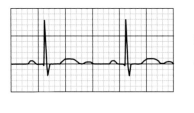

Lead I

QRS amplitude

= 8 − 2 = 6

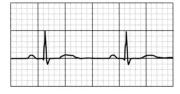

Lead aVF

QRS amplitude

= 5 − 1 = 4

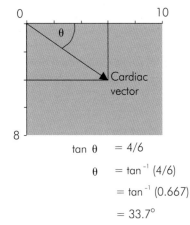

$$\tan \theta = 4/6$$
$$\theta = \tan^{-1}(4/6)$$
$$= \tan^{-1}(0.667)$$
$$= 33.7°$$

Figure 14.13 Calculation of cardiac axis

During cardiac surgery all six of the limb leads are connected for intermittent ST segment examination, and this can increase sensitivity for the detection of ischaemia.

Physiological cardiac arrhythmias

> A **cardiac rhythm** is defined by three characteristics:
> - The anatomical origin – a description of where the rhythm originates anatomically, e.g. SA node, atria, AV node or ventricles
> - The discharge sequence – a description of the pattern of electrical discharge, e.g. sinus rhythm, tachycardia, bradycardia, fibrillation
> - The conduction sequence – a description of abnormalities in conduction of the discharge impulses to the myocardium, e.g. 2:1 SA block, complete AV block

Abnormal cardiac rhythms or arrhythmias can arise as a primary or secondary disorder. Acute arrhythmias occurring during the perioperative period can seriously compromise perfusion. An arrhythmia must be correctly diagnosed and the precipitating causes should be removed before treatment is considered. Acute arrhythmias are more likely to be reversible. Chronic arrhythmias are usually disease-related and relatively stable.

Some departures from a perfectly regular cardiac rhythm occur as a result of normal physiological responses, as opposed to having an underlying pathological cause. These are outlined below:

Sinus rhythm

This is the normal rhythm for the heart. All other rhythms are arrhythmias by definition. In the normal adult heart sinus rhythm originates in the SA node, and has a regular pattern of discharge at a resting rate of between 60 and 80 beats a minute. The conduction sequence occurs on a 1:1 basis from SA node to atria to AV node and to the ventricles. The resting rate for neonates varies between 110 and 180 beats per minute and gradually decreases with increasing age until it reaches the adult rate at about 10 years of age.

Sinus arrhythmia

In healthy young patients with a regular breathing rate, the heart rate increases with inspiration and decreases with expiration. This is a normal finding called sinus arrhythmia. It is caused by an irregular fluctuating discharge of the SA node. During inspiration the stretch receptors in the lungs send impulses via the vagus nerves to inhibit the cardioinhibitory centre in the medulla oblongata. This stimulates the sinus node, increasing the heart rate. This arrhythmia is characterised by normal P–QRS–T complexes with alternating periods of gradually lengthening and shortening P–P intervals.

Sinus bradycardia

This rhythm occurs when the SA node discharges at a rate lower than 60 per minute, with normal P–QRS–T complexes. This is a normal phenomenon in fit young athletes, and may also occur during sleep. Sinus bradycardia can be associated with pathological conditions which include myxoedema, uraemia, glaucoma, and increased intracranial pressure. Various drugs such as β-blockers, digitalis or anaesthetic agents may also cause sinus bradycardia. Occasionally during sinus bradycardia, a ventricular ectopic pacemaker site can take over. This may cause premature ventricular contractions, which will usually disappear when the sinus rate speeds up again. When the heart rate goes below 40 beats per minute it is likely to cause hypotension or decreased perfusion, and should be treated immediately with an antimuscarinic drug (atropine or glycopyrrolate), β-stimulant or pacemaker as required.

Sinus tachycardia

Sympathetic stimuli such as emotion, exercise, pain and fever increase the SA discharge rate to greater than 100 per minute although the P–QRS–T complexes remain normal. It commonly occurs during the perioperative period. Hypovolaemia can often causes a sinus tachycardia through the baroreceptor reflex. Certain pathological conditions such as anxiety, thyrotoxicosis, toxaemia and cardiac failure may also cause it. The administration of drugs like adrenaline, atropine, isoprenaline and many others may lead to sinus tachycardia. When the heart rate exceeds 140 beats per minute there is not enough time for left ventricular filling and the patient becomes hemodynamically compromised. This should be treated first by removal of the cause and thereafter pharmacologically.

Effects of electrolyte changes on the ECG

> The **action potentials** (AP) of the heart depend upon the sodium, potassium and calcium ion distributions across the cell membranes, as well as the resting membrane potentials of the cardiac muscle and pacemaker cells.

Electrolyte abnormalities can often produce ECG changes. Some common electrolyte disturbances are described below with their effects on the ECG.

Hypokalaemia

makes the RMP of the cardiac muscle fibres more negative. The heart becomes less excitable, but automaticity increases. Moderate hypokalaemia (3–3.5 mEq L^{-1}) causes a prolonged PR interval, flattening of the T wave and a prominent U wave. With severe hypokalaemia (2.5 mEq L^{-1}) ST depression can be seen and late T-wave inversion occurs in the precordial leads. The QT interval is often prolonged. None of these changes are exclusively associated with hypokalaemia.

Hyperkalaemia

(> 5.5–6 mEq L^{-1}) is a potentially life-threatening condition, especially when the onset is acute. As the extracellular potassium concentration increases, the RMP of the cardiac cell membrane progressively becomes less negative, moving towards TP. Initially this makes the cardiac muscle more excitable. However, a deterioration of the action potential also occurs, with a reduction in rapid depolarisation and a loss of the plateau phase. This results in poor contraction of the cardiac muscle. At plasma levels of 6–8 mEq L^{-1}, ventricular tachycardia and fibrillation readily occur. As the RMP approaches the TP (plasma levels > 8–10 mEq L^{-1}) the muscle fibres become unexcitable and the heart finally stops in ventricular diastole.

The ECG starts to change when serum potassium level reaches 6.0 mEq L^{-1}. Initially a shortened QT interval and narrow, peaked T wave appears. Further potassium increases produce widening of the QRS complex and PR interval prolongation until the P wave disappears.

Hypocalcaemia

produces a flat prolonged ST segment and QT interval. Advanced stages of hypocalcaemia may lead to increased ventricular ectopic activity and ventricular tachycardia.

Hypercalcaemia

makes the TP of cardiac muscle fibres less negative, decreases conduction velocity and shortens the refractory period. This increases the likelihood of coupled beats, ventricular tachycardia and ventricular fibrillation. In acute hyperkalaemia immediate treatment with an intravenous bolus of calcium opposes the effects of the high potassium levels.

At very high calcium levels (animal experiments) the heart will relax less during diastole and will eventually stop in systole (calcium rigor). ECG changes produced by hypercalcaemia are prolongation of the PR interval, widening of the QRS complex and shortening of the QT interval. The T wave is also broadened.

Hypomagnesaemia

promotes cell membrane depolarisation and tachyarrhythmias, since magnesium is necessary for the normal functioning of the cardiac cell membrane pump. ECG changes produced by hypomagnesaemia include low-voltage P waves and QRS complexes, prominent U waves and peaked T waves.

Hypermagnesaemia

is associated with delayed atrioventricular conduction and therefore presents with a prolonged PR interval, wide QRS complex and T-wave elevation at plasma levels > 5.0 mEq L^{-1}. Levels > 10 mEq L^{-1} may lead to a complete heart block and cardiac arrest.

Hyponatraemia

is characterised by low-voltage ECG complexes.

Alkalosis and acidosis

will produce the same ECG changes as hypokalaemia and hyperkalaemia respectively.

The cardiac cycle

The heart is a pump whose basic functions are to fill with blood, generate a pressure, and displace volume.

> Each **cardiac cycle** consists of a period of relaxation (diastole) followed by ventricular contraction (systole). During diastole the ventricles are relaxed to allow filling. Then in systole the right and left ventricles contract, ejecting blood into the pulmonary and systemic circulations respectively.

The ventricles

The left ventricle (LV) pumps blood into the systemic circulation via the aorta. The systemic vascular resistance (SVR) is 5–7 times greater than the pulmonary vascular

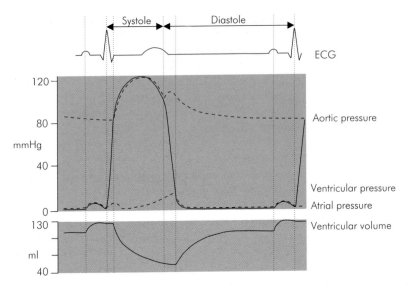

Figure 14.14 Cardiac cycle, showing ventricular volume, ventricular pressure, aortic pressure and atrial pressure

resistance (PVR). This makes it a high-pressure system compared to the pulmonary vascular system. This requires a greater mechanical power output from the LV. The free wall of the LV and the interventricular septum form the bulk of the muscle mass in the heart. A normal LV can develop intraventricular pressures up to 300 mmHg. Coronary perfusion to the LV occurs mainly in diastole when the myocardium is relaxed.

The right ventricle (RV) receives blood from the venae cavae and coronary circulation, and pumps it via the pulmonary vasculature into the LV. Since PVR is a fraction of SVR, pulmonary arterial pressures are relatively low and the wall thickness of the RV is much less than that of the LV. The RV thus resembles a passive conduit rather than a pump. Coronary perfusion to the RV occurs continuously during systole and diastole because of the low intraventricular and intramural pressures.

In spite of the anatomical differences, the RV and LV are very similar in their mechanical behaviour.

The cardiac cycle can be examined in detail by considering the ECG trace, intracardiac pressure and volume curves, and heart valve function (Figure 14.14).

Systolic function

The events during systole are described below in relation to the ventricular pressure, ventricular volume, aortic pressure and atrial pressure curves.

Systole can be broken down into the following stages:

- Isovolumetric ventricular contraction
- Ventricular ejection

Systole commences with a period of isovolumetric contraction initiated by the QRS complex of the ECG. During this brief period the volume of the ventricle does not change, since both the atrioventricular (mitral, tricuspid) and semilunar (aortic, pulmonary) valves are closed (see *The cardiac valves*, below). Isovolumetric contraction ends when the semilunar valve opens and ejection begins.

Left ventricular pressure

Ventricular contraction is initiated by the QRS complex of the ECG. As the pressure in the LV increases during isovolumetric contraction, it comes to exceed the pressure in the aorta. At this point the aortic valve opens and ejection begins. The aortic valve opens at a pressure of approximately 80 mmHg. Ejection continues as long as ventricular pressure exceeds aortic pressure. The total volume ejected into the aorta is the stroke volume. The ventricular pressure increases initially during ejection, but then starts to decrease as the ventricle relaxes. The gradient between ventricle and aorta starts to reverse at this point, since LV pressure has started to fall but aortic pressure is maintained by the momentum of the last of the ejected blood. When the ventricular-to-aortic pressure gradient has reversed, the aortic valve closes and isovolumetric relaxation begins. This point is marked by the dicrotic notch on the aortic pressure curve (see below). The LV pressure normally reaches a systolic maximum of 120 mmHg. At the end of systole the LV pressure is described as the end-systolic pressure, and the LV volume is at its smallest (end-systolic volume), approximately 40–50 mL (see ventricular pressure curve, Figure 14.14).

Right ventricular pressure

This follows a similar course to LV pressure. Events are dictated by the tricuspid and pulmonary valves, with ejection occurring into the pulmonary artery. RV pressure reaches a maximum of approximately 20–24 mmHg during systole.

Ventricular volume

Diastole commences in the left side of the heart with closure of the aortic valve and relaxation of the left ventricle. Since the mitral and aortic valves are both closed at this time the relaxation is described as isovolumetric. The LV contains 40–50 mL of blood at this stage (end-systolic volume). Isovolumetric relaxation ends with opening of the mitral valve, when a period of rapid filling of the ventricle begins, which lasts for the first third of diastole. The initial period of rapid filling is followed by a period of passive filling called diastasis, when flow continues passively into the ventricle providing up to 75% (60 mL) of the filling volume. During the last third of diastole the P wave of the ECG initiates atrial contraction, which contributes the remaining 25% of filling to give an end-diastolic volume of approximately 120 mL. The end-diastolic volume of the ventricle is not always 120 mL, but can vary due to changes in venous return to the heart, contractility and heart rate. A similar sequence of events occurs on the right side of the heart, controlled by the pulmonary and tricuspid valves (see ventricular volume curve, Figure 14.14).

Aortic pressure

Ejection of blood into the aorta begins when the aortic valve opens. During ejection the aortic pressure follows the ventricular pressure curve apart from a small pressure gradient. This gradient is approximately 1–2 mmHg when the aortic valve is normal. As ejection proceeds, aortic pressure increases to a maximum (systolic pressure) and starts to fall as the LV relaxes. When the ventricular pressure has fallen below the aortic pressure, the aortic valve closes and ejection ceases. Following closure of the aortic valve, elastic rebound of the aorta walls gives rise to a small hump in the aortic pressure curve forming the dicrotic notch. This notch marks the beginning of diastole. During diastole the aortic pressure gradually falls to a minimum (diastolic pressure), due to the run-off of blood into the systemic circulation (see aortic pressure curve, Figure 14.14).

Atrial pressure

Normally blood fills the right atrium (RA), via the superior and inferior venae cavae, continuously throughout the cardiac cycle. This flow is returned from the peripheral circulation and is called the venous return to the heart. On the left side of the heart, the left atrium (LA) receives blood from the pulmonary vascular bed via the pulmonary veins.

Passive filling of the atria produces RA pressures of 0–2 mmHg and LA pressures of 2–5 mmHg. During diastole atrial pressures follow ventricular pressures, since the atrioventricular (AV) valves are open and the two chambers are joined. Three waves or peaks are produced in the atrial pressure curve during the cycle. At the end of diastole the atria prime the ventricles by contracting and developing pressures of 0–5 mmHg. Atrial contraction is shown on the atrial pressure curve as a smooth peak immediately preceding systole, the 'a' wave. As systole begins the AV valves close and a brief period of isovolumetric contraction occurs, producing a second low-pressure peak, the 'c' wave. This is due to the AV valve bulging back the atrium.

As blood is ejected during systole the atrium continues to fill with the AV valve closed and atrial pressure increases until early diastole, when the AV valve opens. At this point rapid filling of the ventricles commences, causing a sudden fall in atrial pressure. This gives rise to the 'v' wave (see atrial pressure curve, Figure 14.14).

Diastolic function

Although diastole appears to be a passive part of the cardiac cycle, it has some important functions.

Diastole can be broken down into the following stages:

- Isovolumetric ventricular relaxation
- Rapid ventricular filling
- Slow ventricular filling (diastasis)
- Atrial contraction

- **Myocardial relaxation.** This is a metabolically active phase. One essential process is the reuptake of calcium by the sarcoplasmic reticulum. Incomplete reuptake leads to diastolic dysfunction due to decreased end-diastolic compliance (see *The cardiac pump*, below). Myocardial relaxation can be assessed by the negative slope of the ventricular pressure–time curve during isovolumetric relaxation (dP/dt_{max}). Increased sympathetic tone or circulating catecholamines give rise to an increased dP/dt_{max}. This is known as positive lusitropy.
- **Ventricular filling.** Ventricular filling provides the volume for the cardiac pump. Most of the ventricular filling occurs during early diastole. There is only a small increase in ventricular volume during diastasis. As the heart rate increases, diastasis is shortened first. When the heart rate exceeds approximately 140 beats per minute, rapid filling in early diastole becomes compromised and the volume of blood ejected during systole (stroke volume) is significantly decreased. Ventricular filling depends on several other factors, which are discussed further below.
- **Atrial contraction.** This contributes up to 25% of total ventricular filling in the normal heart. This atrial contribution can become of greater importance in the presence of myocardial ischaemia or ventricular hypertrophy.

- **Coronary artery perfusion.** The greater part of left coronary blood flow occurs during diastole. Coronary artery perfusion is discussed further under *Coronary circulation* in Chapter 15.

The cardiac valves

All the cardiac valves open and close passively in response to the changes in pressure gradient across them. These valves control the sequence of flow between atria and ventricles, and from the ventricles to the pulmonary and systemic circulations. Valve timing in relation to the ventricular pressure curve is illustrated in Figure 14.15.

The atrioventricular (AV) valves are the mitral and tricuspid valves. These prevent backflow from the ventricles into the atria during systole. The papillary muscles are attached to the AV valves by chordae tendinae. They contract together with the ventricular muscle during systole, but do not help to close the valves. They prevent excessive bulging of the valves into the atria and pull the base of the heart toward the ventricular apex to shorten the longitudinal axis of the ventricle, thus increasing systolic efficiency.

The semilunar (SL) valves are the aortic and pulmonary valves. These prevent backflow from the aorta and pulmonary arteries into the ventricles during diastole. The SL valves function quite differently from the AV valves because they are exposed to higher pressures in the arteries. They are smaller (normal aortic valve area is 2.6–3.5 cm^2, whereas

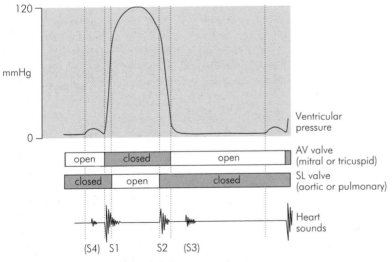

Figure 14.15 Heart sounds and timing

normal mitral valve area is 4–6 cm^2), so the blood velocity through them is greater.

Disease in the cardiac valves may cause them to leak when they are meant to be closed, thus allowing backflow or regurgitation. This situation leads to inefficiency in producing cardiac output, since the work done by the heart has to increase in order to compensate for the backflow and yet maintain adequate cardiac output. Mitral and aortic regurgitation are the most common regurgitant lesions.

Alternatively the orifice of a valve may become narrowed or stenotic. This obstructs the flow of blood through it and requires increased pressure gradients to be generated across the valve in order to achieve adequate blood flows. In mitral stenosis the valve area can be reduced by 50% or more. This causes the left atrium to contract more forcefully in order to maintain ventricular filling. In severe cases a valve area of 1 cm^2 can require the left atrium to produce peak pressures of 25 mmHg in order to produce normal cardiac output. Aortic stenosis obstructs left ventricular output and increases the workload of the left ventricle. The stenosis can multiply the normal pressure gradient across the aortic valve during systole by 10 times or more. When the aortic valve area decreases by 70% (< 0.8 cm^2), the stenosis becomes critical and systolic pressure gradients across the valve of > 50 mmHg may be required in order to produce normal cardiac output.

Differences in timing between left and right sides of the heart

Although the sequence of events on each side of the heart is similar, events occur asynchronously. This disparity in timing reflects differences in anatomy and working pressures between left and right sides of the heart. RA systole precedes LA systole, but RV contraction starts after LV contraction. In spite of contracting later, the RV starts to eject blood before the LV, because pulmonary artery pressure is lower than aortic pressure. Differences of timing also occur in the closure of the heart valves. These differences in valve timing lead to 'splitting' of the heart sounds.

Heart sounds and murmurs

In the normal individual two heart sounds can be heard during each cardiac cycle (Figure 14.15). These sounds are produced by closure of the valves, which causes the ventricular walls and valve leaflets to vibrate, and also produces turbulence of the interrupted blood flow.

The first sound (S1) occurs when the AV valves close at the start of ventricular systole and is best heard over the apex of the heart. The mitral valve normally closes earlier than the tricuspid by 10–30 ms. Thus S1 is split, with the mitral component occurring before the tricuspid component. The second sound (S2) corresponds to closure of the SL valves and is heard at the beginning of diastole. During inspiration the aortic valve closes before the pulmonary valve, due to increased venous return which delays RV ejection. During expiration aortic and pulmonary valve closure is simultaneous, and S2 appears to be a single sound. S2 is louder when the diastolic pressure is elevated in the aorta or pulmonary artery.

Abnormal heart sounds can be heard under pathological conditions. Heart failure can cause a third heart sound (S3) to be heard in mid-diastole. This is due to rapid filling of a dilated non-compliant ventricle following the opening of the AV valves. In conditions where stronger atrial contraction develops to help ventricular filling, a fourth heart sound (S4) may occur immediately before S1 (systole). This is thought to be due to ventricular wall vibration in response to forceful atrial filling.

When the cardiac valves undergo pathological changes abnormal sounds called murmurs can sometimes be heard. Under normal conditions blood flow is not turbulent but remains laminar up to a critical velocity. When blood flows across a narrowed valve, flow velocities are higher and turbulent, giving rise to a murmur. In the case of a 'leaking' or incompetent valve, turbulent regurgitant flow is produced, which also creates a murmur. The most common murmurs occur because of faults in the mitral and aortic valves. The valve involved and the type of lesion (stenotic or regurgitant) can be identified by the timing of the murmur and the site on the chest wall where it is loudest. In normal individuals without cardiac disease (especially children), soft physiological systolic murmurs can often be heard.

Central venous pressure (CVP)

CVP is usually monitored in the large veins feeding the superior vena cava, i.e. the internal jugular or subclavian veins.

Various pathological conditions affect mean CVP or alter the CVP waveform. For example, if the timing of atrial and ventricular contraction become dissociated (as in third-degree block) the right atrium contracts against a closed tricuspid valve and produces prominent or cannon 'a' waves (Figure 14.17).

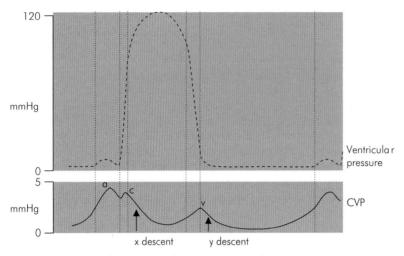

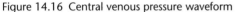

Figure 14.16 Central venous pressure waveform

> The **CVP waveform** reflects right atrial pressure and therefore consists of 'a', 'c' and 'v' waves which correspond to atrial contraction, isovolumetric contraction and opening of the tricuspid valve, as described above for the atrial pressure curve. There are also two labelled downward deflections, the 'x' and 'y' descents, which occur after the 'c' and 'v' waves respectively (Figure 14.16). The 'x' descent reflects the fall in right ventricular pressure when the pulmonary valve opens. The 'y' descent corresponds to the initial drop in atrial pressure caused by rapid ventricular filling when the AV valves open.

The cardiac pump

The ventricular pressure–volume loop

The mechanical performance of the heart as a pump can be summarised using a ventricular pressure–volume loop (PV loop). An example for the left ventricle is shown in Figure 14.18.

The cycle starts at the end-diastolic point (EDP). Isovolumetric contraction follows, represented by a vertical ascending segment which ends with the opening of the aortic valve. The ejection phase segment passes across the top of the loop from right to left. Ejection ends at the end-systolic point (ESP) when the aortic valve closes. Isovolumetric relaxation follows next as a vertical descending segment ending when the mitral valve opens.

Figure 14.17 Some factors affecting the central venous pressure waveform

Factor	Change in CVP
Depleted intravascular volume	↓ mean CVP
Excessive intravascular volume ('overloading' with intravascular fluid)	↑ mean CVP
Cardiac failure	↑ mean CVP
Pericardial tamponade	↑ mean CVP
Bradycardia	More distinct 'a', 'c' and 'v' waves
Tachycardia	Fusion of 'a' and 'c' waves
AV junctional rhythm	Regular cannon 'a' waves
Third-degree AV block	Irregular cannon 'a' waves
Tricuspid regurgitation	Loss of 'c' wave and 'x' descent Prominent 'v' waves

The final lower segment corresponds to ventricular filling and ends when the mitral valve closes at EDP.

This diagram can be used to derive several parameters reflecting ventricular function, including stroke volume

Ventricular
pressure (mmHg)

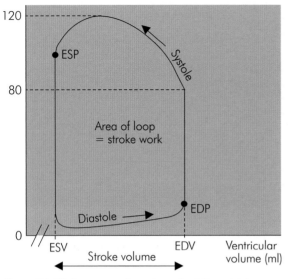

Figure 14.18 Pressure–volume loop for left ventricle

Ventricular
pressure

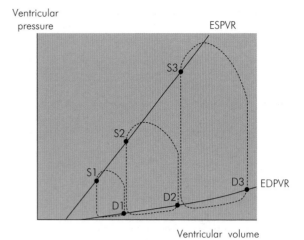

Figure 14.19 End-diastolic and end-systolic
pressure–volume relationship curves

Ventricular
pressure

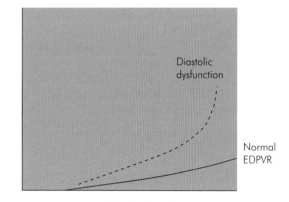

Figure 14.20 Effects of diastolic dysfunction on the
end-diastolic pressure–volume relationship (EDPVR) curve

(SV), stroke work (SW), end-diastolic volume (EDV) and
end-systolic volume (ESV).

Ventricular end-diastolic pressure–volume relationship

On the ventricular PV loop, the end-diastolic point
(EDP) records volume and pressure at the end of
diastole. If different PV loops are plotted for a given
ventricle, different EDPs are obtained (D1, D2 and D3:
Figure 14.19). These points, when plotted, form a
pressure–volume relationship for the ventricle at end
diastole. This is called the end-diastolic pressure–
volume relationship (EDPVR). The EDPVR is a useful
indicator of diastolic function, and in particular ventricular filling performance, since its gradient is equal
to the elastance (or compliance^{-1}), of the ventricle
during filling. The steeper this gradient, the lower the
compliance of the ventricle during filling. Over the
normal range of ventricular filling volumes the EDPVR
gradient is approximately linear and the ventricle is
relatively compliant. As EDV increases and the ventricle becomes more distended at the end of diastole,
the EDPVR gradient becomes steeper, showing a
marked decrease in ventricular compliance to filling.
Pathological conditions such as ischaemic heart disease

and ventricular hypertrophy can shift the EDPVR
up and to the left, demonstrating ventricular diastolic
dysfunction (Figure 14.20).

Ventricular end-systolic pressure–volume relationship

The end-systolic points from several ventricular PV
loops (S1, S2, S3) may be plotted to give an end-systolic
pressure–volume curve (Figure 14.21). This curve is
called the end-systolic pressure–volume relationship

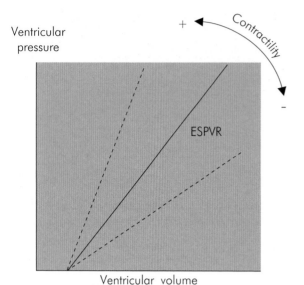

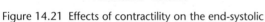

Figure 14.21 Effects of contractility on the end-systolic pressure–volume relationship (ESPVR) curve

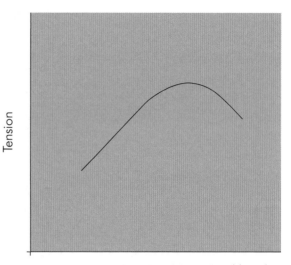

Figure 14.22 Frank curve for isolated muscle fibre

(ESPVR). The gradient of the ESPVR curve represents the elastance of the contracted ventricle at the end of systole. This is partially dependent on how forcefully the ventricle contracts, and hence is related to ventricular contractility. The ESPVR curve is approximately linear under normal conditions. Increased non-linearity is introduced under ischaemic or hypercontractile conditions and appears as a change in gradient and shift in the curve up or down.

The Frank–Starling curve

> The function of the heart as a pump is based on cardiac muscle. The contractile properties of cardiac muscle not only provide the engine to drive the cardiac pump but also give the heart an intrinsic ability to adapt its performance to a continually varying venous return. The mechanism underlying this adaptive ability is the Frank–Starling relationship.

The Frank curve

Frank demonstrated in isolated muscle fibre preparations that the tension developed on contraction was dependent on the initial length of the fibre. As initial length increased from resting value, the tension developed during contraction, increased and reached a maximum. Above this, the tension declined as the sarcomeres became overextended (Figure 14.22).

The Starling curve

The above property of isolated cardiac muscle fibres can be applied to the muscle fibres in the walls of an intact ventricle, where the length of muscle fibres is related to the volume of the ventricle. In this case the tension per unit cross-section (ventricular wall stress, T), developed in the wall during contraction, is dependent on the end-diastolic volume (EDV). Laplace's law relates the wall stress (T) to internal pressure in an elastic sphere (see *Afterload*, below), and thus the Frank relationship for an isolated muscle fibre translates into a relationship between intraventricular pressure and EDV during iso-volumetric contraction. Effectively, the greater the ventricular filling volume, the stronger the contraction of the ventricle. This mechanism gives the intact heart its built-in ability to adjust to varying levels of venous return.

Starling confirmed in ejecting mammalian hearts that with a constant aortic pressure, an increase in EDV produces a more forceful contraction and an increase in stroke volume (SV).

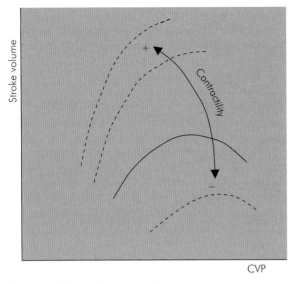

Figure 14.23 Ventricular function curve

Figure 14.24 Force–velocity curve for isolated muscle fibre

The Frank–Starling relationship

In the intact heart, a ventricular function curve (Frank–Starling curve) can be plotted to demonstrate the ability of the ventricle to vary its mechanical output according to its filling volumes. An index of mechanical output (such as SV) can be plotted against a measure of filling pressure (such as CVP) (Figure 14.23).

The Frank–Starling curve and cardiac failure

The normal ventricle never fills to an EDV which would place it on the descending limb of the Frank–Starling curve. This is because of a decreased compliance of the ventricle which occurs at high filling pressures. Sarcomere length at optimum filling pressures ($\approx$ 12 mmHg) is 2.2 μm, but even if filling pressures are increased fourfold (> 50 mmHg) sarcomere length will not increase beyond about 2.6 μm.

If the heart becomes pathologically dilated, as in cardiac failure, ventricular function may then shift to the descending portion of the Frank–Starling curve and cardiac decompensation ensues. Cardiac function can also deteriorate when factors such as hypoxia, acidosis or β-blockers shift the Frank–Starling curve down and to the right, depressing cardiac performance. Alternatively other factors such as endogenous catecholamines or inotropes can shift the Frank–Starling curve upwards and to the left, enhancing cardiac performance and protecting against cardiac failure (Figure 14.23).

The force–velocity curve for cardiac muscle

Starling not only investigated the sarcomere tension–length relationship, but also looked at the interaction between muscle force and velocity. The force–velocity curve demonstrates that the force generated and the velocity of muscle shortening are inversely related. Changes in preload and contractility will influence this relationship by shifting the force–velocity curve (Figure 14.24).

Stroke volume

The stroke volume (SV) is the volume of blood ejected by the ventricle with a single contraction. It can be defined as the difference between the end-diastolic volume (EDV) and the end-systolic volume (ESV).

Stroke volume, SV = EDV − ESV

The normal SV is between 70 and 80 mL, and it can be normalised to take account of body size by dividing by body surface area (BSA). This gives a stroke index (SI) which has a normal value for a 70 kg person (BSA = 1.7 m²) of 30–65 mL beat^{-1} m^{-2}.

Ejection fraction

Stroke volume can be quoted as a percentage of end-diastolic volume. It is then called ejection fraction (EF). The normal EF is approximately 60–65%, and it is a useful index of ventricular contractility.

$$\text{Ejection fraction, EF} = \frac{EDV - ESV}{EDV} = \frac{SV}{EDV} \times 100\%$$

Measurement of stroke volume

Ventriculography

This has been the gold standard for measuring ventricular volumes, to which less invasive measurement methods have been compared. However, it is a cumbersome procedure done in the catheter suite and is not appropriate for repeated estimations. Other techniques to measure LV volume and size include computed tomography, magnetic resonance imaging and radionuclide scans, but none is practical in the perioperative setting.

Echocardiography

The end-systolic and end-diastolic areas can be measured by 2D echocardiography to give an estimate of the stroke volume (SV). The SV is then multiplied by the heart rate to obtain the CO. This technique is limited by the approximation made to transform the two-dimensional images of the ventricular areas into volumes.

Transoesophageal echocardiography

Several studies have found a good correlation between left ventricular (LV) areas measured by transoesophageal echocardiography (TOE) and LV areas or volumes obtained by other techniques. The two-dimensional transgastric short-axis view of LV at the level of the papillary muscles reflects LV filling reasonably well. Modern echocardiography technology includes the automated border detection method, which displays the LV area throughout the cardiac cycle, together with the fractional area change (FAC), where

$$\text{FAC} = \frac{\text{End diastolic area} - \text{End systolic area}}{\text{End diastolic area}}$$

The normal value for FAC varies between 50% and 70%.

Thoracic impedance

A small alternating current of low amplitude and high frequency is introduced between two sets of electrodes around the neck and lower thorax. The resultant electrical impedance between the neck and thoracic electrodes is measured and represents the transthoracic impedance. Changes in thoracic impedance are produced by both ventilation and pulsatile blood flow. Stroke volume (SV) can be estimated by considering the pulsatile cardiac component of the impedance signal only. Cardiac output can then be calculated by measuring the heart rate (HR) and taking the product HR × SV. Although this technique is non-invasive and can provide a continuous reading of cardiac output, a significant degree of inconsistency and inaccuracy is present.

Cardiac output

Cardiac output (CO) gives a measure of the performance of the heart as a pump. It is defined as the volume of blood pumped by the LV (or RV) per minute and is equal to the product of the stroke volume (SV) and heart rate (HR):

$$\begin{aligned}\text{Cardiac output, CO} &= \text{Stroke volume, SV} \\ &\quad \times \text{ Heart rate, HR}\end{aligned}$$

With a normal HR of 70–80 beats per minute and SV of 70–80 mL, the average CO of a 70 kg person varies between 5 and 6 litres per minute under resting conditions. To compare patients of different body sizes, the CO can be divided by the patient's body surface area (BSA) to give a normalised parameter called the cardiac index (CI).

Calculation of cardiac index

$$\text{Cardiac index, CI} = \frac{CO}{BSA}$$

The BSA can be estimated from the height (cm) and weight (kg) of an individual and is quoted in square metres. The average 70 kg adult has a BSA of 1.7 m^2 and a CI of 3–3.5 L min^{-1} m^{-2}.

When the O_2 demand of the body increases during exercise, the CO of a young, healthy individual can increase up to fivefold. The CO should always be evaluated with reference to the oxygen demand at the time.

Cardiac output measurement

In animal models CO can be measured directly by cannulating the aorta, pulmonary artery or any of the great

Figure 14.25 Methods of monitoring cardiac output

Cardiac output (CO) monitor	Method of CO measurement	Advantages	Disadvantages
Pulmonary artery catheter (Swan–Ganz)	Pulmonary artery thermodilution: cold saline bolus injected into PAC, thermodilution principle, measured by thermistor in PAC tip in the pulmonary artery	Continuous PA pressures PACWP measurement Can be used with intra-aortic balloon pump (IABP) Heat dissipation minimised by short travel from injection to catheter tip 'Gold standard' for comparison with newer methods	Invasive – sheath in large vein, catheter through right heart Risk of injury to heart and pulmonary vessels, catheter migration No evident outcome benefit Not continuous
LiDCO	Transpulmonary lithium dilution. Calibration by lithium chloride bolus into CVP or vein while sampling arterial blood past lithium electrode. Continuous CO by arterial wave form analysis	Avoids heat dissipation errors Uses routine CVP and arterial lines Provides continuous CO Various displays target CO to aid management	Requires 24-hourly calibration No pulmonary artery pressures Not used in patients with IABP Cannot be used in patients on lithium
PiCCO	Transpulmonary thermodilution: cold saline bolus injected into CVP line. Thermistor in femoral a-line. CO by continuous arterial wave form analysis	Arterial line is also used for blood sampling Continuous CO	Arterial line in femoral artery Errors due to heat dissipation because of transpulmonary passage between injection point and thermistor
Pulse contour CO Vigileo	Analysis of arterial waveform characteristics and calculate CO from patient demographic data	Arterial line transducer supplied by manufacturer No calibration input	Uses extrapolation from patient demographic data Dependent on quality of a-line trace No use in patient with IABP
Doppler	Oesophageal or sternal notch Doppler probe. Calculation of CO using Doppler signals and patient demographic data	Does not require vascular access No calibration needed	Consistency of monitoring depends on Doppler trace quality Cannot be used in patient with IABP

Author: R. S. Pretorius MB ChB MFamMed MMed (Anaes), Consultant Anaesthetist, University Hospitals of Leicester

veins and then using an electromagnetic or ultrasonic flow meter. However, this is not appropriate in a clinical situation and CO is usually measured by indirect methods (Figure 14.25).

Indicator dilution techniques

Thermodilution This is at present the most commonly used method to measure CO at the bedside. A pulmonary artery catheter (PAC) is inserted, cold saline is injected into the RA, and the change in blood temperature is measured by the PAC-thermistor in the PA. The PAC is connected to an analogue computer, which calculates the CO.

Calculation of CO uses the modified Steward–Hamilton equation:

$$CO = \frac{V\,(T_B - T_I) \times K_1 \times K_2}{\int_0^\infty T_B(t)\,dt}$$

where
V = volume of injectate
T_B = initial blood temperature (°C)
T_I = initial injectate temperature (°C)
K_1 = density constant
K_2 = computation constant
$\int T_B(t)\,dt$ = integral of blood temperature change

The CO is inversely proportional to the area under the temperature–time curve. This technique is popular because multiple CO estimations can be made at frequent intervals without blood sampling. The accuracy of the technique is influenced by several factors, which include intracardiac shunts, tricuspid regurgitation and positive-pressure ventilation.

A modification of this principle is used in the 'continuous' CO monitor. A pulse of electrical current heats up a proximal part of the PAC creating a bolus of warmed blood. The temperature rise is sensed when the warmed blood passes a thermistor in the PA. A computer then calculates the area under the curve and hence the CO.

Dye dilution This was the most popular technique prior to thermodilution. Indocyanine green is injected into a central vein, while blood is continuously sampled from an arterial cannula. The change in indicator concentration over time is measured, a computer calculates the area under the dye concentration curve, and CO is computed. Unfortunately recirculation and build-up of the indicator results in a high background concentration, which limits the total number of measurements that can be taken. The dye is non-toxic and rapidly removed from circulation by the liver.

Fick method The Fick principle states that the amount of a substance taken up by an organ (or the whole body) per time unit is equal to the arterial concentration of the substance, minus the venous concentration (A–V difference),

multiplied by the blood flow. This can be applied to the oxygen content of blood in order to determine the CO.

Application of Fick principle to calculate CO

First the steady-state oxygen content of venous (CvO_2) and arterial blood (CaO_2) are measured. Then oxygen uptake in the lungs is measured over 1 minute ($\dot{V}O_2$). Finally the Fick principle is applied to calculate the blood flowing in 1 minute (CO):

$$Cardiac\ output = \frac{\dot{V}O_2}{(CaO_2 - CvO_2)}$$

This technique is limited by errors in sampling and the inability to maintain steady-state conditions.

Doppler techniques

Ultrasonic Doppler transducers have been incorporated into pulmonary artery catheters, endotracheal tubes, suprasternal probes and oesophageal probes. These probes can then be used to measure mean blood flow velocity through the aorta or any valve orifice. Then, using an estimation for the cross-sectional area of flow, the flow velocity–time integral, heart rate and a constant, the cardiac output can be calculated.

Control of cardiac pump function

Cardiac output (CO) is given by the product of stroke volume (SV) and heart rate (HR). The factors determining CO can thus be divided into those affecting HR and those

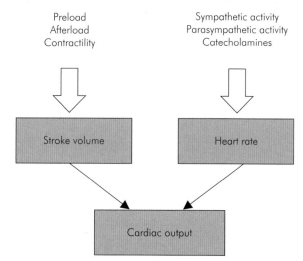

Figure 14.26 Control of cardiac output

which determine SV. Overall control of CO is a combination of the mechanisms controlling SV and HR. This is illustrated in Figure 14.26. The individual control of SV and HR are considered in detail below.

Factors determining stroke volume

> **Three major determinants of SV**
>
> - Preload
> - Afterload
> - Contractility

Overall control of stroke volume is summarised in Figure 14.27. The three main factors, preload, afterload and contractility, are based on physiological concepts arising from the performance of isolated muscle preparations. They have become useful in clinical practice when applied to the intact heart, but are difficult or impractical to measure directly. Hence more easily monitored parameters are used as practical indices.

A summary for each factor precedes a more detailed consideration in the following sections. These summaries consist of:

- Physiological definition – a theoretical definition for the parameter
- Physiological index – a measurement from which the physiological definition can be derived
- Practical concept – a description of the parameter suitable for clinical use
- Practical index – a measurement used clinically for the parameter

Preload

In clinical circumstances the term preload remains loosely defined and has become synonymous with a range of parameters including CVP, venous return and pulmonary capillary wedge pressure (PCWP).

A strict definition for preload can be obtained from the Frank relationship between muscle fibre length and developed tension. Here preload is the initial length of the muscle fibre before contraction. In the intact ventricle the preload would therefore be equivalent to the end-diastolic volume (EDV), since the presystolic length of the myocardial fibres will be directly related to the EDV.

> **Definition of preload**
>
> Physiological definition – Presystolic length of cardiac muscle fibres
> Physiological index – End-diastolic volume (EDV)
> Practical concept – Filling pressure of ventricles
> Practical index – CVP or PCWP

Factors affecting preload

- Total blood volume
- Body position
- Intrathoracic and intrapericardial pressures
- Venous tone and compliance
- Pumping action of skeletal muscles
- Synchronous atrial contribution to ventricular filling
- Ventricular end diastolic compliance

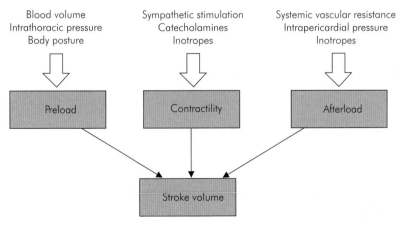

Figure 14.27 Control of stroke volume

Measurement of preload

There are no convenient or practical methods of measuring EDV directly. Because of this, end-diastolic pressure is often used when assessing the filling conditions of the intact ventricle. End-diastolic pressure is related to EDV by the ventricular end-diastolic pressure–volume curve (EDPVR – see Figure 14.20) and is sometimes referred to as the 'filling pressure' of the ventricle. The EDPVR is approximately linear at normal filling pressures, but the gradient (ventricular elastance = compliance^{-1}) gradually increases as filling pressure increases. End-diastolic pressure is therefore only a reasonable index of preload under normal conditions.

In practice end-diastolic pressure can be estimated on the left side of the heart by measuring left atrial pressure (LAP), pulmonary capillary wedge pressure (PCWP) or pulmonary artery diastolic pressure (PADP). On the right side, preload is reflected by right atrial pressure (RAP) or central venous pressure (CVP). All of these measurements can be made using a pulmonary artery catheter, but the most common measurements used are CVP and PCWP as indices of right and left preloads respectively. Interpretation of these estimates is subject to the following limitations.

Limitations of CVP and PCWP as measures of preload

- Ventricular compliance may not be normal, as it can be reduced by factors such as myocardial ischaemia, ventricular hypertrophy or pericardial tamponade. In a non-compliant ventricle, higher than normal filling pressures may be required to provide adequate preload.
- The atrioventricular valve may be abnormal. The presence of mitral stenosis may require higher than normal filling pressures to achieve adequate preload in the left ventricle.
- Positive intrathoracic pressures can be transmitted through to a pulmonary artery catheter and increase the mean PCWP reading. In the case of a ventilated patient, positive end-expiratory pressure (PEEP) and the inspiratory pressure cycles can affect the PCWP signal.
- Placement of the PAC in the dependent part of the lung can add a hydrostatic pressure component to a PCWP signal.

- Increased pulmonary vascular resistance as in pulmonary hypertension can lead to higher than normal pulmonary artery diastolic pressures (PADP). This reduces the accuracy of the PADP as an estimate of left-side preload.

Afterload

In an isolated muscle fibre preparation, the afterload is defined as the tension developed during contraction. Thus the afterload is related to the mechanical resistance to shortening of the muscle fibre. In the intact heart afterload becomes the tension per unit cross-section (or stress), T, developed in the ventricular wall during systole.

Application of Laplace's law to determine ventricular wall tension

This can be related to the intraventricular pressure during systole, by applying Laplace's law for pressure in an elastic sphere:

$$\text{Intraventricular pressure} = \frac{2hT}{r}$$

where h is ventricular wall thickness, and r is the radius of the ventricular cavity.

The afterload is thus a measure of how forcefully the ventricle contracts during systole in order to eject blood.

Definition of afterload

Physiological definition – Ventricular wall stress developed during systole
Physiological index – Systolic ventricular wall stress
Practical concept – Intraventricular pressure developed during systole
Practical index – SVR and MAP, PVR and MPAP

Factors affecting afterload

- Systemic or pulmonary vascular resistance
- Factors stimulating or depressing cardiac contraction
- Intrathoracic pressure or intrapericardial pressure
- Preload
- Ventricular wall thickness

The normal ventricle has an intrinsic ability to increase its performance in response to increases in afterload, in order to maintain stroke volume. If the afterload increases suddenly, it causes an initial fall in stroke volume. The ventricle then increases its EDV in response to the change, which in turn restores the stroke volume. This is called the Anrep effect.

Measurement of afterload

- Arterial pressure or ventricular pressure during systole. These pressures normally follow each other closely during systole and are indirect indices of ventricular wall tension. Arterial systolic pressure is often the available measurement, but its accuracy is limited if there is a significant gradient between aorta and ventricle, e.g. as in aortic stenosis.
- Systemic vascular resistance (SVR) is the most commonly used index of afterload in clinical practice. It can be calculated from mean arterial pressure (MAP), central venous pressure (CVP) and cardiac output (CO), as follows:

$$SVR = \frac{MAP - CVP}{CO} \times 80 \text{ dynes. sec .cm}^{-5}$$

- The normal value for SVR ranges from 900 to 1400 dyne.s.cm^{-5}. The SVR is not a good estimate of afterload, since it is only one component determining afterload, and does not provide any index of intraventricular pressures generated during systole (i.e. how hard the ventricle is contracting). Clearly if the ventricle only generates low intraventricular pressures by contracting softly, the afterload is low irrespective of the value of SVR.
- In a similar manner the pulmonary vascular resistance (PVR) may be calculated as an index of right ventricular afterload, using mean pulmonary arterial pressure (MPAP), pulmonary capillary wedge pressure (PCWP) and cardiac output (CO):

$$PVR = \frac{MPAP - PCWP}{CO} \times 80 \text{ dynes. sec .cm}^{-5}$$

- The normal PVR ranges from 90 to 150 dyne.s.cm^{-5}. The CO, PAP and PCWP have to be obtained with a PAC to calculate SVR and PVR.
- Systemic vascular impedance. The mechanical property of the vascular system opposing the ejection and flow of blood into it is called the vascular impedance. This is composed of two components. One component is the resistive or steady flow component, which is the SVR (see above). This component is mainly due to the frictional opposition to flow in the vessels.

- The other component is the reactive or frequency-dependent component, which is due to the compliance of the vessel walls and inertia of the ejected blood. This component is dependent on the pulsatile nature of the flow and rapidity of ejection. A major part of this reactive component is formed by the arterial elastance (Ea).
- Arterial elastance (Ea). The arterial elastance is the inverse of arterial compliance (Ca), and is a measure of the elastic forces in the arterial system which tend to oppose the ejection of blood into it. Determination of Ea involves plotting a pressure–volume curve for the arterial system using different stroke volumes and recording end-systolic pressures. The slope of the curve then gives the effective elastance (compliance^{-1}) of the arterial system (see Figure 14.31).
- Ventricular systolic wall stress. As noted previously, ventricular wall stress (T) during systole is equal to afterload. A direct measurement of this quantity is impractical under clinical conditions. Since wall stress is force per unit cross-section generated in the muscle on contraction, it is dependent on wall thickness. For a given systolic pressure, the thicker the wall, the larger the cross-section of muscle and the lower the stress. Thus a dilated, thin-walled, 'failing' ventricle will experience a higher afterload (wall stress) than a hypertrophied ventricle.

Contractility

Contractility is a poorly defined term describing the intrinsic ability of a cardiac muscle fibre to do mechanical work when it contracts with a predefined load and initial degree of stretch. In the intact ventricle contractility reflects the amount of work that can be done for a given preload and afterload.

Definition of contractility

Physiological definition – Systolic myocardial work done with given preload and afterload

Physiological index – Ventricular stroke work index. Maximum slope (dP/dt) of ventricular isovolumetric contraction curve

Practical concept – Ejection fraction for given CVP and MAP

Practical index – Ejection fraction

Factors affecting contractility

Contractility can be increased by:

- Increased serum calcium levels
- Sympathetic stimulation
- Parasympathetic inhibition
- Positive inotropic drugs
- Digoxin

Contractility can be decreased by:

- Decreased serum calcium levels
- Parasympathetic stimulation
- Sympathetic blockade – β-blockade, local anaesthetic blockade
- Myocardial ischaemia or infarction
- Hypoxia and acidosis
- Mismatched ventriculoarterial coupling

Ventricular work done during systole

The most direct method of measuring contractility is to measure ventricular work at given preload and afterload values.

The calculation of ventricular work done during systole requires an integral of the ventricular pressure–volume loop area. This is not a practical measurement, but an approximation is stroke work (SW), obtained from the following product:

$$SW = \text{(stroke volume)}$$
$$\times \text{(mean arterial pressure} - \text{filling pressure)}$$

Figure 14.28 illustrates how this value approximates to the PV loop area for the left ventricle. The SV work index (SVWI) is a more useful indicator of contractility, as it is normalised for body surface area (BSA) by using stroke index (SI = SV/BSA) in its calculation.

Calculation of left ventricular stroke work index (LVSWI)

$$LVSWI = \frac{(MAP - PCWP) \times SI}{100}$$
$$\times 1.36 \text{ g.m.m}^{-2}$$

Normal values for LVSWI are 45–60 g.m.m^{-2}

Calculation of right ventricular stroke work index (RVSWI)

$$RVSWI = \frac{(MPAP - CVP) \times SI}{100}$$
$$\times 1.36 \text{ g.m.m}^{-2}$$

Normal values for RSVWI are 5–10 g.m.m^{-2}

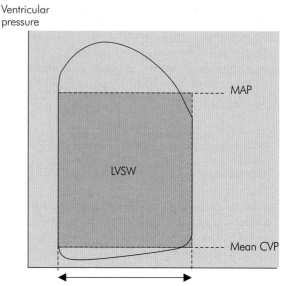

Figure 14.28 Left ventricular stroke work estimate for ventricular pressure–volume loop area

Other methods of measuring contractility

- dP/dt_{max} – This is obtained from the maximum slope of the ventricular pressure curve during isovolumetric contraction. The slope can be measured during cardiac catheterisation.
- Ejection fraction (EF) – This is measured by radio-nuclide ventriculography or transthoracic echocardiography. It is often derived from the fractional area change (FAC) measurement (see *Measurement of stroke volume*, above). EF and FAC are both sensitive to preload and afterload. These latter parameters should also be evaluated with EF or FAC. There is a clear association between EF and prognosis in cardiac patients.
- Ventricular function curves – A ventricular function curve can be plotted between an index of ventricular filling (e.g. CVP or PCWP) and an index of ventricular performance (e.g. cardiac output or stroke volume). Factors increasing contractility will shift the curve upwards and to the left, while those decreasing contractility will shift it downwards and to the right.
- Ventricular end-systolic elastance (Ees). Ees can be obtained from the end-systolic pressure volume relationship (ESPVR) (see Figure 14.21).

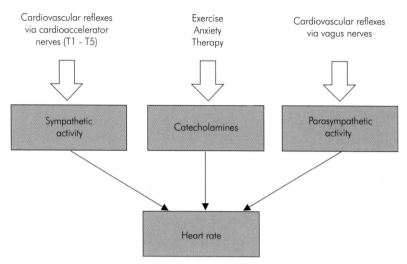

Figure 14.29 Control of heart rate

Heart rate

The heart rate is normally determined by the spontaneous depolarisation rate of the SA node pacemaker cells (see *Physiological cardiac arrhythmias*, above). The normal heart rate of 60–80 beats per minute is much slower than the intrinsic rate of the denervated heart (110 beats per minute). This is because of the dominant parasympathetic tone in the intact cardiovascular system (Figure 14.29).

Autonomic control of pacemaker discharge rate

> In vivo, control of the pacemaker rate is mediated peripherally via the autonomic nervous system. Central control of pacemaker rate lies in parasympathetic and sympathetic nuclei of the medulla. These are responsible for cardiovascular reflexes, and are influenced by higher centres including the posterior hypothalamus and cortical areas.

- Parasympathetic system – Parasympathetic fibres to the heart originate in the dorsal motor nucleus of the vagus and the nucleus ambiguus in the medulla oblongata. These parasympathetic fibres travel to the heart via the right and left vagus nerves. During embryological development the right vagus nerve becomes connected to the SA node, while the left vagus supplies the AV node. Vagal stimulation

(parasympathetic activity) decreases the slope of phase 4 and also increases hyperpolarisation, thus slowing the heart rate.
- Sympathetic system – Sympathetic innervation to the heart originates in the sympathetic chain (T1–T5 fibres), passing via the stellate ganglion to all parts of the heart, with a strong representation to the ventricular muscle. The right side distributes to the SA node, while the left side primarily supplies the AV node. Sympathetic activity increases the slope of phase 4 and hence the heart rate. This effect occurs in exercise, anxiety and febrile illness.
- Direct interconnections exist between the parasympathetic and sympathetic cardiac supplies which enable both systems to inhibit each other directly.

Cardiovascular reflexes

Some recognised cardiovascular reflexes controlling heart rate (HR) include:
- Lung volume stretch receptor reflex – Moderate increases in lung volume increase HR via the vagus nerves.
- Chemoreceptor reflexes – The primary effect of carotid chemoreceptor stimulation is to activate vagal centres in the medulla, leading to a decrease in HR. However, this is modified by a secondary effect exerted by concomitant excitation of respiratory centres in the medulla which oppose the primary effect.
- Atrial stretch receptor reflex (Bainbridge reflex) – Stimulation of atrial stretch receptors by increases in

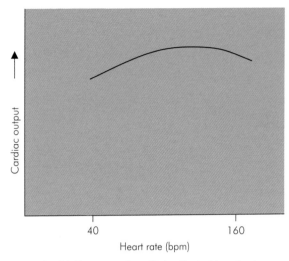

Figure 14.30 Treppe or Bowditch effect of heart rate on cardiac output

venous return or blood volume gives rise to acceleration of the HR. This is mediated via the vagus nerves.

- Baroreceptor reflexes – Stimulation of baroreceptors in the aortic arch or carotid sinus by an increase in blood pressure lead to a decrease in HR. Similarly a drop in blood pressure causes an increase in HR.

Effects of heart rate on cardiac output

Heart rate affects cardiac output (CO) in the following ways:

- An increase in heart rate will lead to a progressive increase in CO up to a rate of about 140 beats per minute. When heart rate increases, stroke volume (SV) decreases due to shorter diastolic filling time, but this only becomes significant at rates > 140 beats per minute.
- When the rate exceeds 150 beats per minute the decrease in diastolic filling time reduces the CO significantly because it encroaches on rapid filling time. Diastolic time is affected by a tachycardia to a much greater extent than systolic time.
- The Bowditch phenomenon ('Treppe' or staircase effect) is increased inotropy in response to increased chronotropy. The increased contractility that occurs at higher heart rates is due to the greater availability of intracellular calcium for excitation–contraction coupling. This follows the reduced diastolic time available for calcium reuptake (Figure 14.30).

- During a tachycardia in a normal heart, the end-diastolic pressure–volume relationship (EDPVR) will move to the left and downwards, i.e. smaller filling volumes at lower end-diastolic pressures. In an ischaemic heart, however, a tachycardia will move the EDPVR to the left but upwards, i.e. smaller filling volumes at higher end-diastolic pressures.
- A tachycardia will increase the ventricular systolic elastance (Ees) due to the increased contractility.
- A pronounced bradycardia below 40 beats per minute will drop CO, because the compensatory increase in SV is not enough to make up for the decrease in ejection rate.

Cardiovascular coupling

In clinical practice, assessment of cardiac function often relies on the available measurements of filling pressures (CVP and PCWP), arterial pressures (pulmonary and aortic), and cardiac output. These measurements are dependent on two sets of characteristics which reflect:

- The contractile performance of the heart
- The elastance (pressure–volume relationship) of the vascular system

Assessing the relative effects of cardiac contractility and vascular system elastance on pressure measurements is important clinically, since it can influence therapeutic decisions.

> Interpretation of pressure and cardiac output measurements is aided by a consideration of the interaction or coupling between the heart and the vascular system. This can be performed at the arterial side (ventriculoarterial coupling) for arterial pressures, or on the venous side of the heart (ventriculovenous coupling) for CVP values.

Ventriculoarterial coupling

Coupling between the ventricle and arterial system is illustrated by plotting the ventricular elastance (Ees) and arterial elastance (Ea) on the same diagram. The end-systolic point (P) then lies at the junction of the curves, which are approximately at right angles to each other. Changes in arterial pressure are reflected by a shift in the position of P. If preload (end-diastolic point) is maintained constant, then the direction of displacement of P identifies the degree to which ventricular contractility or arterial elastance is responsible (Figure 14.31).

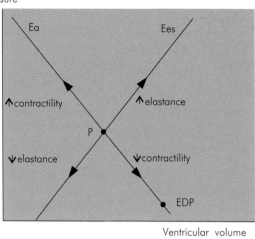

Figure 14.31 Ventriculoarterial coupling diagram

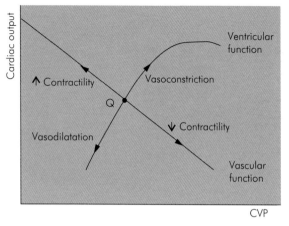

Figure 14.32 Ventriculovenous coupling diagram

The left ventricle (LV) and arterial system can be seen as two elastic chambers with opposing elastances Ees and Ea respectively. The distribution of blood is determined by the individual elastances of the two chambers. Theoretical analysis suggests that the LV will deliver maximal work when Ees = Ea but will work with maximal mechanical efficiency when Ees = 2 × Ea. The implication is that there is an optimum ventriculoarterial coupling ratio for these elastances. If these elastances are mismatched the ventricle may fail, e.g. if the ventricle ejects for a prolonged period of time against a very low afterload.

Ventriculovenous coupling

Description of cardiovascular coupling on the venous side of the heart requires the use of a vascular function curve. This curve describes the changes occuring in CVP as venous return is removed at different rates by the heart. It is obtained by varying the cardiac output (CO) and recording the resulting CVP, at constant intravascular volume. The vascular function curve is a pressure–flow relationship at the venous side of the vascular system, dependent on the balance between vascular tone and intravascular volume. Changes in the gradient reflect alterations in vascular tone. Thus vasodilatation causes a decreased gradient, while an increased gradient is associated with vasoconstriction. Changes in the intercept reflect altered intravascular volume.

A ventriculovenous coupling diagram can be drawn by plotting a vascular function curve and a ventricular function curve on the same axes. The ventricular function curve is

described earlier and in Figure 14.23. These curves intersect at an operating point (Q). When Q becomes displaced by cardiovascular changes, the direction of displacement indicates the relative contributions of vascular tone and ventricular contractility effects to the changes (Figure 14.32).

Ventricular interdependence

Right and left ventricles are situated inside the same non-compliant pericardium. This means that they are both exposed to the same intrathoracic and intra-alveolar pressures. Changes in volume and pressure of one ventricle will directly affect the other. Normally LV pressure is greater than RV pressure and the interventricular septum bows into the RV. However, the thin free wall of the RV makes it more sensitive to increases in afterload than the LV, and any increase in afterload (e.g. pulmonary hypertension) will lead to dilatation of the RV. Under these circumstances the trans-septal pressure gradient can reverse, and the septum can shift to the left, compromising LV filling during diastole. Interaction between the two ventricles occurs during systole and diastole, and is called ventricular interdependence (Figure 14.33).

Cardiac failure

The course of cardiac failure may be acute or chronic. The commonest cause of acute cardiac failure is myocardial infarction, while chronic failure often arises in ischaemic heart disease, hypertension and valvular disease. In acute cardiac failure hypotension without peripheral oedema may occur. While in chronic failure, blood pressure is usually maintained, but signs and symptoms due to congestion develop.

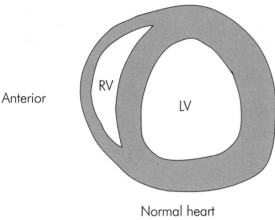

Anterior

RV

LV

Normal heart

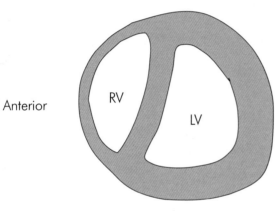

Anterior

RV

LV

Pulmonary hypertension

Figure 14.33 Ventricular interdependence

Cardiac failure is a state of inadequate circulation due to cardiac dysfunction. The condition manifests itself in two ways:

- First, there is a failure to provide adequate arterial pressure and cardiac output into the systemic circulation ('forward failure').
- Second, there is a failure to pump away the venous return, which causes backup or congestion in the pulmonary or systemic venous beds ('backward failure').

Figure 14.34 Signs and symptoms of cardiac failure

Physiological change	Sign or symptom
Congestion in the pulmonary vascular system	Pulmonary oedema Dyspnoea on exertion Orthopnoea Paroxysmal nocturnal dyspnoea
Congestion in the systemic vascular system	Dependent oedema (e.g. ankle) Hepatomegaly Raised jugulovenous pressure
Inadequate systemic circulation	Fatigue Sodium retention Increased intravascular volume

Figure 14.35 Changes in physiological indices in cardiac failure

Change in heart	Change in physiological index
↓ ventricular contractility	↓ Decreased CO ↓ gradient of ESPVR Shift of ventricular function curve down
Ventricular dilatation	↑ CVP ↑ systolic ventricular wall stress ↑ EDV
Ventricular diastolic dysfunction	Shift of EDPVR curve up and left
Altered cardiovascular coupling	Displacement of operating point on ventriculoarterial and ventriculovenous coupling diagrams

Some of the common signs and symptoms of cardiac failure are shown in Figure 14.34.

Many of the physiological parameters and indices reflecting aspects of cardiac performance change in cardiac failure. These include those shown in Figure 14.35.

CHAPTER 15
Physiology of the circulation

Ted Lin

Blood vessels

The circulation can be divided into the systemic and the pulmonary circulation. The systemic circulation receives oxygenated blood from the left side of the heart via the aorta and returns desaturated blood to the right side of the heart in the venae cavae. The desaturated blood is delivered to the pulmonary circulation from the right ventricle via the pulmonary artery to be oxygenated and to exchange carbon dioxide. Oxygenated blood is then returned to the left atrium via the pulmonary veins (Figure 15.1).

Structure and function

Blood vessel walls are basically structured in three layers. The adventitia is the outer layer and is made up of connective tissue with nerve fibres. The middle layer or media is of varying thickness and contains mainly smooth muscle. The innermost layer is the intima and consists of the endothelium, basement membrane and supporting connective tissue (Figure 15.2). The composition of blood vessel walls is mainly a mixture of elastic tissue, fibrous tissue and smooth muscle. This mixture again varies according to the type of vessel. The aorta walls are predominantly elastic and fibrous tissue with little smooth muscle, whereas the vena cava walls consist largely of smooth muscle and fibrous components. The composition of vessel walls reflects their function.

Blood vessel diameter and wall thickness

A major factor determining thickness is mean arterial pressure. Some typical values for vessel diameter, wall thickness and mean arterial pressure are given in Figure 15.4.

Fundamentals of Anaesthesia, 4th edition, ed. Ted Lin, Tim Smith and Colin Pinnock. Published by Cambridge University Press. © Cambridge University Press 2017.

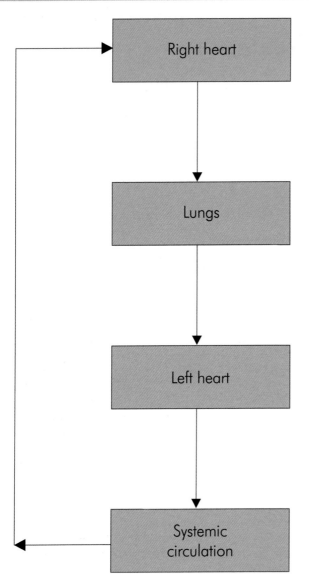

Figure 15.1 Adult circulation system

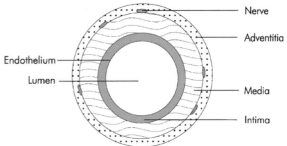

Figure 15.2 Blood vessel structure

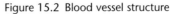

Figure 15.3 Functional aspects of blood vessel wall characteristics

Characteristic	Functional aspect
Wall thickness	Thick walls provide tensile strength to withstand pressure in arteries Thin walls in capillaries allow exchange with interstitial fluid
Elastic component in walls	Smoothing of pulsations, storage of energy to maintain flow in diastole
Smooth muscle component in walls	Control of vessel diameter by autonomic reflex and humoral activity
Fibrous component in walls	Mechanical strength

Blood vessel function

The arteries transport blood under high pressure to the tissues, where they divide into smaller arterioles, which in turn release the blood into capillaries. There the exchange of fluid, nutrients, electrolytes and other substances between the interstitial fluid and the blood takes place. The venules collect blood from the capillaries, and join together into veins to transport the blood back to the heart.

Blood vessels also function to smooth the pulsatile pressure waveform in the aorta, to control pressure at the capillary beds, and to store blood volume. The control of regional perfusion is dependent on reflexes and auto-regulation, which rely on arteriolar control. The functions of the different types of vessel in the circulatory system are summarised in Figure 15.5.

Pressure and flow in the vascular system

Flow and flow velocity

The functioning of organ systems depends on the volume of blood flowing per unit time through them, or the volume flow rate. This is often shortened to the term

Figure 15.4 Blood vessel diameters and mean pressures

Vessel	Diameter	Wall thickness	Mean pressure (mmHg)
Aorta	25 mm	2 mm	100
Artery	4 mm	1 mm	95
Arteriole	20 μm	6 μm	50
Terminal arteriole	10 μm	2 μm	45
Capillary	8 μm	0.5 μm	30
Venule	20 μm	1 μm	20
Vein	5 mm	0.5 mm	8
Vena cava	30 mm	1.5 mm	3

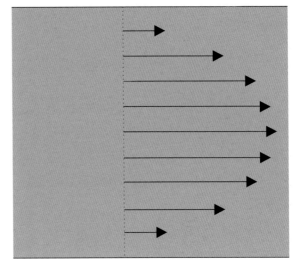

Figure 15.6 Physics of laminar flow

Figure 15.5 Blood vessels and their functions

Vessel	Function
Aorta	Storage of energy to maintain delivery in diastole, and damping of pressure pulses
Arteries	Delivery, distribution and damping of pressure waveform
Arterioles	Resistance to control pressure and distribution to capillaries
Capillaries	Microcirculation and exchange
Venules and small veins	Collection
Large veins and venae cavae	Collection, storage capacitance and delivery of venous return (or portal circulations)

'flow'. Flow can be measured in millilitres per second (or litres per minute). The total flow through the systemic circulation or the lungs is equal to the cardiac output.

Flow should be differentiated from flow velocity. Flow velocity defines how fast fluid is moving at any given point and has units of centimetres per second. In a blood vessel the flow velocity of blood varies between the centre

of the vessel and the vessel wall. If the flow pattern of the blood is described as laminar (i.e. without turbulence) the blood moves smoothly in the direction of the axis of the vessel. The velocity of the blood varies in a predictable pattern, with maximum velocity in the centre of the vessel and minimum velocity next to the wall, as if the blood is moving in concentric layers (Figure 15.6).

Consider a vessel with cross-sectional area A. The mean flow velocity (v) can be taken across the cross-section. The flow (Q) is then related to the mean flow velocity (v) by

$$Q = vA$$

This relationship can be applied to the vascular system as a whole, since the number and diameter of any type of blood vessel determines the total cross-sectional area presented to flow at that stage in the vascular system. The greater the total cross-sectional area of any given generation of vessels, the slower the velocity of blood flow through those vessels. The cross-sectional area of the aorta is about 4.5 cm^2, with peak flow velocities of > 120 cm s^{-1}. In contrast, the flow velocity in the several billion capillaries of the vascular system is usually between 0 and 1 cm s^{-1} due to a total capillary cross-sectional area of > 4500 cm^2 (Figure 15.7). These flow velocities reflect the functions of delivery and distribution in the aorta and arteries, as opposed to perfusion and exchange in the capillaries.

In an individual vessel, if the cross-sectional area is reduced by a constriction such as a valve or an

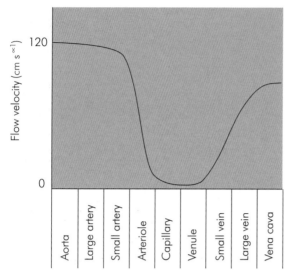

Figure 15.7 Flow velocity in different vessels

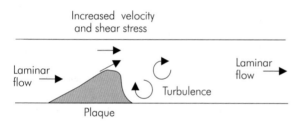

Figure 15.8 Turbulent flow and drag in vessels

There are additional contributions of energy to flow from skeletal muscle contraction and negative intrathoracic pressure during inspiration. These mechanisms create a pressure difference across the vascular system that produces the total flow (cardiac output) through the vascular system.

> A simple electrical analogy can be found in Ohm's law, where a potential difference (V) produces an electrical current (I) through a resistance (R). In this case
>
> $$V = I \times R$$
>
> Thus the pressure difference between mean arterial pressure (MAP) and central venous pressure (CVP) is related to cardiac output (CO) and systemic vascular resistance (SVR) by:
>
> $$MAP - CVP = CO \times SVR$$
>
> This is often approximated to:
>
> $$MAP - CO \times SVR$$

atheromatous plaque, the flow velocity increases through the constriction. Such increases in flow velocity can affect the characteristics of the blood flow, making it turbulent and leading to an increased tendency towards thrombus formation. The motion of blood across the stationary surface of the vessel wall produces a viscous drag or shear stress along the surface of the vessel wall. This shear stress is increased with increased flow velocity, producing a force that tends to pull endothelium and plaques away from the wall, leading to dissection or emboli. Increased flow velocity also produces bruits or murmurs (Figure 15.8).

Flow through the systemic circulation

The energy imparted to blood within the circulation by the heart and the elastic recoil of the great vessels causes it to flow through the systemic and pulmonary circulations.

Vascular resistance

'Vascular resistance' is a clinical term used to represent the effect of all the forces opposing blood flow through a vascular bed. It may be applied to the systemic vascular circulation, the pulmonary circulation or a given visceral circulation. The forces opposing blood flow through a vascular system are composed of two main components. First, there are those which dissipate energy because of frictional effects. This resistance arises as a result of drag between fluid layers and friction between fluid and vessel walls. The viscosity of the blood is a major determinant of this component of resistance.

The second component of opposing forces arises from the conversion of pump work into stored energy. This occurs when potential energy is stored by the elasticity of distended vessel walls or by gravity as blood is pumped to a greater height within the body. In addition, inertial effects store kinetic energy when blood is accelerated. This component is referred to as the 'reactive' component, and it is dependent on the pulsatile component of the pressure waveform. If the pressure difference applied across a vascular bed were constant, the reactive component would be minimal.

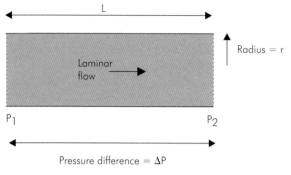

Figure 15.9 The Hagen–Poiseuille law

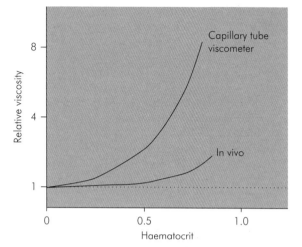

Figure 15.10 Haematocrit related to viscosity

Flow in a single vessel

Blood flow through larger vessels (> 0.5 mm diameter) can be approximated to the case of an idealised or Newtonian fluid (such as water) flowing through a tube. Under laminar flow conditions with a 'steady' pressure gradient, the flow (Q) between any two points, P_1 and P_2, is dependent on the pressure difference, ΔP, between the points, and inversely dependent on the resistance to flow (R):

$$Q = \frac{\Delta P}{R}$$

According to the Hagen–Poiseuille law, which describes laminar flow in tubes, the flow resistance, R, is dependent on the length of the tube and the viscosity of the fluid, but inversely related to the fourth power of the radius (Figure 15.9). The real situation of blood flowing through a vessel differs from this ideal model in the following respects:

- Blood vessels are not uniform in cross-section.
- Blood vessel walls are elastic.
- Pressure gradients pushing blood through vessels are not 'steady' but have a pulsatile component.
- Blood as a fluid behaves differently from a Newtonian fluid because of the cellular components, and its flow properties are not determined solely by viscosity.

Blood viscosity

The rheological properties of blood describe its flow-resistive properties. In a Newtonian fluid these resistive properties are dependent on a constant, the coefficient of viscosity. Blood, however, is a suspension of cells, and although the viscosity can be determined to give an apparent value, this value varies significantly with blood composition and flow conditions. The factors causing this variation in apparent viscosity include:

- Haematocrit – an increase in haematocrit to 0.7 (normal haematocrit = 0.45) can double the apparent viscosity (Figure 15.10).
- Diameter of the vessel – apparent blood viscosity can be measured in vitro using a capillary tube viscometer, and decreases as tube diameter decreases to below about 0.3 mm.

- The functions of different blood vessels are reflected in their structures and flow characteristics.
- Flow velocity is inversely related to the total cross-sectional area of the vascular system, reflecting the functions of the vessels. Lowest flow velocities occur in the capillaries, to allow for exchange of nutrients and metabolites.
- Blood flow in a single vessel may be laminar or turbulent. Laminar flow is governed by the Hagen–Poiseuille law. Turbulence occurs at high flow velocities or irregularities such as branching or valves.
- Vascular resistance depends on blood vessel geometry and compliance. It is also determined by blood viscosity, which varies with flow velocity.

- Red blood cell streaming – in smaller-diameter vessels red blood cells stream centrally along the axis of the vessel. This effectively reduces the haematocrit in these vessels. The haematocrit in capillaries may be 25% of the value in larger vessels (Figure 15.11).
- In vivo – apparent blood viscosity is lower in vivo than in vitro. At normal haematocrit the in vivo blood viscosity may only be half of the equivalent in vitro value.
- Flow velocity – apparent viscosity decreases at higher flow velocities and increases at low flow velocities. This is due to increased red cell aggregation and leucocyte adherence to vessel walls at low flow velocities.

Arterial system

The main function of the arterial system is to distribute and deliver blood to the capillary beds throughout the peripheral vascular system. A secondary arterial function is to convert the high-pressure pulsatile blood flow of the aorta into the low-pressure steady flow of the capillary beds. This modification of the flow and pressure profiles is achieved by the elasticity of the arterial system and is sometimes referred to as hydraulic filtering, or the 'Windkessel' effect

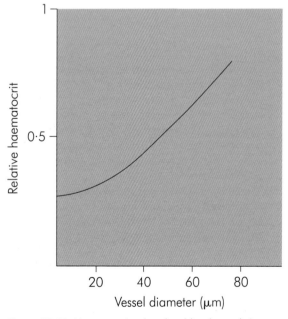

Figure 15.11 Haematocrit related to blood vessel size

(Windkessel – volume of air trapped in a pump reservoir to smooth out pressure variations).

Arterial factors
Flow velocity

In systole, the heart ejects a stroke volume of 70–90 mL blood into the aorta. The heart generates an average flow velocity of 70 cm s^{-1}, with a peak velocity of 120 cm s^{-1}, which makes flow in the aorta turbulent. There is transient backflow at the end of systole until the aortic valve closes. The aorta and arteries distend in systole due to the elasticity of their walls, then subsequent elastic recoil during diastole maintains forward flow distally into the peripheral vascular system.

Pressure wave

In the aorta and arteries the pressure is pulsatile. The maximum pressure is the systolic arterial pressure (about 120 mmHg) and the minimum is the diastolic arterial pressure (about 70 mmHg). The difference between diastolic and systolic is the pulse pressure, normally about 50 mmHg.

The aortic pressure wave changes in magnitude and shape as it travels through the arterial system. The shape of the pressure wave narrows, and high-frequency features such as the incisura (end-systolic notch) become dampened as it moves distally. Initially systolic pressures *increase* as the pressure waves travel from the aorta distally through the large arteries. At the femoral arteries systolic pressures have risen by 20 mmHg, and by the time pressure waves have reached the foot systolic pressures are 40 mmHg higher than in the aorta. Pressure pulsations begin to become attenuated in the smaller arteries and are finally reduced to a steady pressure with a mean level of 30–35 mmHg by the arterioles, ready for the capillary beds (Figure 15.12). The changes in the shape of the pressure waves are mainly due to the viscoelastic properties of the arterial walls. The increases in systolic pressure are thought to be due to factors affecting the propagation of the pressure waves through the vessels, such as reflection, resonance and changes in the velocity of propagation.

Mean arterial pressure

Mean arterial pressure (MAP) is the value obtained when the pressure is averaged over time. As shown above, it can be obtained from the product of cardiac output and systemic vascular resistance. Since the pressure varies

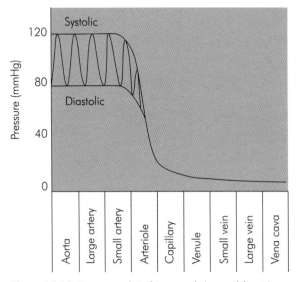

Figure 15.12 Pressure related to vessel size and function

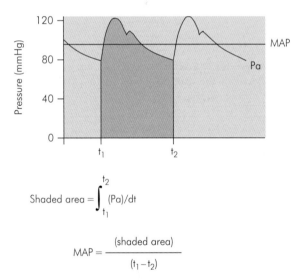

$$\text{Shaded area} = \int_{t_1}^{t_2} (Pa)/dt$$

$$MAP = \frac{(\text{shaded area})}{(t_1 - t_2)}$$

Figure 15.13 Calculation of mean arterial pressure

cyclically, MAP can be determined by integrating a pressure signal over the duration of one cycle (this gives the shaded area shown in Figure 15.13). The mean pressure is then given by the value of this integral divided by time. An estimate of mean arterial pressure may be made by taking the diastolic plus one-third of the pulse pressure.

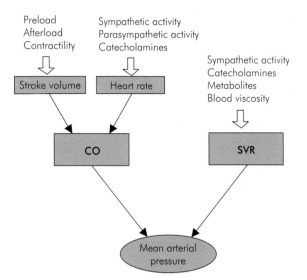

Figure 15.14 Factors affecting mean arterial pressure

Calculation of MAP

For a systolic pressure of 120 mmHg and a diastolic of 70 mmHg:

$$MAP \approx 70 + \frac{(120 - 70)}{3}$$

$$= 86.7 \ \text{mmHg}.$$

The factors affecting MAP are summarised in Figure 15.14.

Compliance

The elasticity of the arterial walls provides an essential mechanism for maintaining forward blood flow during diastole. When the aorta and arteries are distended during systole the elasticity of the walls stores kinetic energy from the ejected blood. This stored energy is then returned in diastole by the recoil of the vessel walls. A useful measure of arterial elasticity is the arterial compliance (Ca). Compliance (as in the respiratory system) is the change in arterial blood volume produced by a unit change in arterial blood pressure. Thus, easily distended arteries have a high compliance, and stiff arteries have a low compliance. The reciprocal relationship between Ca and arterial elastance (Ea) should be noted, as Ea is used in describing left-ventricular performance.

Determination of arterial compliance

- In vitro – The pressure–volume curves of postmortem aorta preparations have been plotted for different age

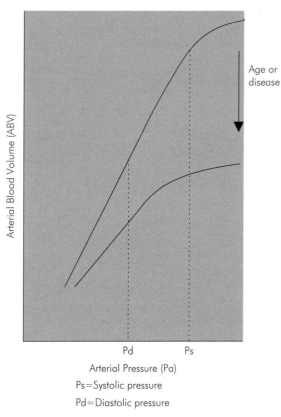

Figure 15.15 Arterial compliance curves

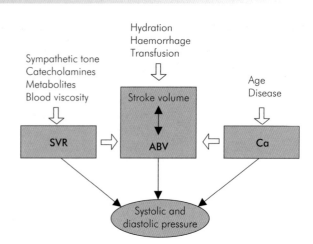

Figure 15.16 Factors affecting systolic and diastolic pressure

- Arterial compliance (Ca)
- Duration of systole

The arterial system can be visualised as a network of elastic vessels containing a varying volume of blood. This volume (ABV) increases with the injection of each stroke volume by the left ventricle (LV) during systole, and decreases with the 'run-off' of blood into the systemic vessels during diastole.

> - During systole, the arterial pressure is dependent on the relationship between SV, Ca and SVR. SV in turn depends on preload and cardiac contractility (see above).
> - During diastole, the arterial pressure falls exponentially and depends on the systolic pressure and the time constant of SVR and Ca. The minimum pressure reached in diastole (diastolic pressure) is therefore also determined by the duration of diastole.

The way in which systolic and diastolic pressures vary with SV, SVR, Ca and duration of diastole is summarised in Figure 15.17.

groups. This is approximately linear in the young normal subject, the gradient of the curve being equal to Ca. With age the arterial walls increase in stiffness and Ca decreases to a fraction of its value in young subjects. In addition, the compliance curve becomes curvilinear in the working arterial pressure range (Figure 15.15).

- In vivo – The end-systolic points from different ventricular pressure–volume loops can be plotted for a given subject. This gives an arterial elastance curve in which the gradient is equal to Ea.

Determinants of systolic and diastolic pressures

The factors determining systolic and diastolic pressures are summarised in Figure 15.16:

- Arterial blood volume (ABV)
- Stroke volume (SV)
- Systemic vascular resistance (SVR)

Technological factors affecting arterial blood pressure

The value obtained for arterial blood pressure is dependent on the method of measurement and the anatomical

Figure 15.17 Changes in systolic and diastolic pressure with SVR, Ca, SV and duration of diastole

	Systolic pressure	Diastolic pressure	Comment
↑ Ca	↓	↓	When arterial compliance is decreased, as with age or disease, the arterial pressure–volume curve becomes non-linear. The effect of this on systolic and diastolic pressures can be seen by comparing the arterial pressure waves produced (P_0 and P_1) by the same stroke volume, using the normal and decreased arterial compliance curves shown in Figure 15.18. Projecting the stroke volume variation on the normal compliance curve produces the pressure signal P_0. Repeating this with the decreased compliance curve gives arterial pressure signal P_1. It can be seen that systolic pressure is increased disproportionately compared with diastolic pressure.
↑ SV	↑	↑	Increasing stroke volume will produce an increase in both systolic and diastolic pressures.
↑ SVR	↓	↓	Increased SVR, as occurs in chronic hypertension, produces non-linearity in the pressure–volume curve, like the effects of age on the arterial compliance curve. This produces similar increases in systolic and pulse pressures. Increased SVR increases the time constant, slowing the rate of diastolic pressure fall.
↑ Duration of diastole		↓	The fall in pressure during diastole is exponential, dictated by the exponential decay constant due to SVR and Ca, so the diastolic pressure will be inversely dependent on duration of diastole.

The arterial system

- The arterial system distributes blood to the capillary vessels.
- Systolic pressure for a given stroke volume is determined by systemic vascular resistance (SVR) and arterial system compliance.
- In systole, when the stroke volume is ejected part of the stroke volume perfuses the peripheral vessels and part expands the elastic vessels.
- In diastole, elastic vessels recoil and help to maintain systemic perfusion.
- Diastolic pressure is determined by SVR as well as arterial elastic recoil and the duration of diastole.

site where pressure is sampled. Arterial blood pressure measurements are often made non-invasively using an occluding cuff, as with the sphygmomanometer or oscillotonometer. Alternatively, intra-arterial cannulation may be performed and the arterial pressure measured using a piezoresistive transducer.

Venous system

The venous system collects blood from the capillary vessels and lymphatic system to return blood flow to the right side of the heart. It also acts as a reservoir for the blood volume and provides the preload for the right heart.

Venous circulation

Venous blood flow is driven primarily by pressure transmitted from the capillary beds. Venous pressure falls from 15–20 mmHg at the venous end of capillaries to

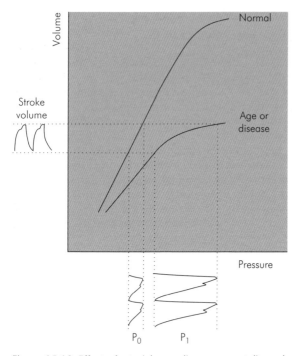

Figure 15.18 Effect of arterial compliance on systolic and diastolic pressures

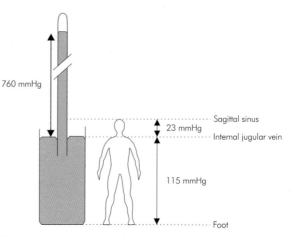

Figure 15.19 Gravity and venous pressure

The **hydrostatic pressure difference** between any two points in the venous system can be calculated by taking the product of the difference in height between the points (h), the density of blood ($\rho = 1.050$ g cm^{-3}), and the acceleration due to gravity ($g = 980$ cm s^{-1}). These figures give a pressure difference equivalent to 0.77 mmHg for every centimetre difference in height.

The venous pressure in the internal jugular vein is normally atmospheric at neck level if the vein is collapsed. Venous pressure above the neck may be less than atmospheric and can be estimated: e.g. 30 cm *above* the neck (sagittal sinus) venous pressure is *less* than atmospheric by $30 \times 0.77 = 23$ mmHg.

Similarly in the foot, 150 cm *below* neck level, venous pressure is *greater* than atmospheric by $150 \times 0.77 = 115$ mmHg.

10–15 mmHg in small veins, and 5–6 mmHg in large extrathoracic veins. Flow in the venules and small veins is continuous. In the great veins, pressure changes due to respiration and the heart beat cause fluctuations in the venous pressure wave. There are three identifiable peaks in the central venous pulse, the 'a', 'c' and 'v' waves, which are related to events in the cardiac cycle. The central venous pulse waveform is described in Chapter 14.

Other secondary mechanisms also assist venous blood flow back to the heart. These are gravity, the thoracic pump and the muscle pump. Unidirectional venous flow is maintained by the presence of valves in the peripheral veins.

Gravity and the venous system

The pressure in the venous system is largely determined by gravity, since the system can be visualised as a simple manometer (Figure 15.19). In the erect position, a hydrostatic gradient is produced from head to toe.

Such hydrostatic pressure differences are reduced significantly by the primary and secondary mechanisms outlined above, and by the presence of valves or venous obstruction. Thus, in the foot venous pressures may only be 80 mmHg when standing and decrease further to < 30 mmHg when walking.

Jugular venous pressure (JVP)

The superior vena cava (SVC) and internal jugular vein effectively form a manometer connected to the right atrium, and are usually collapsed at the level of the neck, being approximately at atmospheric pressure at this point. In the erect position, the level of blood in the internal jugular vein reflects the filling pressure in the right atrium and is not normally visible above the clavicle. The jugular venous pulse may become visible as a pulsatile distension of the internal jugular vein in a reclined or supine position, or when the CVP is increased. The jugular venous pulsations correspond to those of the central venous pulsations as described above. This correlation between jugular venous pulse and central venous pulse is limited if there are any anatomical obstructions to drainage of blood from the superior vena cava.

Cerebral venous pressure and air embolism

In the brain, venous pressure can become subatmospheric (< -20 cmH$_2$O), since the skull is a rigid container and the cerebral veins are held open by surrounding tissue. These veins are therefore susceptible to air embolism during surgery or if punctured by needles or cannulae open to air. The air embolus forms bubbles that are compressible compared with blood. If a large enough volume (> 10 mL) of air becomes trapped in the heart ventricles, cardiac output can be reduced significantly, with serious effects. Small amounts of air may pass through the heart to become trapped in pulmonary capillaries and be eliminated by diffusion without ill effects. On the other hand a few millilitres of air if shunted into the left ventricle and systemic circulation could have disastrous or even fatal effects. Gas embolism may also occur under positive pressure during laparoscopic surgery.

Thoracic pump

Normal respiration produces cyclical changes in intrathoracic pressure which increase the venous return to the heart. During inspiration intrapleural pressure decreases from its resting value of -2 mmHg to -6 mmHg. This increase in negative intrathoracic pressure is transmitted to the central veins, reducing CVP and augmenting the pressure gradient between abdomen and thorax, allowing blood to pool in the pulmonary circulation. Central venous blood flow into the thorax may double during inspiration from its resting expiratory level of about 5 mL s^{-1}. Diaphragmatic displacement caudally during inspiration also contributes to increased venous return by increasing intra-abdominal pressure and consequently the abdominothoracic venous pressure gradient. Pooling of blood in the pulmonary circulation during inspiration produces a small decrease in arterial pressure and increase in heart rate. Forced

inspiration against a closed glottis (Müller manoeuvre) accentuates these changes.

During expiration, which is normally passive, the diaphragm relaxes, intrapleural pressure returns to resting value, pulmonary blood volume is reduced and blood flow in the large veins decreases. Forced expiration against a closed glottis (Valsalva manoeuvre – see below) can produce positive intrathoracic pressures, with marked changes in heart rate and blood pressure.

The venous system

- The venous system collects blood from the capillary vessels and returns it to the heart.
- Venous pressures are mainly determined by gravity.
- Venous return depends on post-capillary pressure, blood volume, muscular and thoracic pump activity (and the venous valvular system), and sympathetic tone.

Microcirculation and lymphatic system

Structure of a capillary network

Capillaries and venules form an interface with a surface area > 6000 m^2 for the exchange of water and solutes between the circulation and tissues. Arterioles feed capillary networks via smaller metarterioles, and the capillaries drain into venules. Metarterioles possess smooth muscle contractile elements in their walls and give rise to capillaries through smooth muscle precapillary sphincters (Figure 15.20). While arterioles are supplied by the autonomic system, the innervation of metarterioles and precapillary sphincters is uncertain, and these vessels may only be responsive to local or humoral agents. Capillary blood flow varies according to the activity of the tissue. At rest the majority of capillary beds is collapsed and arteriovenous anastomoses, allowing direct communication between arterioles and venules, shunt blood away from the tissues. These anastomotic channels are widespread in skin and play a prominent role in thermoregulation.

Capillaries and endothelium

Capillaries contain 6% of the circulating blood volume and measure 5 µm in diameter at their arteriolar end, widening to 9 µm at the venous end. These dimensions are comparable with the 7 µm diameter of red blood cells,

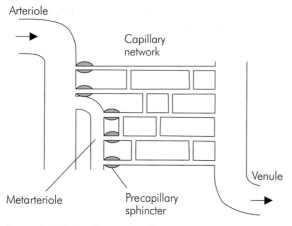

Figure 15.20 Capillary network

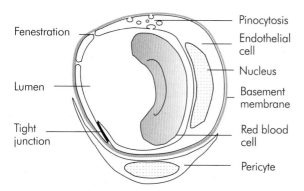

Figure 15.21 Capillaries and pericytes

which decrease in diameter when traversing capillaries. A capillary consists of a tube formed by a single sheet of endothelial cells resting on a basement membrane. Associated with capillaries and venules are interstitial cells called pericytes, akin to renal mesangial cells. These cells release chemicals that mediate capillary permeability and also secrete the basement membrane (Figure 15.21).

Capillary exchange

Capillaries have differing structures and permeabilities according to the tissues they serve. Most capillaries comprise a continuous layer of endothelial cells. Intercellular junctions and small pores representing about 0.02% of the capillary surface area permit the diffusion of small molecules < 8 nm in size. Larger molecules may cross through cell cytoplasm in vesicles and fat-soluble molecules; water, oxygen and CO_2 pass directly across the cell

membrane. Fenestrations, gaps of 20–100 nm diameter, appear in the endothelial cells of endocrine glands, renal glomeruli and intestinal villi to facilitate secretion, filtration and absorption. In the sinusoids of the liver and in the spleen, the endothelium is discontinuous with gaps of > 1000 nm. As a result albumin escapes from hepatic sinusoids much more readily than in other tissues. The exchange of water and solutes depends on both active and passive mechanisms.

> In capillary vessels the exchange of water, gases and solutes across capillary endothelium occurs by diffusion, filtration, pinocytosis and direct passage.

- Diffusion – the main mechanism mediating the exchange of gases, and for the movement of small molecules such as glucose, urea, electrolytes and between circulation and tissues. It occurs at endothelial defects such as pores and fenestrations. Diffusion of gases and lipid-soluble molecules also occurs directly across cell membranes.
- Filtration – the movement of water and small-size solutes across the endothelium under the influence of hydrostatic and osmotic gradients. Transport of substances this way is only a fraction of that occurring by diffusion; however, a significant flow of water circulates between the circulation and interstitial fluid by filtration. About 2% of capillary plasma flow is filtered (20–40 mL min^{-1}).
- Pinocytosis transports larger (> 30 nm) lipid-insoluble molecules across the endothelium. Pinocytotic vesicles form at the cell membrane (endocytosis), migrate across the cell, and expel their contents at the opposite cell membrane (exocytosis). The numbers of pinocytotic vesicles seen varies between tissues, and is greater at the arteriolar end than the venous end of capillaries.
- Direct passage of lipid-soluble compounds and gases occurs by diffusion across cell membranes, through the cells and into the interstitial fluid.

Diffusion across capillary walls

Diffusion is the movement of substances down a concentration gradient. Across the capillary endothelium the diffusion of lipid-insoluble molecules and ions occurs at defects such as intercellular junctions, pores, fenestrations and larger gaps. Gases and lipid-soluble molecules diffuse directly across cell membranes as well as at these endothelial defects.

The **rate of diffusion** of a substance is dependent on concentration gradient ($C_O - C_I$), capillary permeability (k), capillary surface area (A) and capillary wall thickness (D). This is given by Fick's law:

$$\text{Rate of diffusion} = \frac{kA(C_O - C_I)}{D}$$

where
C_O = concentration in the capillary
C_I = concentration in the interstitial fluid

The capillary permeability is a constant combining the various factors that affect the diffusion of different substances, such as:

- Molecular size
- Charge
- Lipid solubility
- Diffusion across membranes as well as pores and fenestrations
- Interactions between solutes

Substances that diffuse readily, such as gases, reach equilibrium close to the proximal end of capillaries, and their exchange rate is said to be 'flow-limited' since it is dependent on the capillary flow rate. In contrast, the movement of substances which diffuse slowly and do not reach equilibrium with the interstitial fluid over the length of the capillary is 'diffusion-limited'. Capillary permeability not only varies between tissues but is also greater at the venous end of the capillaries, and in the venules, than at the proximal end of the capillaries.

Starling forces and filtration

The balance of hydrostatic and colloid osmotic pressures between capillary plasma and interstitial fluid causes fluid to be filtered out of a capillary at the arteriolar end and reabsorbed at the venous end. These forces acting to move fluid in and out of a capillary are sometimes referred to as Starling forces.

In a capillary, hydrostatic pressure (P_C) falls from 33 mmHg at the arterial end to 15 mmHg at the venous end. Interstitial hydrostatic pressure (P_{IF}) can vary from 9 to –9 mmHg, depending on the tissue. In solid tissues it is usually near zero or slightly positive (1 mmHg). Loose

areolar connective tissue, such as in the epidural space, tends to have a negative hydrostatic pressure.

Calculation of proximal and distal transmural pressure gradients in a capillary

Colloid osmotic pressure in the capillaries (π_C) is 25 mmHg, while in the interstitial fluid colloid osmotic pressure (π_{IF}) is usually zero. The Starling forces are summarised in Figure 15.22.

The pressure acting to force fluid out of the capillary is made up of the hydrostatic pressure in the capillary and the colloid osmotic pressure in the interstitial fluid:

Outward pressure $= P_C + \pi_C$

Similarly the pressure acting to force fluid back into the capillary is made up of the interstitial hydrostatic pressure and the colloid osmotic pressure in the capillary:

Inward pressure $= P_{IF} + \pi_C$

The resultant pressure gradient is the difference between outward and inward pressures (Figure 15.22):

Pressure gradient $= (P_C + \pi_{IF}) - (P_{IF} + \pi_C)$

The rate of filtration is proportional to this pressure gradient and is given by:

Rate of filtration $= [(P_C + \pi_{IF}) - (P_{IF} + \pi_C)] \times K$

where
K = filtration coefficient of isotonic fluids (i.e. volume rate filtered per unit of pressure) and is about 0.01 mL $\min^{-1}$ mmHg^{-1} 100 g^{-1} tissue at 37 °C

Assuming an interstitial hydrostatic pressure (P_{IF}) of 1 mmHg, and an interstitial colloid osmotic pressure (π_{IF}) of zero, it can be seen that at the arterial capillary end:

Pressure gradient $= 33 - (1 + 25)$
$= +7 \text{ mmHg}$

Therefore, pressure gradient acts outwards, filtering fluid out of the capillary. While at the venous capillary end:

Pressure gradient $= 15 - (1 + 25)$
$= -11 \text{ mmHg}$

Here the pressure gradient is negative acting inwards, reabsorbing fluid back into the capillary.

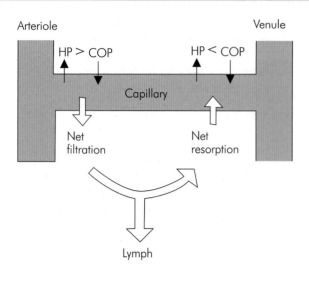

HP = Hydrostatic pressure

COP = Colloid osmotic pressure

Figure 15.22 Starling forces

Figure 15.23 Factors disturbing capillary filtration equilibrium

Change	Effects
Vasodilatation pressure	↑ proximal capillary hydrostatic pressure ↑ filtration
↑ Intravascular volume	↑ proximal capillary hydrostatic pressure ↑ filtration
Vasoconstriction	↓ proximal capillary hydrostatic pressure ↓ filtration
↓ Intravascular volume	↓ proximal capillary hydrostatic pressure ↓ filtration
Hypoalbuminaemia	↓ capillary colloid osmotic pressure ↑ filtration ↓ reabsorption
↑ Venous pressure	↑ distal capillary hydrostatic pressure ↓ reabsorption

The total volume of fluid filtered through the capillaries is dependent on capillary blood flow, but estimates have been made of between 1 and 3 litres per hour. The filtered fluid exceeds the amount of fluid reabsorbed by about 10%, the difference being absorbed by the lymphatic system.

Capillary filtration equilibrium

In a capillary there is normally a dynamic equilibrium between the fluid filtered out, the fluid reabsorbed and the fluid absorbed by lymphatics. Disturbance of this equilibrium either dehydrates tissue or makes it oedematous. The equilibrium can be disturbed by various changes. Some examples are shown in Figure 15.23.

The lymphatic system

The functions of the lymphatic system include:
- Drainage of interstitial fluid – the total lymph drainage for an adult is about 2–4 litres per 24 hours.
- Return of 'leaked' protein in the interstitial fluid to the systemic circulation. Lymph from most tissues contains a protein concentration of 20 g L^{-1}.
- Absorption of particles, proteins and other high-molecular-weight molecules accumulated in inflamed tissues.

- Absorption of protein and fat derived from metabolism and gastrointestinal absorption. The protein concentration is 2–3 times higher in lymph draining from liver and intestine.

Lymphatic vessels

Lymph flows from lymphatic capillaries, with a single layer of lymphatic endothelial cells, into lymphatic vessels that contain smooth muscle in their walls. This smooth muscle contracts in response to distension by the presence of lymph. Valves within lymph vessels maintain unidirectional flow towards the thoracic ducts, which drain into venous blood at the junction of internal jugular and subclavian veins. External compression from adjacent pulsatile arteries and skeletal muscle contractions augment lymph flow through larger lymphatic vessels.

Tissue oedema

The accumulation of abnormal amounts of interstitial fluid results in tissue swelling and is referred to as oedema. The common mechanisms underlying oedema formation include:

- Increased capillary filtration (raised venous pressure, as in congestive heart failure, incompetent venous valves, venous obstruction)
- Decreased capillary colloid osmotic pressure (hypoalbuminaemia from any cause)
- Increased capillary permeability (inflammation, hypersensitivity, systemic inflammatory response syndrome)
- Decreased lymphatic drainage (lymphatic obstruction by lymphadenopathy, Milroy's disease, filiariasis)

Control of the circulation

Control of the circulation ensures that adequate blood flow reaches the tissues to supply their metabolic demands. This is achieved by control of the cardiac pump, the peripheral vascular system and regional perfusion.

Control of the circulation

- Control of the heart varies the cardiac output.
- Control of the peripheral vascular system regulates intravascular volume and venous return to the heart.
- Regional changes in vascular resistance maintain regional perfusion pressure in visceral vascular beds.
- Regional perfusion is controlled by both intrinsic mechanisms (local) and extrinsic mechanisms (autonomic innervation).
- Extrinsic control of the peripheral vascular system is mainly sympathetic, with a smaller parasympathetic influence.

Most areas of the peripheral vascular system are under both intrinsic and extrinsic control. Overall control is predominantly sympathetic, but regional control is dominated by intrinsic mechanisms. Intrinsic control of the circulation in the heart and brain enables regional perfusion to be maintained independently of metabolic disturbances. Extrinsic control enables blood flow to be diverted in order to maintain perfusion of the vital organs such as brain, myocardium and kidneys when sudden decreases in blood pressure occur. In other organ systems intrinsic dominance may be of greater importance, enabling the gastrointestinal system to continue functioning even in the case of spinal cord transection.

Resistance vessels and capacitance vessels

Control of the vascular system is mediated via:

- **Resistance vessels** – these vessels are the arterioles. Increasing or decreasing the tone of the smooth muscle in arterioles (vasoconstriction or vasodilatation) varies the perfusion pressure across a vascular bed. Changes in these vessels also affect flow rates through the capillaries and alter vascular resistance.
- **Capacitance vessels** – these comprise the venous system. Increasing or decreasing the tone of smooth muscle in the venous system (venoconstriction or venodilatation) varies the relative intravascular volume, since the venous system contains > 60% of the blood volume. Changes in these vessels have little effect on vascular resistance.

Arterioles

Resistance vessels, or arterioles, possess a high proportion of smooth muscle in their walls. The smooth muscle fibres are arranged circumferentially in the media, and the effect of varying the muscle tone can range from complete obliteration of the vessel lumen to maximal dilatation.

Vascular smooth muscle

Vascular smooth muscle differs from both skeletal muscle and cardiac muscle, both structurally and functionally. Vascular smooth muscle characteristics include:

- Contractions are mediated by actin–myosin interaction dependent on calcium influx, release from the sarcoplasmic reticulum and reuptake. However, actin and myosin filaments are not arranged to give striations.
- Contractions are relatively slow, develop high forces and are maintained for longer durations when compared with striated muscle fibres.
- There are no action potentials generated. Contraction occurs in response to systemic and locally released agents such as catecholamines, acetylcholine and prostaglandins.
- The majority of vascular smooth muscle is innervated by sympathetic fibres that maintain a basal level of vascular tone. Sympathetic stimulation increases vascular resistance.
- The parasympathetic system supplies a small fraction of visceral vessels, which can produce a decrease in vascular resistance when stimulated.

Intrinsic mechanisms controlling blood flow
Autoregulation

The blood flow to certain organs (e.g. brain or kidney) is adjusted locally to respond to their activity levels and meet their metabolic demands. This process is known as autoregulation, and it is achieved by various mechanisms described below.

Metabolic regulation

This is the most important control mechanism, since it determines the balance of oxygen supply and demand for individual tissues and organs. Exposure of tissue to hypoxia or injury results in the release of factors or accumulation of metabolites, which increase capillary permeability and blood flow. These override central and hormonal control of capillary blood flow. Some examples are:

- Tissue hypoxia or the accumulation of carbon dioxide and hydrogen ions by diffusion around an arteriole causes vasodilatation. Lactic acid, and to a lesser extent pyruvic acid, produced in anaerobic metabolism, vasodilate by reducing tissue pH.
- Adenosine, ATP, ADP and AMP are also strong vasodilators. Adenosine dilates hepatic arteries in response to a fall in flow in the hepatic portal vein.
- The accumulation of potassium and phosphate in exercising muscle augments blood flow to the muscle. This is sometimes referred to as 'active hyperaemia'.
- 'Reactive hyperaemia' occurs when the blood supply to a tissue is occluded, and then the occlusion is released. There follows an immediate vasodilatation and increase in flow to the tissue.
- Local mechanical damage to tissues usually produces localised constriction of vessels associated with serotonin release from platelets at the site of injury.
- An alternative local response to local injury is the 'triple response'. There is an initial red reaction due to arteriolar dilatation caused by the mechanical stimulus. An axon reflex causes a rapid, more widespread brighter red reaction due to further vasodilatation. Later local oedema raises a weal caused by capillary damage.

Mechanical responses of smooth muscle
Myogenic mechanism

Vascular smooth muscle contracts or relaxes in response to changes in transmural pressure. When perfusion pressure in a vessel varies, although blood flow may change initially, the vessel subsequently constricts or dilates in response to the altered transmural pressure, maintaining constant blood flow. Isolated muscle preparations suggest that this local response can maintain constant blood flow over perfusion pressures from 20 to 120 mmHg.

Endothelial mechanism

When flow through a vessel is varied without changes in transmural pressure, increases in flow velocity are associated with dilatation of the vessel. This response may be due to an endothelium-derived factor (e.g. nitric oxide), as it is abolished by removal of the endothelium.

Endothelial factors

Endothelial cells release various local factors that affect blood flow:

- Prostacyclin and thromboxane A_2 – these are arachidonites dependent on the cyclo-oxygenase pathway. Prostacyclin is a vasodilator and inhibits platelet aggregation, while thromboxane A_2 is a vasoconstrictor that promotes platelet aggregation. Regular administration of aspirin causes a predominance of prostacyclin effects, providing prophylaxis against myocardial infarction and stroke.
- Endothelium-derived relaxing factor (EDRF) – the original term for nitric oxide (NO), which has been identified as a potent vasodilator. NO is synthesised from arginine by NO synthase and is inactivated by haemoglobin. NO is released from endothelium by multiple factors such as acetylcholine, bradykinin and various polypeptides. Its role is uncertain but it may act locally to maintain perfusion in different parts of the circulation.
- Endothelins – these polypeptides are potent vasoconstrictors that are produced by endothelium throughout the tissues of the body, including the central nervous system, the kidneys and the gut. The endothelins have multiple physiological effects although their exact role remains uncertain. These effects include contraction of vascular smooth muscle, positive inotropy and chronotropy, reduction of glomerular filtration rate, bronchoconstriction and stimulation of cell growth. Three endothelins have been identified – ET-1, ET-2, and ET-3 – together with two G-protein-coupled receptors.

Intrinsic controls of regional blood flow

- The mechanical response of smooth muscle
- The metabolic response due to the accumulation of metabolites or products of injury
- The release of factors by the endothelium

Extrinsic humoral control of blood flow

Humoral factors affecting the vascular system include both vasodilators and vasoconstrictors. Some examples are shown in Figure 15.24.

Catecholamines

Under physiological conditions the most powerful humoral agents affecting the systemic vessels are the catecholamines. Adrenaline is released from the adrenal medulla and exerts its primary effect on cardiac muscle. It also dilates resistance vessels in skeletal muscle via β-adrenergic fibres at low concentrations. At higher concentrations α-adrenergic effects predominate, causing vasoconstriction. Noradrenaline is a powerful vasoconstrictor and is controlled mainly via its release from sympathetic nerve endings as opposed to its release from the adrenal medulla.

Vasopressin

This 9-amino-acid peptide is also called antidiuretic hormone (ADH), because of its primary action in the kidney of causing the retention of free water from the glomerular filtrate in the collecting ducts. In supranormal doses vasopressin increases blood pressure by systemic vasoconstriction. It also stimulates ACTH secretion from the anterior pituitary and promotes glycogenolysis in the liver.

Angiotensin

The juxtaglomerular apparatus of the kidney synthesises and stores renin. Low renal perfusion stimulates the juxtaglomerular apparatus to release renin, which splits the α_2-globulin angiotensinogen to produce angiotensin I. Angiotensin-converting enzyme (ACE) then cleaves angiotensin I to angiotensin II in the lung. Angiotensin II has central and peripheral vasoconstrictor effects as well as participating in the control of thirst and stimulating the release of aldosterone from the adrenal cortex. Aldosterone increases tubular reabsorption of sodium and, by osmotic effects, water, and stimulates the excretion of potassium and hydrogen ions. Aldosterone also enhances excitability of vascular smooth muscle, augmenting the action of angiotensin II.

Atrial natriuretic peptide (ANP)

This is a 17-amino-acid polypeptide containing a ring formed by a disulphide bond between two cysteine residues. It causes natriuresis, lowers blood pressure and inhibits vasopressin secretion, thus opposing the action of angiotensin II. The rate of release from atrial muscle cells is proportional to the stretch of the atria obtained by changes in central venous pressure.

Kinins

Kinins are peptides originating from the exocrine glands. Bradykinin (9 amino acids) and lysylbradykinin

Figure 15.24 Some endogenous extrinsic vasoconstrictors and vasodilators

Action	Agent	Origin
Vasoconstrictors	Noradrenaline	Adrenal medulla, postganglionic nerve endings
	Adrenaline	Adrenal medulla
	Vasopressin	Posterior pituitary
	Angiotensin II	Conversion of angiotensin I in the lung
Vasodilators	Histamine	Mast cells
	Kinins	Pancreas, salivary glands, sweat glands
	Atrial natriuretic peptide (ANP)	Atria
	Vasoactive intestinal peptide (VIP)	Autonomic nerve endings Gastrointestinal tract nerves

(10 amino acids) are recognised vasodilators. The kinins are formed by kallikreins from protein precursors, and are metabolised by kininases. One kininase is angiotensin-converting enzyme (ACE), which gives this enzyme a pivotal role in the control of blood pressure.

Histamine

This amine is derived from the decarboxylation of histidine, and is produced in the CNS, gastric mucosa and mast cells. Regulation of histamine release is via inhibitory H_1, H_2 and H_3 receptors. Histamine is a potent vasodilator. Hypersensitivity reactions can result in a massive release of histamine, with a disastrous drop in blood pressure due to generalised vasodilatation.

Other polypeptides

Other polypeptides have roles in blood pressure control. At cholinergic neurones, vasoactive intestinal peptide (VIP) causes vasodilatation. Neuropeptide Y causes constriction at sympathetic postganglionic neurones. In association with sensory neurones, substance P causes vasodilatation and increases capillary permeability.

Extrinsic neurological control of blood flow

All blood vessels except capillaries and venules possess smooth muscle in their walls and are supplied by sympathetic motor fibres. The fibres supplying blood vessels form a plexus in the adventitia, and then extend to the outer layers of smooth muscle cells in the media. These sympathetic fibres possess a normal resting firing rate or tone, which may be increased or decreased.

The **vascular smooth innervation** is composed of noradrenergic fibres which mediate their effects through α_1-, α_2-, and β_2-adrenoceptors in the smooth muscle. Activation of α_1 and α_2 receptors produces vasoconstriction, while activation of β_2 fibres produces vasodilatation.

Constriction of arterioles (vasoconstriction) increases systemic vascular resistance, whereas constriction of veins (venoconstriction), especially splanchnic veins, increases the relative intravascular volume, and hence venous return to the heart. Systemic vascular resistance does not change significantly with venoconstriction when compared with vasoconstriction.

Autonomic reflexes mediate neurological control of the peripheral vascular system. In these reflexes peripheral receptors feed impulses into the vasomotor centres in the CNS via afferent pathways. There the sensory information is used to control sympathetic tone, which is relayed back to the peripheral vessels via efferent pathways. Some reflexes are mediated at the spinal level while others involve higher centres.

Vasomotor centres in the CNS

The vasomotor centres are areas of the reticular formation in the medulla oblongata and bulbar parts of the pons. The pressor region is located rostrally in the ventrolateral medulla, and provides a tonic output that maintains a background level of vascular smooth muscle tone. The depressor region is caudal and ventromedial to the pressor area. Sympathetic tone is set by the balance between these two centres, which not only respond to afferents from peripheral reflexes, but are also influenced by central chemoreceptors and higher centres in the brain.

Pressor and depressor responses

- Stimulation of the pressor causes increased vasoconstriction, increased heart rate and increased myocardial contractility.
- Stimulation of the depressor region decreases blood pressure by inhibiting the pressor area and also inhibiting sympathetic outflow directly at the spinal level.

The various influences on the vasomotor centres are summarised in Figure 15.25.

Efferent pathways

The vasomotor centres project directly to preganglionic neurones in the intermediolateral (IML) grey columns of the spinal cord. There is continuous tonic activity in sympathetic noradrenergic but not cholinergic neurones. Preganglionic fibres pass from the IML columns to the paravertebral sympathetic chain, from which postganglionic fibres carry the sympathetic outflow to the heart, vessels and adrenal medullae.

Afferent pathways

Baroreceptors in the carotid sinuses and chemoreceptors in the carotid bodies feed afferent impulses into the CNS via branches (nerve of Hering) of the glossopharyngeal nerves. Cardiac baroreceptors, aortic arch baroreceptors

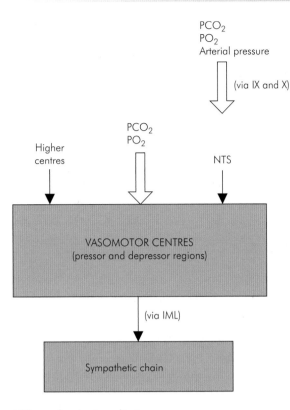

NTS = nucleus tractus solitarius

IML = intermediolateral grey column

Figure 15.25 Factors affecting the vasomotor centre

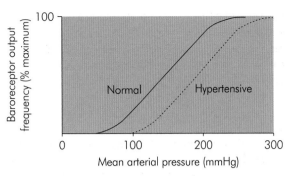

Figure 15.26 Baroreceptor response curve

- Cerebral cortex – stimulation of the motor and pre-motor areas is associated with increased blood pressure and heart rate.
- Limbic system – emotional stimuli can produce depressor responses such as fainting and blushing.

Baroreceptors

Baroreceptors are irregularly branched and coiled nerve endings located in the walls of the carotid sinus, the aorta and the heart. The carotid sinus is an enlargement of the internal carotid artery just above its origin. They respond to the degree of stretch in the vessel or heart wall, and hence to the pressure (or more strictly the transmural pressure) in the vessel or heart. When intraluminal pressure increases, wall stretch increases and the frequency of impulses discharged by baroreceptors increases. If stretch decreases, baroreceptor output frequency decreases. The baroreceptor impulses exert an inhibitory influence on the pressor centre, and baroreceptor control thus represents a negative feedback control system to maintain cardiovascular stability. The baroreceptor response curve is sigmoidal but is linear over a pressure range of 80–180 mmHg (Figure 15.26).

Baroreceptors respond not only to pressure magnitude but also to rate of change of pressure. The impulse discharge rate is thus greater during early systole than diastole. At low pressures there are few discharges during the upstroke of arterial pressure. At higher mean arterial pressures, discharges are present throughout more of the cycle. The frequency remains higher early in the cycle. At very high mean arterial pressures, discharges occur continuously, achieving maximum inhibition of the vasomotor centre (Figure 15.27). The effect of this is that baroreceptors respond not only to changes in pressure but also to changes in pulse pressure and heart rate.

Baroreceptors can reset their working range and sensitivity, or are 'adaptive', in response to sustained

and aortic body chemoreceptors relay afferent impulses centrally in fibres (cardiac depressor nerves) of the right and left vagus nerves. The nucleus tractus solitarius (NTS) is the sensory nucleus for the glossopharyngeal and vagus nerves, and is located in the dorsomedial medulla. Inhibitory connections pass from the NTS to the pressor centre.

Influence of higher centres on vasomotor tone

The vasomotor centres also respond to higher centres in the brain. These include:

- Hypothalamus – stimulation of the anterior hypothalamus decreases blood pressure and heart rate, while stimulation of the posterolateral hypothalamus increases blood pressure and heart rate. The hypothalamus also controls cutaneous vasodilatation and vasoconstriction in response to environmental or body temperature changes.

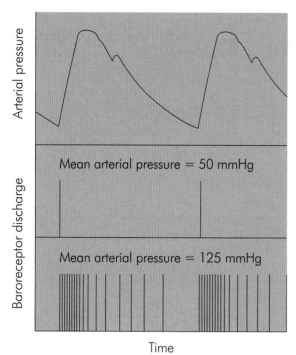

Figure 15.27 Baroreceptor activity during the cardiac cycle

pressure changes. During chronic hypertension, the baroreceptors adapt to higher pressures and the response curve is shifted to the right. These changes are reversible.

Carotid and aortic baroreceptor reflex

Baroreceptors in the carotid sinus and the arch of the aorta monitor arterial pressure, arterial pulse pressure and heart rate. They play a key role in maintaining cardiovascular homeostasis against acute disturbances, such as those that occur in trauma or exercise. Carotid sinus baroreceptors are more sensitive to blood pressure changes than aortic baroreceptors. The carotid baroreceptors also respond to external mechanical stimulation, which increases their firing rate, eliciting an inhibitory vasomotor response. In susceptible individuals this may reduce blood pressure sufficiently to induce syncope. Therapeutically, carotid sinus massage can sometimes be effective in slowing a supraventricular tachycardia.

Cardiopulmonary baroreceptor reflex

Stretch receptors exist in the atria, ventricles and pulmonary vessels. These receptors protect against rapid changes in intravascular volume by varying their tonic discharge, which exerts an inhibitory influence over the medullary pressor centre. They also play a part in controlling heart rate.

There are two types of stretch receptor in the atria. Type A receptors discharge predominantly during atrial systole, while type B discharge during atrial filling, particularly over the later part of diastole. When intravascular volume expands, atrial filling is increased, and both A and B receptors are stimulated. The impulses from these receptors are relayed to the medulla by the vagus nerves, which causes inhibition of the pressor centre and stimulation of the sinus node. This results in vasodilatation, a fall in blood pressure, increased renal blood flow, increased urine output, and a rise in heart rate.

Bainbridge reflex

In 1915 the English physiologist F. A. Bainbridge described the reflex increase in heart rate in response to a rapid intravascular infusion of fluid in anaesthetised animals. The receptors are the atrial A and B receptors described above. The afferent limb of the reflex is the vagus nerves, while the efferent limb consists of sympathetic nerves to the sinus node. Heart rate is thus influenced by the two opposing actions of the arterial baroreceptor reflex and the Bainbridge reflex. Whether the heart rate increases or decreases with a sudden increase in intravascular volume is thought to be dependent on the initial heart rate: if it is high it tends to decrease (arterial baroreceptor reflex), while if the initial heart rate is low it tends to increase (Bainbridge reflex).

Pulmonary stretch receptors

Stretch receptors in the lung, although mainly concerned with respiratory control, also inhibit the vasomotor centres when stimulated. Thus, inflation of the lungs results in systemic vasodilatation and a decrease in blood pressure.

Chemoreceptor reflexes

- Peripheral chemoreceptor reflexes – chemoreceptors are in the carotid and aortic bodies. The carotid bodies are small masses of chromaffin tissue situated on the medial aspects of the carotid sinuses, while the aortic bodies are similar organs located over the anterior and posterior aspects of the aortic arch. The chemoreceptors respond primarily to a reduction in arterial oxygen tension (PaO_2), but are also sensitive to a rise in arterial carbon dioxide tension ($PaCO_2$) or a fall in pH.

Both respiratory and circulatory centres in the brainstem receive the afferent impulses. The main effects of peripheral chemoreceptor reflexes are on the respiratory centre, but a minor effect is exerted on the pressor centre, with hypoxia and hypercapnia producing increases in blood pressure and a transient bradycardia.

- Central chemoreceptor reflexes – the vasomotor centres as well as other medullary receptors respond to changes in $PaCO_2$ and pH. These central reflexes predominate over the peripheral receptors, stimulating the respiratory centres and causing an increase in pressor tone and a decrease in heart rate, following a rise in $PaCO_2$ or a fall in pH. Central chemoreceptors are relatively insensitive to hypoxia, hypoxic reflexes being mediated primarily through the carotid and aortic bodies. Concomitant peripheral vasodilatation often leaves arterial blood pressure unchanged.
- Cushing reflex – a vasomotor centre reflex caused by a direct response of pressor cells to ischaemia. This results in reflex vasoconstriction and decreased heart rate. This increases blood pressure at the expense of cardiac output, but sustains cerebral perfusion pressure.
- The Bezold–Jarisch reflex – a response of coronary artery chemoreceptors to ischaemia causing hypotension and bradycardia but increasing coronary blood flow.
- Pulmonary chemoreceptor reflex – chemoreceptors also exist in the lung, causing apnoea, hypotension and bradycardia when stimulated by ischaemic metabolites.

Chemoreceptor reflexes are mediated centrally by receptors in the medulla, and peripherally by the carotid and aortic bodies.

The chemoreceptors can respond to parameters that reflect hypoxia, hypercapnia, acidaemia or ischaemia.

Chemoreceptor reflexes are mainly directed towards respiratory control but do exert some effects over cardiovascular parameters. Afferent pathways are mainly via the glossopharyngeal or vagus nerves, although coronary and pulmonary chemoreceptors may also possess sympathetic afferents.

Figure 15.28 Distribution of blood in the circulatory system

Location	Volume (%)
Heart	5
Systemic circulation	
• Aorta and arteries	11
• Capillaries	6
• Veins and venules	66
Pulmonary circulation	
• Arteries	3
• Capillaries	4
• Veins and venules	5

Pain reflexes

Cutaneous painful stimuli evoke the somatosympathetic reflex. Afferent impulses stimulate the rostral ventrolateral medulla to cause a rise in blood pressure. Prolonged or severe pain may cause vasodilatation and syncope.

Visceral pain often produces a depressor response due to stimulation of vagal or pelvic parasympathetic afferents. In contrast, large bowel has a significant degree of sympathetic innervation and can produce a pressor response when stimulated.

Blood volume

The volume of blood in the body is about 70 mL kg^{-1} in adults and 80 mL kg^{-1} in infants. Various types of blood vessel contain different proportions of the total blood volume. Distribution of blood volume in the vascular system is summarised in Figure 15.28.

Central venous pressure and blood volume

The venous system contains about two-thirds of the blood volume, and can be visualised as a 'venous reservoir' supplying blood to the heart.

Central venous pressure (CVP) reflects the balance between blood volume, venomotor tone and the demands of the cardiac pump.

CVP is determined by the balance between venous blood volume and venous return to the heart. At any given

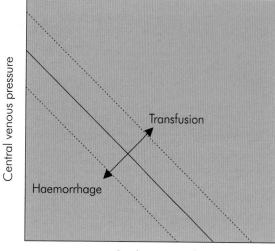

Figure 15.29 Vascular function curve

blood volume, as cardiac output increases, the rate at which blood is removed from the venous reservoir increases and CVP falls. Similarly, when cardiac output decreases, a rise in CVP is produced. This relationship reflects the passive pressure–volume characteristics of the venous system, and is described by the vascular function curve (Figure 15.29), which plots CVP against cardiac output with a fixed blood volume. Alterations in blood volume, e.g. haemorrhage or transfusion, will shift the vascular function curve up or down.

This relationship should be differentiated from the situation in which blood volume is actively increased to increase cardiac output. This is an application of the Frank–Starling relationship, and is described by a ventricular function curve that plots cardiac output against CVP. A combination of the vascular function curve and the ventricular function curve describes ventriculovenous coupling (see Chapter 14), which has a clinical application in balancing the use of IV infusion and inotropes when optimising cardiac output.

Control of blood volume

Cardiovascular function is dependent on the volume of blood in the central venous reservoir. This can either be expressed as a simple volume (in litres) or, more usefully, it can be considered as a 'relative' volume, in relation to the capacity of the venous reservoir. This relative volume determines CVP and venous return, and is controlled

acutely by reflex venoconstriction and redistribution from other areas of the circulatory system (e.g. cutaneous vascular beds, splanchnic vessels, the liver). Longer-term control of blood volume depends on the balance between the intravascular fluid and interstitial fluid compartments, fluid intake and renal loss. These mechanisms are illustrated by the events occurring in response to haemorrhage.

Circulatory control under special circumstances

Haemorrhage

An acute loss of about 5% or more of the blood volume is accompanied by immediate physiological changes, which cause a patient to become pale and sweaty with a rapid thready pulse. A rapid respiratory rate and mild cyanosis may also be present. The underlying physiological changes include:

- Decreased systolic and diastolic blood pressures
- Reduced pulse pressure
- Increased heart rate and contractility
- Increased vasoconstriction and venoconstriction
- Diversion of blood centrally from cutaneous, muscular and splanchnic circulations
- Adrenal medulla stimulation with increased circulating catecholamine levels
- Tachypnoea

These initial haemodynamic changes may reverse over about 20 minutes, depending on the extent of the blood loss. If blood loss is excessive, compensatory mechanisms can only produce transient improvement and haemorrhagic shock ensues, with continued haemodynamic deterioration. Compensation for acute blood loss is mediated via a series of mechanisms:

- The baroreceptor reflex gives rise to selective vasoconstriction of arterioles, which increases systemic vascular resistance and preserves cerebral and coronary blood flow.
- Chemoreceptor reflexes augment the baroreceptor reflex, particularly at lower arterial pressures (< 60 mmHg), where the baroreceptor response is limited by its threshold effect.
- Cerebral ischaemic response. At mean arterial pressures below 40 mmHg cerebral ischaemia is associated with direct stimulation of the adrenal medulla, augmenting the effects produced by baroreceptor and chemoreceptor reflexes.

- Reabsorption of interstitial fluid. Vasoconstriction reduces capillary hydrostatic pressures, which increases net reabsorption of interstitial fluid. About 0.25 mL kg^{-1} tissue fluid can be gained per minute through increased reabsorption. Ultimately fluid is also shifted from the intracellular compartment to the interstitial space, this balance probably being influenced by raised cortisol levels stimulated during haemorrhage.
- Release of catecholamines. Activation of the sympathetic system via the baroreceptor and chemoreceptor reflexes produces stimulation of the adrenal medulla and increased levels of circulating catecholamines.
- Renal conservation of water and salt. Decreased renal perfusion produces secretion of renin from the juxtaglomerular apparatus. The renin converts plasma angiotensinogen to angiotensin I, which in turn becomes angiotensin II, a potent vasoconstrictor. Stimulation of the adrenal cortex also increases aldosterone levels, leading to renal retention of sodium. Reduced intravascular volume decreases firing of atrial stretch receptors and produces increased secretion of vasopressin from the posterior pituitary. This results in the retention of water in the renal collecting ducts. Vasopressin is also a potent vasoconstrictor at higher concentrations. The overall effects are retention of water and sodium, which helps to restore extracellular fluid volume.

Over 6 weeks, increased erythropoietin secretion from the kidney stimulates bone marrow to produce more red blood cells and replace haemoglobin lost during haemorrhage.

Valsalva manoeuvre

A. M. Valsalva (1666–1723) was an Italian anatomist who described a manoeuvre for clearing the Eustachian tubes. The Valsalva manoeuvre is forced expiration against a closed glottis, and provides a good demonstration of autonomic reflex control of heart rate and blood pressure. The manoeuvre produces a square-wave rise in intrathoracic pressure of about 40 mmHg (Figure 15.30). The cardiovascular response can be considered in the following stages:

- Initially there is an immediate increase in arterial blood pressure as the step in intrathoracic pressure is transmitted to the pressure in the aorta. The increased

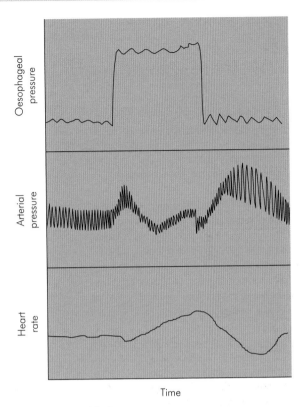

Figure 15.30 Valsalva manoeuvre

intrathoracic pressure also compresses pulmonary veins, forcing their contents into the left atrium and producing a transient rise in cardiac output.
- The sustained increase in intrathoracic pressure is also accompanied by higher intra-abdominal pressure due to contraction of the abdominal wall muscles. Raised pressure in the abdomen and thorax compresses the venae cavae, reducing the venous return to the right and left sides of the heart. This causes a decrease in arterial and pulse pressures.
- The fall in arterial and pulse pressures results in diminished stimulation of baroreceptors, causing a tachycardia and increased systemic vascular resistance. This restores mean arterial and pulse pressures to approximately the resting values recorded before the manoeuvre.
- Opening the glottis releases the positive intrathoracic pressure, producing a sudden fall in aortic pressure. The resulting drop in arterial pressure is maintained briefly as blood fills the pulmonary vessels and central veins, rather than providing venous return to the heart.

Baroreceptor reflexes again respond to this sudden drop in arterial pressure, and act to restore venous return and cardiac output.

- Finally, as venous return to both sides of the heart increases again, cardiac output is restored, but ejects into a peripheral vascular system already constricted by baroreceptor reflexes. Blood pressure thus overshoots its original resting value, until increased stimulation of baroreceptors causes reflex bradycardia and vasodilatation to restore blood pressure to normal once again.

The events described above occur even after sympathectomy, because reflex activity can still be mediated if the vagus nerves remain intact. However, in the case of autonomic neuropathy, a persisting fall in blood pressure is caused by the high intrathoracic pressure, and there is no reflex tachycardia. Then, on release of the intrathoracic pressure, no overshoot of arterial blood pressure occurs.

Exercise

Exercise activates reflex mechanisms that enhance cardiovascular performance. These include:
- Cerebrocortical activation of the sympathetic system due to anticipation of physical activity. This is sometimes referred to as 'central command'.
- Cardiovascular reflexes due to stimulation of muscle mechanoreceptors during contraction. The afferent limb is via small unmyelinated fibres which relay centrally by unidentified connections, to activate sympathetic fibres to the heart and peripheral vessels.
- Local reflexes stimulated by rapid accumulation of metabolites during muscle contraction.
- Baroreceptor reflexes.
- Peripheral chemoreceptors do not play a significant part during exercise, as arterial pH, $PaCO_2$ and PaO_2 remain about normal.
- In addition to the cardiovascular reflexes outlined above, pulmonary reflexes increase the depth and rate of breathing.

Moderate exercise levels
Prior to commencing exercise, anticipation of activity increases sympathetic discharge and inhibits the parasympathetic system. Mild to moderate degrees of exercise lead to graded changes which:
- Increase cardiovascular performance
- Redistribute blood flow to active areas
- Maintain cerebral blood flow
- Increase oxygen consumption
- Increase the efficiency of oxygen extraction

Regional blood flow during exercise
Blood flow is diverted to active muscle from skin, splanchnic regions, kidneys and inactive muscles. Cutaneous blood flow, although decreased initially, gradually increases during exercise with rising body temperature. As exercise severity increases further and oxygen consumption increases to maximum levels, cutaneous vasoconstriction occurs and blood flow to the skin starts to decrease. Myocardial blood flow increases concomitantly according to metabolic demands. Cerebral blood flow remains unchanged during exercise. These changes in the distribution of blood flow are summarised in Figure 15.31.

Skeletal muscle during exercise
Blood flow to the active muscles increases progressively in keeping with the work rate of the tissues. Locally accumulating substances and conditions, such as potassium and adenosine together with a reduction in pH, produce arteriolar dilatation and blood flows at up to 20 times resting values. Capillary recruitment increases dramatically. Net movement of fluid into the interstitial compartment

Figure 15.31 Distribution of blood flow to different organ systems during moderate exercise and rest

Organ system	Blood flow (mL min^{-1})	
	Exercise	Rest
Brain	750	750
Heart	750	250
Skeletal muscle	12,500	1200
Skin	1900	500
Abdominal viscera	600	1400
Kidneys	600	1100
Other	400	600
Total	17,500	5800

occurs and lymph flow increases, aided by muscle contractions. Oxygen extraction can rise by as much as 60 times, outstripping increases in blood flow and leading to greater arteriovenous oxygen differences. This higher degree of extraction is mediated by the right shift in the oxyhaemoglobin dissociation curve, which is associated with the accumulation of lactic acid, decreased pH, increased $PaCO_2$ and increased temperature.

Cardiac output in exercise

The enhanced cardiac output during exercise is achieved mainly through the heart rate, which follows increased sympathetic and decreased parasympathetic drive of the sinoatrial node. At mild to moderate work rates the heart rate increases proportionately to an appropriate level and is then maintained. As work rate is increased further the heart rate plateaus at about 180 bpm. In trained athletes, cardiac output may increase by seven times resting values, but stroke volume may only increase to twice the resting value.

Venous return and blood volume in exercise

The increase in cardiac output during exercise is accompanied by a commensurate increase in venous return. As a result central venous pressure does not change significantly. Thus the Frank–Starling mechanism does not normally play a major part in increasing stroke volume during moderate exercise. However, when exercise becomes maximal, central venous pressure tends to rise and the Frank–Starling mechanism starts to contribute significantly. The mechanisms augmenting venous return include:

- Increased venomotor tone
- Increased muscle pump activity
- Redirection of blood from cutaneous, renal and splanchnic circulations
- Enhanced thoracic pump action due to increased respiratory rate and tidal volume

Intravascular volume is usually slightly reduced during exercise due to increased insensible losses from the respiratory tract and skin. In addition, there is increased net capillary filtration into the interstitial muscle space. As a result there is often a slight rise in haematocrit during exercise.

Arterial pressure

Both systolic and diastolic blood pressures increase during exercise, although systolic pressure increases relatively more than diastolic. This results in an increased pulse pressure, which is attributed to an increased stroke volume and higher ejection velocity from the left ventricle.

This increased arterial pressure occurs in the face of a decreased systemic vascular resistance (mainly due to vasodilatation in active muscle), and reflects the greatly increased cardiac output (up to seven times resting value).

The sympathetic system is important in maintaining blood pressure during exercise, and if it is compromised by drugs (β-blockers) or disease (autonomic neuropathy) effort-induced hypotension or syncope can result. A restricted cardiac output (aortic stenosis) can produce the same effect.

Severe exercise and exhaustion

When exercise is taken to the point of exhaustion, the compensatory reflexes fail and decompensatory changes occur. These include:

- Heart rate rises to plateau of about 180 bpm.
- Stroke volume plateaus and may even decrease.
- Blood pressure begins to fall.
- Dehydration occurs.
- Vasoconstriction due to excessive sympathetic activity.
- Body temperature continues to rise due to decreased heat loss.
- Lactic acid and CO_2 accumulate, giving rise to decreased tissue pH.
- Muscle cramps and pain.
- Subjective feelings of weariness and lack of drive to continue activity.

Special circulations

Cardiac output is distributed between the various organ systems as shown in Figure 15.32.

Circulation to the kidneys, lungs and liver is described in Chapters 16, 17 and 21 respectively. Circulation in the fetus is discussed in Chapter 24. This section discusses the circulations of the heart and brain.

Coronary circulation

In the root of the aorta, the right coronary artery arises behind the right cusp of the aortic valve, and supplies the right atrium and ventricle. The left coronary artery arises behind the posterior cusp of the aortic valve, and divides close to its origin into circumflex and anterior descending branches, before supplying the left atrium and ventricle. Some overlap of the territory supplied by

Figure 15.32 Blood flow to different organ systems at rest

Organ system	Blood flow (mL min^{-1})	% Cardiac output
Brain	750	13
Heart	250	4
Skeletal muscle	1200	20
Skin	500	9
Abdominal viscera	1400	24
Kidneys	1100	20
Other	600	10
Total	5800	100

each main artery usually occurs. Epicardial arteries originate from these main coronary arteries, and branch to form end arteries that penetrate the myocardium. The blood flow through each main artery is equal in 30% of people, but the right coronary artery is dominant in 50%. Two-thirds of coronary blood flow drains into the right atrium via the coronary sinus and anterior coronary veins. The remainder drains directly into the chambers of the heart through small thebesian veins, arteriosinusoidal vessels and arterioluminal vessels. Venous drainage into left-sided chambers constitutes true shunt and makes a small contribution to arterial desaturation.

Coronary blood flow

- Total coronary blood flow at rest is about 250 mL per minute.
- The myocardium normally extracts about 70% of the oxygen content of coronary blood at rest; thus, increasing coronary perfusion is the only way to increase oxygen delivery.
- At rest, the oxygen requirement of the myocardium is 10 mL min^{-1} per 100 g, giving a total basal oxygen requirement of 30 mL min^{-1} for an adult.
- Cardiac muscle is versatile in its use of substrate, normally using 60% fatty acid and 40% carbohydrate as fuel. It may adapt to use different proportions and include ketone bodies as substrate.

Coronary blood flow and its distribution can be studied using:

- Coronary angiography – radiopaque dye is used to outline coronary vessels and radioactive xenon to quantify regional perfusion.
- Thallium scan – radioactive thallium uptake is used as a marker of regional distribution of perfusion in the myocardium.
- Technetium scan – selective uptake of radioactive technetium marks infarcted areas.

Factors determining coronary blood flow

Since the coronary arteries originate in the root of the aorta, aortic pressure provides the main driving force for coronary blood flow. Normally, this pressure is controlled by baroreceptor reflexes, and regulation of coronary blood flow is thus achieved through coronary vasodilatation or vasoconstriction. Coronary vascular resistance is mainly controlled by local factors. Some of the factors affecting coronary blood flow are detailed below:

- Extravascular compression (extracoronary resistance) – This describes the external compression produced by myocardial contraction during the cardiac cycle. Coronary blood flow is reduced to zero in early systole and may even be transiently reversed (Figure 15.33). This 'squeezing' effect is greatest at endocardial levels and least towards the epicardium. However, in the normal heart endocardial and epicardial blood flows are about equal in the cardiac cycle. The bulk of coronary blood flow thus occurs during diastole. However, since diastole decreases as heart rate increases, coronary blood flow can become compromised by tachyarrhythmias. Counterpulsation or 'balloon pumping' assists coronary blood flow by inflating an aortic balloon cyclically during diastole.
- Metabolic demands – The correlation between metabolic activity in the heart and coronary blood flow is fixed. Metabolites or an unidentified vasoactive agent act to increase or decrease the oxygen supply if demand is varied. Alternatively, if the oxygen supply is limited, cardiac activity adapts. Likely substances responsible for this effect include potassium ions and adenosine.
- Autonomic system – Activation of the sympathetic system tends to produce an increase in coronary blood flow. This occurs as a net result of increased metabolic demand in the face of the negative effects of increased contractility and heart rate on coronary blood flow.

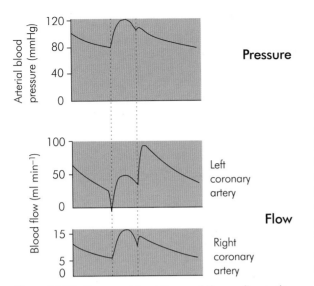

Figure 15.33 Coronary blood flow and the cardiac cycle

Figure 15.34 Summary of factors affecting coronary vascular resistance.

Factor	Effect on coronary vascular resistance
Sympathetic activity	
α-receptors	↑
β-receptors	↓
Vagal activity	↓
Systolic compression	↑
Coronary perfusion pressure	↑ or ↓
Adenosine	↓
Other metabolic factors CO_2, O_2, $H^{\Downarrow}$, $K^{\Downarrow}$	↑ or ↓

Under β-blockade coronary vessels constrict in response to sympathetic stimulation. Stimulation of the vagus nerves produces slight coronary vasodilatation.

- Coronary perfusion pressure (CPP) – This is the pressure across the coronary arteries and equals the difference between aortic pressure and intraventricular pressure. Autoregulation operates over a range of CPP between 60 and 180 mmHg.

If CPP changes suddenly, coronary vessels respond by dilating or constricting to dampen dramatic surges or falls in coronary blood flow.

Cardiac ischaemia

When the oxygen demands of the myocardium outstrip the oxygen supply, myocardial dysfunction and tissue damage follow. The oxygen requirements are related to the cardiac work rate, which in turn is dependent on systolic arterial pressure and cardiac output. Oxygen requirements are increased disproportionately by increases in systolic pressure, compared with cardiac output. Thus, if cardiac work is increased by increasing systolic pressure, oxygen requirements are much greater than if the increase in cardiac work were achieved by increasing cardiac output. 'Pressure' work is therefore more expensive than 'volume' work in terms of oxygen consumption. This is a major factor underlying the mortality associated with aortic stenosis. Clinically, myocardial ischaemia results in the chest pain of angina pectoris and ultimately the tissue necrosis occurring in myocardial infarction.

Myocardial blood flow may be increased in ischaemic heart disease by:

- Coronary vasodilators (glyceryl trinitrate)
- Coronary thrombus dissolution (streptokinase)
- Coronary angioplasty (dilatation by catheter balloon)
- Coronary bypass graft
- Coronary laser endarterectomy

Cerebral circulation

The left and right carotid arteries join the basilar artery to form the circle of Willis, from which the left and right anterior, middle and posterior cerebral arteries arise. The basilar artery is formed by the anastomosis of the two vertebral arteries. Each carotid artery supplies its own side of the brain, and there is no significant perfusion of the opposite side by a carotid. Cerebral venous drainage is via the internal jugular veins, which are fed by the dural sinuses or directly by cerebral veins.

Brain cells are intolerant of hypoxia and require uninterrupted perfusion. Several seconds of total ischaemia can produce unconsciousness, and several minutes may result in irreversible damage. Cerebral vessels are innervated by sympathetic fibres that enter the skull around the carotid arteries. These fibres originate in the superior cervical ganglia. There are also cholinergic fibres from the sphenopalatine ganglia and facial nerve. Cerebral vessels are supplied by sensory fibres originating in the trigeminal ganglia. The stimulation of sensory fibres on vessels by metabolites is thought to cause migraine.

Cerebral blood flow

- Mean cerebral blood flow is about 55 mL 100 g^{-1} min^{-1}, and it is maintained within a relatively narrow range compared with other organs.
- Perfusion varies between the tissues of the brain, with grey matter receiving more than twice (70 mL 100 g^{-1} min^{-1}) the blood flow of white matter (30 mL 100 g^{-1} min^{-1}).
- The brain consumes about 3.5 mL 100 g^{-1} min^{-1} oxygen, leaving the jugular venous blood 65% saturated.
- Structures such as the colliculi and basal ganglia receive much greater blood flows than the brainstem and cerebellum.
- Cortical blood flow is dependent on activity, and perfusion of specific areas reaches high levels ($>$ 130 mL 100 g^{-1} min^{-1}) when activated.

Cerebral blood flow can be estimated by:
- Kety method – an application of the Fick principle that determines the total cerebral blood flow in mL 100 g^{-1} min^{-1}. Nitrous oxide is used as the transported substance because it has a partition coefficient = 1, which ensures that the brain concentration becomes equal to the jugular venous concentration, after an equilibration time of 10 minutes. A subject breathes 15% nitrous oxide for 10 minutes. The total nitrous oxide transferred to 100 g brain tissue per min (Q) can be determined from the final nitrous oxide content of 100 g of jugular venous blood divided by 10. The average arteriovenous difference (D) in nitrous oxide content per mL is determined from arterial and venous samples during equilibration. The blood flow can then be calculated from the ratio Q/D.
- Scintillography – using radioactive tracers (xenon) to trace regional blood flow.
- SPECT scanning – scintillography enhanced by CT or MRI scanning.
- PET scanning – use of 2-deoxyglucose labelled with a positron emitter.
- Doppler – crude but readily available for clinical use in ICU or operating theatre.

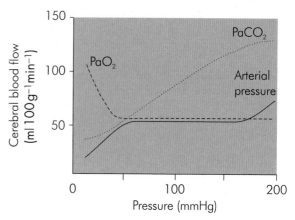

Figure 15.35 Autoregulation of cerebral blood flow

Regulation of cerebral blood flow

Control of cerebral circulation is primarily through autoregulation due to local metabolic factors. Neural control is thought to play a minor role.

Total cerebral blood flow is maintained constant over a range of mean arterial pressure and in the face of varying levels of PaCO$_2$ and PaO$_2$. This is achieved by control of total cerebrovascular resistance and cerebral perfusion pressure (Figure 15.35).

Regional cerebral blood flow, on the other hand, is highly variable and varies according to activity and local metabolic factors. The factors affecting total cerebral blood flow include:
- Cerebral perfusion pressure – pressure across the cerebral vessels, given by the difference between mean arterial pressure and (venous pressure + intracranial pressure). Raised intracranial pressure may reduce cerebral perfusion pressure.
- PaCO$_2$ – arterial CO$_2$ tensions have a marked influence over cerebral blood flow. Low PaCO$_2$ vasoconstricts and raised PaCO$_2$ vasodilates cerebral vessels. Hyperventilation reduces blood volume within the brain and is used to reduce raised intracranial pressure after head injury.
- PaO$_2$ – low PaO$_2$ vasodilates and high PaO$_2$ vasoconstricts, but the effect of oxygen tension on cerebral vessels occurs to a far lesser degree than with PaCO$_2$.
- pH – cerebral vessels are also sensitive to pH independently of PaCO$_2$. A decreased pH causes vasodilatation.

- Metabolites – adenosine and potassium have both been implicated in adjusting local cerebral perfusion. Any event causing decreased PaO_2 or increased oxygen demand produces raised local levels of adenosine in the brain, which are sustained throughout the event. A similar transient rise in potassium ion concentration is also produced. These substances are thought to be instrumental in linking regional blood flow to activity in the brain.

Raised intracranial pressure (ICP)

The skull is a rigid bony enclosure that contains 1400 g brain tissue (80%), 75 mL blood (10%) and 75 mL cerebrospinal fluid (10%). These contents are effectively incompressible; therefore, any increase in one component produces a reciprocal decrease in the others (Monro–Kellie doctrine) and an increase in ICP. Cerebral oedema will thus be accompanied by a reduction in cerebral blood volume and compression of the ventricles. Brain injury secondary to raised ICP occurs when cerebral blood flow is compromised, or when the increase in ICP is asymmetrical and brain shift occurs. Normal ICP is 0–10 mmHg, while > 15 mmHg is considered significantly raised. As ICP continues to rise, cerebral blood flow is increasingly reduced and brain tissue becomes ischaemic. Vital centres respond by increasing systemic arterial blood pressure, slowing the heart rate and respiratory rate. The blood pressure response attempts to restore cerebral blood flow by restoring the cerebral perfusion pressure.

Ultimately herniation of the cerebellar tonsils through the foramen magnum causes compression of the brainstem and death.

Blood–brain barrier

The blood–brain barrier exists between the circulation and the interstitial fluid in the brain. It consists of the ultrafiltration barrier in the choroid plexuses and the barrier around cerebral capillaries. The latter consists of capillary endothelium, basement membrane and a fenestrated layer of astrocyte end feet. Tight junctions, impermeable to solutes, join capillary endothelial cells and form a basic component of the blood–brain barrier. Water, carbon dioxide and oxygen diffuse freely across the blood–brain barrier, but the transport of glucose, the principal brain substrate, and ionised molecules is controlled. Proteins and some drugs cannot cross the endothelium unless it is inflamed. The blood–brain barrier has the following functions:

- To provide tight control over ionic (H^+, Na^+, K^+, Ca^{2+}, Mg^{2+}) concentrations in the interstitial fluid, because brain cells are extremely sensitive to ion changes.
- To protect the brain from transient changes in plasma glucose, the main substrate for the brain.
- To protect the brain from endogenous and exogenous toxins in the plasma.
- To prevent release of central neurotransmitters into the systemic circulation.

CHAPTER 16

Renal physiology

Alexander Ng

Knowledge of the pathway for formation and drainage of urine is required in order to understand the role of the kidney in clinical scenarios which occur in anaesthesia and critical care. These include:

- Anaesthesia as required for surgical interventions on the urinary tract in malignancy, hydronephrosis and urolithiasis
- Renal failure in the perioperative period (pre-renal, renal and post-renal)
- Causes of sepsis involving the kidney and urinary tract (urinary tract infection, haemolytic uraemic syndrome)
- Causes of renal failure after providing an anaesthetic for renal transplantation (arterial blood supply, venous drainage, bladder connections of the new kidney)

Anatomy

There are two kidneys, which are normally 10–12 cm in length. They are enlarged in adult polycystic kidney disease but may be atrophic in chronic kidney disease. The upper pole is located under the eleventh and twelveth ribs in the retroperitoneum. Each kidney has a capsule, cortex and medulla (Figure 16.1a).

Fundamentals of Anaesthesia, 4th edition, ed. Ted Lin, Tim Smith and Colin Pinnock. Published by Cambridge University Press. © Cambridge University Press 2017.

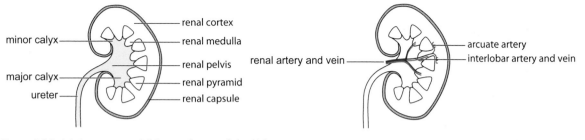

Figure 16.1 (a) Anatomy and (b) vasculature of the kidney

Blood supply of the kidneys

The kidneys receive 20% of cardiac output via the renal arteries. The renal artery to each kidney divides into two upper branches which supply the anterior and posterior upper poles, and one lower branch which supplies the lower pole. These branches then further divide into vessels called interlobar arteries, arcuate arteries, interlobular arteries and afferent arterioles, which lead to the glomerular capillaries of the nephron (Figure 16.1b).

From the glomerular capillaries, efferent arterioles transport blood to the peritubular capillaries and then to the venous circulation via the interlobular veins, arcuate veins, interlobar veins and renal veins. The transport of blood from glomerular capillaries to peritubular capillaries represents a portal system.

Nerve supply of the kidneys

The innervation of the kidney is supplied by autonomic fibres originating at T10–L1, which reach the kidneys by travelling with the renal vessels. Postganglionic sympathetic fibres are distributed to the afferent and efferent arterioles, the proximal and distal tubules and the juxtaglomerular apparatus. Parasympathetic efferents from the vagus nerve also supply the kidneys, but their function is uncertain. Renal nociceptive afferents enter the spinal cord at T10–11 to give referred pain distributed over the flanks.

The nephron

Each kidney contains approximately a million functional units called nephrons, which are located in the cortex. The nephron consists of a knot of capillaries (the glomerulus) and a tubular system with a blind end. The blind end of the tubular system forms a capsule (Bowman's capsule) around the glomerulus, which collects the ultrafiltrate from the glomerular capillaries. The other parts of the nephron are the proximal tubule, the

loop of Henle, distal tubule and collecting duct. The loop of Henle has two limbs, a descending limb and an ascending limb, which are parallel to each other running from the cortex to the renal medulla. Approximately 25% of the nephrons have long loops of Henle, crossing from the cortex deep into the medulla (Figure 16.2).

The glomerular filter

> The function of a **glomerulus** is to produce an ultrafiltrate of the plasma. It is composed of a knot of capillaries fed by an afferent arteriole and drained by an efferent arteriole (Figure 16.3).

Mesangial cells are located between the capillaries, and these have a phagocytic and structural role. The glomerular filtration barrier (Figure 16.4) consists of:

- Fenestrated capillary endothelium – this layer has many circular fenestrations (pores) between adjacent endothelial cells, with a diameter of about 60 nm. The capillary endothelium acts as a screen to prevent blood cells and platelets from coming into contact with the main filter, which is the basement membrane.
- Glomerular basement membrane – this is immediately beneath the glomerular endothelium. It forms a continuous layer, and is the main filtration barrier allowing the passage of molecules according to their size, shape and charge. It consists of collagen and other glycoproteins, including large amounts of heparan sulphate proteoglycan, which is strongly negatively charged.
- Visceral epithelial cells of the Bowman's capsule – these cells are called podocytes and have foot processes (trabeculae) which encircle the

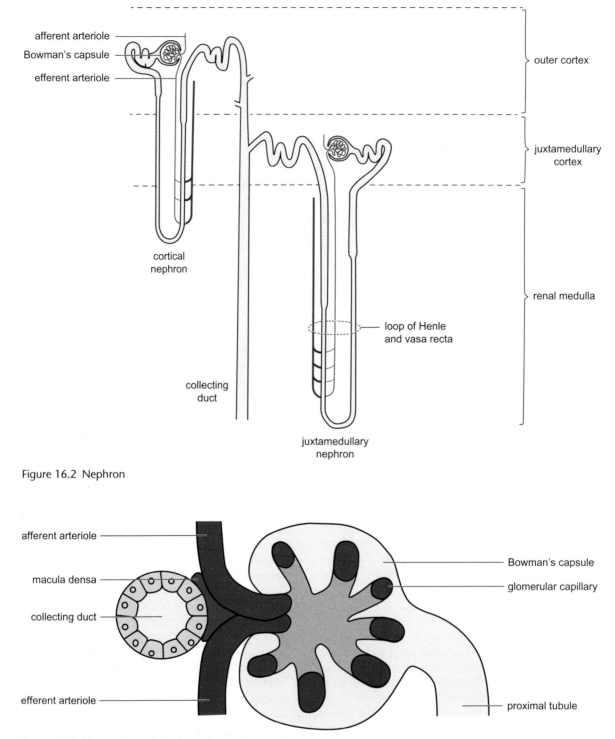

Figure 16.2 Nephron

Figure 16.3 Glomerulus and the juxtaglomerular complex

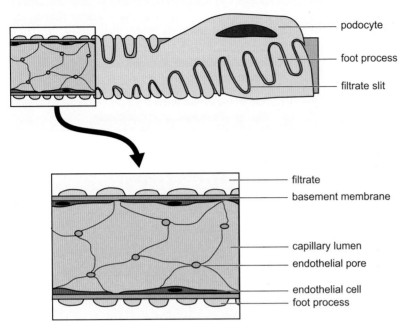

Figure 16.4 Glomerular filtration barrier

basement membrane around the capillary. From the trabeculae, many smaller processes (pedicels) project. Substances pass through the slits (pores) between adjacent pedicels. The podocyte layer also has molecules in the foot processes (integrin, dystroglycan) and slits (nephrin, podocin and CD2-associated protein) which influence its role in maintaining basement membrane integrity and filtration selectivity.

The glomerular ultrafiltrate has a composition echoing that of plasma, which is free from cells and particles of molecular weight > 70,000. Smaller molecules (< 7000) pass freely through the glomerular filter, but permeability to large molecules decreases with size and negative charge.

The tubular system

> The **tubular system** of the nephron determines the final composition of the urine. It functions by actively or passively secreting and reabsorbing substances into the glomerular ultrafiltrate.

The tubular system starts at the Bowman's capsule which surrounds the glomerular capillaries and collects the ultrafiltrate. The ultrafiltrate passes from Bowman's capsule into the proximal tubule, which feeds into the loop of Henle and from there into the distal tubule. From the distal tubule the filtrate enters the collecting duct system consisting of the cortical and medullary collecting ducts.

> It is in the **collecting duct system** that the degree of water reabsorption or excretion by the kidney is determined and ultimately extracellular fluid osmolarity is maintained.

The majority of nephrons have glomeruli in the outer two-thirds of the cortex and possess short loops of Henle only passing a short distance into the medulla. Approximately 15% of nephrons have glomeruli in the inner third of the cortex (juxtamedullary nephrons), with long loops of Henle passing deeply into the medulla.

The urogenital system

The collecting ducts enter the renal papilla and calyces, in the medulla of each kidney. From here urine drains into the renal pelvis, which is a funnel-shaped expansion of each ureter. Urine is then excreted by travelling in the ureter, bladder and urethra. Normal physiological function may be impaired (i.e. post-renal failure) by anatomical factors:

- In the wall, e.g. calculus, malignancy, thrombus
- In the lumen, e.g. stricture
- Outside the wall, e.g. prostate, pelvic malignancy, abdominal aortic aneurysm, retroperitoneal fibrosis

Renal excretion of waste products

Waste products of metabolism such as urea and creatinine are excreted in urine.

Formation of urine involves:

- Filtration of plasma at the glomerulus
- Reabsorption of the majority of the filtrate in the tubules
- Secretion of additional waste products into the tubules

The rate of urine formation has clinical importance, since it is used in determining the severity of acute kidney injury (Figure 16.5).

Glomerular filtration

The glomerular filtration rate (GFR) is about 180 litres a day (125 mL min^{-1}). This is equivalent to filtering the total plasma volume every 20 minutes.

Glomerular filtration of molecules and plasma is determined by:

- Size of molecules filtered
- Charge of the basement membrane
- Hydrostatic pressure gradient
- Renal plasma flow
- Colloid osmotic pressure gradient
- Glomerular capillary coefficient
- Blood pressure

Size of molecules for filtration

Water and ions are filtered, whereas proteins such as albumin, of molecular weight 69,000, are not normally filtered.

Charge of the glomerular basement membrane

The basement membrane is charged negative, and negatively charged molecules are therefore less readily filtered than those which are positively charged.

Figure 16.5 Quantification of reduction in renal function

Acute kidney injury		
Stage	Increase in serum creatinine	Rate of urine output
1	of 26.4 µmol L^{-1} by 150–200%	< 0.5 mL kg^{-1} h^{-1} for > 6 h
2	by 200–300%	< 0.5 mL kg^{-1} h^{-1} for > 12 h
3	of 354.4 µmol L^{-1} by > 300%	< 0.3 mL kg^{-1} h^{-1} for > 24 h 0 mL kg^{-1} h^{-1} for 12 h
Chronic kidney disease		
Stage	Physiological reduction	Glomerular filtration rate, mL 1.73 cm^{-2}
1	Mostly normal (possible urine dipstick, genetic or structural abnormalities)	> 90
2	Mild	60–89
3	Moderate	30–59
4	Severe	15–29
5	End-stage	< 15

The glomerular capillary coefficient (K_F)

K_F is a measure of the resistance to flow of ultrafiltrate across the total glomerular surface, and is given by the ratio:

$$K_F = \frac{(GFR)}{(\text{net pressure gradient})}$$

The coefficient has a value of $12.5 \text{ mL min}^{-1} \text{ mmHg}^{-1}$. Ultrafiltration across glomerular capillaries occurs approximately 10 times more easily than in other capillary beds.

GFR and colloid osmotic pressure gradient

Osmotic pressure gradient $= \pi_G - \pi_B = 32 \text{ mmHg}$

Changes in filtration fraction will alter colloid osmotic pressure, since ultrafiltration from the glomeruli concentrates the plasma proteins in the glomerular capillaries and increases the colloid osmotic pressure. Any increase in the glomerular colloid osmotic pressure will decrease GFR.

> **Colloid osmotic pressure gradient** is determined by the colloid osmotic pressure in the glomerular capillaries (π_G = 32 mmHg), since the colloid osmotic pressure in Bowman's capsule (π_B) is normally zero.
> The colloid osmotic pressure in the glomerular capillaries is dependent on the colloid osmotic pressure in the afferent arterioles, the filtration fraction and renal plasma flow.

GFR and renal plasma flow (RPF)

Renal blood flow is 1100 mL min^{-1}, giving a value for renal plasma flow (RPF) of 600 mL min^{-1}. Approximately 20% of renal plasma flow is filtered in the glomeruli giving a value of 120 mL min^{-1} for GFR. The ratio of glomerular filtration rate (GFR) to renal plasma flow (RPF) is the filtration fraction:

$$\text{Filtration fraction} = \frac{\text{Glomerular filtration rate}}{\text{Renal plasma flow}}$$
$$= \frac{(GFR)}{(RPF)}$$

Changes in filtration fraction affect GFR by altering the colloid osmotic pressure (see above).

> - A decrease in RPF produces an increase in filtration fraction and subsequently a reduction in GFR.
> - Conversely, an increase in RPF will lead to a decrease in filtration fraction and an increase in GFR.

GFR and hydrostatic pressure gradient

The hydrostatic pressure gradient producing the glomerular ultrafiltrate is equal to the difference between the pressure in the glomerular capillaries (P_G = 60 mmHg) and the pressure in Bowman's capsule (P_B = 18 mmHg).

Hydrostatic pressure gradient $= P_G - P_B = 42 \text{ mmHg}$

Glomerular hydrostatic pressure is determined by arteriolar resistance at both the afferent and efferent ends of the glomerular capillaries. A reduction in glomerular hydrostatic pressure causes a decrease in GFR. This occurs as a result of factors which increase afferent arteriolar resistance; these include:
- An increase in activity of the sympathetic nervous system
- Hormones such as noradrenaline, adrenaline and endothelin

An increase in glomerular hydrostatic pressure causes an increase in GFR. This may be caused by factors that:
- Decrease afferent arteriolar resistance, e.g. prostaglandins and nitric oxide
- Increase efferent arteriolar resistance, e.g. angiotensin II

> ### Calculation of net pressure for glomerular filtration
>
> The net pressure for glomerular filtration is the difference in hydrostatic pressure gradient and colloid osmotic pressure gradient (Figure 16.6):
>
> Net filtration pressure = Hydrostatic pressure gradient
> $$\qquad - \text{ colloid osmotic pressure gradient}$$
> $$= (P_G - P_B) - (\pi_G - \pi_B)$$
> $$= (60 - 18) - (32 - 0)$$
> $$= 10 \text{ mmHg}$$

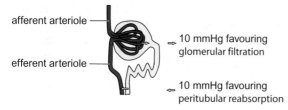

afferent arteriole

efferent arteriole

⇨ 10 mmHg favouring
glomerular filtration

⇦ 10 mmHg favouring
peritubular reabsorption

Figure 16.6 Net filtration pressure in glomerulus and net reabsorption pressure in descending LOH

In addition, an increase in hydrostatic pressure in the Bowman's capsule reduces the hydrostatic pressure gradient and hence glomerular filtration. Factors which may increase hydrostatic pressure in the Bowman's capsule include any cause of obstructive renal failure, e.g. renal stones.

GFR and blood pressure

GFR remains relatively constant in spite of changes in blood pressure. This process of autoregulation is mediated by:

- The myogenic response of blood vessels, which constrict as a result of increases in blood pressure or dilate when blood pressure falls.
- The juxtaglomerular complex for tubuloglomerular feedback, which resists changes in glomerular filtration rate.

The juxtaglomerular complex

The juxtaglomerular complex consists of the juxtaglomerular cells in the walls of the afferent and efferent arterioles, and adjacent epithelial cells in the distal tubule called the macula densa (Figure 16.3). Physiological mechanisms involving the juxtaglomerular complex act to prevent a reduction in GFR when blood pressure falls as follows:

- A reduction in blood pressure reduces glomerular hydrostatic pressure and initially produces a decrease in GFR.
- This decrease in GFR leads to increased absorption of sodium chloride in the loop of Henle, which gives rise to a reduction in the concentration of sodium chloride at the distal tubule and the macula densa.
- A release of renin by the macula densa occurs as a result of the reduced sodium chloride concentration, which stimulates the formation of angiotensin I and II.
- Angiotensin II leads to preferential vasoconstriction of the efferent arterioles, thus maintaining glomerular hydrostatic pressure and GFR.

- In addition, the macula densa causes a reduction in afferent arteriolar resistance, which also acts to maintain glomerular hydrostatic pressure and GFR.

> The **juxtaglomerular complex** provides a feedback mechanism to maintain GFR, by responding to sodium chloride concentration at the distal tubule. It acts by releasing renin, which increases angiotensin II levels.

However, at high angiotensin II levels, GFR is not always maintained because angiotensin II reduces glomerular blood flow, which increases glomerular colloid osmotic pressure and opposes glomerular filtration.

This tubuloglomerular feedback mechanism is driven not only by changes in blood pressure; it is primarily mediated by sodium chloride concentration at the macula densa. For instance, when there is an increase in the delivery of amino acids or glucose to the kidney, a rise in sodium reabsorption in the proximal tubule occurs owing to co-transportation. Under these circumstances tubuloglomerular feedback will also lead to an increase in glomerular hydrostatic pressure and hence in GFR.

Tubular reabsorption and secretion

> Glomerular filtrate is processed in three main tubular regions:
> - The proximal tubule
> - The loop of Henle
> - The distal tubule, collecting tubule and collecting duct system

The proximal tubule

Here, effectively 100% of amino acids and 100% of glucose are reabsorbed. 65% of other ions such as sodium, chloride, bicarbonate (via H^+ secretion) and potassium are reabsorbed (Figure 16.7), while only about 20% of phosphate filtered is reabsorbed. The normal plasma concentration of urea is 2.5–7.5 mmol L^{-1}, of which 50–60% is secreted. Reabsorption of urea occurs passively down its concentration gradient since the the tubular urea concentration tends to increase as sodium chloride and water are reabsorbed from the proximal tubule. The filtrate osmolarity remains similar to plasma, because

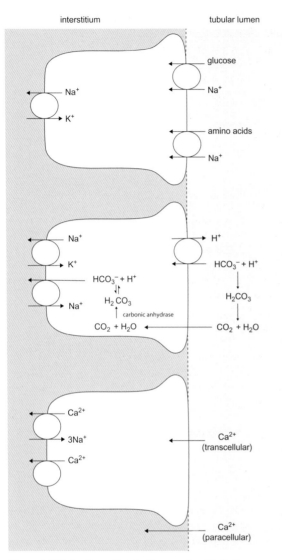

Figure 16.7 Reabsorption in the proximal tubule

tubule. The fluid entering the LOH is initially *isotonic* compared with plasma, but after traversing the loop, the fluid entering the distal tubule is *hypotonic*. Thus the tubular fluid is actually diluted during its passage through the LOH. However, the LOH plays a crucial role in the concentration of urine, by functioning as a countercurrent multiplier.

> The **loops of Henle** do not concentrate the tubular fluid within them, but manufacture a hypertonic interstitial fluid in the renal medulla by a countercurrent mechanism. Urine is then concentrated by osmosis from collecting ducts as they pass through the medulla.

The countercurrent mechanism

A proposed mechanism for countercurrent multiplication was described by Wirz, Hargitay and Kuhn in 1951. The hypertonic interstitium in the renal medulla is produced by a small osmotic pressure difference between the ascending and descending limbs of the loops (i.e. a small transverse gradient). This small difference is then multiplied into a large longitudinal gradient by the countercurrent arrangement (i.e. flow in opposite directions) in the two adjacent limbs of the loop.

- The ascending limb is not uniform in structure but possesses a thin segment and a thick segment. This limb produces an increase in the surrounding interstitium by the extrusion of sodium and accompanying ions. Only the thick segment actively extrudes ions. Here 25% of ions such as sodium, chloride, bicarbonate (via H^+ secretion) and potassium are reabsorbed, and 65% of magnesium is reabsorbed (Figure 16.8).
- Tubular fluid becomes hypo-osmolar because both thin and thick segments are impermeable to water, so that water is unable osmotically to follow the extruded ions. Consequently, the osmolality of the medullary interstitium is increased and the osmolality of the fluid in the ascending limb is decreased.
- The descending limb is permeable to water and, to a lesser extent, is also permeable to NaCl. The fluid within the descending limb will therefore come to osmotic equilibrium with the interstitium. In effect, then, we can consider the transport of NaCl out of the ascending limb as being directed into the descending limb.

60–70% of the water filtered is also reabsorbed. Organic acids, bases and drugs are secreted into the proximal tubular fluid.

The loop of Henle

The loop of Henle (LOH) is continuous with the proximal tubule and originates in the renal cortex. It consists of a descending limb which passes into the medulla and loops round to become the ascending limb which passes back into the cortex. This limb then continues as the distal

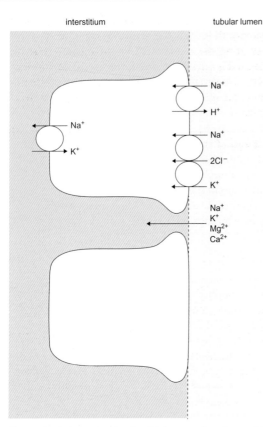

Figure 16.8 Extrusion in the thick ascending loop of Henle

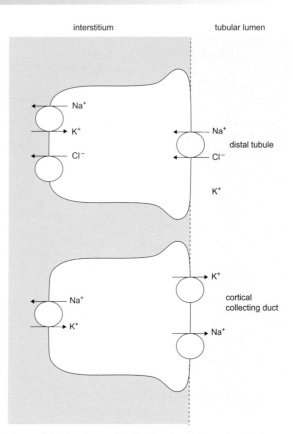

Figure 16.9 Reabsorption in distal tubule and collecting duct cells

Long and short loops of Henle

Only 25% of the nephrons (the juxtamedullary nephrons) have long loops of Henle which pass deeply into the medulla. The remaining 75% of nephrons (cortical nephrons) have short loops of Henle which barely reach the medulla, and these nephrons do not make a significant contribution to the manufacture of medullary hypertonicity. However, the collecting tubules of all the nephrons (both cortical and juxtamedullary) pass through the medulla. Thus only the long-looped nephrons, which form 25% of the total, produce the medullary gradient that concentrates the urine produced by all the nephrons.

The distal tubule

The 'distal tubule', although anatomically defined, is not a distinct section of the nephron in terms of physiological function. Functionally the distal tubule is a segment of the nephron in which the tubule cells undergo transition from ascending-limb-of-Henle-type cells to collecting-tubule-type cells.

The walls of the ascending-limb-of-Henle-type cells have only a very low and essentially constant permeability to water. On the other hand the collecting-tubule-type cells have a variable water permeability, which is regulated by the hormone ADH (antidiuretic hormone, vasopressin).

The collecting tubules have cortical and medullary sections, each section having somewhat different properties. Both are relatively impermeable to water, urea and NaCl, but the water permeability is increased by ADH. Thus, ADH leads to urine concentration by permitting the osmotic abstraction of water into the interstitium.

In the distal tubule and collecting tubules and ducts, variable percentages of sodium, chloride and bicarbonate (via H^+ secretion) may be reabsorbed (Figure 16.9). The osmolarity of the tubular fluid is controlled, and may become high if there is increased water reabsorption and low if there is increased water clearance.

Tubular transport

Transport of substances, ions and water takes place between the tubular filtrate and the peritubular capillaries. The transport path traverses the tubular cells, passing into the interstitium or lateral intercellular spaces (LIS), and from there into the peritubular capillaries. Transport occurs via the following routes:

- Across the tubular cells, via its luminal and basolateral sides (transcellular pathway) and into the LIS
- Between luminal cells (paracellular pathway) into the LIS
- From the LIS across the capillary membrane into the peritubular capillaries

The general mechanisms are the same in both reabsorption and secretion. The difference between reabsorption and secretion lies in the direction of transport.

General mechanisms of transport

- Active transport, an energy-dependent process involving Na^+/K^+ATPase on the basolateral side of the tubular cell. Sodium is actively pumped out of the tubular cell into the interstitium, thus lowering its concentration and creating a negative charge. Other pumps include H^+ATPase and Ca^{2+}ATPase.
- Facilitated diffusion of sodium, a process in which sodium is transported from the tubular lumen into the tubular cell, on a carrier protein, along its electrochemical gradient.
- Co-transport of sodium with other substances, e.g. glucose, amino acids, hydrogen, chloride and potassium ions, on carrier proteins. These substances undergo secondary active transport as they move against a concentration gradient.
- Reabsorption of water by osmosis.

Water reabsorption

There is no active water reabsorption. Water reabsorption in the nephron follows solute absorption and can be both transcellular and paracellular.

It has become clear in recent years that much of the water movement through epithelia is transcellular, and occurs via specific water channel proteins, termed aquaporins (AQP). Several different aquaporins have been identified:

- AQP1 (also called CHIP-28, or 28-kilodalton channel-forming integral protein) is abundant in the apical and basal membranes of renal proximal tubule cells, and the cells of the thin descending limb of Henle, as well as in many extrarenal tissues.
- AQP2 is the vasopressin (ADH)-sensitive channel, discussed in more detail later (see Figure 16.11).
- AQP3 is in the basolateral membranes of the collecting duct principal cells, where it provides an exit route for water.
- AQP4 is abundant in the brain, and may be important in the hypothalamic osmoreceptor cells.

Rates of tubular reabsorption

Transport mechanisms for some substances and in some parts of the tubular system may become saturated, resulting in a maximum reabsorption rate called the transport maximum. An example is the transport maximum for glucose in the proximal tubule in diabetic patients, when the filtered glucose cannot be reabsorbed completely and an excess appears in the urine. Similarly there is a maximum value for the reabsorption of sodium in the distal tubule.

Alternatively a maximum value for reabsorption may not occur, as in the case of sodium transport in the proximal tubule. This transport mechanism does not appear to reach saturation, but continues to increase as the sodium load increases. The transport mechanism here is dependent on the electrochemical gradient of sodium and time.

The maximum reabsorption rate of some substances, such as Na^+, is also affected by leakage from the LIS back into the tubular lumen (or 'backflux'). This in turn is affected by the rate of peritubular capillary uptake.

Peritubular capillary reabsorption

Reabsorbed fluid returns to the circulation by uptake of fluid from the LIS into the peritubular capillaries (Figure 16.6). The overall reabsorption rate is 124 mL min^{-1}, just less than the glomerular filtration rate of 125 mL min^{-1}.

Peritubular capillary uptake is dependent on:

- Colloid osmotic pressure gradient of 17 mmHg, arising from the difference between 32 mmHg in the peritubular capillary and 15 mmHg in the LIS fluid. This pressure gradient favours reabsorption into the capillaries.
- Peritubular hydrostatic pressure gradient of 7 mmHg, arising from the difference between 13 mmHg in the peritubular capillary and 6 mmHg in the LIS. This pressure gradient resists fluid reabsorption into the capillaries.

- Filtration coefficient ($K_F = 12.4$ mL min^{-1} mmHg^{-1}) for the peritubular capillaries, determined by the product of the permeability of the capillary walls and their total surface area.

Calculation of peritubular capillary reabsorption rate

Net reabsorption pressure = (Colloid osmotic pressure gradient)
$$- \text{(Hydrostatic pressure gradient)}$$
$$= (32 - 15) - (13 - 6)$$
$$= 10 \text{ mmHg}$$

Peritubular reabsorption rate $= K_F \times$ Net reabsorption pressure
$$= 12.4 \times 10$$
$$= 124 \text{ mL min}^{-1}$$

These pressure gradients explain the phenomenon of glomerulotubular balance, a process in which a rise in glomerular filtration and hence tubular load leads to increased peritubular capillary reabsorption. This physiological mechanism occurs because:

- A rise in glomerular filtration rate or a reduction in plasma flow, e.g. due to angiotensin II, leads to an increase in filtration fraction.
- The increase in filtration fraction causes an increase in peritubular colloid osmotic pressure, which favours reabsorption.

This process acts to ensure that the distal tubule, cortical collecting tubule and medullary collecting duct receive a relatively constant volume of filtrate. However, this mechanism is attenuated by high blood pressure, which leads to an increase in peritubular capillary hydrostatic pressure, which decreases peritubular reabsorption.

Maximum rate of reabsorption

The overall transport maximum from tubular lumen to peritubular capillary is a result of the transport maximum from tubular lumen into LIS, the backflux, and the rate of uptake from the LIS into the peritubular capillaries.

Measurement of renal function

Filtration fraction is the ratio of glomerular filtration rate to renal plasma flow, and so it may be estimated by measurement of these factors.

In clinical practice, **glomerular filtration rate** is the most useful measure for quantifying renal function.

Glomerular filtration rate (GFR)

Glomerular filtration rate can be measured by administering a substance (e.g. inulin) which is filtered with no reabsorption and no secretion. In such a case, the mass of the substance filtered per unit time is equal to the mass of substance excreted per unit time in the urine.

Calculation of glomerular filtration rate (GFR)

Consider a substance X in the plasma that is only filtered and is not secreted or reabsorbed, where

Plasma concentration of X $= P_X$

Urine concentration of X $= U_X$

Urine flow rate $= V$

Mass of substance filtered per unit time $= P_X . \text{GFR}$

Mass of substance excreted per unit time $= U_X . V$

Then:

$$P_X . \text{GFR} = U_X . V$$
$$\text{GFR} = \frac{U_X . V}{P_X}$$

In clinical practice, creatinine is used to estimate glomerular filtration rate (although it should be noted that creatinine is not solely filtered but is also secreted to a small extent). Clinically, both creatinine levels and glomerular filtration rate are utilised to grade the severity of acute kidney injury (AKI) and chronic kidney disease (CKD) (Figure 16.5). Abnormal glomerular function occurs as a result of several pathophysiological mechanisms, which are summarised in (Figure 16.10).

Renal clearance

Historically the concept of 'renal clearance' has been used as a measure of renal function. This was defined by:

Figure 16.10 Pathophysiology in the glomerulus

Type of dysfunction	Structural changes
Minimal change glomerulonephritis	Effacement and fusion of the foot processes of the podocytes
Membranous glomerulonephritis	Thickened capillary loops and subepithelial deposits
Focal segmental glomerulosclerosis	Reduction of proteins called nephrin, podocin and α-actinin at the foot processes of the podocytes Occurrence in some glomeruli and parts of each glomerulus
Mesangiocapillary glomerulonephritis	Mesangial cell proliferation and deposition of immune complexes in the subendothelium, subepithelium and basement membrane
Diffuse proliferative glomerulonephritis	There is proliferation of capillaries, which may occur as a result of formation of immune complexes and complement activation at the basement membrane and subendothelium Occurrence in the whole of all glomeruli
Crescentic glomerulonephritis	The glomerular capillaries are compressed by a crescent-shaped inflammatory mass

The clearance of any substance excreted by the kidney is the volume of plasma which is cleared of the substance in unit time. Thus the units of clearance are those of volume per unit time (usually mL min^{-1})

In fact clearance only represents a theoretical volume of plasma, since no aliquot of plasma is completely cleared of any substance during its passage through the kidney. In the case of a substance which is neither reabsorbed or secreted (e.g. inulin) the renal clearance is equal to the GFR.

Renal plasma flow

Renal plasma flow can be estimated using the administration of a substance which is completely cleared from plasma. The substance not only has to be filtered but must also be secreted, since glomerular filtration accounts for only 20% of renal plasma flow. Assuming complete clearance, the mass of substance cleared from plasma per unit time is equal to the mass of the substance excreted in the urine per unit time.

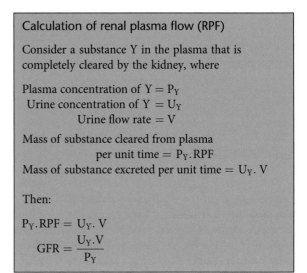

Calculation of renal plasma flow (RPF)

Consider a substance Y in the plasma that is completely cleared by the kidney, where

Plasma concentration of $Y = P_Y$
Urine concentration of $Y = U_Y$
Urine flow rate $= V$

Mass of substance cleared from plasma
per unit time $= P_Y . RPF$
Mass of substance excreted per unit time $= U_Y . V$

Then:

$$P_Y . RPF = U_Y . V$$

$$GFR = \frac{U_Y . V}{P_Y}$$

In the kidney, para-aminohippuric acid is 90% cleared and may be used to estimate 90% of renal plasma flow. The measured value would have to be divided by 90% to avoid underestimating true renal plasma flow.

Renal control of extracellular osmolarity

Cells of the body are surrounded by extracellular fluid (ECF), which is compartmentalised into interstitial fluid, plasma and lymphatics. The osmolarity of ECF of approximately 282 mOsm L^{-1} is determined by solutes and water. By controlling the degree of water reabsorption or water clearance, change in ECF osmolarity may be prevented.

The mechanism for water reabsorption in the distal tubule, cortical collecting tubule and medullary collecting ducts involves:

- Generation of a hypertonic medullary interstitium
- Control of tubular permeability by antidiuretic hormone (ADH)

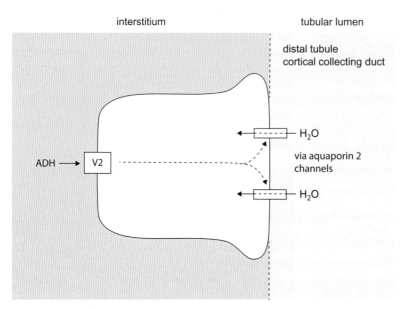

interstitium

tubular lumen

Figure 16.11 ADH binding onto V_2 receptors in distal tubule and collecting duct cells

Hyperosmolar medullary interstitium

The medullary interstitium is hyperosmolar as a result of the accumulation of sodium chloride and urea. There is a gradient of osmolarity, increasing from outer medulla to inner medulla. This environment is created by the juxta-medullary nephrons, which have long loops of Henle and which represent 25% of all nephrons. The arrangement of the peritubular blood supply of the medulla, called vasa recta, prevents solute loss and hence dilution.

Sodium chloride

The high concentration of sodium chloride in the medulla originates from the active transport of sodium out of the tubular lumen by the thick ascending limb of the loop of Henle. The $Na^+K^+ATPase$ pumps on the basolateral side of the tubular cells actively transport sodium into the interstitium. This process generates an electrochemical gradient for co-transport of sodium from the luminal side of the tubular cells via sodium–potassium-chloride and also sodium–hydrogen co-transporters, and establishes a small osmotic gradient of $200\,mOsm\,L^{-1}$, between the fluid in the tubular lumen and that in the medullary interstitium.

The countercurrent mechanism

This small transverse osmolarity difference (200 mOsm L^{-1}) between tubular lumen and interstitium is multiplied

several times over to produce a larger longitudinal gradient between the outer medulla and the inner medulla ($> 1000\,mOsm\,L^{-1}$), by a countercurrent system formed by the opposing flows in the descending and ascending limbs of the loops of Henle (LOH).

This countercurrent system operates as follows:

- The descending limb of the LOH is permeable to water and thus water will be reabsorbed from the descending lumen, into the interstitium due to the small hyperosmolarity gradient established by the thick ascending limb.
- This passage of water from the lumen of the descending limb causes the filtrate osmolarity to gradually increase from 280 mOsm L^{-1} at the outer medulla to 1200 mOsm L^{-1} deep in the medulla.
- The hyperosmolar filtrate in the descending limb of the LOH then reverses direction deep in the medulla by passing into the ascending limb of the LOH.
- As the filtrate passes back to the outer medulla in the ascending limb its osmolarity gradually decreases as sodium chloride is pumped out into the interstitium.
- Water cannot follow the extruded sodium, since the ascending limb is impermeable to water.
- By the time the filtrate reaches the distal convoluted tubule in the outer medulla it is slightly hypotonic.

The countercurrent system formed by the descending and ascending limbs of the LOH establishes an increasing osmolarity gradient from outer medulla to inner medulla, which enables the final concentration of urine to take place in the collecting ducts.

Urea

Urea accounts for approximately 40% of the total osmolarity of 1200 Osm L^{-1} in the inner medullary interstitium. The collecting ducts help to maintain the hyperosmolarity of the medullary interstitium by recirculating urea. This process is mediated initially by the facilitated diffusion of urea from the medullary collecting ducts into the interstitium, via urea transporters UT-A1 and UT-A3. UT-A3 is activated by ADH.

The concentration of urea in the medullary collecting ducts is high because of ADH-dependent water reabsorption from the distal tubules and the cortical collecting ducts.

Urea recirculates from the medullary interstitium by entering the descending and ascending limbs of LOH, from where it passes back to the medullary collecting ducts. The urea is then returned from the collecting ducts to the interstitium by facilitated diffusion.

Vasa recta

The countercurrent exchange performed by the vasa recta involves the movement of solute and water across the capillary membrane as plasma flows in opposite directions in each limb of the vasa recta, and provides the blood supply to the medulla without disturbing the osmolarity gradient necessary for urine formation.

The blood supply to the medulla occurs via the vasa recta (or peritubular capillaries) which accompany the limbs of the LOH from the juxtamedullary nephrons. The vasa recta thus form descending and ascending limbs. Plasma from the efferent arterioles flows from outer medulla to inner medulla in the descending limbs of the vasa recta, and then from inner medulla to outer medulla in the ascending limbs of the vasa recta. Plasma flowing in the descending limbs becomes progressively concentrated as the hyperosmolar interstitium causes water to exit and solutes to enter the vessel. This concentrated plasma then passes through the ascending vasa recta, gradually becoming less concentrated as water enters from the decreasingly hyperosmolar interstitium, and solute returns to the interstitium.

Control of water reabsorption by antidiuretic hormone

The reabsorption of water in the collecting duct system in the kidney is controlled by antidiuretic hormone (ADH). As the filtrate flows from distal tubule to cortical collecting tubule and medullary collecting duct, water is reabsorbed into an increasingly hyperosmolar medulla for reuptake into the circulation via the peritubular capillaries.

ADH controls water reabsorption by the following pathway:

- A rise in osmolarity in the extracellular fluid is detected in the anterior hypothalamus, at the supraoptic and paraventricular nuclei. It is also detected in the third ventricle at the subfornical organ and the organum vasculosum of the lamina terminalis.
- ADH is synthesised in the supraoptic and paraventricular nuclei. It is transported in the neurones of these nuclei to the posterior pituitary gland, where it is released in response to a rise in ECF osmolarity.
- ADH binds to V_2 receptors in the distal tubule, cortical collecting tubule and medullary collecting duct (Figure 16.11).
- A G-protein-coupled mechanism leads to deposition of aquaporin-2 (AQP2) channels on the luminal side of these tubules.
- These channels increase the permeability of the tubules to water, which, when reabsorbed, prevents change in ECF osmolarity.
- The main stimulus for release of ADH is ECF osmolarity. Subsidiary factors which favour release of ADH include: hypovolaemia, hypotension, hypoxia and nausea.
- Conversely, water reabsorption is reduced when there is a decrease in osmolarity or a rise in blood pressure or blood volume. There is a reduction in ADH and in water permeability, leading to increased water clearance and formation of dilute urine.

In clinical practice, excessive water absorption occurs when there is excessive release of ADH owing to:

- Drugs, e.g. opioids, chlorpromazine
- Respiratory disease, e.g. pneumonia
- Central nervous pathology, e.g. head injury and Guillain–Barré syndrome
- Malignancy of lung, prostate, pancreas
- Metabolic disease, e.g. porphyria

Water clearance

Calculation of water clearance

Water clearance can be defined as:

Water clearance = urine volume per unit time (V_U)
— volume of plasma cleared
of solutes per unit time (V_P)

Assuming that :

Rate of solute clearance from plasma
= Rate of solute appearance in the urine

Let Osmolarity of the plasma = C_P

Rate of solute clearance from plasma = $V_P.C_P$

And if Osmolarity of the urine = C_U

Rate of solute appearance in the urine = $V_U.C_U$

Then:

$V_P.C_P = V_U.C_U$

Volume of plasma cleared of solutes per unit time

$$V_P = \frac{V_U.C_U}{C_P}$$

Water clearance = $V_U - V_P$

$$= V_U - \frac{V_U . C_U}{C_P}$$

From the equation of water clearance, we find that if urine volume per unit time is:

- greater than volume of plasma cleared of solute per unit time, then free water clearance is positive.
- less than volume of plasma cleared of solute per unit time, then free water clearance is negative, indicating that there is water reabsorption.

Water clearance is an index of body hydration obtained by relating the osmolarity and volume of urine produced per unit time to the plasma osmolarity.

- If the urine is *hypo-osmolar* compared with plasma, then the plasma filtered is being diluted by free water, and the water clearance is *positive*. Thus a relatively well-hydrated or overhydrated state exists.
- If the urine is *hyperosmolar* compared with plasma, then the free water clearance is *negative*, and a relatively underhydrated state exists.

Renal control of sodium

Sodium salts are the main osmotically active solutes in the ECF. Control of body sodium content is a vital function of the kidneys, since it is a major determinant of body fluid volume. Humans are able to conserve sodium (Na^+) very effectively, and urinary losses can be less than 1 mmol L^{-1}. However, maximal sodium reabsorption can increase the excretion of K^+ and H^+, and so may disturb acid–base balance. Changes in Na^+ excretion are normally brought about by changes in tubular reabsorption.

When disturbances of body fluid osmolality occur, disturbances in body sodium content and consequently in body fluid volume may take hours or even days to correct. This contrasts with the more rapid ADH release in response to disturbances.

Primary control of sodium reabsorption is mediated by the release of the systemic hormones renin, angiotensin and aldosterone. The effects of these hormones are modified by other mechanisms, and also depend on changes in effective circulating volume.

Regulation of sodium reabsorption

Sodium reabsorption is complex, being influenced by:

- Systemic hormones (renin, angiotensin, aldosterone)
- Starling forces in the peritubular capillaries
- Neurological reflexes
- Renal prostaglandins
- Atrial natriuretic peptide
- Dopamine

> **Renin** is an enzyme which is synthesised and stored in the granular cells of the juxtaglomerular apparatus. It is released into the plasma when the body sodium content decreases.

Renal control of extracellular fluid volume

> Control of total body fluid volume is dependent on the regulation of the extracellular fluid (ECF) volume. The role of the kidney in controlling ECF volume depends on the control of water reabsorption by ADH and the regulation of sodium reabsorption or secretion.

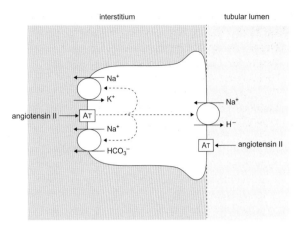

Figure 16.12 Angiotensin II binding in tubular cells

Reduction in extracellular fluid volume

In the presence of a sudden reduction in ECF volume (e.g. haemorrhage) and hence blood pressure, there is a rise in sympathetic stimulation to maintain blood pressure and also ECF volume via the following physiological sequence:

- An immediate increase in venoconstriction, heart rate, contractility of the heart and arteriolar vasoconstriction.
- A subsequent reduction in stress relaxation of the vascular system and an increase in capillary fluid shift of interstitial fluid into the blood compartment
- A slow renal response involving sympathetically mediated release of renin from juxtaglomerular cells in the afferent arterioles of the glomeruli. Renin catalyses the conversion of angiotensinogen, a plasma peptide, to angiotensin I. In the lungs, angiotensin-converting enzyme catalyses the conversion of angiotensin I to angiotensin II.

Renal effects of angiotensin II

As well as stimulating systemic vasoconstriction, angiotensin II produces efferent arteriolar constriction in the kidney. This results in increased tubular reabsorption of sodium and water as a result of the following changes:

- Reduced peritubular capillary pressure increasing the reuptake of sodium and water from the interstitium.
- An increase in filtration fraction leading to increased peritubular capillary colloid osmotic pressure with increased uptake from the interstitium.

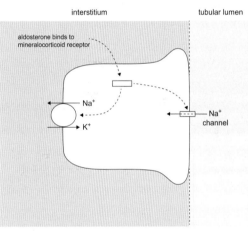

Figure 16.13 Aldosterone binding in tubular cells

- Sodium and water reabsorption in the proximal tubule, loop of Henle, distal tubule and cortical collecting tubule by stimulating $Na^+K^+ATPase$, co-transport of sodium and bicarbonate, and sodium–hydrogen exchange (Figure 16.12).
- Aldosterone release from the adrenal cortex. Aldosterone binds to cortical collecting tubular mineralocorticoid receptors intracellularly, and leads to increased sodium and water reabsorption as a result of stimulating Na^+/K^+ pumps in the distal tubal and collecting duct via nuclear mineralocorticoid receptors (Figure 16.13).

Nephrotic syndrome

In nephrotic syndrome, there is a reduction of extracellular fluid volume and blood volume due to:

- Proteinuria. In health, there should be < 150 mg of protein per 24 hours, in urine. In nephrotic syndrome, proteinuria occurs at a rate of 3500 mg per 24 hours. Proteinuria is likely when the albumin-to-creatinine ratio is > 30 mg mmol^{-1} or the protein-to-creatinine ratio is > 50 mg mmol^{-1}.
- Reduction in colloid osmotic pressure in tissue capillaries.
- Reduction in reabsorption fluid and hence loss of fluid into tissue, causing oedema.

There is compensatory activation of the sympathetic activity as well as sodium and water retention via the renin–angiotensin–aldosterone pathway.

In the presence of liver cirrhosis, similar compensatory mechanisms for low blood volume occur as a result of:

- Decreased plasma protein synthesis by the liver and hence low colloid osmotic pressure for reabsorption of tissue fluid
- Portal hypertension and loss of blood volume in ascitic fluid.

Increase in extracellular fluid volume

An increase in ECF volume may occur acutely as a result of transfusion or more gradually by an increased intake of water or both salt and water. Following expansion of the ECF there is a concomitant increase in blood volume, cardiac output and blood pressure (Figure 16.14). The increase in blood pressure leads to a renal response which involves excretion of sodium and water via a reduction in renin–angiotensin–aldosterone stimulation. This results in a restoration of normal ECF volume, blood volume and cardiac output.

Chronic increases in sodium and water intake enhance the kidney's ability to excrete salt and water. This ability of the kidney to compensate for persisting changes in ECF volume leads to almost no long-term changes in blood pressure (Figure 16.14).

Hypertension

In hypertensive patients who have renal pathology, the compensatory mechanism in the kidney is obtunded. In these patients, an initial increase in ECF volume may be corrected by enhanced excretion of sodium and water. However, blood pressure ultimately rises after increased salt and hence water intake

The blood pressure may then continue to be elevated despite restoration of ECF volume, blood volume and

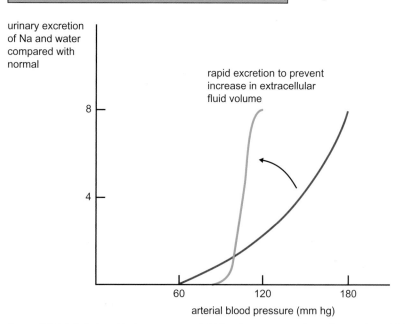

Figure 16.14 Relationship between arterial blood pressure and renal excretion of Na and H$_2$O

hence cardiac output to normal. In these patients, hypertension continues as a result of high systemic vascular resistance rather than increased ECF volume.

Renal control of acid–base balance

In conjunction with the lungs, the kidneys keep body pH constant. Normal blood pH is kept within the range 7.35–7.45, although life may remain viable over a range of 7.0–7.8. Most of the enzyme reactions in the body have a pH optimum at which they are most efficient.

The pH notation is an inverse logarithmic representation, so the pH range of 7.0–7.8 will correspond to a variation in H^+ concentration between 100 and 15 nmol L^{-1}.

The body pH continually trends towards acidity because of H^+ produced by intermediate metabolism, and the kidney is the final pathway which eliminates H^+ via the urine. In order to maintain the body pH within viable limits, systems of different buffers exist which combine with or 'buffer' the free H^+ in the body.

Figure 16.15 The main physiological buffer systems

Body compartment	Buffer
Blood	Bicarbonate/CO_2 Haemoglobin (HHb/Hb^- and HHbO$_2$/HbO$_2$) Plasma proteins (H^+-protein/protein$^-$) Phosphate ($H_2PO_4^-$ / HPO_4^{2-})
Extracellular fluid	Bicarbonate/CO_2 Plasma proteins (H^+-protein/protein$^-$) Phosphate ($H_2PO_4^-$ / HPO_4^{2-})
Intracellular fluid	Plasma proteins (H^+-protein/protein-) Phosphate ($H_2PO_4^-$ / HPO_4^{2-}) Organic phosphates Bicarbonate/CO_2

Definition of pH and normal [H⁺] values

Let concentration of H^+ = $[H^+]$
By definition pH = $-\log [H^+]$
But normal pH = 7.4. Therefore:

$$-\log [H^+] = 7.4$$
$$[H^+] = \log^{-1}(-7.4)$$
$$= \log^{-1}(-8) + \log^{-1}(0.6)$$
$$= 10^{-8} \times 3.98$$
$$= 39.8 \times 10^{-9} \text{mol } L^{-1}$$
$$= 39.8 \text{ nmol } L^{-1}$$

Physiological buffers

Intermediate metabolism generates a continuous load of H^+. This is buffered by the blood buffer systems, which prevent excessive levels of free H^+, but become depleted as their base reserves combine with the H^+. Thus the buffer bases need to be constantly regenerated.

A buffer solution minimises the change of pH, when acid or base is added to it. Buffer solutions consist of a weak acid and the conjugate base of that acid.

Thus in solution:

(acid) $\leftrightarrows$ (hydrogen ion) + (conjugate base)

$HA \leftrightarrows H^+ + A^-$

The Henderson–Hasselbalch equation and buffers

In any buffer system consisting of a dissociating weak acid HA, the pH of the buffer solution is dependent on the ratio of conjugate base concentration $[A^-]$ to undissociated acid concentration $[HA]$.

(acid) $\leftrightarrows$ (hydrogen ion) + (conjugate base)

$HA \leftrightarrows H^+ + A^-$

Rearranging the equation for K from the above definition of pK for a buffer:

$$[H^+] = \frac{K[A^-]}{[HA]}$$
$$\left[\frac{1}{H^+}\right] = \frac{1}{K} \cdot \frac{[HA]}{[A^-]}$$
$$-\log[H^+] = -\log K + \log \frac{[A^-]}{[HA]}$$
$$pH = pK + \log \frac{A^-}{[HA]}$$
$$pH = pK + \log \frac{[\text{conjugate base}]}{[\text{acid}]}$$

which is known as the Henderson–Hasselbalch equation.

When hydrogen ions are added to the buffer solution, the above reaction is driven to the left and the hydrogen ions (H^+) are 'neutralised' by combination with the conjugate base (A^-).

In the body fluids, there are several buffer systems. These are summarised in Figure 16.15.

Definition of pK for a buffer

The equilibrium constant (K) for the above dissociation reaction is given by

$$K = \frac{[H^+][HA^-]}{[HA]}$$
$$pK = -\log K$$

From the above, and using the definition of pH, it can be seen that pK is the pH at which $[A^-] = [HA]$, i.e. when the weak acid, HA, is half dissociated.

The bicarbonate buffer system

The most important buffer is bicarbonate, since H^+ is readily neutralised by plasma HCO_3^- to give carbonic acid, which is easily excreted as CO_2 in the lungs. The bicarbonate reserve is regenerated continually by the reabsorption process in the kidney.

The reaction sequence for this system is:

$$CO_2 + H_2O \leftrightharpoons H_2CO_3 \leftrightharpoons H^+ + HCO_3^-$$

The importance of this system stems from the regulation of the body CO_2 levels by the lungs, which excrete CO_2, and the maintenance of bicarbonate levels by the kidneys, through reabsorption of bicarbonate. These actions continually drive the above reaction sequence to the left, neutralising H^+ as it is produced by intermediate metabolism.

The bicarbonate system, chemically, is a poor buffer, but physiologically it is extremely effective because of the physiological control over $[HCO_3^-]$ and pCO_2. Since bicarbonate is regulated by the kidneys and pCO_2 by the lungs, it is apparent that body pH depends on the activity of both organs.

From the Henderson–Hasselbalch equation (below) it can be seen that acidosis occurs when the bicarbonate-to-carbon dioxide ratio decreases. Conversely, alkalosis occurs when this ratio increases. The kidney controls pH by altering the bicarbonate component of this equation.

The bicarbonate buffer system and the Henderson–Hasselbalch equation

For the bicarbonate buffer system (pK = 6.3), we can write the Henderson–Hasselbalch equation as follows :

$$pH = 6.3 + \log \frac{[HCO_3^-]}{[H_2CO_3]}$$

$[H_2CO_3]$ is proportional to the PCO_2 (partial pressure of CO_2 in mmHg) and has a value of approximately 2.0 mmol L^{-1}. Assuming a normal value of $[HCO_3^-]$ of 25 mmol L^{-1}, substitution in the above equation gives:

$$pH = 6.3 + \log 25/2$$
$$= 7.39$$

This illustrates how the bicarbonate buffer system determines normal pH for the body fluids, by fixing its [conjugate base] : [acid] ratio. This pH will then determine the [conjugate base] : [acid] ratio for all the other buffer systems in the body.

Renal mechanisms for pH control

The main role of the kidney in pH control can be seen as the conservation of the HCO_3^- buffer base and the generation of additional HCO_3^- as required.

Renal mechanisms involved in pH control (Figure 16.16) include:
- Reabsorption of filtered bicarbonate
- Generation of bicarbonate by the reabsorption of CO_2
- Secretion of H^+ in exchange for sodium
- Secretion of H^+ buffered by ammonia
- Secretion of H^+ buffered by hydrogen phosphate
- Metabolism of glutamine

Reabsorption of filtered bicarbonate

Reabsorption of filtered bicarbonate occurs in the proximal tubule (85%) and the thick ascending limb of the

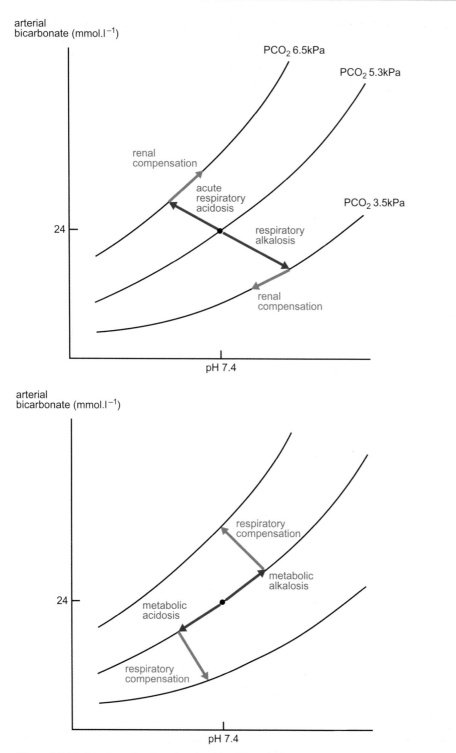

Figure 16.16 Renal mechanisms involved in pH control

loop of Henle (10%), as well as in the distal tubule and collecting duct (4.9%). Some bicarbonate (approximately 25 mmol L^{-1}) is filtered, and is reabsorbed directly.

Generation of bicarbonate in the tubular cells

The secretion of H^+ into the tubular lumen takes place in exchange for sodium via a $Na^+K^+ATPase$ pump. In the tubular lumen the H^+ is buffered by free bicarbonate in the filtrate, forming CO_2, which passes back into the tubular cells, where it generates more bicarbonate by the action of carbonic anhydrase.

Secretion of H^+ in exchange for sodium

In the proximal tubule sodium reabsorption is favoured by the electrochemical gradient and occurs in exchange for H^+. In the distal tubule and collecting duct there is active secretion of H^+ via the hydrogen ATPase pump. The secreted H^+ may be buffered by bicarbonate, ammonia or the phosphate buffer systems. A total of 80 mmol of hydrogen ions is excreted per day, and urinary pH can decrease as far as 4.5.

H^+ buffering by ammonia

Excess nitrogen from protein metabolism circulates as glutamine and glutamic acid, which are the main source of NH_4^+. The ultimate fate of NH_4^+ is to be excreted by the kidney either as ammonia or as urea. Ammonia (NH_3) is formed in the tubular cells, from where it diffuses freely between tubular cells, the interstitium and the tubular lumen. In the urine it buffers H^+ secreted by the tubular cells:

$$NH_3 + H^+ \leftrightharpoons NH_4^+$$

H^+ buffering by phosphate

In the plasma there are two phosphate salts, disodium hydrogen phosphate (alkaline phosphate, Na_2HPO_4) and sodium dihydrogen phosphate (acid phosphate, NaH_2PO_4). The ratio of alkaline phosphate to acid phosphate in plasma is approximately 4:1. These phosphate salts are filtered in the glomeruli and form an additional buffer system in the urine:

$$HPO_4^{2-} + H^+ \leftrightharpoons H_2PO_4^-$$

Metabolism of glutamine

Bicarbonate is also generated by the deamination of glutamine, which is a source of NH_4 in the tubular cells. This reaction occurs in the proximal tubule, thick ascending limb of the loop of Henle and distal tubule.

Renal changes occurring in acidosis and alkalosis

In acidosis the body pH may decrease from normal (pH 7.4) to pH 7.0. Lower pH levels (pH < 7.0) may become incompatible with life. A clinical index of the degree of acidosis present may be calculated as the anion gap.

Definition of anion gap

The anion gap is the calculated difference between the measured primary cations and anions. It represents unmeasured anions present in the plasma and will be raised in acidosis.

Anion gap $= Na^+ - HCO_3^- - Cl^-$

The mechanisms returning pH to normal include:

- Reabsorption of all filtered bicarbonate (Figure 16.17)
- Increased H^+ secretion, which is facilitated by phosphate and ammonia buffers
- Increased bicarbonate generation due to increased metabolism of glutamine and an increase in hydrogen ions and carbon dioxide
- A decrease in extracellular fluid volume
- Aldosterone release with sodium reabsorption and hypokalaemia

In contrast, when alkalosis is present there is:

- Incomplete reabsorption of filtered bicarbonate
- Decreased generation of bicarbonate
- Decreased ammonium excretion in urine
- Decreased excretion of acid bound to hydrogen phosphate

Persisting acidosis

A persisting acidosis can occur when there is:

- Acid secretion in the collecting duct
- Potassium secretion in the distal tubule, which leads to reduced exchange of hydrogen for secretion in the collecting duct
- Bicarbonate reabsorption by the proximal tubule

In this situation, there is inadequate acidification of urine (pH > 5.3) and metabolic acidosis, called renal tubular acidosis (Figure 16.18). Also, there is hyperchloraemia, a normal anion gap and variable serum potassium. The anion gap is normal because there is chloride retention to compensate for the reduction in bicarbonate during acidosis.

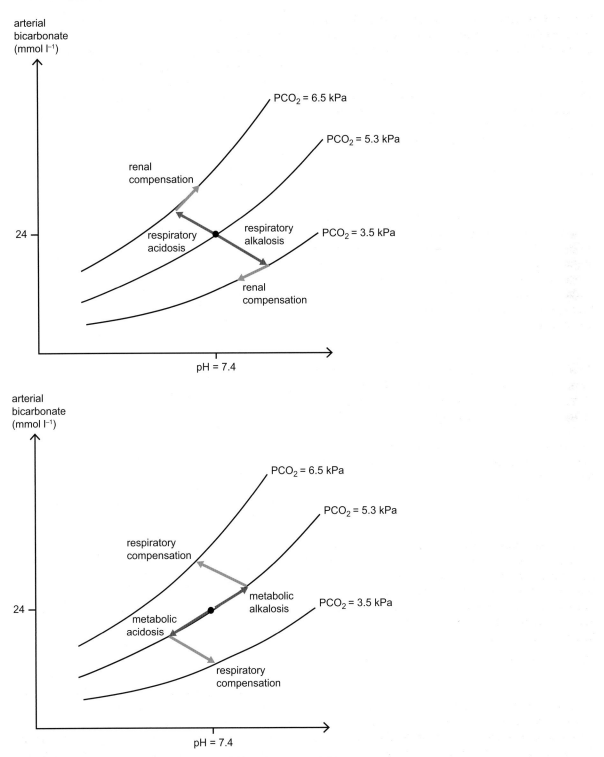

Figure 16.17 Relationship between pH, arterial bicarbonate and CO_2

Figure 16.18 Renal tubular acidosis

Physiological mechanism	Aetiological factors	Associated features
Reduced acid secretion by α intercalated cells in the collecting duct (type 1 distal renal tubular acidosis) owing to defective function of one or more of: • Hydrogen ATPase • Bicarbonate and chloride anion exchange • Carbonic anhydrase	Genetic Drugs, e.g. amiloride, lithium, trimethoprim, amphotericin, ifosfamide Pregnancy Sickle cell disease Autoimmune diseases, e.g. systemic lupus erythematosis, rheumatoid arthritis	Hypokalaemia Urine pH > 5.3 Nephrocalcinosis Urinary tract infection Plasma HCO_3^- < 10 mmol L^{-1}

Renal control of extracellular potassium

Extracellular potassium is approximately 4.1 mmol L^{-1}. Any change in extracellular potassium is resisted by redistribution with the intracellular compartment and by altering potassium secretion in the kidney. Over 90% of the potassium filtered at the glomerulus is reabsorbed in the proximal tubule and the ascending limb of LOH. Regulation of potassium secretion occurs in the distal tubule and collecting duct, where potassium is secreted down an electrochemical gradient. This enables correction of disturbances in extracellular potassium.

Secretion of potassium in the distal nephron depends on:

- The concentration of potassium in the tubular cells
- The activity of $Na^+K^+ATPase$ on the basolateral membrane of the tubular cells (Figure 16.13)
- The potassium permeability of the tubular cells' luminal membrane
- The filtrate flow rate in the distal tubule – the faster the flow rate the lower the filtrate potassium concentration

---

In hyperkalaemia

Excretion of potassium is stimulated by:
- The rise in extracellular potassium, which stimulates $Na^+K^+ATPase$ and increases release of aldosterone
- Aldosterone, which enhances $Na^+K^+ATPase$ and increases the permeability of the luminal membrane for potassium secretion (Figure 16.19)
- An increase in distal tubular flow associated with increased intraluminal sodium, sodium ingestion and fluid intake

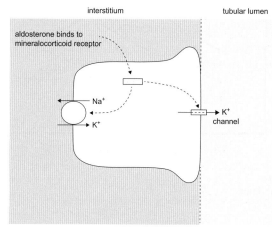

Figure 16.19 Excretion of potassium by $Na^+K^+ATPase$ pump

- Increased sodium and fluid loss due to diuretics or reduced proximal tubular absorption in chronic acidosis

In hypokalaemia

Excretion of potassium is decreased by reversal of the above changes. In addition, the acute acidosis which may accompany hypokalaemia inhibits the sodium–potassium pump, leading to reduced potassium secretion.

Renal control of calcium and phosphate metabolism

Calcium regulation

99% of filtered calcium is reabsorbed in the kidneys. The majority is reabsorbed in the proximal tubule (65%). The remainder is reabsorbed in the thick ascending limb of the loop of Henle as well as in the distal tubule and cortical collecting tubule. Most of the calcium reabsorption follows a paracellular pathway, in which calcium diffuses through the tight junctions. Approximately 30% of calcium reabsorption, particularly in the distal areas, occurs via the transcellular pathway (Figure 16.8), which is stimulated by parathyroid hormone and to a lesser extent by 1,25-dihydroxycholecalciferol.

> **The kidney takes part in calcium regulation by:**
> - Converting 25-hydroxycholecalciferol to 1,25-dihydroxycholecalciferol in the proximal tubule
> - Adjusting reabsorption of filtered calcium

The transcellular pathway for calcium is an energy-dependent pathway consisting of:
- Ca^{2+} ATPase and sodium–calcium counter-transport, in the basolateral membrane
- Calcium channels in the luminal membrane of the tubular cell

Phosphate reabsorption
80% of filtered phosphate reabsorption is in the proximal tubule, while 10% occurs in the distal tubule. The phosphate reabsorption pathway is transcellular, via a sodium-phosphate co-transporter on the luminal side of the tubular cell. Control of reabsorption is via parathyroid hormone.

Hypocalcaemia
The presence of reduced extracellular calcium is detected by calcium-sensing receptors in the parathyroid glands, leading to an increase in parathyroid hormone. Parathyroid hormone stimulates hydroxylation of 25-hydroxycholecalciferol to 1,25-dihydroxycholcalciferol.

Actions of 1,25-dihydroxycholecalciferol
- Increases renal reabsorption of calcium and phosphate
- Increases intestinal absorption of calcium and phosphate
- Increases bone mineralisation

Actions of parathyroid hormone
- Increases renal reabsorption of calcium
- Increases formation of 1,25-hydroxycholecalciferol
- Increases renal excretion of phosphate
- Increases calcium release from bone

Calcium and phosphate in chronic kidney disease

> In chronic kidney disease there is failure of hydroxylation of 25-hydroxycholecalciferol, leading to hypocalcaemia. This causes an increase in parathyroid hormone levels, resulting in secondary hyperparathyroidism.

The actions of increased parathyroid hormone in chronic kidney disease:
- Releases calcium from bone, causing osteomalacia or rickets.
- Stimulates compensatory phosphate excretion and so corrects hyperphosphataemia which is present as a result of reduced renal excretion of phosphate in renal failure. Renal excretion of phosphate is also augmented by fibroblast growth factor 23.

In severe cases, autonomous release of parathyroid hormone occurs, i.e. production that is independent of calcium levels. This state of tertiary hyperparathyroidism leads to:
- Hypercalcaemia
- Excessive intestinal absorption of calcium
- Excessive calcium resorption from bone

Hypercalcaemia may also occur in malignancy, which causes an increase in parathyroid hormone. In this state of primary hyperparathyroidism, there is hypercalcaemia and hypophosphataemia. There may be metastatic calcification and nephrolithiasis.

Pathophysiological mechanisms in the nephron
Renal failure occurs as a result of pre-renal, renal and post-renal factors. In this section, renal failure as a result of physiological dysfunction in the glomeruli, the tubules and the interstitium is considered.

Glomerular disease
In clinical practice, normal glomerular function is reduced in several pathophysiological states (Figure 16.10). Glomerulonephritis has variable presentations including systemic illness, nephrotic syndrome and nephritic syndrome. Nephrotic syndrome comprises proteinuria (> 3500 mg 24 h^{-1}), hypoalbuminaemia, oedema and

possible hypercholesterolaemia. Nephritic syndrome presents with haematuria, hypertension, acute renal failure and possible oedema. The aetiology of these syndromes may be primary or attributable frequently to infection, malignancy, autoimmunity and drugs. In membranous nephropathy, for example, NSAIDs, ACE inhibitors, gold and penicillamine are implicated. A special case of immunity and renal failure is the acute humoral-mediated rejection of a transplanted kidney, as described below.

Acute tubular necrosis

Tubular cells are susceptible to hypoxaemic conditions. They have high metabolic rate and high oxygen consumption, and their blood supply originates from the peritubular capillaries, which are the second set of capillaries, in series, after the glomeruli. When there is hypotension and efferent arteriolar vasoconstriction, hypoxemia and hence acute tubular necrosis are likely to occur.

In addition, during rhabdomyolysis, myoglobin, which is filtered freely at the glomerulus, forms myoglobin casts which may cause acute tubular necrosis. Aetiological factors, many of which occur in anaesthetic practice, include:

- Muscle trauma, e.g. prolonged muscle compression, electrocution and crush syndrome
- Drug toxicity, e.g. cocaine, ecstasy, amphetamines, alcohol
- Medications, e.g. muscle relaxants, statins, antipsychotic drugs
- Metabolic emergencies, e.g. diabetic ketoacidosis, hypothyroidism
- Infection
- Autoimmune muscular diseases, e.g. polymyositis, dermatomyositis
- Disorders of muscle energy supply, e.g. phosphofructokinase deficiency

Acute tubulointerstitial nephritis

Acute tubulointerstitial nephritis is characterised by eosinophilia, oedema, necrosis, fibrosis and atrophy. While many causes are due to infection, others are attributable to drugs utilised in anaesthetic practice. Examples include:

- Non-steroidal anti-inflammatory drugs
- Aspirin
- Proton pump inhibitors
- H_2 antagonists
- Diuretics
- Antibiotics (penicillin, gentamicin, erythromycin)

Acute cellular rejection

Acute cellular rejection of a transplanted kidney involves injury in the tubules and interstitium, 1–12 weeks after surgery. Alloantigens are presented to alloreactive CD4 T cells, which become activated and produce cytokines such as IL-2, IL-4 and IFN-8, which stimulate B cells. These B cells release antibodies which bind to antigens on the graft endothelial cells, leading to the following physiological response:

- Phagocytosis
- Activation of the classical complement cascade
- Platelet activation
- Thrombus formation
- Neutrophil infiltration of the glomeruli and endothelialitis

Chronic tubulointerstitial nephritis

Chronic tubulointerstitial nephritis, in which there is tubular atrophy and scarring, may also be caused by drugs such as analgesics, immunosuppressants (e.g. ciclosporin) and lithium. Other reasons for its occurrence include:

- Infection (chronic pyelonephritis, obstruction, vesicoureteric reflux)
- Toxins (e.g. lead)
- Malignancy
- Autoimmunity
- Radiation
- Metabolic diseases (uric acid and calcium)

Renal stones

Renal stones may form as a result of one or more of the following physiological factors:

- Stagnant conditions
- Presence of foreign bodies
- Urine acidity
- Excess biochemical substrates

Types of stones include:

- Triple phosphate stones, i.e. containing calcium, ammonium and magnesium, which form during stagnant conditions and the presence of foreign bodies.
- Uric acid stones, which occur as a result of uricosuria, particularly when there is hyperuricaemia and acidic urine, e.g. ileostomy, chronic diarrhoea and proximal renal tubular acidosis.

Figure 16.20 Interactions between drugs and the kidney

Physiological action of diuretics

Physiological mechanism	Drug group	Example
Inhibition of Na^+ K^+ $2Cl^-$ cotransport in the luminal membrane of the thick ascending limb of the loop of Henle	Loop diuretics	Frusemide
Inhibition of Na^+ Cl^- co-transport in the luminal membrane of the distal tubule	Thiazide diuretics	Bendroflumethiazide
Inhibition of action of aldosterone on mineralocorticoid receptors in cells of collecting tubules	Aldosterone antagonist	Spironolactone
Inhibition of Na^+ transport in luminal channels in the collecting tubules	Sodium channel blocker	Amiloride
Inhibition of carbonic anhydrase for reabsorption of bicarbonate	Carbonic anhydrase inhibitors	Acetazolamide
Increase osmolarity of tubular fluid and decrease reabsorption of water and solutes	Osmotic diuretics	Mannitol

Drugs to manage physiological features of kidney injury

Physiological dysfunction	Drug treatment	Example
Anaemia	IV iron therapy Erythropoietin	
Hypocalcaemia	1-hydroxycholecalciferol, which is hydroxylated in the liver to 1,25-dihydroxycholecalciferol	Alfacalcidol
Hyperphosphataemia	Phosphate binders	Aluminium hydroxide Calcium carbonate (Calcichew) Sevelamer
Hypertension	β-Blockers Calcium antagonists ACE inhibitors (omitted when there is hyperkalaemia and rising creatinine) α-Blockers	Bisoprolol Amlodipine Ramipril Doxazocin
Failure to acidify urine, hypokalaemia, and metabolic acidosis	Neutralise hypokalaemia and acidosis	Bicarbonate Potassium

Suppression of immune response to a transplanted kidney

Physiological category	Mechanism of drug action	Example
Lymphocyte depletion	Anti-CD52 antibody	Alemtuzumab

Figure 16.20 (*cont.*)

Anti-inflammatory actions	Corticosteroids for lysosomal membrane stabilisation. There is also reduction in release of lysosomal proteolytic enzymes, T-cell formation, IL-1 release, and capillary permeability	Methyprednisolone Prednisolone
Cytokine blockade	Anti-CD25 antibody for induction	Basiliximab Daclizumab
	Reduction in IL-2 via activation of nuclear factor of activated T cells by calcineurin inhibitors	Ciclosporin Tacrolimus
	Reduction of protein synthesis and proliferation	Sirolimus
Antiproliferation	Inhibition of DNA synthesis in lymphocytes	Mycophenolate mofetil Azathioprine

- Calcium oxalate stones, which arise in the presence of hypercalciuria and hyperoxaluria. While hypercalciuria occurs as a result of hypercalcaemia (e.g. in malignancy, hyperthyroidism, sarcoidosis and acromegaly), it may be precipitated by drugs (e.g. loop diuretics, corticosteroids) as well as Cushing's or Conn's syndrome, when there is normocalcaemia. Hyperoxaluria may be autosomal recessive or secondary to increased absorption of oxalate in Crohn's disease or during ingestion of tea, chocolate and spinach.
- Cystine stones during cystinuria.

Micturition

Micturition occurs as a result of the following factors:

- Micturition reflexes increase in frequency, duration and pressure when there is a rise in intravesical pressure detected by stretch receptors in the wall of the bladder and posterior urethra. This mechanism occurs at the level of the spinal cord in the sacral region: afferent sensory impulses travel in the parasympathetic splanchic nerves to the spinal cord. From there, motor impulses travel in the parasympathetic nerves to stimulate contraction of the detrusor muscle.
- The micturition reflexes occur and then disappear.

- When the bladder is sufficiently full, these micturition reflexes overcome inhibitory signals from the brain. Then there is relaxation of the external sphincter in the urogenital diaphragm via motor impulses travelling in the pudendal nerve (S2, S3), and the bladder empties.

In the presence of sacral spinal cord damage:
- The afferent limb of the micturition reflex is damaged.
- The bladder fails to empty.
- Overflow incontinence occurs.

In contrast, when there is brain or higher spinal cord injury:
- The effect of the micturition reflex is uninhibited.
- The bladder is in an uninhibited neurogenic state.
- There is frequent micturition.

Drugs and the kidney

Drugs affect renal function and vice versa (Figure 16.20). The main categories include:
- Diuretics.
- Drugs to manage physiological problems in kidney injury.
- Drugs for immunosuppression in patients requiring anaesthesia for renal transplantation.

CHAPTER 17

Respiratory physiology

Bal Appadu and Ted Lin

Functional anatomy

The primary function of the respiratory system is the exchange of oxygen and carbon dioxide between the body and the environment. In addition, the lungs also have a metabolic role, act as a filter for small emboli in the circulation, play a part in acid–base balance and contribute to the immune defences of the body. These functions are all reflected in the anatomy of the components of the respiratory system.

Upper airway and larynx

In respiration, the function of the nose, mouth and pharynx is to conduct fresh gas to the larynx, which marks the entrance to the conducting airways. These structures also warm, humidify and filter the gases.

During quiet nasal breathing this section of the airway can provide two-thirds of the total resistance to airflow of the respiratory system. Since the pharynx is a muscular tube without rigid structures to maintain its patency, it

Fundamentals of Anaesthesia, 4th edition, ed. Ted Lin, Tim Smith and Colin Pinnock. Published by Cambridge University Press. © Cambridge University Press 2017.

Figure 17.1 Conducting and gas exchange airways of the respiratory system (after Haefeli-Bleuer & Weibel 1988)

Generation	Structure	Anatomy	Function
1	Trachea	11 cm length × 18 mm diameter Ciliated columnar epithelium Many goblet cells Mechano- and chemoreceptors	Gas conduction
2–4	Major bronchi	Right main bronchus 25° angle of deviation from trachea Left main bronchus 45° angle of deviation from trachea	
5–11	Small bronchi	Large increase in total cross-sectional area with lower flow velocities	
12–16	Bronchioles	Diameter < 1 mm No cartilage, with high proportion of smooth muscle in walls	
17–19	Respiratory bronchioles	Intermittent alveolar outpockets Cuboidal epithelium	Gas exchange
20–23	Alveolar ducts and alveolar sacs	Continuous alveoli form walls of ducts Alveolar sacs are blind ended Total surface area 50–100 m^2	

can increase the flow resistance considerably, even to the point of total obstruction, depending on the tone of its muscular wall, the associated muscles and the transmural pressure.

The larynx has three main functions:

- Regulation of expiratory airflow (expiratory braking). This is important for vocalisation, coughing and control of end-expiratory lung volume.
- Protection of the lower airway. Vocal cord closure prevents aspiration of foreign material or objects, and expiratory braking enables the cough reflex to expel foreign material and secretions.
- Vocalisation.

Conducting airways

The respiratory system is traditionally divided into gas-conducting and gas-exchanging components. The conducting system begins with its smallest cross-sectional area at the level of the larynx, which leads into the trachea and undergoes irregular dichotomous branching for about 23 generations. The 23 generations are called Weibel's classification, after E. R. Weibel, an anatomist from Bern in Switzerland (Figure 17.1).

Adult trachea (generation 1)

The trachea is lined with columnar ciliated epithelium containing many mucus-secreting goblet cells. It also contains a number of receptors that are sensitive to mechanical or chemical stimuli. These mediate respiratory and cough reflexes.

Major bronchi (generations 2–4)

The major bronchi are named after the lobe or segment supplied. Circumferential cartilage rings support them. The right bronchus is wider than the left and leaves the trachea at about 25° from the tracheal axis, while the angle of the left bronchus is about 45°. Inadvertent endobronchial intubation or aspiration of foreign material is, therefore, more likely to occur in the right lung than the left. The right upper-lobe bronchus branches posteriorly at about 90° to the right main bronchus. Thus, foreign bodies or fluid aspirated by a supine subject usually enter the right upper lobe.

Small bronchi (generations 5–11)

These are smaller versions of the major bronchi, and their mucosa tends to be more cuboidal than columnar towards the periphery. As the number of bronchi increases, the total cross-sectional area increases markedly, with a reduction in the velocity of gas flow and a decrease in airway resistance.

Bronchioles (generations 12–16)

Bronchioles typically have diameters < 1 mm. They are devoid of cartilage and have a high proportion of smooth muscle in their walls in relation to intraluminal diameter. There are 3–4 bronchiolar generations, the final generation being the terminal bronchioles. Goblet cells are not found in bronchioles, and there is a continued gradual transition from ciliated epithelial cells to cuboidal epithelium.

Respiratory areas of the lung

Gas exchange begins in the smaller bronchioles and extends throughout the succeeding generations of airways to the most peripheral spaces, which are the alveoli.

Respiratory bronchioles (generations 17–19)

These are characterised by intermittent alveolar outpockets. Their cuboidal epithelium is thinning and a muscle layer is still present, forming 'sphincters' around openings to alveoli.

Alveolar ducts and sacs (generations 20–23)

These are formed from the alveoli that line and form their walls. The sacs differ from the ducts in being blind-ended. The alveolus is the basic unit of gas exchange, being a thin-walled pocket, about 0.3 mm in diameter. There are 300 million alveoli, with a total surface area of 50–100 m^2.

Three types of cells cover the alveolar surface:

- Type I alveolar cells occupy 80% of the surface for gas exchange. They provide a very thin layer of cytoplasm, spread over a relatively wide area (50 times that of a type II cell). Type I cells are derived from type II cells and are highly differentiated and metabolically limited, which makes them susceptible to injury.
- Type II alveolar cells have extensive metabolic and enzymatic capacity and manufacture surfactant. Both type I and II alveolar cells have tight intracellular junctions, providing a relatively impermeable barrier to fluids.

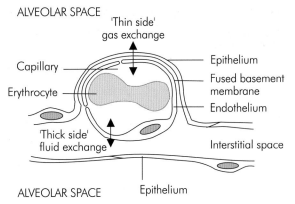

Figure 17.2 Alveolar–capillary membrane

- Type III alveolar cells are alveolar macrophages and form an important part of lung defences. They contain proteolytic enzymes, which may be released during lung injury, thus contributing to pulmonary damage.

Alveoli have holes in their walls called pores of Kohn (8–10 μm in diameter), which permit collateral ventilation between neighbouring alveoli. Similarly, larger-diameter (30 μm) ducts allow collateral ventilation between respiratory bronchioles.

Alveolar–capillary membrane

The alveolar–capillary membrane or 'blood–gas barrier' exists between the alveolar space and the capillary lumen, and consists of:

- Alveolar epithelium, which is a thin layer of type I alveolar cell cytoplasm
- Interstitial tissue, consisting of fused alveolar and endothelial basement membranes
- Pulmonary capillary endothelium

In order to allow gas exchange and fluid exchange, the capillaries are located asymmetrically in the alveolar walls, which gives them a 'thick side' and a 'thin side'. The 'thick side' is used for fluid exchange with the interstitium, while the 'thin side' forms the blood–gas barrier (Figure 17.2).

> **The alveolar–capillary membrane performs two conflicting functions:**
>
> - Gas exchange across the blood–gas barrier
> - Fluid exchange between alveolar interstitial tissue and the capillary lumen

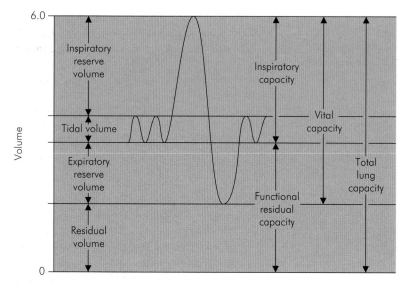

Figure 17.3 Spirometer trace of lung volumes

Blood vessels and lymphatics

The lung is divided into lobes, each supplied by its own artery, vein and bronchus. The arterioles form densely packed sheets of capillaries in the walls of the alveoli, thus matching the large ventilated surface area with an equivalent perfused area. Bronchi receive their own blood supply via bronchial arteries originating directly from the aorta.

Lymphatic drainage is important in the lung because of the magnitude of the perfused area and the effect accumulating interstitial fluid would have on gas exchange. Pulmonary lymphatics travel with blood vessels to the hila, ultimately draining into the thoracic duct.

Lung volumes

The lung can be divided into various volumes. These are identified either by measurements made during lung function testing, or according to the function of the lung in gas exchange.

Lung volumes derived from spirometry

During quiet breathing a small volume of gas is moved in and out of the lungs repeatedly. If a maximal inspiration is taken, followed by a maximal expiration, the volume changes occurring can be recorded using a spirometer. Figure 17.3 shows a typical spirometer trace of these changes.

Lung volumes vary with age, sex and body size (height more so than weight). The lung volumes are:

Figure 17.4 Values for lung volumes (mL)

Lung volume	Male	Female
TLC	6000	4200
V_T	500	500
IRV	3300	1900
ERV	1000	700
RV	1200	1100

- Total lung capacity (TLC) – volume of gas present in the lungs at the end of maximal inspiration
- Tidal volume (V_T) – amount of gas inspired and expired during normal quiet breathing
- Inspiratory reserve volume (IRV) – extra volume of gas that can be inspired over and beyond the normal V_T
- Expiratory reserve volume (ERV) – amount of gas that can be forcefully expired at the end of normal tidal expiration
- Residual volume (RV) – amount of gas remaining in the lungs at the end of a maximum forced expiration
- Vital capacity (VC) – maximal volume of gas which can be expelled after a maximal inspiration
- Functional residual capacity (FRC) – lung volume following expiration during quiet breathing

Some typical values for the above volumes are given in Figure 17.4.

Figure 17.5 Factors affecting FRC

Factor	Change in FRC
Age	Decreased
Posture	
Anaesthesia	
Surgery	
Pulmonary fibrosis	
Pulmonary oedema	
Obesity	
Abdominal swelling	
Thoracic wall distortion	
Reduced muscle tone	
Positive intrathoracic pressure	Increased
Emphysema	
Asthma	

Vital capacity

Apart from body size, the major factors that determine VC are the strength of the respiratory muscles, and chest and lung compliance.

> **Vital capacity** is an important clinical measure of respiratory sufficiency, particularly in patients with restrictive diseases.
> $VC < 10$ mL kg^{-1} is indicative of impending respiratory failure.

Functional residual capacity

From the spirometry trace in Figure 17.3 it can be seen that FRC is the lung volume at the end of normal quiet expiration, and is also equal to the sum of ERV + RV. The thoracic cage normally has a resting volume > FRC, while the normal lung has a volume < FRC.

> **FRC** represents the equilibrium point between the tendency of the lungs to collapse and of the thoracic cage to expand. It is not a fixed volume, and it varies with normal respiration as well as depending on gravity and other factors.

FRC is decreased by 20–25% in the supine position and is further decreased by the head-down posture and induction of anaesthesia. Some of the factors affecting FRC are shown in Figure 17.5.

Measurement of FRC

Spirometry does not give a value for FRC, nor for TLC and RV. The latter two can be derived if FRC is measured. Two common methods of determining FRC are:

- Helium dilution – used to obtain FRC using a spirometer, and an analyser to measure helium concentration. The subject is connected to the spirometer containing a known volume of fresh gas mixture (V_1) with a known initial concentration of helium (C_1). Normal breathing is allowed to take place through the spirometer until the helium becomes diluted and mixed in the larger combined volume (V_1 + FRC) of the spirometer and the respiratory system of the subject. Oxygen is fed into the spirometer to keep the spirometer reading constant, thus compensating for the difference between oxygen consumption and CO_2 production. Helium is used because it is virtually insoluble and not metabolised. FRC can be derived by measuring final helium concentration (C_2) and using the expression for the amount of helium present before and after as follows:

$$\text{Amount of helium} = V_1 \times C_1(\text{before})$$
$$= (V_1 + \text{FRC}) \times C_2(\text{after})$$

- Body plethysmograph – obtains FRC by placing the subject in a closed chamber and measuring the pressure and volume changes occurring when the subject makes an inspiratory effort. Boyle's gas law can be applied before and after the inspiratory effort to derive FRC.

Closing capacity

Closing capacity (CC) is the volume at which airway collapse and closure occurs during expiration.

> **Closing capacity** (CC) is important because it can affect gas exchange by virtue of its relationship to FRC. Under normal circumstances FRC is always > CC.

If FRC decreases or CC increases, for example due to loss of lung elasticity from disease, then airway closure may occur at the end of normal expiration in the dependent areas of the lung. Plate-like areas of atelectasis develop in dependent areas of the lungs shortly after induction of anaesthesia. The difference between FRC and CC is also reduced in infants and the elderly.

Dynamic lung volumes

Lung function can also be measured by its dynamic performance during active inflation or deflation. A common test is the recording of expired volumes during forced expiration of a maximal breath. The forced vital capacity (FVC) is the total volume of gas that can be forcibly expired after maximal inspiration. During forced expiration, dynamic compression of the intrathoracic airways occurs, limiting both the rate of expiration and the total amount of gas that can be expelled. The limiting effect may be seen from the expiratory curve of a VC breath, which is linear rather than exponentially declining and is described by the mid-expiratory flow rate, which applies to the gas volume expired between 25% and 75% of the total ($MEFR_{25-75}$). In clinical practice the volume expired in the first second (FEV_1) is often measured as part of an FVC measurement. The ratio (FEV_1/FVC) can then be derived, which is a useful index of obstructive airways disease (Figure 17.6).

> Normally the (FEV_1/FVC) ratio is $> 95\%$, but it declines with age, and 85% may be acceptable in an elderly subject.

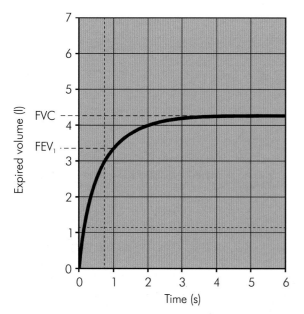

Figure 17.6 Vitalograph trace

Ventilation

Ventilation describes the process of fresh gas reaching the areas of the lung where gas exchange takes place. Gas exchange is dependent on the volume of gas moved in and out of the lungs per minute. This is referred to as total ventilation (minute ventilation).

> **Calculation of total expired ventilation**
>
> Let respiratory rate (n) = 10 breaths per minute
>
> Tidal volume = V_T = 0.5 L
>
> Total ventilation = respiratory rate × tidal volume
> $$= n \times V_T = 5\,L\,min^{-1}$$

> **Dead space and alveolar space**
>
> Not all of the gas moving in and out of the lungs takes part in gas exchange, since there are two main parts of the lung: **dead space**, which does not take part in gas exchange, and **alveolar space**, in which gas exchange does take place.

Dead space

Dead space refers to the volumes of the lungs which are ventilated but do not take part in gas exchange.

> Dead space can be subdivided into **anatomical dead space**, which corresponds to the conducting airways, and **alveolar dead space**, which consists of those parts of the lung which are ventilated but not perfused.

The sum of the anatomical and alveolar dead space is the physiological dead space.

Anatomical dead space

This is about 2 mL kg^{-1} (150 mL in an adult). Early measurements of the volume were obtained by taking casts of the conducting airways, but it may be measured non-invasively by Fowler's method.

In Fowler's method the patient takes a single VC breath of 100% oxygen and exhales through a rapid nitrogen analyser. Expired N_2 concentration is then plotted against expired volume (Figure 17.7). The initial gas from the dead space (phase I) is free of nitrogen, being pure oxygen, and thereafter the nitrogen concentration increases with the introduction of alveolar gas (phase II) until an 'alveolar' plateau is achieved (phase III). The dead

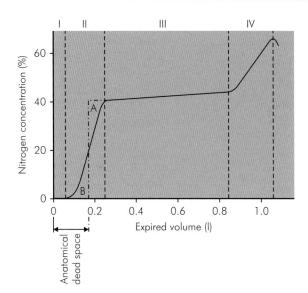

Figure 17.7 Fowler's method of dead space measurement

Physiological dead space

Under normal circumstances, physiological dead space differs very little from the anatomical and may be estimated with Bohr's equation:

$$\frac{V_D}{V_T} = \frac{P_A CO_2 - P_{\bar{E}} CO_2}{P_A CO_2}$$

In practice, the partial pressure of the mixed expired gas ($P_{\bar{E}} CO_2$) can be measured from a collection of mixed expired gas in a large bag, and the partial pressure in the alveoli ($P_A CO_2$) can be taken as being equal to that in the arteries ($PaCO_2$).

space is found by dividing phase II by a vertical line such that area A = area B and measuring the volume from zero.

Anatomical dead space will vary with changes in bronchial muscle tone and also with changes in position of the head and neck or the placing of an endotracheal tube. A functional decrease in anatomical dead space occurs at low V_T, when gas flow in the airways is laminar.

Alveolar dead space
Alveolar volume

Only fresh gas reaching the alveoli takes part in gas exchange. In each breath, only a portion of each V_T will reach the alveoli, because of anatomical dead space (V_D). This portion is the alveolar volume (V_A).

Alveolar ventilation

Alveolar ventilation is the volume of gas per minute reaching the alveolar spaces. It can be calculated from the respiratory rate (n) and alveolar volume (V_A).

Calculation of alveolar volume and alveolar ventilation

for $V_T = 500$ mL and $V_D = 150$ mL and
n = 15 breaths min^{-1} alveolar volume V_A
= $V_T - V_D$
= 350 mL alveolar ventilation
= $n \times V_A$
= 15×350
= 3250 mL min^{-1}

Derivation of Bohr's equation

The total volume of CO_2 expired in one breath ($V_T CO_2$) may be expressed in two ways.

First, as the product of the alveolar volume and the fractional concentration of CO_2 in the alveolar gas ($F_A CO_2$):

$$V_T CO_2 = V_A \times F_A CO_2$$

Second, as the product of V_T and the concentration of CO_2 in the mixed expired gas ($F_{\bar{E}} CO_2$):

$$V_T CO_2 = V_T \times F_{\bar{E}} CO_2$$

Thus

$$V_A \times F_A CO_2 = V_T \times F_{\bar{E}} CO_2$$

Substituting, as

$$V_A = V_T - V_D$$

gives

$$(V_T - V_D) \times F_A CO_2 = V_T \times F_{\bar{E}} CO_2$$

Rearrange to give

$$\frac{V_D}{V_T} = \frac{F_A CO_2 - F_{\bar{E}} CO_2}{F_A CO_2}$$

As the barometric pressure is the same for expired gas and alveolar gas, the partial pressures in the alveoli ($P_A CO_2$) and mixed expired gas ($P_{\bar{E}} CO_2$) may be substituted instead, yielding

$$\frac{V_D}{V_T} = \frac{P_A CO_2 - P_{\bar{E}} CO_2}{P_A CO_2}$$

Physiological dead space is dependent on both ana-tomical and alveolar dead space. Anatomical dead space varies as noted above. Alveolar dead space will be increased whenever areas of the lung become better ven-tilated than perfused.

Respiratory mechanics

> The movement of gas in and out of the lungs is a mechanical process, which is dependent on the following factors:
> - The respiratory muscles and their actions
> - The compliance of the chest wall and the lungs
> - The gas flow in the airways

The respiratory muscles and their actions
Respiration can be divided into inspiration and expir-ation. Inspiration is normally active while expiration is passive.

Inspiration
During inspiration the lungs can be expanded with two degrees of freedom (Figure 17.8):
- Displacement of the abdominal contents by contrac-tion of the diaphragm
- Radial expansion of the thoracic cage by the accessory respiratory muscles

Diaphragm
This is the principal muscle of breathing, accounting for about 75% of the air that enters the lungs during spon-taneous inspiration. Contraction of the diaphragm moves abdominal contents downward and forward during each inspiration. Two-thirds of the diaphragmatic fibres are slow twitch, making it relatively resistant to fatigue.

Accessory respiratory muscles
These comprise the external intercostal and strap muscles (sternocleidomastoid, anterior serrati, scalenes). During quiet breathing their contribution to inspiration is small. They act mainly to stabilise the upper rib cage and prevent indrawing. As respiration deepens, the contribution of these muscles increases by elevating the rib cage and expanding it in the lateral and anteroposterior directions.

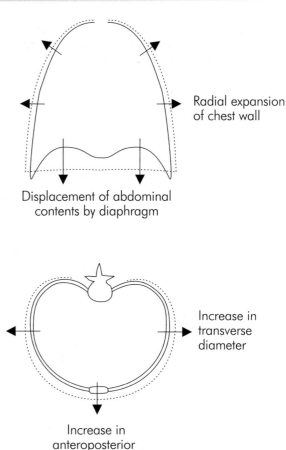

Radial expansion of chest wall

Displacement of abdominal contents by diaphragm

Increase in transverse diameter

Increase in anteroposterior diameter

Figure 17.8 Movement of the chest wall during inspiration

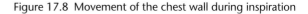

Expiration
In contrast with inspiration, the diaphragm relaxes during exhalation and the elastic recoil of the lungs, chest wall and abdominal structures compresses the lungs. Forced expiration for a cough or when airway resistance is increased requires the abdominal muscles and the internal intercostals. Paralysis of abdominal muscles produced by regional anaesthesia does not usually influence alveolar ventilation.

Compliance of the chest wall and lungs
Mechanically the respiratory system consists of two main components, the lungs and thoracic cage (including the diaphragmatic surface), which expand and contract together. Thus, the lungs and chest wall move together

as a unit. The lung expands in response to a pressure gradient produced across its surface, called the transpulmonary pressure. The transpulmonary pressure is equal to the difference between the airway pressure in the lungs and the pressure on the lung surface, i.e. in between the lung and chest wall. This pressure is the intrapleural pressure.

Intrapleural pressure
The resting position of the lungs and chest wall occurs at FRC. If isolated, the lungs, being elastic, would collapse to a volume < FRC. However, the isolated thoracic cage would normally have a volume > FRC. Since the chest wall is coupled to the lung surface by the thin layer of intrapleural fluid between parietal and visceral pleura, opposing lung and chest wall recoil forces are in equilibrium at FRC. This produces a pressure of about −0.3 kPa in the pleural space. Normal inspiration reduces intrapleural pressure further to −1.0 kPa, but with forced inspiration it can reach negative pressures of −4.0 kPa or more. Intrapleural pressure may be measured by an intrapleural catheter or from a balloon catheter placed in the mid-oesophagus.

Transpulmonary pressure
Normally, during spontaneous respiration, airway pressures in the lung can be approximated to atmospheric pressure. The pressure on the lung surface is the intrapleural pressure, which may reach −1.0 kPa during inspiration. This is equivalent to a distending transpulmonary pressure of +1.0 kPa.

Lung compliance
The lungs expand in response to the transpulmonary pressures produced by the respiratory muscles. The amount of expansion for a given transpulmonary pressure represents the ease with which the lungs expand. This property is measured by the lung compliance, which is the change in lung volume produced by unit change in transpulmonary pressure.

Definition of lung compliance

$$\text{Lung compliance} = \frac{\text{Change in volume}}{\text{Change in transpulmonary pressure}}$$

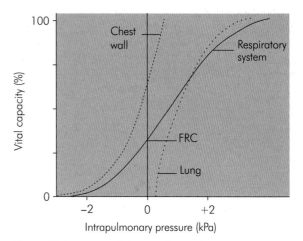

Figure 17.9 Lung and chest wall compliance

A value for compliance can be obtained from the pressure–volume curve for a normal isolated lung undergoing inflation, as shown in Figure 17.9. It can be seen that the curve is approximately linear over the 'working range' of the lung centred around FRC. At FRC, lung compliance is about 200 mL cm^{-1} H$_2$O. However, compliance is reduced at high lung volumes because the elastic fibres are fully stretched close to their elastic limit, while at low lung volumes compliance is reduced because airway and alveolar collapse occurs, requiring greater pressures to open up the airways and alveoli. Lung compliance may also be reduced by other factors (see below).

Chest wall compliance
If a pressure–volume curve is plotted for the isolated thoracic cage (Figure 17.9) the chest wall compliance can be obtained from the gradient, and this is also about 200 mL cm^{-1} H$_2$O at FRC. The chest wall compliance can be reduced by disease, as in ankylosing spondylitis, in which the chest wall can become virtually rigid, giving an extremely low compliance value.

Total respiratory system compliance
In the respiratory system the lungs and chest wall move together during inspiration and expiration. The respiratory system compliance is, therefore, the combination of chest wall and lung compliances.

Combining lung and chest wall compliances

If lung compliance (C_L) = 200 mL cm^{-1} H$_2$O, and chest wall compliance (C_W) = 200 mL cm^{-1} H$_2$O, then respiratory system compliance (C_R) is given by

$$\frac{1}{C_R} = \frac{1}{C_L} + \frac{1}{C_W}$$

$$\frac{1}{C_R} = \frac{1}{200} + \frac{1}{200} = \frac{1}{100}$$

$$C_R = 100 \text{ mL cm}^{-1}\text{H}_2\text{O}$$

The effect of combining lung and chest wall compliances to give the overall respiratory system pressure–volume curve is shown in Figure 17.9. Here it can be seen how the respiratory system compliance at FRC (gradient of the curve) is less than the individual gradients for lung or chest wall.

Measurement of respiratory system compliance

Compliance can be obtained from the gradient of a pressure–volume curve plotted for the respiratory system. However, this leads to two different values depending on the measurement technique.

Static compliance

To obtain static compliance a pressure–volume curve is plotted by applying known distending pressures to the respiratory system, and measuring the corresponding changes in volume produced. Appropriate time must be allowed between measurements for equilibration of the lung, when all gas movement has ceased. The static compliance is then given by the gradient of this pressure–volume curve based on static measurements.

Dynamic compliance

To measure dynamic compliance a pressure–volume curve is plotted continuously during spontaneous breathing or mechanical ventilation. In this case the changes in volume and pressure are recorded continuously as analogue signals with no pause between measurements. The dynamic compliance is derived from the gradient of the continuous pressure–volume curve.

The value for dynamic compliance is usually lower than the static compliance.

This is because:

- Airflow may not have ceased completely within the lung in response to pressure changes, particularly in diseased lungs. Further volume increases can follow gas movement from less distensible areas of the lung to more distensible areas ('pendelluft').
- Relaxation of tissues occurs with applied pressures that are sustained. This is due to the so-called 'viscoelastic' nature of tissues. This property of tissues, which mimics the action of hydraulic dampers in mechanical systems, means that when stretching forces are applied to real tissues they do not respond instantaneously, but stretch gradually in a viscous manner.
- The intrapulmonary pressure will be less than the applied airway pressure, because of airway resistance and inertia of the respiratory system. This causes an underestimation of the compliance.

The resultant effect of making dynamic measurements is that airway pressures in the dynamic case will be greater than those in the static case at any given lung volume. This means that the value for dynamic compliance will always be less than the static compliance.

Factors decreasing respiratory system compliance

Respiratory system compliance is usually maximum or optimal at FRC, and is decreased by both physiological factors and disease. Disease may affect both lung compliance (C_L) and chest wall compliance (C_W). Some examples of these factors are shown in Figure 17.10.

Pressure–volume loop for the respiratory system

If a pressure–volume curve for the respiratory system is plotted through a cycle of inspiration and expiration a 'loop' is obtained, as the inspiratory and expiratory limbs of the curve do not exactly coincide (Figure 17.11). This 'loop' effect is known as hysteresis. The area of the loop represents wasted energy, which occurs as a result of viscous losses during the stretching and recoil of the tissues, and also the frictional losses due to airway resistance. A factor that reduces this wasted energy and hence improves the efficiency of the breathing cycle is the lining of surfactant in the alveoli.

The area of the inspiration–expiration loop for the respiratory system represents the energy expended or 'wasted' as heat, as the lungs expand and deflate through the inspiratory–expiratory cycle.

Figure 17.10 Factors decreasing respiratory system compliance (C_R)

Factor	Change in C_R
FRC	
• Normal	Maximum
• High	Decreased
• Low	Decreased
Posture	
• Standing	Maximum
• Supine	Decreased
Age	
• Infant	Decreased
• Elderly	Decreased
• Pregnancy	Decreased
Disease	
• ARDS	Decreased ($\downarrow C_L$)
• Pulmonary oedema	Decreased ($\downarrow C_L$)
• Ankylosing spondylitis	Decreased ($\downarrow C_L$ and $\downarrow C_W$)

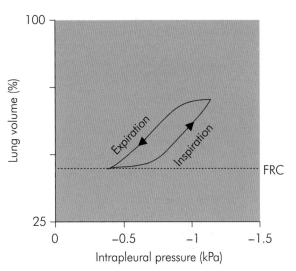

Figure 17.11 Inspiration–expiration loop, showing hysteresis

Surfactant

> **Surfactant** is a phospholipid-based substance secreted by the alveolar type II cells, which lines the alveoli and acts by markedly reducing surface tension.

Surfactant has the following effects:

- Reduction of surface tension, which helps to even out the distribution of compliance and hence ventilation. Without surfactant, alveoli with low resting volumes are significantly more difficult to expand than those with larger resting volumes. This effect is important in neonates, in whom deficiency of surfactant is associated with infant respiratory distress syndrome.
- Stabilisation of small alveoli. In a bubble wall, surface tension acts to shrink or collapse the bubble. A similar effect is seen in an alveolus. The smaller the alveolus

the greater the tendency to collapse. Because of this, small alveoli tend to collapse by forcing their gas into larger communicating alveoli. The reduction of surface tension by surfactant decreases this effect.

- Reduction of the energy expended as heat during each inspiratory–expiratory cycle, i.e. the hysteresis area of the pressure–volume loop is decreased.
- Surfactant also keeps the alveoli dry by reducing the 'suction' effect created by surface tension as it tries to collapse alveoli. Surface tension creates negative interstitial pressures as it tries to shrink alveoli, thus drawing fluid from capillaries into the air spaces.

Distribution of ventilation

When inspiration occurs the fresh gas entering the lung is not evenly distributed. Traditional teaching has upheld for decades that ventilation is distributed unevenly, with the majority of fresh ventilation passing to the more dependent regions of the lung. This model is based on the assumption of gravitationally determined distribution of lung perfusion, which indirectly determines local lung compliance and leads to ventilation inequalities. Thus both ventilation ($\dot{V}$) and perfusion ($\dot{Q}$) become gravitationally determined, ensuring optimum ventilation/perfusion ($\dot{V}/\dot{Q}$) matching.

More recent work, however, challenges this simple model of ventilation distribution by demonstrating significant variations in distribution in sections at the same

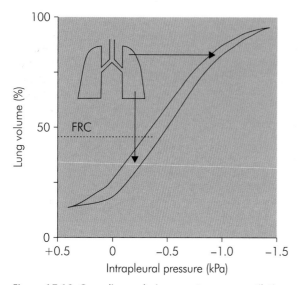

Figure 17.12 Compliance during spontaneous ventilation

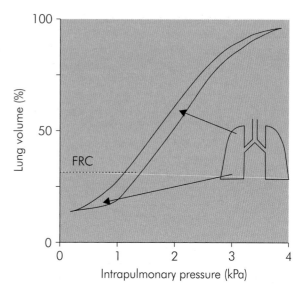

Figure 17.13 Compliance during mechanical ventilation

vertical level, i.e. in areas subject to the same gravitational effect. In addition, the dependence of perfusion on gravitational effects is also challenged. This leads to a different concept of ventilation and perfusion distribution and matching that is based on the structural heterogeneity of the lung.

Gravitational model for distribution of ventilation and perfusion

The mechanism determining the preferential distribution of ventilation to the most dependent regions of the lung during spontaneous breathing depends on the basic assumption of a gravitationally defined distribution of perfusion throughout the lung. Effectively the lung behaves as a continuous volume of fluid with a hydrostatic pressure gradient increasing from apex to base in the upright position. In the upright adult the intrapleural pressure at the base of the lung is approximately 0.7 kPa greater than the pressure at the apex. This variation in intrapleural pressure means that the alveoli will also vary in degree of distension, and correspondingly the alveoli will vary their position on the pressure–volume curve for the lung (Figure 17.12). The more dependent alveoli will be less distended, and located on the linear part of the pressure–volume curve, compared with the apical alveoli, which are over-distended and situated on the top part of the pressure–volume curve. Thus at the base of the lung the alveolar compliance (gradient of the pressure–volume

curve) is greater than that at the apex. Consequently, during inspiration, greater expansion of alveoli in the lower parts of the lung occurs, and ventilation is preferentially directed to the base. The end result is to direct ventilation to the areas of the lung with the most perfusion. In addition to the effects of gravity, airway resistance also plays a part in directing ventilation preferentially to the bases, since airway resistance is lower to the dependent areas of the lung.

This distribution of ventilation during spontaneous breathing contrasts with the situation when a patient is undergoing artificial ventilation. Under these circumstances the FRC is reduced, and this causes a reversal of the distribution of alveolar compliances, producing preferential ventilation of non-dependent areas (Figure 17.13).

Structural model for distribution of ventilation and perfusion

The traditional model for distribution of ventilation, as described above, is based on gravity being the most important determinant of local perfusion and hence indirectly regional ventilation. The use of enhanced CT scanning techniques suggests that regional variation of ventilation follows a more centripetal pattern rather than the vertical gravitationally determined distribution described above. Similarly, studies under variable and zero gravity conditions refute the predominant effect of gravity in determining local perfusion and ventilation, and offer the following observations:

- Significant heterogeneity of ventilation and perfusion occurs at the same vertical level (iso-height), i.e. where gravitational effects are excluded.
- The variability in perfusion and ventilation at iso-height level may be much greater than that observed over a vertical (gravitational) gradient.
- Heterogeneity of perfusion and ventilation occurs under zero gravity conditions.
- Postural changes fail to produce predicted changes in ventilation and perfusion, e.g. total lung perfusion in the dependent lung when in the left lateral position is less than in the non-dependent lung.

A more recent concept suggests that the main determinant of regional perfusion differences is regional vascular resistance, which will be largely influenced by changes in lung volume. Ventilation and perfusion remain matched in the lungs by virtue of their development as a twinned system of branching airways and pulmonary vessels. In this way, although regional variations in perfusion may occur independently of gravity, the distribution of ventilation will tend to vary in parallel since the main determinant of regional ventilation will be local airways resistance. The variability of perfusion and ventilation throughout the lung is attributed mainly to the asymmetrical branching nature of the airways and vascular trees, rather than to the gravitational gradient of the traditional model.

Summary of ventilation and perfusion distribution

- Traditional concepts suggest that both ventilation and perfusion are gravitationally determined, with optimum ventilation and perfusion occurring in the lung bases.
- More recent ideas suggest that ventilation and perfusion follow a centripetal distribution because of histological architecture.

Gas flow in the airways

The movement of gas in and out of the lungs is produced by the transpulmonary pressure and is conducted through the airways. The ease with which gas moves through the airways depends on:

- Airway resistance
- Pattern of gas flow

Airway resistance

The gas flow (F, in mL s^{-1} or L min^{-1}) through an airway is determined by the pressure difference between the ends of the airway (ΔP), and the resistance of the airway to gas flow (R). This is loosely analogous to the flow of electrical current through a conductor with electrical resistance. The case of laminar gas flow in an airway can be approximated to fluid (i.e. gas or liquid) flow in a tube, in which

$$\text{Flow, F} = \frac{\Delta P}{R}$$

This is modified in the Hagen–Poiseuille law, which substitutes factors for the resistance R. These factors include radius, viscosity and length. R is inversely proportional to (radius)^4, but dependent on the viscosity of the gas and the length of the tube.

Pattern of gas flow

Gas flow through an airway can occur in a smooth fashion, behaving as if in circumferential layers sliding across each other in the direction of flow. This is laminar flow, which occurs with a 'cone'-shaped gas velocity profile across the airway cross-section, the velocity being faster in the centre than at the periphery (cf. Chapter 15: Figure 15.6).

Alternatively, gas flow can be disorderly, with random eddies and whirls occurring across the overall direction of flow. This is turbulent flow, which moves with a relatively flat velocity profile in the direction of flow. Both laminar and turbulent flow exist within the respiratory tract, usually in mixed patterns.

Turbulent flow

In a given airway with a known gas and flow velocity, the likelihood of turbulent flow can be predicted from an index known as Reynolds number (Re).

Calculation of Reynolds number (Re)

$$Re = \frac{2rv\rho}{\eta}$$

where
r = airway radius
v = average velocity of gas flow
ρ = gas density
η = viscosity of the gas

Re < 1000 is associated with laminar flow, while Re > 2000 results in turbulent flow.

The pressure–flow relationship for turbulent flow is different from that in laminar flow, because the pressure gradient producing the flow is:

- Proportional to (flow velocity)^2
- Dependent on gas density and independent of viscosity
- Inversely dependent on (radius)^5

The resultant effect of turbulence is to increase the effective resistance of an airway compared with laminar flow.

Turbulent flow occurs at the laryngeal opening, in the trachea and in the large bronchi (generations 1–5) during most of the respiratory cycle. It is usually audible and almost invariably present when high resistance to gas flow is encountered.

Location of airway resistance

The principal sites of resistance to gas flow in the respiratory system are the nose and the major bronchi rather than the small airways. Since the cross-sectional area of the airway increases exponentially as branching occurs, the velocity of the airflow decreases markedly with progression through the airway generations, and laminar flow becomes predominant below the fifth generation of airway.

Measurement of airway resistance

Airway resistance can be measured during spontaneous breathing by simultaneous recording of air flow and the pressure gradient between mouth and alveoli. In practice the alveolar pressure is difficult to obtain, since it must be derived using a body plethysmograph. Intrapleural pressure can be used instead, but this will include the pressure gradient required to overcome lung tissue resistance and inertial properties. Thus, this technique measures not only the resistance to air flow, but also the viscous resistance due to the lung tissue and the inertia of the lung. Under normal circumstances, these additional factors are negligible, but tissue viscous resistance may become more significant in pulmonary oedema and fibrosis. Inertia of the lung may be of importance during high-frequency ventilation.

In clinical practice airway resistance can be assessed using forced expiratory flow rates such as FEV_1, peak expiratory flow rate (PEFR), and mid-expiratory flow rate. These indices are more easily measured, but they rely upon expiratory muscle activity in addition to airway resistance, and are affected by patient technique.

Factors affecting airway resistance

- Lung volume – the main factor affecting airway resistance. Increasing lung volume decreases airway resistance, and thus patients with high airway resistance often increase their FRC by position or pursed-lip breathing.
- Bronchial smooth muscle tone – airway smooth muscle is primarily under parasympathetic (vagal) control. Reflex constriction occurs with stimulation of the larynx, trachea or bronchi. Sympathetic influence is mediated mainly by β-receptors in the airway smooth muscle.
- Histamine release – H_1 receptors cause bronchoconstriction, while H_2 receptors cause bronchodilatation. However, the predominant effect of histamine is bronchoconstriction.
- Properties of inspired gas – flow resistance dependent on the density and viscosity of the inspired gas. Use of a helium–oxygen mixture improves ventilation in some cases of severe bronchospasm.
- Lower airway obstruction, which may be due to mucosal oedema, mucous plugging, epithelial desquamation or foreign bodies.
- Upper airway obstruction secondary to decreased conscious level, drugs, position of head, neck or jaw, tonsils or adenoids.
- Anaesthesia – airway resistance doubles during anaesthesia, due mainly to a reduction in FRC but also to increased upper airway resistance in some patients. Inappropriate selection of breathing systems may also contribute to increased total airway resistance. It is often forgotten that the upper airway contributes significantly to total airway resistance.

Work of breathing

Work is normally expended in inspiration, expiration being passive.

The work of inspiration can be subdivided into:

- Work required to overcome the elastic forces of the lung (compliance), which is stored as elastic energy
- Work required to overcome airway resistance during the movement of air into the lung
- Work required to overcome the viscosity of the lung and chest wall tissues (tissue resistive work)

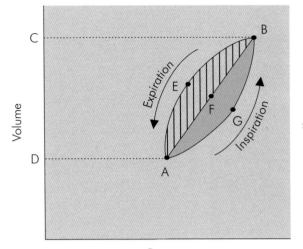

Figure 17.14 Work of breathing loop

During quiet breathing, most of the work performed is elastic. This inflates the lungs but provides a store of elastic energy to be returned during expiration. Since the energy is stored and returned to maintain the respiratory cycle, this is 'useful' work done.

The energy expended in overcoming tissue resistance and airway resistance is dissipated as heat and can be viewed as wasted energy. Figure 17.14 shows an idealised pressure–volume loop, with inspiration occurring along the path AGB and expiration along BEA. The following points illustrate the relationship between the wasted work done and the useful work done:

- In an ideal elastic lung, with no tissue or airway losses, the work stored in inspiration would be completely returned in expiration. Inspiration and expiration would then occur along the straight line AFB, with equal amounts of inspiratory work and expiratory work, represented by the area AFBCD.
- In the real lung, with tissue and airway losses, inspiration occurs along curve AGB. The inspiratory work done (AGBCD) is thus greater than the ideal case (by the shaded area AGBF). This wasted work is only a fraction of the inspiratory work.
- In the real lung, expiration occurs along BEA. The expiratory work returned (BEADC) is thus less than the ideal case (by hatched area BEAF).
- The total 'wasted' energy due to tissue and airway losses is thus the sum of the shaded and hatched areas, or the area of the loop.

In lung diseases all three types of work are increased. Compliance work and tissue resistive work are greatly increased during restrictive diseases such as fibrosis of the lungs, whereas airway resistance work is increased in pulmonary obstructive diseases.

Expiration does not normally entail active work, but this may be necessary in forced breathing or when airway resistance or tissue resistance are increased. In some circumstances, expiratory work may be greater than inspiratory work, for example in asthma.

Gas exchange

The oxygen tension in air (at sea level) is about 20 kPa, falling to 0.5 kPa in the mitochondria, where it is utilised. The transport of oxygen down this concentration gradient is described as the oxygen cascade (Figure 17.15). It involves different transport mechanisms, convection, diffusion through gas and liquid media and transport bound to Hb. The same process occurs in the reverse direction for CO_2.

Calculation of the partial pressure of oxygen in inspired gas (P_IO_2)

The fractional concentration of oxygen in dry ambient air ($F_{AMB}O_2$) is 0.21, and at sea level with a barometric pressure (P_B) of 101.3 kPa the partial pressure of oxygen ($P_{AMB}O_2$) is given by

$$P_{AMB}O_2 = F_{AMB}O_2 \times P_B$$
$$= 0.21 \times 101.3$$
$$= 21.3 \text{ kPa}$$

The addition of saturated water vapour ($P_{SVP} = 6.3$ kPa) by the upper airway mucosa reduces the oxygen partial pressure by a small amount to give:

$$P_IO_2 = F_{AMB}O_2(P_B - P_{SVP})$$
$$= 0.21(101.3 - 6.3)$$
$$= 20 \text{ kPa}$$

Alveolar oxygen tension

The alveolar oxygen tension (P_AO_2) is less than the inspired oxygen tension (P_IO_2) because some oxygen is absorbed in exchange for CO_2 excreted. Thus, the P_AO_2 is determined by:

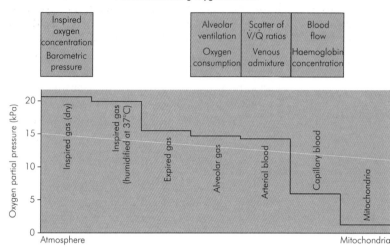

Figure 17.15 Oxygen cascade

- The rate at which oxygen is introduced into the alveoli (dependent on alveolar ventilation and inspired oxygen concentration)
- The rate of removal by absorption into pulmonary capillary blood (oxygen consumption)
- The rate of delivery of CO_2 ($\dot{V}CO_2$) by pulmonary capillary blood

The decrease in oxygen tension caused by oxygen absorption is estimated by using the tension of CO_2 excreted (approximately P_ACO_2), which must be corrected by the respiratory quotient (because less CO_2 is excreted than O_2 absorbed). This forms the basis of the alveolar gas equation, which can be used to calculate alveolar oxygen tension (P_AO_2).

The importance of P_AO_2 in clinical practice is that it determines the partial pressure gradient driving oxygen across the alveolar–capillary membrane. It is not easily measured directly, but an awareness of its value in clinical practice is useful in patient management. The following points should be noted:

- P_AO_2 is most easily increased by increasing inspired oxygen fraction (F_IO_2).
- P_AO_2 will fall with hypoventilation, but it only falls rapidly below alveolar ventilation levels of about 4 litres per minute, assuming normal oxygen consumption (about 250 mL min^{-1}). Figure 17.16a illustrates how varying alveolar ventilation rate affects P_AO_2.

- Hypermetabolic states (sepsis, malignant hyperthermia) will significantly increase the susceptibility to hypoxaemia by increasing oxygen consumption ($\dot{V}O_2$), and by increasing the rate of CO_2 delivery into the alveoli. Thus, both F_IO_2 and alveolar ventilation may need to be increased in such patients.
- P_AO_2 can be decreased iatrogenically by sodium bicarbonate infusion, since this increases body CO_2 levels and hence CO_2 delivery to the alveoli.

The alveolar gas equation

$$P_AO_2 = P_IO_2 - \frac{P_ICO_2}{RQ}$$

where RQ is the respiratory quotient, and

$$RQ = \frac{\dot{V}CO_2}{\dot{V}O_2}$$

Thus P_AO_2 is intermediate between the inspired oxygen tension (P_IO_2) and the arterial oxygen tension (PaO_2), due to oxygen being absorbed in exchange for CO_2.

For example, in a normal subject on a mixed diet with RQ = 0.8, P_IO_2 = 20 kPa and P_ACO_2 = 5 kPa:

$$P_AO_2 = 20 - (5 \div 0.8)$$
$$= 13.8 \, kPa$$

(a)

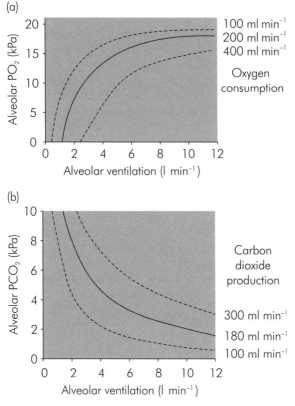

(b)

Figure 17.16 Variation of alveolar gas tensions with alveolar ventilation

- P_AO_2 can be used to calculate the alveolar–arterial PO_2 difference, which is a useful index of gas-exchange efficiency in the lungs.

Alveolar carbon dioxide tension

Alveolar CO_2 tension (P_ACO_2) is determined by the balance between:
- Rate of delivery of CO_2 ($\dot{V}CO_2$) into the alveoli by pulmonary capillary blood
- Rate of removal by alveolar ventilation

Alveolar CO_2 tension (P_ACO_2) can be varied by controlling alveolar ventilation. This effect is most noticeable at rates of alveolar ventilation below about 6 litres per

minute, given normal rates of CO_2 production (about 200 mL min^{-1}). Hyperventilation above this level produces a more gradual reduction in P_ACO_2. Figure 17.16b illustrates the variation of P_ACO_2 (which correlates well with $PaCO_2$ in the normal subject) with alveolar ventilation.

Gas diffusion from alveoli to blood

Gases diffuse between alveoli and pulmonary capillary blood across the blood–gas barrier. The rate of diffusion is determined by Fick's law.

The **blood–gas barrier** is effectively a membrane with a total surface area about 70 m^2. Over this membrane about 60–140 mL blood is spread as a thin sheet. The rate of gas transfer across this membrane will depend on:

- Properties of the gas (solubility and molecular weight)
- Properties of the membrane (surface area, A, and thickness, D)
- Partial pressure gradient (ΔP) across the membrane

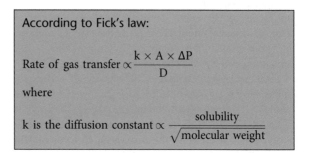

According to Fick's law:

$$\text{Rate of gas transfer} \propto \frac{k \times A \times \Delta P}{D}$$

where

k is the diffusion constant $\propto \dfrac{\text{solubility}}{\sqrt{\text{molecular weight}}}$

The lower molecular weight of oxygen and its greater alveolar-to-capillary partial pressure gradient favour its diffusion compared with CO_2. However, the higher blood/gas solubility coefficient of CO_2 (24 times that of O_2) causes CO_2 to diffuse more readily than oxygen, in spite of a lower partial pressure gradient.

Nevertheless, the efficiency of oxygen diffusion across the alveolar–capillary membrane is such that a red cell is fully oxygenated in < 50% of the transit time through the pulmonary capillary bed. Any factor that increases the thickness of the membrane, such as pulmonary oedema, interferes with the diffusion of oxygen more than with that of CO_2.

Oxygen transport in the blood

> Most of the oxygen (97%) in the blood is transported in combination with haemoglobin (Hb). Once the Hb is saturated, oxygen content can only be marginally increased (3%) by dissolved oxygen.

Dissolved oxygen is a linear function of P_AO_2 and is 0.023 mL kPa^{-1} per 100 mL plasma. Thus, for $P_AO_2 = 13$ kPa, only 0.3 mL oxygen (3%) is carried in a dissolved state. Even breathing pure oxygen, where it is possible to increase P_AO_2 to about 80 kPa, the dissolved arterial oxygen content would be only about 2.0 mL per 100 mL blood.

Haemoglobin

Oxygen is transported and delivered to the tissues by haemoglobin. Hb is a conjugated protein with a molecular weight of 66,700 daltons, and is composed of four haem subunits. Each subunit has a central ferrous (Fe^{2+}) atom and is conjugated to a polypeptide chain. The four polypeptide chains collectively form the globin moiety. Different forms of Hb exist, identified by their polypeptide chains. Normal adult Hb consists of HbA_1 (98%) containing two α and two β polypeptide chains, and HbA_2 (2%) containing two α and two δ chains.

Fetal erythrocytes contain HbF with two α and two γ chains. HbF is also modified by having a lower affinity for binding 2,3-diphosphoglycerate (2,3-DPG) than adult forms of Hb. 2,3-DPG is a highly anionic intermediate of glycolysis. It binds to the deoxygenated form of Hb, significantly reducing the affinity of Hb for oxygen. This facilitates the 'unloading' of oxygen in tissues with low oxygen tensions. HbF thus has an increased affinity for oxygen, which adapts its transport and delivery characteristics to the lower oxygen tensions in the placentofetal circulation. After birth the production of β chains starts, and HbA replaces HbF during the first year of life.

Oxygenation of haemoglobin

Each molecule of Hb can bind four molecules of oxygen. This is not a chemical reaction as in oxidation, but is a readily reversible bond. The following are characteristics of Hb oxygen binding:

- It is determined primarily by local oxygen tension (PaO_2).
- It is affected by local tissue conditions (e.g. pH, temperature) and local concentrations of substances (e.g. 2,3-DPG, CO_2).
- It produces an allosteric change in the structure of Hb to a 'Relaxed' form, while deoxygenated Hb has a 'Tense' form. This switching between R and T forms underlies the oxygenation and delivery mechanisms.
- It is 'cooperative', meaning that binding O_2 at each site promotes binding at the remaining sites due to allosteric changes. This increases the amount of O_2 delivered under physiological conditions, compared with a carrier having independent binding sites.
- Deoxygenation of Hb increases the affinity of several proton-binding sites on its molecule. This enhances its ability to transport CO_2 from the tissues to the lungs (Haldane effect) and underlies the role of Hb as a major buffer in acid–base regulation.

Oxyhaemoglobin dissociation curve

The percentage of Hb saturation with oxygen (SO_2) at different partial pressures of oxygen in blood is described by the oxyhaemoglobin dissociation curve (ODC) (Figure 17.17).

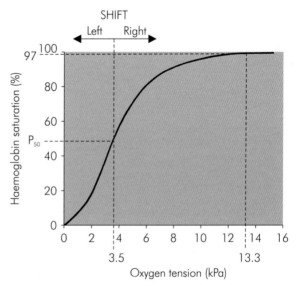

Figure 17.17 Oxyhaemoglobin dissociation curve

The **oxyhaemoglobin dissociation curve** (ODC) is a sigmoid curve whose shape is due to the cooperativity of the oxygen binding process. The position of the curve is best described by the P_{50}, which is the PO_2 at which Hb is 50% saturated (normally 3.56 kPa).

- Various factors can increase the affinity of Hb for O_2, 'shifting' the ODC to the left.
- Alternatively, factors decreasing the affinity between Hb and O_2 cause a shift of the ODC to the right.

'Left shift' of the ODC

This represents an *increase* in the affinity of Hb for oxygen in the pulmonary capillaries, requiring lower tissue capillary PO_2 to achieve adequate oxygen delivery. P_{50} is reduced by factors causing a left shift, which include:

- Alkalosis
- Decreased PCO_2
- Decreased concentration of 2,3-DPG
- Decreased temperature
- Presence of HbF rather than adult forms of Hb

'Right shift' of the ODC

This represents a *decrease* in the affinity of Hb for oxygen. In this situation P_{50} is increased, requiring higher pulmonary capillary saturations to saturate the Hb, but enhancing delivery at the tissues. Factors causing a right shift of the ODC include:

- Acidosis
- Increased PCO_2
- Increased concentration of 2,3-DPG
- Increased temperature

Bohr effect

The shift in position of the ODC caused by CO_2 entering or leaving blood is known as the Bohr effect.

The **Bohr effect** enhances the 'unloading' of oxygen in tissues, where PCO_2 levels are high compared with that in the pulmonary capillaries. The Bohr effect reverses in the pulmonary capillaries, enhancing the uptake of oxygen.

In the tissues CO_2 enters the red cells, combining with water and dissociating into H^+ and HCO_3. The increased $[H^+]$ shifts the ODC to the right, facilitating the release of oxygen from Hb. The HCO_3 diffuses out of the cells and is matched by an inward movement of chloride. This change reverses in the lungs.

Oxygen content of blood

The oxygen content of blood is the volume of oxygen carried in each 100 mL blood. It is determined by the blood's oxygen carrying capacity and oxygen saturation.

The theoretical maximum oxygen carrying capacity is 1.39 mL O_2 g^{-1} Hb, but direct measurement gives a capacity of 1.34 mL O_2 g^{-1} Hb.

Calculation of oxygen content of blood

(O_2 carried by Hb) + (O_2 in solution)
$$= (SO_2 \times 1.34 \times Hb \times 0.01) + (0.023 \times PO_2)$$

where
SO_2 = percentage saturation of Hb with oxygen
Hb = Hb concentration in grams per 100 mL (g dL^{-1})
PO_2 = partial pressure of oxygen

For a normal male adult the oxygen content of arterial blood can be calculated as follows:

Given arterial oxygen saturation (SaO_2) = 100%, Hb = 15 g dL^{-1}, and arterial partial pressure of oxygen (PaO_2) = 13.3 kPa, then oxygen content of arterial blood (CaO_2):

$$CaO_2 = 20.1 + 0.3 = 20.4 \text{ mL per } 100 \text{ mL}$$

Similarly, the oxygen content of mixed venous blood can be calculated. Given normal values of mixed venous oxygen saturation ($S\bar{v}O_2$) = 75%, and venous partial pressure of oxygen ($P\bar{v}O_2$) = 6 kPa:

$$C\bar{v}O_2 = 15.1 + 0.1 = 15.2 \text{ mL per } 100 \text{ mL}$$

Oxygen delivery ($\dot{D}O_2$) and oxygen uptake ($\dot{V}O_2$)

Oxygen delivery ($\dot{D}O_2$) is the amount of oxygen delivered to the peripheral tissues per minute.

$\dot{D}O_2$ is calculated by multiplying the arterial oxygen content (CaO_2) by the cardiac output ($\dot{Q}$). For $CaO_2 = 20.1$ mL per 100 mL and $\dot{Q} = 5$ litres per minute

$$\text{Oxygen delivery}(\dot{D}O_2) = 1005 \text{ mL min}^{-1}$$

Oxygen uptake ($\dot{V}O_2$) is the amount of oxygen taken up by the tissues per minute.

$\dot{V}O_2$ can be calculated from the difference between oxygen delivery and the oxygen returned to the lungs in the mixed venous blood.

The oxygen return is given by the product of mixed venous oxygen content ($C\bar{v}O_2$) and cardiac output ($\dot{Q}$). For $CaO_2 = 15.2$ mL per 100 mL and ($\dot{Q}$) = 5 litres per minute:

$$\text{Oxygen return} = 760 \text{ mL min}^{-1}$$

thus

$$\text{Oxygen uptake}\,(\dot{V}O_2) = (\text{oxygen delivery}) - (\text{oxygen return})$$
$$= 1005 - 760 = 245 \text{mL min}^{-1}$$

The primary goal of the cardiorespiratory system is to deliver adequate oxygen to the tissues to meet their metabolic requirements, a balance between $\dot{V}O_2$ and $\dot{D}O_2$.

The balance between oxygen uptake by the body tissues and oxygen delivery to them is assessed by:
- The oxygen content of mixed venous blood, which is normally about 15 mL per 100 mL
- The oxygen extraction ratio, which is the ratio of $\dot{V}O_2$ to $\dot{D}O_2$ expressed as a percentage. Normally the extraction ratio is about 25%, but it can double to 50% if tissue demand increases

Both of the above indices are dependent on mixed venous saturation and cardiac output.

Increased tissue demand due to exercise or disease is normally compensated for by increased oxygen delivery. This has to be mediated by increasing cardiac output, since the ability to increase SaO_2 and Hb is limited. However, under extreme conditions (severe exercise, sepsis, malignant hyperthermia) tissue demand can increase 12-fold (requiring a $\dot{V}O_2$ of up to 3000 mL O_2 min^{-1}). Cardiac output can usually be increased by a maximum of up to seven times, and thus under extreme conditions tissue demand can outstrip the body's capacity to increase delivery. In such a case $S\bar{v}O_2$ falls, extraction ratios increase and tissue hypoxia ensues. This susceptibility towards tissue hypoxia will be greatly increased in conditions where cardiac output is limited or compromised.

Carbon dioxide transport

CO_2 diffuses passively down its concentration gradient from the mitochondria to the capillaries. Although partial pressure gradients are low between tissues and blood, transfer is rapid because of the high solubility of CO_2.

Partial pressures of CO_2 (PCO_2) in the tissues equilibrate with capillary blood to produce a venoarterial PCO_2 difference of about 0.7 kPa. This corresponds to a CO_2 content difference of about 4 mL per 100 mL blood, depending upon RQ.

The 4 mL CO_2 that is added to each 100 mL arterial blood as it passes through the tissues consists of (Figure 17.18):
- 2.8 mL (70%) that enters erythrocytes to form carbonic acid (H_2CO_3). This reaction is catalysed by carbonic anhydrase, which, if inhibited, produces a marked increase in the alveolar–capillary PCO_2 gradient. The H_2CO_3 formed dissociates to give H^+ and HCO_3^-.

  As noted above, deoxygenation of Hb activates H^+ acceptor sites, increasing its buffering capacity. This encourages the dissociation of H_2CO_3 and as a result enhances the 'loading' of CO_2 in the tissues. The HCO_3^- formed diffuses out of the erythrocytes in exchange for chloride (Cl^-), which enters the red cells to maintain electroneutrality (the 'chloride shift'). The increase in osmotically active ions and Cl^- in venous red blood cells leads to an increase in their size. This is probably the reason for the venous haematocrit being about 3% greater than that of arterial blood.
- 0.9 mL (22%) carried as carbamino compounds, which are formed by reactions of CO_2 with terminal and side chain amino groups of proteins. Haemoglobin provides most of the amino groups, reduced Hb having at least three times more active sites than oxyhaemoglobin.
- 0.3 mL (8%) carried in solution.

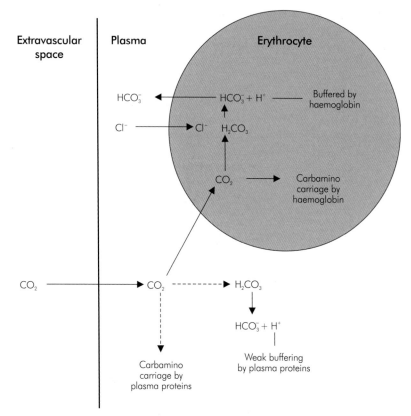

Figure 17.18 CO_2 transport in blood

Haldane effect

The Haldane effect describes the way in which CO_2 carriage in red blood cells varies according to the oxygenation state of haemoglobin. In the tissues, deoxygenation of Hb enhances carriage of CO_2, by activating proton binding and carbamino formation sites. Correspondingly, oxygenation of Hb causes the reverse effect, displacing H^+ and CO_2, thus facilitating the 'unloading' of CO_2 in the lungs.

> The dependency of CO_2 carrying capacity on the oxygenation state of Hb is known as the **Haldane effect**.

Body stores of oxygen and carbon dioxide

The total body oxygen of 1.5 litres is held as:

- 50% in combination with Hb
- 30% in the lungs
- 20% in combination with myoglobin

Not all stored oxygen is available for use, since severe hypoxaemia occurs before even half of the oxygen stored in combination with Hb and myoglobin is released. These available stores will last only for 3–4 minutes of apnoea, assuming air breathing and normal oxygen consumption. Breathing 100% O_2 increases the oxygen stores to about 4.25 litres, mainly by increasing the O_2 contained in the lungs.

In contrast, total body stores of CO_2 are about 120 litres. During apnoea, $PaCO_2$ increases by about 1 kPa in the first minute. This initial rise in $PaCO_2$ then decreases to a rate of 0.4 kPa min^{-1}, as alveolar PCO_2 levels build up and CO_2 elimination by diffusion through the airways increases.

> The **oxygen stores** of the body are relatively small in comparison to the consumption (around 250 mL min^{-1} for an adult). Total body oxygen is about 1.5 litres. Total body CO_2 stores are approximately 120 litres.

Pulmonary circulation

The pulmonary circulation is a low-pressure, low-resistance system in series with the right ventricle. The cardiac output from the right ventricle passes through the lungs into the left atrium. The cardiac output from the right ventricle is almost the same as that from the left ventricle.

Blood passes through pulmonary capillaries in about 0.5–1.0 seconds, depending on the cardiac output, during which time it is oxygenated and excess CO_2 is removed. The distributions of blood flow and ventilation throughout the lungs are generally very well matched, but this may vary markedly during anaesthesia or disease.

The pulmonary artery is a thin-walled structure which arises from the right ventricle and divides immediately into left and right branches and then divides successively, following a similar pattern to the conducting airways down to the terminal bronchioles. These small branches give rise to a dense capillary network, which may be viewed as a sheet of blood broken up by 'pillars' of connective tissue that maintain the stability of the alveoli. The oxygenated blood is collected by venules that run between the lobules and then unite to form the four pulmonary veins that drain into the left atrium.

> The **pulmonary vascular system** is a low-pressure, low-resistance system in series with the right ventricle. Pressures in the pulmonary circulation are about 20% of those in the systemic circulation.

The innervation of the pulmonary vasculature is supplied by the sympathetic nervous system, with α-adrenergic fibres producing vasoconstriction and β-adrenergic fibres vasodilatation. The vagus supplies parasympathetic fibres that produce vasodilatation.

Bronchial arteries from the thoracic aorta supply oxygenated blood to the supporting tissue of the lung, including connective tissue, septa and bronchi, and drain into the pulmonary veins, contributing to the anatomical shunt. An average of 1–2% of the total cardiac output passes through the bronchial arteries, thus making the left ventricular output slightly greater than the right.

Normal pulmonary arterial pressure has a systolic value of 25 mmHg, a diastolic value of 8 mmHg, and a mean of 15 mmHg. The mean pulmonary capillary pressure is 10 mmHg, with a pulmonary venous pressure of 4 mmHg at heart level. Pulmonary arterial and right ventricular pressures are not greatly influenced by increases in cardiac output in normal subjects, demonstrating the distensibility of the pulmonary vasculature.

Pulmonary vascular resistance

Pulmonary vascular resistance (PVR) is influenced by the following factors:

- Autonomic innervation – vasomotor tone is minimal in the normal resting state and pulmonary vessels are maximally dilated. The autonomic system exerts a relatively weak influence on PVR, increases in sympathetic tone giving rise to vasoconstriction.
- Nitric oxide (NO) – an important mediator of pulmonary vascular tone causing vasodilatation (it is also active in systemic vessels). Nitric oxide has been identified as endothelium-derived relaxing factor (EDRF), which also mediates other processes by the relaxation of smooth muscle. It is derived from L-arginine and increases intracellular concentrations of cyclic guanosine monophosphate (cGMP). Its actions as a potent vasodilator have led to its use in severe acute lung disease, where inhaled concentrations of 5–80 ppm can improve oxygenation.
- Prostacyclin (prostaglandin I_2) – an arachidonate, which is a potent vasodilator also of endothelial origin.
- Endothelins – potent vasoconstrictor peptides released by the pulmonary endothelial cells.
- Vascular transmural pressure – important in the pulmonary circulation because the thinner vessel walls make them more prone to collapse when alveolar pressure exceeds intravascular pressure. During controlled ventilation, high positive alveolar pressures can cause increased PVR and decrease perfusion in some areas of the lung.
- Lung volume – which also determines the calibre of the vessels embedded in the lung parenchyma. PVR is least at FRC. As the lung increases in volume, the vessels become narrowed and elongated; as it decreases in volume, the vessels become tortuous.
- Lung disease – both acute and chronic lung disease can result in significant increases in PVR. Long-term increases in PVR due to chronic disease can lead to right-sided heart failure.
- Hypoxic vasoconstriction – a powerful physiological reflex which diverts perfusion away from hypoxic areas of the lung.

Figure 17.19 Drugs modifying the HPV reflex

Drugs	Effect on HPV
Volatile anaesthetic agents Nitrates Nitroprusside Calcium channel blockers Bronchodilators	Attenuate HPV
Cyclo-oxygenase inhibitors Propranolol Almitrine	Potentiate HPV

Figure 17.20 Causes of pulmonary hypertension

Mechanism	Clinical condition
Intracardiac shunt	Atrial septal defect Ventricular septal defect
↑ left ventricular end-diastolic pressure	Mitral stenosis Constrictive pericarditis
Obliteration	Pulmonary fibrosis
Obstruction	Pulmonary embolism
Vasoconstriction	Sleep apnoea syndrome High altitude
Idiopathic	Primary pulmonary hypertension

> • Various factors affect PVR, including physiological mechanisms such as endothelium-derived relaxing factor (nitric oxide) and hypoxic pulmonary vasoconstriction.
> • Pathology or drugs can also affect PVR and may result in pulmonary hypertension.

Hypoxic pulmonary vasoconstriction

Hypoxic pulmonary vasoconstriction (HPV) is an important mechanism that improves the match between perfusion and ventilation by diverting blood from poorly ventilated areas to better ventilated areas. HPV maintains this balance of ventilation to perfusion on a breath-to-breath basis. The predominant site of HPV lies in the small pulmonary arteries (30–50 μm), with the remaining resistance arising from the capillary bed and venous system.

HPV may also affect the pulmonary vessels in general rather than on a regional basis. Low PaO_2 levels are responsible for generalised HPV in the fetus, reducing blood flow through the pulmonary vascular bed to about 10–15% of the fetal cardiac output. This generalised response also causes a significant increase in PVR at high altitude.

The exact mechanism of HPV is unknown. It is potentiated by acidosis and modified by various drugs (Figure 17.19).

> HPV improves ventilation/perfusion mismatch by diverting perfusion from poorly ventilated areas to better ventilated areas.

Pulmonary hypertension

Increased pulmonary arterial pressures can be caused by various pathological mechanisms. These are listed in Figure 17.20, together with examples of associated clinical conditions.

Distribution of perfusion

As outlined above, the pulmonary vascular resistance (PVR) is influenced by various factors. Although PVR determines the overall blood flow through the lungs, this blood flow is not evenly distributed throughout each lung.

> Two contrasting models exist for the distribution of perfusion within the lung (see *Distribution of ventilation*, above):
>
> • A traditional model based on a **gravitational gradient** from apex to base
> • A more recent **structural** model

Functional zones of the lung

The gravitational model for the distribution of ventilation and perfusion has led to a lung model based on 'functional zones' defined by the pressure difference across the walls (transmural pressure) of the pulmonary blood vessels (arteries, capillaries and postcapillary veins). When the extravascular pressure is greater than the hydrostatic

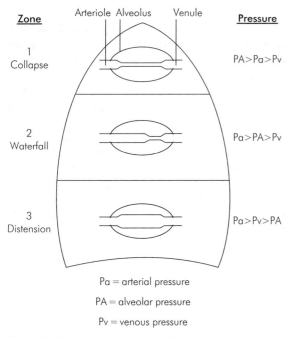

Zone	Arteriole Alveolus Venule	**Pressure**
1 Collapse		PA>Pa>Pv
2 Waterfall		Pa>PA>Pv
3 Distension		Pa>Pv>PA

Pa = arterial pressure

PA = alveolar pressure

Pv = venous pressure

Figure 17.21 Functional zones of the lung

pressure in the vessel, the vessel collapses, obstructing flow. If the transmural pressure is reversed (intravascular greater than extravascular pressure) the vessel remains patent.

In the lung, gravity gives rise to an intravascular hydrostatic pressure gradient that increases from the top of the lung to the base. Thus the arterial (Pa) and venous (Pv) pressures in the base are greater than those in the apex by about 23 mmHg. In contrast, extravascular pressure is effectively equal to alveolar pressure (P_A), which is approximately atmospheric pressure and is the same throughout the lung.

The relative magnitudes of P_A, Pa and Pv define the following functional zones in the lung (Figure 17.21).

Zone 1

In zone 1 alveolar pressure (P_A) is greater than the arteriolar pressure (Pa) and venular pressure (Pv). Both arterioles and venules will collapse, obstructing blood flow completely. In this case:

$P_A > Pa > Pv$

Arterial pressures (Pa) are minimal in the lung apex, and are just adequate to provide perfusion to these areas. In practice, Pa in the apical areas, although low, is not normally less than alveolar pressure (P_A), and zone 1 does not exist. Usually this can only occur under conditions of reduced pulmonary arterial pressure (e.g. hypovolaemia, decreased cardiac output) or increased alveolar pressure (e.g. controlled ventilation of the lungs, positive end-expiratory pressure). In such a case, perfusion to this part of the lung is zero and alveolar dead space increases significantly.

Zone 2

In zone 2 alveolar pressure is greater than the venous pressure but less than the arterial pressure. The veins collapse but the arteries remain patent, and blood flow will be partially obstructed. In this case:

$Pa > P_A > Pv$

Below the apical regions of the lung, alveolar pressure is less than arterial pressure, but greater than the venous pressure. In these areas the postcapillary veins are collapsed, offering high resistance to flow. The collapsed vessels can open up during systole or if pulmonary arterial pressure increases. This model of a collapsible tube with variable flow resistance due to downstream occlusion by external pressure is sometimes referred to as the Starling resistor or 'waterfall' effect.

Zone 3

Alveolar pressure is less than venous pressure in zone 3, and both arteries and veins will remain patent and blood flow will be unobstructed. In this case:

$Pa > Pv > P_A$

In the more dependent regions of the lung, arteries, capillaries and veins are patent and pulmonary blood flow is continuous. This zone extends from about 7–10 cm above the heart to the lowermost portions of the lung. There is some increase in perfusion moving down the zone, as pulmonary arterial pressure increases due to the gravitational pressure gradient. This increase in blood flow is achieved by:

- Recruitment of closed pulmonary vessels
- Perfusion of open but not perfused vessels
- Dilatation of vessels already perfused

These mechanisms enable zone 3 blood flow to increase in response to increases in pulmonary arterial pressure. Their overall result is a decrease in pulmonary vascular resistance.

Delineation of the functional zones is variable and affected by different conditions, which alter the relationship between Pa, Pv and P_A. In the supine position, nearly all portions of the lung become zone 3, with pulmonary blood flow being more evenly distributed. During exercise, pulmonary artery pressures increase and recruit previously under-perfused capillaries, thus converting most of the lung to a zone 3 pattern of pulmonary blood flow.

A zone 4 is sometimes described for regions in the most dependent parts of the lung, where intravascular pressures are highest but blood flow is reduced.

> - Three functional zones in the lung are defined by the relative magnitudes of alveolar pressure (P_A), pulmonary arterial pressure (Pa) and pulmonary venular pressure (Pv).
> - The delineation of these functional zones is variable and affected by posture and exercise.

Ventilation/perfusion ratio ($\dot{V}/\dot{Q}$)

Efficient gas exchange in the lung requires the gas flow in and out of each functional unit to be matched by the blood flow through it, i.e. ventilation ($\dot{V}$) must match perfusion ($\dot{Q}$). At rest the overall ratio of total alveolar ventilation (about 5250 mL min^{-1}) to total pulmonary blood flow (about 5000 mL min^{-1}) is about 1. Thus, it is normally assumed that the optimum ventilation/perfusion ($\dot{V}/\dot{Q}$) ratio for any unit of lung tissue is also 1.

When a unit of lung tissue is inadequately ventilated (< 1), some of the pulmonary capillary blood perfusing it effectively bypasses the lungs, since there is too much perfusion for the blood gases to equilibrate adequately with alveolar gas. This increases the 'shunt' effect in the lungs (see below).

When a lung unit is under-perfused (> 1), the expired gas from the unit contains a lower than normal concentration of CO_2, since excess fresh gas is supplied which does not exchange gases with pulmonary capillary blood. This increases the 'alveolar dead space' effect in the lungs.

> Ventilation/perfusion ($\dot{V}/\dot{Q}$) ratio for any area of lung tissue is an index that reflects the efficiency of gas exchange in that region. It has an optimum value of 1.
> In an area of lung tissue:
>
> - If < 1, it increases the 'physiological shunt'.
> - If > 1, it increases the 'alveolar dead space'.

Distribution of $\dot{V}/\dot{Q}$ ratios in the lung

In the normal lung, although ventilation and perfusion are both distributed to favour the dependent areas, the ratios are not uniform and vary from the lung apices to the bases. At the top of the lung ratios have been estimated to be about 3.3, and this value decreases passing down the lung to the bottom, where the ratios are about 0.6. $\dot{V}/\dot{Q}$ ratios vary in three dimensions, so that a distribution of values will be found across a horizontal section of the lung as well as from apex to base.

In diseased lungs $\dot{V}/\dot{Q}$ ratios vary over a wider range, as there is greater non-homogeneity of the lung tissue. The effect on gas exchange of increased mismatch is reflected by a deterioration in the following indices from their normal values, so there is:

- An increase in shunt fraction
- An increase in the alveolar–arterial PO_2 difference ($P_AO_2–PaO_2$)
- An increase in alveolar dead space
- A decrease in PaO_2 or an increase in $PaCO_2$

Alveolar–arterial PO_2 difference

In the normal lung there is a small alveolar–arterial partial pressure gradient for oxygen ($P_AO_2–PaO_2$) of 0.5–1.0 kPa.

> The ($P_AO_2–PaO_2$) difference is the sum of the PO_2 gradient across the alveolar–capillary membrane and the effect of admixture of shunted blood.

Any increase in the thickness of the diffusion barrier (e.g. pulmonary oedema or fibrosis) or the shunt effect due to $\dot{V}/\dot{Q}$ mismatch in the lungs will, therefore, produce an increase in this value.

Physiological shunt (venous admixture, shunt fraction)

Arterial blood may be less well oxygenated than blood leaving the alveoli for several reasons:

- Venous blood may bypass the lungs entirely (e.g. intracardiac shunts, thebesian veins, bronchial circulation).
- Blood may pass through parts of the lung which are not ventilated adequately, in which case $\dot{V}/\dot{Q} < 1$ (e.g. pneumonia).
- Blood may pass through areas of the lung which are not ventilated at all, in which case $\dot{V}/\dot{Q} = 0$. This is sometimes referred to as 'true' shunt.

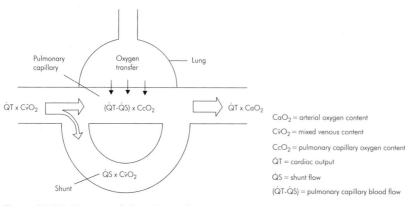

$\dot{Q}T \times C\bar{v}O_2$ $(\dot{Q}T\text{-}\dot{Q}S) \times CcO_2$ $\dot{Q}T \times CaO_2$

$\dot{Q}S \times C\bar{v}O_2$

CaO_2 = arterial oxygen content
$C\bar{v}O_2$ = mixed venous content
CcO_2 = pulmonary capillary oxygen content
$\dot{Q}T$ = cardiac output
$\dot{Q}S$ = shunt flow
$(\dot{Q}T\text{-}\dot{Q}S)$ = pulmonary capillary blood flow

Figure 17.22 Diagram of shunt in the lung

Shunt equation

Physiological shunt can be calculated as a fraction of total pulmonary blood flow (cardiac output).
Figure 17.22 shows the flows and oxygen contents of systemic, pulmonary capillary and shunt circulations.
Thus if

CaO_2 = arterial O_2 content

$C\overline{v}O_2$ = mixed venous O_2 content

CcO_2 = pulmonary capillary O_2 content

$\dot{Q}_T$ = cardiac output

$\dot{Q}_S$ = shunt flow

$(\dot{Q}_T - \dot{Q}_S)$ = capillary flow

The total O_2 content of blood leaving the lungs is

= (cardiac output × arterial O_2 content)

= $\dot{Q}_T \times CaO_2$

But the total oxygen content is also

= (shunt flow × mixed venous O_2 content)
+(pulmonary capillary flow
×pulmonary capillary O_2 content)

= $(\dot{Q}_S - C\overline{v}O_2) + (\dot{Q}_T - \dot{Q}_S) \times CcO_2$

So

$\dot{Q}_T \times 2CaO_2 = (\dot{Q}_S \times C\overline{v}O_2) + (\dot{Q}_T - \dot{Q}_S) \times CcO_2$

This can be rearranged to give the 'shunt' equation as follows:

$$\frac{\dot{Q}_S}{\dot{Q}_T} = \frac{(CcO_2 - CaO_2)}{CcO_2 - C\overline{v}O_2}$$

The effect of physiological shunt on arterial blood gases is shown in Figure 17.23, which illustrates an 'iso-shunt' diagram. Shunt fractions up to 10% are not considered clinically significant, but when greater than 30% they are associated with poor survival. The iso-shunt diagram is helpful in following clinical progress and in adjusting oxygen therapy.

Physiological shunt

Shunt effectively reduces oxygen content of pulmonary capillary blood due to admixture of venous blood which has bypassed the lungs.
  The 'shunt' equation assesses the shunt as a fraction of the total flow, and can be stated as:

$$\frac{\text{(shunt flow)}}{\text{(total flow)}} = \frac{\text{(reduction in oxygen content due to shunt)}}{\text{(total oxygen content added by lungs)}}$$

This fraction is usually quoted as a percentage, and it is a useful clinical index of oxygenation efficiency in critically ill patients.

Control of ventilation

Respiratory control is mediated by neurological and chemical reflexes that involve control centres in the central nervous system, the lungs, respiratory muscles and specialised receptors (Figure 17.24).
  The primary goal of respiratory control is to maintain homeostasis of blood gases. In addition, reflexes also modify the respiratory pattern in order to:

- Allow speech
- Enable coughing, sneezing, yawning

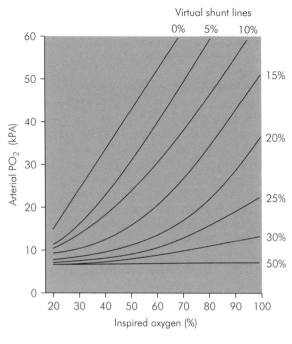

Virtual shunt lines

Conditions
Hb 10–14 gd l^{-1}
PaCO$_2$ 3.3–5.3 kPa
a-v oxygen content difference 5 ml 100 ml^{-1}

Figure 17.23 Iso-shunt diagram

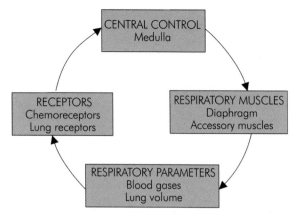

Figure 17.24 Central control of ventilation

- Protect the airway during eating, drinking and vomiting
- Minimise the work of breathing

Central control of ventilation

Centrally, ventilation is controlled by centres at different levels:
- In the medulla, there are inspiratory and expiratory pools of neurones.
- At the pontine level, there are the pneumotaxic and apneustic centres.
- Above the brainstem, control is exerted by the limbic system and at the cortical level.

Medullary centres

The medulla contains two pools of ventilatory control neurones, an inspiratory pool and an expiratory pool.

These inspiratory and expiratory neurones function by a system of reciprocal innervation. As activity increases in one centre, a rising level of inhibitory activity is relayed from the opposite centre, resulting in a reversal of the ventilatory phase.

- The inspiratory pool is located in the dorsal medullary reticular formation and is the source of basic ventilatory rhythm (i.e. it is the pacemaker for the respiratory system). The rhythmic activity persists even when all connections to these neurones are blocked. During inspiration, activity in the inspiratory pool leads to increased output to the muscles of inspiration, principally the diaphragm. At the same time, increasing inhibitory activity from the expiratory centre is relayed to the inspiratory neurones, until inspiratory activity ceases and expiration begins.
- The expiratory pool is found in the ventral medullary reticular formation. During inspiration, gradually increasing activity is relayed from the expiratory pool, inhibiting the inspiratory pool until expiration begins. At the same time, inhibitory activity is relayed to the expiratory neurones from the inspiratory pool, until expiration ceases and inspiration begins.

Pontine centres

- The pneumotaxic centre is a region in the upper pons which 'fine-tunes' ventilatory rate and V$_T$ to minimise respiratory work. It controls V$_T$ by switching off the inspiratory centre during the inspiratory phase, which limits V$_T$. This control of the inspiratory phase also varies the respiratory rate. Even in the absence of the pneumotaxic centre a basic ventilatory rhythm is maintained by the medullary inspiratory group.

- The apneustic centre is in the lower pons and is thought to prolong the inspiratory phase by acting on the medullary inspiratory pool of neurones. This also provides some control over the ventilatory rate and pattern. The section immediately above this centre gives rise to 'apneustic' breathing, with prolonged inspiration and brief expiratory efforts.

Respiratory control by higher centres

The cerebral cortex also affects breathing pattern, although precise neural pathways are not known. Voluntary hyperventilation and hypoventilation can be performed and maintained to the extent of producing changes in arterial blood gases. The limbic system and hypothalamus can also affect the respiratory pattern, as seen in emotional states.

Reflexes in the control of ventilation

The primary goal of ventilatory control is to maintain homeostasis of PaO_2 and $PaCO_2$. Various reflexes are integrated to produce the responses of the respiratory system to disturbances of arterial blood gases, or to the increased demands of exercise. Other reflexes protect the airway by coordinating breathing with eating, drinking or talking, and enabling coughing and sneezing. An example is the protective reflex that inhibits inspiration momentarily during swallowing, which is usually followed by a single large breath and a brief increase in ventilation. Similarly, it is advantageous to inhibit inspiration during vomiting, because of the risk of aspirating gastric contents.

Reflexes controlling ventilation are mediated by specialised receptors including:

- Central and peripheral chemoreceptors
- Chemical and pressure receptors in the airways
- 'J' receptors and stretch receptors in the lungs
- Golgi tendon organs and muscle spindles in the respiratory muscles

---

Chemoreceptors

- The central chemoreceptors are situated bilaterally 0.2 mm beneath the ventral surface of the medulla and are highly sensitive to changes in hydrogen ion concentration.
- The peripheral chemoreceptors are found in the carotid bodies located bilaterally at the bifurcation of the common carotid artery, and in the aortic bodies located along the arch of the aorta. The afferent nerve fibres of the carotid bodies pass through Hering's nerves to the glossopharyngeal nerves, and those of the aortic bodies pass through the vagi to the dorsal respiratory area. The chemoreceptors have a very high oxygen consumption and respond both to decreases in oxygen content of the arterial blood and to decreases in blood flow. They therefore act as oxygen delivery sensors to the brain, an organ which is particularly vulnerable to hypoxaemia, with limited ability to increase oxygen extraction.

The effect of CO_2 and hydrogen ion concentration on the peripheral receptors is much less than the direct effects of both these factors on the respiratory centre itself. However, the peripheral stimulation occurs as much as five times more rapidly than the central effect, so that peripheral receptors will increase the rapidity of the response to CO_2 at the onset of exercise.

Chemical and irritant receptors

These exist in the mucosa of the upper airways and trachea, and help protect the lungs from inhalation of injurious substances, such as gastric acid. These reflexes initiate laryngeal closure, apnoea, hyperpnoea and bronchoconstriction. Similar receptors respond to impending closure of the upper airway during inspiration by increasing pharyngeal dilator activity.

Pressure-sensitive receptors

These are located within the smooth muscle of all airways, and help to control the depth of respiration.

'J' receptors

'J' receptors are found in the alveolar walls close to the capillaries. Their stimulation causes rapid, shallow breathing or apnoea. They are thought to be involved in the tachypnoea observed in pulmonary oedema and irritation of the lungs.

Pulmonary stretch receptors

These are believed to lie in the smooth muscle of the airways. They inhibit inspiration in response to lung distension, and slow ventilatory rate by increasing expiratory time. This reflex was first reported by Hering and Breuer in 1868, who noted that lightly anaesthetised, spontaneously breathing animals would cease or decrease ventilatory effort during sustained lung distension. This response is abolished by bilateral vagotomy.

The Hering–Breuer reflex is only weakly present in humans, who can continue to breathe spontaneously with continuous positive airway pressures (CPAP) in excess of 40 cmH$_2$O. This reflex in humans is not activated until $V_T > 1.5$ L, and it is probably a protective mechanism for preventing excess ventilation, rather than an important component of the normal ventilatory control.

Golgi tendon organs

Golgi tendon organs are particularly plentiful in the intercostal muscles, and are also involved in the pulmonary stretch reflex. When the lungs are distended, the chest wall is stretched and these receptors send signals to the brainstem that inhibit further inspiration.

Muscle spindles

Muscle spindles in the inspiratory muscle and diaphragm contribute to control of depth and effort during inspiration. These receptors are thought to activate when particularly intense respiratory efforts are required, as in airway obstruction. They are also thought to be responsible for the sensation of dyspnoea.

Response of ventilation to carbon dioxide tension

Figure 17.25 shows the effect of PaCO$_2$ on alveolar ventilation. Increasing PaCO$_2$ from normal produces an increase in alveolar ventilation, which is effectively linear. Alveolar ventilation goes up by 1–2 litres per minute for each 0.1 kPa increase in PaCO$_2$. Decreasing CO$_2$ levels produce a fall in alveolar ventilation, but cease to have effect below a PaCO$_2$ of about 4 kPa. Various factors can displace this line to the left or right, and also alter its gradient. Some examples include:

- Sleep – reduces the gradient of the line and displaces it slightly to the right. These effects represent a decrease in the sensitivity of the ventilatory response to CO$_2$.

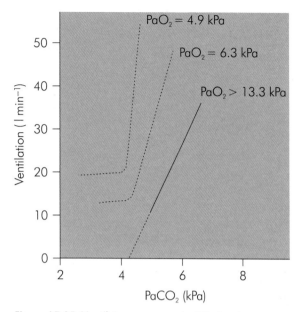

Figure 17.25 Ventilatory response to CO$_2$ tension

- Morphine – also reduces the gradient of the line and displaces it to the right, by central depression of the respiratory centres. Other opioid drugs and barbiturates have a similar effect.
- Work of breathing – increased work of breathing can reduce the response to CO$_2$. This does not appear to depress the respiratory centres, but reduces the peripheral response to central drive. This effect may be noted in some patients with bronchospasm, whose CO$_2$ response may increase with broncodilator therapy.
- Very high levels of CO$_2$ – thought to produce central depression and thus a reduction in CO$_2$ response curve gradient, followed by narcosis and respiratory depression.
- Age, genetics and race.

The effect of increased CO$_2$ levels on ventilation is mediated mainly by the central response to increased [H$^+$]. The central chemoreceptors attempt to maintain the PaCO$_2$ levels within normal range and increase alveolar ventilation. There is some additional response to increased PaCO$_2$ and [H$^+$] due to peripheral chemoreceptors, but the main effect is central.

The response to CO$_2$ is maximal over the first few hours and gradually declines to about only 20% of the

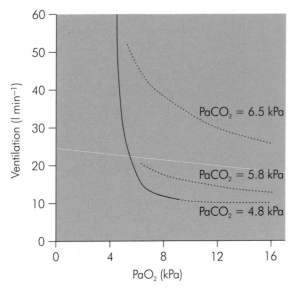

Figure 17.26 Ventilatory response to oxygen tension

Below this level an exponential increase in ventilation is produced as PaO_2 decreases further. Oxyhaemoglobin saturation and oxygen content start to decrease rapidly at this PaO_2. Thus, the peripheral chemoreceptors play a role in safeguarding cerebral oxygen delivery as well as monitoring PaO_2. At high altitude, hypoxaemia produces a marked increase in ventilatory drive.

Hypoxaemia has virtually no specific effect on central chemoreceptors but does produce a general depression of cerebral function. Periodic respiration (Cheyne–Stokes breathing) may be induced at moderate levels of hypoxaemia, but the mechanism is unknown.

Simultaneous changes in $PaCO_2$ have a marked effect on the ventilatory response to oxygen levels. Increases in $PaCO_2$ from normal exaggerate the ventilatory response to oxygen levels. Thus, when $PaCO_2$ levels are greater than normal, increasing hypoxaemia produces increased levels of ventilation. In the response to altitude, the hyperventilation due to hypoxaemia is initially blunted by the decrease in $PaCO_2$ produced. With acclimatisation, the $PaCO_2$ returns towards normal and the ventilatory response increases.

The hypoxic ventilatory drive becomes important in some patients suffering from chronic lung disease, who retain higher than normal levels of CO_2. If these patients compensate for their hypercarbia by retaining bicarbonate and producing a normal body pH, they become dependent on hypoxic ventilatory drive to maintain their breathing pattern. Caution is often advised in the administration of high F_IO_2 mixtures to such patients for fear of depressing their endogenous drive.

The hypoxic ventilatory drive is reduced or abolished by the same drugs and situations that impair hypercapnic ventilatory drive. The volatile anaesthetic agents are implicated even at subanaesthetic concentrations.

initial effect over the next 48 hours. This decline is due partly to the renal readjustment of [H^+] back toward normal by reabsorption of bicarbonate ions. More importantly, over a period of time bicarbonate ions slowly diffuse across the blood–brain and blood–CSF barrier, reducing the cerebral [H^+] back to normal.

Ventilation response to CO_2 level

- Increased levels of CO_2 in the body are associated with an increase in ventilation.
- This is mainly mediated by central chemoreceptors responding to [H^+].
- Peripheral chemoreceptor reflexes also contribute to ventilatory control by responding to $PaCO_2$ levels.

Response of ventilation to oxygen tension

The effect of PaO_2 on ventilation is shown in Figure 17.26. These curves are measured with $PaCO_2$ held constant (isocapnic responsiveness). It can be seen that increasing PaO_2 to supranormal levels produces virtually no effect on ventilation. Decreasing oxygen levels from normal also has little effect on ventilation, until PaO_2 is below about 8 kPa.

Ventilation response to O_2 level

Changes in oxygen levels mediate their effect on ventilation mainly through the peripheral chemoreceptors.

- Supranormal oxygen levels have little effect on ventilatory drive
- Subnormal oxygen levels also have little effect on ventilatory drive until the PaO_2 decreases to below 8 kPa.

Non-respiratory lung functions

Defence mechanisms

The lungs are continuously exposed to particulate matter and infectious material, which demands that they possess well-developed defence mechanisms. These include:

- Filtration – large particles are physically filtered out by the hairs and lining of the nasal passages.
- Sneeze and cough reflexes, which remove foreign bodies or particulate matter physically by the explosive airway pressure and air flow generated.
- Mucociliary clearance – smaller particles that are inhaled become impacted on a thin layer of mucus secreted by goblet cells. This is moved up and out of the respiratory tract by the rhythmic 'beating' of ciliated epithelial cells. The cilia may be paralysed by inhaled toxins or anaesthetic drugs.
- T and B lymphocytes – T cells produce pro-inflammatory peptides (interleukins, interferon γ, tumour necrosis factor) that cause multiplication of cytotoxic lymphocytes and recruitment of neutrophils. B lymphocytes secrete IgG and IgA in the airways. IgA promotes clearance of microorganisms, while IgG opsonises bacteria and fungi for phagocytosis.
- Macrophages and neutrophils, which engulf particles and microorganisms reaching the terminal airways and alveoli. Macrophages arise from blood monocytes and are capable of secreting a host of substances that are important for lung defence (Figure 17.27).

Blood filtration

The pulmonary vasculature acts as a filter in the circulation. Since the diameter of the pulmonary capillaries is about 8 μm, particles greater than this are filtered or slowed during their passage through the lungs.

The lung also filters out small clots, which are then dissolved by the fibrinolytic system. Pulmonary endothelium secretes a plasmin activator converting plasminogen to plasmin, which activates the fibrinolysis. The lung is also a rich source of endogenous heparin and produces a variety of thromboplastins, which play a role in the overall control of coagulation.

Larger clots may obstruct branches of the pulmonary arteries, producing an increase in pulmonary arterial pressure and tachypnoea. The rise in pulmonary artery pressure is due to reflex vasoconstriction via sympathetic nerve fibres. However, the pulmonary vascular bed has

Figure 17.27 Secretory products of alveolar macrophages

Type of secretion	Substance secreted
Enzymes	Elastase Plasminogen activator Acid hydrolases
Oxidative radicals	Hydrogen peroxide Superoxide anion Singlet oxygen
Complement components	
Enzyme inhibitors	α_1-antitrypsin
Platelet activating factor	
Leukotrienes	LTB_4, LTC_4, LTD_4, LTE_4
Interferon γ	
Cytokines	Interleukin 1 Tumour necrosis factor

an intrinsic ability to compensate for blocked vessels by opening new channels.

Metabolic functions of the lung

The lung is an important site for the metabolism of both endogenous and exogenous substances. Some of these metabolic functions are shown in Figure 17.28.

Abnormal metabolic responses of the lungs to drugs, infection or physical injury may lead to lung damage. Among these are:

- Lung injury due to bleomycin, cyclophosphamide and amiodarone. The mechanism suggested is the production of oxidative radicals or the impairment of antioxidant activity.
- Lung injury in acute respiratory distress syndrome is also thought to involve abnormal actions of oxidative radicals and elastases on lung tissue.

Lung function at high altitude

The most important environmental change at high altitude is the decrease in barometric pressure, because this gives a proportional reduction in inspired oxygen tension (P_IO_2).

Figure 17.28 Metabolic functions of the lung

Function	Substances
Extracellular metabolism by endothelium	Bradykinins Adenine nucleotides
Intracellular metabolism by endothelium	Noradrenaline, serotonin Prostaglandins E and F Atrial natriuretic peptide
Activation	Angiotensin I, enkephalin
Synthesis	Somatostatin, cholecystokinin Opioid peptide, substance P Prostaglandin E and F, prostacyclin Nitric oxide
Systemic release	Prostaglandins, histamine Kallikreins, eosinophil chemotactic factor of anaphylaxis, platelet activating factor
Production of surfactant	
Uptake and metabolism of anaesthetic agents	

Barometric pressure at an altitude of 5500 m is reduced to about half the value at sea level, i.e. about 50 kPa.

Inspired oxygen tension (P_IO_2) at high altitude

P_IO_2 at an altitude of 5500 m can be calculated by:
- Correcting for humidification, by subtracting saturated vapour pressure of water (about 6.3 kPa)
- Multiplying by the normal fractional oxygen concentration in air (about 0.21)

This gives $P_IO_2 = 9.2$ kPa instead of the normal value at sea level of about 20 kPa.

Alveolar oxygen tension (P_AO_2) is reduced from this inspired oxygen tension by saturated vapour pressure, gas exchange and hyperventilation, and may reach levels of 1 kPa.

Alveolar oxygen tension at high altitude

Applying the alveolar gas equation, the P_AO_2 at 5500 m can be estimated. The alveolar gas equation is given by:

$$P_AO_2 = P_IO_2 - \frac{P_ACO_2}{RQ}$$

Then for $P_IO_2 = 9.2$ kPa (see above), assuming a normal value for $P_ACO_2 = 5.3$ kPa and respiratory quotient (RQ) = 0.8:

$$P_AO_2 = 9.2 - 6.6 = 2.6 \, kPa$$

Thus, if P_ACO_2 levels remain normal at an altitude of 5500 m, the P_AO_2 would only be 2.6 kPa, which would result in a loss of consciousness in a few minutes. In practice, a marked hyperventilation response occurs at altitude, which increases P_AO_2.

Hyperventilation at altitude

Physiological changes occur at high altitude which enable survival. These changes are called acclimatisation.

Hyperventilation is one of the most important features of acclimatisation, and is produced by the low PaO_2, which causes a left and upward shift of the ventilation–$PaCO_2$ curve.

At high altitude alveolar ventilation can increase by four or five times to give alveolar ventilation rates greater than 20 litres per minute. This can reduce the P_ACO_2 to levels of about 1 kPa. In such a case the new P_AO_2 can be found by substituting this value in the above equation. Thus, at 5500 m

$$P_AO_2 = 9.2 - 1.2 = 8.0 \, kPa$$

Although this is less than the normal P_AO_2 at sea level (about 15 kPa), it is compatible with survival, particularly in combination with the other features of acclimatisation, which help to increase oxygen carriage to the tissues.

The hyperventilation response at high altitude is biphasic. Alveolar ventilation increases rapidly initially, over the first 2 hours or so, but then a slow steady rise is recorded over the following several days. The initial hyperventilatory phase is the result of a balance between hypoxic stimulation of chemoreceptors and inhibition due to reduced CO_2 levels and respiratory alkalosis. The second more gradual increase occurs because of renal elimination of bicarbonate, bicarbonate shift out of the cerebrospinal fluid compartment, and desensitisation of the chemoreceptors.

Acclimatisation

Acclimatisation describes the adaptive physiological changes that occur when a person moves from sea level to high altitude. There are physiological differences between people who live their whole lives at high altitude and those who live at sea level, which are referred to as 'adaptation'. The main changes occurring in acclimatisation are:

- Hyperventilation – an immediate and sustained response
- Polycythaemia – Hb levels reach 20 g dL^{-1} or more, increasing the oxygen content of blood to > 22 mL O_2 dL^{-1}
- Right shift of the oxyhaemoglobin dissociation curve – due to increased levels of 2,3-DPG
- Increased capillary density – in peripheral tissues, particularly muscle
- Increased mitochondrial density – and increased concentration of respiratory chain enzymes
- Increased pulmonary arterial pressures – due to hypoxic vasoconstriction
- Increased ventilatory capacity – aided by the decreased density of air. Maximum ventilation rates of 200 litres per minute or more may occur
- More even distribution of perfusion

Ventilation/perfusion matching at altitude

The distribution of perfusion is more even throughout the lung due to higher pulmonary arterial pressures and lower alveolar pressures. This has the effect of reducing the transmural pressure of the capillaries and postcapillary venules in perfusion zones 1 and 2. As described above, perfusion in these zones is dependent on the Starling resistor effect of these vessels, which is reduced by the changes at high altitude.

High-altitude disease

Additional physiological changes to those described in acclimatisation may develop. These include:

- Right ventricular hypertrophy
- Muscle atrophy and catabolism
- Antidiuresis and oedema formation
- Increased thyroid activity
- Sleep disturbance and periodic breathing
- Impaired central nervous system performance

These changes may develop into acute and chronic mountain sickness, pulmonary oedema and cerebral oedema.

References and further reading

Haefeli-Bleuer B, Weibel ER. Morphometry of the human pulmonary acinus. *Anat Rec* 1988; **220**: 401–14.

West JB. *Respiratory Physiology: the Essentials*. Philadelphia, PA: Lippincott Williams & Wilkins, 2008.

Lumb A. *Nunn's Applied Respiratory Physiology*, 7th edn. Edinburgh: Churchill Livingstone, 2012.

CHAPTER 18
Physiology of the nervous system

Peter Featherstone, Anand Sardesai and Arun Gupta

Structure and function of neurones

The main excitable cell in the nervous system is the neurone. Non-excitable cells or glial cells support neurones and perform various other functions (Figure 18.1). Neurones specialise in processing and transmitting information. The human nervous system contains between 10^{11} and 10^{12} neurones. Functionally, neurones are classified as sensory, motor and interneurone. Structurally, a typical neurone is made up of three parts: a cell body, an axon and terminal buttons (Figure 18.2). The cell body consists of intracellular organelles by which the cell maintains its functional and structural integrity. The axon

originates from the cell body and divides into terminal branches; each branch terminates in enlarged endings called terminal buttons. The axon is a long projection surrounded by supporting cells (oligodendrocytes or Schwann cells). When there is a layer of lipid–protein complex deposited within the Schwann cell membrane, the neurone is said to be myelinated, otherwise it is unmyelinated. Myelination allows saltatory conduction with an accompanying increase in speed of propagation of a nerve impulse. Mammalian neurones have varying fibre diameters and speeds of conduction, as summarised in Figure 18.3.

Fundamentals of Anaesthesia, 4th edition, ed. Ted Lin, Tim Smith and Colin Pinnock. Published by Cambridge University Press. © Cambridge University Press 2017.

The ionic basis of membrane potential

Membrane potential at rest

As in other excitable tissues in the body, the electrical potential of a neurone in the resting state is more negative on the inside of the cell than on the outside. This polarity is maintained by the active transport of Na^+ ions out of the cell, together with the active transport of K^+ ions into the cell. However, there is a tendency for both ions to diffuse passively down their concentration gradient through leaky ion channels. In its resting state, the membrane is more permeable to K^+ than to Na^+ ions, and therefore more K^+ ions leak out of the neurone than Na^+

ions enter the cell. At the same time, the resting membrane is impermeable to anions. The result is that the interior of the neurone is more electronegative (–70 mV) than the outside. This is the resting membrane potential.

Resting membrane potential

- The resting membrane potential in a neurone is –70 mV, the inside of the membrane being negative with respect to the outside.
- This is due to the K^+ permeability in the resting neurone membrane being greater than Na^+ permeability.

Figure 18.1 Functions of different cells in the nervous system

Cell	Function
Neurones	Generation, transmission and processing of potentials
Astrocytes	Support neurones and contribute to blood–brain barrier
Oligodendrocytes	Insulate neurones in the CNS
Microglial cells	Mediate immune responses in the CNS
Ependymal cells	Line ventricles and spinal cord
Schwann cells	Insulate axons in the PNS

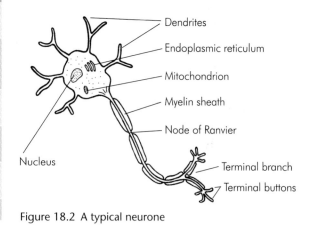

Figure 18.2 A typical neurone

Figure 18.3 Classification of mammalian neurones

Fibre type	Function	Fibre diameter (mm)	Conduction speed (ms^{-1})
Aα	Proprioception, somatic motor	12–20	70–120
Aβ	Touch, pressure	2–12	30–70
Aγ	Muscle spindle motor	3–6	15–30
Aδ	Pain, temperature, touch	2–5	12–30
B	Preganglionic ANS	< 3	3–15
C dorsal root	Pain, temperature, mechanoreceptors, reflex responses	0.4–1.2	0.5–2
C sympathetic	Postganglionic ANS	0.3–1.3	0.7–2.2

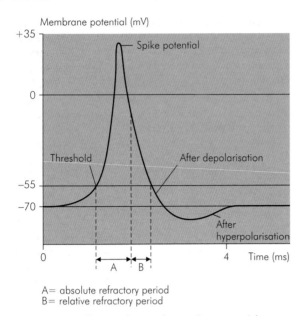

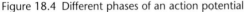

A= absolute refractory period
B= relative refractory period

Figure 18.4 Different phases of an action potential

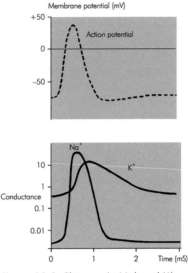

Figure 18.5 Changes in Na$^+$ and K$^+$ conductance during the course of an action potential

Characteristics of the action potential

Neurones respond to a stimulus by transiently producing changes in ion permeability or conductance in the cell membrane. Ion conductance is defined as the reciprocal of electrical resistance of the membrane to a given ion, and it therefore reflects permeability. When the stimulus is below the threshold potential, the changes produced remain localised. However, when the stimulus reaches the threshold, the membrane becomes depolarised. When this depolarisation is propagated along the axon, it gives rise to an action potential. The latter can be divided into a number of phases (Figure 18.4).

At the beginning of an action potential, the rate of depolarisation increases so that the inside of the cell becomes increasingly positive until it rises to a peak, then falls when repolarisation begins. This sharp rise and decline is called the spike potential, and it is due to an increase in Na$^+$ conductance, so that Na$^+$ ions diffuse down their electrical and concentration gradients.

However, there are three factors which limit the depolarisation process:

- The Na$^+$ channels open only very transiently.
- As the inside of the cell becomes increasingly more electropositive, the initial gradients which facilitate Na$^+$ influx disappear.
- K$^+$ conductance also increases. The rate of repolarisation slows down when the process is about 70% complete; this phase is known as after-depolarisation.

During the final recovery phase, there is a slight but prolonged overshoot after the resting potential is reached. This is due to the slow return of K$^+$ conductance to normal (Figure 18.5). This phase is called the after-hyperpolarisation.

A neurone is said to be in the absolute refractory period when it is totally unresponsive to any stimulus regardless of its strength. This corresponds to the period between the threshold being reached and when repolarisation is one-third completed. The relative refractory period starts at this point until the beginning of after-depolarisation. During this period, a stronger than normal stimulus may lead to excitation.

Action potentials (AP)

- APs are produced by transient changes of ion permeability in the neurone cell membrane.
- An AP is initiated by a marked increase in Na$^+$ permeability.

Synaptic transmission

Nerve impulses are transmitted from one neurone to another through junctions known as synapses. Synapses are formed between the terminal buttons of a neurone and the cell body or axon of another neurone. The number of terminal buttons forming synapses with a neurone varies from one to several thousand. Synapses almost invariably allow unidirectional impulse conduction, i.e. from the presynaptic to the postsynaptic neurone. This ensures nerve impulses are transmitted in an orderly fashion. Most synaptic transmissions are chemical in nature; others are either electrical or mixed. In electrical synapses, the membranes between the presynaptic and postsynaptic neurones meet to form gap junctions, which contain channels that facilitate diffusion of ions.

Structure of a synapse

Chemical synapses consist of a small gap known as a synaptic cleft. The synaptic cleft measures about 20 nm in width and contains extracellular fluid across which the neurotransmitters diffuse. There are three essential structures that can be found in the cytoplasm of the terminal button: synaptic vesicles, mitochondria and endoplasmic reticulum (Figure 18.6). The synaptic vesicles, containing the neurotransmitters, are usually found in large concentrations in the release zone adjacent to the synaptic cleft. The endoplasmic reticulum is responsible for the production of new vesicles, and recycling the used ones. Mitochondria provide the energy required for chemical transmission and the formation of synaptic vesicles by the endoplasmic reticulum.

Synaptic mechanism

When an action potential is transmitted down an axon, the depolarisation opens the voltage-gated calcium channels, allowing an influx of Ca^{2+} ions into the terminal button. In the release zone the Ca^{2+} ions bind with groups of protein molecules in synaptic vesicle membranes. These protein molecules spread apart, allowing fusion between vesicle and terminal button membranes. This releases neurotransmitter into the synaptic cleft. The amount of neurotransmitter released is directly proportional to the Ca^{2+} influx. The postsynaptic receptors are activated by the binding of neurotransmitters, which leads to the opening of ion channels, resulting in postsynaptic potentials.

Postsynaptic potentials are transient in action because of three mechanisms. The first is transmitter reuptake; this is the predominant mechanism, and is performed by the presynaptic terminal buttons, which rapidly and actively take up neurotransmitters at the end of transmission. The second mechanism is enzymatic deactivation by enzymes in the synaptic cleft. Finally autoreceptors on the presynaptic membrane inhibit the continued release of neurotransmitter. Figure 18.7 summarises the different types of neurotransmitter found in the central nervous system (CNS).

The events following the generation of postsynaptic potentials depend mainly on two conditions: first, the amount of neurotransmitter released, and, second, the type of ion channel that is being opened. Not all postsynaptic potential changes are propagated as action potentials in the postsynaptic neurone. When an insufficient amount of neurotransmitter becomes bound to the postsynaptic receptor, the change in membrane potential may not reach the firing threshold of the neurone, thus giving rise only to local potential changes. When sodium channels are open, there is a sudden influx of Na^+ ions down its concentration and electrical gradients, producing an excitatory postsynaptic potential (EPSP). However, when K^+ or Cl^- channels are open, K^+ and Cl^- ions move down their concentration gradients, making the inside of the neurone more electronegative with respect to the outside of the neurone, i.e. hyperpolarised, resulting in an inhibitory postsynaptic potential (IPSP). When the postsynaptic potential reaches threshold an action potential occurs.

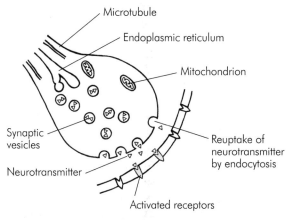

Synaptic vesicles · Microtubule · Endoplasmic reticulum · Mitochondrion · Reuptake of neurotransmitter by endocytosis · Neurotransmitter · Activated receptors

Figure 18.6 Structure of a chemical synapse

Synapses

- Synapses are junctions between the terminal buttons of one neurone and the body or axon of another.
- A neurone may have between one and several thousand synapses contacting it.
- Transmission across the synapse is unidirectional and is usually chemical but may be electrical.

Figure 18.7 Locations and functions of different types of neurotransmitter

Neurotransmitter	Location	Function
Acetylcholine	Cerebral cortex, thalamus, limbic system	Likely to be involved in memory, perception, cognition, attention and arousal functions
Noradrenaline	Locus coeruleus	Descending pain pathway
	Cerebellum	Inhibits Purkinje cells
	Hypothalamus	Regulates secretion of anterior pituitary hormones
Adrenaline	Medulla	Functions uncertain
Dopamine	Substantia nigra	Control of motor functions
	Hypothalamus	Regulates prolactin secretion
Serotonin	Neocortex and limbic system	Alters mood and behaviour
	Hypothalamus	Increases prolactin secretion
	Nucleus raphe magnus and spinal cord	Pain modulation

Sensory receptors

Sensory receptors are specialised structures that receive and transmit information from the external and internal environment to the CNS. A sensory receptor may be part of a neurone, such as nerve endings, or a separate structure that is capable of generating and transmitting action potentials to a neurone. They are essentially transducers that respond to different forms of energy, such as mechanical or thermal energy, and convert them into electrical signals. Special sense organs such as the eye are a collection of sensory receptors supported by highly organised structural and connective tissue.

Sensory receptors may be classified according to whether they perceive visceral or somatic sensory changes:

- Visceral receptors are primarily concerned with perceiving changes in the internal environment; such information does not usually reach consciousness. These include chemoreceptors which are sensitive to changes in glucose level, oxygen tension, osmolality and acidity in the plasma. Stretch receptors in the lungs and pressure receptors in the carotid sinus are other examples of visceral receptors.
- Somatic receptors are sensory receptors that respond to external stimuli such as temperature, light touch, and pressure. Pain is initiated by noxious or potentially damaging stimuli; pain receptors are, therefore, also known as nociceptors. Information from the somatic

receptors usually reaches consciousness and is represented at the cerebral level, giving rise to a variety of sensations. Sensory pathways are multisynaptic and thus involve a first-order neurone such as a dorsal root ganglion (DRG) which then synapses with a central chain of second-order and third-order neurones, as outlined in Figure 18.8.

Organisation of the nervous system

The nervous system is divided into two main parts: the central nervous system, consisting of the brain (cerebral cortex, basal ganglia, cerebellum, brainstem) and the spinal cord (Figure 18.9), and the peripheral nervous system, which includes the cranial and spinal nerves and their ganglia. The autonomic nervous system also forms an important part of the nervous system, and can be subdivided into the sympathetic and parasympathetic nervous systems.

Coverings of the central nervous system

A fibrous membrane, comprising three layers known collectively as the meninges, surrounds the entire CNS. Outermost is the **dura mater**, which covers the brain and is composed of two layers – an inner or meningeal layer of cerebral dura and an outer endosteal layer, which at the foramen magnum merges with

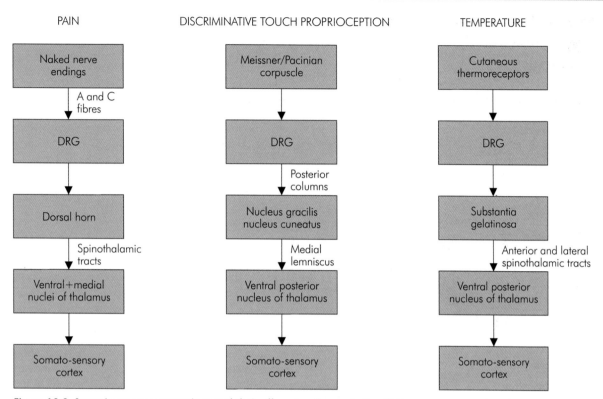

Figure 18.8 Somatic sensory perceptions and their afferent pathways to the CNS

the periosteum of the skull. The cerebral dura is represented in the vertebral canal by its periosteum, while the inner layer continues down to cover the spinal cord. The dural sac usually ends at the level of the second sacral vertebra in adults. Dura covering the spinal cord is attached to the edges of the vertebral canal except posteriorly, where it is completely free. The middle meningeal layer is called the **arachnoid mater** and closely lines the dural sheath. The innermost layer is known as the **pia mater** and is in contact with the neural tissues of the brain and the spinal cord. The trabeculated space between the arachnoid and pia mater contains cerebrospinal fluid (CSF).

Cortex

The cerebral cortex is topographically the highest level of the central nervous system, and always functions in association with the lower centres. The surface of the cerebral cortex is thrown into convolutions called gyri, which are separated by the sulci.

The cortex is divided into various lobes, namely frontal, temporal, parietal and occipital, which have different functions.

- The **frontal lobe** lies in front of the central sulcus and is divided into the precentral area and prefrontal cortex. The precentral area is further divided into anterior and posterior regions. The posterior region is referred to as the primary motor area or Brodmann's area 4, and the anterior region is known as the premotor area. The supplemental motor area is also situated in the frontal lobe. The rest of the frontal lobe, the prefrontal cortex, is divided into superior, middle and inferior frontal gyri. Broca's speech area is situated in the inferior frontal gyrus of the dominant hemisphere. The prefrontal cortex is concerned with personality, initiative and judgement. The frontal cortex controls motor function of the opposite side of the body, insight and control of emotions.
- The **temporal lobe** contains primary and secondary auditory areas. The ability to locate the source of sound

is impaired with the destruction of the primary auditory area. Bilateral destruction leads to complete deafness. The secondary auditory area is necessary for the interpretation of sounds. Wernicke's area, which is the sensory speech area, is located in the categorical (dominant) hemisphere and is associated with comprehension of speech.

- The **parietal lobe** houses the primary sensory area in the postcentral gyrus. The majority of sensations reach the cortex from the contralateral side of the body, although some signals from the oral region go to the same side, and those from the pharynx, larynx, and perineum go to both sides. A secondary sensory area is situated in the wall of the Sylvian fissure. Loss of the primary sensory cortex leads to inability to judge shape or form (astereognosis), degree of pressure or weight of an object. Problems occur with position sense and in localising different sensations occurring in different parts of the body. The secondary sensory area is involved in receiving information and relating it to past experience so that the information can be interpreted.

- The **occipital lobe** contains the primary visual area (area 17) close to the occipital pole. The macula lutea of the retina is represented on the cortex in the posterior part of area 17 and accounts for a third of the visual cortex. Lesions of the occipital pole produce central scotomas.

Higher functions of the cerebral cortex
Consciousness

There are different levels of consciousness, ranging from alertness to coma. The level of consciousness is determined by activities of both the cerebral cortex and the reticular activating system (RAS). The latter is a diffuse network of neurones situated in the brainstem reticular formation. It receives sensory information from ascending sensory tracts as well as auditory, visual, olfactory and trigeminal tracts. The reticular formation projects to the cerebral cortex directly and indirectly via the thalamic nuclei. RAS activity is closely related to the electrical activity of the cerebral cortex.

Electrical activity of the cerebral cortex can be recorded by scalp electrodes as an electroencephalogram (EEG). Various EEG rhythms can be identified (Figure 18.10).

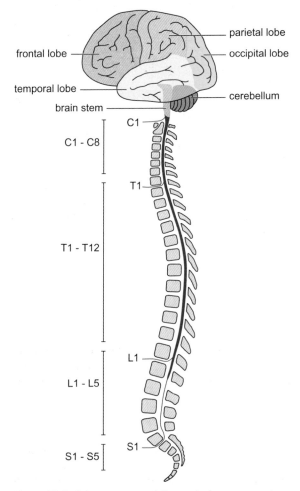

Figure 18.9 Gross anatomy of the central nervous system

Figure 18.10 EEG rhythms

α **rhythm**	Seen in an adult human at rest with eyes closed. It is more common in parieto-occipital areas and has a frequency of 8–12 Hz with an amplitude of 50–100 mV.
β **rhythm**	Lower-amplitude wave with a frequency of 18–30 Hz. It is seen over the frontal region in a normal alert adult.
θ **rhythm**	Large amplitude with a frequency of 4–7 Hz. It is normally seen in the very old and very young.
δ **rhythm**	Consists of large slow waves with a frequency of less than 4 Hz.

Two basic sleep patterns are seen: rapid eye movement sleep (REM) and non-rapid eye movement sleep (NREM). NREM has four stages. From stage 1 to 4 there is progressive slowing of the EEG with associated increase in EEG amplitude. Stage 1 sleep occurs at the beginning of sleep, while stage 4 sleep represents deep sleep. In stage 2 bursts of α-like rhythm known as sleep spindles are seen. In REM sleep the NREM pattern of EEG is replaced by fast low-voltage electrical activity similar to that seen in alert individuals. However, sleep is not disturbed and in fact the threshold for arousal is increased. This kind of sleep is associated with rapid eye movements, hence the name. In REM sleep, large phasic potentials are seen, there is a decrease in muscle tone, and it is also associated with dreaming.

Language

Wernicke's area in the categorical hemisphere receives auditory and visual information and is concerned with comprehension of this information. It communicates via the arcuate fasciculus with Broca's area, which is concerned with output of speech. It processes the information from Wernicke's area to produce appropriate movements of the vocal apparatus.

Memory

Memory is the process of retention and storage of acquired information, and can be divided into **explicit** and **implicit** memory.

- Explicit memory involves hippocampus and medial temporal lobes of the brain. It requires conscious retrieval or awareness and can be further divided into **episodic** memory (memory of events) and **semantic** memory, which is memory of words, rules, language and the world around us.
- Implicit memory does not require conscious awareness and is not processed in the hippocampus. It is associated with skills required for day-to-day activities and habits. When learning certain tasks, such as driving or cycling, explicit memory is used, but once the tasks are well learned then implicit memory is used to perform them.

Both forms of memory can also be divided into **short-term** and **long-term** memory. Information is processed in the hippocampus as a short-term memory, and then stored as a long-term memory, which lasts for years. Short-term memory lasts from a few seconds to hours, and is easily affected by drugs and trauma.

It is thought that short-term memory is a transient store of limited capacity which permits instantaneous encoding and retrieval, but when the material is no longer the focus of conscious attention, only some of this material may pass on to long-term memory. The latter represents a long-term storage of indefinite capacity that requires effortful encoding and retrieval. The more elaborate and effortful the encoding process, the better the memory of the material.

At the cellular level, it is thought that information is stored in the short-term memory as reverberating electrical activity in the brain, whereas long-term memory is stored in a more robust form. It is thought that memory formation may lead to an alteration in the transmission of electrical signals through parts of the brain. However, it is not clear whether this is the result of facilitation of existing synapses or due to the formation of new synapses. In both situations, however, protein synthesis is thought to be ultimately involved in the formation of long-term memory, and this is brought about through either structural or enzymatic changes in the neurones. The hippocampus is primarily involved in memory storage, since pathological lesions in this area result in both anterograde and retrograde amnesia.

Higher cerebral function

- Conscious level depends on the activity levels of the reticular activating system (RAS) and the cortex.
- Sleep may either be associated with dreaming and rapid eye movement (REM), or non-rapid eye movement (NREM) sleep.
- Memory is associated with the hippocampus and temporal lobes. It may be explicit (conscious) or implicit (unconscious).

Basal ganglia

The basal ganglia consist of interconnected deep nuclei including the caudate, globus pallidum, substantia nigra and putamen. The basal ganglia are involved in control of posture and movement.

Cerebellum

The cerebellum consists of two cerebellar hemispheres and a central structure. In contrast to the cerebral hemispheres, the cerebellar hemispheres control the structures on the same side of the body. The central cerebral structures control gait and maintain balance, including when seated.

Brainstem

Included in the brainstem are the midbrain, pons and medulla. The brainstem contains the reticular formation, which maintains consciousness, and the nuclei of all the cranial nerves except I and II. It also has ascending and descending tracts from cerebral structures and spinal cord. The corticospinal tract (one of the main descending tracts) and the dorsal columns, which are the ascending tracts, cross over in the medulla. Thus a lesion in the brainstem can produce cranial nerve lesions on the same side but limb signs on the other side.

The brainstem contains control centres for respiration, cardiovascular homeostasis, gastrointestinal function, balance, equilibrium and eye movements. Irreversible brainstem lesions are therefore frequently incompatible with life without artificial support.

Cerebral circulation

The arterial blood supply to the brain is derived from the right and left internal carotid arteries (ICAs) and the vertebrobasilar system (Figure 18.11). Each ICA gives rise to a posterior communicating artery (PCoA) before dividing into an anterior cerebral artery (ACA) and middle cerebral artery (MCA). The basilar artery (formed by the fusion of the vertebral arteries) lies on the ventral surface of the brainstem before dividing to form the two posterior cerebral arteries (PCAs). The anastomoses between the internal carotid and vertebrobasilar systems form the circle of Willis.

Venous drainage occurs through a series of sinuses which lie between folds of dura mater and empty into the internal jugular vein.

Regulation of cerebral blood flow

The brain has the highest metabolic requirement of any organ, accounting for 20% of basal oxygen consumption (50 mL min^{-1}) and 25% of total body glucose consumption. Cerebral blood flow (CBF) is approximately 700 mL min^{-1} (14% of cardiac output) in the resting adult. While this equates to a mean blood flow of approximately 50 mL per 100 g tissue per minute, flow is variable, with grey matter (110 mL 100 g^{-1} tissue min^{-1}) receiving on average five times that of white matter (22 mL 100 g^{-1} tissue min^{-1}). The pressure required to maintain CBF is the cerebral perfusion pressure (CPP).

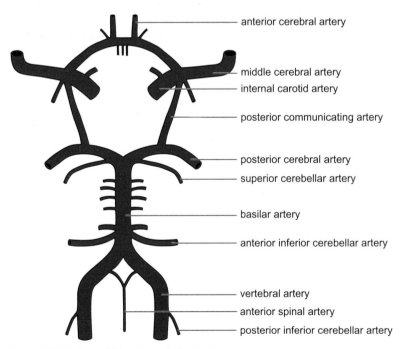

anterior cerebral artery

middle cerebral artery
internal carotid artery

posterior communicating artery

posterior cerebral artery
superior cerebellar artery

basilar artery

anterior inferior cerebellar artery

vertebral artery
anterior spinal artery
posterior inferior cerebellar artery

Figure 18.11 Arterial blood supply to the brain

Cerebral perfusion pressure (CPP)

CPP = Mean arterial pressure (MAP)
  − Intracranial pressure (ICP)
  − Venous pressure (VP)

CBF is usually tightly regulated to ensure constant delivery of glucose and oxygen to the brain. Four major factors control CBF:

- Pressure autoregulation
- Flow–metabolism coupling
- PaO_2
- $PaCO_2$

Pressure autoregulation

Autoregulation is the process by which the cerebral circulation maintains a constant blood flow despite alterations in CPP.

Cerebral blood flow autoregulation

When cerebral perfusion pressure (CPP) varies, autoregulation maintains cerebral blood flow (CBF) by changes in cerebrovascular resistance (CVR). This is mediated by the myogenic response to changes in intramural pressure, since:

CBF = CPP/CVR

As shown in Figure 18.12, as MAP (or CPP) increases the cerebral vasculature constricts to maintain CBF. Conversely as MAP (or CPP) decreases cerebral vasodilatation occurs and CBF is maintained. Cerebral blood volume increases but vascular resistance decreases with vasodilatation. Classically, CBF remains relatively constant in healthy adults between CPP values of 50 and 150 mmHg. Chronic hypertension shifts the autoregulatory curve to the right. The presence of intracranial pathology and a number of drugs utilised in anaesthetic practice may impair autoregulation. For example, volatile anaesthetic agents cause dose-dependent vasodilatation of the cerebral vasculature and hence impair autoregulation. Hypocapnia is thought to augment autoregulation by increasing vascular tone.

Flow–metabolism coupling

The precise mechanism of flow–metabolism coupling remains unknown, although acetylcholine, nitric oxide, serotonin and substance P have been described as mediators of the process. Pyrexia and convulsions increase metabolic activity, which causes a global increase in cerebral metabolic rate (CMR) and therefore a rise in CBF. Conversely anaesthetic drugs (specifically propofol, thiopental, etomidate and benzodiazepines) reduce electrical activity of the brain, thereby reducing metabolism and CBF. Hypothermia further reduces the energy required to maintain cellular homeostasis, resulting in a reduction in CMR and hence CBF.

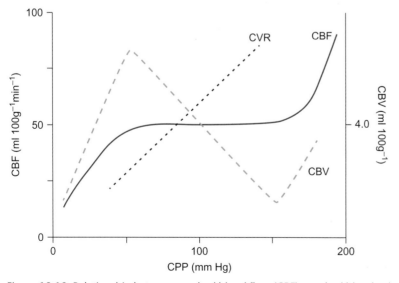

Figure 18.12 Relationship between cerebral blood flow (CBF), cerebral blood volume (CBV) and cerebrovascular resistance (CVR) over a range of perfusion pressures

> ### Flow–metabolism coupling
>
> Increased neuronal activity causes an increase in cerebral metabolic rate (CMR) and a compensatory increase in CBF to meet oxygen demand – a process known as flow–metabolism coupling.

Arterial blood gases

Carbon dioxide tension Carbon dioxide is a potent vasodilator. Within the physiological range there is an approximately linear relationship between $PaCO_2$ and CBF (Figure 18.13). Outside the normal range a 1 kPa rise in $PaCO_2$ increases CBF by approximately 30%. These changes are believed to be driven by changes in the extracellular or interstitial H^+ ion concentration. However, after 6–8 hours, the CBF returns to baseline values because CSF pH gradually normalises as a result of the extrusion of bicarbonate. Above a $PaCO_2$ of 10 kPa there is no further increase in CBF due to maximal vasodilatation. Below 2.5 kPa there is no further vasoconstriction.

Arterial oxygen tension While it is widely believed that there is little alteration in CBF in response to changes in arterial oxygen tension within the normal physiological range, and blood flow remains relatively constant until PaO_2 falls below 6.7 kPa (50 mmHg) (Figure 18.13), studies in human volunteers have demonstrated the onset of hypoxic vasodilatation once arterial saturations fall below 92%.

> ### Arterial blood gases and cerebral blood flow (CBF)
>
> - Increasing $PaCO_2$ causes cerebral vasodilatation. Within the physiological range there is an approximately linear relationship between $PaCO_2$ and CBF.
> - Decreasing PaO_2 does not alter CBF until arterial saturations fall below 92%, when hypoxic vasodilatation occurs.

Neurogenic regulation

The autonomic nervous system mainly affects the larger cerebral vessels. β_1-Adrenergic stimulation results in vasodilatation whereas α_2-adrenergic stimulation causes vasoconstriction. Significant vasoconstriction can be produced by extremely high concentration of catecholamines.

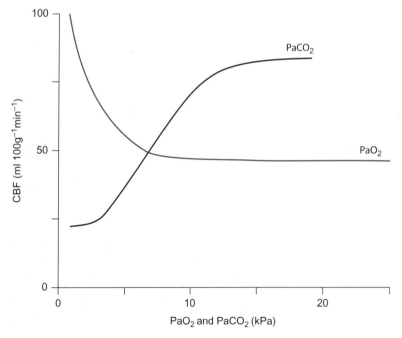

Figure 18.13 Effect of arterial blood gas tensions on cerebral blood flow

Spinal cord

The spinal cord extends from the lower part of the medulla. At birth it ends at the lower border of the third lumbar vertebra, and in the adult between the first and second lumbar vertebral bodies. The spinal cord is an elongated cylinder with cervical and lumbar enlargements corresponding to the origins of the brachial and lumbosacral plexuses. The spinal cord tapers into the conus medullaris. Owing to the arrangement of the meninges around the spinal cord, the following compartments are formed:

- **Subarachnoid space.** This contains the cerebrospinal fluid, and is traversed by three incomplete trabeculae – a single posterior subarachnoid septum and the ligamentum denticulatum on either side.
- **Subdural space.** This is a potential space only between the arachnoid and the dura mater, and contains a thin film of serous fluid.
- **Extradural space.** A space between the dura and the spinal canal which extends from the foramen magnum downwards as the dura covering the spinal cord fuses with the edges of the foramen magnum. It ends at the sacral hiatus and contains fat, lymphatics, arteries, and veins which are valveless and form the venous plexus of Bateson communicating between the pelvic veins and cerebral veins.

Anterior and posterior spinal roots emerge at the lateral surface of the spinal cord and are covered by the pia and arachnoid mater. They then pierce the dura mater and are subsequently covered by the dura, which fuses with the epineurium of the spinal nerve. Spinal nerves then travel through the epidural space and come out through the intervertebral foramen into the paravertebral space. Paravertebral spaces on either side of the vertebral column are in communication with each other through the epidural space.

Structure of the spinal cord

The spinal cord has an anterior median fissure and a posterior median sulcus which extends as a posterior median septum into the spinal cord. Posterior roots emerge along the posterolateral sulci, which are on either side of the posterior median sulcus. Anterior roots emerge as a series of nerve tufts at the front of the cord.

The spinal cord has a central canal, which is the continuation of the fourth ventricle and contains the CSF. An H-shaped zone of grey matter, which contains nerve cells,

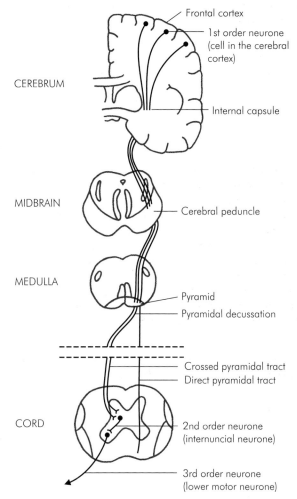

Figure 18.14 Descending tracts of the spinal cord

surrounds the central canal. It has an outer zone of white matter, which contains myelinated nerve cells and forms ascending and descending tracts (Figures 18.14 and 18.15).

Descending tracts

Descending pathways, which start in the cerebral cortex, are usually made of three neurones (Figure 18.14). The first-order neurone lies in the cells of the cerebral cortex. The axons of these cells synapse on the second-order neurone situated in the anterior grey column of the spinal cord. The second-order neurone is known as the internuncial neurone, the axon of which is shorter than the axon of the first-order neurone. It synapses with the

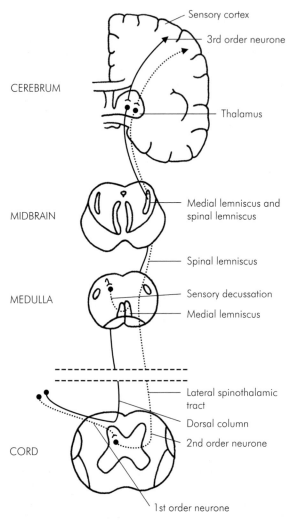

CEREBRUM

Sensory cortex

3rd order neurone

Thalamus

MIDBRAIN

Medial lemniscus and spinal lemniscus

Spinal lemniscus

MEDULLA

Sensory decussation

Medial lemniscus

Lateral spinothalamic tract

Dorsal column

2nd order neurone

CORD

1st order neurone

Figure 18.15 Ascending tracts of the spinal cord

third-order neurone, known as the lower motor neurone. The lower motor neurone also lies in the anterior grey column of the spinal cord. The axon of this lower motor neurone innervates the skeletal muscle through the anterior root and the spinal nerve. Figure 18.16 gives examples of descending tracts.

Ascending tracts

Like the descending tracts, ascending tracts have three neurones (Figure 18.15). The first-order neurone lies in the posterior root ganglia. The peripheral process of this neurone receives the sensory information from the sensory receptor. The central process of this neurone enters the spinal cord via the posterior root and synapses with the second-order neurone. The axon of the second-order neurone crosses the midline and synapses with the third-order neurone in the thalamus. The third-order neurone projects to the sensory cortex. Figure 18.17 details important ascending tracts.

Spinal cord transection
Complete transection

In humans, cord transection is followed by a variable period of spinal shock. In this period all spinal reflexes are profoundly depressed or absent. All muscles innervated by spinal nerves below the level of the cord lesion become paralysed. The initial phase of spinal shock is followed by recovery of reflex function, but the voluntary control is lost forever. The time of reflex recovery is variable, and can be delayed for up to 6 weeks, although the most frequent interval is about 2 weeks from initial injury. The first reflexes to return are flexor responses to touch and anogenital reflex responses. Reflex responses are hyperactive in the early recovery phase. Tendon reflexes are the slowest to recover. Hyperactivity of tendon reflexes can be accompanied by clonus. In paraplegic patients over time, a mass reflex response develops. This can occur even after a minor noxious stimulus is applied to the skin. This results in evacuation of bladder and bowel, along with signs of autonomic hyperactivity such as sweating, pallor and swings in blood pressure. In complete transection there is total loss of sensation in the dermatomes supplied by the cord below the level of injury.

Hemisection of the spinal cord (Brown-Séquard syndrome)

This affects the pyramidal tracts and posterior columns of the ipsilateral side, while the spinothalamic tracts which have crossed over from the opposite side are also affected. Thus there is paralysis of muscles on the same side along with loss of touch, pressure, joint and vibration sense. The pain and temperature fibres coming from the opposite side are also affected.

Blood supply of the spinal cord

> Blood supply of the spinal cord arises from a single anterior spinal artery and two small posterior spinal arteries.

Figure 18.16 Detail of descending tracts of the spinal cord

Tract	Detail
Corticospinal tract (pyramidal tract)	First-order neurones originate in the pyramidal cells of the motor cortex. Axons descend, enter the medulla and group to form the pyramid. At the junction of medulla and cord 80% decussate to form the lateral corticospinal tract, the remainder continuing as the anterior corticospinal tract. The axons synapse in the anterior grey column with internuncial neurones, which in turn synapse with lower motor neurones that innervate skeletal muscle.
Reticulospinal tract	Originates in the reticular formation, pons and medulla. Fibres synapse in the anterior grey column and influence α and γ motor neurones. The reticulospinal tract also carries descending autonomic fibres.
Tectospinal tract	Arises in the superior colliculus of the midbrain. Axons decussate and end in the anterior grey column in the cervical cord. Mediates reflex postural movement secondary to visual stimuli.
Rubrospinal tract	Originates in the red nucleus of the midbrain and decussates. Affects α and γ motor neurones in the anterior grey columns of the cord to facilitate flexor groups of muscles and inhibit extensors.
Vestibulospinal tract	Associated with posture and balance, having a facilitation of extensor muscle groups and inhibition of flexors.
Olivospinal tract	Originates in the olivary nucleus in the pons.
Descending autonomic fibres	Minor significance only.

Figure 18.17 Detail of ascending tracts of the spinal cord

Tract	Detail
Spinothalamic tract	Originates from free nerve endings in the skin carrying pain and temperature sensation. First-order neurones are Aδ and C fibres which enter the cord and synapse with second-order neurones in the posterior grey columns. Second-order neurones cross to the opposite side within one segment and ascend as the lateral spinothalamic tract. Fibres synapse with third-order neurones in the ventral posterolateral nucleus of the thalamus. Termination is the sensory area of the postcentral gyrus.
Gracile and cuneate tracts	Fibres from receptors for touch, vibration and joint proprioceptors enter the cord via the posterior root ganglia and travel in the posterior white columns of the ipsilateral side. Descending branches affect intersegmental reflexes. Ascending fibres synapse with cells in the posterior grey horn, internuncial neurones and anterior horn cells before travelling up as the gracile and cuneate tracts. Fibres synapse with second-order neurones in the gracile and cuneate nuclei of the medulla, which then decussate to travel as the medial lemniscus. The third-order neurones lie in the ventral posterolateral nucleus of the thalamus and terminate in the postcentral gyrus of the sensory cortex.
Anterior and posterior spinocerebellar tracts	Relay information from muscle and joints to the cerebellum.
Spinotectal tract	Transmits pain, temperature and touch sensation to the superior colliculus of the midbrain. Facilitates spinovisual reflexes.
Spinoreticular tract	Relays various information to the reticular formation. Affects consciousness.
Spino-olivary tract	Minor afferent path to cerebellum.

The anterior spinal artery is formed by the union of a branch from each vertebral artery and runs along the midline of the cord, supplying the anterior two-thirds of the spinal cord. Thrombosis of this artery can cause anterior spinal artery syndrome, in which there is paralysis due to ischaemia of the pyramidal tract, although there is sparing of the posterior columns so that sensation conveyed by these columns remains intact.

The two smaller posterior spinal arteries lie on each side of the cord posteriorly. They are derived from posterior inferior cerebellar arteries and supply the posterior third of the spinal cord. Blood vessels known as vasa coronae communicate between the anterior and posterior spinal arteries. Various radicular arteries (which arise from deep cervical, intercostal and lumbar arteries) supply the anterior and posterior spinal arteries along the spinal canal. The arteria radicularis magna (major anterior radicular artery) is the principal arterial blood supply of the lower two-thirds of the spinal cord (usually found between T11 and L3). In case of occlusion of the anterior spinal artery the blood supply of the lower two-thirds of the spinal cord may be compromised.

Anterior and posterior spinal arteries do not anastomose with each other except within the spinal cord itself.

The reflex arc

Stimulation of the reflex arc by a specific sensory stimulus produces a repetitive, specific response. The reflex arc begins with a sense organ (e.g. muscle spindle), which transmits information via the afferent neurone to the spinal cord, entering via the dorsal root or cranial nerve. The ganglia of these neurones act as a central

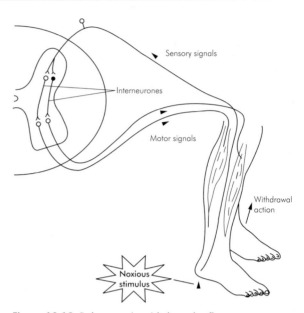

Figure 18.19 Polysynaptic withdrawal reflex

coordinating station. The efferent nerve leaves the central station via the ventral roots or a motor cranial nerve and innervates an effector organ such as a voluntary muscle. The activity in this reflex arc is influenced by the central nervous system.

The reflex arc can be monosynaptic, with a single synapse between the afferent and efferent neurone (Figure 18.18), or polysynaptic, where two or more synapses occur between afferent and efferent neurones (Figure 18.19).

Monosynaptic stretch reflex

The stretch reflex is an example of a monosynaptic reflex. The sense organ for this reflex is the muscle spindle. Skeletal muscle consists of two types of muscle fibres, namely the extrafusal and intrafusal fibres. Contraction of the extrafusal fibres is controlled by motor neurones located in the anterior horn of the spinal cord. These contractions result in contraction of a muscle. The number of muscle fibres controlled by a single motor neurone varies according to the precision of the movement involved. The finer the movement the smaller the number of extrafusal fibres: in the case of muscles controlling finger movement a neurone controls fewer than 10 fibres, whereas for lower limb muscle there may be several hundred extrafusal fibres per neurone.

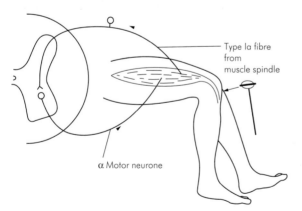

Figure 18.18 Monosynaptic stretch reflex

Polysynaptic withdrawal reflex

When a noxious stimulus is applied to a limb, the signal is first transmitted via sensory fibres to the interneurone(s) in the spinal cord and then on to the motor neurones (Figure 18.19). The neuronal circuitry involves not only activation of muscle(s), which carry out the withdrawal, but also the inhibition of the antagonist muscles. Other muscle groups may also be stimulated or inhibited so that the withdrawal of the limb and movement of the rest of the body are coordinated to move safely away from the noxious stimulus.

Monosynaptic and polysynaptic reflexes

- The stretch reflex is an example of a monosynaptic reflex.
- The withdrawal reflex is polysynaptic. Contraction of flexor muscles and relaxation of the extensors in response to a painful stimulus result in withdrawal of the stimulated part.

Structure of muscle spindles

The intrafusal fibres form specialised sensory organs called muscle spindles, which are arranged in parallel with the extrafusal fibres. These spindles respond to the change in length of surrounding extrafusal fibres and form part of the control system for maintaining posture and limb position. Each spindle consists of up to a dozen intrafusal fibres whose ends are attached to the extrafusal fibres. Each intrafusal fibre consists of two portions: the central non-contractile region and a contractile muscle fibre portion at either end. The efferent control of these contractile portions is supplied by the γ motor neurones. The central portion of the intrafusal fibres can take two forms, either a nuclear bag or a nuclear chain. The former consists of an expanded central portion containing a collection of nuclei whereas the latter consists of nuclei arranged in a chain. Two types of sensory nerve fibres innervate the central portion of the intrafusal fibres: type Ia (or annulospiral) and type II fibres. Type Ia fibres innervate both the nuclear bag fibres and nuclear chain fibres, but the type II fibres only innervate the nuclear chain fibres (Figure 18.20).

Function of muscle spindles

The central portion of the muscle spindle detects the change in length of the muscle. When the whole muscle contracts, the muscle spindle relaxes, and firing in its afferent axon stops. However, the opposite occurs when the muscle relaxes or is stretched passively. One of the most basic functions of the muscle spindle, therefore, is to maintain muscle length. Furthermore, the sensitivity of the muscle spindle is adjustable. When the muscle spindles are relaxed, they are relatively insensitive to stretch. However, when the motor neurones are active, they become shorter and much more sensitive to changes in muscle length. Therefore by establishing a rate of firing in the motor system, the higher centres control the length of the muscle spindles and, indirectly, the length of the entire muscle.

During normal movements, both the α and γ motor neurones are activated at the same time. If little resistance is encountered, both the extrafusal and intrafusal muscle fibres will contract at approximately the same rate, and as a result the central portion of the muscle spindle retains its original length before the contraction and little change in activity will be detected in the afferent axons of the

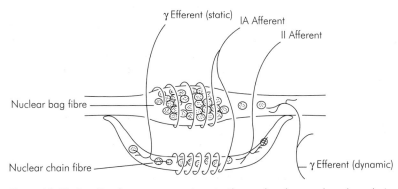

Figure 18.20 Details of nerve connections to the nuclear bag and nuclear chain muscle spindle fibres

spindle. If, however, the limb meets with resistance, the intrafusal muscle fibres will shorten more than the extrafusal muscle fibres, the centre of the muscle spindle becomes stretched, and the rate of firing in the afferent axons increases. This will stimulate the motor neurone and thereby increase contraction of the motor unit.

The inverse stretch reflex implies that the harder a muscle is stretched, the stronger is the reflex contraction. If the muscle tension increases excessively, the Golgi tendon organs, which are attached in series with the muscle, inhibit the activity of the motor neurone, providing an inhibitory feedback mechanism to prevent muscle damage. The relaxation in response to strong stretch is called the inverse stretch reflex.

Muscle spindles and Golgi tendon organs

- The muscle spindle acts as a muscle length detector. It should not be confused with the Golgi tendon organ, which is a stretch receptor within a tendon and responds to tension, not length.
- The muscle spindles and the Golgi tendon organs work hand in hand to make sure that length and tension in a muscle are appropriate to perform a particular task.

The resistance of a muscle to stretch is known as tone. When a motor nerve is cut, the muscle it supplies becomes flaccid. The muscle is hypotonic if the rate of efferent discharge is low and hypertonic when it is high. Another phenomenon seen in the hypertonic state is clonus. This occurs when a sustained and sudden force is applied to a muscle, resulting in regular rhythmic contractions of the stretched muscle.

Motor function

The structures involved in the control of movement are the cerebral cortex, cerebellum and basal ganglia.

Cerebral cortex

The motor cortex is situated in the frontal lobe. It is divided into three parts:

- The **primary motor cortex** is situated in the precentral gyrus. Different areas of the body are represented in the primary cortex. Parts of the body performing the finer functions have the largest representation. The facial area is represented bilaterally.

- The **premotor area** lies anterior to the primary motor cortex immediately superior to the Sylvian fissure. It is concerned with postural adjustment at the beginning of a voluntary movement.
- The **supplemental motor area** is concerned with the planning of complex movements.

Motor signals are transmitted directly from the cortex to the spinal cord through the corticospinal tract, and indirectly through multiple accessory pathways that involve the basal ganglia, the cerebellum, and the various nuclei of the brainstem.

Cerebellum

The cerebellum is situated in the posterior fossa and has two lateral lobes that are joined in the centre by the vermis. It is functionally divided into three parts:

- The **vestibulocerebellum** has connections with the vestibule of the middle ear and maintains the body's equilibrium during motion.
- The **spinocerebellum** is mainly concerned with proprioception. It receives information from the whole body as well as the motor cortex. Voluntary movements are coordinated here, depending on the sensory information received. The central portion of the cerebellum is concerned with axial and proximal limb muscles, while the lobes control the distal musculature.
- The **neocerebellum** is involved in planned execution of voluntary movements. Fast coordinated activity is affected in cerebellar disease. Dysdiadochokinesia (the inability to perform rapid alternating movements) is a feature of cerebellar dysfunction. Other signs of cerebellar dysfunction include ataxia, scanning speech and intention tremor.

Basal ganglia

The term basal ganglia refers to the following structures: caudate nucleus, putamen, globus pallidus, subthalamic nucleus and substantia nigra.

The caudate nucleus and putamen are together called the striatum. The basal ganglia form a loop with the cortex (Figure 18.21). The cortex projects to the striatum via the corticostriate projections, the striatum sends efferents to the globus pallidus, and this in turn sends efferents to the thalamus. The thalamus then communicates with the primary motor cortex via accessory motor areas.

Command for voluntary action originates in the cortical association area. It is further planned in the cortex, basal ganglia and lateral portion of the cerebellar cortex.

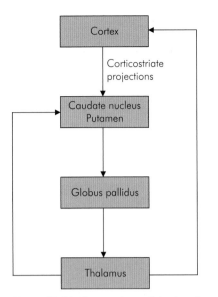

Figure 18.21 Connections of the basal ganglia

The efferents to muscle travel in the corticospinal tract (pyramidal system) and bring about the voluntary action. The cerebellum and basal ganglia both influence voluntary action. The cerebellum enhances the stretch reflex, fine-tuning of rapid movements preventing oscillations, and the basal ganglia help by carrying out various subconscious movements which are required to carry out a voluntary activity.

Control of posture
The maintenance and control of posture is essential for performing voluntary actions, which require smooth coordinated activity in different muscle groups. The postural reflexes involved are coordinated at the level of the spinal cord and are influenced by higher centres. When the influence of these higher centres is experimentally removed at different levels it is possible to understand the postural reflexes involved.

Spinal cord components
The stretch reflex contributes to posture control at the spinal level and has been described in detail earlier. Additionally, proprioceptors in opposing flexor and extensor muscles contribute to the maintenance of an upright stance. Placing a foot on the ground stiffens the leg so that the body can be supported. This is the positive supporting reaction. The disappearance of this is known as the negative supporting reaction.

Brainstem components
These components can be studied by transection of the brainstem at the superior border of the pons. This is known as decerebration, and it causes increased rigidity. In the brainstem there are areas that facilitate and inhibit stretch reflexes. After decerebration the influence of the inhibitory area is reduced while that of the facilitatory area is increased, resulting in increased efferent discharge. This facilitates the stretch reflex and causes rigidity. Spasticity produced by decerebration is most marked in the extensor group of muscles, as these are the antigravity muscles helping the animal to maintain its posture. In humans decerebrate rigidity causes extension in all four limbs.

The scale of rigidity of the limbs in a decerebrate animal is position-related. In the prone position the rigidity is minimal, while if the animal is on its back the rigidity is maximal. This is known as the tonic labyrinthine reflex. The receptors for this reflex are in the otolithic organs.

When the head of the decerebrate animal is turned to one side, the limbs on that side become more rigidly extended and the limbs on the opposite side become less rigid. Flexion of the neck causes flexion of the forelimbs and hindlimbs. The reverse happens with the extension of the head. This is known as the tonic neck reflex, and it is initiated by the stretch receptors in the neck.

Midbrain components
Midbrain components can be studied by interrupting the neural pathways at the superior border of the midbrain. In the midbrain animal, the phasic postural reflexes are intact so that the animal can stand, walk and correct its position. Rigidity is seen only when the animal is at rest, as it is due to static postural reflexes.

The righting reflexes, such as the labyrinthine righting reflex, body on head righting reflex, neck righting reflex, and body on body righting reflex, are essential for maintaining the normal position of the animal. These reflexes are coordinated by the nuclei in the midbrain.

Cortical components
Removal of the cerebral cortex is called decortication. In the decorticate animal there is loss of the cortical area that inhibits γ-efferent discharge. The increased (γ) efferent discharge causes facilitation of the stretch reflex, leading to rigidity. This is only seen at rest, due to the presence of phasic postural reflexes. Postural reactions like hopping and the placing reaction are seriously affected by decortication.

Control of posture

Posture-regulating mechanisms involve structures in the spinal cord, the brainstem and the cerebral cortex.

- Basic musculoskeletal reflexes are coordinated at the spinal level.
- Tonic reflexes related to head and neck position are mediated in the midbrain.
- Phasic postural reflexes are dependent on cortical input.

Cerebrospinal fluid (CSF)

Most (50–70%) of the CSF is produced in the choroid plexuses of the lateral, third and fourth ventricles, which are highly vascular invaginations of pia mater, covered by single-layered ependymal epithelium. It is formed by secretion and filtration of plasma. Formation of CSF is not affected by intracranial pressure, but removal of CSF increases with increasing pressure. CSF from the lateral ventricles drains into the third ventricle via the foramina of Monro. From the third ventricle it travels to the fourth ventricle via the aqueduct of Sylvius. It enters the cerebral subarachnoid space through the median foramen of Magendie and lateral foramina of Luschka. CSF is absorbed into the venous sinuses by the arachnoid villi. Arachnoid villi are projections of arachnoid into the venous sinuses which are covered by a single-layered endothelium of the venous sinuses. The composition and circulation of the CSF is covered in more detail in Chapter 11.

Larger-molecular-weight substances do not pass from blood into the CSF or the interstitial spaces of the brain due to the presence of 'tight junctions' between the endothelium of cerebral capillaries. This blood–brain barrier is highly permeable to water, carbon dioxide, oxygen and most lipid-soluble substances such as volatile anaesthetic agents. The barrier is impermeable to plasma proteins and large-molecular-weight substances.

Cerebrospinal fluid (CSF)

- CSF is present in the cerebral ventricles and the subarachnoid space.
- The total volume of CSF is about 150 mL.
- Approximately 550 mL of CSF is produced per day in an adult.

Intracranial pressure (ICP)

Intracranial pressure (ICP)

This is the pressure inside the cranial vault relative to atmospheric pressure. Normal intracranial pressure ranges between 5 and 15 mmHg, although this varies with arterial pulsation, breathing, coughing and straining.

Intracranial compartments

Intracranial contents can be divided into four compartments: solid material ($\approx$ 10%), tissue water ($\approx$ 75%), CSF (150 mL, $\approx$ 10%), blood (50–75 mL, $\approx$ 5%). These compartments are all contained within the rigid cranial vault.

The Monro–Kellie doctrine

A change in volume of one intracranial compartment is accompanied by a reciprocal change in another compartment

---

Factors affecting ICP

Raised ICP causes brain damage by reducing cerebral perfusion pressure or by focal compression of brain tissue due to distortion and herniation of intracranial contents. Control of ICP depends on compensatory mechanisms involving the four compartments described above.

The relationship between ICP and volume

This is illustrated in Figure 18.22. With an increase in intracranial volume, compensatory mechanisms maintain ICP within the normal range (between point 1 and point 2 on the figure). At point 2, further increases in volume cause a slight rise in ICP. As volume increases, there is a steady decline in compliance, which increases the ICP even more (point 3) until a small rise in volume is associated with a marked rise in ICP, causing a fall in the perfusion pressure and ultimately cerebral ischaemia (between points 3 and 4).

Cerebrospinal fluid (CSF)

The CSF plays a major part in compensating for an increase in intracranial volume. As a space-occupying lesion expands, it will cause progressive reduction of the CSF space (reduced size of the ventricles and basal cisterns). CSF outflow into the spinal canal increases, and its

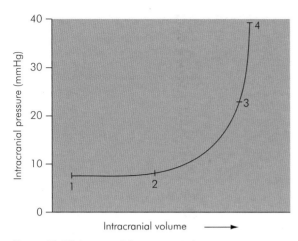

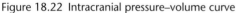

Figure 18.22 Intracranial pressure–volume curve

absorption into the venous system is also increased. Rapid rises in intracranial volume (e.g. acute intracranial haematoma) exhaust spatial compensation quickly, resulting in a rapid rise of ICP.

Cerebral blood volume

Another important compensatory mechanism is provided by changes in cerebral blood volume (CBV). Most of the intracranial blood volume is contained in venous sinuses and the pial veins, and only a small change in CBV can have a profound effect on ICP. A rise in ICP decreases cerebral perfusion pressure (CPP), which in turn causes vasodilatation to maintain a constant cerebral blood flow (CBF) (see Figure 18.12). This results in a rise in CBV and consequently a rise in ICP in a non-compliant or swollen brain. Conversely, a rise in mean arterial pressure will within autoregulatory limits cause cerebral vasoconstriction, resulting in a reduction in CBV and ICP.

Arterial blood gases

Arterial blood gas values also make a major contribution to CBF and CBV. Both CBF and CBV increase with raised $PaCO_2$, but the CBV response curve is flatter than the CBF curve. A reduction in $PaCO_2$ from 5.3 to 2.7 kPa results in a 65% reduction in CBF but only a 28% reduction in CBV. This small decrease in intracranial volume will cause a significant reduction in ICP in the presence of intracranial hypertension, because the system operates on the steep part of the pressure–volume curve. A reduction in arterial oxygen tension causes cerebral vasodilatation, resulting in a rise in CBV.

Cerebral metabolism

Increased metabolic demand increases CBF, CBV and ICP due to flow metabolism coupling. Reduction in cerebral metabolism (using intravenous anaesthetic agents, for example) will reduce CBV, and this is a useful therapeutic intervention in patients with raised ICP.

Control mechanisms in raised intracranial pressure

Auto-regulatory:

- Reduction in the volume of CSF spaces
- Reduction in cerebral blood volume (CBV)
- Cerebral vasoconstriction causing reduction of cerebral blood flow (CBF) and CBV
- Increase in arterial pressure (within auto-regulatory limits) causing cerebral vasoconstriction

Therapeutic:

- Reduction of cerebral metabolic rate
- Reduction in $PaCO_2$ causing cerebral vasoconstriction
- Maintenance of PaO_2 avoiding cerebral vasodilatation
- Avoiding raised jugular venous pressure

Jugular venous pressure

Venous distension is a common cause of increased cerebral venous volume and can occur from jugular venous obstruction, increased intrathoracic pressure, raised central venous pressure, head-down tilt etc. For details see Chapter 15.

Special senses
Vision
Structure of the eye

Before reaching the photoreceptors on the retina, light must pass through the optical apparatus that is made up of the cornea, aqueous humour, lens and vitreous humour (Figure 18.23). The globe is protected by the sclera, which becomes transparent in the anterior part of the eye known as the cornea. Aqueous humour is produced by the ciliary processes and catalysed by the action of carbonic anhydrase; it passes from the posterior chamber through the pupil into the anterior chamber of the eye. It is then drained into a vein via the canal of Schlemm (located at the angle of the anterior chamber).

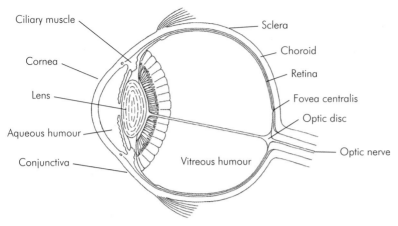

Figure 18.23 Structure of the eye

Pupillary size is determined by the activities of the smooth muscle fibres in the iris: the circular fibres constrict (miosis) while the radial fibres dilate (mydriasis) the pupil. The interior surface of the globe is lined by the retina, except where the optic nerve leaves the eye and where the ciliary muscle begins. The ciliary muscle changes the tension of the suspensory ligaments, which alters the convexity of the lens and thereby achieves accommodation.

The retina
The retina is made up of photoreceptors – rods and cones. These are located along the outer surface of the retina adjacent to the pigment epithelium. The blood supply of the photoreceptors is derived from the choroid and not from blood vessels on the inner retinal surface. There are about 120 million rods and only 7 million cones in each eye. Rods are uniformly distributed throughout the retina and are responsible for night and monochromatic vision. They contain the pigment rhodopsin. Cones, however, are concentrated in the fovea and are responsible for bright and colour vision. Cones contain opsins that are sensitive to red, green and blue.

The visual pathway
Electrical potential is generated when light reaches the photoreceptors on the retina. This potential is then transmitted to the ganglion cells via the bipolar and/or the horizontal and amacrine cells. Axons from the ganglion cells converge at the blind spot of the optic disc to form the optic nerve. The axons coming from the nasal half of the retina decussate at the optic chiasm, while those situated on the temporal half remain on the ipsilateral side (Figure 18.24). These then synapse in the lateral geniculate nuclei. From here, synaptic connections are made via the optic radiation to the primary visual cortex, giving rise to a topographical projection of the visual field around the calcarine fissure. Some fibres of the optic tracts relay to the superior colliculi, which are involved in the control of eye movements or posture. Lesions in the visual pathway will give visual field defects according to their position. Thus, as shown in Figure 18.24, the following lesions will give rise to their corresponding defects:

- Lesion 1 – right-eye blindness
- Lesion 2 – bitemporal hemianopia
- Lesion 3 – right homonymous hemianopia

Hearing
Structure of the ear
The ear is divided into external, middle and internal compartments. The external compartment consists of the pinna, which directs sound waves via the external auditory meatus to the tympanic membrane. Vibrations of the tympanic membrane transmit sound energy to the middle ear, which contains the three ossicles: malleus, incus and stapes. The last of these stimulates the inner ear through the oval window. The middle ear is air-filled and is connected to the pharynx via the Eustachian tube, which allows equilibration of pressure to occur between the middle ear and the environment. The inner ear consists of the cochlea, which is a bony coiled tube divided lengthwise into three canals by two membranes: the scala vestibuli and scala media (or cochlear duct) are separated by Reissner's membrane, while the scala media and scala tympani are separated by the basilar membrane

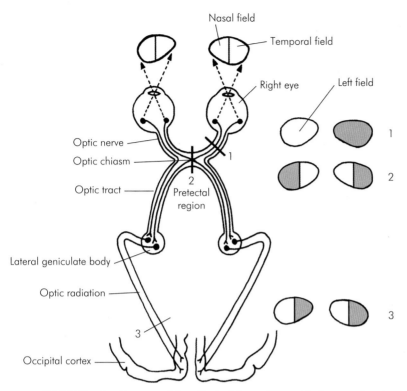

Figure 18.24 Visual pathway and the effect of three different lesions on the visual field

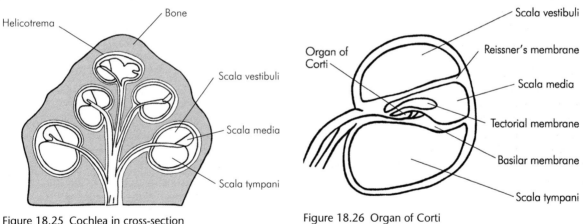

Figure 18.25 Cochlea in cross-section

Figure 18.26 Organ of Corti

(Figure 18.25). The scala tympani communicates with the middle ear via the round window.

The inner ear is fluid-filled: the scala media is filled with endolymph, while the scala vestibuli and tympani, being joined at the helicotrema, are filled with perilymph. The sound receptors are found in the organ of Corti

(Figure 18.26), which is located on the basilar membrane within the cochlear duct. The organ of Corti is made up of an epithelium of hair cells and supporting cells. Each hair cell is anchored on the basilar membrane and has a bundle of hairs projecting from its tip into the scala media. Directly opposite to these hair cells is the tectorial membrane.

The hair cells synapse with dendrites of the ganglion cells, which in turn synapse with fibres from the cochlear nerve. The latter traverses the subarachnoid space and enters the brainstem at the pontomedullary junction.

Mechanism of hearing

Sound waves produce vibrations of the tympanic membrane that lead to movements of the ossicles. Movements of the footplate of the stapes in the oval window are converted to pressure waves in the scala vestibuli. These pressure waves are then transmitted in the endolymphatic canal to reach the basilar membrane. Such oscillations cause displacements of the tectorial membrane with respect to the basilar membrane. The hair cells situated on the latter are thus stimulated and become depolarised. The resulting receptor potential is then transmitted via the underlying ganglion cells to the cochlear nerve. All the cochlear nerve fibres terminate at the cochlear nucleus in the brainstem. From here, second-order fibres project mainly to the contralateral (and to a lesser extent to the ipsilateral) inferior colliculus via the lateral lemniscus. From the inferior colliculus, connections are projected, via the medial geniculate body, to the primary auditory cortex in the temporal lobe.

Taste and olfaction

Taste

Taste buds are made up of specialised epithelial cells (taste cells) and supporting cells, which are located on the surface of the tongue, soft palate and oropharynx.

Most taste buds are found on protuberances called papillae at the back of the tongue. Taste cells have a half-life of about 2 weeks and are constantly being replenished by division of the underlying basal cells. There are four basic tastes: sweet, sour, salty and bitter. All complex tastes are thought to be composed of different combinations of the basic tastes. Nearly all tastes are the combined result of taste and smell. The transduction process of taste is poorly understood: it is thought that chemicals in food interact with chemoreceptors on the surface membrane of taste cells to induce a change in membrane permeability to Na^+ ions. This leads to depolarisation of taste cells, which then leads to the production of generator potentials in the afferent nerve fibres. Taste buds are innervated by the chorda tympani (anterior two-thirds of the tongue), glossopharyngeal (posterior third of the tongue), vagus (epiglottis), and greater petrosal (soft palate) nerves. These then relay in the tractus solitarius in the medulla before projecting to the thalamus and cortex.

Olfaction

Olfactory cells are specialised bipolar neurones found in the olfactory epithelium in the roof of the nasal cavity. The olfactory epithelium also contains basal and supporting cells. Olfactory cells are the only neurones in the body known to be replaced continually by division of the underlying basal cells. Situated at the apical region of these cells are long cilia embedded in a layer of mucus, produced by the supporting cells. Odoriferous compounds reach the olfactory epithelium by diffusion, which is facilitated by sniffing to increase the airflow. These compounds must first dissolve in the mucus; the chemical interactions between odoriferous chemicals and the chemoreceptors on the cilia trigger changes in ion conductance in the olfactory cell, resulting in the generation of action potentials in the olfactory neurones. The axons of the olfactory nerve pass through the cribriform plate and enter the olfactory bulb. Here there is complex signal processing in that there is marked convergence of afferent inputs and also the presence of interneurones. From here second-order neurones project to the olfactory cortex and also to other regions such as the thalamus and the limbic system.

Autonomic nervous system

Visceral activity is controlled by a combination of the autonomic nervous system (ANS) and both systemic and local hormones. For example, one cannot consciously increase cardiac output, but when physical threat is detected, the ANS will initiate changes in various systems of the body which enable the individual to deal with the physical demand. The ANS is controlled mainly by centres in the brainstem and hypothalamus. Sensory inputs are relayed to these areas and reflex responses are effected in the visceral organs. Acting in concert with the hypothalamus and the endocrine system, the ANS is largely responsible for the control of the internal environment of the body.

There are two subdivisions, the sympathetic and the parasympathetic nervous system (Figure 18.27). In general, the two systems are antagonistic to each other. It is not always predictable whether sympathetic or parasympathetic stimulation will produce inhibition or excitation in a particular organ, but most organs are predominantly controlled by one or the other system. This background activity is known as the sympathetic or parasympathetic tone. For example, arteriolar smooth muscle has a predominant sympathetic tone, whereas the basal tone in the gut is mainly parasympathetic.

Parasympathetic system   **Sympathetic system**

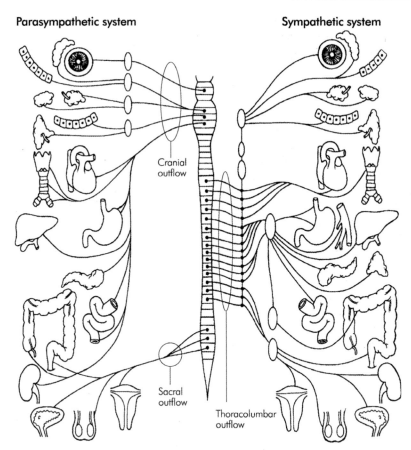

Figure 18.27 Distribution of the autonomic nervous system

The autonomic nervous system (ANS) is that part of the nervous system which provides neurological control over the visceral activities of the body. This control is involuntary and enables the body to adjust to varying physiological demands.

Sympathetic nervous system

Neurones of the sympathetic nervous system originate in the thoracic and lumbar segments (from T1 to L2) of the spinal cord, the so-called thoracolumbar outflow. These synapse in a paired chain of ganglia, the sympathetic ganglia, situated on either side of the vertebral column. The nerve fibres which run from the spinal cord to the sympathetic ganglia are known as preganglionic fibres, while those which leave the ganglia to reach their effector organs are known as postganglionic fibres. A few of the preganglionic fibres pass through the sympathetic chain without forming synapses until they arrive at a more peripheral location in the coeliac and mesenteric ganglia or the adrenal medulla. The adrenal medulla is unique in that it is innervated by sympathetic preganglionic fibres but has no postganglionic nerve fibres.

Parasympathetic nervous system

The parasympathetic nervous system leaves the central nervous system via cranial nerves (III, VII, IX and X) and sacral nerves (S2, 3, 4). This is called the craniosacral outflow. Approximately three-quarters of all parasympathetic fibres are located in the two vagus (X) nerves. Like the sympathetic pathway, the parasympathetic system has both preganglionic and postganglionic neurones. However, the cell bodies of the parasympathetic ganglia are located within the effector organs themselves, so the preganglionic fibres travel long distances from the spinal cord and the postganglionic fibres are relatively short.

Neurotransmitters and receptors in the autonomic nervous system

The sympathetic and parasympathetic nerve fibres release either acetylcholine or noradrenaline in the nerve endings. All preganglionic fibres are cholinergic in both the sympathetic and parasympathetic ganglia. Nearly all the postganglionic neurones of the parasympathetic system are also cholinergic, but a few may release vasoactive intestinal polypeptide (VIP). Most of the postganglionic sympathetic fibres are noradrenergic, except in sweat glands, piloerector muscles and a few blood vessels, where they are cholinergic.

Sympathetic stimulation to the adrenal medulla releases adrenaline and noradrenaline into the circulation. In general, about 80% of the secretion is adrenaline and 20% is noradrenaline, but this proportion may change considerably depending on physiological conditions. There are two major types of adrenoceptors, α and β. Noradrenaline acts predominantly on α-receptors, whereas adrenaline acts on both α- and β-adrenoceptors. α-Receptors can also be divided into two types: α_1 and α_2, and there are three subtypes of β-adrenoceptors.

There are two types of cholinergic receptors: nicotinic and muscarinic. Nicotinic receptors are found in both the sympathetic and parasympathetic ganglia. On the other hand, muscarinic receptors are located in the postganglionic parasympathetic synapses. Although five distinct subclasses of muscarinic receptors have been identified by gene cloning, functionally there are three subtypes: M_1 receptors are found mainly in the CNS; M_2 receptors are located in the heart; M_3 receptors are found in exocrine glands and vascular endothelium.

Sympathetic and parasympathetic systems

- The sympathetic supply is provided via the thoracolumbar outflow originating from levels T1 to L2.
- The parasympathetic supply occurs via some cranial nerves (III, VII, IX and X), and sacral nerves S2, 3 and 4.
- All autonomic preganglionic fibres are cholinergic.
- The majority of parasympathetic postganglionic fibres are cholinergic.
- The majority of the sympathetic postganglionic fibres are noradrenergic.

Figure 18.28 'Stress' responses due to sympathetic mass discharge

Tachycardia
Raised arterial pressure
Sweating
Pupillary dilatation
Increase in blood glucose concentration
Increase in glycolysis and gluconeogenesis
Redistribution of blood flow from splanchnic to cerebral and coronary circulation
Increase in cellular metabolism throughout the body
Increase in mental alertness

Consequences of autonomic stimulation

In life-threatening situations, the sympathetic nervous system discharges almost as a complete unit, a phenomenon known as mass discharge. This may occur when the hypothalamus is activated by fear, noxious stimulus or severe pain. There is stimulation of different systems and organs simultaneously to prepare the individual for survival. The resulting sympathetic 'stress' response is summarised in Figure 18.28.

The parasympathetic nervous system, on the contrary, is more organ-specific. For example, stimulation of the heart by the parasympathetic system is quite separate from that of gastric secretion. Nevertheless, there is some association between closely related functions; for example, although salivary secretion can occur separately from gastric secretion, they are often coordinated and occur together.

Limbic system

The limbic system is made up of a number of cortical and subcortical structures situated around the basal regions of the cerebrum. It is principally involved in the control of instinctive and learned behaviour, emotions, sexual and motivational drives. The limbic system has extensive neuronal connections with the frontal and temporal cortex. The most important components of the limbic system are the hypothalamus, amygdala and hippocampus (Figure 18.29).

Hippocampus and amygdala

As with other structures within the limbic system, stimulation of different areas of the hippocampus also leads to

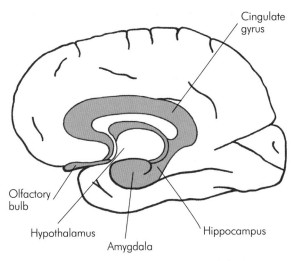

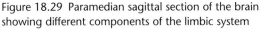

Figure 18.29 Paramedian sagittal section of the brain showing different components of the limbic system

behavioural and emotional changes such as increased sex drive, rage and placidity. In addition, when the hippocampi have been surgically excised, the end result is anterograde amnesia and some degree of retrograde amnesia. It is therefore suggested that the hippocampus may be involved in both short- and long-term memory processes. Due to the extensive neuronal connections between it and various areas of the brain, stimulation of the amygdala not only causes effects similar to that of the hypothalamus, but also widespread behavioural patterns. It is thought that the amygdala projects into the limbic system the current behavioural status in relation to both the surroundings and the thoughts of the individual. It is believed to help pattern the behavioural response of the individual so that it is appropriate for each occasion.

Hypothalamus

The hypothalamus is situated just rostral to the brainstem in the basal region of the brain. Inferior to it is the pituitary gland. It has extensive neuronal connections to the brainstem, pituitary gland and cerebrum. Together with other limbic structures and the endocrine system, the hypothalamus controls the vegetative and endocrine functions of the body as well as many aspects of emotional behaviour. The hypothalamus maintains homeostatic control of the internal environment, and as such it plays a central role in the control of body temperature, pituitary secretion, osmolality of body fluids and the drive to eat and drink (Figure 18.30).

Figure 18.30 Functions of the hypothalamus

| Control of body temperature |
| Control over endocrine system via pituitary gland |
| Regulation of water balance |
| Control of food intake |
| Behavioural and emotional influence |

Figure 18.31 Hypothalamic releasing and inhibiting hormones

| Adrenocorticotropic hormone releasing hormone (corticotropin releasing hormone) |
| Thyrotropin releasing hormone |
| Growth hormone releasing hormone |
| Luteinising hormone releasing hormone |
| Follicle-stimulating hormone releasing hormone |
| Prolactin releasing hormone |
| Prolactin inhibiting hormone |

Control of body temperature

The hypothalamus receives and processes information from both the central thermoreceptors, situated in the preoptic (anterior) part of the hypothalamus itself, and the peripheral thermoreceptors found on the skin. Physiological changes are initiated in response to temperature changes so that a nearly constant body temperature is maintained. For example, in response to cold the hypothalamus will initiate peripheral vasoconstriction and shivering. At the same time, behavioural changes also occur, so that a lowering of environmental temperature will lead to an increase in muscular activity to generate heat, and extra layers of clothes may be added to conserve heat.

Control of pituitary secretion

Anterior pituitary secretion is controlled by releasing and inhibiting hormones carried in the portal hypophyseal vessels from the hypothalamus to the pituitary gland. These chemical agents are secreted by nerve endings in the median eminence of the hypothalamus. These nerve endings are in close proximity to the capillary loops from which the portal vessels are formed. There are seven hypothalamic releasing and inhibiting hormones, as summarised in Figure 18.31.

The posterior pituitary gland secretes the hormones oxytocin and vasopressin. They are synthesised in the neurones in the supraoptic and paraventricular nuclei of the hypothalamus and are transported down the axons to their endings in the posterior pituitary, where they are released into the circulation. Oxytocin is released when the breast is suckled and is responsible for milk ejection. It also causes contraction of the uterine smooth muscle. The release of vasopressin depends on the osmolality of the plasma. Even small changes in osmolality may cause significant changes in vasopressin release. The main effect of vasopressin is water retention by the kidneys. It increases the permeability of the collecting ducts of the kidney so that more water is reabsorbed.

Water balance

The hypothalamus maintains water balance by controlling both water intake and water loss. Electrical stimulation or injection of hypertonic saline into the anterior hypothalamus leads to the desire to drink. Drinking is regulated by changes in plasma osmolality and extracellular fluid (ECF) volume. Depletion in ECF volume leads to thirst. The thirst sensation is mediated partly by vasopressin release from the hypothalamus and also via the renin–angiotensin system. When an individual is dehydrated, plasma osmolality increases and the volume of the ECF (therefore plasma volume) decreases. As a consequence, the hypothalamic osmoreceptors and stretch receptors in the large vessels are stimulated and vasopressin is released from the hypothalamus. However, the stimuli for vasopressin release as a result of changes in plasma osmolality and plasma volume may override one another. For instance, during haemorrhage the resulting hypovolaemia increases vasopressin release even when the plasma is hypotonic.

Food intake

Two hypothalamic centres, the feeding centre and the satiety centre, control food intake. Animal studies suggest that the two centres are antagonistic. Electrical stimulation of the feeding centre results in feeding behaviour, while stimulation of the satiety centre stops feeding behaviour. It is also suggested that the feeding centre is constantly active and its activity is only temporarily inhibited by the satiety centre after food intake. The level of blood glucose probably controls the activity of the satiety centre. After a meal, blood glucose rises and the satiety centre is activated, inhibiting the feeding centre.

Behavioural functions

Apart from the functions described above, animal studies suggest that stimulation of or lesions in the hypothalamus lead to significant changes in behaviour. For instance, stimulation in the ventromedial hypothalamus leads to placidity and satiety whereas stimulation in the lateral hypothalamus leads to increased rage, restlessness and fighting behaviours. Stimulation of the extreme anterior and posterior areas of the hypothalamus increases sexual drive. Destructive lesions such as tumours usually lead to the opposite effects.

CHAPTER 19

Physiology of pain

Ted Lin

Pain has been defined as 'an unpleasant sensory and emotional experience associated with actual or potential tissue damage' by the International Association for the Study of Pain (IASP), which has become the parent organisation for many national pain societies. This definition has arisen because pain is a multimodal experience.

Nociception

Nociception is the sensory modality by which noxious stimuli are detected peripherally and transmitted centrally to the central nervous system. Noxious stimuli may or may not be associated with tissue damage. The pathway by which nociception is mediated (Figure 19.1) consists of:

- Nociceptors
- Dorsal root ganglia containing the body of the nociceptor
- The primary synapse
- The dorsal horn of the spinal cord
- Ascending tracts
- Thalamus and higher centres

Dimensions of the pain experience

- Pain has a protective function and may or may not be associated with tissue damage.
- Pain should not be equated to nociception. Nociception is often a component of pain symptoms but not necessarily so.
- Intrinsic modulatory mechanisms exist in the body which attenuate the intensity of the pain experience.
- Sensitisation mechanisms exist which intensify pain symptoms, resulting in the phenomenon of hyperalgesia.
- Pain possesses a subjective and affective element as a result of connections between the pain system, cortical centres and the limbic system.
- Pain levels are also influenced by past experience and anticipation due to interaction between the pain system and the prefrontal cortex.
- Pain can affect visceral and neuroendocrine function as a result of interconnections with medullary centres and the hypothalamus.

Fundamentals of Anaesthesia, 4th edition, ed. Ted Lin, Tim Smith and Colin Pinnock. Published by Cambridge University Press. © Cambridge University Press 2017.

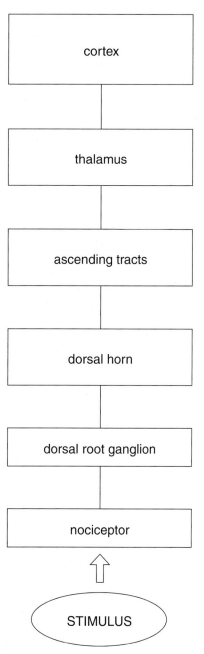

Figure 19.1 The nociceptive pathway

Nociceptors

The primary afferent neurones for pain are referred to as 'nociceptors', which possess specialised nerve endings in almost all tissues of the body. These primary afferents respond to different types of noxious stimuli. Such stimuli are most commonly mechanical, thermal or chemical.

> **Nociceptor characteristics**
>
> - The type of stimuli they are sensitive to
> - The class of nerve fibre serving the receptor
> - The receptor response characteristics – slow or fast, short or long latency
> - The ion channel proteins expressed on the receptor cell membrane

Unimodal receptors respond to mechanical distortion, thermal receptors to heat, and polymodal receptors to mechanical distortion, heat, cold or chemical stimuli. The majority of receptors are polymodal, being sensitive to mechano-heat (MH) stimuli. Some receptors are only sensitive to mechanical stimuli and are referred to as mechanically sensitive afferents (MSA) while others are insensitive to mechanical stimuli (mechanically insensitive afferents, MIA).

There are two main types of nociceptor fibre which transmit nociceptor signals to the central nervous system, C fibres and Aδ fibres.

- **C nociceptors** are unmyelinated, with conduction velocities < 2 m s^{-1}. They evoke slow-response burning pain and dull aching pain. They are mostly polymodal, responding to heat, mechanical and chemical stimuli. These nociceptors may be referred to using the nomenclature CMH (C mechano-heat nociceptors). Some C-fibre nociceptors are mechanically insensitive afferents, and are referred to as C-fibre MIAs.

- **Aδ nociceptors** are connected centrally by myelinated fibres with conduction velocities between 15 and 55 m s^{-1}. Aδ fibres evoke sharp fast-response pains of a burning, stabbing, pricking and aching nature. There are two types of Aδ nociceptor. Type I have higher conduction velocities (> 25 m s^{-1}) and are found in hairy and glabrous skin (palms of hands and soles of feet). These Aδ nociceptors may be referred to as AMHs (A mechano-heat nociceptors). Type II are slower, with conduction velocities of around 15 m s^{-1}, and are distributed in hairy skin only. An outline of their contrasting responses to stimuli is shown in Figure 19.2.

Figure 19.2 Responses of type I and type II Aδ nociceptors

Response	Type I	Type II
Mechanical	Usually sensitive (MSA)	Usually insensitive (MIA)
Heat	Insensitive (high threshold) initially with increasing response to prolonged stimulus (> 5 s)	Sensitive (low threshold) initially with decreasing response to prolonged stimulus
	Long latency	Short latency
Chemical	Sensitive	Sensitive

Cellular functions of nociceptors

> **Nociceptor functions**
>
> - Transducing and encoding noxious stimuli to generate afferent action potentials
> - Synthesising and releasing neuropeptides such as calcitonin gene-related peptide (CGRP) and substance P, both peripherally and centrally
> - Synthesising and releasing neurotrophins such as glial cell-line-derived neurotrophic factor (GDNF) and nerve growth factor (NGF), which modulate gene expression in the nociceptor
> - Synthesising and releasing neurotransmitters at the primary synapse, e.g. glutamate
> - Synthesising and releasing inflammatory mediators which sensitise the nociceptive pathway centrally and peripherally

Nociceptor ion channels

Nociceptors possess families of ion channels in their cell membranes which initiate their functions and have the following properties:

- They are usually specific for sodium, potassium, calcium or hydrogen ions (acid-sensing ion channels, ASICs). However, non-specific ion channels also exist.
- Transient receptor potential (TRP) channels in the nociceptor membrane transduce noxious physical or chemical stimuli to initiate action potentials.
- TRP channels can be sensitised or activated by inflammatory mediators released from damaged tissue or by the nociceptors themselves. This results in hyperalgesia.

- Voltage-gated channels are opened at different thresholds of membrane potential. Such channels can be triggered by the transient changes in membrane potential produced when TRP channels are activated. TRP channels can thus initiate an action potential. In this way a stimulus can be encoded into action potentials with a rate which varies according to the intensity of the stimulus.
- Up to nine different voltage-gated sodium channels have been identified in a single nociceptor cell membrane. Individual members of such families of ion channels are identified by established nomenclature: e.g. ion channels specific to nociceptors have been identifed as Nav 1.8 and 1.9 (Na, sodium; v, voltage-gated; '1' gene subfamily; '8' isoform).

> Nociceptor functions are initiated by **ion channels** and receptors in the nociceptor cell membrane. Each nociceptor possesses different types of ion channel. They include transient receptor potential (TRP) ion channels, ligand-gated ion channels and voltage-gated ion channels.

Nociception and inflammatory mediators

When a noxious stimulus is applied, chemical mediators such as prostaglandins, hydrogen ions and kinins are released by the nociceptor or as a result of tissue damage. These substances not only initiate nociception, but also produce hyperalgesia. In addition, these agents mediate the inflammatory process by inducing the following changes:

- Increases in local blood flow and vascular permeability
- Activation and migration of immune cells
- Release of growth and trophic factors from surrounding tissues

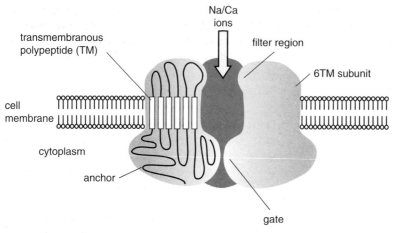

Figure 19.3 Transient receptor potential (TRP) channel

Transient receptor potential (TRP) channels

- TRP channels are the 'transducer' channels in the plasma membranes of a wide variety of animal and human cells (Figure 19.3).
- They are activated by different physical and chemical stimuli (pressure, temperature, osmotic pressure, vibration, H^+, capsaicin, cannabinoids).
- When activated, the TRP channels produce a transient drop in resting membrane potential to trigger action potentials and thus mediate sensory modes such as heat and pressure sensation, vibration sense and pain.
- At least seven subfamilies of TRP channel have been identified.
- A prominent TRP channel in hyperalgesic conditions is the TRPV1 (vanilloid 1) channel, which is a calcium/sodium channel. The TRPV1 channel can also be potentiated by heat and H^+, and is inhibited by glycine or intracellular phosphatidylinositol biphosphate (PIP_2).

There are different mechanisms by which inflammatory mediators influence nociceptor function:

- Activation of membrane ion channels, e.g. lipid metabolite activation of TRPV1 channels, proton activation of ASICs, ATP activation of purinergic (P2X) channels.

- Activation of G-protein-coupled receptors which increase the activities of second messengers such as cyclic adenosine monophosphate (cAMP) or inositol triphosphate (IP_3). These in turn may lead to structural changes in membrane ion channels or changes in the activity of intracellular enzymes affecting membrane excitability.
- Activation of cytokine receptors by interleukins (IL-1) or tumour necrosis factor α (TNF-α).
- Activation of tyrosine kinase receptors TrkA, TrkB, by specific neurotrophic factors such as NGF (which activates TrkA), and brain-derived neurotrophic factor (BDNF) (which activates TrkB)

Some examples of inflammatory mediators and their origins are shown in Figure 19.4.

The dorsal root ganglion

The dorsal root ganglion (DRG) contains the cell bodies for all primary afferents including the nociceptors. The primary afferent fibres are classified according to conduction velocity. Aα and Aβ fibres are the fastest group with large cell bodies, forming about 40% of the DRG cells. Aδ and C fibres are slower with small cell bodies, and account for about 60% of the DRG population. Nociceptors form the majority of the small cells. They can be further classified into peptidergic if they contain peptides (CGRP, substance P, somatostatin) or non-peptidergic. Approximately 50% of C and 20% of Aδ fibres are peptidergic. Although nociceptors are mainly small-cell-bodied, some nociceptors also exist in the faster larger-neurone groups. Specific populations of DRG neurones can be identified by the expression of different neurotrophin receptors on their cell membranes.

The DRG is situated in the lateral foramen between neighbouring vertebral bodies and is in close relationship to the sympathetic chain (Figure 19.5). This anatomical relationship becomes significant in chronic pain conditions such as complex regional pain

syndrome (CRPS), in which abnormal overgrowth of the DRG by fibres from the sympathetic chain is thought to be responsible for the sympathetically maintained symptoms and trophic changes in the affected areas.

The dorsal horn

Nociceptors terminate almost exclusively in the dorsal horn of the spinal cord. The grey matter of the spinal cord was divided into 10 laminae (numbered I to X) by Rexed in 1952. The dorsal horn is composed of laminae I to VI (Figure 19.6). The majority of nociceptor fibres (Aδ and C) terminate in two areas, which are laminae I/II (marginal layer and substantia gelatinosa) and lamina V. It should be noted that in addition to Aδ and C fibres, a small fraction of Aβ afferent fibres are nociceptive with high-threshold mechano-heat characteristics. The nociceptive fibres synapse with second-order neurones or interneurones within the dorsal horn.

The second-order neurones in the dorsal horn may be excited or inhibited by different configurations of the nociceptors and interneurones. Sensitisation of the primary synapse by the descending modulatory system or interneurones can also occur in hyperalgesic states (Figure 19.7). Similarly, various configurations of the descending modulatory system and interneurones may occur to inhibit transmission in the primary synapse (Figure 19.8).

Figure 19.4 Some inflammatory mediators and their origins

Mediator	Source/origin
Bradykinin	Damaged tissue
Arachidonites	Arachidonic acid
Serotonin	Platelet and mast cells
Histamine	Mast cells
Cytokines (TNF-α, IL-1)	Immune system
Intracellular molecules (ATP, NO)	Damaged tissue
Neurotrophins (NGF, GDNF, BDNF)	Nociceptors

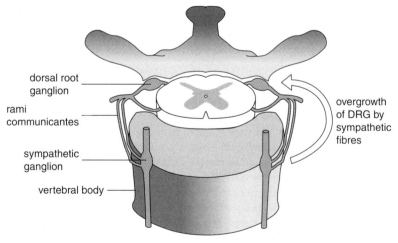

dorsal root ganglion

rami communicantes

sympathetic ganglion

vertebral body

overgrowth of DRG by sympathetic fibres

Figure 19.5 Anatomy of a dorsal root ganglion

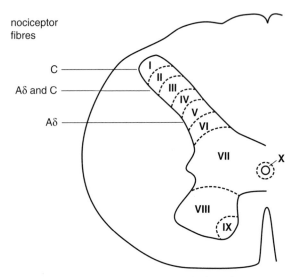

nociceptor fibres

C
Aδ and C
Aδ

I
II
III
IV
V
VI
VII
VIII
IX
X

Figure 19.6 Dorsal horn laminae in spinal cord

(a)
nociceptor — dorsal horn neurone
+

(b)
nociceptor — interneurone — dorsal horn neurone
+ +

(c)
descending modulatory system — sensitisation
nociceptor — dorsal horn neurone
+ +

Figure 19.7 Excitatory connections in the dorsal horn

Contents of the dorsal horn

The dorsal horn contains the following neuronal elements which participate in nociception:

- Primary afferent axons and their synapses connecting with secondary neurones or interneurones
- Secondary neurones which project afferent information to the brain via ascending tracts
- Interneurones which form interconnection circuits at one level, or can ascend and descend to interconnect in other segments
- Descending axons from supraspinal centres modulating nociception

- Gating of nociceptive signals (see The 'gate control' theory, below)
- Sensitisation of the primary synapse
- Presynaptic inhibition of primary afferents
- Relaying primary afferent signals to the appropriate ascending tracts

Interneurone function

Interneurones form at least 90% of the neurones in the dorsal horn. They perform multiple functions including sensitisation and inhibition of transmission in the primary synapse, as well as gating and relaying nociceptive signals.

Interneurones

The great majority of neurones in the dorsal horn are interneurones. Inhibitory and excitatory interneurones exist. Excitatory interneurones release glutamate as the neurotransmitter into the primary synapse. Inhibitory neurones use γ-aminobutyric acid (GABA) and glycine as their neurotransmitters, and may be stimulated by primary afferents, the descending modulatory system or non-nociceptive primary afferents such as Aβ fibres. The interneurones form interconnection circuits which participate in the following aspects of dorsal horn activity:

The primary synapse

Nociceptors are the primary afferent neurones of the pain system; they stimulate action potentials in the dorsal horn neurone via the primary synapse. The primary synapse is central to the mechanism by which the pain system controls its sensitivity. The main excitatory neurotransmitter in the primary synapse is glutamate (Figure 19.9).

Primary afferents can also inhibit action potentials in dorsal horn neurones by stimulating inhibitory interneurones. The main inhibitory neurotransmitters are GABA and glycine (Figure 19.10).

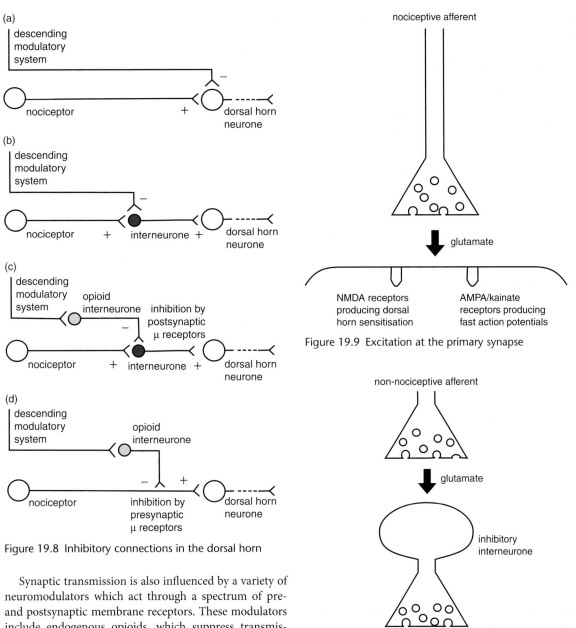

Figure 19.8 Inhibitory connections in the dorsal horn

Figure 19.9 Excitation at the primary synapse

Synaptic transmission is also influenced by a variety of neuromodulators which act through a spectrum of pre- and postsynaptic membrane receptors. These modulators include endogenous opioids, which suppress transmission, but other modulators can enhance transmission. Neuromodulators in the pain system are described further below.

Descending control of the primary synapse is exerted by supraspinal centres which form the descending modulatory system. This system not only can inhibit synaptic transmission but may also facilitate it, leading to sensitisation.

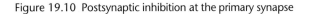

Figure 19.10 Postsynaptic inhibition at the primary synapse

Figure 19.11 Some examples of neurotransmitters in the pain system

Neurotransmitter	Location	Comments
Excitatory neurotransmitters		
Glutamate	Widespread throughout CNS. Primary afferents	Main excitatory transmitter in CNS. > 50% of DRG neurones. The main excitatory transmitter in nociception, acting via ionotropic receptors (AMPA, NMDA and kainite receptors)
Substance P	Primary afferents	30% of DRG neurones, mainly small sensory afferents. Small peptide agonist for neurokinin (NK1) receptor. Excitatory role in 'wind up'
Calcitonin gene-related peptide (CGRP)	Dorsal root ganglion cells	50% of DRG neurones, both small and large pain fibres. Released by thermal and mechanical stimuli. Excitatory role in 'wind up'
Inhibitory neurotransmitters		
γ-Aminobutyric acid (GABA)/ glycine	Descending modulation system, dorsal and ventral horn	Potent inhibition of spinal cord neurones. Act through ligand-gated channels
Noradrenaline	Dorsal horn and descending modulation system	Dorsal horn inhibition
Serotonin	Dorsal horn and descending modulation system	Dorsal horn inhibition
Glutamate	Dorsal horn	Inhibitory effects in dorsal horn exerted via metabotropic receptors

Control of transmission in the primary synapse

Control of synaptic transmission in the dorsal horn is therefore a result of complex interactions between afferent, descending, ascending and interneurone fibres (Figures 19.7 and 19.8).

Neurotransmitters in the pain system

Many different synapses exist in the pain pathways of the CNS. It is recognised that each synapse operates with multiple transmitters. Some examples of known neurotransmitters in the pain system are presented in Figure 19.11.

Receptors in the primary synapse

The presynaptic and postsynaptic membranes of the primary synapse possess different families of receptor proteins (Figure 19.12). Some receptors (*ionotropic*) control associated ion channels. Others, such as tyrosine kinase (Trk) receptors, signal intracellular pathways, resulting in the synthesis and release of peptides, neurotransmitters or neurotrophic factors. These are *metabotropic* receptors.

Primary synapse receptors

Primary synapse receptors may be classified into metabotropic receptors and ionotropic receptors:

- **Metabotropic receptors** activate intracellular pathways when triggered by an agonist.
- **Ionotropic receptors** alter the conductivity of an associated ion channel.

The main excitatory transmitter is glutamate, which activates three different subtypes of ionotropic receptor

Figure 19.12 Examples of primary synapse receptors

Receptor	Location	Comments
NMDA	Postsynaptic membrane	Important in producing long-lasting sensitisation by allowing calcium influx into the projecting dorsal horn neurones. Normally suppressed by Mg^{2+}, may also be blocked by ketamine
AMPA	Postsynaptic membrane	Produce fast excitatory postsynaptic action potentials. The main receptor responsible for transmission between primary afferents and dorsal horn neurones. Mainly sodium ionophores
Kainate	Postsynaptic membrane	Produce slow postsynaptic potentials associated with activation of high-threshold primary afferents. Sodium and potassium ionophores
NK1		Metabotropic receptors activated by substance P. Activate nociceptive dorsal horn neurones and produce hyperalgesia. Increase intracellular Ca^{2+}
CGRP receptors	Postsynaptic membrane	Produce facilitation of the dorsal horn response
Opioid δ, κ, μ	Postsynaptic and presynaptic membranes	Inhibition of dorsal horn neurones
$GABA_A$, $GABA_B$	Postsynaptic membrane	Inhibition of dorsal horn neurones $GABA_A$ increases Cl^- conductance and stabilises postsynaptic membrane potential $GABA_B$ decreases Ca^{2+} conductance and causes postsynaptic membrane hyperpolarisation
$α_2$	Presynaptic membrane	Selective inhibition of nociceptive primary afferents leading to analgesia
Serotonin receptors	Postsynaptic membrane, NMDA receptors	Inhibition of dorsal horn transmission. Some serotonin receptors associated with excitatory action

on the postsynaptic membrane. These are NMDA (N-methyl-D-aspartate), AMPA (α-amino 3-hydroxy 5-methyl 4-isoxazolepropionic acid) and kainate receptors (Figure 19.9). The NMDA receptor has a prominent role in chronic pain conditions, while the AMPA receptor mediates the transmission of fast action potentials.

In addition to these ionotropic receptors there are modulatory receptors on the postsynaptic membrane which can facilitate or inhibit action potential formation.

The main inhibitory receptors are γ-aminobutyric acid (GABA) and glycine receptors (Figure 19.8). Other inhibitory receptors include μ and κ opioid receptors and adenosine receptors, which are G-protein coupled.

The presynaptic nociceptor membrane has a range of receptors which include opioid (μ, δ and κ), nicotinic and muscarinic receptors. These also function to modulate synaptic transmission (Figure 19.13).

Ascending tracts

The signals generated by nociception ascend to the brain by sensory-discriminative pathways and affective pathways. The sensory-discriminative pathways enable a nociceptive stimulus to be localised and its different qualities to be distinguished. The affective pathways relay the nociceptive signals to visceral, neuroendocrine and affective centres in the brain to produce the multidimensional nature of the pain response.

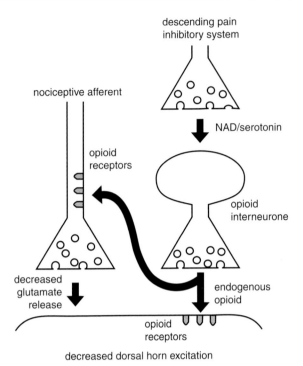

Figure 19.13 Presynaptic inhibition at the primary synapse

Sensory discriminative pathways

- The spinothalamic tract (STT) is formed by fibres from dorsal horn neurones which cross the midline and carry touch, pinprick, pain and temperature sensations from below the neck, to the thalamus. It is monosynaptic and phylogenetically the most recent of the nociceptive pathways. It is sometimes referred to as the 'neospinothalamic' pathway.
- The STT terminates in the ventral posterior nucleus (VPN) of the thalamus, and is divided into an anterior portion mainly responsible for touch sensation and a lateral portion responsible for pain, temperature and pinprick modes.
- The trigeminothalamic tract – this pathway is responsible for pain, temperature, pinprick and touch sensations in the head and neck, to the thalamus. Fibres from the contralateral spinal trigeminal nucleus form this tract and again terminate in the VPN.

Both pathways tend to lie laterally in the spinal cord and ascend to the contralateral VPN of the thalamus, from which they are projected to the cortex (Figure 19.14).

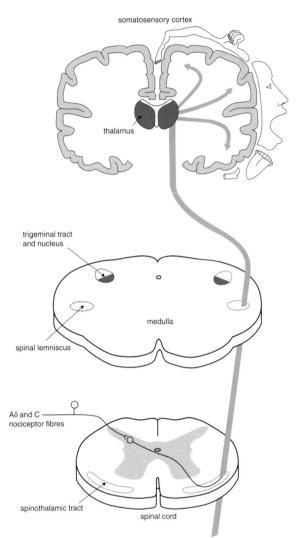

Figure 19.14 Sensory discriminative pain pathway

Affective pathways

- These pathways are the spinoreticular tracts, which are multisynaptic and thought to be phylogenetically the more primitive of the ascending tracts. They are sometimes referred to as 'palaeospinothalamic' projections.
- Initially they project to brainstem areas including the reticular formation, the parabrachial nuclei, catecholamine cell groups and the periaqueductal grey matter.
- Spinoreticular tracts function by integrating incoming pain signals with visceral nuclei

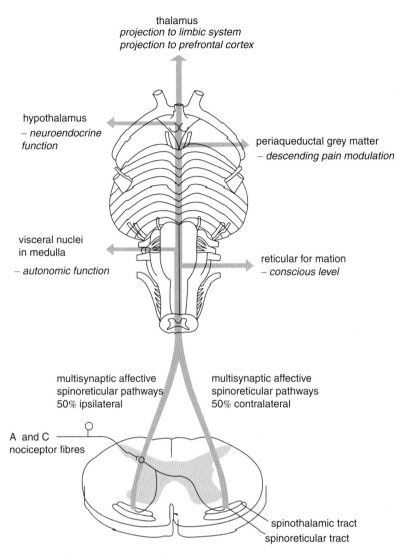

thalamus
projection to limbic system
projection to prefrontal cortex

hypothalamus
– neuroendocrine
function

periaqueductal grey matter
– descending pain modulation

visceral nuclei
in medulla

– autonomic function

reticular for mation
– conscious level

multisynaptic affective
spinoreticular pathways
50% ipsilateral

multisynaptic affective
spinoreticular pathways
50% contralateral

A and C
nociceptor fibres

spinothalamic tract
spinoreticular tract

Figure 19.15 Affective pain pathways

(e.g. nucleus tractus solitarius), the limbic system and the descending inhibitory system. They therefore mediate the emotional autonomic responses to pain.

• Spinohypothalamic pathways ultimately connect incoming nociceptive signals through to the hypothalamus, and these are also relayed to the prefrontal cortex. These hypothalamic connections are reflected by the disturbance of neuroendocrine

function such as ACTH and vasopressin activity, produced by pain. The prefrontal cortex is concerned with the highest cerebral activities such as abstract thought, decision making and anticipation. Such connections enable the prefrontal cortex to influence the response to nociceptive input.

The affective pathways assume a position medial to the spinothalamic tract in the spinal cord (Figure 19.15).

Ascending pain pathways

Two types of ascending pathway transmit nociceptive signals to the brain:

- The **sensory discriminative pathway** is monosynaptic with cortical projection, enabling somatosensory localisation of the noxious stimulus. This is phylogenetically more recent.
- The **affective pathways** are phylogenetically more primitive. They are polysynaptic, projecting to subcortical centres and mediating affective and autonomic dimensions of the pain response.

The thalamus

The right and left thalami are large oval masses of neurones which are located deep in the brain, forming the lateral walls of the third ventricle. Lateral to the thalamus on each side is the internal capsule, and above the thalamus is the floor of the lateral ventricle. The thalamus is a complex collection of nuclei with multiple connections to the cortex and other basal ganglia.

The thalamus and pain

Although no single function can be attributed to the thalamus, because of its complexity, one of its primary functions is the projection of somatosensory signals from the spinothalamic tracts and the trigeminal nuclei, which mediates the localisation and discrimination of painful stimuli.

The afferent nociceptive signals are received by the ventral posterior nucleus (VPN) of the thalamus, which is somatotopically arranged. This 'mapping' of the sensory signals is maintained in the thalamic projection to the cortex, and corresponds to the 'homunculus' representation on the postcentral gyrus (S1 somatosensory area).

Spinoreticular projections from the brainstem are received in the reticular, intralaminar and some medial areas of the thalamus. These are thought to exert an inhibitory influence on the VPN via interconnections. Disruption of these interconnections may underlie 'central' or 'thalamic' pain conditions. Part of the thalamic projection also goes to the secondary somatosensory area

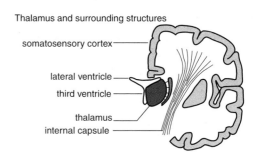

Thalamus and surrounding structures

somatosensory cortex

lateral ventricle
third ventricle

thalamus
internal capsule

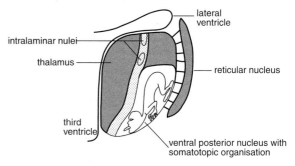

Ventral posterior nucleus of thalamus

lateral ventricle

intralaminar nulei

thalamus

reticular nucleus

third ventricle

ventral posterior nucleus with somatotopic organisation

Figure 19.16 Thalamus and surrounding structures

of the cortex (S2) at the foot of the postcentral gyrus (Figure 19.16).

Cortical sites of pain projection

Nociception not only activates subcortical structures such as the thalamic and brainstem nuclei, but also activates a network of cortical centres which is sometimes referred to as the 'cortical pain matrix'.

Imaging studies have consistently demonstrated activation of the following cortical areas during acute and chronic pain:

- The primary somatosensory cortex (postcentral gyrus, SI)
- The secondary somatosensory cortex (S2)
- The insular cortex (IC)
- The anterior cingulate cortex (ACC)

Activation of the somatosensory areas, S1 and S2, is thought to play a role in perceiving the location and duration of pain. The ACC, which is part of the limbic system, and the IC, which is close to the limbic system, are thought to be important in the emotional, affective and motivational aspects of pain (Figure 19.17).

(a) Lateral aspect of cerebral hemisphere

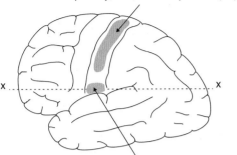

(b) Horizontal section of brain (xx)

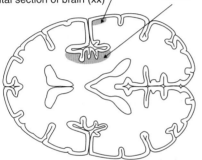

(c) Medial aspect of cerebral hemisphere

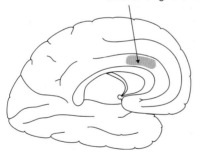

Figure 19.17 Cortical matrix for pain

The prefrontal cortex, which is responsible for higher cortical thought processes such as anticipation, prediction and modelling based on past experience, is also activated by noxious stimuli and can exert an enhancing or suppressive effect on the intensity of pain experienced. It is thought to play a part in placebo analgesia.

> ### The cortical pain matrix
>
> This is the network of cortical centres activated by ascending nociceptive signals. It provides a cortical dimension to the pain experience, enabling accurate somatic localisation of noxious stimuli as well as predictive and affective dimensions to the pain experience. The response of the cortical matrix can be enhanced to increase the intensity of the pain experience, as in hyperalgesia.

Sensitisation of the pain system

One of the characteristic features of pain which distinguishes it from other sensory modalities is the ability of the pain pathways to sensitise themselves. This can be regarded as a form of positive feedback control, in contrast to the familiar negative feedback control of homeostatic physiological systems. Sensitisation is recognised as occurring both peripherally at nociceptor level and centrally in the dorsal horn.

> **Sensitisation** is a neurophysiological term used to describe an enhanced response of nociceptors (peripheral sensitisation) or an enhanced efficacy of the primary synapse in the dorsal horn (central sensitisation). It should not be confused with the clinical term 'hyperalgesia', which refers to the overall pain response experienced and may involve supraspinal mechanisms as well as sensitisation. Sensitisation is mediated by chemical factors acting through various cellular mechanisms outlined below.

Peripheral sensitisation

Nociceptors, like other sensory receptors, are characterised by a response–stimulus curve. These receptors are sensitive to thermal, mechanical and chemical stimuli, but only respond above a certain threshold of stimulus intensity. Peripheral sensitisation usually occurs when tissue damage takes place, producing a shift of the nociceptor response curve to the left so that the nociceptor response is enhanced at any given stimulus intensity (Figure 19.18). It is dependent on the release of various substances such as inflammatory mediators, prostaglandins and cytokines.

Peripheral sensitisation can also occur in neuropathic pain conditions, owing to peripheral sympathetic–sensory coupling. Such conditions are referred to as sympathetic-ally maintained pain (SMP). The underlying mechanisms in SMP are thought to be increased adrenergic sensitivity of sensory neurones and proliferation of sympathetic nerve endings. Proliferation of sympathetic nerve endings around the dorsal root ganglion has also been suggested as a site of sympathetic–sensory coupling in chronic pain conditions such as complex regional pain syndrome.

Central sensitisation

A number of mechanisms operate to sensitise nociception in the dorsal horn.

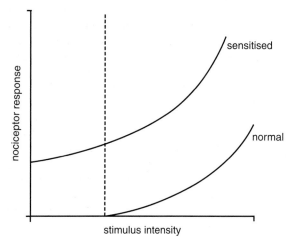

Figure 19.18 Nociceptor response-curve shift in hyperalgesia

- Short-term homosynaptic potentiation ('wind-up') – Dorsal horn cells can produce progressively increasing outputs in response to prolonged C-fibre nociceptor inputs. When dorsal horn neurones are repetitively stimulated by C fibres at low frequencies, the postsynaptic potentials may steadily increase in amplitude with each stimulus. This type of sensitisation only manifests itself in the primary synapse fed by the stimulated primary afferent (homosynaptic) and only occurs over the duration of the nociceptive stimulus.

- Long-term homosynaptic potentiation – This is a prolonged increase in the efficacy of primary synapses which have already been activated by a period of high-intensity nociception. NMDA receptors (Figure 19.19) play a key role in a cascade which leads to AMPA receptor sensitisation on the postsynaptic membrane. Other mechanisms include presynaptic sensitisation via tyrosine kinase receptors (Trk) which increase the release of glutamate. This type of potentiation may outlast the noxious stimulus by hours or longer.

- Heterosynaptic sensitisation – When a nociceptive stimulus is maintained for a period of minutes, synapses outside the directly activated path (heterosynaptic) will also become sensitised. This sensitisation includes non-nociceptive (low-threshold) afferents, such as Aβ fibres serving areas neighbouring the area receiving the noxious stimulus. Heterotopic sensitisation contributes to secondary hyperalgesia and can also be associated with the production

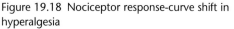

Figure 19.19 NMDA channel

of muscular, joint and visceral pains, and headache. This form of sensitisation may also outlast the nociceptive stimulus by hours.

- Transcription-dependent sensitisation – Intense prolonged nociceptive stimulation, such as that produced by inflammation or nerve injury, produces increased levels of factors including substance P and BDNF. These factors activate gene transcription centrally in dorsal horn cells and the primary afferents themselves. This process switches on genes in dorsal horn neurones, leading to an increase in levels of receptors such as NK1 and TrkB (i.e. the receptors for substance P and BDNF). The gene activation is mediated by an intracellular kinase (extracellullar signal-regulated kinase, ERK) which can enter the nucleus and promote transcription. In some chronic inflammatory conditions the promotion of Cox-2 transcription contributes to the systemic effects of muscular aches and pains, anorexia and headaches experienced.

- Loss of inhibition – As described above, primary afferents not only activate secondary dorsal horn neurones but also inhibit them via inhibitory GABAergic interneurones. Sustained stimulation of Aδ fibres or peripheral nerve injury results in long-term loss of inhibitory activity. In the case of nerve injury this loss of inhibition involves death of the GABAergic inhibitory neurones. GABA mimetics such as gabapentin can thus compensate for this reduction of inhibition in neuropathic pain conditions. Long-term loss of inhibition may also involve resorption of AMPA receptors by dorsal horn neurones. Thus long-term sensitisation occurs via degenerative changes in the dorsal horn in neuropathic pain conditions.

- Changes in synaptic architecture – Allodynia following nerve injury is mediated by non-nociceptive Aβ fibres and associated changes in dorsal horn architecture. In particular, low-threshold Aβ afferents sprout and reconnect from their normal position in laminae III and IV to dorsal horn nociceptive neurones in lamina II. This abnormal reorganisation of dorsal horn architecture can be prevented by treatment with neurotrophins (NGF, BDNF).

- Glial cell activity – There is substantial evidence that activation of glial cells (astrocytes and microglia) follows tissue injury and results in facilitation of primary synapses in the dorsal horn, thus leading to hyperalgesia.

> **Central sensitisation** involves changes in the primary synapse (synaptic plasticity) and plays a significant part in the production of neuropathic pain. These changes occur at the cellular level in the expression of presynaptic and postsynaptic receptors, in the inhibitory mechanisms modulating synaptic transmission, in dorsal horn architecture and in glial cell (astrocyte and microglia) function.

Modulation of pain

Pain is essential for the survival of an animal. It functions by aiding the animal to avoid harmful external influences and it ensures that an animal takes the appropriate actions to immobilise and protect injured tissue, thus promoting recuperation and healing. Prolongation and sensitisation of the pain response beyond the immediate occurrence of tissue injury or damage is required to fulfil these functions.

However, under certain circumstances survival may be advantaged by transiently suppressing the pain response. This might occur in order to allow escape in the face of threat, to ensure victory in combat, or to protect offspring.

Pain modulation can thus suppress the pain experience or intensify it, and it is thought to occur at cortical, brainstem and spinal levels. A number of mechanisms are discussed in further detail below.

> ### Pain modulating mechanisms
>
> - **Gate control** – This is one of the earliest pain modulation mechanisms proposed
> - **Descending modulatory system** – These pathways originate in the midbrain and medulla and descend to suppress nociception in the dorsal horn. They are not only known to exert an antinociceptive effect, but can also have a pronociceptive effect, enhancing nociception. Nociceptive sensitivity is therefore a resulting balance of this bidirectional control.
> - **Neuromodulators** – These modify neurotransmission both supraspinally and in the dorsal horn. Many modulators have been identified, both enhancing and suppressing neurotransmission. They include endogenous opioids, orphanins and cholecystokinins.

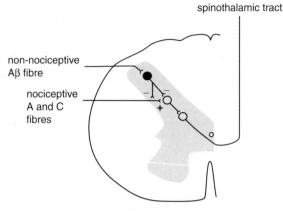

Figure 19.20 Gating mechanism

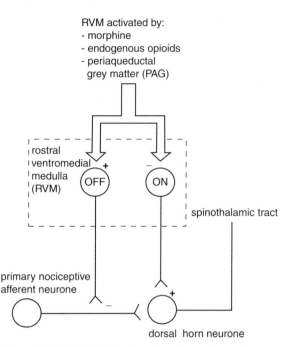

Figure 19.21 PAG–RVM axis in the descending pain modulatory system

The 'gate control' theory

The 'gate control' theory was first proposed by Melzack and Wall in 1965. It describes how synaptic transmission between primary nociceptive neurones and secondary nociceptive neurones can be modulated or 'gated' by internuncial neurones. In particular, inhibitory interneurones in the substantia gelatinosa can exert presynaptic inhibition on primary afferent neurones and postsynaptic inhibition on secondary neurones, thus closing the 'gate' and decreasing the pain response to a nociceptive stimulus (Figure 19.20). These inhibitory interneurones may be activated by alternative non-nociceptive primary afferents (e.g. Aβ mechanoreceptor afferents). This enables activated pain fibres to be 'gated' out by other sensations, such as rubbing or pressure, applied to the affected area.

Examples of 'gating' at spinal level
- 'Rubbing a sore spot'
- Transcutaneous electrical nerve stimulation (TENS)
- Dorsal column electrodes

Descending modulatory system

Descending modulation of nociception is mediated by a network of pathways. It centres around an axis between the periaqueductal grey (PAG) region of the midbrain and the rostral ventromedial medulla (RVM).

The PAG is believed to be the main descending inhibitory control over nociception. It receives inputs from the hypothalamus, thalamus, limbic system and cortex and delivers its main projections to the RVM. The RVM is central in a network of medullary nuclei, and exerts

bidirectional control over nociceptive transmission in the dorsal horn via 'on' and 'off' cells (Figure 19.21).

The **descending pain modulatory system** consists of:

- The nucleus raphe magnus
- The locus coeruleus
- The dorsolateral pontine tegmentum
- The nucleus reticularis gigantocellularis

These components are illustrated in Figure 19.22.

Descending modulation therefore results from the integration of multiple inputs enabling diverse cerebral functions such as prediction, anticipation, affect and emotion, as well as the neuroendocrine axes and autonomic function, to modulate the intensity of pain. This concept has implications in the management of both acute and chronic pain conditions.

Neuromodulators in the pain system

The neurotransmitters in the pain system are outnumbered by families of neuromodulators, which suppress or enhance synaptic transmission in the pain system.

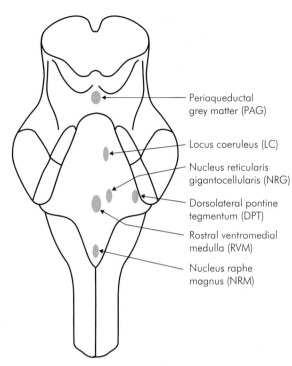

Figure 19.22 Components of the descending pain modulatory system

- Periaqueductal grey matter (PAG)
- Locus coeruleus (LC)
- Nucleus reticularis gigantocellularis (NRG)
- Dorsolateral pontine tegmentum (DPT)
- Rostral ventromedial medulla (RVM)
- Nucleus raphe magnus (NRM)

- Excitatory and inhibitory modulators operate in the primary synapses and are responsible for producing hyperalgesic states or analgesic states at the dorsal horn level.
- Different neuromodulators also act at the supraspinal level and ultimately enhance or suppress nociception in the dorsal horn via descending connections.
- Spinal and supraspinal interaction is important in determining the effect of some modulators.
- A modulator released supraspinally may have the opposite effect on nociception if released at the spinal level.
- Simultaneous excitation of spinal and supraspinal areas may be essential to produce some analgesic effects.

Thus the clinical effects of neuromodulators depend on their properties and location of action. Properties of some of the recognised neuromodulators in the pain system are summarised in Figure 19.23.

> **Families of neuromodulators** exist which up-regulate or down-regulate synaptic transmission in the pain system, forming the basis by which the intensity of pain is endogenously controlled.
> In the primary synapse, neuromodulators released by the descending pain modulatory system or by interneurones control the ascending pain signals to supraspinal centres.

Endogenous opioids

Endogenous opioids are peptides which are released supraspinally and spinally. They have a recognised inhibitory effect on the pain response and exert their effects by their selective affinities for a number of receptors. These receptors are the classically described μ, δ, κ receptors together with the more recently discovered ORL_1 ('opioid-receptor like') type.

The opioid receptors are G-protein-coupled receptors with seven transmembrane regions and six extracellular loops (Figure 19.24). When activated, they decrease neuronal excitability by inhibiting voltage-dependent sodium channels and activating potassium and calcium channels. Some properties of endogenous opioids are summarised in Figure 19.25.

Clinical aspects of pain

The complex nature of pain conditions has led to the introduction of different methods of characterising pain. Pain has been described by its

- Temporal variation – phasic, acute or chronic
- Physiological and pathological mechanisms
- Anatomical localisation
- Qualitative descriptors

Phasic pain, acute pain and chronic pain

A number of terms are applied as clinical descriptions of the course of pain symptoms.

Phasic pain

This term is used to describe the short-duration often high-intensity pain when the immediate impact of trauma or tissue injury is experienced. It is usually accompanied by reflex verbal or non-verbal (facial) expression, withdrawal or protective action.

Figure 19.23 Neuromodulators in the pain system

Neuromodulator	Location	Comments
Excitatory modulators – enhancing nociception		
Cholecystokinin 8	Dorsal horn Supraspinal centres – RVM	Endogenous antiopioid
Prostaglandins	Dorsal horn	Reduce the inhibitory action of glycine and cause hyperalgesia. Suggest a role for cyclo-oxygenase inhibitors in hyperalgesic conditions
Dynorphin 1–17	Dorsal horn	May be implicated in hyperalgesic and allodynic conditions
Orphanin FQ/ nociceptin	Supraspinal inhibition of opioid action	Endogenous agonist for ORL$_1$ receptor. Reverses opioid analgesia when released at supraspinal sites
Inhibitory modulators – suppressing nociception		
Opioids	Mesencephalon – PAG Basal ganglia – thalamus, amygdala Descending inhibitory pain system – locus coeruleus (LC) Dorsal horn – primary synapse	Some opioids may have excitatory effects producing hyperalgesic conditions. Analgesic effects may depend on synergistic concurrent action at two sites e.g. PAG and LC
Cannabinoids	Wide distribution of cannabinoid receptors (CB1 and CB2) in CNS, including limbic system, descending pain inhibitory system, thalamus and spinal cord	Analgesic effects of cannabinoids probably dependent on complex interaction between supraspinal and spinal sites
Orphanin FQ/ nociceptin	Dorsal horn inhibition	Gives analgesia when released at spinal sites
Acetylcholine	Dorsal horn inhibition	Inhibition of nociception mediated by muscarinic and nicotinic receptors in laminae I–II of the dorsal horn

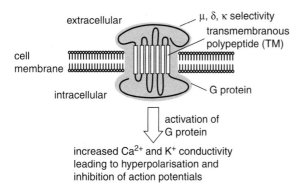

Figure 19.24 Opioid receptor

Acute pain

This is applied to the pain provoked by tissue damage; it consists of a phasic component of short duration and a tonic component which is of longer variable duration (hours to days). Acute pain occurs in the period initially following trauma or surgery.

Chronic pain

This is pain persisting beyond the period of time normally expected for healing and recovery from trauma or tissue injury. A chronic pain condition may therefore exist in the absence of active tissue injury or damage, and can be recognised as early as 6 weeks after trauma. Such

Figure 19.25 Summarising endogenous opioid receptor affinities

Opioid	Number of amino acids	Receptor affinity
Leu-enkephalin	5	$\delta > \kappa >> \mu$
Met-enkephalin	5	$\delta > \mu >> \kappa$
β-endorphin	30	$\delta = \mu >> \kappa$
Dynorphin	17	κ
Endomorphin 1	4	μ
Endomorphin 2	4	μ
Nociceptin	17	ORL_1

conditions, however, are usually diagnosed some months after a precipitating injury, and are frequently associated with depression, social and behavioural dysfunction as well as functional impairment. They may run a progressively deteriorating course over many years.

Chronic pain conditions

Some commonly recognised chronic pain conditions are outlined in Figure 19.26.

Physiological and pathological pain

Underlying mechanisms can be used to divide pain into:
- **Physiological (normal) pain** – occurring within the bounds of normal physiological function
- **Pathological (abnormal) pain** – pain outside the bounds of normal physiology

Physiological pain

This term describes pain caused by a noxious stimulus in the absence of actual tissue or nerve damage. Physiological pain therefore simply warns of impending injury, and can be described as *nociceptive*, warning of potential tissue damage (e.g. painful heat sensation without occurrence of burns). In physiological pain no sensitisation of the pain system occurs.

Examples of physiological pain include muscle cramp, tourniquet pain and abdominal colic.

Pathological pain

When tissue or nerve damage occurs, pain becomes pathological. Thus pathological pain may be classified as nociceptive or neuropathic. When tissue or nerve injury occurs, sensitisation of the pain system is mediated through the various mechanisms described above. An *adaptive* function of sensitisation is thought to be the optimisation of conditions for healing. Pain sensitisation may persist and pain may be experienced long after healing has occurred. This type of sensitisation is *mal-adaptive*. Sensitisation results in the clinical phenomena of hyperalgesia and allodynia.

Hyperalgesia

Hyperalgesia is an inevitable companion of injury, and can be defined as follows:

Hyperalgesia – a clinically used term describing the enhanced pain response resulting from sensitisation. It may arise from both peripheral and central mechanisms.

Primary hyperalgesia is localised in the zone of injury and occurs in response to both mechanical and thermal stimuli. Secondary hyperalgesia is produced in areas neighbouring the primary zone and only occurs in response to mechanical stimuli. It is contributed to by 'heterotopic sensitisation' (see *Sensitisation of the pain system*, above).

Two distinct forms of hyperalgesia are recognised, differing in the type of mechanical stimulus employed:
- *Punctate hyperalgesia* occurs in response to pressure from a fine probe (e.g. blunt pin) and is thought to be mediated by small-diameter nociceptive fibres.
- *Allodynia* (stroking hyperalgesia) is a hyperalgesic response to light stroking touch, and is mediated by low-threshold mechanoreceptors.

Hyperalgesia, allodynia and sensitisation

- Hyperalgesia describes the enhanced pain response resulting from sensitisation.
- Allodynia is a hyperalgesic response to light touch.
- Sensitisation is a neurophysiological term used to describe an enhanced nociceptor response (peripheral sensitisation) or an enhanced efficacy of the primary synapse in the dorsal horn (central sensitisation).

Figure 19.26 Common chronic pain conditions

Condition	Signs/symptoms
Complex regional pain syndrome Type I (reflex sympathetic dystrophy) – no nerve injury Type II (causalgia) – nerve injury	Accompanied by abnormal perfusion, localised oedema and abnormal sweating in the affected limb or area. Trophic changes in skin, hair and nails also occur. Impaired limb function is accompanied by muscle wasting and loss of bone density.
Trigeminal neuralgia	Unilateral severe shooting/stabbing pains in the territory of one branch of the trigeminal nerve. Background constant burning, gnawing pain may be present.
Phantom limb pain	Phantom sensations are felt by virtually all amputees. Severe pain only persists in 5–10%. Stump pain also develops in 5–10%. The role of pre-emptive analgesia is uncertain.
Post herpetic neuralgia	This pain syndrome follows shingles (herpes zoster infection). Peripheral sensitisation of nociceptors and central sensitisation of the dorsal horn occur. Hyperalgesia, allodynia and spontaneous pain result, together with numbness and loss of temperature sensation. Symptoms may persist for years.
Low back pain (LBP)	LBP affects a significant proportion of the population, but only 5–10% of these become chronic LBP sufferers. Serious consequences include reduction of individual quality of life, disability and socioeconomic costs. A specific underlying pathology can be found in only 10% of LBP patients.
Painful neuropathies	The most common cause of painful neuropathy is diabetes. Other causes include hypothyroidism, alcohol, beriberi and drug toxicity (isoniazid, cytotoxics). Distal symmetrical peripheral neuropathy is present, with associated numbness, paraesthesia, hyperalgesia and burning pain. Symptoms are often most distressing at night.

Neuropathic pain

The concept of pathological pain gives rise to the term *neuropathic pain*. Neuropathic pain is defined by the IASP as:

Pain initiated or caused by a primary lesion or dysfunction of the nervous system

Neuropathic pain does not necessarily imply physical damage or destruction of nerves but may be due to reorganisation or dysfunction of the intact nervous system. Most chronic pain conditions will have a significant neuropathic pain component.

Pain descriptors and localisation

Somatic pain occurs in structures such as skin, muscle and joints. Visceral pain occurs in internal organs. Consideration of the underlying mechanisms of these pains can be useful in their management.

Joint pain
- Inflammatory changes in the synovium, periosteum and surrounding capsule.
- Stretching and distortion of the periosteum.
- Inflammatory changes in tendons (tendinitis) and their insertions (enthesopathies).

Muscular pain
- Deep, intense, unpleasant sensation associated with ischaemic muscular damage.
- Localised tenderness with referred distribution of pain characteristic of myofascial 'trigger points'.
- Distributed diffuse tenderness and pain associated with chronic conditions such as fibromyalgia.

Visceral pain
- Diffuse and poorly localised because of sparse innervation and spread of spinal input over several segments.

- Convergence of spinal input with somatic afferents which leads to referred pain in somatic structures such as skin and muscle.
- Viscerovisceral convergence may also occur, leading to referred pain in neighbouring viscera and the diffuse nature of visceral pain.
- Associated with autonomic symptoms because visceral afferents often traverse prevertebral and paravertebral autonomic plexuses, giving rise to dual afferents.
- Stronger emotional and autonomic associations than with somatic pain.

Headache

- Primary neurovascular headaches caused by activation of the trigeminocervical complex by changes in intracranial vasculature, e.g. migraine and cluster headaches.
- Associated with head or neck trauma, e.g. whiplash involving myofascial trigger points in neck, cranial and shoulder musculature.
- Headache associated with raised intracranial pressure/intracranial infection involving mechanical or inflammatory meningeal irritation.
- Tension type headache is the most common type of headache. The underlying mechanism remains uncertain.

Qualitative descriptors of pain

Descriptors are commonly used by pain patients and may be suggestive of underlying mechanisms (Figure 19.27).

Psychology of pain

The supraspinal connections of the nociceptive system project via somatosensory and affective pathways to the cortex, limbic system and reticular formation. These projections not only affect the intensity of the pain experienced but also stimulate psychological responses, which include:

- An emotional response
- A cognitive reponse
- A behavioural response

These psychological processes are inextricably interwoven with the physiological process of nociception. They are important because they play a significant part in determining the intensity of pain perceived and the effect of pain on a patient's life, particularly in the context of chronic pain symptoms. Clinically, good management

Figure 19.27 Qualitative descriptors

Type of pain	Characteristics
Sharp pain	Localised, sharp sensation transmitted by Aδ fibres. Rapid-response pain
Dull pain/ aching	Diffuse, dull, intense sensation transmitted by C fibres. Slow-onset pain
Burning pain	Mediated by TRPV receptors on C and Aδ fibres
Pinprick	Mediated by Aδ fibres – mechano-heat sensitive nociceptors
Itching	A nocifensive sensation which provokes a characteristic scratch reflex. Is subject to peripheral and central sensitisation, as in chronic pain conditions.

of these psychological responses can not only reduce the intensity of pain symptoms but also help patients to reduce the impact of pain on their lives.

Emotional response

A person's emotional response can have a significant effect on physiological parameters as well as analgesic requirements in the context of acute pain. In chronic pain patients, the emotional response can often lead to long-term depression and anxiety, which can seriously affect their quality of life. Pain can produce the basic emotions of anxiety, fear, depression, anger and guilt. It is commonly believed that depression and anxiety not only accompany pain symptoms but also increase their intensity. Such a causal relationship remains controversial, but it is recognised that the treatment of depression and anxiety are an important part of pain management.

Cognitive response

The cognitive response refers to the information-processing functions of the brain and involves the interaction of variables such as a patient's pain beliefs, pain memories and degree of attention to pain symptoms. Maladaptive cognitive responses include catastrophising and lack of self-efficacy (low self-confidence). Use of the patient's cognitive responses to produce coping strategies is a useful part of a pain management programme.

Behavioural response

This refers to the learned patterns of behaviour resulting from the emotional and cognitive responses. Behavioural responses can be adaptive or maladaptive, producing either a beneficial or a detrimental effect on a patient's quality of life. Manipulation of behavioural responses may be useful in managing patients with chronic pain.

Pain management

The management of pain is multidisciplinary, corresponding to the multiple physiological and psychological mechanisms which determine the intensity of pain experienced.

In the clinical setting, pain management divides into acute pain and chronic pain management. Acute pain usually focuses on postoperative pain, and is increasingly being managed outside the recovery room by an acute pain team. Chronic pain on the other hand is managed by the multidisciplinary team of a pain management service, which will operate through pain clinics, day-case procedure lists, specialist nurse-led clinics and a pain management programme.

Acute (postoperative) pain management

The mechanisms underlying acute pain are mainly those of nociception, with a limited degree of sensitisation peripherally and centrally. Supraspinal effects are minimal, with anxiety and fear contributing to the pain experienced to a limited extent. Pain management techniques rely on modifying the nociceptive process and involve the use of drugs administered by the oral and parenteral routes together with local anaesthetic techniques.

Chronic pain management

In chronic pain conditions, the effect of central sensitisation at the dorsal horn level, and of supraspinal mechanisms, is more pronounced. A multidisciplinary team is essential, and pain management may involve multiple inputs in order to achieve a satisfactory result. The approaches used may include:

- Pharmacology
- Local anaesthetic techniques
- Physiotherapy
- Complementary therapies
- Psychological techniques

Pharmacology

The range of drugs used in the pharmacological approach to chronic pain management reflects the diverse physiological factors that determine chronic pain levels. Many exert their effects by multiple actions. They include those listed in Figure 19.28.

Local anaesthetic techniques

These methods include spinoaxial blockade, peripheral nerve blocks and sympathetic blockade. In some cases neurolytic blockade may be useful, either with a chemical agent such as phenol or using radiofrequency (RF) lesioning.

Physiotherapy

Physiotherapy remains an essential component of chronic pain management. It reduces pain levels and improves function. In order to reduce pain, physiotherapy employs techniques such as massage and manipulation, injections, acupuncture and acupressure, ultrasound and the application of heat and ice. Active management of rehabilitation is crucial in minimising the impact of injury and pain on a patient's life, and is a major part of the physiotherapist's role.

Complementary techniques

These methods include:

- Osteopathy – a system of medicine based on the principle that many disease conditions can be improved by musculoskeletal manipulation, which reverses dislocations and malalignments in the body's musculoskeletal framework, thus allowing the body to heal itself. This is essentially a holistic approach to the patient.
- Chiropractic – an alternative system of treatment by musculoskeletal manipulation which focuses on treating 'subluxations' and 'malpositioning' of vertebral segments in order to allow the body to heal itself. In common with osteopathy, chiropractic is also a holistic approach to the patient.
- Acupuncture – has been imported from traditional Chinese medicine and is based on restoring the flow of 'chi' (interpreted as 'energy') through a system of 14 meridians in the body by dry needling. The success of acupuncture has led to extensive research into its mechanisms over the past 30 years or more but the picture still remains incomplete, although endorphin release is believed to form an integral part of the process.

Figure 19.28 Some useful drugs in chronic pain management

Type of drug	Example	Comment
Opioids	Morphine, oxycodone, buprenorphine	Action by opioid receptors
Non-steroidal analgesics	Ibuprofen, diclofenac, celecoxib	Ibuprofen and diclofenac are non-selective COX inhibitors Celecoxib is a selective COX-2 inhibitor
Tricyclic antidepressants	Amitriptyline, imipramine	Inhibit presynaptic uptake of serotonin and noradrenaline in descending inhibitory system Block sodium and calcium ion channels Block postsynaptic muscarinic and histamine receptors
Anticonvulsants	Carbamazepine, phenytoin	Both block voltage-dependent sodium channels Carbamazepine also has serotonergic effects
GABA mimetics	Gabapentin, pregabalin	Increase GABA concentrations in some areas of the brain Modulation of voltage-gated calcium channels
Antispasmodics	Buscopan, baclofen	Both relax smooth muscle spasm Baclofen also decreases skeletal muscle tone
Anxiolytics	Diazepam, temazepam	Also relax skeletal muscle spasm
α_2-Agonists	Clonidine, tizanadine	Systemic effect in reducing neuropathic pain Local effect, reducing allodynia
NMDA antagonists	Ketamine	Has been used to treat chronic pain state by infusion
Combination	Tramadol	Opioid action, and increases serotonin and noradrenaline activities in the descending inhibitory system

- Reflexology – a system of treating patients by stimulating nerves on the feet, hands, and ears. Again the practitioners operate on the basis of restoring balance to the flow of 'chi' in the patient's body. It is believed that the body has a topographical representation over the soles of the feet, as well as on the hands and the ears.
- Homeopathy – a holistic system of medicine based on treating 'like with like', using medicines in which the active ingredient has been diluted to virtually undetectable levels. The active ingredient if given in adequate concentrations is thought to reproduce the original patient's symptoms. The dilution process producing the medicines involves vigorous shaking of the solutions ('succussion') which is thought to leave an 'imprint' of the solute molecules in the aqueous solution. Homeopathy is generally accepted as being a safe form of treatment and is compatible with other forms of therapy, but mechanisms of action remain unproven.

The underlying mechanisms of complementary therapies remain uncertain, but they may succeed in cases where other therapies fail. Although such complementary therapies are accepted by many workers in chronic pain management, their use remains controversial due to difficulties in evaluating their effects objectively. The possibility of the placebo effect being the primary underlying mechanism is questioned by the successful application of many of these techniques in veterinary practice.

Psychological techniques and pain management programmes

Clinical psychologists are an integral part of the pain management team. As seen throughout this chapter, pain levels are influenced significantly by the activity of cortical centres and the limbic system. Psychological techniques have long been recognised as playing an important part in helping patients to cope with chronic pain symptoms. This is particularly so in the context of pain management programmes, which provide a structured course of training for patients in psychological and physical methods.

CHAPTER 20

Gastrointestinal physiology

Matthew Faulds and Nick Morgan-Hughes

The gastrointestinal (GI) tract extends from the mouth to the anus. It represents a series of organs with specialised roles, motor patterns and secretory functions. Its primary purpose is the absorption of water and nutrients. Food is moved along its length and mixed with secretions that aid digestion. Nutrients are absorbed across the gut wall and waste products and indigestible residue excreted as faeces.

Gastrointestinal motility

For most of its length the GI tract has three layers of smooth muscle: the outer longitudinal layer, the middle circular layer and the inner submucosal layer. The enteric nervous system (ENS) comprises the myenteric plexus located between circular and longitudinal layers and the submucosal plexus found between circular and submucosal layers (Figure 20.1).

Patterns of motility
Basal electrical rhythm (BER)

Distal to the oesophagus, smooth muscle cells exhibit spontaneous variations in transmembrane potential, between −70 and −40 mV, termed basal electrical rhythm (BER). This rhythm is controlled by the interstitial cells of Cajal, pacemaker cells with an intrinsic frequency. As in the myocardium, the pacemaker with the highest frequency dominates.

BER determines the maximum rate at which contractions can occur. When the transmembrane potential crosses the threshold voltage, approximately −40 mV, ion channels open. The resultant influx of sodium and calcium ions is seen as spike-burst activity, and this is associated with smooth muscle contraction (Figure 20.2). Gap junctions between neighbouring cells allow electrical activity to propagate such that smooth muscle cells act as a syncytium and contract in a coordinated manner.

The frequency and amplitude of BER varies along the bowel and is modulated by nervous system control, hormones and drugs. Acetylcholine stimulates contraction by raising the cell membrane potential, thus increasing spike-burst activity. Conversely, adrenaline is inhibitory, hyperpolarising the cell membrane and reducing spike-burst activity.

> **Basal electrical rhythm (BER)** determines the maximum rate at which contractions can occur. The frequency and amplitude of BER varies along the bowel and is modulated by nervous system control, hormones and drugs.

Peristalsis

Peristalsis is a reflex response to gut wall stretch that occurs throughout the GI tract. When luminal contents

Fundamentals of Anaesthesia, 4th edition, ed. Ted Lin, Tim Smith and Colin Pinnock. Published by Cambridge University Press. © Cambridge University Press 2017.

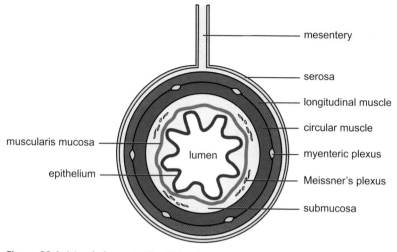

mesentery

serosa

longitudinal muscle

circular muscle

muscularis mucosa

myenteric plexus

lumen

epithelium

Meissner's plexus

submucosa

Figure 20.1 Muscle layers in the GI tract

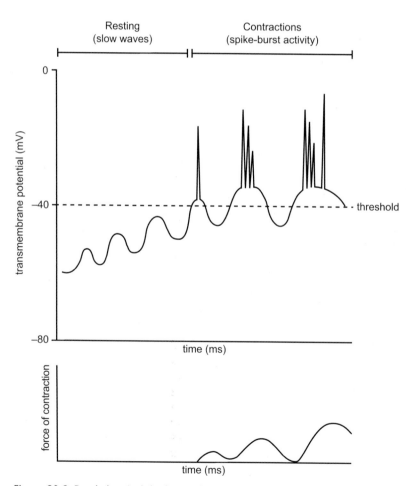

Figure 20.2 Basal electrical rhythm without and with spike potentials and relationship to muscular contraction

stretch the wall, a contraction forms behind that point and a relaxation is generated in front of it. Contents are then moved along the bowel by a wave of radially symmetrical contraction and relaxation of smooth muscle, similar to the mechanism used by earthworms to drive locomotion. It is a manifestation of two reflexes within the enteric nervous system (ENS). Mechanical distension stimulates afferent enteric neurones which synapse with two sets of interneurones. One group of interneurones activates excitatory motor neurones proximal to the bolus and stimulates contraction of smooth muscle. The other group of interneurones activates inhibitory motor neurones that stimulate relaxation of smooth muscle beyond the bolus.

Regulation mechanisms

Gut motility is modulated by neural and chemical control mechanisms which are complex and often work simultaneously on secretory function (Figure 20.3). Several gut reflexes, such as peristalsis, rely on the integrity of the myenteric plexus and although modulated by extrinsic nerve supply will continue in isolated bowel. Extrinsic neural input is predominantly involuntary via the autonomic nervous system through sympathetic and parasympathetic fibres. Somatic (voluntary) control is present only during the initial stages of swallowing and in external anal sphincter control of defecation.

Swallowing

Swallowing moves food from the mouth to the stomach without aspiration into the trachea. It is a reflex with voluntary and involuntary components which cannot be interrupted once initiated. Swallowing is coordinated by the swallowing centre located in the reticular system of the medulla and lower pons. This receives sensory inputs from the trigeminal, glossopharyngeal, superior laryngeal, recurrent laryngeal and vagus nerves, with motor efferents mainly carried by the vagus.

Oral stage

The oral or voluntary stage is the only part of the swallowing reflex where conscious control is possible. Masticated food is pushed into the pharynx by upward and backward pressure of the tongue against the hard palate.

Pharyngeal stage

Sensory receptors on the tonsillar pillars detect pressure from the food bolus and transmit signals to the swallowing centre, which then initiates the involuntary stages of the swallowing reflex. The soft palate is elevated, closing off the nasopharynx, and respiration is halted. The vocal cords are closed and the larynx moves anteriorly and cephalad, allowing the epiglottis to cover the glottis. This movement opens the upper oesophagus and contributes to upper oesophageal sphincter relaxation. The superior constrictor muscle of the pharynx initiates a wave of smooth muscle contraction that propels the bolus into the oesophagus.

Oesophageal stage

The primary peristaltic wave started in the pharynx moves the food bolus down the oesophagus where lower oesophageal sphincter (LOS) relaxation allows entry to the stomach. If primary peristalsis fails, secondary peristalsis is initiated by the continued stimulation of oesophageal stretch receptors.

Figure 20.3 Autonomic nervous supply to the GI tract

Modality	Nerves/ganglia	Sensory afferents	Secretomotor efferents	Motor efferents
Parasympathetic	Vagus and sacral fibres; preganglionic	Pain, distention, toxins	↑ gastrin ↑ salivary production ↑ pancreatic and bile secretion	↑ motility ↑ tone ↑ force of contraction ↑ gastric emptying
Sympathetic	Coeliac, mesenteric and pelvic ganglia; postganglionic	Pain, distention	↑ salivary production	↓ motility ↓ gastric emptying vasoconstriction

Oesophagus

The oesophagus is 30 cm long in the adult and has upper and lower sphincters. The oesophagus differs from the rest of the GI tract in that the upper 6 cm consists of striated skeletal muscle with no spontaneous contractile activity.

The upper oesophageal sphincter consists of the cricopharyngeal and pharyngeal constrictor muscles. It is innervated by the vagus and is usually in a state of tonic contraction to prevent entrainment of air during respiration.

The lower oesophageal sphincter (LOS) is a functional zone of increased intraluminal pressure in the lower 2–4 cm of the oesophagus (Figure 20.4). The intrinsic component of the LOS is formed from semicircular oesophageal muscle fibres on the left and gastric sling fibres on the right. The external component is formed from the crural diaphragm. The LOS is usually closed but briefly relaxes during swallowing to allow the bolus to pass into the stomach.

Barrier pressure

Barrier pressure is the pressure difference between the LOS and the intragastric pressure, normally 15–25 mmHg. When there is a fall in LOS tone or an increase in intragastric pressure, reflux of stomach contents into the oesophagus can occur, which encourages regurgitation, the passive transit of gastric contents into the pharynx (Figure 20.5). The acute angle where the oesophagus joins the stomach and the encircling diaphragmatic muscle results in a flutter-valve action below the diaphragm that helps to prevent reflux when intragastric pressure is raised.

Stomach

The stomach has three main types of contraction. Firstly, during the 'fed' state, the proximal stomach (fundus and upper body) exhibits slow sustained contractions that generate a basal intragastric pressure facilitating gastric emptying. As food enters the stomach the proximal stomach relaxes, minimising any further increase in intragastric pressure (receptive relaxation). Secondly there are rhythmic synchronised contractions in the lower part of the stomach (antral systole) which mix food with acid, mucus and pepsin, grinding it down to a fine paste called chyme. Chyme splashes against a contracted pyloric sphincter which allows the controlled passage of liquid and small food particles into the duodenum. Thirdly, between meals, there are occasional bursts of very strong, synchronised contraction that are accompanied by opening of the pyloric sphincter. These are called 'housekeeper' waves because their function is to sweep any indigestible material out of the stomach. They are initiated by motilin and halted by eating.

Gastric emptying

The pylorus does not close completely during antral systole, and small amounts of liquid chyme are squirted into the duodenum with each contraction. This emptying is regulated to optimise small bowel performance via complex control mechanisms. Gastric emptying is reduced with pain, anxiety and stress mediated by activation of the sympathetic nervous system. Distension of the stomach leads to the stimulation of vagal and local enteric reflexes and the release of gastrin. As a result there is increased secretion of acid and antral peristaltic activity, thereby increasing gastric emptying and the production of chyme.

The composition of the chyme reaching the duodenum also regulates gastric emptying. If the stomach empties too quickly, duodenal receptors may be activated by stretch, increasing acidity, osmolarity or concentration of fatty or amino acids. This initiates reflex arcs that reduce gastric emptying. As a result, carbohydrate-rich meals leave the stomach within a few hours, protein more slowly, and fatty food the slowest.

If small bowel contents rich in fat reach the ileum, an inhibitory reflex termed the 'ileal brake' reduces gastric emptying, pancreatic secretion and small bowel transit to improve digestion and absorption. This is hormonally mediated by peptide YY.

Small and large bowel

The small bowel is around 5 m long in the adult. Several motility patterns occur which contribute to transit times that are longer in the fed state compared with the fasted state, thus encouraging absorption.

The large bowel is important for absorption of water and electrolytes, the production of vitamins such as vitamin K by colonic bacteria, and the storage of faeces. The motility characteristics of the colon maximise contact with the mucosa and facilitate mass movement for defecation.

Secretory functions

Salivary glands

The three paired salivary glands produce 0.5–1.5 L of saliva a day. The constituents include water, mucus, digestive enzymes and electrolytes.

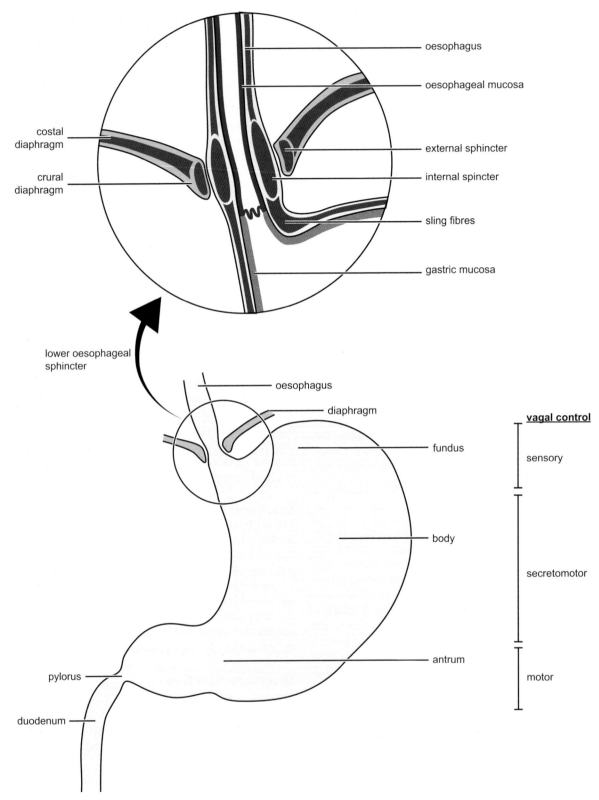

Figure 20.4 The lower oesophageal sphincter and the stomach

Figure 20.5 Factors and drugs affecting LOS tone

Increased LOS tone	Decreased LOS tone
Cholinergic stimulation (suxamethonium, neostigmine) Dopaminergic inhibition (metoclopramide, prochlorperazine) Gastrin α-adrenergic stimulation β-adrenergic blockade Motilin Prostaglandin F_2 Cyclizine	Antimuscarinics (atropine, glycopyrrolate) Dopamine Cholecystokinin α-adrenergic blockade β-adrenergic stimulation Secretin Prostaglandin E_1 Thiopental Alcohol

Figure 20.6 Glandular cell types in the stomach

Cell types	Location	Secretion
Mucous (surface and neck)	Throughout stomach	Mucus and bicarbonate
Parietal (oxyntic)	Body and fundus	Hydrochloric acid and intrinsic factor
Chief (peptic)	Body and fundus	Pepsinogens and gastric lipase
G cells	Antrum	Gastrin
D cells	Distal antrum	Somatostatin
Enterochromaffin-like cells	Fundus	Histamine

Functions of saliva

- Lubrication to aid swallowing and speech
- Solvent for molecule transfer to taste buds
- Buffering and dilution of irritants
- Antimicrobial properties
- Digestion of starch by salivary amylase
- Digestion of fats by salivary lipase

Gastric secretion

The stomach secretes about 1.2–2.5 L of gastric juice a day and maintains a pH between 1 and 3.5. Numerous pits in the mucosal surface, around 100 gastric pits mm^{-2}, are connected to a variety of secretory glands depending on location in the stomach (Figure 20.6).

Functions of gastric secretions

- Aid protein digestion
- Activate pepsinogen to pepsin
- Provide optimal pepsin pH
- Improve solubility of dietary iron
- Antimicrobial activity
- Stimulate biliary and pancreatic secretions

Constituents of gastric secretion
Hydrochloric acid

Gastric acid is secreted from the apical surface of parietal cells via an $H^+K^+ATPase$ (proton pump). Gastrin, acetylcholine and histamine stimulate acid secretion via gastrin, M_1 muscarinic and H_2 histamine receptors located on the basolateral parietal cell membrane (Figure 20.7). Acid secretion generates bicarbonate, which moves into the gastric venous blood in sufficient amounts to produce alkaline urine (the alkaline tide). H^+ ions are produced by the action of carbonic anhydrase on water and CO_2. At times of peak acid production net gastric consumption of CO_2 gives the stomach a negative respiratory quotient.

Pepsinogens

Pepsinogens are pro-enzymes which are converted to the active enzyme, pepsin, in acid conditions. Pepsinogens are stored in secretory granules within the chief cells and are released from the apical membrane. Stimuli that activate acid secretion also stimulate pepsin secretion.

Mucus

Mucus is secreted from the entire mucosa and consists of complex glycoproteins mixed with water, electrolytes and sloughed cells. In the normal stomach, the epithelium is covered by a thin layer of mucus that is continually eroded and replaced. Stimulation from the vagus, gastrin and prostaglandin E_2 and I_2 increases production of mucus. Failure of the mucus barrier or hypersecretion of acid can result in ulceration.

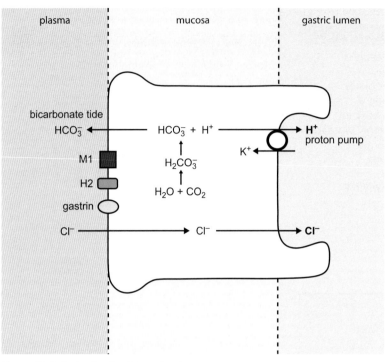

Figure 20.7 Parietal cell acid production

Intrinsic factor

Intrinsic factor is a glycoprotein secreted by parietal cells and is essential for the absorption of vitamin B_{12} in the terminal ileum.

Phases of gastric secretion

During fasting there is very little gastric secretion and the volume of the stomach may be as low as 30 mL. However, food ingestion rapidly increases secretion in three phases:

- **Cephalic** – triggered by the anticipation, sight, taste or smell of food and contributes around 30% of gastric secretions. Vagal stimulation increases gastric motility and causes the release of gastrin and histamine, thereby leading to increased gastric acid production.
- **Gastric** – lasting around 30 minutes and resulting in 60% of secretions. Stomach distension or an increase in luminal peptides promotes local and vagal reflexes which release gastrin and therefore increase acid secretion. When the pH reaches 2.0, acid secretion is stopped by somatostatin.
- **Intestinal** – the intestinal phase is inhibitory and only adds 10% of gastric secretions. When chyme reaches the duodenum many feedback mechanisms including

the release of somatostatin inhibit gastric secretions. There is also a decrease in stimulatory factors.

Pancreatic secretion
Pancreatic juice

Normally the pancreas produces about 1500 mL a day of alkaline fluid containing inactive pro-enzymes. The pro-enzymes are stored in zymogen granules in the cells of the exocrine pancreas before being released into the pancreatic ducts (Figure 20.8).

Control of pancreatic secretion

Pancreatic secretory patterns are closely related to food ingestion and dietary content. Control is predominantly hormonal via two main secretory hormones with additional neural input. Somatostatin reduces exocrine secretions (Figure 20.9).

Biliary secretion
Bile

The liver produces 500–1000 mL of bile a day, of which 30–60 mL can be stored and concentrated in the gallbladder.

Figure 20.8 Examples of pancreatic enzymes and their substrates

Enzyme	Pro-enzyme	Activator	Substrate
Trypsin	Trypsinogen	Enteropeptidase, trypsin	Protein and polypeptides
Chymotrypsin	Chymotrypsinogen	Trypsin	Protein and polypeptides
Carboxypeptidase	Procarboxypeptidase	Trypsin	Protein and polypeptides
Phospholipase A_2	Pro-phospholipase A_2	Trypsin	Ribonucleic and deoxyribonucleic acids
Elastase	Proelastase	Trypsin	Elastin
Pancreatic amylase	–	Chloride	Carbohydrates
Pancreatic lipase	–	–	Triglycerides

Figure 20.9 Control of biliary and pancreatic secretion

Agent	Production	Stimulus	Pancreatic effect	Biliary effect
Secretin	S cells in upper small intestine	Acid in duodenum	Production of bicarbonate-rich fluid; augments CCK	Production of watery, bicarbonate-rich bile
Cholecystokinin (CCK)	Duodenal mucosa	Amino acids, peptides and fats	Release of zymogen granules via phospholipase C	Gallbladder contraction and relaxation of the sphincter of Oddi
Acetylcholine	Vagus	Cephalic phase of secretion	Similar to CCK	Gallbladder contraction (Sphincter of Oddi relaxation via NO/VIP)
Bile salts	Liver and enterohepatic circulation	Increasing concentrations of bile salts in portal circulation	–	Potent choleretic – increases secretion of bile

Bile is a solution of bile salts, pigments and other organic and inorganic compounds. Bile salts emulsify fats by decreasing their surface tension. The daily production and reserves of bile salts are low, with a total pool of around 3.5 g. Recycling of bile salts via the enterohepatic circulation is essential, with the entire pool being recirculated twice per meal.

Control of biliary secretion

Like pancreatic secretion, biliary secretion is related to diet and feeding. Eating causes relaxation of the sphincter of Oddi and initial gallbladder contraction via the vagus. There are also ENS reflexes that stimulate gallbladder contraction in response to gastric distension. Further control is modulated by hormones and bile salts (Figure 20.9).

Digestion and absorption

Digestion is the chemical breakdown of ingested food by enzymes into smaller units that can then be absorbed from the intestines into the lymph or blood. The majority of these processes occur across the large surface area of the small intestine.

Carbohydrate

Carbohydrates are only absorbed in the small bowel and must be broken down into one of three monosaccharides: glucose, galactose or fructose.

Glucose and galactose are actively absorbed via the type 1 sodium-dependent glucose co-transporter (SGLT1).

Fructose undergoes facilitated absorption via the type 5 glucose transporter (GLUT5). Fructose absorption is increased in the presence of glucose, with a maximum absorption of up to $50 \, g \, h^{-1}$, around half the maximum for glucose at $100 \, g \, h^{-1}$. This 1-to-2 absorption ratio is recognised by some manufacturers of sport energy drinks. The

majority of monosaccharides are produced by the action of small bowel brush border enzymes, which have a huge functional reserve to cope with variations in diet (Figure 20.10).

Cellulose is a complex polysaccharide with β-glucose linkages indigestible to human enzymes and therefore forms dietary fibre.

Protein

Ingested proteins are initially broken down by stomach pepsins to smaller polypeptides. More powerful pancreatic and brush border enzymes in the small intestine produce absorbable peptides and amino acids. Epithelial cells of the small intestine absorb these products, with the peptides further hydrolysed by intracellular peptidases. This system is extremely efficient, with only 2–5% of protein escaping absorption (Figure 20.11).

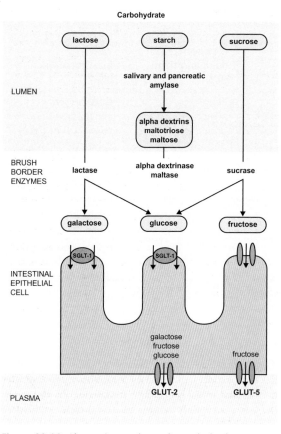

Figure 20.10 Absorption pathway for carbohydrate

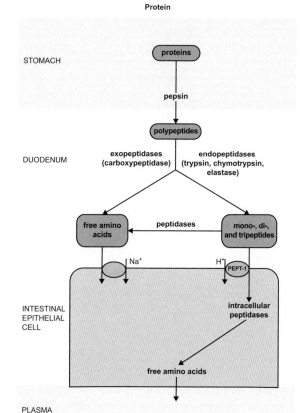

Figure 20.11 Absorption pathway for protein

Lipid

95% of dietary fat is absorbed in the adult. The majority of this fat is triglyceride. The predominant enzyme acting on fat is pancreatic lipase, which hydrolyses triglycerides to free fatty acids and monoglycerides in the duodenum.

Bile salts emulsify the relatively insoluble fats, bringing them into contact with the water-soluble lipases. The subsequently released free fatty acids and monoglycerides combine with the bile salts to form water-soluble lipid aggregates called micelles. Phospholipids are metabolised by pancreatic phospholipase A_2 to free fatty acids and lysophospholipids, which are taken up into micelles. Micelles then fuse with the epithelial cells. Small free fatty acids are actively transported directly into the circulation but larger free fatty acids and monoglycerides are re-esterified into triglycerides, which are then incorporated into large lipoproteins called chylomicrons consisting of a hydrophobic core and a hydrophilic shell. The chylomicrons enter the extracellular fluid by pinocytosis and then pass into the lymphatic system (Figure 20.12).

Digestion

- Carbohydrates are absorbed as monosaccharides in the small bowel.
- Proteins are absorbed as small polypeptides in the small bowel.
- Lipids are primarily absorbed as micelles containing triglycerides, monoglycerides and free fatty acids.

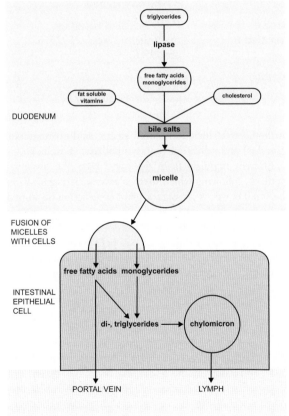

Figure 20.12 Absorption pathway for lipids

Fluid and electrolytes
Water absorption

A large volume of water, up to 10 L, is handled by the intestine each day yet only 200 mL is excreted in the faeces, the majority being absorbed in the small intestine and about 1500 mL in the colon. Water moves freely in and out of the intestine along osmotic gradients driven by solute absorption, particularly sodium and glucose.

Sodium and chloride

The intestine absorbs 25–35 g sodium a day, which accounts for about 15% of the total body sodium. Most of this sodium is reabsorbed from intestinal secretions, with dietary sodium contributing about 5–8 g. Chloride ions are absorbed throughout the intestine.

In addition to its renal effects, the mineralocorticoid aldosterone has effects on sodium and water absorption in the intestine, particularly the colon. Aldosterone increases the number of sodium channels on the epithelium and the number of Na^+K^+ pumps on the basolateral membrane, therefore increasing sodium and water absorption.

Vitamins and minerals

The absorption of the fat-soluble vitamins depends on bile salts and micelle uptake. Water-soluble vitamins and minerals are absorbed in a variety of ways (Figure 20.13).

Figure 20.13 Absorption of water-soluble vitamins and selected minerals

Substance	Site	Mechanism	Special information
Water-soluble vitamins (6 out of 9)	Proximal small bowel	Sodium co-transport	–
Vitamin C	Small bowel	Active and passive transport	–
Folic acid	Whole small bowel	Active, sodium-independent transport	–
Vitamin B$_{12}$	Terminal ileum	Active, sodium-independent transport (pinocytosis)	Cofactors: R-factor in stomach; **intrinsic factor** in duodenum
Iron	Duodenum and jejunum	Pinocytosis	Gastric secretions dissolve dietary iron; 3–6% absorbed
Calcium	Duodenum	Active and passive transport; facilitated by protein	Regulated by 1,25-dihydroxycholecalciferol; 30–80% absorbed
Magnesium	Small and large bowel	Active and passive transport; facilitated by protein	Finely adjusted based on magnesium status; 25–75% absorbed
Trace elements (zinc, selenium etc.)	Small bowel	Active and passive transport	

Nausea and vomiting

Nausea is an unpleasant sensation associated with the impulse to vomit. Physiologically, nausea is preparation for the act of vomiting, which is the active and forceful expulsion of the contents of the upper GI tract. It is a reflex coordinated by the vomiting centre, which is not one discrete area but rather a number of interconnected areas in the brainstem receiving input from a wide range of stimuli and pathways (Figure 20.14).

Vomiting reflex

Once sensory input to the vomiting centre reaches a threshold, the vomiting reflex is activated, coordinating GI, respiratory, cardiovascular, somatic and autonomic nervous systems. The reflex can be divided into two phases, pre-ejection and ejection.

Pre-ejection

Pre-ejection begins with the sensation of nausea followed by signs of sympathetic up-regulation. Secretory changes in the GI tract include reduced gastric acid (sympathetic stimulus) and salivation (parasympathetic stimulus).

Efferent impulses from the vagus relax the proximal stomach, following which there is reverse peristalsis from the small bowel. A retrograde giant contraction beginning in the mid-small intestine propels small bowel contents back into the stomach in preparation for ejection.

Simultaneous to the reverse peristalsis, the upper airway is prepared for vomiting with protective measures including a deep inspiratory breath and closure of the glottis.

Ejection

Ejection is often preceded by retching. The initial phase of ejection is identical to retching and involves synchronised contraction of the abdominal wall and diaphragm to produce a rapid rise in intra-abdominal pressure. When retching, the peri-oesophageal diaphragm contracts, compressing the oesophagus tightly and preventing reflux of gastric contents into the oesophagus. With ejection this

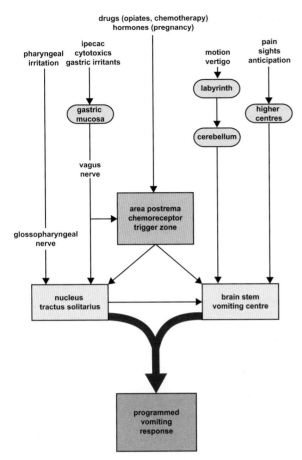

Figure 20.14 Causes of nausea and vomiting

area of the diaphragm relaxes, the stomach empties into the oesophagus and vomit is expelled out of the mouth. Respiration temporarily ceases, to further protect the airway from aspiration.

References and further reading

Barrett KE, Barman SM, Boitano S, *et al. Ganong's Review of Medical Physiology*, 24th edn. New York: McGraw-Hill, 2012.

Jentjens RLPG, Moseley L, Waring RH, Harding LK, Jeukendrup AE. Oxidation of combined ingestion of glucose and fructose during exercise. *J Appl Physiol* 2004; **96**: 1277–84.

Jolliffe DM. Practical gastric physiology. *Contin Educ Anaesth Crit Care Pain* 2009; **9**: 173–7.

Levy DM. Pre-operative fasting: 60 years on from Mendelson. *Contin Educ Anaesth Crit Care Pain* 2006; **6**: 215–18.

CHAPTER 21
Metabolism and temperature regulation

Smita Gohil and Ted Lin

Nutrition

Food provides basic energy requirements, and provides the structural building blocks to maintain metabolic integrity.

> **Nutrients**
>
> A normal diet consists of six classes of nutrient: carbohydrates, proteins, fats, water, vitamins and minerals.

Nutritional status may be assessed by measurement of skin-fold thickness with callipers (the area overlying the triceps muscle is often used) or by calculation of the body mass index (BMI). BMI is obtained by dividing weight (kg) by the square of the height (m^2). Values between 20 and 24 are normal, with > 30 indicating obesity and > 40 severe obesity. BMI is also called Quetelet's test after Adolphe Quetelet (1796–1874), a Belgian mathematician who came up with the concept of the 'average' man.

The average calorific requirement for 24 hours in a fit 70 kg man is about 2000 kcal to meet basal demands, and 500–2500 kcal more depending on occupation. In a balanced diet, approximately 55% of energy is derived from carbohydrates, 15% from protein and 30% from fat.

Fundamentals of Anaesthesia, 4th edition, ed. Ted Lin, Tim Smith and Colin Pinnock. Published by Cambridge University Press. © Cambridge University Press 2017.

Carbohydrates

Dietary carbohydrates may be in the form of simple or complex carbohydrates. Complex carbohydrates, mainly plant starches, are acted upon by salivary amylase to produce oligosaccharides. The intestinal mucosa secretes maltase, lactase and sucrase to complete the conversion of these oligosaccharides to simple hexoses. The products of carbohydrate digestion are rapidly absorbed in the small intestine. Pentoses are absorbed by diffusion, although glucose utilises a sodium-driven active transport mechanism, with a limit of around 120 g per hour. The average daily requirement of carbohydrate for an adult is between 5 and 10 $g\,kg^{-1}$.

Proteins

Dietary proteins may be classed as grade I (containing all the essential amino acids, usually of animal origin) and grade II (lacking one or more of the essential amino acids, almost always of plant origin). Essential amino acids are not more important than others, but cannot be created de novo in the body and therefore must be included in the diet.

Pepsin in the stomach and trypsin and chymotrypsin in the small intestine break down protein into peptides. The peptides are then further degraded to free amino acids by peptidases in the small intestine, where they are absorbed. The average daily requirement of protein is 0.5–1 $g\,kg^{-1}$; however, newborns require about five times as much protein for growth. Amino acids are used to produce new protein or replace damaged protein. Excess amino acids can be converted to glucose through gluconeogenesis. Since there is no storage provision for protein or amino acids the surplus is excreted in the urine.

Lipids

Dietary lipids are usually in the form of neutral fats (fatty acids condensed with glycerol to produce an uncharged triglyceride) but may also include phospholipids and cholesterol. Ingested fats are digested by pancreatic lipase to produce free fatty acids (FFAs), mono- and diglycerides. These are absorbed by simple diffusion, and reconstituted within the mucosal cell. Some lipid crosses the mucosal barrier by uptake as small lipid micelles. Reformed triglycerides, carrier proteins, phospholipids and cholesterol are then combined as chylomicrons. The average intake of fat in the diet is 1–2 $g\,kg^{-1}$, although much lower intakes are well tolerated. A small percentage of the lipid intake must consist of essential fatty acids, which cannot be synthesised by the body. These include linoleic, linolenic and arachidonic acids.

Vitamins and minerals

Vitamins are organic molecules essential for life, but which can no longer be synthesised by higher organisms. Vitamins are only required in small amounts, but fulfil key functions. They are divided loosely into the water-soluble (C, B complex) and fat-soluble vitamins (A, D, E and K). The latter are poorly absorbed in the absence of bile or pancreatic lipase.

Minerals are single elements also essential to life. They include calcium, phosphorus, magnesium, zinc, iron and iodine, all of which have minimal recommended daily intakes for an adult.

In addition, there are also minute quantities of other elements essential to life, such as copper, cobalt, manganese, nickel, molybdenum and chromium, which are known as trace elements.

Deficiencies of vitamins or minerals can produce a wide range of clinical syndromes. Some of these are outlined in Figure 21.1.

Energy balance

Energy in the body is obtained by breaking down the larger molecules of digested food or alternatively using stored carbohydrate, fat or protein from body reserves. The degradation of these larger molecules is referred to as catabolism, and it is accompanied by the release of energy as the chemical bonds are broken. The energy released is either used to perform work or appears as heat. Approximately 60% of the energy released during catabolism appears as heat; only 40% produces useful work. The work done may be external work, such as that performed by skeletal muscles. Alternatively, internal work may be done, either mechanically, as in cardiac contraction, or biochemically, in the synthesis of larger molecules and high-energy compounds such as adenosine triphosphate (ATP). Cellular processes, such as the active transport of substances across membranes and mucosa, also use energy internally.

Energy balance

The energy balance in the body can be summarised as:

Total energy expenditure = Heat produced by the body
+ External work done
+ Internal work done
+ Energy stored

Figure 21.1 Vitamin and mineral deficiencies

Substance	Function or coenzyme derivative	Deficiency
Water-soluble vitamins		
Vitamin C (ascorbic acid)	Antioxidant maintaining collagen integrity	Scurvy
Vitamin B_1 (thiamine)	Thiamine pyrophosphate	Beri-beri, congestive heart failure
Vitamin B_2 (riboflavin)	Flavine adenine dinucleotide	Angular stomatitis
Vitamin B_3 (niacin)	Nicotinamide adenine dinucleotide	Pellagra dermatosis, mental disorders
Vitamin B_4 (pyridoxine)	Pyridoxal phosphate	Peripheral neuropathy, convulsions
Pantothenic acid	Coenzyme A	Fatigue, sleep disturbance
Biotin	Carboxylases	Fatigue, depression, dermatitis
Folate	Tetrahydrofolate	Macrocytic anaemia, stomatitis, diarrhoea
Vitamin B_{12} (cyanocobalamin)	Cobamide coenzymes	Macrocytic anaemia, optic neuritis
Fat-soluble vitamins		
Vitamin A	Retinal precursor	Night blindness, xerophthalmia
Vitamin D	Regulation of calcium metabolism	Rickets, osteomalacia
Vitamin E	Antioxidant	Anaemia
Vitamin K	Coagulation cascade	Bleeding diathesis
Minerals and trace elements		
Iron	Component of haemoglobin, myoglobin, cytochromes	Microcytic, hypochromic anaemia
Zinc	Alcohol dehydrogenase Alkaline phosphatase Carbonic anhydrase Superoxide dismutase	Growth restriction, hypogonadism
Copper	Cytochrome c oxidase Superoxide dismutase	Microcytic, hypochromic anaemia

Basal metabolic rate (BMR)

The energy requirements of an individual are met by internal metabolism and reflected by total heat production (thermogenesis). The metabolic rate is the energy used by an individual per unit time, a measurement of power ($kcal\ h^{-1}$ or watts).

BMR is dependent on various factors, which include:
- Age (increased in childhood and declines with age)
- Sex (testosterone causes increase)
- Height, body weight and body surface area (core body temperature more effectively maintained in obesity, therefore lower BMR)

- Pregnancy, menstruation and lactation (all cause increase in BMR)
- Body temperature or environmental temperature (increase of 1 °C causes 10% increase in BMR)
- Muscular activity
- Emotional state (anxiety and pain increase BMR, depression lowers it)
- Circulating levels of hormones, e.g. thyroxine and adrenaline
- Recent ingestion of food (protein-rich meal raises BMR more than lipid-rich content)
- Conscious level
- Presence of sepsis or other disease (uncontrolled diabetes can increase BMR)
- Malnutrition (causes decrease in BMR)

The **basal metabolic rate** (BMR) is the total energy expended over 24 hours, by a subject under standardised conditions at mental and physical rest, in a comfortable environmental temperature and fasted for 12 hours. For an average young adult the BMR is approximately 2000 kcal 24 h^{-1} (96 watts).

Measurement of BMR

Under the specified steady-state conditions BMR can be measured directly, using a whole-body calorimeter. The subject is placed in a calorimeter chamber, and the heat produced causes a temperature rise in a steady flow of water through the calorimeter.

The BMR can be estimated indirectly by measuring the oxygen consumption of a subject at rest. The oxygen consumption per hour is multiplied by 4.8 kcal of heat produced per litre of oxygen, to give the heat produced per hour. This is an empirical figure representative of heat production regardless of substrate used. The oxygen usage can be measured using a modified spirometer containing oxygen and a carbon dioxide absorber.

Respiratory quotient (RQ)

The respiratory quotient is a dimensionless number used in calculations of BMR. It is the ratio, at steady state, of CO_2 expired to O_2 consumed. The energetic equivalent of

Figure 21.2 RQ and calorie equivalent of O_2 for different substrates

Nutrient	RQ	Calorie equivalent of oxygen (kcal L^{-1} O_2)
Glucose	1	5.01
Fat	0.7 (pure fat)	4.7
Protein	0.8–0.9	4.6
Ethyl alcohol	0.66	4.86

O_2 is the amount of energy released from food for each mole of O_2 consumed, and this varies for different substrates (Figure 21.2). The RQ of individual organs is of interest in drawing inference about the metabolic process occurring within them. For example, the RQ for the brain is regularly 0.97–0.99, indicating that its principal (but not its only) fuel is carbohydrate.

Respiratory quotient (RQ)

$$RQ = \frac{\text{volume of } CO_2 \text{ eliminated}}{\text{volume of } O_2 \text{ consumed}}$$

The volume of CO_2 expired can vary with various non-metabolic states, such as hyperventilation following exercise or compensation for metabolic acidosis, which in turn will increase the RQ.

Metabolism

This term is used to describe the complex mass of biochemical reactions which break down the absorbed products of digestion to extract chemical energy, synthesise substances for structural maintenance and growth, and synthesise or detoxify waste products.

Organisation

The organisation of metabolism can be visualised as being composed of three sets of interlinked pathways. These deal with the three main types of molecule fed into the system, and are often referred to separately as carbohydrate metabolism, protein metabolism and fat metabolism. The three areas of metabolism are linked by the main energy-producing machinery, which comprises the citric

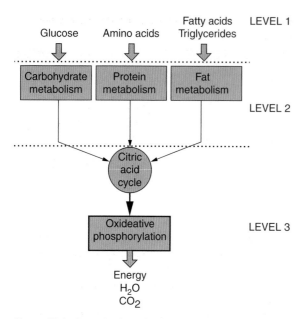

Figure 21.3 Organisation of metabolism

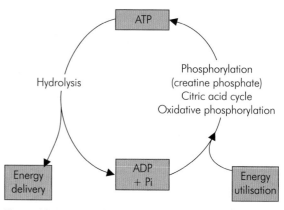

Figure 21.4 ATP cycle

acid cycle and the oxidative phosphorylation cascade (Figure 21.3).

The extraction of energy is a primary function of metabolism and provides the driving force that determines the direction taken by the different biochemical pathways. The universal energy currency used to move and supply energy to various pathways is a high-energy compound, adenosine triphosphate (ATP). Figure 21.3 also shows how there are three levels of reactions involved in harvesting energy:

- Level 1 – breakdown of carbohydrates, proteins and fats into their simple molecules of glucose and other sugars, amino acids, and fatty acids and glycerol. No energy is produced at this level.
- Level 2 – degradation of these simpler molecules to a common smaller molecule, acetyl coenzyme A (acetyl-CoA). A small amount of ATP is produced at this stage.
- Level 3 – passage of acetyl-CoA through the citric acid cycle, and an oxidative phosphorylation pathway, which generates > 90% of the finally harvested ATP.

In general terms, metabolism tends to proceed spontaneously in the direction of catabolism, oxidation and the production of protons. The processes and reactions reversing these trends – i.e. anabolism, reductive reactions

and the maintenance of acid–base balance – require energy. Thus, the supply of chemical energy for these reactions is the key to maintaining the life process.

Chemical energy is supplied in different forms, which are outlined below.

Adenosine triphosphate (ATP)

The majority of reactions and processes requiring chemical energy to drive them use it in the form of ATP. This compound is used in processes such as the myosin–actin interaction in muscle or the active transport of substances across cell membranes, and is sometimes referred to as the common energy currency of metabolism. ATP delivers its energy when it is hydrolysed to adenosine diphosphate (ADP), since its usable energy is carried in a high-energy phosphoryl bond (Figure 21.4). The ADP is 'recharged' by various reactions including the citric acid cycle, oxidative phosphorylation and phosphorylation by creatine phosphate. There is a continuous turnover of ATP, and at rest an adult can use 40 kg ATP in 24 hours.

Activated carriers

Although ATP has a universal role in supplying energy to drive reactions, other compounds also have the ability to drive reactions that require energy. The energy in these cases may be carried in the form of a high-potential electron or an activated group. In the case of an electron carrier, donation of an electron to one of the reagents constitutes a chemical reduction, which reverses the spontaneous tendency of the metabolic pathways towards

Figure 21.5 Activated carriers

Carrier molecule	Group carried
Adenosine triphosphate (ATP)	Phosphoryl
Nicotinamide adenine dinucleotide (NADH)	Electrons
Nicotinamide adenine dinucleotide phosphate (NADPH)	Electrons
Flavine adenine dinucleotide (FADH$_2$)	Electrons
Co-enzyme A	Acyl
Thiamine pyrophosphate (TPP)	Aldehyde
Creatine phosphate	Phosphoryl

Figure 21.6 Compartmentation of metabolic reactions between cytoplasm and mitochondria

Reaction site	Reaction pathway
Cytoplasm	Glycolysis Pyruvate oxidation Glycogenolysis Fatty acid synthesis
Mitochondria	Citric acid cycle Oxidative phosphorylation β-oxidation

oxidation. ATP can be regenerated with the use of a major electron carrier, nicotinamide adenine dinucleotide (NADH). Figure 21.5 shows some of the known activated carriers operating in metabolic pathways.

Control of metabolism

Metabolic pathways are carefully regulated, to ensure that the production of energy and intermediates meets the needs of the individual cell. The control of metabolic pathways must be flexible enough to enable adaptation to varying conditions, such as periods of starvation, exercise and stress.

The main mechanisms of metabolic control

- Availability of substrate
- Allosteric control of enzymes
- Hormonal control

Metabolic reactions are regulated via three basic mechanisms:

The availability of substrates – Substrate levels intracellularly can be controlled by hormones that affect the transport of substrates across cell membranes. An example of this mechanism is the action of insulin in promoting glucose entry into cells.

Enzyme activity and allosteric control – An allosteric modulator binds to a regulatory site on an enzyme.

This is distinct from the catalytic site. A positive allosteric modulator increases enzyme activity and stimulates the pathway, e.g. 2,3-DPG. A negative allosteric modulator inhibits the pathway (see Chapter 10, Figure 10.25).

Hormonal control – Various hormones such as the catecholamines, insulin, cortisol and thyroxine produce their physiological responses through wide-ranging changes in the metabolism of different tissues. Some examples are outlined below, while a summary of endocrine effects on metabolism is given in Chapter 22.

Additional control of metabolism is provided by maintaining separate synthetic and degradative pathways. This may be achieved by physical separation of the pathways, as in intracellular compartmentation. In such a case, for example, fatty acid breakdown (β-oxidation) occurs in mitochondria while fatty acid synthesis takes place in the cytoplasm (Figure 21.6).

Systemic control of metabolic responses is mainly mediated by hormones. Various hormones such as the catecholamines, insulin, cortisol and thyroxine produce their physiological responses through wide-ranging changes in the metabolism of different tissues. Examples include insulin, glucagon, adrenaline and noradrenaline (see below). A summary of endocrine effects on metabolism is given in Chapter 22.

Insulin

Insulin secretion is stimulated by glucose and amino acid uptake as well as by parasympathetic innervation. Within the liver it increases glycogen synthesis, prevents gluconeogenesis and stimulates the glycolytic production of fatty acid precursors, with resultant increase in fat storage. In the gut it increases the uptake of branched-chain amino acids, and is a stimulant to the formation of protein.

Amylin, co-secreted with insulin, may promote lactate transfer back to the liver, and support generation of fat stores.

Glucagon

Glucagon is released by the pancreas in response to hypoglycaemia. It acts on the liver to inhibit glycogen synthesis and promote gluconeogenesis and glycogen breakdown. In adipose tissue it results in the activation of lipases and fatty acid mobilisation.

Adrenaline and noradrenaline

Secreted as a response to stress or hypoglycaemia, these catecholamines promote glycogenolysis (greater in muscle than in liver) while reducing muscle uptake of glucose. Fatty acids are mobilised from adipose tissue to provide fuel for the increase in muscle activity.

Carbohydrate metabolism

Carbohydrate metabolism is mainly concerned with the generation of energy and the storage of carbohydrate as glycogen. The transportable form of carbohydrate throughout the body is the hexose sugar glucose (six-carbon, termed C6), which can be thought of as a universal fuel for all cells. The circulating levels of this are derived from:

- Dietary intake of carbohydrate
- Breakdown of stored carbohydrate in the form of glycogen, i.e. glycogenolysis
- Synthesis from smaller precursor molecules derived from other pathways, i.e. gluconeogenesis

The energy produced by the metabolism of one mole of glucose can be measured by the number of moles of ATP produced. Under aerobic conditions there is a net gain of 38 moles ATP per mole glucose. Each ATP molecule provides the energy from one activated phosphoryl group (7.6 kcal), which gives a total yield of 288 kcal chemical energy per mole glucose. If 1 mole glucose undergoes complete combustion in a calorimeter, it liberates about 686 kcal heat. The efficiency of carbohydrate metabolism is therefore 42%.

The main pathways in carbohydrate metabolism
- Glycolysis
- Gluconeogenesis
- Glycogenolysis and glycogenesis
- Pentose phosphate pathway (PPP) or hexose monophosphate (HMP) shunt

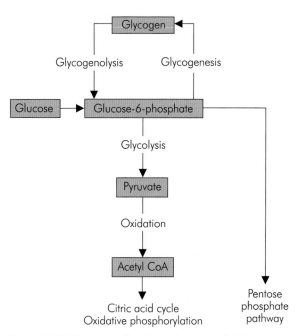

Figure 21.7 Overview of carbohydrate metabolism

These pathways and their relationship to each other are illustrated in Figure 21.7, and their functions are outlined below.

Glycolysis

Glycolysis (also called the Embden–Meyerhof pathway) breaks down glucose (C6) to the triose, pyruvate (C3). Its main function is to produce pyruvate for oxidation to acetyl-CoA to feed the citric acid cycle. Glucose is activated to glucose 6-phosphate to enter the pathway. This activated form may also be utilised to generate glycogen or for conjugation, but most enters into glycolysis (Figure 21.8).

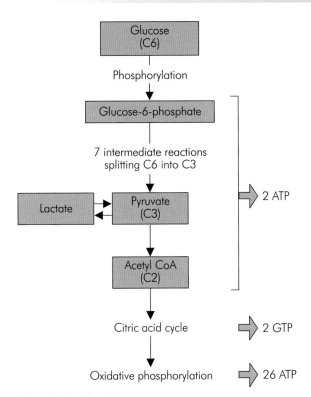

Figure 21.8 Glycolysis

is no net increase in production of ATP from this step, but the 2,3-DPG produced has an important allosteric effect. It fits into the space between the two β chains of deoxygenated haemoglobin and has a stabilising effect on the molecule, reducing its affinity for oxygen. This is important in enhancing the 'offloading' of oxygen in adaptation at altitude or during exercise, and for smokers or COPD sufferers.

Increased affinity for oxygen occurs in fetal haemoglobin, which does not have any β chains and therefore a low affinity for 2,3-DPG. Stored blood without additives (e.g. saline, adenine, glucose and mannitol) would have a low concentration of 2,3-DPG and therefore a high affinity for oxygen. Such red blood cells when transfused would have a reduced ability to offload oxygen.

Glycogenolysis

Glycogen is a branched polymer of glucose and is how carbohydrate is stored in the body. Total body reserves are about 325 g, and these are distributed between skeletal muscle and liver in the ratio of 3:1. The pathways for the breakdown of glycogen (glycogenolysis) and its synthesis (glycogenesis) are different, employing different enzymes and controls. They are illustrated in Figure 21.7. In glycogenesis glucose is activated by phosphorylation and combination with uridine triphosphate. It is then added to a pre-existing glycogen chain by glycogen synthetase. Branching of the glycogen chains requires a branching enzyme. Glycogenolysis requires a phosphorylase to activate and split off the terminal glucose unit from a glycogen chain. A debranching enzyme is also required to deal with branching points in the glycogen polymer. The enzymes in the glycogenesis and glycolytic pathways are distinct and respond individually to hormonal control. Storage of glucose as glycogen is highly efficient. The energy cost of storage and retrieval is a little over 3% of the total energy available from glucose.

Gluconeogenesis

Gluconeogenesis is the generation of glucose from substrates such as pyruvate and lactate. These in turn may be produced from amino acids by deamination, and consequently muscle mass also serves as a large potential glucose source. This occurs predominantly in the liver, and to some extent in the renal cortex. The much smaller mass of the kidney means that the overall renal contribution is small. Through gluconeogenesis plasma glucose levels can be maintained for those tissues

This pathway uses up 2 ATP, but generates 4 ATP and 2 NADH per molecule of glucose. Thus overall there is a net gain of 2 ATP and 2 NADH. Under aerobic conditions, the 2 NADH can be oxidised through oxidative phosphorylation to generate further ATP.

Glycolysis can also proceed under anaerobic conditions, but the net energy gain is then only 2 ATP, and lactate accumulates. Anaerobic glycolysis is important to the white muscle fibres of skeletal muscle. These are capable of intense activity disproportionate to their oxygen supply, which incurs an 'oxygen debt' in the form of the accumulated lactate. Lactate itself can be used as a substrate by some tissues. Pyruvate is oxidised to acetyl-CoA, which enters the citric acid cycle (also known as the Krebs cycle, after the biochemist who elucidated it) or can be used in other pathways.

Rapoport–Leubering shunt
The Rapoport–Leubering shunt is active in red blood cells and produces 2,3-diphosphoglycerate (2,3-DPG) from the 1,3-DPG produced in the main glycolytic pathway. There

Amino acid metabolism

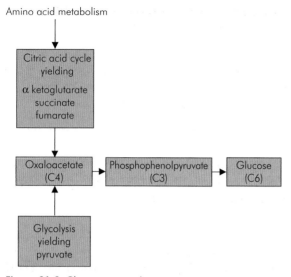

Figure 21.9 Gluconeogenesis

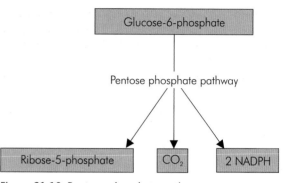

Figure 21.10 Pentose phosphate pathway

The cyclic process involves the transfer of a C2 fragment between pentoses (C5), and also provides a source of ribose 5-phosphate, an aldopentose required in the production of nucleic acids (Figure 21.10).

Oxidation of pyruvate to acetyl-CoA

This step in carbohydrate metabolism occurs inside the mitochondria, and it is important because it irreversibly funnels pyruvate (C3) into the citric acid cycle. The net reaction is:

$$Pyruvate + CoA + NAD^+ = acetyl - CoA + CO_2 + NADH$$

It is a complex reaction requiring pyruvate dehydrogenase (an enzyme complex composed of three different types of enzyme) and several cofactors (including TPP and NAD). This key reaction is subject to feedback control, in which the presence of high levels of energy in the form of NADH, ATP and acetyl-CoA 'switch off' the pyruvate dehydrogenase complex. There is thus a net energy gain in this step in the form of NADH, which can be converted to ATP through oxidative phosphorylation.

Citric acid cycle

The citric acid cycle and the oxidative phosphorylation process both form the core of the energy-producing machinery in metabolism. They take place in the mitochondria and are not exclusive to carbohydrate metabolism, but form a common end pathway for the products of carbohydrate, lipid and protein metabolism. Carbohydrate metabolism and the breakdown of lipids feed acetyl-CoA into the cycle, while protein metabolism can feed into the cycle via several intermediates, including oxaloacetate (C4), α-ketoglutarate (C5) and fumarate (C4).

that preferentially use glucose as an energy source. An outline of the gluconeogenesis pathway is shown in Figure 21.9. Gluconeogenesis from pyruvate is not simply a reverse of glycolysis, since the energetics so greatly favour pyruvate formation from the breakdown of glucose. Instead, pyruvate is converted to oxaloacetate at the cost of a single ATP by pyruvate carboxylase, and then phosphorylated and decarboxylated using guanosine triphosphate (GTP) as an energy source, to give phosphoenolpyruvate. The net cost of glucose synthesis from pyruvate is 6 ATP, whereas only 2 ATP are generated in glycolysis.

Pentose phosphate pathway

The pentose phosphate pathway (PPP) or hexose monophosphate (HMP) shunt is an alternative pathway for the activated form of glucose, glucose 6-phosphate. It is important in tissues that require reductive power for anabolic processes such as cell membrane repair, the synthesis of amino acids, fatty acids and steroids, and the production of nucleic acids.

The PPP is a cyclic pathway that takes in activated glucose units and produces CO_2, ribose 5-phosphate and NADPH (nicotinamide adenine dinucleotide phosphate). The NADPH is important as an activated reducing agent in certain tissues such as the liver, adipose tissue, erythrocytes and the testes.

The main entry to the citric acid cycle is via acetyl-CoA, which is essentially an activated C2 (acetyl) group bound to a carrier (coenzyme A). This C2 fragment is loaded onto a C4 molecule (oxaloacetate) to form citrate (C6), which passes around a cycle of intermediate compounds. Two decarboxylation reactions take place to regenerate the oxaloacetate (C4).

> **Energy production from each citric acid cycle**
>
> - Three NADH
> - One high-energy phosphoryl bond in GTP
> - One $FADH_2$

The NADH and $FADH_2$ are high-potential electron carriers, and enter the oxidative phosphorylation process to generate ATP (Figure 21.11).

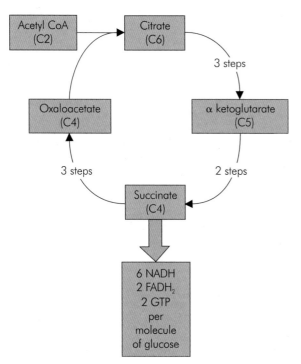

Figure 21.11 Citric acid cycle

Oxidative phosphorylation

Oxidative phosphorylation is the process of generating ATP by passing high-potential electrons carried by NADH and $FADH_2$ down through the low-potential carriers of the *respiratory chain* on the inner mitochondrial membrane. *High potential* refers to the tendency for electrons to be transferred from these activated carriers to a cascade of lower-potential carriers (NADH-Q reductase, cytochrome reductase and cytochrome oxidase). These mitochondrial membrane carriers are basically proton pumps activated by the flow of electrons through them. They pump H^+ out of the inner mitochondrion to give an H^+ gradient across the inner membrane. This H^+ gradient then generates ATP by driving H^+ back across the inner membrane through channels of ATP synthase. The passage of H^+ through these channels catalyses the synthesis of ATP (Figure 21.12).

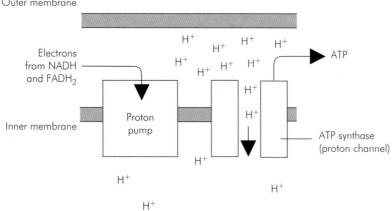

Figure 21.12 Oxidative phosphorylation

Oxidative phosphorylation

The generation of ATP in the mitochondria, by the passage of high-potential electrons down the respiratory chain.

Defects in carbohydrate metabolism

Inborn errors in the metabolism of carbohydrates can be grouped as follows:
- Intestinal defects
- A deficiency of an enzyme in the intermediary metabolic pathways, with accompanying lactic acidosis
- A deficiency of an enzyme in the intermediary metabolic pathways, without accompanying lactic acidosis
- Glycogen storage disease

Some examples are shown in Figure 21.13.

Protein metabolism

The basic building block of a protein is the amino acid. Amino acids are characterised by the presence of carboxyl and amine groups on a carbon atom. Also attached is a group R, as shown below:

$$H_2N - \overset{\overset{\displaystyle H}{|}}{\underset{\underset{\displaystyle R}{|}}{C}} - COOH$$

R may be simple, as in glycine, where R = H; or complex, as in glutamic acid, where R = $(CH_2)_2COOH$.

Amino acids can be condensed into chains to form peptides, and these chains can increase in size to form proteins. Protein chains can form a secondary structure by winding and twisting together. Such twisted chains can form more complex molecules by assuming a tertiary structure, resulting in sheets or fibres. In a quaternary structured protein, the amalgamation of several tertiary proteins or subunits forms a final complex protein molecule. Examples of such quaternary structures are haemoglobin (formed by four globin subunits connected to a haem core) and apoferritin (20 subunits arranged to form a hollow sphere).

Amino acid pool

Body proteins undergo a continual turnover by being broken down into amino acids and resynthesised from the same amino acids. This creates a metabolic *amino acid pool*, which provides not only precursors for protein synthesis but also many other compounds and pathways, including:
- Purines and pyrimidines
- Hormones
- Neurotransmitters
- Creatine
- Gluconeogenesis
- Fatty acid synthesis
- Citric acid cycle

Figure 21.13 Examples of defects in carbohydrate metabolism

Disease	Biochemical defect	Clinical features
Intestinal defect		
Lactose intolerance (non-familial type)	Gastrointestinal lactase deficiency	Diarrhoea, flatulence, abdominal discomfort
Enzyme deficiency with lactic acidosis		
von Gierke disease	Glucokinase deficiency	Large liver and kidneys, stunted growth, 'doll's face', lactic acidosis
Enzyme deficiency without lactic acidosis		
Galactosaemia	Galactokinase deficiency	Cataracts, hepatomegaly, mental retardation
Glycogen storage disease		
Pompe disease	Lysosomal debranching enzyme deficiency	Infantile cardiomegaly, hepatomegaly, hypotonia

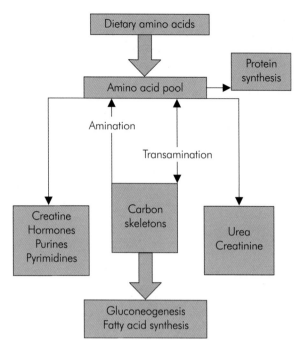

Figure 21.14 Overview of protein metabolism

Figure 21.15 Conversion of some amino acids to metabolic intermediates

Amino acid	Intermediate
Isoleucine Leucine Tryptophan	Acetyl-CoA (C2)
Alanine Cysteine Glycine Serine	Pyruvate (C3)
Aspartate Phenylalanine Tyrosine	Fumarate (C4)
Methionine Threonine Valine	Succinyl-CoA (C4)
Arginine Glutamate Histidine Proline	α-Ketoglutarate (C5)

Interconversion of different amino acids, or between amino acids and intermediates of carbohydrate and lipid metabolism, enables specific pathways to link into the amino acid pool. These interconversions occur via transamination, amination or deamination reactions, which are active in many tissues. The metabolic amino acid pool is replenished by the absorbed products of ingested protein.

Excess amino acids from the amino acid pool have their amino groups removed, leaving carbon skeletons. These residues enter other pathways (such as the citric acid cycle), while the excess amino groups are ultimately excreted as urea and creatinine. Figure 21.14 gives a simple overview of protein metabolism.

Transamination and deamination

Transamination is the transfer of an NH_2 group to another molecule, usually a keto acid. This common reaction allows excess amino acids to be degraded to intermediates that can be metabolised to give energy. Alternatively these intermediates can be used in gluconeogenesis or the synthesis of fatty acids. An example is the transfer of NH_2 from alanine to α-ketoglutarate:

alanine $+ \alpha -$ ketoglutarate $\rightarrow$ pyruvate $+$ glutamate

Pyruvate can then be oxidised to acetyl-CoA and enter the citric acid cycle.

Deamination is the removal of the amino group from an amino acid to leave a carbon skeleton that can be metabolised. An example of deamination occurs with serine, which can be deaminated to give pyruvate:

serine $\rightarrow$ pyruvate $+ NH_4^+$

In this way many of the amino acids can be converted to relatively few intermediate molecules (Figure 21.15).

Defects in amino acid metabolism
Congenital syndromes are recognised that are due to the disruption of specific amino acid pathways. These are usually rare but illustrate the importance of individual amino acids. Some examples are shown in Figure 21.16.

Nitrogen balance
Although amino acids are continually recycled from the amino acid pool, a daily loss occurs from the gastrointestinal tract and in the urine. Therefore, protein intake is required to compensate for these losses. The intake and losses of

Figure 21.16 Examples of defects in amino acid metabolism

Condition	Biochemical defect	Clinical features
Phenylketonuria	↓ conversion of phenylalanine to tyrosine	1 in 10,000 births Mental retardation
Homocystinuria	↓ levels of cysteine and cystine ↑ levels of homocystine and methionine	Tall, thin body, subluxation of lens, mental retardation
Alkaptonuria	↑ levels of homogentisic acid	Ochronosis (pigmented connective tissues), arthritis

protein may be assessed by their nitrogen content, and these should be balanced in the healthy adult. Normal nitrogen requirements for an adult are a daily intake of about 10 g (approximating to 46 g protein).

Negative balance occurs if losses exceed intake, as in the case of hypermetabolic and hypercatabolic states such as starvation, in sepsis or illness, and particularly in burns. Positive balance, when intake is greater than losses, occurs in growth, convalescence or the use of drugs such as anabolic steroids. Urinary nitrogen losses are mainly contained in the excreted urea, although small amounts of nitrogen are also excreted as creatinine, uric acid and amino acids. A positive nitrogen balance can also occur in hepatic or renal dysfunction, since the capacity of the body to produce and excrete urea is compromised. Dietary intake should be decreased in the presence of these conditions.

Nitrogen balance is helpful in calculating nutritional requirement as well as in assessing nutritional response.

Urea cycle

Excess amino acids are deaminated to release NH_4^+. This reaction occurs mainly in two tissues:

- The kidneys, where the NH_4^+ dissociates into NH_3 and H^+ for excretion into the urine.
- The liver, where the NH_4^+ is converted to carbamyl phosphate, which then contributes to the formation of urea.

The formation of urea is a cyclic process that takes place in the mitochondria. In a normal adult, about 30 g urea is produced daily. In hepatic failure, this

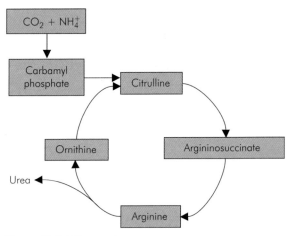

Figure 21.17 Urea cycle

conversion is less likely to occur, and an accumulation of ammonia occurs. The formation of urea is illustrated in Figure 21.17, which shows how urea, which has two nitrogen atoms, obtains one from carbamyl phosphate and the other by transamination from aspartate. The synthesis of one molecule of urea requires the energy from 3 ATP. This process is sometimes referred to as the ornithine cycle.

Creatine and creatinine

Creatine is present in muscle, brain and blood. It is particularly important in its phosphorylated form as an immediate store of high-energy phosphoryl bonds for the generation of ATP from ADP. The chemical energy for the first few seconds of muscle contraction is supplied by ATP generated from this source. Creatine is phosphorylated by creatine kinase. The serum levels of this enzyme are used as a marker of muscle damage following trauma or myocardial infarction – although creatine kinase activity may also be raised simply as a result of violent exercise.

Creatinine is the anhydride of creatine and is formed as a metabolite for excretion in the urine. The 24-hour urinary excretion of creatinine is relatively constant for any given individual, while renal tubular reabsorption is small. This means that the value for creatinine clearance can be used as an approximation to glomerular filtration rate.

Purines and pyrimidines

These substances are ring-based structures that occur widely throughout the body. They form the base components in the ribonucleotides and deoxyribonucleotides, i.e. the 'alphabet' triplets that code RNA and DNA strands. Purines and pyrimidines occur throughout the tissues as carriers of high-energy phosphoryl bonds, e.g. adenosine triphosphate (ATP), guanosine triphosphate (GTP) and uridine triphosphate (UTP). These molecules are also ubiquitous as the functional parts of many cofactors.

Purines

Purines are double-ringed molecules with six- and five-membered nitrogenated rings, commonly occurring examples being adenine and guanine. When metabolised, purines ultimately give rise to uric acid, which is excreted in the urine. The average excretion rate for an adult is between 400 and 600 mg over 24 hours. Uric acid and sodium urate are found in the plasma and urine. They have relatively limited solubility at body pH and urine pH, and it requires only a moderate increase in uric acid levels to precipitate the deposition of urate crystals in the tissues or the kidneys. The clinical syndrome of gout is associated with hyperuricaemia and deposition of urate in soft tissues and joints. The underlying defect is usually a combination of overproduction and increased breakdown of purines, but the cause may range from an enzyme deficiency to a hypercatabolic state.

Pyrimidines

Pyrimidines are based on a six-membered nitrogenated ring. Common pyrimidines in the body are cytosine, thymine and uracil. Breakdown of pyrimidines occurs in the liver and results in highly soluble products, β-alanine and β-aminoisobutyric acid.

Protein metabolism

This general term is used to describe the many interwoven pathways providing the continual synthesis and breakdown of nitrogen-containing compounds in the body. These centre around the amino acid pool and include:

- Protein synthesis
- Synthesis of creatinine, peptides, purines and pyrimidines
- Deamination, transamination and amination pathways
- Synthesis of urea and creatinine for excretion

Lipid metabolism

The lipids occurring in the body can be classified into the following groups:

- Fatty acids – chains of saturated or unsaturated carbon atoms with a terminal carboxyl group. These form the body's main energy store, and are also components of many structural molecules.
- Triglycerides – storage form for fatty acid chains, in which three chains are attached to a glycerol (C3) mole by ester linkages. Triglycerides are not free in the plasma but are transported as lipoproteins in chylomicra.
- Plasma lipoproteins – 95% of plasma lipids are transported in combination with protein to make them soluble. These lipoproteins have different roles and are targeted to specific tissues.
- Phospholipids and glycolipids – form building blocks for membranes and tissues.
- Cholesterol – precursor of steroid hormones and a component of membranes.

Free fatty acids (FFAs)

Free fatty acids form only 5% of the lipids in plasma, but this group of lipids is the most active metabolically. They are stored as triglycerides and metabolised to yield energy by β-oxidation in the mitochondria. The energy yield from fatty acid oxidation is about 9 kcal g^{-1}, compared with 4 kcal g^{-1} for carbohydrates and protein. In addition, because triglycerides are hydrophobic they are effectively anhydrous compared to glycogen, which

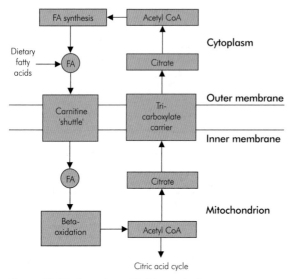

Figure 21.18 Overview of lipid metabolism

binds twice its weight in water. This means weight for weight triglycerides contain more than six times the energy of carbohydrates. A 70 kg man possesses about 11 kg triglycerides, representing a reserve of 100,000 kcal stored energy, compared with 25,000 kcal stored as protein and only 600 kcal stored as carbohydrate. The synthesis of fatty acids takes place in the cytoplasm by using acetyl-CoA to elongate fatty acid chains in C2 steps. An overview of lipid metabolism is shown in Figure 21.18.

Beta-oxidation of fatty acids

The breakdown of fatty acid chains to give energy is a cyclic process called β-oxidation, which takes place in the mitochondrial matrix. Free fatty acids in the cytoplasm are first activated by esterification with acetyl-CoA. The activated fatty acid is then loaded onto a carrier protein called carnitine at the outer mitochondrial membrane. This complex is transported across the inner mitochondrial membrane into the mitochondrial matrix, where it is unloaded by recombination with acetyl-CoA. This is performed by an inner membrane protein called carnitine acyltransferase. Carnitine is then returned to the outer membrane, where it is available to pick up more activated fatty acid. This cyclic process is sometimes known as the *carnitine shuttle*. In the matrix C2 fragments are split off from the fatty acid in repeated steps, each C2 fragment producing acetyl-CoA to feed into the citric acid cycle. In this way a molecule of a C16 fatty acid (palmitoyl) can produce 106 molecules of ATP.

Fatty acid synthesis

Fatty acid synthesis takes place in the cytoplasm, in contrast to β-oxidation, which is mitochondrial. This is also a cyclic process that builds up fatty acid chains by the addition of activated C2 fragments (acetyl-CoA). These C2 fragments are obtained from the mitochondria and are transferred out to the cytoplasm by a citrate carrier. The acetyl-CoA is removed from the citrate in the cytoplasm, leaving the citrate, which is then converted to pyruvate. The pyruvate passes back into the mitochondria, where it is re-converted back to citrate.

Reducing power in the form of NADPH is required for fatty acid synthesis. Some of this is generated by the citrate–pyruvate carrier cycle, while the pentose phosphate pathway provides the rest.

Fatty acid synthesis is regulated by a key enzyme, acetyl-CoA carboxylase, to ensure that synthesis and degradation occur appropriately for the body's needs. This control responds to biochemical feedback as well as hormones such as insulin and the catecholamines.

Free fatty acids are synthesised from acetyl-CoA and broken down by the β-oxidation spiral. FFAs have the following important functions:

- Fuel molecules
- Components of phospholipids and glycolipids
- Components of hormones and intracellular messengers

Plasma lipoproteins

Plasma triglycerides and cholesterol combine with proteins to form a range of lipoprotein particles, the largest being chylomicrons (100–1000 nm diameter), while the smallest are the high-density lipoproteins (7.5–20 nm diameter). These macromolecular aggregates have different lipid contents and are metabolised by specific tissues. Their basic structure consists of a lipid core coated with protein and phospholipid to solubilise them. Specific apoproteins in the particle coatings act as cellular signals for target tissues. The lipoproteins are classified according to density and have different metabolic functions (Figure 21.19).

Cholesterol

Cholesterol is a component of all cell membranes and produces membrane fluidity by its interaction with membrane phospholipids. It possesses a steroid-based

Figure 21.19 Plasma lipoproteins

Lipoprotein	Major core lipid	Function
Chylomicrons	Dietary triglyceride	Carries dietary triglycerides to tissues for fuel (e.g. muscle)
Chylomicron remnants	Dietary cholesterol	Taken up by liver for metabolism
Very-low-density lipoprotein (VLDL)	Endogenous triglyceride	Exported form of excess triglyceride and cholesterol from liver
Low-density lipoprotein (LDL)	Endogenous cholesterol	Major carrier of cholesterol to peripheral tissues for metabolism
High-density lipoprotein (HDL)	Endogenous cholesterol	Cholesterol from dying cells and membrane repair, for recycling

structure and is also a precursor of the steroid hormones. Cholesterol is, therefore, essential for the growth and viability of the tissues. Tissues outside the liver obtain cholesterol from the plasma low-density lipoprotein (LDL) particles, using membrane LDL receptors to mediate uptake. Normal plasma levels of cholesterol are $2.5\text{–}3.5\ \mathrm{mmol\ L}^{-1}$, and are contributed to by both diet (normal daily intake is about 1 g) and endogenous synthesis. Abnormally high levels of cholesterol result in disease due to deposition of cholesterol in soft tissues and formation of cholesterol-containing plaques in arteries (atherosclerosis).

Eicosanoids

The eicosanoids are C20 unsaturated fatty acids containing a five-carbon ring. They are derived from arachidonic acid, which is synthesised from linoleic acid, one of the essential fatty acids. The eicosanoids include the following compounds:

- Prostaglandins
- Leukotrienes
- Thromboxanes
- Prostacyclin

These substances are local hormones with short-lived and highly localised effects, depending on the tissue in which they are released. Their effects are wide-ranging and include stimulation of the inflammatory response, regulation of local blood flow, control of membrane transport, modulation of synaptic transmission and modulation of platelet adhesion. A key step in the synthesis of prostaglandins is cyclo-oxygenase, which can be inhibited by non-steroidal anti-inflammatory drugs (NSAIDs) such as aspirin.

Ketones

When excessive levels of acetyl-CoA are present, the acetyl-CoA is diverted to form acetoacetate and γ-hydroxy-butyric acid. These compounds are known as ketone bodies, and accumulation of ketone bodies results in the clinical syndrome of ketosis or ketoacidosis (Figure 21.20).

Acetyl-CoA represents a crossroads between major metabolic pathways. It can be produced either by glycolysis or by β-oxidation. Normally glycolysis is responsible for supplying the acetyl-CoA for the citric acid cycle, but if the glycolytic pathway fails, as in uncontrolled diabetes or starvation, acetyl-CoA is obtained from β-oxidation. Under such circumstances excessive levels can result because of:

- Insulin deficiency, leading to increased free fatty acid levels
- Increased glucagon levels, which stimulate β-oxidation
- Decreased levels of oxaloacetate, due to increased gluconeogenesis

Starvation

Starvation is a complete absence of dietary intake, and can result in death after about 60 days. This should be differentiated from malnutrition, in which some calorific intake may be present, but which follows a more protracted course accompanied by the effects of chronic lack of protein, fats and essential vitamins and minerals.

(a) Normal metabolism

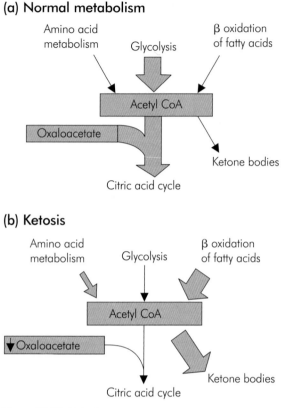

(b) Ketosis

Figure 21.20 Ketosis

Fed state

Insulin signals the well-fed state and brings about energy storage and glycolysis.

At rest, the brain accounts for 70–80% of the glucose utilised, and erythrocytes account for most of the remainder. Resting muscle utilises fatty acids for its metabolism.

Initial 12–24 hours

In starvation, glucose supplies to the brain are a priority, since it is largely dependent on glucose as an energy substrate. Glucagon signals starvation (as well as stress/exercise/hypoglycaemia), instigating glycogenolysis to maintain fuel levels. However, as glycogen reserves are depleted over 12–24 hours, blood glucose falls to subnormal levels. This is followed by an increase in basal levels of other stress hormones: noradrenaline, cotrisol, growth hormone, thyroxine and oestrogen. See Figure 21.21 for effects of stress hormones in starvation.

24 hours to 4 days

With the depletion of glycogen, gluconeogenesis increases, using amino acid residues derived from the breakdown of muscle protein and glycerol from lipolysis and oxaloacetate. These processes occur in the liver. The use of these substrates leads to the accumulation of acetyl-CoA and hence the formation of ketone bodies. Thus starvation is associated with ketosis. Protein catabolism is quite rapid in early starvation. However, since most tissues, including the brain, can ultimately adapt to the use of ketone bodies as a fuel source, the body shifts to the use of ketone bodies and the rate of protein breakdown decreases. After 3 days approximately a third of the brain's energy requirements are derived from ketone bodies, and ultimately this proportion increases to a half. The total reserves of an average adult are sufficient to provide the calorie requirements for about 3 months.

The 'protein-sparing effect' occurs as a result of ketone utilisation that prevents gluconeogenesis from muscle protein. The amount of ATP derived from β-oxidation depends on the fatty acid chain but is comparable to that derived from glucose, e.g. oxidation of D-3-oxybutyrate has a net yield of 22 ATP, compared with a net yield of 38 ATP from 1 molecule of glucose.

After 4 days

Ketoadaptation gradually occurs, allowing a decrease in protein consumption. This relatively slow process is complete by 2 weeks as it is hormone-dependent. However, erythrocytes, the renal medulla and 50% of the CNS still continue to require glucose as their primary energy substrate, which continues to be provided by gluconeogenesis from amino acids and glycerol.

Once fat stores are depleted, death follows as a result of protein malnutrition.

Exercise

The entry of glucose into skeletal muscle is increased during exercise in the absence of insulin by causing an insulin-independent number of type 4 glucose transporters (GLUT4) in the muscle cell membrane. This increase in glucose entry persists for several hours after exercise, and regular exercise training can produce prolonged increases in insulin sensitivity.

The demands of active muscle are initially met by glycogenolysis with increased glucose uptake, but plasma glucose levels may fall with prolonged strenuous exercise. Similar to starvation, gluconeogenesis ensues, with a fall

Figure 21.21 Effects of stress hormones in starvation

	Insulin	Glucagon	Cortisol	Catecholamines	Growth hormone	Progesterone and oestrogen	Thyroxine
Gluconeogenesis	↓	↑ (in liver only)	↑	↑ (in liver only)	–	–	↑
Glycogenolysis	↓	↑ (in liver only)	↓ (maintains glycogen stores, contrary to other hyperglycaemic hormones)	↑ (in liver and skeletal muscle)	↑ (in liver only)	–	↑
Protein breakdown	↓	↑	↑	–	↓	–	↑
Lipolysis	↓	↑ (including ketoacid formation)	↑	↑ (mobilisation of FFA)	↑	–	↑
Peripheral glucose utilisation	↑	↑	↓ (except brain or heart)	↓	–	↓ (hence gestational diabetes)	Increases glucose uptake from gut
Other	Signals well-fed state and promotes anabolism and glycolysis Also increases potassium uptake by cells	Stimulates release of insulin, growth hormone and somatostatin	Cortisol effect takes hours to days, promotes ketoadaptation in preparation for prolonged starvation	.	Anabolic hormone, similar to insulin Promotes ketoadaptation		

in plasma insulin levels and rise in glucagon, adrenaline and growth hormone that is proportional to intensity of exercise.

Exercise is also associated with extensive alterations in circulatory and respiratory systems which are largely similar to those seen in the stress response.

Glucose transporter type 4 (GLUT4)

This glucose transporter protein, found mainly in striated muscle (skeletal and cardiac) and adipose tissue, enhances the entry of glucose into cells. The expression of GLUT4 on the plasma membrane is increased by insulin but may also be stimulated by exercise.

The temperature increase seen is due at least in part to the inability of the heat-dissipating mechanisms to handle the great increase in heat production. If it is not dissipated effectively, this will impair enzyme function and contribute to fatigue.

The liver

Structure
The liver weighs 1.5–2 kg and is divided into right and left lobes, the right lobe being much larger than the left (up to six times its size). The functional unit of the liver is the hepatic lobule. These are roughly hexagonal in cross-section and possess a central vein from which cords of hepatocytes radiate outwards (Figure 21.22). In between the lobules are portal spaces through which run a bile duct and branches of the hepatic artery and portal vein. The radial spaces between the hepatocytes are called sinusoids; these carry a mixture of arterial and portal blood, supplied by the vessels in the portal spaces, towards the centre of the lobule, where it drains into the central vein. The central veins join to form the hepatic vein, which drains into the inferior vena cava.

As the blood flows through the sinusoids it is exposed over a large surface area to the hepatocytes, which are highly active metabolically. The walls of the sinusoids are also lined by macrophages known as Kupffer cells, which are an active part of the reticuloendothelial system.

The cords of hepatocytes are closely apposed to bile cannaliculi, which drain centrifugally towards the bile ducts in the portal spaces. These carry the bile secreted by the hepatocytes to the gallbladder and common bile duct. For details of bile formation and content see Chapter 20.

Metabolic functions
The metabolic functions of the liver may be divided into:

- Storage – of iron, copper, glycogen, vitamins A, D, E and K
- Metabolism – of fat, carbohydrates, proteins, bile, hormones and coagulation factors
- Excretion and detoxification – excretion of bilirubin, formation of urea, biotransformation of drugs, filtration of blood and degradation of endotoxins
- Immunological – synthesis of immunoglobulins and phagocytic action of Kupffer cells

Protein synthesis
The major proteins synthesised by the liver include albumin, globulins and clotting factors.

Albumin
This is synthesised at about 200 mg kg^{-1} per day in a normal adult. This is about 4% of the total body albumin pool. Plasma albumin correlates well with liver synthetic activity, but with a half-life of about 20 days it is a poor marker for acute liver injury. Albumin is important in the maintenance of plasma colloid oncotic pressure, and in the transport of drugs, bilirubin and some hormones.

Globulins
These are a range of lipo- and glycoproteins with transport functions (e.g. ferritin, caeruloplasmin). The liver is the principal site for synthesis and recycling of haptoglobin, which serves to bind and conserve free haemoglobin.

Clotting factors
Most clotting factors are synthesised exclusively by the liver. Half-lives of these clotting factors vary widely, ranging from about 4 hours for factor VII to 28 days for prothrombin. Coagulopathies may occur either due to failure of hepatic synthesis directly or because of failure of bile excretion leading to a reduction in the absorption of vitamin K, necessary for the synthesis of factors II, VII, IX and X.

Protein catabolism
The liver is involved in protein catabolism either directly, in turnover of proteins in the hepatocyte, or indirectly, in handling the products of the absorption of dietary proteins or amino acids from peripheral protein turnover. Amino acids or dipeptides from portal or systemic circulations are absorbed by the liver. They may be used as

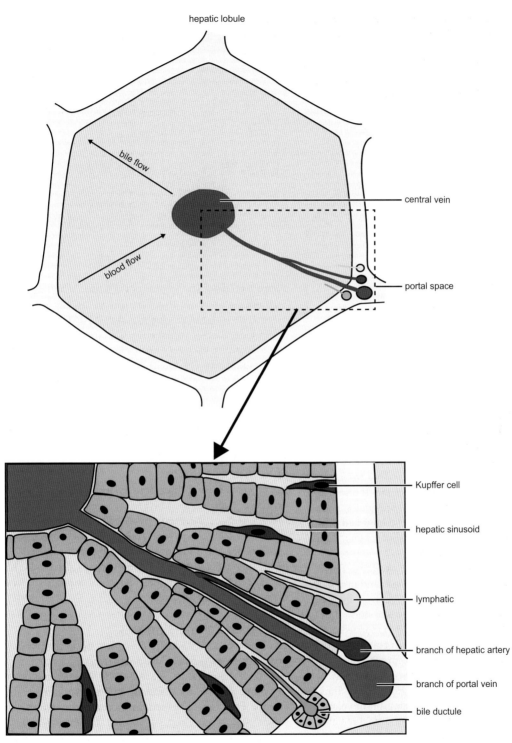

Figure 21.22 Structure of the liver

substrates for new protein synthesis, or used for gluco-neogenesis. The conversion of amino acids to carbon skeletons may involve transamination, deamination or modification to primary amines. The by-product from deamination is ammonia, which may be converted by the ornithine cycle to urea. In a normal adult, about 30 g of urea is produced daily. In hepatic failure, this conversion is less likely to occur, and an accumulation of ammonia occurs.

Carbohydrate metabolism

The liver's main role in carbohydrate metabolism is in maintaining glucose homeostasis during periods of fasting. It accomplishes this by glycogenesis, storing glycogen, and glycogenolysis. When glycogen reserves are depleted it is the site of gluconeogenesis.

Lipid metabolism

The liver synthesises fatty acids and lipoproteins for export. It is also a major site of endogenous cholesterol and prostaglandin synthesis.

Detoxification

The liver has a major function in the detoxification of steroid hormones. The mechanisms for detoxification are also used for the metabolism of exogenous substances, in particular therapeutic drugs.

Drug metabolism

Drug metabolism in the liver is divided into two phases:
- Phase 1 – covers modification of the drug to increase its polar nature and make it hydrophilic. It also provides reactive end groups to act as conjugation sites.
- Phase 2 – involves conjugation of the modified drug with hydrophilic groups to increase its solubility and aid renal excretion.

Phase 1 metabolism is almost entirely oxidative. There is a little reductive metabolism in the gut, and in isolated hepatocytes, as most of the liver is relatively hypoxic, with periportal hepatocytes running at a normal PO_2 of about 3 kPa. This oxidative activity is carried out by a diverse enzyme superfamily known collectively as cytochrome P450 (CYP), which occurs in many tissues. A large part of first-pass metabolism may be due to cytochrome activity in the gut mucosa. Similarly, nephrotoxicity after the metabolism of volatile anaesthetic agents may be due to intrarenal metabolism by cytochromes, rather than a consequence of elevated plasma fluoride levels.

Figure 21.23 Hepatic metabolism of drugs

Phase	Reaction
Phase 1	Oxidation Hydrolysis Hydration Dealkylation Reduction N-oxidation Isomerisation
Phase 2	Glucuronidation Sulphation Acetylation Glutathione conjugation

Phase 2 metabolism is conjugative. Drugs that have been modified by phase 1 metabolism are usually left with reactive end groups (such as hydroxyl). These groups provide sites for conjugation with more hydrophilic compounds, such as glucuronic acid, acetate, sulphate or glutathione (Figure 21.23).

The overall result of phase 1 and 2 metabolism is to produce a modified drug structure that is hydrophilic and rapidly eliminated by the kidneys.

Body temperature and thermoregulation

Many enzyme and transport systems cannot tolerate excessive temperature changes. Therefore, considering that 40–60% of the energy released during oxidation of glucose is released as heat and is not used by cells to perform specific functions, body temperature needs to be tightly regulated. Body temperature may also be altered by various factors including exercise, feeding, thyroid disease, infection and drugs.

Physiological mechanisms

The body can be thought of as having a core and a peripheral compartment. Normothermia is defined as a core body temperature of 36.5–37.1 °C, and it is kept to within 0.2 °C to maintain optimal conditions for enzyme reactions. The peripheral compartment acts as a heat sink, absorbing or releasing thermal energy to maintain the core, its temperature varying between 36 and 28 °C.

Normal variations of core body temperature are due to:

- Circadian variation of up to 0.7 °C from core temperature, with the minimum temperature before waking, when cortisol levels are at their lowest, and the maximum in the evening.
- Menstrual cycle produces a rise in temperature at ovulation (luteal phase) by as much as 1 °C.

Like many physiological systems in the body, the maintenance of homeostasis relies on multiple levels of positive and negative feedback. Afferent thermal sensing comes from hypothalamus, spinal cord, deep thoracic and abdominal viscera and skin. As core compartment temperature is more tightly regulated than the peripheral, core tissues contribute 80% of the input. The hypothalamus integrates information and produces efferent responses that are broadly classified as behavioural, hormonal and neuronal (Figure 21.24). The response pattern is proportional to the temperature deviation from the norm.

Thermoregulatory responses

If the **warm threshold** is exceeded, heat-loss responses are initiated, which include:

- Behavioural modification – e.g. removal of clothes.
- Cutaneous vasodilatation – can increase capillary blood flow up to about 7 litres per minute, causing heat loss by conduction and convection.
- Sweating – increases evaporative losses. In stressed athletes sweating can account for the loss of about 2 litres per hour, with heat loss increased by a factor of 10.
- Hairs lie flat to the skin – this increases the flow of air next to the skin, increasing heat loss by convection.

If the **cold threshold** is exceeded, thermogenic activities are initiated. These include:

- Behavioural – in the conscious adult this is the major regulator of heat loss (e.g. turning on heat sources, adding more clothes).
- Exercise – increases BMR and hence increases heat production.
- Cutaneous vasoconstriction – skin blood flow is a combination of capillary flow and extracapillary shunts.
- Shivering – causing increased oxygen consumption and increased BMR by up to 600%. The effectiveness of this heat source is reduced by the fact that muscle

activity also increases blood flow to peripheral tissues, dissipating the heat generated.

- Non-shivering thermogenesis – adrenaline and noradrenaline can uncouple oxidative phosphorylation in cellular metabolism, so that heat is produced instead of generating the metabolic fuel ATP. This can increase heat production by 10–15% in adults. However, brown fat contains large numbers of specialised mitochondria for this form of chemical thermogenesis. It is prevalent in the neonate and can increase the rate of heat production by about 100%.
- Piloerection – erection of the hair of the skin due to contraction of the tiny arrectores pilorum muscles that elevate the hair follicles above the rest of the skin and move the hair vertically, trapping an insulatory layer of air.

Disturbances of thermoregulation
Fever
This is one of the most common manifestations of disease. It is due to the production of endogenous pyrogens, which are most likely to include certain interleukins, interferons and tumour necrosis factor (TNF). These cytokines are thought to act by causing the local release of prostaglandins in the hypothalamus. The antipyretic effect of aspirin and other NSAIDs is due to the inhibition of cyclo-oxygenase, a key enzyme in prostaglandin synthesis.

Malignant hyperpyrexia
A genetic condition that causes widespread persistent muscle contraction when triggered by stress or specific anaesthetic agents. The result is massive heat production and a rapid uncontrolled rise in body temperature with metabolic acidosis and myoglobinuria. The underlying lesion is a defect in the gene coding for the ryanodine receptors in the sarcoplasmic triads, which leads to excessive Ca^{2+} release.

Other causes of hyperpyrexia
The drug MDMA ('ecstasy') can cause hyperpyrexia and sudden death in predisposed individuals. Certain lesions in the brain following a stroke, particularly in the region of the pons, can cause disordered thermoregulation.

Hypothermia
Hypothermia is said to be present when body core temperatures are less than 36 °C. It may be associated with:

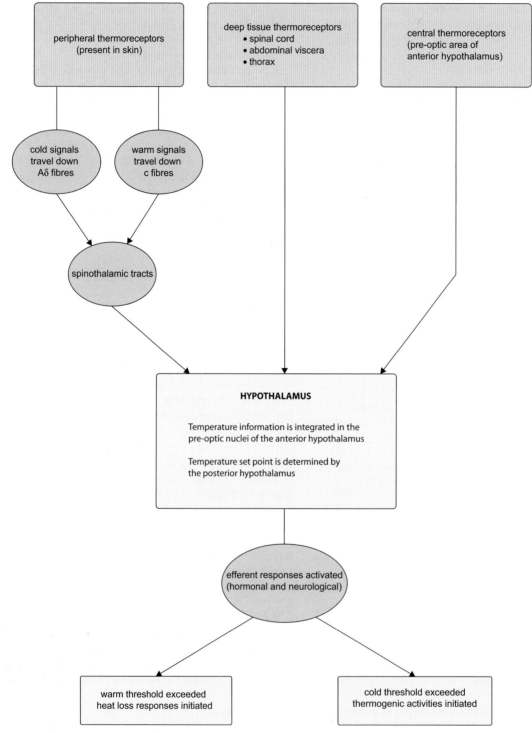

Figure 21.24 Temperature homeostasis

Figure 21.25 Effects of hypothermia on major organ systems

Central nervous system	Below 35 °C cognitive impairment begins Loss of consciousness at 30 °C Cerebral autoregulation impaired Neuroprotective – equivocal evidence to date
Cardiovascular system	Depressed myocardial contractility and reduced myocardial oxygen uptake Reduced inotropic effect of catecholamines Enhanced negative effect of volatiles Vasoconstriction Bradycardia, prolonged conduction, with longer PR, QT and QRS complexes Cardiac output reduced by ~1/3 Arrhythmias more common at 32 °C J waves appear on the ECG in at least 80% of patients below 30 °C Life-threatening ventricular arrhythmias occur, ventricular fibrillation at 28 °C, which is difficult to reverse unless the heart is rewarmed
Respiratory system	Reduced oxygen delivery and increased uptake Shift of ODC to left Gases more soluble Increased peripheral vascular resistance Increased tidal volumes Apnoea at 24 °C
Haematological	Increased blood viscosity (4–6% for each 1 °C reduction) Thrombocytopenia and leucopenia due to sequestration Impaired coagulation as enzymatic processes affected Poor wound healing Thrombogenic
Immune	Immunosuppression
Metabolic	Decreased metabolic rate, by 8–10% per 1 °C fall in body temperature Shivering increases oxygen uptake by up to 800% Reduced tissue perfusion causing metabolic acidosis Increased circulating catecholamines Hyperglycaemia Reduced drug metabolism and decreased hepatic blood flow Intracellular shift of K^+ Increased protein catabolism and decreased synthesis
Other	Reduced renal blood flow and oliguria

- Exposure
- Near-drowning
- Old age
- Hypothyroidism
- Prolonged surgery

There is progressive reduction in all normal metabolic and physiological processes, resulting in hypotension, bradycardia, bradypnoea and loss of consciousness. It is not until core temperature reaches 30 °C that life-threatening changes start to appear. Causes of death are systole and ventricular fibrillation below 30 °C, and apnoea at 24 °C (Figure 21.25).

Re-warming can be active or passive, and with adequate physiological support humans can be resuscitated from 20–25 °C without permanent sequelae.

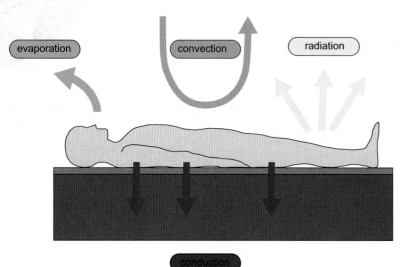

Figure 21.26 Heat loss during anaesthesia and surgery

Hypothermic effects of anaesthesia and surgery
Anaesthesia and surgery have a significant impact on thermoregulation:

- Behavioural responses are totally abolished under anaesthesia.
- Hyperthermic thresholds are increased by about 1 °C, while hypothermic thresholds are markedly reduced, by up to 3–4 °C. These broadened thresholds can remain altered for up to 6–12 hours postoperatively, prolonged even further by concomitant opioid use. The body does not initiate hormonal or neuronal responses to restore core temperature until the new thresholds are reached.

- Cutaneous vasoconstriction is antagonised by vaso-dilator anaesthetics. This effect also appears to be dose-dependent.

The physical mechanisms that lead to heat loss during anaesthesia and surgery are summarised in Figure 21.26.

References and further reading

Guyton AC, Hall EJ. *Textbook of Medical Physiology*, 12th edn. Philadelphia, PA: Elsevier, 2011.

Lim MY, Roach JN. *Metabolism and Nutrition.* Mosby Elsevier, 2007.

Salway JG. *Metabolism at a Glance.* Oxford: Blackwell, 2004.

Buggy DJ, Crossley AWA. Thermoregulation, mild perioperative hypothermia and post anaesthetic shivering. *Br J Anaesth* 2000; **84**: 615–28.

Endocrine physiology

Jo James

Endocrine physiology is the study of hormones, the glands that produce them, and the effects that hormones have on their target organs. Endocrine function is necessary to maintain homeostasis, and is associated with the unconscious and subconscious functions of the body. It is closely linked with areas in the brain and nervous system that control homeostasis, especially the hypothalamus.

> The main **effects of hormones** on the body are in the control of metabolism, nutrition and growth; the development of sexual characteristics and reproduction; and the control of blood pressure and temperature.

The classical concept of a gland releasing a hormone into the bloodstream, in which it travels to the target organ to produce an effect, describes a relatively slow process. It is now recognised that the physiology is more complex. In paracrine secretion, hormones such as histamine and prostaglandins act on neighbouring cells.

Alternatively, as in autocrine secretion, the hormones may even act on the secreting cell itself. These latter pathways produce effects much more rapidly than the classical pathway.

Classification of hormones

The more common hormones are listed in Figure 22.1.

Polypeptides

Examples – vasopressin, oxytocin, prolactin, insulin, glucagon. These are usually produced as a prohormone which undergoes conversion to its active form. These hormones are stored in granules and secreted by exocytosis into the bloodstream.

Glycoproteins

Examples – TSH, FSH, LH. These are polypeptide hormones linked to carbohydrate residues. Polypeptides and glycoproteins are hydrophilic and unbound in the bloodstream.

Fundamentals of Anaesthesia, 4th edition, ed. Ted Lin, Tim Smith and Colin Pinnock. Published by Cambridge University Press. © Cambridge University Press 2017.

Figure 22.1 List of more common hormones

Polypeptides	Glycoproteins	Steroids	Amines	Fatty acid derivatives
Vasopressin	FSH	Aldosterone	PIH (dopamine)	Prostaglandins
Oxytocin	LH	Corticosteroids	Adrenaline	Vitamin D
ACTH	TSH	Testosterone	Noradrenaline	
FSH-RH		Oestrogen	Thyroxine	
LH-RH		Progesterone	Tri-iodothyronine	
ACTH-RH				
TRH				
PTH				
Calcitonin				
Insulin				
Glucagon				
Somatostatin				

Note that ACTH (adrenocorticotropic hormone) is sometimes still referred to as corticotropin, and ACTH-RH (adrenocorticotropic hormone releasing hormone) is also frequently called CRH (corticotropin releasing hormone) or CRF (corticotropin releasing factor). We have chosen to use the terms ACTH and ACTH-RH in this text.

Steroids

Examples – corticosteroids, aldosterone, sex hormones. Steroids are synthesised in the cell mitochondria, from cholesterol. These hormones are not stored in secretory granules, but are produced by the cell as and when required. Steroid hormones are lipophilic and highly bound to proteins in the bloodstream en route to the target organ.

Amines

Examples – thyroxine, adrenaline. All the amine hormones are synthesised from the amino acid tyrosine. They are stored in follicles (thyroxine) or granules (catecholamines). Some (e.g. thyroid hormones) may be converted to a more active form nearer to the site of action.

Indole and fatty acid derivatives

Examples – prostaglandins. These produce effects either in the cell where they are secreted or in adjacent cells.

Cellular action of hormones

Hormones exert their cellular effects by initially binding to receptors, which then produce secondary effects to change cellular function.

Hormone receptor-mediated secondary effects include:

- Changes in membrane permeability
- Release of second messengers
- Changes in intracellular protein synthesis

Hormone receptors

Hormone receptors may be on the cell membrane (or transmembranous) or inside the cell. They increase and decrease in number depending on external stimuli. When there is an excess of hormone the number of receptors decreases (down-regulation); conversely, when there is a deficit of hormone the number of receptors increases (up-regulation). Sometimes down-regulation occurs when the receptors change their chemical structure and become less responsive. The hydrophilic hormones have receptors in the cell membrane, and the lipophilic hormones (e.g. thyroid and steroid hormones) have receptors within the cell, either cytoplasmic or nuclear.

Some hormones require the presence of small amounts of other hormones in order for their receptors to be fully active. This is known as permissiveness. Small amounts of glucocorticoids, for example, are necessary for catecholamines to produce their lipolytic effects.

Mechanisms of hormonal action
Direct effects on cell membranes

The hormone alters the permeability of the membrane to certain ions, e.g. K^+ and Ca^{2+}, via G proteins. This effect is very rapid.

Effects via second messengers

Hormones bind with receptors in the cell membrane and cause intracellular effects via second messengers.

Figure 22.2 Common hormones and their mechanism of action

Affecting permeability	Via G proteins increasing cAMP	Via G proteins decreasing cAMP	Via PIP$_2$, IP$_3$ and DAG	Via mRNA
GH Prolactin Insulin	Oxytocin Vasopressin LH FSH TSH ACTH Adrenaline (β-receptors) PTH Glucagon	Somatostatin Adrenaline (α$_2$)	Adrenaline (α$_1$) Vasopressin	Thyroxine Tri-iodothyronine Steroid hormones

The second messenger cyclic adenosine monophosphate (cAMP) phosphorylates proteins within the cell. Hormones may increase or decrease levels of cAMP. When a hormone reacts with the receptor within the cell, guanylyl nucleotide regulatory proteins are activated within the cell membrane. These may be stimulatory (Gs) or inhibitory (Gi) to the production of cAMP.

Other hormones activate different second messengers, such as inositol triphosphate (IP$_3$) and diacylglycerol (DAG). The hormone receptor complex activates an enzyme which breaks down a membrane phospholipid, phosphatidylinositol diphosphate (PIP$_2$), to IP$_3$ and DAG. IP$_3$ releases Ca^{2+} from intracellullar stores, such as the endoplasmic reticulum, while DAG activates protein kinase C, which increases cell division and multiplication. This latter reaction is enhanced by the released Ca^{2+}.

Effects on protein synthesis

Thyroid and steroid hormones, being highly lipophilic, cross the cell membrane rapidly to bind with intracellular receptors. Once bound with their receptor they cross to the nucleus, where they bind with DNA. This increases mRNA synthesis and via ribosomes leads to an increase in protein production. This process is relatively slow.

Figure 22.2 shows the mechanism of action of common hormones.

Control of hormone production

Various mechanisms control hormone secretion. These include levels of inorganic ions (e.g. sodium-dependent release of vasopressin), organic molecules (e.g. glucose stimulating insulin release) and direct physical and chemical stimulation (e.g. as in the case of gut hormones).

> The most important regulator of hormone production is the negative feedback loop.

In the negative feedback system high levels of a substance produced by the hormone suppress the secretion of that hormone, ensuring that the level of the substance itself remains relatively constant.

Negative feedback can be direct or indirect. An illustration of direct negative feedback is the effect of circulating glucose on insulin production. An example of indirect negative feedback is the effect of circulating glucocorticoids on ACTH-RH, which in turn affects levels of ACTH.

Hypertrophy and atrophy

If the level of a specific hormone in the blood remains very low despite maximal production and release, there will be a large increase in the level of the relevant tropic hormone, and the other cells in the producing gland will enlarge and multiply in order to compensate. This is seen as a thyroid goitre in iodine deficiency. Conversely, if there are very high circulating levels of hormone produced by medication (e.g. steroids), the tropic hormones will fall to very low levels and the gland will atrophy. Tropic hormones, therefore, influence both hormone production from the cell and the size of the gland producing the hormone.

Pituitary gland

Anatomy

The pituitary gland is made up of the anterior lobe (adenohypophysis) and posterior lobe (neurohypophysis), and is connected to the hypothalamus by the pituitary stalk. It weighs less than 1 g, and is located at the base of the brain in the sella turcica.

Embryological development of the pituitary

The anterior and posterior lobes develop quite separately from each other. The anterior lobe develops from Rathke's pouch, an outgrowth from the roof of the mouth. The posterior lobe develops as an extension from the hypothalamus, an evagination of the floor of the third ventricle. The two join together. The part of the anterior lobe which fuses with the posterior lobe is known as the intermediate lobe, and it is rudimentary in humans. The remains of Rathke's pouch form the residual cleft (Figure 22.3).

Anterior lobe of pituitary

The anterior and posterior lobes have independent functions, but both are connected to the hypothalamus by the pituitary stalk. The anterior lobe is connected to the hypothalamus by the portal circulation, which transports releasing hormones into the lobe, stimulating the production of tropic hormones into the bloodstream.

The portal circulation is a network of capillaries which arises from the superior hypophyseal artery. The primary capillary plexus, located on the floor of the hypothalamus (known as the median eminence), absorbs releasing factors; the blood then passes via the portal veins in the pituitary stalk to the secondary capillary plexus, where they are released into the anterior lobe. The tropic hormones are then secreted into the plexus and into the bloodstream (Figure 22.4). The anterior lobe hormones are found in five types of secretory cell:

- Somatotropes (50%) produce growth hormone (GH).
- Lactotropes (10–30%) produce prolactin.
- Corticotropes produce adrenocorticotropic hormone (ACTH).
- Thyrotropes produce thyroid-stimulating hormone (TSH).
- Gonadotropes produce follicle-stimulating hormone (FSH) and luteinising hormone (LH).

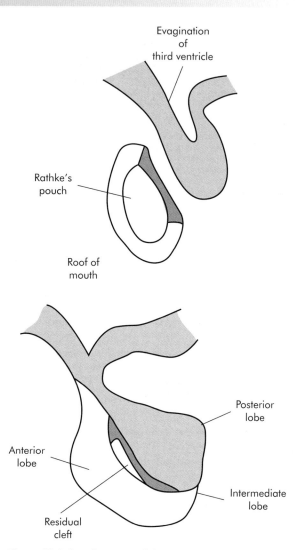

Figure 22.3 Development of the pituitary gland

Posterior lobe of pituitary

Posterior lobe hormones are produced in neurosecretory cells in the hypothalamus, in the so-called median eminence. These form granules which pass down the axons through the pituitary stalk and are stored in the posterior lobe, later to be released into the bloodstream when stimulation occurs.

Vasopressin is produced in the supraoptic nucleus of the hypothalamus, and oxytocin from the paraventricular nucleus, within the median eminence (Figure 22.5).

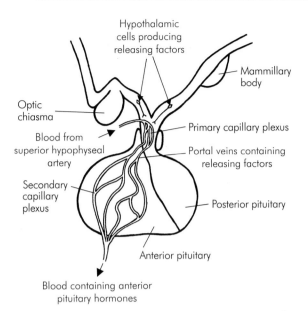
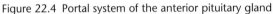

Figure 22.4 Portal system of the anterior pituitary gland

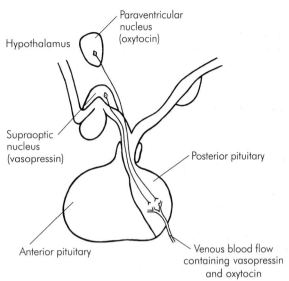

Figure 22.5 Secretion of vasopressin and oxytocin by the posterior pituitary

Pituitary hormones

> **Anterior pituitary hormones**
> - Thyroid-stimulating hormone (TSH, thyrotropin)
> - Adrenocorticotropic hormone (ACTH, corticotropin)
> - Growth hormone (GH, somatotropin, STH)
> - Prolactin (PRL)
> - Follicle-stimulating hormone (FSH)
> - Luteinising hormone (LH)
>
> **Posterior pituitary hormones**
> - Vasopressin (antidiuretic hormone, ADH)
> - Oxytocin

Functions of individual hormones
Thyroid-stimulating hormone (TSH)
Stimulates the production of thyroid hormones from the thyroid gland, and growth of the gland itself.

Adrenocorticotropic hormone (ACTH)
Stimulates the adrenal cortex to produce corticosteroid hormones (mainly cortisol) and also binds to melanotropin receptors in the melanocytes in the skin, which produce melanin and pigmentation. There is significant diurnal variation in its secretion, which is higher in the morning and lower in the evening.

Growth hormone (GH)
Stimulates the growth of tissues in the body by promoting protein synthesis, lipolysis and a rise in blood glucose. It is especially active in childhood, and causes an increase in length of the long bones until the epiphyses fuse. Not all of its effects are direct. Some of the effects on target tissues are mediated through polypeptide substances produced by the liver and other tissues, called somatomedins. These are closely related to insulin. Insulin-like growth factor 1 (IGF-1) is involved with skeletal and cartilage growth. IGF-2 also exists and is thought to be involved in fetal growth.

Lack of GH in childhood leads to dwarfism, and excess to gigantism. The patients in these cases are respectively either very small or very tall, but are in proportion. Excess GH in the adult leads to acromegaly. As this occurs after the epiphyses have fused there is little increase in height, but there is overgrowth of the skull, facial bones and hands and feet. Reduced glucose tolerance in such cases is common.

Prolactin
Prolactin is structurally similar to GH. This hormone stimulates the development of milk-producing breast tissue and milk production post partum. It also suppresses

ovulation. Excess production of prolactin can cause lactation and infertility.

Follicle-stimulating hormone (FSH)
Stimulates ovulation in females and spermatogenesis in males.

Luteinising hormone (LH)
Stimulates ovulation and luteinisation of ovarian follicles in females. It also stimulates testosterone secretion in males. FSH and LH together are involved in the regulation of the menstrual cycle.

Vasopressin (antidiuretic hormone, ADH)

> Vasopressin causes water retention by increasing water absorption from the distal tubules and collecting ducts of the kidney.

The secretion of vasopressin is stimulated by the following changes:
- A rise in osmotic pressure in the plasma (via osmoreceptors in the anterior hypothalamus)
- A decrease in extracellular volume
- A rise in angiotensin II levels
- Pain, stress and exercise
- Nausea and vomiting
- Smoking

Its secretion is reduced by:
- A decrease in plasma osmotic pressure
- An increase in extracellular volume
- Alcohol

There are several types of vasopressin receptors, V_{1a}, V_{1b} and V_2, which are all G-protein coupled. The antidiuretic effects are mediated through V_2 receptors, which open aquaporin 2 (AQP2) water channels in the collecting ducts of the kidneys. Vasopressin also has a powerful vasoconstrictor effect in vitro on vascular smooth muscle, although this is small in vivo. This is mediated through receptors found in the area postrema in the brain, and the mechanism is very sensitive to haemorrhage. Vasopressin receptors are also found in the liver, where they stimulate glycogenolysis, and in the brain. Figure 22.6 shows how these are arranged. V_3 is an alternative classification for V_{1b}.

Figure 22.6 Classification of vasopressin receptors

Type	Location	Function
V_{1a}	Smooth muscle and heart	Vasoconstrictor effect
V_{1b}/V_3	CNS	Mediate release of ACTH-RH
V_2	Collecting ducts	Permit water reabsorption

Deficiency of vasopressin leads to diabetes insipidus, in which there is polyuria and polydypsia due to water loss. It can be primary, due to disease of the gland, or secondary, where the kidneys are unable to respond to vasopressin.

Excess of vasopressin (inappropriate secretion) leads to fluid retention with low plasma osmolarity and hyponatraemia. Vasopressin-secreting malignant lung tumours are one cause.

Oxytocin
Oxytocin is structurally similar to vasopressin, and causes milk ejection from glands in the breast, stimulated by suckling and via touch receptors. It also causes uterine contraction during labour and in the immediate postpartum period, as well as being involved in sexual arousal.

Deficiency and excess of pituitary hormones
Pituitary deficiency can be caused by tumours and cysts which press on the pituitary gland. Acute failure may also occur in an enlarged pituitary gland following severe hypovolaemia. This may occur in women who have experienced severe bleeding and hypovolaemia during childbirth leading to pituitary necrosis (Sheehan's syndrome). The changes which develop depend on the location of damage in the gland.

Pituitary excess can be produced by secreting tumours, which may arise from the gland itself or from other sites in the body.

Control of pituitary hormones
The hypothalamus is intimately connected to the pituitary gland, and is responsible for a number of so-called releasing hormones. These polypeptides are produced in the median eminence of the hypothalamus, and pass into the portal system to the anterior lobe, where they stimulate or inhibit production of the tropic hormones.

Hypothalamic releasing factors include:

- Thyrotropin releasing hormone (TRH)
- Adrenocorticotropic hormone releasing hormone (ACTH-RH)
- Growth hormone releasing and inhibiting hormones (GH-RH and GH-IH) (GH-IH is somatostatin, also produced in pancreatic islet cells)
- Prolactin releasing and inhibiting hormones (PRH and PIH – dopamine)
- Gonadotropin releasing hormone (Gn-RH) – stimulates production of FSH and LH

Some releasing factors have an effect on other hormones. TRH stimulates prolactin production, and GRH inhibits TSH, for example.

The hypothalamus has many inputs which are concerned with vegetative regulation, and it is also connected to other parts of the central nervous system, and its output is affected by stress, diurnal rhythm and emotional factors.

The function of the anterior lobe is under negative feedback control. When the levels of hormones which are produced in the target organs increase, the production of both the tropic hormones and the releasing factors is reduced. Conversely, when the target-organ hormone levels decrease there is increased production of both the tropic hormones and the releasing factors. This keeps the hormone levels relatively constant (Figure 22.7).

When steroids are given as medication over a period of time, the anterior pituitary and the hypothalamus produce minimal stimulation of endogenous cortical adrenal steroids, and the adrenal gland atrophies. This can have serious consequences if the steroids are suddenly stopped, especially if the patient is undergoing a stressful procedure such as surgery.

The pituitary hormones are summarised in Figure 22.8.

Thyroid gland

The **thyroid gland** secretes hormones which control the basal metabolic rate, enabling the body to function optimally.

The thyroid hormones affect carbohydrate, lipid and protein metabolism, also affecting growth and maturation, and body temperature.

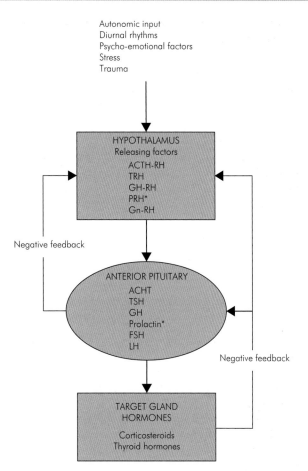

*Main control of prolactin is by PIH

Figure 22.7 Feedback control of pituitary hormones

Anatomy

The embryonic origin of the thyroid gland is from the floor of the pharynx. The thyroglossal duct marks the path of the gland from the tongue to its final site, and sometimes this persists in adults. The gland is situated in the neck at the level of the second and third tracheal rings. It comprises two lobes on either side of the trachea, joined by the thyroid isthmus. Each lobe has an upper and lower pole. Sometimes there is a third lobe, the pyramidal lobe, which arises anteriorly from the thyroid isthmus. The gland is highly vascular, its arterial supply coming from the superior and inferior thyroid arteries, and its venous drainage via the superior, middle and inferior thyroid veins. The parathyroid glands are located within the thyroid gland.

Figure 22.8 Pituitary hormones: their production, control and action

Part of pituitary	Hormone	Main stimulus and control	Action
Anterior lobe	TSH	+ve TRH, −ve thyroid hormones	Thyroid gland to produce thyroid hormones
	ACTH	+ve ACTH-RH, −ve corticosteroid hormones	Adrenal gland to produce corticosteroid hormones
	GH	+ve GH-RH, −ve GH-IH	Increase growth of body tissue especially bone
	Prolactin	+ve PRF, −ve PIH	Milk production, suppression of ovulation
	FSH	+ve Gn-RH	Breast development, milk secretion, spermatogenesis
	LH	+ve Gn-RH	Stimulation of ovulation, testosterone secretion
Posterior lobe	Vasopressin	+ve osmolarity, thirst, pain, haemorrhage	Water reabsorption from distal tubules
	Oxytocin	+ve touch receptors in breast and genitalia	Ejection of milk from breast, uterine contraction

The gland itself comprises many follicles (acini). The follicles are lined by the thyroid epithelial cells, and within the follicle itself is a variable amount of colloid, which mainly contains thyroglobulin and iodine. There are also parafollicular (C or clear) cells which secrete calcitonin. The thyroid cells rest on a basal membrane, which separates them from the capillaries.

When the gland is inactive the follicles are large and contain substantial amounts of colloid. The cells are small and flattened. When the gland is active, the follicles reduce in size; there is little colloid, and the cells become enlarged and columnar or cuboid. The edge of the colloid develops a scalloped appearance due to reabsorption lacunae at the tips of the cells (Figure 22.9).

Thyroid hormones

The most important hormones secreted by the thyroid gland are tri-iodothyronine (T_3) and thyroxine (tetra-iodothyronine, T_4). Both are produced from tyrosine found in thyroglobulin, which combines with iodine in the colloid, and is then secreted by the thyroid cells into the bloodstream.

Iodine is required for synthesis of thyroid hormones. Iodine is ingested from dietary sources. It is converted to iodide (I^-) in the gut and passes into the bloodstream. It is taken up principally by the thyroid gland, but also by the kidney, which excretes it.

The thyroid cell membranes which lie next to the capillaries absorb iodide via a sodium and iodide pump which concentrates iodide levels in the cell 20- to 40-fold. Energy for this is supplied by $Na^+K^+ATPase$. The iodide is secreted into the colloid and oxidised back to iodine.

Synthesis of thyroid hormones

Thyroglobulin is a large glycoprotein, containing about 10% carbohydrate. It is produced by the thyroid cells and secreted onto the colloid by exocytosis. It contains 123 tyrosine residues. In the colloid, iodine combines with 4–8 of these residues to form mono-iodotyrosine (MIT) and di-iodotyrosine (DIT). MIT combines with DIT to form tri-iodothyronine (T_3) and DIT combines with DIT to form tetra-iodothyronine (T_4) (Figure 22.10). MIT and DIT also combine to form isomeric reverse tri-iodothyronine (rT_3), which is inactive.

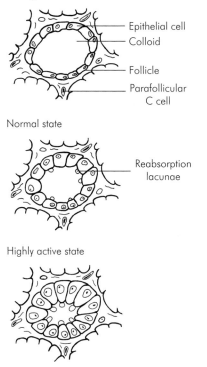

Resting state

— Epithelial cell
— Colloid

— Follicle

— Parafollicular
  C cell

Normal state

Reabsorption
lacunae

Highly active state

Figure 22.9 Follicular structure of the thyroid gland

Alanine is produced in all these coupling reactions as the side chain making up the outer ring of the molecule is eliminated. These reactions are catalysed by the enzyme thyroid peroxidase, which also oxidises iodide to iodine in the colloid (Figure 22.11).

The hormones are held bound to thyroglobulin until they are secreted. They then pass into the thyroid cell by endocytosis, and are secreted by the cells into the bloodstream. The removal of the hormones from the colloid adjacent to the cells creates the reabsorption lacunae seen in active cells.

The thyroid cell has three main functions:
- Absorption and concentration of iodide, and secretion into the colloid
- Production of thyroglobulin and thyroid peroxidase and secretion into the colloid
- Absorption of thyroid hormones from the colloid and secretion into the bloodstream

---

Secretion, transport and metabolism of thyroid hormones

Secretion is controlled by circulating levels of thyroid-stimulating hormone (TSH). Normal plasma levels for the active unbound (free) hormone are about 5 pmol L^{-1} for T_3, and 15 pmol L^{-1} for T_4. Ninety per cent of total secretion per day is of T_4, the remainder being T_3 and a small amount of rT_3, which is inactive. T_3 is, however, up to five times as potent as T_4, which is considered to be a prohormone of T_3. Thirty-three per cent of T_4 is converted to T_3, and much of the remainder to rT_3. The difference in activity is due to differing binding at the intracellular receptors.

Thyroid hormones are transported in the blood by a variety of proteins, including albumin, thyroxine-binding prealbumin (TBPA or transthyretin) and thyroxine-binding globulin (TBG). Albumin has the greatest capacity, but TBG the greatest affinity, such that most of the hormone (70%) is bound to TBG. Less than 1% of the hormone remains unbound. If there is a fall or rise in the total level of the binding proteins the level of the free unbound hormone will remain the same. It is the level of unbound hormone which stimulates or reduces the plasma levels of TSH.

The hormones are deiodinated in the kidney, liver and other tissues, and 33% of T_4 is converted to T_3. Both hormones are also partly broken down to DIT, and also conjugated in the liver to form sulphates and glucuronides, which are excreted in the bile.

Control of thyroid hormone secretion

The main control is the negative feedback system operating via TSH from the anterior pituitary gland, and releasing factor (TRH) from the hypothalamus.

TSH increases secretion of T_3 and T_4 by releasing the hormones from thyroglobulin, from where they are secreted into the thyroid cells and thence into the blood. TSH also increases the size and number of the cells in the thyroid gland itself, which when excessive may lead to goitre. There is also an increase in iodide binding, an increase in T_3 and T_4, release of thyroglobulin into the colloid, and increased endocytosis of colloid by the cells.

Other factors which affect hormone production are trauma, stress and warmth, which decrease it, and cold, which increases it.

Mechanism of action of thyroid hormones

T_3 and T_4 both enter cells and bind with receptors in the nuclei, T_3 more avidly. The hormone receptor complex

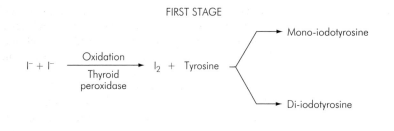

FIRST STAGE

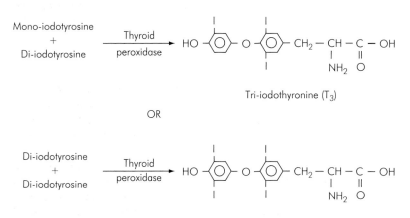

Figure 22.10 Thyroid hormone synthesis

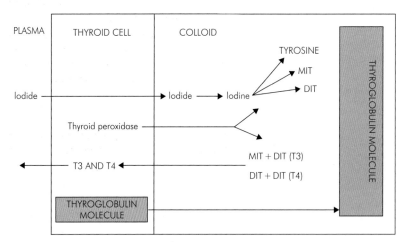

Figure 22.11 Outline of thyroid hormone formation in cell and colloid

Figure 22.12 Summary of main effects of thyroid hormones

Effect	Mechanism
Catabolic	Increased protein breakdown in muscle
	Increased lipolysis in adipose tissue
Metabolic	Increased absorption of carbohydrate from gut
Developmental	Normal skeletal growth
	Normal brain development
Cardiovascular system	Increase β-adrenoceptors in heart
	Increased sensitivity to catecholamines
	Inotropic and chronotropic effects, reduced peripheral resistance
Heat production	Increased metabolic rate in active tissues

then binds with DNA, leading to new mRNA and protein synthesis. The number of mitochondria increases, and there is an increase in metabolic rate, with increased oxygen utilisation, energy production and heat.

There is a catabolic effect, with a stimulation of lipolysis and increased protein breakdown. Absorption of carbohydrate from the gut is increased.

In the cardiovascular system, there is an increase in the number of β-adrenergic receptors in the heart, which also becomes more sensitive to the effect of catecholamines. This leads to a rise in the pulse rate, a decrease in peripheral resistance and an increase in contractility of the heart muscle.

Thyroid hormones are also necessary for normal skeletal and nervous system development. The effects of thyroid hormones are summarised in Figure 22.12.

Deficiency and excess of thyroid hormones
Deficiency (hypothyroidism)
This may be caused by pituitary or hypothalamic failure, disease of the thyroid gland itself, or iodine deficiency.

In adults it may lead to myxoedema. Symptoms and signs include lethargy, slow mental processes and sometimes severe mental symptoms (myxoedema madness). Metabolism is slow; there may be weight gain and intolerance to cold. The voice becomes husky, and the skin and subcutaneous tissues become thickened and stiff, due to reduced breakdown of proteins which accumulate in those sites. In iodine deficiency there may be goitre due to the increased levels of TSH stimulating gland growth.

Children with hypothyroidism develop cretinism. They are mentally retarded, and have the characteristic signs of dwarfism, pot bellies and large protruding tongues.

Excess (hyperthyroidism)
This may be caused by excess production of TSH, for instance from a pituitary tumour, or due to disease of the thyroid gland itself. Solitary adenomas, toxic multinodular goitres and thyroiditis may all lead to excess hormone production.

Graves' disease is an autoimmune disorder in which there are thyroid auto-antibodies which stimulate the TSH receptors and produce excess thyroid hormone that stimulate the receptors themselves. In 50% of patients there is also deposition of tissue behind the eyeball, giving the characteristic appearance of exophthalmos, which can cause severe eye problems. There is also a goitre. The condition is more common in women.

Symptoms and signs of hyperthyroidism include nervousness, tremor, weight loss, sweating and heat intolerance. There may be a tachycardia and a widened pulse pressure. Atrial fibrillation may occur.

Thyroid storm occurs rarely when patients are sick, and can occur during surgery. There may be severe hyperthermia, tachycardia and other arrhythmias, vomiting, diarrhoea, coma and possibly death if untreated.

Parathyroid glands
The parathyroid glands secrete parathyroid hormone (PTH) which is essential for maintaining normal levels of serum calcium.

- Calcium is necessary for normal cell function, in which it acts as a second messenger intracellularly.
- It is needed for coagulation of blood, transmission of nervous impulses and muscular contraction.

Calcium is provided by various dietary sources, and plasma levels are altered by varying absorption in the gut, mobilisation from bone and excretion by the kidney.

Anatomy

There are four disc-like parathyroid glands, two embedded in the upper poles of the thyroid gland, and two in the lower, though their location and number can be variable.

The cells within the gland are of two types. The so-called chief cells have abundant Golgi apparatus and endoplasmic reticulum, and contain secretory granules that produce PTH. The oxyphil cells are fewer but larger, and their function is unknown.

Parathyroid hormone

PTH is a polypeptide produced in the chief cells. It is converted from a preprohormone to a prohormone and thence to PTH, which is stored in the secretory granules before release into the bloodstream.

Action and regulation

PTH has three main actions:

- Mobilisation of Ca^{2+} from bone, raising the plasma Ca^{2+} level.
- Increased reabsorption of Ca^{2+} in the distal tubules, raising the plasma level of Ca^{2+}, and decreased reabsorption of phosphate in the proximal tubules, increasing phosphate excretion. PTH causes an increase of phosphate absorption from the gut and from bones, so there is overall only a small net decrease in plasma phosphate.
- Increased production of 1,25-dihydroxycholecalciferol, which increases Ca^{2+} absorption from the intestine.

There are at least three types of PTH receptors. The main mechanism of action appears to be activation of adenylyl cyclase via G proteins, increasing cAMP levels.

PTH levels are regulated via a negative feedback linked to Ca^{2+} levels. Low levels of Ca^{2+} stimulate PTH secretion and raise Ca^{2+}; high levels of Ca^{2+} reduce PTH production and lower Ca^{2+}, thus maintaining homeostasis. Magnesium is also necessary for the proper function of the parathyroid glands.

Other hormones affecting calcium levels

> Two other hormones, apart from parathyroid hormone, have a direct effect on calcium levels. These are vitamin D and calcitonin.

Vitamin D

Vitamin D refers to a group of sterol compounds which are closely related.

- Cholecalciferol (vitamin D_3) is synthesised in the skin by the action of ultraviolet light on ingested 7-dehydroxycholesterol.
- 25-cholecalciferol (calcidiol) is formed by the conversion of cholecalciferol in the liver. Less than 10% of ingested vitamin-D-related sterols are converted directly to 25-cholecalciferol in the liver, bypassing conversion to cholecalciferol in the skin (Figure 22.13).
- 1,25-dihydroxycholecalciferol (calcitriol) is much more active than 25-cholecalciferol, and is formed by conversion of 25-cholecalciferol in the kidney.

Like other steroid hormones, 1,25-dihydroxycholecalciferol acts by binding to the cell nucleus receptor, exposing DNA binding sites and altering transcription of mRNA. It raises Ca^{2+} and phosphate levels by increasing absorption from the gut, and increases Ca^{2+} absorption in the kidneys. It increases the activity of osteoblasts, laying down Ca^{2+} in the bone matrix.

Vitamin D appears to have effects on immune function, and there is some evidence that low levels may be associated with malignancy and multiple sclerosis.

Calcitonin

Calcitonin is produced by the parafollicular cells (C cells) of the thyroid gland. It reduces Ca^{2+} and phosphate levels in the plasma by reducing bone reabsorption, and is stimulated by high levels of calcium. The function in humans is unclear. Low levels of calcitonin, which occur following thyroidectomy, do not appear to cause any deficiency syndromes. It may be involved with skeletal development and control of Ca^{2+} levels after meals.

Glucocorticoids and others

Glucocorticoids lower Ca^{2+} by inhibiting bone breakdown by osteoclasts, but may cause osteoporosis in the long term. Thyroid hormones cause a rise in plasma calcium but also increase excretion in the kidney. Growth hormone

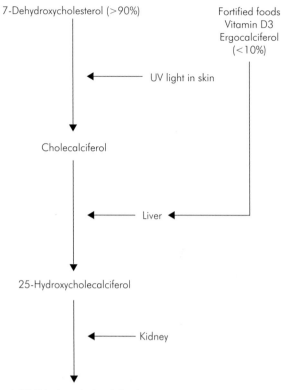

7-Dehydroxycholesterol (>90%)

Fortified foods
Vitamin D3
Ergocalciferol
(<10%)

UV light in skin

Cholecalciferol

Liver

25-Hydroxycholecalciferol

Kidney

1,25-Dihydroxycholecalciferol

Figure 22.13 Formation of 1,25-dihydroxycholecalciferol

Figure 22.14 Summary of main effects of hormones on calcium and phosphate levels

Hormone	Ca^{2+}	Phosphate
PTH	Increase	Decrease
1,25-dihydroxycholecalciferol	Increase	Increase
Calcitonin	Decrease	Decrease
Glucocorticoids	Decrease	Decrease
Thyroid hormones	Variable	Variable
Growth hormone	Increase	Increase

increases absorption of calcium from the gut and has a lesser effect on the kidney, causing increased excretion.

The effects of hormones on calcium and phosphate levels are summarised in Figure 22.14.

Deficiency and excess of parathyroid hormones

Deficiency

Deficiency of PTH, which may occur following thyroid surgery, can cause hypocalcaemia and hyperphosphataemia, leading to increasing neuromuscular excitability and possible tetany.

In pseudohypoparathyroidism, the levels of PTH are normal, but there is a receptor abnormality leading to a similar picture.

Lack of vitamin D can lead to rickets in children and osteomalacia in adults.

Excess

Excess PTH may be produced by a secreting parathyroid adenoma. There is hypercalcaemia and hypophosphataemia, but the patient is often asymptomatic. There may be associated kidney stones or mental symptoms.

In chronic kidney disease the kidney cannot form 1,25-dihydroxycholecalciferol. This leads to a chronically low Ca^{2+}. The parathyroid glands hypertrophy in response to the low Ca^{2+}, leading to secondary hyperparathyroidism.

Excess consumption of vitamin D leads to a rise in both Ca^{2+} and phosphate in the blood.

Adrenal glands

The adrenal glands are found on the upper poles of both kidneys. They comprise two functionally distinct parts, the adrenal cortex and the adrenal medulla.

The cortex is divided into three parts or zones:
- The zona glomerulosa (15% of the gland) secretes mineralocorticoids, which maintain sodium balance and extracellular fluid (ECF) volume.
- The zona fasciculata (50%) secretes glucocorticoids, which have widespread effects on metabolism.
- The zona reticularis (7%) secretes androgenic hormones.

The adrenal medulla (28%) secretes catecholamines, which are produced in 'fight or flight' situations. Both the zona glomerulosa and the zona reticularis are necessary to sustain life. The other parts of the adrenal gland are not.

Adrenal cortex

The zona glomerulosa is situated on the outside layer of cortex, the zona fasciculata in the middle, and the

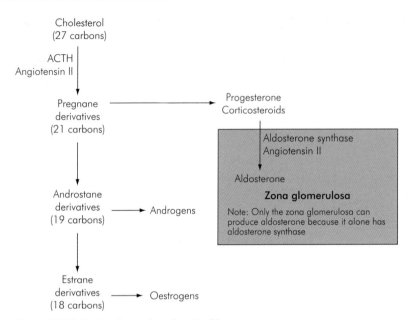

Figure 22.15 Synthesis of adrenal cortical hormones

zona reticularis in the inside, next to the adrenal medulla.

All the cortical cells contain large amounts of endoplasmic reticulum, and large amounts of lipid. There is some overlap of hormone production between the three zones, although mineralocorticoids are only produced in the zona glomerulosa. The latter zone is also able to generate new cells for the other zones should they be damaged or removed.

All the cortical hormones are synthesised from cholesterol, and therefore they all have similar chemical structures based around a steroid nucleus. Aldosterone can be produced only in the zona glomerulosa, because the enzyme which converts corticosteroids to aldosterone, aldosterone synthase, is only found in that zone.

As with all steroid hormones, they bind to intracellular cytoplasmic receptors, the resulting complex then moving to the nucleus. This process produces increased DNA transcription, with increased mRNA synthesis, leading to the formation of proteins and enzymes (Figures 22.15, 22.16).

Mineralocorticoids

Aldosterone is the most important mineralocorticoid as it provides 95% of the total mineralocorticoid activity in the

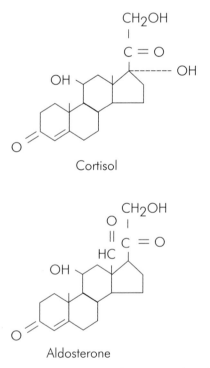

Figure 22.16 Chemical structures of cortisol and aldosterone

body. The remainder is provided by the glucocorticoids. Its production is essential for the maintenance of sodium levels and ECF volume.

> Aldosterone production is stimulated by:
>
> - Increased plasma Na^+
> - Decreased plasma K^+
> - Reduced ECF volume
> - Trauma, stress, surgery, anxiety

Mineralocorticoids increase reabsorption of sodium from the kidneys, stomach, sweat, saliva and intestine. In the kidneys water is also absorbed, while K^+ and H^+ are excreted in exchange into the urine.

Aldosterone is produced in very small amounts, is only slightly protein-bound, and has a very short half-life of about 20 minutes.

> Control of aldosterone secretion is mediated by:
>
> - Angiotensin II
> - ACTH (very little effect in vivo)

Angiotensin II is the most important controlling factor for aldosterone. Low Na^+ levels or reduced perfusion at the juxtaglomerular apparatus cause the production of renin, and via the renin–angiotensin system produce increased angiotensin II levels.

Glucocorticoids

> The most important glucocorticoid produced is cortisol (hydrocortisone). Less important ones include corticosterone and cortisone.

Glucocorticoids have far-reaching effects on the body and are essential to sustain life. Their effects are summarised in Figure 22.17.

Cortisol is bound in the plasma to an α-globulin, transcortin, and to albumin to a lesser extent. The half-life in plasma is about 100 minutes, but the effects of the hormone last much longer.

The level of free unbound hormone activates the feedback control linked to ACTH. If the amount of binding globulin rises, more hormone is bound, which reduces

Figure 22.17 Summary of main effects of glucocorticoid hormones

Metabolism	Catabolic ↑ Protein breakdown
	↑ Gluconeogenesis
	↑ Lipolysis
	Anti-insulin effect (not in brain or heart)
Water	Allows body to excrete a water load (mechanism not understood)
Vascular reactivity and blood pressure control	Allows vascular smooth muscle to respond to circulating catecholamines
	Facilitates conversion of noradrenaline to adrenaline in adrenal medulla
Blood cells	↑ Red cells, platelets, neutrophils
	↓ Neutrophils, basophils, eosinophils
Mineralocorticoid effect	↑ Na^+ ↓ K^+ ↓ H^+ (effect normally small)
Anti-inflammatory	Only at high levels

plasma levels. ACTH production is stimulated and more unbound fraction is formed until a new equilibrium is reached.

Control of cortisol secretion is via the negative feedback system linked with ACTH from the anterior pituitary gland. ACTH is itself controlled by a negative feedback system by ACTH-RH, secreted from the hypothalamus.

Circadian rhythms in the body cause a fluctuation in cortisol levels because of the effects of these on the hypothalamus and ACTH-RH production. Cortisol levels tend to be higher in the morning. Likewise, stress and trauma will stimulate ACTH-RH via the hypothalamus, stimulating ACTH and increasing cortisol production.

Adrenocortical androgenic hormones

The main hormones secreted are dehydroepiandrosterone (DHEA) and androstenedione. The latter is converted to testosterone and oestrogens in peripheral tissues and fat. The androgenic effects of the cortical hormones are small unless they are secreted in excess. There is a sensitive negative feedback system linked with ACTH.

Adrenal medulla

In essence the adrenal medulla is a large sympathetic ganglion which has lost its postganglionic fibres and become purely secretory. About 90% of the cells secrete adrenaline and 10% secrete noradrenaline. Small amounts of dopamine and opioid peptides are also produced.

Extra-adrenal medullary sites are found along the course of the aorta.

Catecholamines are produced in the cells from tyrosine by hydroxylation and decarboxylation (Figure 22.18). Noradrenaline is converted to adrenaline by the enzyme N-methyl transferase (more specifically called phenyl-ethanolamine N-methyl transferase, PNMT), which has to be induced by adequate levels of glucocorticoids.

The catecholamines are metabolised by monoamine oxidase (MAO) and catechol-O-methyl transferase (COMT).

The effects of adrenaline and noradrenaline are mediated through two classes of G-protein-coupled receptor, α and β, which are subdivided into α_1 and α_2 receptors, and β_1, β_2 and β_3 receptors. The effects are summarised in Figure 22.19.

Stimulus and control of medullary hormones

Secretion of medullary hormones is very low during basal states, but is stimulated via the sympathetic nervous system when preparing the individual for 'fight or flight'. Situations which may stimulate secretion include hypoglycaemia, myocardial infarction, heavy exercise, trauma and surgery.

Secretion by the adrenal medulla may be important in the control of blood pressure when changing from a lying to a standing position.

Glucocorticoids are necessary for the secretion of the hormones, as they activate the enzyme which converts noradrenaline to adrenaline.

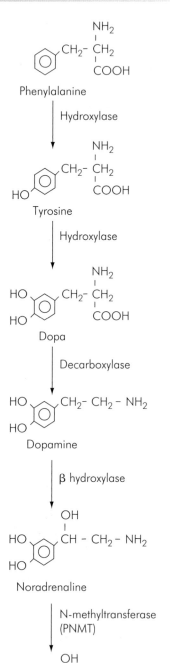

Figure 22.18 Synthesis of adrenaline and noradrenaline

Figure 22.19 Summary of effects of adrenaline and noradrenaline

Metabolic effects	Glycogenolysis in liver and muscle Mobilisation of free fatty acids Stimulation of metabolic rate, increased heat production	
Nervous system	Stimulation	
Cardiovascular system	Adrenaline	Noradrenaline
Heart rate	↑	↓
Cardiac output	↑	↓ low dose ↑ high dose
Peripheral resistance	↓ low levels	↑
Mean arterial pressure	↑ low levels	↑

Abnormalities of adrenal gland function

These manifest themselves in different ways, depending on which part of the adrenal gland is affected.

Adrenal insufficiency

Congenital deficiency in steroid hormone production may evolve into adrenogenital syndrome later in life. The pituitary gland produces large amounts of ACTH, which stimulates growth of the adrenal gland and produces a relative excess of androgens. This can cause virilisation in the female and precocious puberty in the male. Basal production of glucocorticoids and mineralocorticoids is enough to sustain life.

Adrenal insufficiency may be due to disease of the adrenal gland itself or to deficiency of ACTH production. This gives rise to *Addison's disease*, in which a lack of mineralocorticoids and glucocorticoids results in:

- Loss of Na^+ and water, and retention of K^+ and H^+
- Hypotension and weakness, hypoglycaemia, weight loss, loss of resistance to infection and trauma
- Inability to excrete a water load, with water retention
- In severe cases, collapse and coma (Addisonian crisis)

In the primary disease there is increased production of ACTH. This can cause increased pigmentation due to its stimulating effect on melanocytes in the skin. The primary disease is usually more serious than the secondary form.

Adrenal excess

This can affect mineralocorticoid or glucocorticoid hormones, and can be primary or secondary.

Primary aldosteronism is commonly caused by an adenoma of the zona glomerulosa. Excess secretion of mineralocorticoids leads to retention of Na^+ and depletion of K^+, with hypertension, tetany and hypokalaemic alkalosis (Conn's syndrome).

Secondary hyperaldosteronism is due to high renin production, found in cirrhosis, heart failure and some forms of renal disease. Hypertension is a common presenting sign, and hypokalaemia may be severe.

Cushing's syndrome – in this condition excess glucocorticoid production gives rise to the following:
- Muscle wasting, thin hair, poor skin and subcutaneous tissue, and bruising, due to protein catabolism
- Redistribution of body fat to face ('moon face'), abdominal wall and upper back ('buffalo hump'), with numerous striae in the skin
- Hyperglycaemia, which may lead to insulin-resistant diabetes mellitus
- Hyperlipidaemia
- Sodium and water retention due to the mineralocorticoid effects of the glucocorticoids, with accompanying hypertension
- Osteoporosis due to decreased bone formation and increased bone reabsorption
- Mental effects, including increased appetite, insomnia, euphoria and toxic psychosis
- If due to excess production of ACTH there may be hyperpigmentation

Phaeochromocytoma occurs when excess catecholamines are produced by a tumour of the chromaffin cells of the adrenal medulla. These tumours produce varying quantities of adrenaline and noradrenaline. Some may arise from extra-adrenal sites. Patients present with severe hypertension, headaches, sweating and cardiac pathology including arrhythmias and myocardial infarcts.

Pancreas

The **pancreas** is a gland that has both exocrine (secretion of digestive enzymes) and endocrine (secretion of insulin and glucagon) functions.

The pancreas is divided by connective tissue septa into lobules, each of which contains an exocrine secretory unit called an acinus. The acini secrete digestive enzymes which are collected by a duct system and delivered into the duodenum. Lying between the acini and ducts are groups of cells known as the *islets of Langerhans*, which are associated with the endocrine function of the pancreas.

The islets of Langerhans

The islets of Langerhans make up about 2% of the pancreas, and produce hormones which regulate the intermediary metabolism of glucose, fat and protein. The hormones are:

- Insulin, produced by the B cells of the islets (60–75%), which is anabolic, increasing storage of glucose, protein and fat
- Glucagon, produced by the A cells (20%), which is catabolic, opposing the effects of insulin
- Somatostatin, produced by the D cells, which helps regulate islet function
- Pancreatic polypeptide, produced by the F cells, the function of which is little understood

It is perhaps worth noting that B, A and D cells are still often referred to as β, α and δ.

Insulin

Insulin is a polypeptide hormone made of two chains of amino acids, the A and B chains, linked by two pairs of disulphide bridges. It is produced in the endoplasmic reticulum and then transported to the Golgi apparatus, where it is stored in granules, and secreted by exocytosis into the capillaries.

It is synthesised from a preprohormone, preproinsulin, which is a much bigger molecule. When this enters the endoplasmic reticulum part of it splits off, and the remaining molecule folds in two and is joined by the disulphide bonds to form proinsulin. The C-peptide part of the molecule, which facilitates the folding, is then removed, leaving insulin.

There is very little difference between insulin produced by different species, which has allowed bovine and porcine preparations to be given in the past, with little antibody production. It is more common nowadays, however, to give human insulin produced by recombinant DNA technology.

Insulin has far-ranging effects on cells throughout the body, the most obvious one being the effect on uptake of glucose.

There is a specific receptor for insulin on certain cells. This is a tetramer of 340,000 daltons which has two α and two β subunits. The α units occupy an extracellular position and directly bind insulin. The β units are membrane-spanning, and their intracellular portion activates a second messenger system via tyrosine kinase.

Glucose enters most cells by facilitated diffusion (although in the intestine and kidney the process is by secondary active transport with sodium), utilising a group of seven distinct glucose transporter proteins. When insulin binds to a receptor on an insulin-sensitive cell a pool of intracellular transporter-containing vesicles moves to the cell membrane and fuses with it, thus actually inserting transporters into the cell membrane. This process is mediated by phosphoinositol 3-kinase. After the action of insulin ceases, the portions of the membrane containing the transporters are endocytosed, in preparation for the process to begin again.

Although insulin is known to facilitate the entry of potassium ions into the cell, it is not known exactly how this occurs. It may be an effect that increases the activity of the $Na^+K^+ATPase$ pump in a relatively non-specific manner.

The principal anabolic effects of insulin are summarised in Figure 22.20.

Glucagon

Glucagon is a polypeptide hormone produced by the A cells of the islets, firstly as a preprohormone, preproglucagon, which undergoes processing to glucagon and a number of other peptides, some with glucagon-like activities. In a similar fashion to insulin, it is stored in secretory granules and secreted by exocytosis.

Glucagon is a catabolic hormone, and most of its effects are therefore opposite to those of insulin. Glucagon receptors lie in the cell wall. They are G-protein-coupled and therefore exert their effect by activation of adenylyl cyclase and increased intracellular cAMP.

The main effect of glucagon is to raise blood glucose. It does this by:

- Glycogenolysis in the liver (not muscle)
- Gluconeogenesis
- Lipolysis and ketogenesis

Somatostatin

This hormone is produced by the D cells of the islets. Two forms are secreted, SS14 and SS28, but the latter is more active. It is the same hormone as that produced

Figure 22.20 Main actions of insulin on muscle, adipose tissue and liver

	Muscle	Adipose tissue	Liver
Glucose	↑ Glucose entry ↑ Glycogenesis	↑ Glucose entry	↑ Glycogenesis
Protein	↑ Amino acid uptake ↑ Protein synthesis ↓ Protein catabolism ↑ Retention of gluconeogenic amino acids	↑ Protein synthesis	
Fat		↑ Fatty acid synthesis ↑ Activation of lipoprotein lipase	↑ Lipid synthesis
Other	↑ K^+ uptake ↑ Ketone uptake Increased cell growth	↑ K^+ uptake	↓ Ketogenesis

by the hypothalamus which is termed growth hormone inhibiting factor (GH-IH). The effects of somatostatin are:

- Inhibition of insulin
- Inhibition of glucagon
- Inhibition of pancreatic polypeptide

The release of somatostatin is stimulated by a rise in plasma glucose, and it generally slows down propulsive movement in the gastrointestinal tract.

Pancreatic polypeptide

This polypeptide hormone is produced in the F cells of the islets. Its function is uncertain, but it may act to smooth out blood levels of glucose and amino acids after a meal. Its effects can be summarised as follows:

- It is stimulated by a protein meal, and by fasting, exercise and hypoglycaemia.
- It is suppressed by somatostatin and hyperglycaemia.
- It slows absorption of food from the intestine.

Role of the pancreatic hormones in metabolism

The role of the separate hormones has been described. The hormones work together to achieve the following:

- Storage of absorbed nutrients (mainly mediated by insulin)
- Mobilisation of energy reserves during times of stress and hunger (mainly mediated by glucagon)

Figure 22.21 Main factors affecting release of insulin and glucagon

	Stimulating	Inhibiting
Insulin	↑ Glucose (main) Glucagon Selective β-receptor agonists Acetylcholine Sulphonylureas	Adrenaline Somatostatin β-Blockers α-Agonists Thiazides
Glucagon	↓ Glucose Hunger, stress, trauma, exercise, infection Selective β-agonists	↑ Glucose Somatostatin Insulin Ketones Free fatty acids Selective α-agonists

- Maintenance of a steady level of blood glucose (mediated via both insulin and glucagon, with a smoothing effect of somatostatin and possibly pancreatic polypeptide)
- Promotion of growth (insulin)

The stimulating and inhibiting factors acting on insulin and glucagon are summarised in Figure 22.21.

Role of other hormones in carbohydrate metabolism

- Adrenaline causes glycogenolysis followed by a rise in hepatic glycogen production. It also decreases peripheral glucose utilisation.
- Thyroid hormones tend to cause hyperglycaemia due to increased absorption from the intestine. They also cause increased glycogenolysis in the liver, and possibly increased degradation of insulin.
- Adrenal glucocorticoids cause hyperglycaemia, and in excess can produce a diabetic picture (see above). They are needed for glucagon to produce its gluconeogenic effect during fasting; a deficit can lead to hypoglycaemia and collapse.
- Growth hormone causes hyperglycaemia by decreasing glucose uptake in cells, increased glycogenolysis and decreasing binding of insulin. The rise in blood glucose produced when the hormone is produced in excess may stimulate insulin production and exhaust the B islet cells.

Deficiency and excess
Deficiency of insulin
This results classically in diabetes mellitus.

Type 1 (formerly known as insulin-dependent diabetes, IDDM) commonly develops in childhood and is thought to be an autoimmune disease affecting islet B cells only. Patients tend to be thin and have a high incidence of ketosis and acidosis. There may be B-cell antibodies, but it is thought the disease may be mediated via T lymphocytes. The evidence that the disease is autoimmune is supported by the fact that sufferers may be susceptible to other autoimmune conditions such as Graves' disease, Addison's disease and myasthenia gravis.

Type 2 (formerly known as non-insulin-dependent diabetes, NIDDM) usually develops in older, often obese patients. There is also often a family history. There is normal or high insulin production but increased insulin resistance. As the B cells become exhausted the insulin levels may fall. Ketosis and acidosis are rare.

Secondary diabetes may occur when there is overproduction of glucocorticoids or growth hormone, or when there is disease of the pancreas.

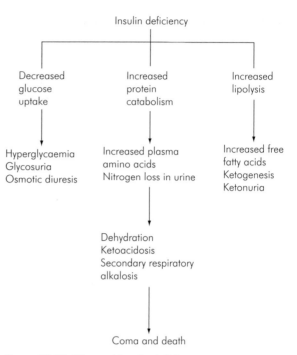

Figure 22.22 Effects of insulin deficiency

The effects of diabetes mellitus

- Glucose – hyperglycaemia leads to an osmotic diuresis with loss of water, Na^+ and K^+. This may lead to severe dehydration. There is reduced uptake of glucose into cells, which may lead to hunger. Glycogen stores are reduced.
- Protein – increased protein catabolism leads to a rise in amino acids in the blood and loss of nitrogen in the urine. This can lead to muscle wasting and reduced resistance to infection.
- Fat – increased catabolism of fat leads to an increase in free fatty acids. Metabolism of these fatty acids produces acidosis, ketosis and ketonuria.
- In the severe acute form of the disease the dehydration may lead to coma and death.
- Over a period of time diabetic patients may develop secondary changes in other organs. Microvascular changes can occur in the eye and kidney. Macrovascular changes can lead to strokes and ischaemic heart disease. Peripheral and autonomic neuropathy can also occur. The neuropathy, in combination with the atherosclerosis, can lead to chronic ulceration and gangrene, especially in the feet.

An overview of the effects of insulin deficiency is shown in Figure 22.22.

Excess of insulin

This can occur with overtreatment of diabetes with insulin or with sulphonylureas and biguanides. Rarely, a tumour of the islet cells, known as an insulinoma, can produce insulin excess.

The manifestations of insulin excess are those that occur because of the effect in the central nervous system, which uses glucose primarily as its source of energy. In milder forms there may be anxiety, palpitations and sweating. As the glucose level falls there may be confusion, fits, coma and death.

References and further reading

Hall GM, Hunter JM, Cooper MS, eds. *Core Topics in Endocrinology in Anaesthesia and Critical Care*. Cambridge: Cambridge University Press, 2010.

Mitchell SLM, Hunter JM. Vasopressin and its antagonists: what are their roles in acute medical care? *Br J Anaesth* 2007; **99**: 154–8.

CHAPTER 23
Physiology of pregnancy

Mary Mushambi

Pregnancy

Normal pregnancy involves major physiological and anatomical adaptations by maternal organs. It is important that anaesthetists involved in the care of the pregnant woman understand these changes in order to provide safe maternal anaesthetic care which is compatible with safe delivery of the baby.

Cardiovascular system

Changes occur in the cardiovascular system during pregnancy, and many of these are compensatory changes designed to cope with the growing fetus, uterus and placenta. They are summarised in Figure 23.1. Although the majority of changes occur during pregnancy, significant changes also occur during labour and immediately following delivery of the baby.

Cardiac output

Cardiac output continues to increase throughout the trimesters of pregnancy, resulting in a rise of 35–40% by the end of the first trimester, increasing to 50% by the end of the second trimester. Cardiac output then remains at 50% above non-pregnant levels throughout the third trimester (Figure 23.2).

Patient posture has been found to influence cardiac output measurements during pregnancy (Figure 23.3). Measurements performed in the lateral position, to avoid aortocaval compression, demonstrate an increase in cardiac output by 5 weeks gestation.

A further transient rise in cardiac output occurs during labour, at delivery and in the immediate period after delivery as a result of uteroplacental transfusion of 300–500 mL of blood from the intervillous space into the maternal intravascular volume (autotransfusion). Cardiac output increases by a further 45% during contractions, a further 60% in the second stage, and up to a further 80% immediately after delivery when compared with the pre-delivery state.

- **Cardiac output** increases throughout pregnancy, to reach a level of 50% greater than in the non-pregnant state during the last trimester.
- The increase in cardiac output in pregnancy is produced by a combination of increased heart rate, reduced systemic vascular resistance (SVR) and increased stroke volume.

Heart rate and stroke volume

Heart rate (HR) is increased above non-pregnant values by 15% at the end of the first trimester. This increases to 25% by the end of the second trimester, but there is no further change in the third trimester.

Stroke volume (SV) is increased by about 20% at 8 weeks and by up to 30% by the end of the second trimester, after which it remains level until term (Figure 23.2). Stroke volume and heart rate both increase during labour and immediately post delivery.

Fundamentals of Anaesthesia, 4th edition, ed. Ted Lin, Tim Smith and Colin Pinnock. Published by Cambridge University Press. © Cambridge University Press 2017.

Figure 23.1 Changes in haemodynamic parameters during pregnancy

	Parameter	Change
Heart	Cardiac output	↑ by 50%
	Stroke volume	↑ by 30%
	Heart rate	↑ by 25%
	Ejection fraction	↑ by 20%
	Left ventricle mass	↑ by 50%
	Left ventricular end-diastolic volume	↑ by 10%
Systemic circulation	Systemic vascular resistance	↓ by 20%
	Pulmonary vascular resistance	↓ by 34%
	Systolic blood pressure	↓ by 6–8%
	Diastolic blood pressure	↓ by 20–25%

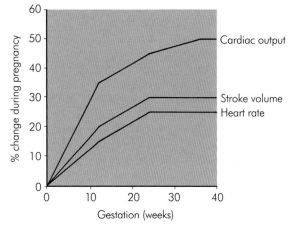

Figure 23.2 Changes in cardiac output through the trimesters of pregnancy

Figure 23.3 The effect of position on cardiac output during pregnancy

Position	Change in cardiac output
Supine	Baseline
Left lateral	↑ by 13.5%
Lithotomy	↓ by 17%
Steep Trendelenburg	↓ by 18%

Distribution of the cardiac output during pregnancy is different from that of the non-pregnant state, with increased blood flow to the uterus, kidneys and skin. Uterine blood flow varies from 500 to 700 mL min^{-1} (about 10–12% of the cardiac output) at term, of which > 80% perfuses the placenta. The flow to the kidneys is increased, as is the flow to the skin due to peripheral vasodilatation. Flow to the liver and brain remains unchanged.

Blood pressure

Blood pressure falls during pregnancy and returns towards the baseline near term. Systolic blood pressure is minimally affected, with a maximum decline of 8% during early and mid-gestation, returning to non-pregnant levels at term. Diastolic blood pressure falls to a greater extent, with early and mid-gestational decreases of 20–25%, and returns to normal at term. In the supine position, 70% of mothers have a fall in blood pressure of at least 10%, and 8% have decreases of 30–50%.

Aortocaval compression

Compression of the inferior vena cava (IVC) and aorta by the gravid uterus occurs during pregnancy and reduces cardiac output. The severity of this effect is dependent on:
- Patient position
- Gestation
- Systemic blood pressure
- Presence of sympathetic block

In the supine position during pregnancy, IVC obstruction occurs and venous blood bypasses this obstruction

Systemic vascular resistance and blood flow to organs

Systemic vascular resistance (SVR) is reduced during pregnancy. The average SVR in pregnancy is about 980 dyne.s.cm^{-5}, compared with about 1150 dyne.s.cm^{-5} in non-pregnant women. The decrease in the SVR results from the development of a low-resistance vascular bed (the intervillous space) and vasodilatory effects of oestrogens, prostacyclin and progesterone.

primarily via vertebral venous plexuses which empty into the azygos vein. IVC compression develops as early as 13–16 weeks gestation, causing a 50% increase in femoral venous pressures. Near term, women in the supine position may experience a 10–20% reduction in stroke volume and cardiac output. This effect becomes maximal between 36 and 38 weeks, after which it may decline as the fetal head descends into the pelvis. Moving from a supine to a lateral position reduces the femoral and IVC pressures, but these are still elevated above those of the non-pregnant woman, indicating that the compression of the IVC is not completely relieved by lateral positioning. In the supine position, 15–20% of pregnant women experience a substantial drop in blood pressure (supine hypotension syndrome), and the patients develop systemic signs of shock, i.e. pallor, sweating, nausea, vomiting and syncope.

Obstruction of the aorta in the supine position has been demonstrated angiographically, but the higher pressures in the aorta prevent total obstruction. This does not cause maternal hypotension but causes arterial hypotension in the lower extremities and in the uterine arteries, which can lead to inadequate uterine blood flow resulting in fetal asphyxia and bradycardia.

> **Aortocaval compression** can reduce cardiac output by up to 20% during pregnancy when the mother is supine at term. The left lateral position can correct this reduction by 60%.

Electrocardiogram (ECG) and echocardiogram

The ECG in pregnancy may show the following changes:
- Sinus tachycardia, reduced PR interval and reduced uncorrected QT interval
- Rotation of the electrical axis of the heart to the left
- ST segment depression
- T wave flattening

However, these changes are thought to be of no clinical significance.

Echocardiographic studies during pregnancy have shown:
- Left ventricular hypertrophy from 12 weeks gestation.
- A 50% increase in left ventricular mass at term. This is due to increase in the size of cardiomyocytes.

- A 12–14% increase in tricuspid, pulmonary and mitral valve annular diameters. The majority of pregnant women have tricuspid and pulmonary regurgitation, and 27% have mitral regurgitation.

Studies have demonstrated a high incidence of asymptomatic pericardial effusion during normal pregnancy.

Heart sounds

The apical impulse moves to the fourth intercostal space and mid-clavicular line. Most pregnant women develop a loud and sometimes split first heart sound. A third heart sound is common, and 16% of women have a fourth heart sound. A grade I–II early to mid-systolic heart murmur is commonly heard at the left sternal edge. This may be due to tricuspid regurgitation resulting from dilatation of the tricuspid valve.

Venous pressure

In the absence of IVC compression by the uterus, central venous pressure (CVP) and venous pressure in the upper limbs are normal. However, during late pregnancy when in the supine position, IVC compression by the gravid uterus occurs and CVP may decrease dramatically. IVC compression can also cause increased venous pressure in the lower limbs.

During labour various factors can cause an increase in CVP, including:
- Contractions – can increase CVP by about 5 cmH$_2$O.
- Expulsive efforts of the second stage – can create a major rise in CVP by up to 50 cmH$_2$O.
- IV ergometrine 0.25 mg after delivery of the baby can produce a rise in CVP of 8 cmH$_2$O, which can last up to 60 minutes.

There are no observed changes in pulmonary capillary wedge and pulmonary artery pressures during pregnancy.

Haematology

The haematological changes found at term are summarised in Figure 23.4.

Blood volume

Plasma volume (PV), total blood volume (TBV) and red blood cell volume (RBCV) all increase during pregnancy. The development of these changes through the trimesters is illustrated in Figure 23.5. Plasma volume rises by 15% during the first trimester and can reach 50% above non-

Figure 23.4 Haematological changes at term, compared with non-pregnant values

	Parameter	Change
Blood volumes	Total blood volume	↑ by 45%
	Plasma volume	↑ by 50%
Blood cells	Red blood cell volume	↑ by 18%
	White cell count	↑
	Haematocrit	↓ by 15%
	Haemoglobin	↓ by 15%
Plasma proteins	Total plasma protein	↓ by 18%
	Albumin	↓ by 14%
	Globulin	↓ or ↑
	Plasma cholinesterase	↓ by 20–25%
	Colloid osmotic pressure	↓ by 18%
Coagulation	Platelets	↓ by 0-5%
	Prothrombin time	↓ by 20%
	Bleeding time	↓ by 10%
	Partial thromboplastin time	↓ by 20%
	Antithrombin III	↓ by 10%
	Fibrinogen	↑ from 2.5 to 4.6 g L^{-1}
	Fibrin degradation	↑ by 100%
	Products	
	Plasminogen	↑
	Fibrinolysis	↑
	Thromboelastography	Hypercoagulable state
Clotting factors	I	↑ by 100%
	VII	↑ by 100%
	VIII	↑ by 150%
	IX	↑ by 100%
	X	↑ by 30%
	XII	↑ by 30%
	XI	↓ by 40–50%
	XIII	↓ by 50%
	Antithrombin III	↓ by 10%
	II	← →
	V	← →

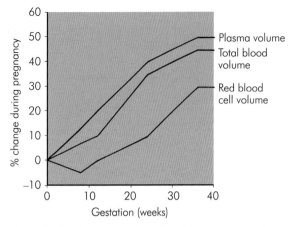

Figure 23.5 Changes in PV, TBV and RBCV through the trimesters of pregnancy

$9-11 \times 10^9$ L^{-1}. This is predominantly an increase in polymorphonuclear cells. There is a further leucocytosis to about 15×10^9 L^{-1} during labour. White cell count returns to normal by 6 days post delivery. Serum levels of IgA, IgG and IgM remain unchanged.

Immunity during pregnancy

In spite of a leucocytosis during pregnancy, depressed neutrophil chemotaxis and adherence leads to reduced polymorphonuclear leucocyte function. This may account for the increased incidence of infection during pregnancy and the reduced incidence of symptoms in women with autoimmune diseases such as rheumatoid arthritis.

---

pregnant values by 32 weeks; it then remains at this level unchanged. Plasma volume returns to non-pregnant levels by 6 days post delivery. There is often a sharp rise of up to 1 litre in plasma volume 24 hours after delivery. This is of significant importance in patients with cardiac disease, such as those with fixed cardiac output. Such patients may develop pulmonary oedema during this period.

RBC volume falls during the first 8 weeks of pregnancy, increasing back to non-pregnant levels by 16 weeks and then rising to 30% above non-pregnant levels by term. This increase in RBC volume is due to raised erythropoietin levels that occur from 12 weeks gestation.

The **physiological anaemia of pregnancy** arises from the increase of only 30% in RBC volume, relative to an increase of 50% in plasma volume in the last trimester. This results in overall reductions of about 15% in haemoglobin (Hb) and haematocrit.

The above changes combine to give total blood volume increases of 10%, 30% and 45% at the end of the first, second and third trimester respectively (Figure 23.5). Oestrogens and progesterone appear responsible for the increase in plasma volume through their effect on the renin–angiotensin–aldosterone systems.

Immune system

The white blood cell (WBC) count rises progressively during pregnancy from non-pregnant levels to

Coagulation

Pregnancy is associated with enhanced platelet turnover, clotting and fibrinolysis (Figure 23.4). Thrombocytopenia (platelets $< 100 \times 10^9$ L^{-1}) occurs in 0.8–0.9% of normal pregnant women, while increases in platelet factor and β-thromboglobulin suggest elevated platelet activation and consumption. Since there is no change in platelet count in the majority of women during pregnancy, there is probably an increase in platelet production to compensate for the increased consumption. Platelet function, however, remains normal during pregnancy.

The concentrations of most coagulation factors (I, VII–X and XII) are increased, and a few (XI and XIII) are reduced. The levels of factors II and V remain the same during pregnancy. There are increases in fibrin degradation products (FDP) and plasminogen concentrations which indicate increased fibrinolytic activity during pregnancy.

Plasma proteins

The plasma concentration of albumin is reduced to 34–39 g L^{-1}, but fibrinogen levels are increased. Globulin is reduced in the first trimester then increases to 10% above the pre-pregnancy level at term. These reductions in plasma proteins are associated with the following changes (Figure 23.4):

- Total colloid osmotic pressure is reduced by 5 mmHg.
- Drug-binding capacity of the plasma is altered, with consequent changes in pharmacokinetics and dynamics (e.g. a reduction in plasma α-acid glycoprotein concentration reduces the lidocaine binding capacity).

Figure 23.6 Respiratory changes at term during pregnancy.

	Parameter	Change
Anatomy	Capillary engorgement	↑
	Upper airway	↑ swelling
	Airways	Dilated
	Diaphragm	Elevated
	Thoracic circumference	↑ by 5–7cm
Lung volumes	Tidal volume	↑ by 45%
	Inspiratory reserve volume	↑ by 5%
	Expiratory reserve volume	↓ by 25%
	Residual volume	↓ by 20%
	Functional residual capacity	↓ by 30%
	Total lung capacity	↓ by 0–5%
	Vital capacity	Nil
	Closing capacity	Nil
Ventilation	Minute ventilation (MV)	↑ by 50%
	Alveolar ventilation (AV)	↑ by 70%
	Respiratory rate (RR)	↑ by 0–15%
	Dead space	↑ by 45%
Lung mechanics	Diaphragm movement	↑
	Chest wall movement	↓
	Total pulmonary resistance	↓ by 50%
	Lung compliance	nil
	FEV_1	nil
	FEV_1/VC	nil
	Flow volume loop	nil
Arterial blood gases	$PaCO_2$	↓ to 3.7–4.2kPa
	PaO_2	↑ to 13.3–14.6 kPa
	pH	↑ to 7.44
	HCO_3	↓ to 18–21 mmol L^{-1}

- Plasma concentration of plasma cholinesterase is reduced by 20–25% at term.
- Erythrocyte sedimentation rate (ESR) and blood viscosity are increased.

Fluid compartments

As described above, plasma volume increases by up to 50% in pregnancy. Extravascular interstitial water also increases, but this increase is variable, from

1.7 litres in women without oedema to 5 litres in women with oedema.

Oedema and plasma protein levels in pregnancy

- Extravascular interstitial fluid volume increases by a variable amount during pregnancy depending on the presence of oedema.
- Total plasma protein concentration falls to 65–70 $g L^{-1}$.

Respiratory system
Anatomical changes
Capillary engorgement and oedema of the mucosa of nasal cavity, pharynx and larynx begin early in the first trimester. This may explain why many pregnant women complain of difficulty in nasal breathing, have more episodes of epistaxis and experience voice changes. The thoracic cage increases in circumference by 5–7 cm because of the increase in both the anteroposterior and transverse diameters from flaring of the ribs. Flaring of the ribs begins early in pregnancy, and is therefore not entirely due to pressure from the enlarging uterus. The enlarging uterus displaces the diaphragm upwards in the later weeks of pregnancy, but the internal volume of the thoracic cavity remains unchanged (Figure 23.6).

Lung mechanics and volumes
Inspiration is mainly as a result of diaphragmatic movement, since flaring of the ribs reduces chest wall movement. Bronchial smooth muscle relaxation decreases airway resistance but lung compliance remains unchanged. Factors contributing to airway dilatation include direct effects of progesterone, cortisone and relaxin.

Forced expiratory volume at 1 second (FEV_1), the ratio of FEV_1 to forced vital capacity (FVC), and the flow–volume loop remain unchanged, demonstrating that large airway function is not impaired during pregnancy.

The following changes in lung volumes occur during pregnancy, relative to non-pregnant values:
- Tidal volume (TV) increases steadily from the first trimester, by up to 45% at term (Figure 23.7).
- Functional residual capacity (FRC) is decreased by 20–30% at term due to reductions of 25% in expiratory reserve volume (ERV) and 15% in residual volume (Figure 23.6).

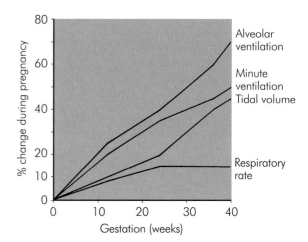

Figure 23.7 Progression of AV, MV, TV and RR changes through the trimesters of pregnancy

- Closing capacity can encroach on FRC, increasing ventilation/perfusion mismatch and leading to the ready occurrence of hypoxia, particularly in supine and Trendelenburg positions.
- Inspiratory capacity increases by 15% at term due to increases in inspiratory reserve and tidal volumes.

Minute ventilation (MV)
MV is increased by up to 50% above non-pregnant values at term. Since respiratory rate remains unaltered, this increase is due to larger tidal volumes. The increased MV levels are stimulated by the high progesterone levels and increased carbon dioxide production occurring during pregnancy.

Dead space is greater by 45% due to dilatation of large airways, but the concomitant increase in tidal volume leaves the ratio of dead space to tidal volume unchanged (Figure 23.6).

Diffusing capacity
Diffusing capacity of the lungs for carbon monoxide (DLCO) is increased during the first trimester, but then decreases until 24–27 weeks gestation, after which it remains unchanged until term.

Blood gases
$PaCO_2$ decreases to 3.7–4.2 kPa by the end of the first trimester and remains at this level until term (Figure 23.8). This is due to alveolar hyperventilation and gives rise to various compensatory mechanisms in an attempt to

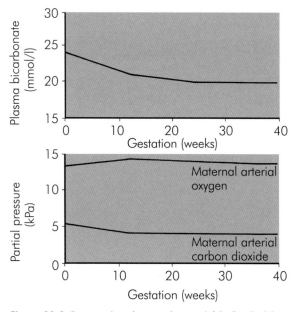

Figure 23.8 Progressive changes in arterial PaO_2, $PaCO_2$ and bicarbonate through pregnancy

maintain normal pH. Metabolic compensation for the respiratory alkalosis reduces the serum bicarbonate concentration to about 18–21 mmol L^{-1}, the base excess (BE) by 2–3 mmol L^{-1}, and the total buffer base by about 5 mmol L^{-1}. Metabolic compensation is not complete, which explains the elevation of maternal blood pH by 0.04 units.

PaO$_2$ in upright pregnant women is in the region of 14.0 kPa, higher than that in non-pregnant women (Figure 23.8). This is due to lower PaCO$_2$ levels, a reduced arteriovenous oxygen difference and a reduction in physiological shunt. The small progressive decline in the PaO$_2$ during the second and third trimesters is due to an increase in arteriovenous oxygen difference.

When PaO$_2$ is determined in the supine position, the values after mid-gestation are often < 13.3 kPa. This occurs because:

- FRC is less than the closing volume in up to 50% of supine pregnant patients.
- Aortocaval compression reduces cardiac output, which increases arteriovenous oxygen difference and reduces mixed venous oxygen content.

Dyspnoea during pregnancy
About 60% of normal pregnant women with no history of cardiorespiratory disease experience dyspnoea. Dyspnoea during pregnancy is therefore not always an indication of organic disease. It commonly occurs in the first and second trimesters, and it is probably a result of lowered PaCO$_2$ levels.

Pulmonary circulation
Pulmonary vascular resistance is reduced from 119 dyne.s.cm^{-5} in the non-pregnant woman to 78 dyne.s.cm^{-5} in the pregnant woman at term. Pulmonary blood flow is increased in pregnancy due to increased cardiac output, and pulmonary blood volume is also greater, as demonstrated by increased vascular markings on chest x-ray. The normal woman can cope with these changes, and the pressures in the right ventricle, pulmonary artery and pulmonary capillaries are not raised.

Oxygen consumption
Oxygen consumption is increased in pregnancy by 30–60% because of the metabolic demands of the fetus, uterus and placenta. The decreased FRC and increased metabolic rate predispose the mother to the rapid onset of hypoxia during induction of anaesthesia or airway obstruction.

Respiratory changes during pregnancy

Tidal volume increases by up to 45%, with associated increases in minute ventilation, and a respiratory alkalosis. Also oxygen consumption increases and FRC decreases during pregnancy.

Gastrointestinal system
Pregnant women have been regarded for many years as being at higher risk of acid aspiration because of the reduction in barrier pressure, increased gastric secretion, reduced gastric pH and delayed gastric emptying.

Barrier pressure
Barrier pressure is reduced significantly in pregnancy compared with the non-pregnant state, because of increased intragastric pressure and reduced lower oesophageal sphincter (LOS) pressure (Figure 23.9). LOS pressure appears to return to normal by 48 hours post delivery. Heartburn occurs in 55–80% of pregnant women and may occur at < 20 weeks gestation. This is thought to be due to gastro-oesophageal reflux that occurs when barrier pressure is reduced. Lowered barrier pressure can be asymptomatic.

Figure 23.9 Gastrointestinal tract changes during pregnancy compared with non-pregnant state

Parameter	Value (non-pregnant value in brackets)
LOS pressure	15.7 cmH$_2$O (15.2)
Gastric pressure (supine)	11.1 cmH$_2$O (5.7)
Barrier pressure	4.6 cmH$_2$O (9.5)
Heartburn	↑
Gastric acid secretion	↓
Gastric emptying	no change or ↓

Figure 23.10 CNS changes during pregnancy compared with non-pregnant state

Increased	Decreased	No change
β-Endorphins Epidural space pressure CSF pH Sensitivity to LA	MAC of volatile anaesthetic agents Epidural space volume LA dose requirements CSF volume	CSF pressure CSF composition

MAC, minimum alveolar concentration; CSF, cerebrospinal fluid; LA, local anaesthetic

Causes of reduced barrier pressure include:

- The altered position of the stomach, which displaces the intra-abdominal part of the oesophagus into the thorax and lowers LOS pressure.
- The relaxant effect of progesterone.
- Elevation of intragastric pressure in the last trimester in both standing and supine positions.
- Intragastric pressure is raised in the lithotomy position (increased by 5.6 cmH$_2$O) and the Trendelenburg position (increased by 8.8 cmH$_2$O).

> **Barrier pressure** = Lower oesophageal sphincter (LOS) pressure − Gastric pressure
>
> This is significantly reduced during pregnancy.

Gastric secretion

The changes in gastric acid secretion in pregnancy and labour are less clear. Commonly used criteria to assess the risk of acid aspiration as high is when gastric pH is < 2.5 and gastric volume is > 25 mL. Some studies have suggested that the total acid content of the stomach is reduced during pregnancy. Gastric pH has been shown to be lower in non-labouring pregnant women (pH 2.4) undergoing elective Caesarean section when compared with non-pregnant women undergoing gynaecological surgery (pH 3.0). Gastric volume is increased during labour.

Gastric emptying

Gastric emptying is not delayed during pregnancy but becomes delayed during labour, particularly if opioids are administered. When labour is conducted with no analgesia or with epidural using local anaesthetics, gastric emptying is not delayed. The use of systemic opioids (e.g. intramuscular pethidine), epidural opioids as a bolus (100 µg fentanyl) and intrathecal opioids (25 µg fentanyl) reduce gastric emptying compared with patients with no opioids, but the effect of low-dose epidural opioid infusions is less clear. Provided that opioids have not been used during labour, gastric emptying returns to normal within 24–48 hours post delivery.

Central nervous system

There are substantial pressure and volume changes in the epidural and subarachnoid spaces, which have important effects on the spread of solutions within these compartments (Figure 23.10).

Epidural space

Compression of the IVC by the gravid uterus results in increased venous pressure below the level of the obstruction. Venous blood is then diverted through vertebral plexuses within the epidural space, and this causes epidural veins to become engorged. Consequently, the epidural volume is reduced and any solutions injected into the lumbar epidural space will spread more extensively.

Pressure in the epidural space of non-pregnant patients is usually negative (−1 cmH$_2$O), but in the pregnant woman it is slightly positive. During contractions, the epidural pressure rises by 2–8 cmH$_2$O, while during expulsion it ranges between 20 and 60 cmH$_2$O.

Subarachnoid space

There are no changes in the constituents or the specific gravity of cerebral spinal fluid (CSF) during pregnancy. CSF pressure is increased by aortocaval compression and by uterine contractions during labour. Baseline pressure in labour between contractions is 28 cmH$_2$O. It is 22 cmH$_2$O when the uterus is displaced laterally to relieve aortocaval compression. During painful contractions, the pressure is increased, and it may reach 70 cmH$_2$O in the second stage.

Sympathetic nervous system

There is increased sympathetic nervous system activity throughout pregnancy, and it is maximal at term. The effect is primarily on the venous capacitance system of the lower extremities, which counteracts the adverse effects of uterine compression of the IVC. Hence, sympathetic block due to either epidural or spinal anaesthesia can result in marked decrease in blood pressure in pregnant women compared with non-pregnant patients.

Drugs and the nervous system

The minimal alveolar concentration (MAC) of inhalational anaesthetic agents is reduced by 40%, which may be related to gestational increase in progesterone levels. β-Endorphin levels in the mother are increased during gestation, labour and delivery.

Epidural drugs during pregnancy

There are reduced requirements for local anaesthetics when administering spinal or epidural anaesthesia during pregnancy. This may be due to decreased volumes of the epidural and subarachnoid spaces, or increased nerve-fibre sensitivity to local anaesthetics.

Endocrine system
Melanocyte-stimulating hormone

Hyperpigmentation of the face, neck and abdominal midline (linea nigra) is due to the effects of increased levels of melanocyte-stimulating hormone (MSH).

Thyroid gland

The thyroid gland increases in size during pregnancy. A goitre may develop as a result of increased blood flow and follicular hyperplasia. Iodine uptake by the thyroid gland increases. Thyroid-binding globulin levels double, which leads to an increase in total tri-iodothyronine (T$_3$) and thyroxine (T$_4$), but free plasma T$_3$ and T$_4$ remain at the non-pregnant level or fall, so that the mother remains euthyroid.

Adrenal gland

The maternal adrenal gland remains the same size but the width and secretion of the zona fasciculata are increased. Plasma cortisol and other corticosteroids increase to 3–5 times the non-pregnant level by term. The half-life of cortisol is prolonged.

Pituitary gland

The pituitary gland increases in weight, making the anterior pituitary very sensitive to haemorrhage and hypotension because its blood supply does not come directly from arterial vessels, but from a portal system whose pressure is below that of the systemic arteries.

Pancreas

The number of B cells increases during pregnancy (causing the islets of Langerhans to enlarge), as does the number of receptor sites for insulin. However, there is a resistance to the action of insulin, possibly due to the presence of human placental lactogen, prolactin and other pregnancy hormones. Human placental lactogen (hPL) and cortisol increase the tendency to hyperglycaemia and ketosis, which may unmask or exacerbate pre-existing diabetes mellitus. The pregnant woman adapts rapidly to starvation. When feeding is withheld, there is early activation of fat metabolism. Fatty acids are utilised and glucose is saved for the fetus.

The upper limit of normal blood glucose in the glucose tolerance test is 7.5 mmol L^{-1} in the second trimester, rising to 9.6 mmol L^{-1} in the third trimester.

Renal function

Renal function changes from early pregnancy. An increase in glomerular filtration rate (GFR) presents the tubules with more urine volume and they lose some of their reabsorptive capacity. Glucose, uric acid and amino acids are not completely reabsorbed, and there is an increased loss of protein of up to 300 mg a day (Figure 23.11).

The activities of renin–angiotensin, aldosterone and progesterone are increased, leading to sodium and water retention and a reduction in plasma osmolality. The changes in renal physiology increase volume of

Figure 23.11 Renal changes during pregnancy compared with non-pregnant state

Increased	Decreased
Renal plasma flow	Renal tubular reabsorption
Glomerular	Plasma urea concentration
filtration rate	Plasma creatinine
Urine volume	concentration
Glycosuria	Plasma osmolality
Proteinuria	Reabsorption of protein
Creatinine	and glucose
clearance	
HCO_3^- excretion	
Urinary stasis	
Renin–angiotensin	
activity	

distribution for drugs. Progesterone helps to conserve potassium during pregnancy.

Progesterone induces ureteric smooth muscle relaxation, which can lead to urinary stasis, making pregnant women prone to urinary tract infections. The collecting system including the renal pelvis dilates, and hydronephrosis occurs in about 80% of women in the second trimester.

Increase in minute ventilation during pregnancy leads to respiratory alkalosis, and the kidney is involved in maintaining acid–base status. There is an increase in the renal excretion of bicarbonate and hence a reduction in the serum bicarbonate levels.

Renal function in pregnancy

Renal plasma flow increases to 30–50% above the non-pregnant level by 30 weeks, then declines gradually. The glomerular filtration rate (GFR) increases to about 150 mL per minute in the second trimester and falls towards term. As a result the plasma concentrations of urea and creatinine decrease.

Liver and biliary system

There are no changes in the liver size or blood flow during pregnancy. However, there are a few minor changes in the liver enzymes (Figure 23.12). The total alkaline phosphatase (ALP) activity is increased by up to 4 times because of the placental secretion of ALP. Other liver enzymes such as alanine aminotransferase (ALT) , aspartate aminotransferase (AST) and lactic dehydrogenase (LDH) remain within

Figure 23.12 Changes in the liver and biliary system during pregnancy compared with non-pregnant state

Parameter	Change
Plasma concentration of ALP	↑
Plasma concentration of ALT	nil
Plasma concentration of AST	nil
Plasma concentration of LDH	nil
Gallstones	↑

ALP, alkaline phosphatase; ALT, alanine aminotransferase; AST, aspartate aminotransferase; LDH, lactic dehydrogenase

normal range but with a tendency to the upper normal levels. Progesterone appears to inhibit the release of cholecystokinin, which reduces the contractile function of the gallbladder resulting in an increase in the incidence of gallstones in pregnancy. There is an increase in the total bile acids. A mild decrease in serum albumin is due to the expanded plasma volume, and as a result plasma oncotic pressure is reduced. A 25–30% decrease in plasma cholinesterase activity is present at term, but this rarely produces clinically significant prolongation of suxamethonium.

Musculoskeletal system

Placental production of the hormone relaxin stimulates generalised ligamentous relaxation. This results in widening of the pubic symphysis and increased mobility of the sacroiliac, sacrococcygeal and pubic joints. As a result, about 49% of pregnant women experience low back pain at 36 weeks.

Relaxin also changes the nature of connective tissue, allowing more fluid to be absorbed. This may contribute to the increased incidence of carpal tunnel syndrome during pregnancy.

Back pain in pregnancy

Back pain is common during pregnancy, and this may be due to changes in the lumbar lordosis as well as the effects of the hormone relaxin. As the uterus enlarges, lumbar lordosis is enhanced to maintain the woman's centre of gravity over the lower extremities.

Weight gain

Weight increases by 10–12 kg owing to increases in maternal body water and fat, the fetus, placenta, amniotic fluid and the uterus. At term, 40% of the weight gained is often in the fetus, amniotic fluid, placenta and uterus. Breast enlargement is typical in normal pregnancy, due to human placental lactogen secretion. Enlarged breasts may be a cause of difficult intubation, and using a short-handle laryngoscope or polio blade may help to overcome this problem.

The placenta

> The **placenta** is critical in the development and maintenance of a healthy fetus. It consists of maternal and fetal tissues and is composed of projections of fetal tissue (villi) that lie in maternal vascular spaces (intervillous spaces). Although the placenta appears as a physical barrier between maternal and fetal tissues, it brings the maternal and fetal circulation into close apposition for physiological exchange across a large area. Fetal wellbeing depends on good placental function for the supply of nutrients and the removal of waste products.

Embryology and anatomy

The ovum is fertilised in the Fallopian tube and enters the uterine cavity, where it rapidly converts to a blastocyst with an inner and outer cell mass. The outer cell layer of the blastocyst then proliferates to form the trophoblastic cell mass. At implantation, the trophoblast erodes into the surrounding decidua of the endometrium and its associated capillaries until the blastocyst is surrounded by circulating maternal blood (trophoblastic lacunae).

The placental tissue develops from the chorion, which consists of the trophoblast and mesoderm of the developing blastocyst. The trophoblast differentiates into two layers, the thick outer syncytiotrophoblast and the thin inner cytotrophoblast. In the second week of development, the (inner) cytotrophoblast layer begins to proliferate and extend cellular fingers into the (outer) syncytiotrophoblast (Figure 23.13). The cytotrophoblast cell columns and their covering syncytiotrophoblast extend as villous stems into the lacunae of maternal blood within the decidua. A mesodermal core appears within the villous stems. These villous stems form the framework from which the villous tree will later develop. Cellular differentiation of the villous mesoderm results in the

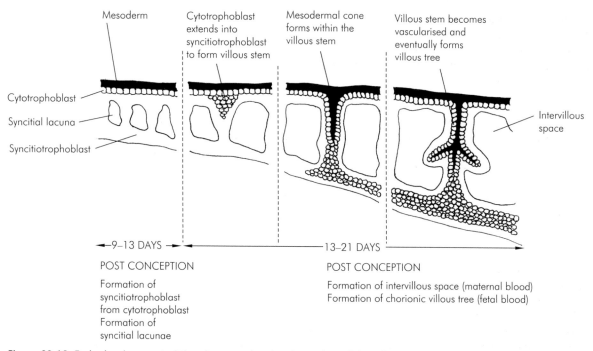

Figure 23.13 Early development of the placenta, showing formation of the villous tree and the intervillous space

formation of blood cells and blood vessels and forms the villous vascular network. With development, the villi branch out extensively into the lacunae (intervillous spaces), forming the villous tree and thereby increasing their surface area.

Cytotrophoblastic cells grow into the lumens of the maternal spiral vessels within the decidua, where they replace the endothelial cells, invading and destroying the musculoelastic medial tissue. As a result of the destruction of the smooth muscle, the walls of the spiral vessels in the decidua become thin and their vasoconstrictor activity is reduced. This wave of trophoblastic invasion starts at 10 weeks and is complete by 16 weeks. A second wave of vascular trophoblastic invasion occurs between 16 and 22 weeks and extends more deeply into the myometrial portions of the spiral arteries. These vessels are easily dilated as maternal flow to the placenta increases. Failure of this physiological change is found in

pre-eclampsia and intrauterine growth retardation. This means that these vessels still respond to vasoconstrictor stimulation, and there is reduced flow to the intervillous space. Further maturation of the villi results in a marked reduction in the cytotrophoblast component and decreases the diffusional distance between the fetal villi and maternal intervillous blood. At term in humans, only a single layer of fetal chorionic tissue (syncytiotrophoblast) separates maternal blood and fetal capillary endothelium. Hence, the human placenta is classified as a haemomonochorial villous placenta.

The placenta is connected to the developing embryo by a connecting stalk that subsequently becomes the umbilical cord containing the umbilical vessels. The placenta is supplied with maternal blood from the uterine blood vessels. Blood enters the intervillous space from the open ends of the uterine spiral arteries (Figure 23.14). The intervillous space is a large cavernous expanse into which

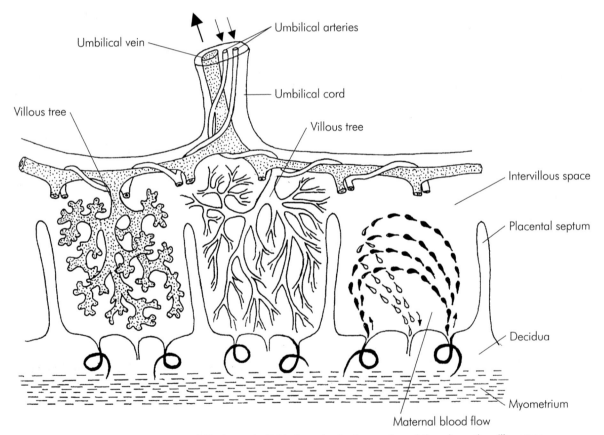

Figure 23.14 Placental circulation. Umbilical vessels divide into chorionic vessels and then form the villous tree (fetal blood). Blood in spiral arteries flows into the intervillous spaces (maternal blood).

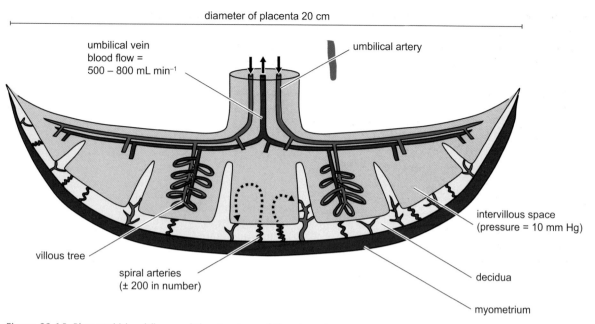

Figure 23.15 Placental blood flow and the structure of the placenta

the villous trees reach. Blood enters the intervillous spaces and flows into loosely packed areas, then into densely packed intermediate and terminal villi. It then empties into collecting veins. However, the relative direction of the blood flow is haphazard and behaves like a concurrent system, though with maternal blood flow exceeding fetal blood flow. The area of densely packed terminal villi is where placental exchange occurs. Maternal placental blood flow is a low-pressure system; the pressure in the intervillous space is on average 10 mmHg. The increasing demands of the growing fetus require 100–200 spiral arteries to feed directly to the placenta (Figure 23.15). The maternal circulation through the intervillous space is fully developed by 20 weeks. Blood flow will increase from 50 mL min^{-1} at 10 weeks to 500–800 mL min^{-1} at term.

Two umbilical arteries arising from the fetal internal iliac arteries carry deoxygenated fetal blood via the umbilical cord to the placenta, and a single umbilical vein returns oxygenated blood to the fetus. The umbilical arteries divide into chorionic arteries, which feed the multiple placental lobules, and these in turn subdivide into the villous trees, which end as capillaries in the terminal villi (Figure 23.15). Fetal sinusoids formed within the terminal villi provide a large endothelial surface area and make it the ideal region for maternal–fetal exchange. Each villous tree drains into a large vein that perforates the chorionic plate to become

chorionic veins. Each of the venous tributaries courses towards the umbilical cord attachment site, where they empty into one umbilical vein.

The placenta grows dramatically from the third month of gestation until term. There is direct correlation between growth of the fetus and that of the placenta. By term, the mature placenta is oval and flat with an average weight of 500 g, average diameter of 20 cm and thickness of 3 cm.

Uterine blood flow

> **Uterine blood flow** is influenced by intrinsic and extrinsic factors. Chronic regulation of uterine blood flow occurs mainly through intrinsic factors. These include prostaglandins (prostacyclin), nitric oxide and oestrogens. Extrinsic factors are more involved in the acute changes of uterine perfusion.

In general, uterine blood flow (UBF) is related to perfusion pressure and vascular resistance according to the following formula:

$$UBF = \frac{Uterine\ arterial\ pressure - Uterine\ venous\ pressure}{Uterine\ vascular\ resistance}$$

Figure 23.16 Factors which reduce uteroplacental blood flow

1. Maternal arterial hypotension due to:
   - Hypovolaemia
   - Aortocaval compression
   - Sympathetic block

2. Increased uterine venous pressure due to:
   - Contractions
   - IVC compression as part of aortocaval compression
   - Valsalva manoeuvre (such as when pushing in second stage of labour)

3. Increased vascular resistance due to:
   - Maternal hypertension
   - Pre-eclampsia
   - Endogenous and exogenous vasoconstrictors

Any factors that alter uterine blood flow will affect placental perfusion (Figure 23.16). Uterine arterial pressure is reduced by systemic hypotension. Uterine venous pressure is increased by IVC compression, uterine contractions and Valsalva manoeuvre (i.e. pushing in the second stage of labour).

Uterine vascular resistance is affected by endogenous and exogenous vasoconstrictors. Endogenous vasoconstrictors such as catecholamines are increased by stress and pain during labour.

Functions of the placenta

- Placental transfer of products between maternal and fetal blood
- Transfer of immunity by transfer of immunoglobins from the mother
- Endocrine function
- Detoxification of drugs and substances transferred from the mother

Placental transport
Mechanisms of placental transport
Cellular membrane transport mechanisms in the placenta include:
- Simple diffusion
- Facilitated transport
- Secondary active transport

Figure 23.17 Blood gas tensions in maternal and fetal blood

Location	PO_2 (kPa)	PCO_2 (kPa)
Maternal artery	13.3	3.9
Fetal umbilical artery	2.0	5.9
Fetal umbilical vein	3.9	4.7

- Active transport
- Pinocytosis
- Bulk transport

Substances crossing the placenta
The placenta acts as a barrier between maternal and fetal tissues. However, it is an imperfect barrier, and most substances will cross the placenta, as detailed below.

Oxygen
Oxygen crosses the placenta by simple diffusion, depending mainly on the difference between the oxygen tension of the maternal blood in the intervillous space and that of the fetal blood in the umbilical artery. The PO_2 of blood in the intervillous space varies greatly but will be dependent on maternal arterial PO_2 (Figure 23.17). The placenta is a metabolically active organ, using 30% of the total oxygen delivered to it.

Other factors affecting oxygen transfer include the shape of the fetal oxyhaemoglobin dissociation curve (ODC) and the Bohr effect. The fetal oxyhaemoglobin dissociation curve (P_{50} = 2.5–2.8 kPa) lies to the left of the maternal curve (P_{50} = 3.6 kPa). This favours the transfer of oxygen from the mother to the fetus.

A rise or fall in CO_2 tension (with corresponding fall or rise in pH) leads to right or left shift response in the dissociation curve and also affects oxygen transfer (the Bohr effect) (Figure 23.18). At the gas exchange interface, fetal blood gives up carbon dioxide, becomes more alkaline (left shift) and develops a greater affinity for oxygen. The maternal blood on the other hand takes up carbon dioxide, becomes more acidic (right shift) and promotes release of oxygen. This is referred to as the double Bohr effect, and it accounts for 2–8% of the transplacental transfer of oxygen.

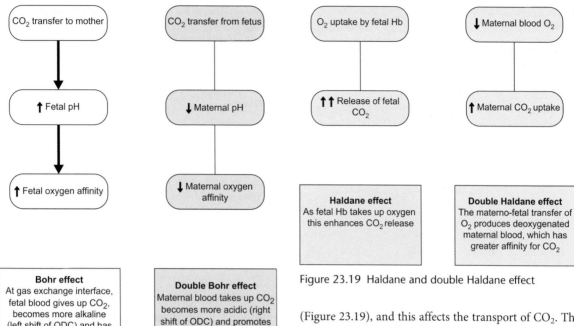

Figure 23.19 Haldane and double Haldane effect

Figure 23.18 Bohr and double Bohr effect

Factors determining oxygen transfer across the placenta

- High materno-fetal oxygen concentration gradient
- Double Bohr effect
- The shape of the fetal oxyhaemoglobin dissociation curve
- High fetal haemoglobin concentration
- Functional status of the placenta
- Uterine blood flow and placental perfusion

Carbon dioxide

CO_2 crosses the placenta by simple diffusion. It is present as dissolved CO_2 (8%), bicarbonate ion (62%), and carbamino haemoglobin (30%), with very small quantities as carbonic acid (H_2CO_3) and carbonate ion CO_3^{2-}. Dissolved CO_2 is the form that crosses the placenta. The placental membrane is highly permeable to CO_2, which is 20 times more diffusible than oxygen.

A rise or fall in oxygen tension leads to a reduced or increased affinity for CO_2 (the Haldane effect) (Figure 23.19), and this affects the transport of CO_2. The materno-fetal transfer of oxygen produces deoxyhaemoglobin in the maternal blood that has a greater affinity for CO_2 than oxyhaemoglobin. As the fetal blood takes up oxygen, it enhances CO_2 release. This is known as the double Haldane effect, and it may account for as much as 46% of the transplacental transfer of CO_2. HCO_3^- is not a major contributor to this process because of its ionised form, but it does act as a source of CO_2 through the carbonic anhydrase reaction that keeps CO_2 and HCO_3^- in equilibrium.

Glucose

Glucose crosses the placenta by facilitated transport, which is stereospecific for the D-isomer. The placenta uses most of the glucose absorbed from the maternal surface.

Amino acids

Amino acids cross the placenta by means of secondary active transport. Much of the transplacental transfer of amino acids occurs by way of linked carriers for both amino acids and sodium. The transport of sodium down its concentration gradient drags amino acids into the cells. The process is stereospecific.

Fatty acids

Fatty acids probably cross the placenta by simple diffusion.

Electrolytes and water

Sodium and water cross the placenta by simple diffusion and bulk transport. Iron, iodine, calcium and phosphate require active transport.

Proteins

The placenta is relatively impermeable to plasma proteins. However, some immunoglobulins, particularly IgG, cross the placenta by pinocytosis.

Hormone secretion

The placenta produces the following hormones:

- Human chorionic gonadotropin (hCG)
- Human placental lactogen (hPL)
- Hypothalamic releasing factors
- Hypothalamic inhibitory factors
- Oestrogens
- Progesterone
- Thyroid-stimulating hormone (TSH)
- Prostaglandins

hCG rises rapidly in early pregnancy, and it forms the basis of the routine pregnancy test. This rapid rise in hCG production in early pregnancy stimulates the corpus luteum to secrete progesterone, which is required to maintain the viability of the pregnancy. Peak excretion is at 8–10 weeks. The role of hCG in late pregnancy is not clear.

Progesterone is secreted by the corpus luteum until the 8th week. After the 8th week, it is secreted by the placenta. It is responsible for many of the maternal physiological changes.

The concentration of human placental lactogen (hPL) increases during pregnancy. Its functions include increased lipolysis, increased gluconeogenesis and anti-insulin effect.

Four types of oestrogens are secreted by the placenta (oestrone, oestradiol, oestriol and oestretol). Oestrogens stimulate uterine expansion to accommodate the growing fetus.

It is likely that the interaction between these placental peptides is important in the control of growth and development of the fetus.

Immunological functions of the placenta

The placenta modifies the immunological system in the fetus and the mother so that the fetus is not rejected. The mechanism for this is not well understood, but during pregnancy there is a reduction in cell-mediated immunity and activity of T-cytotoxic cells, increased neutrophils and reduced IgG. IgG (but not IgA or IgM) is transferred across the placenta. The placenta forms a barrier against transfer of some infections to the fetus but does not protect against others such as HIV and rubella.

Placental transfer of drugs

Measurement of placental drug transfer

Feto-maternal (F/M) concentration ratios of drugs are frequently used as an index of placental transfer of drugs, but they are influenced by several factors, such as:

- Site of fetal sampling
- Time interval between drug administration and sampling
- Whether drug is given as bolus or infusion

Factors affecting placental drug transfer

Most drugs, given enough time, will cross the placenta. The rate of transfer is dependent on:

- Lipid solubility
- Degree of ionisation
- pH of maternal blood
- Protein binding
- Molecular weight of drug
- Materno-fetal concentration gradient
- Placental blood flow

Lipid solubility

Lipophilic molecules diffuse readily across lipid membranes, of which the placenta is one.

Degree of ionisation

Only the non-ionised fraction of a partly ionised drug crosses the placental membrane. Most drugs used in anaesthesia, analgesia and sedation are poorly ionised in the blood and their placental transfer is almost unrestricted. Muscle relaxants are highly ionised, and therefore their transfer is almost negligible.

pH of maternal blood

The pH of maternal blood can alter the degree of ionisation of a drug. This effect is dependent on the pK_a of the drug. If the pK_a is near the pH of blood, then small changes in blood pH (such as may occur during labour) produce large changes in drug ionisation.

Protein binding

The diffusibility of a protein-bound drug is negligible compared with that of free drug. Protein binding is influenced by blood pH and concentration of plasma proteins. Acidosis reduces the protein binding of local anaesthetic, and low serum albumin in pre-eclampsia will cause a higher proportion of unbound drug and therefore promote transfer of drugs across the placenta.

Molecular weight of drug

Drugs with molecular weight of 600 daltons or less readily diffuse across the placenta. Most drugs used in anaesthetic practice have molecular weights < 600, and therefore diffuse readily.

Materno-fetal concentration gradient

When a drug is transferred by simple diffusion, its rate of transfer is determined by Fick's law of diffusion.

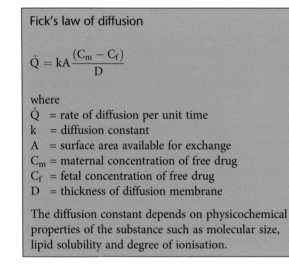

Fick's law of diffusion

$$\dot{Q} = kA \frac{(C_m - C_f)}{D}$$

where
$\dot{Q}$ = rate of diffusion per unit time
k = diffusion constant
A = surface area available for exchange
C_m = maternal concentration of free drug
C_f = fetal concentration of free drug
D = thickness of diffusion membrane

The diffusion constant depends on physicochemical properties of the substance such as molecular size, lipid solubility and degree of ionisation.

Placental blood flow

With poorly diffusible drugs, the concentration in maternal and fetal blood changes little during placental transit, and hence blood flow has little impact on transplacental gradient. With highly diffusible drugs, concentration gradient falls significantly as a result of transfer, and hence blood flow has a marked effect on gradient.

Placental transfer of individual drugs
Opioids

All opioids cross the placenta in significant amounts. Pethidine is commonly used during labour. It is about

Figure 23.20 Half-lives for pethidine and norpethidine in mother and neonate

	Half-life (hours)	
	Pethidine	*Norpethidine*
Mother	4	21
Neonate	19	62

50% plasma protein-bound and has almost unrestricted placental transfer. The drug can be detected in umbilical venous blood as early as 90 seconds after maternal administration, and the maximum uptake by fetal tissue occurs 2–3 hours after a maternal IM dose, which is when neonatal respiratory depression is most likely to occur. The F/M ratio may exceed 1 after 2–3 hours. Maternal levels fall rapidly because of the greater capacity for maternal metabolism. Longer half-lives for pethidine and its active metabolite norpethidine in the neonate, compared with the mother, mean that there is a risk from cumulative side effects in the neonate (Figure 23.20).

Morphine is poorly lipid-soluble and weakly plasma protein-bound, but readily crosses the placenta. Its F/M ratio is about 0.61. Fentanyl is highly lipid-soluble, crossing the placental membrane rapidly, but is largely albumin-bound (74%). The F/M ratio after maternal epidural administration is between 0.37 and 0.57. Alfentanil is less lipophilic than fentanyl but is more highly bound to plasma protein. Its F/M ratio is 0.30. Administration of remifentanil has been associated with rapid placental transfer and has potential to produce respiratory depression in the newborn. Fetal blood concentrations of remifentanil are generally about half of that of the mother just before delivery. The umbilical artery/umbilical vein (UA/UV) ratio is about 30%, suggesting rapid metabolism by the neonate.

Local anaesthetic agents

Local anaesthetic agents cross the placenta by simple diffusion. Commonly used local anaesthetics have molecular weights ranging from 234 daltons (lidocaine) to 288 (bupivacaine). They are weak bases and have relatively low degrees of ionisation and high lipid solubility at normal pH. Local anaesthetic accumulation in the fetus can occur if the fetus is acidotic, due to 'ion trapping'. This occurs when reduced pH in the fetus produces increased ionisation of the local anaesthetic and resultant lower diffusibility.

Drugs that are highly plasma protein-bound (bupivacaine, etidocaine) will have reduced placental transfer and lower F/M ratios compared with those with lower plasma protein binding (lidocaine, mepivicaine).

Transfer to the fetus is also affected by other factors, which include dose, site of administration and effects of adjuvants such as adrenaline. Higher doses result generally in higher maternal and fetal blood concentrations. The vascularity of the site of injection will determine the rate of absorption of the drug. For example, absorption from a paracervical injection is greater than from epidural injection. Addition of adrenaline to local anaesthetic solutions affects the rate of absorption from the site of injection, but the true effect of adrenaline on the various local anaesthetics is still unclear. The addition of adrenaline is thought to reduce absorption of lidocaine but not of bupivacaine.

Inhalational agents
The high lipid-solubility and low molecular weight of these agents facilitate rapid transfer across the placenta. Halothane rapidly crosses the placenta (F/M ratio = 0.87) and can be detected in umbilical venous and arterial blood within 1 minute. Enflurane and nitrous oxide also cross rapidly (F/M ratio = 0.6 and 0.83 respectively), but there is limited information on isoflurane. Diffusion hypoxia may occur in a neonate exposed to nitrous oxide immediately before delivery.

Induction agents
Sodium thiopental is a highly lipophilic weak acid and it is 75% bound to plasma albumin. It rapidly crosses the placenta (F/M ratio = 0.4–1.1), and so do ketamine (F/M ratio approximately 1.3) and propofol (F/M ratio 0.65–1.15). However, the pharmacokinetics of propofol are yet to be investigated fully. Propofol is highly protein-bound, and therefore placental transfer is affected by maternal plasma protein concentration.

Muscle relaxants
These drugs are fully ionised and poorly lipid-soluble, and therefore do not readily cross the placenta.

Anticholinergics
The placental transfer rates of anticholinergic drugs correlate directly with their ability to cross the blood–brain barrier. Atropine is detected in umbilical circulation within 1–2 minutes of maternal IV injection. In contrast, glycopyrrolate is poorly transferred.

Vasopressors
Vasopressors are often used to treat hypotension secondary to regional anaesthesia. Ephedrine appears to cross the placenta easily and has an F/M ratio of 0.7.

Benzodiazepines
Diazepam readily crosses the placenta. It is highly non-ionised and very lipophilic. The F/M ratio reaches 1 within minutes of injection and reaches 2 an hour after injection. Midazolam has an F/M ratio of 0.76, but it has a short half-life.

References and further reading

Frolich MA. Maternal and fetal physiology and anesthesia. In Butterworth JF, Mackey DC, Wasnick JD, eds., *Morgan and Mikhail's Clinical Anesthesiology*, 5th edn. Columbus, OH: McGraw-Hill, 2013, pp. 825–42.

Gaiser R. Physiologic changes of pregnancy. In Chestnut DH, Wong CA, Tsen LC, *et al.*, eds., *Chestnut's Obstetric Anesthesia: Principles and Practice*, 5th edn. Philadelphia, PA: Elsevier Saunders, 2009, pp. 15–38.

CHAPTER 24
Fetal and newborn physiology

Andrew Wolf

As the fetus develops from a single dependent cell into a fully formed neonate capable of sustained life outside the womb, the physiology of individual organs and the integrated systems of the body undergo substantial developmental changes. Although physiology in the early stages may be crude, and significantly different from that observed in maturity, it usually reflects functional differences that allow the fetus to cope with the challenges of the intrauterine environment, and also with the sudden, extreme changes needed for adaptation to extrauterine life. For example, the presence of fetal haemoglobin in utero allows oxygen to be extracted from the placenta in a very low-oxygen environment compared to after birth. In considering developmental physiology (ontogeny) it is necessary to see fetus, preterm newborn, neonate, infant, child and adolescent as stages of development that merge into each other.

Fetal circulation

The fetus and placenta encompass a unit in which the placenta enables the fetus to eliminate carbon dioxide and metabolic waste products in exchange for oxygen and nutrients from the maternal circulation (Figure 24.1). Blood leaves the placenta in the single umbilical vein with an oxygen saturation of approximately 80%. The ductus venosus shunts half of the oxygenated umbilical venous blood through the liver to enter the inferior vena cava (IVC).

The mixed IVC blood, with a saturation of 65%, enters the right atrium, but only one-third passes into the right ventricle. The majority is directed through the foramen ovale to the left atrium and left ventricle to supply the heart, brain and upper body with relatively oxygenated blood. Venous blood from the superior vena cava, with low saturation (25%), is directed preferentially to the right ventricle and pulmonary artery. In the fetus, pulmonary vascular resistance (PVR) is high, and less than 10% of cardiac output passes through the lungs. This is achieved by intense vasoconstriction in the pulmonary arterioles and patency of the ductus arteriosus, which allows the majority of blood passing into the pulmonary artery to join the aorta. This mixed aortic and ductal blood flow supplies the lower body with blood with a saturation of approximately 55%. Blood returns to the placenta via two umbilical arteries arising from the internal iliac arteries. Placental blood flow is large, comprising 60% of the fetal cardiac output.

Newborn circulation

At birth, with onset of spontaneous ventilation in the lungs and loss of the placenta, the circulation changes dramatically. The first breath generates a negative pressure of approximately 50 cmH_2O, drawing in about 80 mL of air and expanding the functional residual capacity. Pulmonary vascular resistance (PVR) falls rapidly, allowing blood to flow from the right ventricle through the lungs. As placental flow ceases with clamping of the umbilical cord, systemic vascular resistance (SVR) rises. The result is a reversal of right-to-left flow through the ductus arteriosus. Exposure to oxygenated blood and reduced prostaglandin-E_2 production stimulates ductal constriction, with functional closure in the majority of

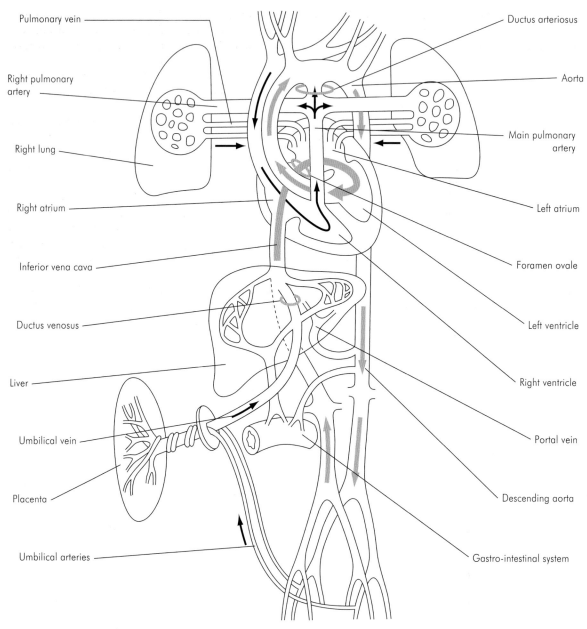

Figure 24.1 Fetal circulation

newborns by 24 hours. A shunt murmur may be audible prior to closure. Histological obliteration occurs by 3 weeks in most normal term infants. Preterm babies have a higher incidence of patent ductus arteriosus, and may require medical treatment with indomethacin, or surgical ligation. The ductus venosus closes passively, due to absent blood flow.

After the first breath, pulmonary venous blood returns to the left atrium, causing pressure in the left atrium to exceed that in the right. This effect on raised left atrial pressure is enhanced by the sudden rise in SVR from loss of the placental blood flow. The valve-like foramen ovale closes, thus preventing deoxygenated blood from the right atrium crossing to the left.

Although the PVR is reduced after birth, it continues to fall for several days after birth, and the pulmonary arteriolar medial walls remain very muscular. This muscle layer reduces considerably over the first few months and becomes thin-walled and elastic with little muscle by 6 months. However, immediately after birth, resistance in the pulmonary circuit is higher than in adults and the pulmonary arterioles remain very reactive. If the neonate becomes hypoxic, hypercapnic or acidotic, pulmonary vasoconstriction can lead to raised right-sided pressures and significant shunting through the foramen ovale, and reversion to a fetal-type circulation. This condition is called persistent pulmonary hypertension of the newborn (PPHN). Oxygen, hyperventilation or nitric oxide may be needed to reverse the condition, and extracorporeal membrane oxygenation (ECMO) has been successfully used in severe and persistent cases.

In addition, calcium metabolism is immature in neonatal myocytes. Consequently there is a relatively flat Starling curve, and while inadequate preload is poorly tolerated, overloading results in early cardiac failure.

Ventricular end-diastolic volume increases from 40 mL m^{-2} body surface area at birth to 70 mL m^{-2} in children over 2 years of age. Normal heart rate at birth ranges from 100 to 170 beats per minute, decreasing with age and reaching adult values by puberty (Figure 24.2). The preterm neonate has significantly lower blood pressure than the term infant, and adult levels are not reached until adolescence.

Autonomic innervation of the heart and blood vessels is incomplete in the newborn, with a relative lack of sympathetic supply. This is highlighted by the relatively small falls in blood pressure associated with high spinal blockade when using regional anaesthesia. Moreover, neonates are also less sensitive to the effects of catecholamines, needing much larger doses than older children or adults to achieve an increase in blood pressure and heart rate.

Fetal and newborn circulation

- The placenta supplies oxygen and nutrients to the fetus via an umbilical vein, and removes carbon dioxide and waste via two umbilical arteries.
- Fetal circulation depends on three shunts to direct the best oxygenated blood to the upper body (foramen ovale), to bypass the underdeveloped liver (ductus venosus), and to bypass underdeveloped lungs (ductus arteriosus and foramen ovale).
- Following delivery and the first breath, PVR decreases rapidly, allowing blood to flow through the lungs, from the RV to LA. This reverses the pressure gradient across the foramen ovale and closes it.
- SVR increases after delivery, reversing the pressure gradient and flow in the ductus arteriosus.
- Blood flow through the liver increases, and the flow is decreased through the ductus venosus, which closes spontaneously.

The fetal heart

- In the fetus, the two ventricles are effectively in parallel, with the dominant right ventricle pumping approximately two-thirds of the combined ventricular output via the pulmonary artery, through the ductus arteriosus and into the aorta.
- In the newborn, stroke volume is relatively fixed, and increases in cardiac output are achieved largely by increases in heart rate.
- Both ventricles weigh the same at birth, although the right ventricle is the dominant ventricle in fetal life, possessing a thicker wall at the time of delivery.
- The left ventricle enlarges rapidly after birth, and by age 6 months reflects the adult ratio. This is mirrored in the ECG, which shows right axis deviation at birth, with an axis of up to $+180°$, changing to $+90°$ by 6 months.

The heart

The newborn heart consists of cardiac myofibrils that are poorly organised and lack the structured architecture of the mature heart. The increased ratio of connective tissue to contractile tissue compared to adults results in limitation in myocyte contractility and ventricular compliance.

Pulmonary function

The fetal lung is filled with fluid essential for lung maturation and development. Irregular breathing movements are made in utero, which helps development of respiratory muscles, including the diaphragm and intercostal muscles. As full term approaches, catecholamines and triiodothyronine (T_3) stimulate the reabsorption of pulmonary fluid by reversal of the chloride pump mechanism.

Figure 24.2 Normal cardiovascular values in childhood

Age	Systolic BP (mmHg)	Diastolic BP (mmHg)	Heart rate (beats min^{-1})
Preterm 750 g[a]	45	25	> 120
Birth	60	35	> 120
Neonate	70–80	40–50	120–150
3–6 months	80–90	50–60	120–140
1 year	90–100	60–80	110–130
5 years	95–100	50–80	90–100
12 years	110–120	60–70	80–100

[a] Mean arterial BP $\leq$ gestational age in weeks is a good rule of thumb for preterm infants.

Final reabsorption is stimulated by the physical passage through the birth canal. This stage is less effective in babies born by Caesarean section, and can lead to a condition called transient tachypnoea of the newborn (TTN). Type II pneumocytes produce surfactant under hormonal stimulation (cortisol) from 26 weeks gestation. Surfactant stabilises alveoli by reducing surface tension, and artificial surfactant administration may be needed in preterm infants to prevent them developing respiratory distress syndrome (RDS). Term babies may also be surfactant-deficient if they suffer severe acidosis or hypoxia, or if they are born to mothers with diabetes mellitus.

The bronchial tree is fully developed at birth, in contrast to the alveoli, which continue to expand in both size and number, thus increasing the surface area of the lung by up to 25 times. Newborn infants have extremely compliant chest walls with compressible, horizontally aligned ribs. The diaphragm is the major muscle of ventilation in infancy, but can fatigue more easily in the neonate. In the first year of life, the percentage of type I, slow-twitch muscle fibres, which fatigue more slowly, increases from 10% to 25% (the adult level).

Newborn ventilatory control

- Newborn infants show ventilatory responses to changes in PaO_2 and $PaCO_2$, but these are less responsive and affected by other factors such as gestational and postnatal age, temperature, wake–sleep cycles and drugs.
- Neonates react to hypoxia with a brief period of hyperpnoea followed by centrally mediated respiratory depression. In the weeks that follow, as chemoreceptors mature, the infant develops a predominantly hyperpnoeic response to hypoxia.

- In sleeping infants the arousal response to hypoxia (normal in adults) is much diminished, and often completely absent during rapid eye movement (REM) sleep.
- Intercostal muscle activity is inhibited during REM sleep, and can lead to inefficient ventilation as the chest wall recesses on inspiration.
- Periodic respiration, where rapid shallow breathing alternates with apnoeas of up to 10 seconds, is normal in many infants.

Renal function

In the developing embryo, the first nephrons form during week 5, are functional from week 8 and have reached their full complement by week 36. After this there is merely growth in size and number of cells in existing nephrons rather than new nephron formation. Renal blood flow comprises 5% of cardiac output at birth, but with reduced renal vascular resistance this increases to 20% by 1 month of age, with increasing flow to cortical areas. The glomerular filtration rate (GFR) is correspondingly low at birth (30 mL min^{-1}), and is even lower in preterm infants (3 mL min^{-1}). By 2 years GFR has increased to near adult levels (110 mL min^{-1}). Low GFR and immature tubular function limit the neonate's ability to deal with water and solute loads, notably sodium and glucose, and they are unable to effectively excrete hydrogen ions or retain bicarbonate as a compensation for acidosis.

Hepatic function

During intrauterine life, the fetus excretes fat-soluble unconjugated bilirubin via the placenta and maternal liver. There is a physiological rise in bilirubin soon after birth, due to both an increased bilirubin load and immaturity of neonatal hepatic enzymes. The peak occurs on day 3–4 of postnatal life, due to immature oxidation–reduction reactions (phase I), with levels dropping in the second week of life as the conjugating enzymes needed for glucuronidation mature (phase II). This drop takes longer in preterm babies, and the risk of kernicterus (damage to basal ganglia and auditory pathways) from unconjugated bilirubin entering the brain via an immature blood–brain barrier is significant. Infants handle hepatically excreted drugs differently to older children and adults. Immature enzyme systems play a role, but so does the difference in blood supply to the liver. Infants receive a higher proportion of their hepatic blood supply via the portal vein than via the hepatic artery. Any increase in intra-abdominal pressure, e.g. after abdominal surgery, reduces clearance of hepatically excreted drugs such as fentanyl.

Thermoregulation

Neonatal heat loss

Neonates lose heat readily because of their higher ratio of surface area to body weight, and relative paucity of subcutaneous fat. Preterm infants have particularly thin skins, needing higher ambient temperatures and humidity. Heat loss occurs by evaporation, radiation, convection and to a lesser extent conduction, as well as by insensible losses such as through respiration.

Infants are seldom able to increase heat production enough to compensate for heat loss, and newborns need to be nursed in a thermoneutral environment (at an ambient temperature that minimises oxygen consumption and heat loss).

Unlike older children and adults, who generate heat involuntarily by shivering, newborns rely on non-shivering thermogenesis to increase their basal metabolic rate and thereby retain heat. This is a function of their unique brown fat, present in the first few weeks of life as an adaptive, protective entity. These specialised adipose cells are situated around the kidneys and adrenals, in the mediastinum and around the scapulae. They are abundant in mitochondria and have a rich blood and autonomic nerve supply. Noradrenaline in sympathetic nerve endings stimulates the hydrolysis of triglycerides to fatty acids and glycerol, resulting in oxygen consumption and heat production.

Nociception

Circumstantially, even the most preterm neonates respond to painful stimuli similarly to an adult, in terms of cardiovascular, stress and behavioural responses, but the presence or absence of pain as a conscious event can never be proven.

Pain in the fetus and neonate

Little can be inferred about the actual experience of pain in the fetus or neonate, or the attendant emotions, if any, relating to it. Much depends on the nature of self-awareness, consciousness and the development of 'self' in fetal life. Given the impossible task of making judgements on the nature of pain perception in the fetus and neonate, the term nociception is more appropriate.

Nociceptive pathways develop early in gestation, and even early in development they can produce complex protective responses to painful stimuli. Dorsal horn cells in the spinal cord have formed synapses with developing sensory neurones by 6 weeks gestation, and peripheral nerves migrate to the skin of the limbs by 11 weeks, achieving a density of nociceptive nerve endings similar to that of the adult by birth. The first appearance of transmitter vesicles is seen at 13 weeks gestation, and further synaptic connections and organisation of the dorsal horn structure continues up to 30 weeks.

The fetal neocortex has a full complement of cells by 20 weeks, and thalamocortical tracts can be shown to synapse with dendritic processes of the cells in the neocortex by 24 weeks gestation. Myelination of some ascending nociceptive tracts is seen by 30 weeks, but thalamocortical radiations are not myelinated until 37 weeks and some nociceptive tracts are myelinated much later. However, lack of myelination does not imply lack of function: transmission of nerve impulses within the central nervous system still takes place in unmyelinated nerves, albeit at a reduced velocity. Noxious stimuli can produce both haemodynamic and stress responses in a human fetus as young as 18 weeks gestation, and these responses can be reduced by pretreatment with analgesic drugs. Visual and auditory evoked potentials are present by 30 weeks gestation, by which time a complex EEG reactive to external influences has developed.

Overall, even the very preterm infant has complex interneuronal connections capable of integrated responses to tactile or nociceptive input. These infants show inconsistent responses to external stimuli, which may reflect the late functional connections of sensory afferents (particularly C fibres) within the spinal cord. However, the combination of larger receptive fields, recruitment of non-nociceptive afferents and reduced inhibitory controls results in 'under-damped' responses (long-lasting, exaggerated and poorly localised) once afferent stimuli have achieved central activation above a threshold level. Inconsistency of response to more complex noxious stimuli may also reflect the profound effects that conscious state and other external responses have on behaviour.

Surgical stress in the neonate

Although newborn infants often have short-lived behavioural and stress responses to noxious stimuli, there is evidence in this age group that surgical trauma or injury can have long-term consequences for sensory and pain behaviour in infancy. It is clear that in neonates repeated noxious stimuli produce hypersensitivity to further stimulation, and that poor operative analgesia can be associated with long-lasting hyperalgesia and behavioural changes such as irritability, reduced attentiveness and poor orientation, which may continue long after the expected duration of pain.

CHAPTER 25
Physical chemistry

Tim Smith

Intermolecular and interatomic bonds

The two main types of intermolecular bond are ionic and covalent, with weaker bonds providing intermolecular interactions and determining structural conformation. The structure of the component atoms determines the type of bonds within the molecule.

Atomic structure

Knowledge of the basic structure of atoms is important in understanding the types of intermolecular bond and their functions. A number of key terms are defined in Figure 25.1, and a schematic view of atomic structure is shown in Figure 25.2.

Each atom has a nucleus (central core) of neutrons and protons, surrounded by a cloud of negatively charged electrons. Figure 25.3 shows the properties of these components. The charge of an atom is the number of protons minus the number of electrons. It is clear that almost all the mass of an atom is in the nucleus. The number of protons (the atomic number) defines the element, and the atomic mass is close to the combined masses of protons and neutrons in the atom. Elements may exist with different numbers of neutrons in the nucleus while having the same atomic number. These

Figure 25.1 Important terms relating to atomic structure

Atom	The smallest part of an element that can take part in chemical reactions
Atomic number	The number of protons in each atom of an element
Element	A group of atoms all having the same atomic number
Molecule	A combination of atoms which is the smallest unit of a chemical substance that can exist while still retaining the properties of the original substance
Atomic mass	The mass of one mole of an element
Mole	A constant number (the Avogadro constant: 6.022×10^{23}) of atoms or molecules

are called isotopes, and those that release particles (radioactive) are called radioisotopes. Carbon provides an example: it has atomic number 6, and therefore six protons,

Fundamentals of Anaesthesia, 4th edition, ed. Ted Lin, Tim Smith and Colin Pinnock. Published by Cambridge University Press. © Cambridge University Press 2017.

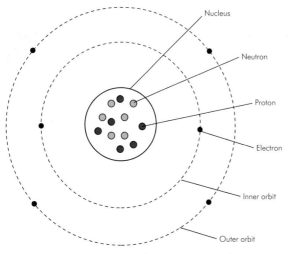

Figure 25.2 Two-dimensional representation of atomic structure

Figure 25.3 Properties of atomic particles

	Nucleus		Electron
	Proton	Neutron	
Mass number	1	1	1/1836
Charge	+1	0	−1

Figure 25.4 Capacities of electron shells

Shell	Maximum number of electrons
K	2
L	8
M	18
N	32

though ^{12}C (carbon 12) has six protons and six neutrons, while ^{14}C (carbon 14) has six protons and eight neutrons (radioactive). Conventionally, the mass number is shown as a prefix superscript and the atomic number is shown as a prefix subscript, for example $^{12}_{6}C$ for carbon and $^{23}_{11}Na$ for sodium (11 protons and 12 neutrons).

Electrons are arranged in orbital shells around the nucleus, from the innermost K shell outwards to L, M, N, O, P and Q shells (Figure 25.4). These are not precise concentric rings, but the conceptual model helps to predict molecular behaviour. Shells are filled in their alphabetical order. Complete electron shells, pairs and octets of electrons confer stability. Each orbital shell has a maximum number of electrons, and some stability is conferred when this is achieved.

Valency

Valency may be defined as the number of atoms of hydrogen that one atom of an element can combine with or replace.

Each element has at least one valency state, and the valency is used to establish possible intermolecular bonds. Each group in the periodic table has a characteristic valency. For example, group IA elements have a valency of +1. The valency can be predicted from the electron shell configuration, as shown in Figure 25.5. Atoms of a particular element lose or gain electrons to achieve the stability described above. This loss or gain of electrons may be complete (in ionic bond) or by sharing with other atoms (in covalent bond). In this way, they adopt the electron configuration of the closest (by atomic number) rare or inert gas (for example helium, neon, argon). The inert gases are already at their most stable and do not gain or lose electrons. Consequently, they have minimal interaction with other atoms and exist as gases. Carbon is the single most important element in organic chemistry because it is chemically versatile – it can either lose or gain electrons to achieve electron stability.

Ionic bonds

The ionic bond (also termed an electrostatic bond) relies on the fact that certain elements (termed electrovalent) have a tendency to lose or gain electrons to form charged atoms or molecules called ions. Like charges repel, but opposite charges attract, and therefore create a bond. This is illustrated by the formation of sodium chloride in Figure 25.6.

With respect to the process shown in Figure 25.6, the movement of an electron from the sodium atom to the chlorine atom results in both ions having stable outermost shells. The sodium ion now has the electron configuration of neon, and chloride that of argon. The resultant change in charge causes a strong attraction between the sodium and chloride ions (the ionic bond) which is sufficient to maintain the precise crystalline structure of solid sodium chloride. Figure 25.7 shows another example of ionic bonding with the relevant electron configurations.

Figure 25.5 Arrangement of electrons in orbital shells

Element	Protons	Neutrons	Electrons in shell					Valency
			K	L	M	N	O	
Hydrogen	1	0	1					1
Helium	2	2	2					0
Carbon	6	6	2	4				4
Nitrogen	7	7	2	5				3
Oxygen	8	8	2	6				2
Sodium	11	12	2	8	1			1
Magnesium	12	12	2	8	2			2
Chlorine	17	18	2	8	7			1
Argon	18	18	2	8	8			0
Potassium	19	20	2	8	8	1		1
Calcium	20	20	2	8	8	2		2
Xenon	54	77	2	8	18	18	8	0

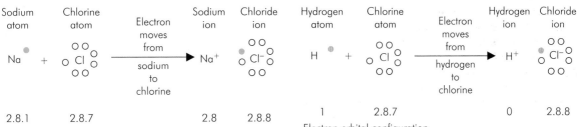

2.8.1   2.8.7   2.8   2.8.8

Electron orbital configuration

Figure 25.6 Ionic bonding illustrated by the formation of sodium chloride. In Figures 25.6, 25.7, 25.8 and 25.10 the colouring of electrons enables identification of their origin when considering the end result.

1   2.8.7   0   2.8.8

Electron orbital configuration

Figure 25.7 Ionic bonding illustrated by the formation of hydrochloric acid

Covalent bonds

Covalent bonds are similar to ionic bonds in that they depend on forming stable electron shells. In contrast with ionic bonding, the atoms share electrons rather than donate them completely. Carbon, nitrogen, hydrogen and oxygen frequently behave in this way. The electron configuration of carbon is 2.4 (see Figure 25.5). Stability is achieved either by losing four electrons or by gaining four electrons, resulting in a pair or an octet of electrons in the outer shell, respectively. Covalent bonds may be single, double or triple, depending on the number of electron pairs

that are shared. Methane is an example of covalent bonding with four single covalent bonds (Figure 25.8). The carbon atom of methane adopts the electron configuration of neon (2.8) while hydrogen adopts the configuration of helium, both being inert gases with stable atomic configurations.

A comparison of the properties of ionic and covalent bonds is given in Figure 25.9.

Dative bonds

The dative bond is a type of covalent bond in which both electrons of the shared pair are from the same atom. This bond is a feature of atoms that have

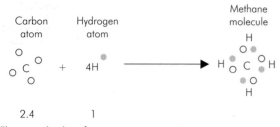

2.4   1

Electron orbital configuration

Figure 25.8 Covalent bonding illustrated by the formation of methane

Figure 25.9 A comparison of the properties of ionic and covalent bonds

Ionic	Covalent
No sharing of electrons, therefore non-directional bond, therefore no particular shape	Electrons shared, therefore directional bond, therefore definite shape, so isomerism and stereoisomerism possible
Usually solid (crystalline)	Usually highly volatile liquids or gases
Not easily vaporised	Easily vaporised
Fused state	
Melt form is a conductor	Poor conductor
Readily dissolves in water	Not readily soluble in water
Forms electrolyte in water	

complete pairs of electrons in their outer shells in the non-combined state. Typical examples are oxygen, nitrogen, phosphorus and sulphur. The formation of ammonium chloride from ammonia and hydrogen chloride illustrates this bond, as well as ionic and covalent bonds (Figure 25.10).

Van der Waals forces

Because electrons are not rigidly fixed relative to the nucleus, but move in characteristic orbitals, the resulting electron cloud has a characteristic shape. Highly

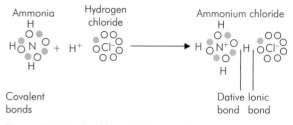

Figure 25.10 Mixed bonds illustrated by the formation of ammonium chloride

electronegative atoms such as oxygen attract electrons so that the distribution of the electron cloud of the molecule is uneven. This produces dipoles where component atoms of a molecule are not electrostatically neutral. The value of these charges is much less than the +1 or –1 of ions, and the molecule may have a polarity. Van der Waals forces are the attraction and repulsion of these weakly charged areas to similar areas in neighbouring molecules. Graphite is an example of sheets of covalently bonded carbon in which the layers are held together by van der Waals forces, and they are also essential in receptor and enzyme bonding.

Hydrogen bonds

A hydrogen bond is a weak electrostatic bond between the positive nucleus of a covalently bonded hydrogen atom in one molecule and the unshared pair of electrons of a highly electronegative atom of another molecule. Oxygen, sulphur and nitrogen are highly electronegative atoms, and water provides an example of hydrogen bonding (Figure 25.11). The hydrogen bonding in water is responsible for the relatively high boiling point (compared with non-polar liquids) and the structure of ice crystals.

Hydrophobic bonds

In water, individual molecules are attracted to each other by hydrogen bonds. Any molecules added to the water will disrupt this loosely held 'structure'. If the electron distribution of the additive is not uniform (it has polarity) or if it is readily ionised, then it too will form bonds with the water molecules. This will allow it to spread readily and evenly throughout the containing vessel. If, however, the electron distribution is even, then the energy required to break the hydrogen bonds of water will be greater than that released by the formation of the new bonds. In this case, the most stable arrangement exists when the additive collects together, leaving as much of the water

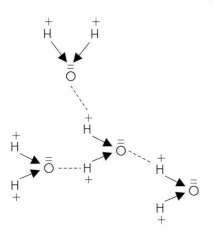

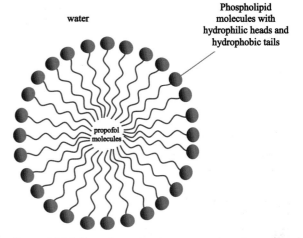

Figure 25.12 Two-dimensional representation of emulsion micelle

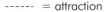 = attraction

——▶ = electron shift within covalent bond

+ /– = dipolar non uniformity of electrostatic charge

Figure 25.11 Hydrogen bonding in water. Dotted lines represent hydrogen bonds and arrows represent covalent bonds, with the arrow head showing direction of electron donation

Figure 25.13 The strengths of intermolecular bonds

Bond	Bond energy (kcal mol^{-1})
Covalent	50–150
Ionic	5–10
Hydrogen	2–5
van der Waals	0.5

together as possible. This is easily seen when oil is added to water, and is a feature of lipids. Its density relative to water determines where the oil subsequently distributes. Vigorous mixing will provide the energy to break the hydrogen bonds and disperse the fat molecules, temporarily. This is the basis of the hydrophobic bond, which is very important physiologically, occurring at a local level around proteins and other molecules. Areas of membranes and proteins that do not have polarity do not attract water molecules. The water molecules therefore tend to maintain bonds with other water molecules, leaving these hydrophobic areas vacant. This promotes the movement of non-polar hydrophobic molecules to these sites. Looking at this situation in overview gives the impression that the hydrophobic areas and molecules are attracted to each other, but in fact there is little or no attraction at all between the two. It is, in effect, the result of displacement of the hydrophobic molecules by the attraction of water and other hydrophilic molecules.

Emulsions
Emulsions are used in pharmacology to provide solutions of fat-soluble drugs such as propofol. An emulsion is a mixture of two (or more) immiscible liquids. This means that one exists in the form of miscoscopic particles within the other. In propofol the drug is dissolved in the lipid of the emulsion. Using water alone provides insufficient propofol to achieve an effective dose (see *Phenols* in Chapter 30). In the case of propofol the lipid is contained within small envelopes (micelles) formed by a layer of molecules (e.g. phospholipid) that have both a hydrophilic end and a hydrophobic end (Figure 25.12).

Strength of intermolecular bonds
The strengths of the main intermolecular bonds are shown in Figure 25.13. The stronger the bond the higher the energy required to break it. Covalent bonds are thus very difficult to break without a catalyst or enzyme. In physiological and pharmacological systems, therefore, covalent bonds are effectively irreversible. They are 'reversed' by metabolism of the receptor–agonist or enzyme–substrate complex and replacement of the enzyme or receptor.

Examples of pharmacological covalent bonding include phenoxybenzamine to α-adrenoceptors, organophosphates to acetylcholinesterase and monoamine oxidase inhibitors to monoamine oxidase.

The strength of ionic and other bonds decreases with the distance between the molecules such that the force of attraction is given by the following formulae:

Ionic bond : $\qquad$ force $\alpha \dfrac{1}{\text{distance}^2}$

van der Waals force : force $\alpha \dfrac{1}{\text{distance}^7}$

In the latter, neighbouring groups of electrons cause repulsion once the distance decreases below a critical level.

Oxidation and reduction

Chemically, the loss of electrons is referred to as oxidation, and it involves the use of an electron acceptor (such as oxygen) which is correspondingly reduced. Oxidation can therefore include the binding of oxygen molecules to a molecule, as in the conversion of acetaldehyde to acetic acid:

$$2CH_3CHO + O_2 \rightarrow CH_3COOH$$

In the formation of the new molecule the oxygen accepts an electron from the acetaldehyde in order to complete the formation of a new covalent bond.

Serial oxidations and reductions occur in the mitochondrial release of energy in the cytochrome oxidase electron chain. Anaerobic dehydrogenases facilitate the removal of hydrogen.

In pharmacology, local anaesthetic agent ionisation by the acceptance of a proton (H^+) also constitutes oxidation.

Diffusion

Simple diffusion

Diffusion is a property of gas mixtures and solutions. Molecules of gases can move freely and tend to distribute themselves equally within the limits of the containing vessel (Figure 25.14). In a similar way, molecules and ions in solution move freely throughout a solvent, so that the distribution (and therefore the concentration) becomes uniform throughout the solution. Ions and molecules, therefore, move down the concentration gradient and any electrical gradient until those gradients disappear. The result is an even distribution of all the ions and molecules in the container, so that any selected volume,

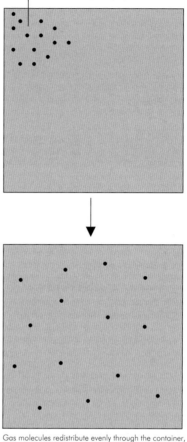

Gas molecules added to container

Gas molecules redistribute evenly through the container, resulting in uniform concentration throughout

Figure 25.14 Effect of diffusion on gas molecule distribution

regardless of shape, size or location, will have identical composition. Diffusion of molecules in a gaseous or liquid state can also occur between the molecules of a solid. This property of permeability may differ for each solid/gas or solid/liquid combination.

Graham's law describes gaseous diffusion as follows:

$$\text{Rate } \alpha \frac{1}{\sqrt{\text{density}}}$$

The rate of diffusion of a gas at a given temperature and pressure is inversely proportional to the square root of its density. Thus the rate of diffusion increases with rising temperature as the speed of molecular movement increases.

Non-ionic diffusion

Most drugs are categorised as weak acids or weak bases, which implies that they are encountered in a partly ionised form. A higher degree of ionisation confers water solubility and thus is desirable for admixture, for example. In contrast, the un-ionised form of a drug is required for lipid membrane penetration and hence delivery to the target. The proportion of a drug present in ionised form is dependent on environmental pH. A drug that is a weak acid will dissociate in the following way:

$$HA \leftrightharpoons H^+ + A^-$$

The relationship between dissociation and pH can be obtained by applying the Henderson–Hasselbalch equation:

$$pH = pK_a + \log_{10} \frac{[A^-]}{[HA]}$$

pK_a is the negative logarithm of the dissociation constant, and is the pH at which the drug is 50% ionised. For a practical application of this concept consider thiopental (pK_a 7.8), which is deliberately made up in an alkaline solution, pH about 11, to render it more ionised and therefore water-soluble. After injection parenterally, into an environment of pH 7.4, the proportion of un-ionised drug form will become greater, enabling membrane penetration of the CNS.

Solubility and partition coefficients

The partition coefficient of a substance can be defined as a numerical constant that is the ratio at equilibrium of the concentrations of that substance in two adjacent compartments separated by an interface through which the substance readily passes.

When two or more compartments exist together then there will be movement of particles through the interface (permeable) between the compartments. The interface may be a physical boundary such as a cell membrane, or a liquid–gas interface. In contrast to the case of simple diffusion, the two compartments in a physiological system are likely to have different affinities for the particles. The resulting equilibrium will therefore have different concentrations of particles in the compartments. Solubility and partition coefficients can be determined for a pair of compartments for a given diffusing molecule. The coefficient is a dimensionless ratio describing the relative concentrations at equilibrium.

Partition coefficients are routinely used to describe the properties affecting distribution of volatile anaesthetic

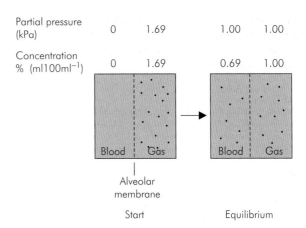

Figure 25.15 Distribution of sevoflurane between blood and gas

agents. The Ostwald partition coefficients used are specified for a given agent at body temperature (37 °C). Gases and vapours travel down their partial pressure gradient until the partial pressures are equal. The concentration for a given partial pressure in a particular compartment is determined by the affinity of the constituents of the compartment for the specified molecule. The total amount of the molecule in any compartment will also depend on the volume of the compartment. At equilibrium, the partial pressures will be equal but the concentrations will not. Figure 25.15 shows these features using sevoflurane as an example. Sevoflurane has a blood/gas partition coefficient = 0.69. This means that at equilibrium the ratio of sevoflurane concentration in the two compartments is 0.69 in the blood for every 1.00 in the gas phase. Solubility coefficients may also be between different solvents, such as oil and water. A highly oil-soluble molecule such as isoflurane will have a high oil/water solubility coefficient (174). A highly water-soluble molecule such as sodium chloride will have a low oil/water solubility coefficient. In general, ions are more soluble in water whereas isoelectric and non-polar molecules are more soluble in oils.

Osmosis

Osmosis is the passage of a solvent through a semipermeable membrane that separates two compartments having different concentrations of a solute (or solutes) to which the membrane is impermeable. A pure semipermeable membrane is one that is freely permeable to the solvent but impermeable to the solute. The glomerular membrane is an example of a functional semipermeable

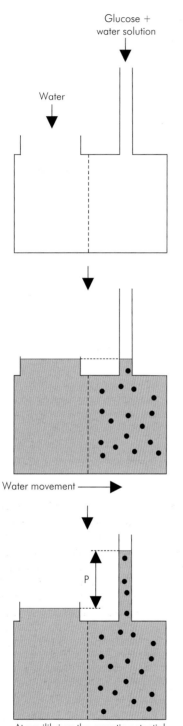

Water movement ⟶

At equilibrium the osmotic potential
of the solution is P cm solution

Figure 25.16 Osmosis

membrane: it is freely permeable to water and smaller molecules but impermeable to larger molecules (molecular weight > 69,000 daltons).

In osmosis, an imbalance in the concentration of non-permeable molecules on two sides of a semipermeable membrane causes movement of the freely permeable solute towards the side of higher concentration. The solute tends to move, equalising concentration gradients. The osmotic pressure or potential is the pressure required to prevent this passage of solvent. Figure 25.16 shows the effect of osmosis on fluid distribution. Osmotic activity continues until the hydrostatic pressure balances the osmotic potential. All solutions have an osmotic potential for a given semipermeable membrane and concentration. The solvent (e.g. water) moves towards the compartment with the highest concentration of solute and the pressure is, by definition, negative.

Osmotic potential may be the result of a single solute, but is usually due to many different molecules. Osmotically active particles in a solution are those to which the membrane is impermeable. Cell membranes are semi-permeable, although ionic transport systems make this picture rather complex.

The difference between osmolarity and osmolality is:

Osmolarity = concentration by volume of solution (in $mOsm\ L^{-1}$)

Osmolality = concentration by mass of solvent (in $mOsm\ kg^{-1}\ H_2O$)

Pharmacological aspects of osmosis

Drugs affecting the distribution of solutes between compartments will have an osmotic effect. Diuretics interfere with membrane transport of ions and other solutes through the renal cells and in the renal lumen and renal circulation. This manipulates the ionic concentrations in the medulla, and therefore water follows ionic concentrations in the tubules and urine output is increased. Mannitol is a drug used specifically for its osmotic effects. It is a high-molecular-weight alcohol that remains extracellular, and this produces a negative osmotic potential in the extracellular space that pulls water out of the intracellular space. It is also an osmotic diuretic because it passes readily through the glomerular membrane but is not reabsorbed.

Drug isomerism

Isomers are chemical compounds that have the same empirical molecular formula (and so the same molecular weight) but differing physical or chemical properties.

Structural isomerism

Structural (or constitutional) isomerism is the presence of different structures with the same empirical molecular formula. The formula $C_{18}H_{23}NO_3$ is common to both dobutamine and hydrocodeine, but the atoms are arranged in an entirely different order.

Chain isomerism

In chain isomerism the carbon skeleton varies between isomers while retaining the same functional group. Example: butane $CH_3CH_2CH_2CH_3$ and isobutane (2-methyl butane) $CH_3CH(CH_3)CH_3$.

Position isomerism

In position isomerism the component atoms or functional group are in different positions on an identical carbon skeleton. Example: enflurane and isoflurane (Figure 25.17). It is also of note that these two molecules each have a chiral centre, so they form enantiomers (see *Stereoisomerism*, below).

Functional group isomerism

In this form of isomerism the functional group changes. For example the movement of the oxygen of an alcohol into the carbon chain produces an ether. Example: propanol $CH_3CH_2CH_2OH$ and methyl ethyl ether $CH_3OCH_2CH_3$.

Dynamic isomerism

Dynamic isomerism (tautomerism) is a variant of functional group isomerism in which two isomers exist in dynamic equilibrium obeying the law of mass action. The barbiturates thiopental and methohexital exist in two forms (keto and enol), and the = S/-SH and = O/-OH groups in thiopental and methohexital respectively are in a dynamic equilibrium, the relative proportions of each being determined by the pH of the solution (see also Figure 30.4). Nitrous oxide is another tautomer (see Figure 29.4).

Stereoisomerism

Stereoisomerism (spatial isomerism) is another form of molecular rearrangement. Stereoisomers have the same molecular formula, carbon skeleton and structure but have a different spatial arrangement. Each atom in the molecule bonds to the same atoms as in the other stereoisomers. There are two types, optical and *cis–trans*.

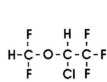

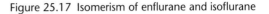

Figure 25.17 Isomerism of enflurane and isoflurane

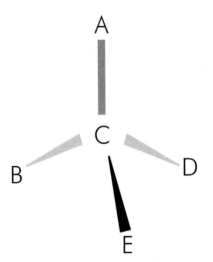

Figure 25.18 Asymmetry about a single carbon atom

Optical isomerism

Optical stereoisomerism requires atoms which are at least tetravalent (having the potential for four bonds), with different groups of molecules on each bond. Carbon is the most important tetravalent atom, and has four hybridised covalent links with neighbouring molecules. Figure 25.18 shows the principles of optical stereoisomerism. The carbon atom in the chiral centre has four different groups attached to it. It can be seen that if two of these groups are interchanged then the resulting arrangement is a non-superimposable mirror image of the original. These are called enantiomers. Enantiomers often have different crystalline structures. Characteristically, they rotate polarised light in opposite directions. The amount of rotation is a feature of the molecular structure. Molecules with multiple chiral centres will not form simple superimposable mirror images unless every chiral centre is mirrored

Figure 25.19 Classification of stereoisomers

	Right	Left
Handedness	**R** (D)	**S** (L)
Rotational (of polarised light)	+ (*d*)	− (*l*)
Contemporary terms typically used in pharmacology: R, S, +, −		
Traditional terms typically used in physiology are shown in brackets		

concurrently. Non-superimposable stereoisomers are called diastereomers, and these include isomers with multiple chiral centres and *cis–trans* isomers.

Classification

Several methods exist for classifying optical isomers, and it can seem confusing. Simply put, isomers may be described according to the actual molecular configuration about the chiral centre(s), and also by the direction in which polarised light is rotated (Figure 25.19).

The molecular arrangement is described as either right- or left-handed, based on prioritising the groups attached to the chiral atom by atomic number of the attached atoms and molecules. The details of this are beyond the scope of this book. Right-handed isomers are classified as D (from the Latin *dexter*) or R (from the Latin *rectus*), both terms referring to the right. Left-handed isomers are classified as L (from the Latin *laevus*) or S (from the Latin *sinister*), both terms referring to the left.

The optical rotation may be clockwise (to the right) or anticlockwise (to the left). Clockwise rotation is said to be dextrorotatory and is represented by (+) or *d*. Anticlockwise rotation is said to be laevorotatory and is represented by (−) or *l*.

Chiral molecules are variously classified in texts, using a mixture of the above terms. It is sufficient to use either handedness or optical rotation to define the enantiomer, but for completeness both terms are often used, especially with drugs. *d* and *l* have largely been superseded by (+) and (−). D and L are still used for physiological components, but R and S are usually used for drugs.

Physiological stereoisomers

Glucose exists naturally as D(+)glucose (which is why it is also referred to as **dextr**ose). Its right-handedness is by comparing carbon-5 with the configuration of D-glyceraldehyde. The mirror image is L(−)glucose, which is a mirror image of all the chiral carbons of glucose. Most naturally occurring carbohydrates are right-handed. Alterations in the chirality about carbon atoms (2, 3, 4) within the carbohydrate ring (interchanging hydrogen and hydroxyl group) result in epimers. Examples include D-galactose and D-mannose. D(−)fructose has the same configuration, but in fructose this rotates light to the left, as denoted by the (−). The hexoses are further complicated by their dynamic isomerism into cyclic forms, with variation about carbon-1 leading to α and β forms of D-glucose.

Conversely, the amino acids in proteins (except glycine, which has no chiral atom) all have an absolute configuration similar to that of L-glyceraldehyde. They rotate light in different directions (for example L(+)alanine and L(−)leucine). Some D-amino acids do occur naturally, for example in bacterial cell walls.

Pharmacological considerations

Different enantiomers often have different potencies (stereoselectivity), and may be responsible for different side effects. The manufacture of most stereoisomeric drugs results in equal amounts of each stereoisomer. This is called a racemic mixture, and the rotational effects on light cancel out. Where multiple chiral atoms exist, the number of stereoisomers increases greatly.

The naturally occurring receptors are often stereospecific and will interact mainly or entirely with one racemate (e.g. R(+)etomidate). The rest of the drug may be redundant. As the chemical properties are usually identical, the measurement of drug levels will not distinguish between the species. This affects pharmacokinetic calculations. The elimination of the drug may also be different for each racemate, as will be the activity of any metabolites, so each racemate will have a different pharmacokinetic profile. Unfortunately the 'redundant' stereoisomer (e.g. R-bupivacaine) may be responsible for unwanted effects, and may preclude the drug's use and further development unless the desired stereoisomer can be isolated. This requires special techniques that are costly. Specific manufacture of stereoisomers is advantageous.

Cis–trans (geometric) isomerism

Cis–trans (or geometric) isomerism refers to the possible atomic orientational variants about a double bond. Figure 25.20 shows an example of this. These stereoisomers are a type of diastereomer (have a non-superimposable mirror image) and are also referred to as *E–Z* isomers.

The main parts of each half are in the same plane in the *cis* (Latin: same side) or (*E*) isomers and in opposite planes in *trans* (Latin: other side) or (*Z*) isomers.

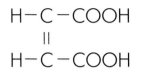

H−C−COOH
||
H−C−COOH

cis form (maleic acid)

H−C−COOH
||
COOH−C−H

trans form (fumaric acid)

Figure 25.20 An example of *cis–trans* isomerism

Mivacurium contains two such bonds, and the resultant isomers (*cis–cis*, *cis–trans* and *trans–trans*) have different pharmacokinetic profiles (see Chapter 32). *Cis*-atracurium is now available, to minimise the undesirable effects such as histamine release thought to be caused by the *trans* isomers.

Protein binding

Protein binding depends on the structure of the protein. A protein may have up to four levels of structure (Figure 25.21):

- Primary structure – the chemical formula of the protein, which is usually simplified by using the component amino acids to describe it. It concerns the covalent bonds, excluding cross-linking disulphide and hydrogen bonds.
- Secondary structure – the relative spatial positions of neighbouring covalently bonded molecules to each other. Free rotation occurs about single covalent bonds (but not double bonds). This rotation allows the molecule to settle into its most stable orientation.

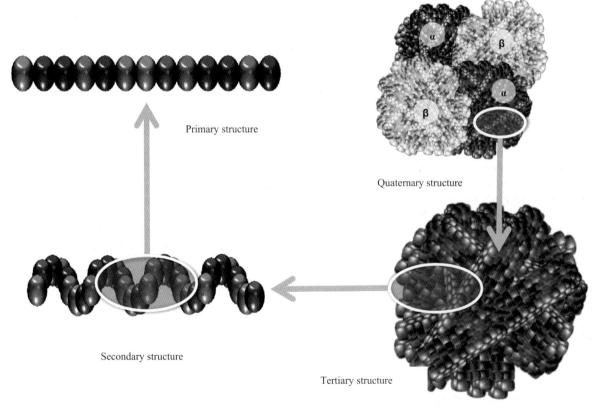

Primary structure

Quaternary structure

Secondary structure

Tertiary structure

Figure 25.21 Levels of protein structure

The secondary structure refers to the one-dimensional regular ziz-zag or coil produced. A representation of the α helix is shown in Figure 25.21; this is found in fibrous proteins and in sections of globular proteins.

- Tertiary structure – the shape in which the α helix is subsequently arranged, which may be long and straight or may curl around itself.
- Quaternary structure – the interrelationship between individual protein molecule subunits when more than one subunit constitutes the protein. Subunits are held together by weak bonds such as hydrogen bonds and van der Waals forces. Figure 25.21 is a representation of haemoglobin.

Proteins are highly complex molecules and potentially have multiple areas or sites with individual properties. These sites vary in size, shape, electrostatic charge and their relationship to other sites. They have the potential to attract molecules of a suitable size, shape and charge in a similar manner to a three-dimensional jigsaw or key. Plasma proteins act in this way to transport poorly soluble molecules to other locations in the body. The bound molecules are generally in equilibrium with their unbound molecules, and are released as the free concentration falls.

Enzymes are specific proteins that bind molecules and then facilitate the formation or destruction of covalent bonds within molecules, allowing synthesis of new molecules and destruction of other molecules. Receptors are usually proteins or glycoproteins that bind or receive specific molecules (agonists and antagonists), producing a conformational change in the receptor that is responsible for the effect. The effect of the agonist–receptor complex may be to open an ion channel in a membrane, for example.

Drugs may interact with binding sites in the following ways:

- Agonist drugs have a similar structure to the intended molecule, bind to the receptor site and mimic the endogenous agonist.
- Antagonist drugs have a similar structure to the intended molecule, bind to the receptor site without causing any change but prevent the endogenous agonist binding to the receptor.
- Drugs may bind to another part of the protein and cause a configuration change that prevents the receptor site from binding to the agonist.
- Drugs may bind to another part of the protein and prevent the configuration change necessary for the physiological effect.

Figure 25.22 Drug affinity for plasma proteins

	Predominantly bound to	
	Albumin	**Globulin**
Basic	Bilirubin Fatty acids Tryptophan	Chlorpromazine Lidocaine Bupivacaine Propranolol Opioids
Acidic or neutral	Salicylates Warfarin	

- Drugs may bind to the protein and prevent ions reaching the opened channel.

Plasma protein binding

The degree of drug binding to plasma proteins is relevant to the transport of poorly soluble drugs, and also in determining dose requirements.

Features of plasma proteins

The main plasma proteins involved in drug transport are albumin and globulin. Other molecules, such as α_1-acid glycoprotein, which binds basic drugs, and specific carriers for cortisol and thyroxine, contribute to the transport system. These molecules are large (albumin has a molecular weight of 69,000 daltons) and have multiple, relatively non-specific binding sites. As with all binding sites, the shape and charge of the site are important. The bonds are a combination of any of the relatively weak bonds (hydrogen bonds, hydrophilic bonds and van der Waals forces), which allows rapid dissociation of drugs (determined by concentration) at the site of action and for elimination. A drug will bind to a protein binding site to produce a complex in the following manner:

Drug + protein binding site ⇆ Drug–protein complex.

According to the law of mass action, as the concentration of free drug falls due to diffusion at locations with a low drug concentration, so the balance of the equation will shift to the left. Figure 25.22 shows the different protein binding affinities of some important drugs.

Factors affecting binding

Changes in drug or protein nature alter the amount of protein binding. The amount of protein in the plasma will alter the number of available binding sites, as will abnormalities in the protein structure. Surgery and other trauma, myocardial infarction, carcinoma and rheumatoid arthritis increase the concentration of α_1-acid glycoprotein. Changes in pH may alter the ionisation of some groups on the protein and drug, resulting in either increased or decreased attraction between the molecules as well as increased or decreased activity of the drug. The presence of other drugs having an affinity for the same binding sites on the protein creates competition and displacement so that less of each drug will be bound. This is particularly relevant when a new drug is added after a patient has been stabilised on the first drug, and can cause toxicity from excessive plasma levels of the first drug.

Effects of changes in binding

Changes in binding alter the amount of free drug. There is considerable inter-patient variation in the degree of protein binding for a given drug. Only the unbound drug is available to diffuse and attach to a site of action for pharmacological effect, and the bound portion is effectively inactive. If protein binding for a particular drug is low then the majority of the drug is free to have its effect. Any change in protein binding will need to be large before any significant change in plasma levels of free drug is seen. If, however, the proportion of bound drug is high then even small changes in the proportion of drug bound will have a pronounced effect. Depending on the direction of the effect, these changes can reduce or enhance the therapeutic effect but, more importantly, may permit toxic effects of overdose to develop. Protein binding might appear from this to be a disadvantage. In fact, it is particularly important for the transport of lipophilic drugs, which may not dissolve in aqueous media in sufficient concentration to provide an effective concentration at the target site. There is also a degree of 'buffering' of the administered dose.

Protein binding affects the pharmacokinetic properties of a drug. The greater the degree of binding, the less drug there is available for diffusion into other tissues, and more remains in the plasma. This shows as a low volume of distribution. A low volume of distribution results in higher elimination of the drug.

References and further reading

Otter C, Stephenson K. *Salter's Advanced Chemistry: Chemical Ideas*, 3rd edn. Harlow: Heinemann, 2008.

CHAPTER 26

Pharmacodynamics

Tim Smith

Pharmacodynamics is the study of the quantitative effects of drug concentration on the activity and response at specific receptor sites. In simple terms, this is often expressed by the phrase 'what the drug does to the body'.

Both endogenous ligands and exogenously administered drugs interact with receptor sites to produce an effect. Drugs can act in a number of different ways, depending on their characteristics (Figure 26.1).

This chapter considers the key mathematical model used to explain pharmacodynamic principles and its expansion to describe the interactions of agonists (full, partial and inverse) and antagonists. Variations and clinical examples are considered. This key mathematical model is represented by the equation

$$R = \frac{E[D]}{K_D + [D]}$$

which is graphically demonstrated in Figures 26.4, 26.5 and 26.6.

In this chapter the steps in the derivation of this and other equations are shown in boxes.

In this chapter the term 'drug' is used for molecules binding to receptors, although the model applies equally to other molecules (ligands) that bind to receptors.

Initial terms used

$\Rightarrow$ implies that
$\propto$ proportional to
Square brackets [ ]   are used to indicate a concentration
[D]   concentration of free drug
[R]   concentration of unoccupied receptors
[DR]   concentration of drug-occupied receptors
k_1 constant that defines the rate of the association (forward) reaction
k_2 constant that defines the rate of the dissociation (backward) reaction
K_D constant (the dissociation constant) that defines the equilibrium point of the whole interaction

Concentration–effect relationships

Drug–receptor kinetics

The essential pharmacodynamic interaction is that of a drug binding reversibly to a receptor to form a drug–receptor complex.

Figure 26.1 Drug properties

Agonism	Drug binds to the receptor and can produce a maximal response
Partial agonism	Drug binds to the receptor and causes a similar but less than maximal response
Antagonism	Drug may prevent binding by the agonist or interfere with the response outcome

Fundamentals of Anaesthesia, 4th edition, ed. Ted Lin, Tim Smith and Colin Pinnock. Published by Cambridge University Press. © Cambridge University Press 2017.

We will use the interaction of noradrenaline (nor-epinephrine) with an α_1-adrenoceptor to illustrate the concept (see Chapter 28 for details on receptor binding sites).

Drug + Receptor $\rightleftharpoons$ Drug–receptor complex

$$D + R \underset{K_2}{\overset{K_1}{\rightleftharpoons}} DR$$

The law of mass action states that the velocity of a chemical interaction is proportional to the molecular concentrations of the reacting components.

Development of Key equation 1 from the drug–receptor interaction

Forward (association) reaction	$\propto$	$[D]$
and also	$\propto$	$[R]$, so
Forward (association) reaction	$\propto$	$[D] \times [R]$, and
Backward (dissociation) reaction	$\propto$	$[DR]$

For clarity the multiplication sign is usually omitted, and $[D] \times [R]$ is written as $[D][R]$.

The next step is to insert the constants to convert $\propto$ to $=$, which results in the two terms:

Forward reaction $= k_1 [D][R]$

Backward reaction $= k_2 [DR]$

At equilibrium, there is no net change in the balance of concentrations and the rate of association reaction equals the rate of the dissociation reaction, so
$k_1[D][R] = k_2[DR]$

This can be rearranged as:

$$\frac{k_2}{k_1} = \frac{[D][R]}{[DR]}$$

In any equation, constants can be combined as a single constant. In this case, the ratio of the two constants k_1 and k_2 is called the equilibrium or dissociation constant, which is termed K_D.

The final step is to substitute one constant for two, which leads to Key equation 1:

$$K_D = \frac{[D][R]}{[DR]}$$

Key equation 1

$$K_D = \frac{[D][R]}{[DR]}$$

Key points
- K_D is called the **dissociation** (or equilibrium) **constant**.
- K_D is a constant for a particular drug–receptor interaction and defines that interaction.
- K_D permits quantitative comparisons of the equilibrium points of different drug–receptor combinations (e.g. noradrenaline with α_1-receptor, noradrenaline with α_2-receptor and adrenaline with α_1-receptor all have different values for K_D).
- The reciprocal of the dissociation constant is called the affinity of the drug for the receptor. In other words:

$$\text{Affinity} = \frac{1}{K_D}$$

- The higher the affinity of the receptor for the drug then the more associated (less dissociated) it is, so the lower the dissociation constant and vice versa.

Example
An example K_D for noradrenaline and the α_1-adrenoceptor is 10^{-7} molar (100 nanomoles L^{-1}).

While the dissociation constant is very important, the equation itself is of limited use. What is required is the relationship of occupancy (the proportion of receptors occupied by the drug) to drug concentration.

Additional terms used
r   receptor occupancy
R_T total number of receptors

So, occupancy $r = \dfrac{[DR]}{[R_T]}$

Key equation 2

$$r = \frac{[D]}{K_D + [D]}$$

This equation relates occupancy to drug concentration and the dissociation constant for the drug–receptor combination.

Development of Key equation 2

To derive Key equation 2 the receptor term [R], not featuring in occupancy (r), must be substituted in Key equation 1.

The total number of receptors is the sum of free and drug-bound receptors

$$[R_T] = [R] + [DR] \Rightarrow [R] = [R_T] - [DR]$$

Substituting [R] from Key equation 1 gives

$$K_D = \frac{[D]([R_T] - [DR])}{[DR]}$$

⇓ Rearrange

$$\frac{K_D[DR]}{[D]} = [R_T] - [DR]$$

⇓ Divide both sides by [DR]

$$\frac{K_D[DR]}{[D][DR]} = \frac{[R_T] - [DR]}{[DR]}$$

⇓ Simplify

$$\frac{K_D}{[D]} = \frac{[R_T]}{[DR]} - 1$$

⇓ Rearrange

$$\frac{K_D}{[D]} + 1 = \frac{[R_T]}{[DR]}$$

⇓

$$\frac{K_D + [D]}{[D]} = \frac{[R_T]}{[DR]}$$

⇓ Take the reciprocal

$$\frac{[D]}{K_D + [D]} = \frac{[DR]}{[R_T]}$$

Substitute the term for occupancy (r)

$$\frac{[D]}{K_D + [D]} = r$$

This is Key equation 2:

$$r = \frac{[D]}{K_D + [D]}$$

Key points

- When the drug concentration is zero, occupancy will be zero.
- When the drug concentration is equal to K_D then occupancy will be ½.
- As drug concentration rises the dissociation constant becomes very small **in relation to** the concentration, so occupancy will reach close to 100%.

These features will become apparent in the charts later in the chapter.

In our example using noradrenaline, at a noradrenaline concentration of 100 nmol L^{-1} at any particular time **at equilibrium**, half of the α_1-receptors will be occupied as a drug–receptor complex.

In the model, the occupancy relationship is important for explaining how pure agonists behave, but it also applies equally to partial agonists, competitive antagonists and inverse agonists.

To make full use of the model, a term to describe the effect that is produced is required.

Additional terms used

R   response (not the same as [R] in earlier equations)
E   efficacy (a constant for a drug–receptor complex)

The receptor response produced by an agonist binding with the receptor is a function of the occupancy and the effect (efficacy) of the agonist on that receptor. For the purpose of this model, response (R) is proportional both to occupancy (r) and to the efficacy (E) of the drug–receptor complex:

$$R = E\,r$$

Derivation of Key equation 3

A simple substitution of r from Key equation 2 creates Key equation 3:

$$R = \frac{E[D]}{K_D + [D]}$$

Key equation 3

$$R = \frac{E[D]}{K_D + [D]}$$

Key points
- When the drug concentration is zero, response will be zero.
- When the drug concentration is equal to K_D then response will be ½ that of the efficacy.
- As drug concentration rises the dissociation constant becomes very small **in relation to** the concentration, so response will reach close to 100% of maximum.

These features will also become apparent in the charts later in the chapter.

In our example using noradrenaline, **at equilibrium** at a noradrenaline concentration of 100 nmol L^{-1} the **response** from the α_1-receptors will be half of the maximal response.

Figure 26.2 Classification of drug–receptor interaction

Type of drug–receptor interaction	Efficacy	Response maximum from that drug
Pure agonist	1	Full
Partial agonist	Between 0 and 1	Some response but never maximal
Reversible competitive antagonist	0	No response
Inverse agonist	Negative value	Opposite effect

Efficacy and drug–receptor interactions

Graphical plots based on Key equation 3 are used to demonstrate and explain the features of the drug–receptor interactions. These are classified in Figure 26.2. Non-competitive and non-reversible antagonists produce no response. The plots are purely a graphical demonstration of Key equation 2 or Key equation 3 above.

In this section A and B are introduced to represent different pairs of drugs, and so the following additional terms are used:

[B]	concentration of antagonist
[BR]	concentration of receptors occupied by the antagonist
[D_A]	concentration of agonist
[D_B]	concentration of antagonist
r_A	occupancy of receptor by agonist
r_B	occupancy of receptor by antagonist
K_A	equilibrium constant for defining the agonist–receptor interaction (**replaces K_D from previous section**)
K_B	equilibrium constant for defining the antagonist–receptor interaction

Do not confuse the terms K_A and K_B with the terms K_a and K_b used in acid–base calculations.

Figure 26.3 lists the values used in the graphical examples that follow. Note that the values for equilibrium constants are not actual ones but represent concentrations for the purposes of illustration.

Agonists

An agonist is an agent that reversibly binds to a receptor site to produce a conformational change in the receptor, which mediates a response. A pure agonist produces the maximum response that the receptor is capable of mediating, and is therefore said to have an efficacy of 1 (E = 1).

Figure 26.3 Values used for the various ligands in the ensuing graphs

Ligand	Abbreviation	Dissociation constant	Efficacy
Agonist 1	A_1	50	1
Agonist 2	A_2	25	1
Agonist 3	A_3	100	1
Partial agonist 1	P_1	50	0.75
Partial agonist 2	P_2	500	0.75
Reversible competitive antagonist	B	450	0
Irreversible competitive antagonist	I		0

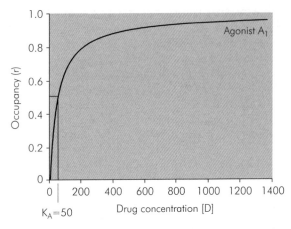

Figure 26.4 Plot of occupancy against drug concentration

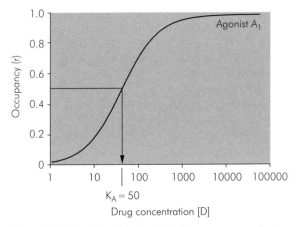

Figure 26.5 Semilogarithmic plot of occupancy against drug concentration

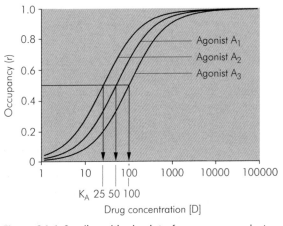

Figure 26.6 Semilogarithmic plot of occupancy against drug concentration, showing the effect of changes in equilibrium constant

Figure 26.4 plots receptor occupancy (r) against drug concentration and demonstrates the characteristic shape often described as a rectangular hyperbola. This shows that as the drug concentration increases so the initially high increase in occupancy reduces progressively as more receptors become occupied. The most rapid increase in occupancy occurs when the concentration is low and the number of unoccupied receptors is at its highest. The rate of increase in occupancy rapidly falls off as the agonist concentration rises and unoccupied receptors fall in number. A working model of the mechanics of this may be thought of as a decrease in opportunity for binding as

fewer free receptors are left. However, it is important to remember that drug–receptor bonds are constantly being made and broken. The important points to identify on the graph are:

- Zero occupancy with zero agonist concentration
- Maximal occupancy (always 1 with competitive binding)
- Concentration at 0.5 (50%) occupancy (this is K_A)

For a pure agonist (efficacy = 1) the y-axis can also be labelled as response. At this point maximal occupancy and response are by definition both 1, but antagonists and partial agonists alter this finding, and thus identifying the maximal response becomes important.

The shape of the plot makes it difficult to identify the maximum or the equilibrium constant accurately using a single plot even if a relatively small concentration range is used. The plot is useful to demonstrate the pharmacodynamic basis of the drug–receptor interaction but does not lend itself easily to comparisons and predictions with other agonists and antagonists or their interactions.

To address these problems the semilogarithmic plot is used. This plots occupancy on a linear scale against drug concentration on a logarithmic scale. This is the basis of Figures 26.5 to 26.10. Figure 26.5 uses the same agonist profile (A_1) as Figure 26.4 and shows the characteristic sigmoid shape. The occupancy is plotted as a proportion of full receptor occupancy, and for a pure agonist this equates with response. The 0.5 occupancy point that determines the concentration value for K_A ($K_A = [D]$) is on the 'straight' part of the plot where the direction of curvature changes from upwards to downwards.

Figure 26.6 shows two more full agonists (A_2 and A_3) with K_A half and double that of the original example ($K_A = 50$). Changing K_A has the following effects:
- Parallel shift to right or left
- No change in maximal occupancy

K_A defines the affinity of the ligand for the receptor (= 1/affinity), so the lower the affinity the higher the equilibrium constant. When the affinity is doubled the K_A is halved, and vice versa. The occupancy profiles for pure agonists, partial agonists and reversible competitive antagonists with identical K_A are identical, but variations in efficacy alter the responses proportionally.

Example

In comparison with noradrenaline, which has a K_D of 10^{-7} molar (100 nanomoles L^{-1}) at the α_1-adrenoceptor, phenylephrine has a K_D of 2×10^{-5} molar (20 micromoles L^{-1}) at the same receptor. So the phenylephrine plot is parallel and to the right of the noradrenaline plot.

Receptors with multiple molecular binding sites

Consider 'n' to represent the number of molecules that must bind to each receptor to mediate a response. Frequently each receptor has one binding site for a particular molecule, but this is not always so. The nicotinic acetylcholine receptor has two binding sites for acetylcholine, one on each α subunit. For a response, both sites must be simultaneously occupied by the agonist. Key equation 4 shows this relationship.

Key equation 4

$$[D]^n = \frac{r}{1-r} K_A$$

If the logarithm of the whole equation is taken the formula below results:

$$n \log[D] = \log\left(\frac{A}{1-r}\right) + \log K_A$$

This formula provides a means of determining 'n'.

Partial agonists

A partial agonist is an agent that reversibly binds to a receptor site to produce a conformational change in the receptor that mediates a response which is less than the

---

Derivation of Key equation 4

Key equation 4 is derived in the same way as Key equation 1.

$$nD + R \rightleftharpoons D_n R$$

From this modification it follows that the forward reaction $\propto [D]^n \times [R]$, and therefore

$$K_D = \frac{[D]^n [R]}{[D_n R]}$$

This may be rearranged to produce an expression for $[D]^n$ as follows:

$$[D]^n = \frac{[D_n R]}{[R]} K_A$$

If top and bottom of the resulting fraction are divided by the total number of receptors, Key equation 4 is obtained:

$$[D]^n = \frac{r}{1-r} K_A$$

---

maximum possible. Examples include buprenorphine and buspirone (5-$HT1_A$). It is, therefore, said to have an efficacy of between 0 and 1.

Figure 26.7 shows a comparison of the drug–response profile of partial agonists (P_1 and P_2) with that of the standard agonist (A_1). A partial agonist is one that does not elucidate a maximal response regardless of concentration, and it therefore has an efficacy (E) of < 1 but > 0. A partial agonist with the same affinity for the receptor (P_1) has the same K_A as the agonist (A_1). Characteristically, however, partial agonists also have a lower affinity for the receptor (K_D higher), as demonstrated by P_2, although buprenorphine has a higher affinity for the receptor (K_D lower).

The following features are apparent:
- Sigmoid-shaped curve
- Response curve shifts downwards
- Shift not parallel
- Maximal response < 1
- Response maximum = efficacy (E)

A partial agonist has the same occupancy profile for a given K_A as a full agonist. The K_A of the partial agonist is a feature of **occupancy** and not response. It is calculated by appreciating that the point of half-maximal occupancy is achieved at half-maximal response. In Figure 26.7 the maximal response of each partial agonist is 0.75 of that of the pure agonist, so the K_A concentration is read off at a response (R) of 0.375, as indicated by the line labelled X.

Figure 26.8 shows the effect on response of the addition of a partial agonist in the presence of various constant concentrations of agonist. For a given concentration of a pure agonist, addition of increasing amounts of partial agonist will eventually result in the observed effect approaching that of the partial agonist alone. At receptor level, competition ensures that the partial agonist displaces the pure agonist from an increasing proportion of the receptor pool until it occupies (almost) all receptors.

Reversible competitive antagonists

A reversible competitive antagonist is an agent that reversibly binds to a receptor site without mediating a response. A pure antagonist, therefore, has an efficacy = 0. These agents act by preventing the bonding of an agonist with the receptor, and therefore preventing any subsequent response. The occupancy profile of a reversible competitive antagonist is the same as that for an agonist or partial agonist for a given dissociation constant. However, as E = 0 for the antagonist, response will be zero **irrespective of drug concentration**. Examples include naloxone and non-depolarising muscle relaxants, the latter only having to block one of the two receptors on the acetylcholine receptor to prevent a response (see *Receptors with multiple molecular binding sites*, above).

Figure 26.9 shows the effect of adding fixed concentrations of a reversible competitive antagonist on the agonist dose–response plot. Occupancy is similarly affected. The important features are:

- A parallel shift to the right
- Antagonist overcome by increasing agonist concentration
- No change in maximal response

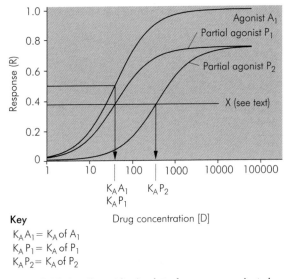

Key
$K_A A_1 = K_A$ of A_1
$K_A P_1 = K_A$ of P_1
$K_A P_2 = K_A$ of P_2

Figure 26.7 Semilogarithmic plot of response against drug concentration, showing the effect of the reduction in efficacy which a partial agonist displays

The effect of the reversible competitive antagonist can always be overcome by increasing the concentration of the agonist. K_A does not change, but the effect is similar to

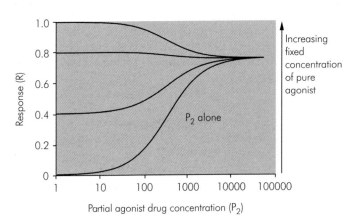

Figure 26.8 Semilogarithmic plot of combined response against partial agonist drug concentration. Each line represents the response in the presence of a fixed concentration of pure agonist

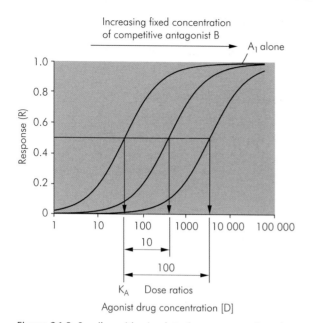

Figure 26.9 Semilogarithmic plot of response against drug concentration, showing the effect of introducing increasing doses of competitive antagonist possessing no intrinsic activity

that of a change in agonist affinity. The dose ratio is the quantitative measure of this effect. This is the ratio of the concentration of agonist in the presence of the antagonist at a given level of response (usually 0.5) to the concentration of agonist alone that produces the same response. In other words, the dose ratio is the factor by which the agonist concentration must be increased to achieve the same effect as in the absence of the antagonist. Using Figure 26.9 as an example, $K_A = 50$ and the concentration with drug B is 500, producing a dose ratio of 10.

The dose ratio is dependent on antagonist concentration and antagonist receptor affinity, but independent of agonist affinity. The antagonist binds with the receptor in a similar manner to the agonist, and the equations for occupancy derived above apply. Thus for a competitive antagonist:

Antagonist + Receptor $\rightleftharpoons$ Antagonist–receptor complex

$$[B] + [R] \rightleftharpoons [BR]$$

In a similar manner to the agonist binding, this produces the following definition of antagonist affinity for the receptor:

$$\text{Antagonist affinity} = \frac{1}{(K_B)}$$

The antagonist is only effective in the presence of the agonist with which it competes for the binding sites.

Derivation of Key equation 5

Key equation 5 is a simple modification of Key equation 1 in which the concentrations are represented by their ratio to the equilibrium constant (K_A). A similar ratio for the antagonist, relative to its own equilibrium constant with the receptor (K_B), may be added. This will have the same effect as increasing K_A, because of its mathematical position in the equation. Dividing the terms of Key equation 1 by K_A gives

$$r_A = \frac{[D_A]/K_A}{[D_A]/K_A + K_A/K_A} = \frac{[D_A]/K_A}{[D_A]/K_A + 1}$$

and adding the ratio for the antagonist B gives Key equation 5:

$$r_A = \frac{[D_A]/K_A}{[D_A]/K_A + [D_B]/[K_B + 1]}$$

Key equation 5

$$r_A = \frac{[D_A]/K_A}{[D_A]/K_A + [D_B]/[K_B + 1]}$$

This predicts that the addition of antagonist B necessitates an increase in the concentration of drug A to achieve the same receptor occupancy with drug A as in the absence of the antagonist. Taking the term that has replaced K_A/K_A in the equation provides a ratio relative to this which describes the effect of the antagonist on the agonist–receptor interaction. This is the dose ratio:

$$\text{Dose ratio} = [D_B]/K_B + 1$$

This is not constant but is proportional to antagonist concentration and increases linearly. The affinity of the antagonist is defined by the K_B, and the potency pA_2 is derived from this. In a similar way to pH, pA_2 is the negative logarithm of the concentration of reversible competitive antagonist that has a dose ratio of 2. pA_2 is constant for a particular antagonist–receptor interaction. Substituting 2 for dose ratio enables calculation of pA_2, thus:

$$2 = [D_B]/K_B + 1$$

⇓ Rearrange

$$1 = [D_B]/K_B$$

⇓ Take logarithms

$$\log 1 = 0 = \log[D_B] - \log K_B$$

⇓ Rearrange

$$-\log D_B = -\log K_B = PA_2 \text{ (as dose ratio is 2)}$$

Therefore, potency as an antagonist is defined by receptor affinity (K_B). Competitive antagonism involves direct competition for the receptor in exactly the same way as the pure agonist and partial agonists.

The competition exists between agonist and antagonist or partial agonist, and there is only space for one drug molecule at each receptor binding site at any time. The balance that results from this competition is determined by the relative affinities of the competing molecules.

Irreversible competitive antagonists

The irreversible competitive antagonist competes with the agonist for receptor sites but once attached it dissociates only very slowly or not at all because of the strength of the bond, which is usually covalent. There is no change in agonist affinity, and the equilibrium constant for the agonist in the presence of antagonist is unchanged, so the concept of pA_2 is inappropriate.

Figure 26.10 shows the effect of adding fixed concentrations of an irreversible competitive antagonist with

zero efficacy on the dose–response plot. Occupancy is similarly affected. The important features are:

- A downward shift
- Antagonism is not overcome by increasing agonist concentration
- Reduced maximal response

The maximal response is reduced in proportion to the reduction in receptors not occupied by the antagonist represented by r_B. A simple modification to Key equation 1 to produce Key equation 6 is all that is required to illustrate this point.

Key equation 6

$$r_A = \frac{D_A}{D_A + K_A}(1 - r_B)$$

Key equation 2 states that the maximum occupancy (and response) cannot be > 1. Key equation 6 predicts the maximum occupancy, and therefore the maximum response, to be $1 - r_B$. In receptor terms the concentration–effect relationship is based on the interaction of the agonist with the remaining unoccupied receptors. At any given concentration, therefore, the effect will be a constant proportion of the maximal response with that level of antagonist. The equation predicts that the overall effect is similar to that of a partial agonist alone.

Lineweaver–Burk plot

The double reciprocal plot in Figure 26.11 is a form of concentration–effect graph to convert a sigmoid curve

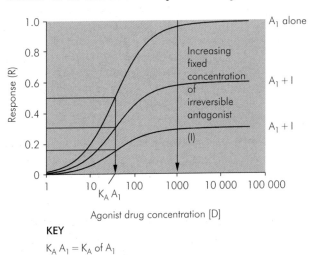

Agonist drug concentration [D]

KEY

$K_A A_1 = K_A$ of A_1

Figure 26.10 Semilogarithmic plot of response against drug concentration, showing the effect of introducing increasing doses of an irreversible competitive antagonist possessing no intrinsic activity

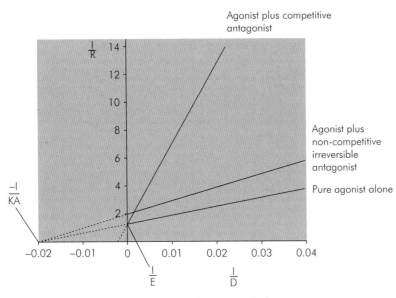

Figure 26.11 Lineweaver–Burk or double reciprocal plot

into a straight line. It is used to determine the type of drug–receptor interaction and the equilibrium constants. The intersection with the y-axis (1/R) gives the reciprocal of efficacy. The intersection with the x-axis gives the negative reciprocal K_A for a single drug.

Variations from predictions

Occupancy–response inconsistencies

Receptor occupancy produces a response at the receptor (R = E r). However, the response is not necessarily identical to the occupancy, even for a pure agonist, because many receptor systems have silent receptors. Silent receptors represent a proportion of the total receptor pool that must be occupied before there is any response at all. This is a conceptual model, and the silent receptors are not a discrete subgroup. Interactions between receptors can also alter the shape of the plots from the theoretical.

Hysteresis

Hysteresis is a feature of changes in a dynamic system in which the response to a stimulus in one direction does not follow the same path when in the opposing direction. The binding of a drug to a receptor confers a degree of stability, and energy must be supplied to break this bond. A rise in drug concentration results in diffusion of drug towards receptors, which facilitates binding. During decreases in drug concentration, there is a lag phase before drug–receptor bonds will break, and thus the system demonstrates hysteresis.

General variation

Within biological systems there is variation between individuals, which usually has a normal distribution. A single individual may also exhibit temporal variation. There are a number of pharmacological terms that use a representative sample of the total population to describe the response. For example:

ED_{50} – dose causing the specified effect in 50% of the sample population

LD_{50} – dose causing a lethal effect in 50% of the sample population

Ratio of $ED_{50} : LD_{50}$ – therapeutic index

Some of these variations originate from identifiable physiological differences such as age, sex and race, but most are the result of pharmacokinetic differences.

Interactions of drugs with similar effects

When two drugs with similar effects are given they may compete, as with partial agonists, competitive antagonists and inverse agonists as described above, or they work independently by different mechanisms. The outcome of the combination may be simply additive, or there may be

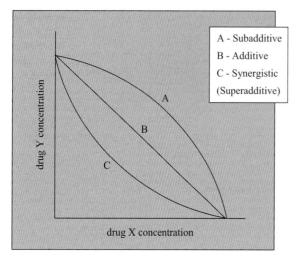

Figure 26.12 Isobologram examples

A - Subadditive
B - Additive
C - Synergistic
(Superadditive)

an enhanced response (synergism or superadditive) or a reduced response (subadditive). An isobologram is a graphical plot of this effect (Figure 26.12). The concentration of one drug is shown on the x-axis, and the other drug on the y-axis. A line is plotted for drug combinations that produce an identical response. Line B in Figure 26.12 illustrates a linear relationship between the concentrations of the two drugs. It is arranged so that when only one drug is used the same effect is achieved with either drug X or drug Y. In combination, the same effect is achieved with ½ that amount of drug X and ½ the amount of drug Y, or ¼ of X and ¾ of Y, and so on. Line C illustrates a combination of two drugs that reduces the proportions of each drug to achieve equipotency, so that the total proportion is less than 1. The drugs work better together, and this is called synergism. Line A shows the opposite effect (subadditive).

For example, volatile anaesthetic agents are considered to be additive, and this is used when calculating the MAC for combinations such as nitrous oxide and isoflurane. Clonidine and morphine act synergistically.

Pharmacogenetics

Genetic variation can alter drug metabolism. For example, the metabolism of warfarin and phenylbutazone varies much less between identical twins than in the rest of the population. Another example concerns the drug suxamethonium, which is metabolised by plasma cholinesterase. Abnormal and deficient plasma cholinesterase result from abnormalities in the gene responsible for transcription of this enzyme, leading to the inherited deficiencies described in more detail in Chapter 4.

Fast and slow acetylators exist for the metabolism of such drugs as hydralazine, procainamide and isoniazid. Slow acetylators may show a higher incidence of unwanted effects for a given dose. Slow acetylators receiving hydralazine are more likely to develop SLE syndrome, for example.

Enzymes

Enzymes are closely related to receptors in their structure and related functional properties. Many receptors have enzymatic actions (e.g. Na^+K^+ATPase in the cell membrane). They possess binding sites that bind substrates with low-energy bonds. Enzymes are proteins, sometimes linked with coenzymes such as vitamins or ions. They provide a low-energy pathway that facilitates a reaction so that equilibrium is reached more rapidly. Enzymes do not alter the final product, nor do they alter the position of the equilibrium. The effects of an enzyme are similar to those that might result from energy provided in another way, such as thermal energy, but avoid the obvious tissue damage that this would entail. Enzymatic processes may be synthetic or destructive. Enzyme kinetics bear a strong resemblance to receptor kinetics, as outlined below.

For a synthetic reaction:

$$xA + yB \rightleftharpoons A_xB_y$$

The law of mass action indicates that the reaction rate in each direction is proportional to the product of the concentrations on each side. x and y represent numbers of substrate molecules A and B; A_xB_y is the product of the reaction. The relative concentrations at equilibrium are defined by the equilibrium constant (K_{eq}):

$$K_{eq} = \frac{A_xB_y}{[A]^x[B]^y}$$

The equilibrium constant is a feature of the reaction itself, regardless of whether or not an enzyme is present. Therefore, an additional concept is required to compare enzymatic function. This is the initial velocity of the enzyme-catalysed reaction, the velocity of the reaction when negligible substrate has reacted.

The equation for initial velocity is based on the reaction

Substrate (S) + Enzyme $\rightleftharpoons$ Product (P) − Enzyme

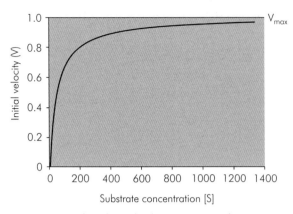

Figure 26.13 Plot of initial velocity against substrate concentration

which may be expressed as follows:

$$V = \frac{V_{max}[S]}{K_m} = [S]$$

where
V = initial velocity
V_{max} = maximum initial velocity
K_m = concentration at which the initial velocity is half the maximum initial velocity

Note that this is identical in structure to Key equation 3 describing receptor interactions, and therefore describes a rectangular hyperbola (Figure 26.13).

Some caution should be exercised when alluding to the similarities. While drug and substrate concentrations are comparable terms, and V_{max} and the initial velocity of the substrate–enzyme interaction might be compared with the efficacy and response of the drug–receptor interaction, K_m is not an equilibrium constant. With this in mind, the equations and plots used in the drug–receptor interactions described above can be used to understand the inhibition of enzyme reactions and their plots. Semilogarithmic plots could be used in exactly the same way as with the receptor interactions, and similar features would be apparent, but by convention the double reciprocal (Lineweaver–Burk) plot is favoured.

Enzyme inhibition may be competitive (reversible) or non-competitive, which may be reversible or irreversible. Neostigmine provides an example of a competitive enzyme inhibitor. Ecothiopate and monoamine oxidase inhibitors are non-reversible enzyme inhibitors.

False substrates compete for the binding site and in addition have a product, so they are reversible and competitive. Methyldopa is a false substrate for the enzyme dopamine decarboxylase. Inhibition of the enzyme will be the result of more prolonged binding to the enzyme during the reaction. Although neostigmine is a competitive inhibitor of acetylcholinesterase and is hydrolysed by plasma cholinesterase, of which it is a substrate, it is also slowly hydrolysed by the acetylcholinesterase and is therefore a false substrate for this enzyme.

CHAPTER 27
Pharmacokinetics

Tim Smith

Pharmacokinetics is the study of the movement of a drug through the compartments of the body and the transformations (activation and metabolism) that affect it. Pharmacokinetics is often referred to as 'what the body does to the drug'. Figure 27.1 shows an overview of these processes.

Drug administration

Drugs are administered by many different routes. The aim of drug administration is to achieve therapeutic levels of the drug at its site (or sites) of action. In general, this is achieved using the vascular compartment as the transport mechanism for redistribution. Drug administration is, therefore, designed to produce suitable drug levels within the blood. The choice of route for a particular drug takes into account physical properties, target site of action, consideration of possible toxic effects and the practicalities of administration. The routes are summarised in Figure 27.2 in a practical classification. The enteral and topical routes are most easily accessible, but require absorption across a barrier or membrane to establish their effect.

Absorption

Absorption is the process of taking the drug from the site of administration to the blood. This is necessary for all enteral and parenteral routes except for intravenous (IV) administration. Systemic absorption may occur from topically administered drugs, but this is not the intended route. Absorption involves the crossing of barriers between administration site and vascular compartment with subsequent movement across the physical distance between the two. The distance within any local compartment is traversed by simple passive diffusion down the concentration gradient. Most barriers are made up of cells closely linked by tight junctions. The cell thus acts as both a filter and a device for active uptake, so the drug must pass into and then out of the cell to cross the barrier. The main principles affecting absorption include:

- Simple passive diffusion
- Facilitated diffusion
- Active uptake
- Pinocytosis

The rate of diffusion is shown by the following formula:

$$\text{Rate of diffusion} \propto \frac{CAP}{T}$$

where
C = concentration difference either side of membrane
A = area of membrane
P = membrane permeability
T = membrane thickness

Fundamentals of Anaesthesia, 4th edition, ed. Ted Lin, Tim Smith and Colin Pinnock. Published by Cambridge University Press. © Cambridge University Press 2017.

INPUT

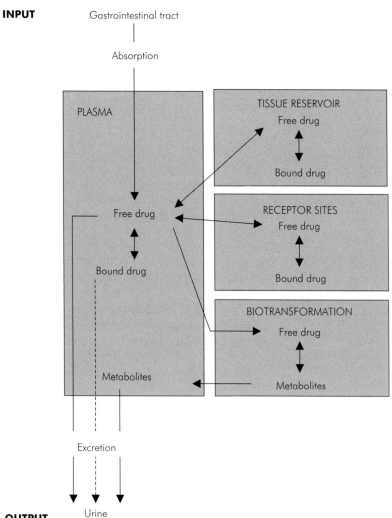

Figure 27.1 Overview of pharmacokinetic processes

The ability of a drug (or any molecule) to pass through a membrane is influenced by:

- Solubility in the membrane (lipid solubility)
- Degree of ionisation
- pH
- Size of molecule
- Carrier processes
- Pinocytosis
- Partition coefficient across the membrane

Enteral administration

Enteral administration encompasses any route that requires the gastrointestinal (GI) tract. Where a patient is incapacitated, access to the stomach and small intestine can still be achieved using a nasogastric tube or an endo-scopically sited nasoduodenal small-bore feeding tube. Most enterally administered drugs have sites of action distant from the GI tract and therefore require absorption first. This exposes them to the first-pass effect, which is elimination during passage through the liver via the hepatic portal vein. The hepatic portal vein receives blood from the GI tract from oesophagus to upper rectum. Oral and nasogastric administrations imply that the drug enters the stomach, but absorption may occur throughout the length of the GI tract. Buccal administration, and to a degree rectal administration, bypass the liver and so avoid

Figure 27.2 Routes of drug administration

Enteral	Oral
	Buccal
	Rectal
Parenteral	Intravenous
	Intramuscular
	Subcutaneous
	Intradermal
	Transdermal
	Inhalational
	Transtracheal
Topical	Skin
	Eyes
	Ears
	Intranasal
	Vaginal
	Urethral

the first-pass effect. Enterally administered drugs may also be subjected to other effects before absorption, including neutralisation of alkaline drugs by gastric acid and enzymatic action in the intestinal lumen or wall. The advantages and disadvantages of enteral administration are as follows:

Advantages
- Easy to give
- Special equipment not required
- Patient can self-administer

Disadvantages
- May not be appropriate route
- Patient may be unable to swallow
- Drug may be destroyed in the GI tract lumen
- May have excessively high first-pass effect
- Drug may be irritant to GI tract
- First-pass effect and bioavailability variable
- Effective dose unpredictable

Most drugs administered enterally require absorption followed by distribution via the blood to the effector sites. It is difficult to measure effector levels of drug, but blood levels can be used as a predictor of achievement of an effective level. Absorption is therefore the mechanism for achieving an effective plasma level, and absorption and uptake are essential to this aim. For IV administration, however, this stage is bypassed. IV administration involves administration of a bolus of drug that rapidly becomes distributed throughout the whole circulating volume.

First-pass effect
Enterally administered drugs absorbed from the stomach, small intestine or colon enter the hepatic portal vein. The whole of the absorbed drug dose passes through the liver and is therefore potentially subjected to hepatic metabolism and extraction (elimination) before entering the systemic circulation. This is termed the first-pass effect.

Bioavailability
Bioavailability is the amount of drug administered by a given route that reaches the systemic circulation. IV administration therefore achieves 100% bioavailability. Bioavailability is usually taken to refer to oral administration (oral bioavailability), but other routes also have a bioavailability. Bioavailability is reduced by destruction in the lumen, poor absorption and metabolism. Oral bioavailability is greatly influenced by the first-pass effect, so that a high first-pass effect produces a low bioavailability.

Parenteral administration
By definition, parenteral administration uses routes other than the GI tract. Following absorption, the drug is transported in the blood. This may be in the plasma or the red blood cells or both, and may involve protein binding. The absorption process is generally simpler than enteral absorption but still entails some degree of variability between patients, sites and drugs. The advantages and disadvantages of parenteral administration are as follows:

Advantages
- Unaffected by first-pass metabolism
- Plasma levels may be more predictable
- Does not require functioning GI tract
- Does not require patient assistance

Disadvantages
- Administration requires training
- Not usually self-administered
- Administration usually requires injection
- Requires special equipment

Intramuscular
Intramuscular (IM) injection is one of the commonest methods of parenterally administering drugs, avoiding the need to cannulate a vein and slowing the onset of the effect, which may confer a safety advantage. The absorption profile means that the drug will be absorbed

slowly over a period and will last longer than the same drug administered intravenously.

The factors affecting absorption from an IM injection are:

- Drug solubility in blood
- Tissue binding
- Protein binding
- Blood flow to site

Transdermal

Fentanyl and glyceryl trinitrate (GTN) are examples of drugs that may be administered transdermally. The method avoids the first-pass effect, and provides a slow absorption and therefore a prolonged effect without significant peaks and troughs in plasma levels. Transiderm-Nitro 5 has a reservoir of 25 mg GTN with a contact surface area of 10 cm^2, which achieves an average 24-hour absorption of 5 mg. A plateau in the plasma level of glyceryl trinitrate is achieved within 2 hours of application. This plateau level is directly proportional to the surface area of the permeable membrane of the patch. It is important, therefore, that the patch makes good contact with the skin. Transiderm-Nitro 10 achieves double the transfer (10 mg per 24 hours) by doubling the contact surface area to 20 cm^2.

Inhaled

Inhaled anaesthetic agents are covered elsewhere (Chapter 29). Their effect depends on achieving sufficient brain concentration of the drug (which is produced from an alveolar concentration) secondary to an inhaled dose at the nose or mouth.

Inhaled bronchodilators act in a topical manner, but systemic absorption also occurs.

Distribution

Once a drug is absorbed into the circulation it undergoes distribution. An overview of mass drug movement is shown in Figure 27.3.

The distribution to individual tissues depends on the solubility of the drug in those tissues and its delivery to them. The factors determining the uptake of the drug and speed of distribution to an individual tissue are:

- Plasma protein binding
- Blood flow to tissue
- Mass of tissue to which distributed
- Tissue/blood partition coefficient
- Tissue protein binding
- Facilitated transport
- Drug ionisation
- Drug molecular size

Blood flow to tissues

Blood flow determines the speed of distribution and the amount of drug reaching the tissue capillaries, and therefore the amount available for uptake into that tissue.

Three compartments are generally used to explain pharmacokinetic principles: the vessel-rich group (VRG), the muscle group (MG) and the fat group (FG). The vascularity of these tissue groups varies, and the

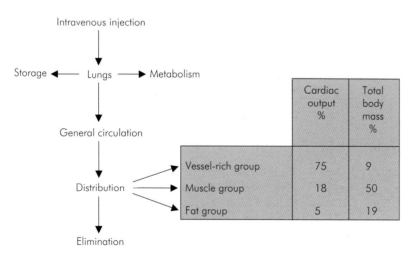

	Cardiac output %	Total body mass %
Vessel-rich group	75	9
Muscle group	18	50
Fat group	5	19

Figure 27.3 Overview of drug distribution

proportion of cardiac output received by them is shown in Figure 27.3.

Drug uptake by tissues

Uptake depends on the drug concentration in tissue and blood, and the partition coefficient. The blood concentration will change as it flows through the capillaries provided that tissue and blood are not at equilibrium. The drug will pass into (or out of) the tissue towards equilibrium. The commonest mode of transit is diffusion, but carrier-facilitated diffusion and active transport systems also occur. The partition coefficient indicates the ratio of drug concentration in neighbouring tissue compartments at equilibrium, and drug movement will occur towards this equilibrium point. As blood concentration falls due to redistribution and elimination, then the balance will be restored by movement out of the tissue back into the blood. The speed of transfer to and from compartments depends on the degree of deviation from the equilibrium partition coefficient and the ease of molecular movement. The mass of tissue involved will alter the rate at which equilibrium is reached and so in turn will alter the rate of uptake. For a given partition coefficient, a large volume of tissue will increase both total uptake and rate of uptake of the drug, but will reduce the speed of achievement of equilibrium.

The ease of transfer between compartments is influenced by:

- Ionisation (determined by pH and pK_a)
- Membrane components
- Molecular size

Figure 27.4 shows the temporal relationship of drug distribution within various compartments following an IV bolus administration of a typical IV induction agent.

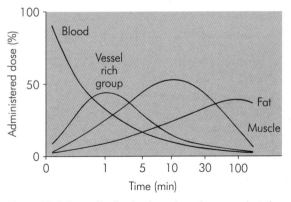

Figure 27.4 Drug distribution in various tissues against time following IV bolus administration of thiopental

Drug distribution causes the blood concentration to fall. The VRG then has more drug than plasma, so movement is reversed and the drug moves from the tissue back into the blood. At this early stage, the blood concentration is higher than that in either the muscle group or the fat group. There is a net redistribution from VRG to MG and FG. Later the same effect will occur from MG to FG, and much later the drug in FG will return to the blood and be eliminated. All redistribution processes require the blood as an intermediary phase.

Active transport

Penicillin is a drug that is actively transported. This is a unidirectional process regardless of the concentration gradient. Probenecid blocks active transport in the liver, kidney and choroid plexus, which increases the proportion in the blood, and so the apparent volume of distribution is reduced.

Protein binding

Protein binding alters the concentration of free drug as a proportion of the total. Different proteins have different affinities for drugs. Albumin mostly binds acidic drugs such as aspirin, whereas α_1-glycoprotein is more important for basic drugs. The amount of drug bound is influenced by plasma pH (which alters the ionisation of the drug), age and certain disease states. Hypoalbuminaemia is a common finding in chronic disease, and in hepatic (reduced synthesis) and renal (increased loss) failure in particular. Such conditions reduce the amount of albumin available for drug binding, and therefore increase the amount of free drug. Note that α_1-glycoprotein is increased in:

- Obesity
- Trauma
- Burns
- Postoperative period
- Myocardial infarction
- Carcinoma
- Inflammatory diseases

Placental transfer

Most drugs cross the placenta to some degree. Transfer is favoured by high lipid solubility and a high un-ionised proportion. Placental blood flow and metabolism also influence transfer. The ratio of concentrations in fetal and maternal placental blood is called the feto-maternal concentration ratio (Figure 27.5).

Figure 27.5 Examples of feto-maternal (F/M) concentration ratios

Induction agents	Propofol	0.65–0.85
	Thiopental	0.4–1.1
Volatile agents	Isoflurane	0.7–0.91
	Nitrous oxide	0.83
Opioids	Alfentanil	0.3
	Fentanyl	0.1–1
	Morphine	0.92
	Pethidine	1
Muscle relaxants	Suxamethonium	0.04
	Atracurium	0.05–0.2
	Vecuronium	0.11–0.12
Local anaesthetic agents	Bupivacaine	0.2–0.4
	Lidocaine	0.5–0.7
	Ropivacaine	0.2

Elimination

Elimination is the removal of active drug from the body, and it has two components, biotransformation and excretion. It may thus occur simply as excretion of the unchanged active form of the drug, or after inactivation. Many drugs require biotransformation to enable excretion. Alternatively, an irreversibly inactivated enzyme or receptor (e.g. inhibited monoamine oxidase) may need to be replaced by fresh, unaffected protein.

Enterohepatic circulation

Hepatocytes possess active transport systems that concentrate certain drugs (e.g. digoxin) and conjugates (e.g. morphine) within the bile. In the gut, the glucuronide becomes hydrolysed and active drug is reabsorbed into the hepatic portal vein. Enterohepatic circulation prolongs the half-life of a drug.

Biotransformation

There are two basic phases of biotransformation, I and II.
- Phase I reactions are simple chemical reactions such as oxidation, reduction and hydrolysis, and they tend to be destructive. Oxidation and reduction are mainly hepatic functions in which cytochrome P450 is

particularly important. Hydrolysis is widespread and may take place in the plasma by free enzymes such as plasma cholinesterase.
- Phase II reactions are important for the removal of substances that are not readily water-soluble. They are more complex synthetic reactions that add molecular groups (such as acetylation or glucuronide conjugation), and biotransformation often involves several of these reactions before final products are excreted.

Biotransformation predominantly occurs in the liver, but other sites in the body such as lungs, plasma and kidney are also involved.

Extraction ratio

The extraction ratio (ER) is a measure of the effectiveness with which a substance is removed or processed by an organ. Hepatic extraction is the most useful to consider, this being the proportion of drug delivered to the liver which is extracted and does not appear in the hepatic vein. Note that this is a dimensionless ratio, which may be expressed as:

$$ER = \frac{C_a - C_v}{C_a}$$

where
C_a = arterial concentration of a substance
C_v = venous concentration of a substance

The extraction of a drug depends on:
- ER
- Enzyme activity
- Drug–protein binding
- Red blood cell partitioning
- Perfusion

Clearance (see Chapter 16) represents a volume of blood completely cleared of drug in unit time. For example, in the case of hepatic clearance

$$\text{Hepatic clearance} = \dot{Q}_{hep} \times ER$$

where
$\dot{Q}_{hep}$ = hepatic blood blow

Hepatic clearance of a drug with a high ER is highly dependent on liver blood flow because most of the delivered drug is extracted. Enzyme activity, protein binding and red cell partitioning, therefore, have less influence on hepatic extraction. Conversely, clearance of a drug with a low ER is relatively unaffected by blood flow but highly dependent on the other factors.

Excretion

Excretion involves the removal of active drug and its metabolites from the body. The main routes of excretion are in urine and bile, but the lungs, faeces and sweat represent other routes. Excretion of a substance relies on it being soluble in the solvent being excreted (usually water). Biotransformation to a water-soluble form is therefore essential for the excretion of highly lipid-soluble drugs. Excretion via the lungs primarily applies to inhaled volatile anaesthetic agents. However, substances administered by other routes, such as ethanol, are also eliminated partially in expired gases.

Molecules presented to the glomerulus in the renal plasma will cross the basement membrane into the renal tubules, but there is a 'cutoff' at a molecular weight of about 69,000 daltons, depending on shape and charge. In effect, this applies mainly to water-soluble compounds, because highly lipid-soluble substances will only be present free in the plasma in very low concentrations. Similarly, protein binding will reduce the amount of free drug available to cross the glomerulus. If the drug in the filtrate is not reabsorbed as much as the water in the kidney tubule then the concentration of the drug will increase by the time it reaches the renal pelvis. However, it is the amount of drug excreted that is important in elimination and not the concentration, although the two are interdependent. Tubular reabsorption occurs to a limited extent, and this is affected by ionic charge, which is in turn altered by pH. A high filtration rate will facilitate elimination, so good renal blood flow is desirable, but the absolute volume of urine produced is less important.

Active transport systems exist for some drugs (such as penicillin), which are actively secreted into the tubules. Probenecid may be used to block this penicillin transport and thus prolong the half-life of the drug.

Pharmacokinetic models

Measurement of drug levels in blood and other fluids is relatively easy when compared with the measurement of tissue drug levels. Models are created to help to describe, understand and predict the pharmacokinetic behaviour of drugs, and mathematical relationships are used to describe these interrelationships.

Compartment models

Compartment models are based on the body behaving as if it is divided into a number of hypothetical interlinked spaces or compartments. Each compartment has specific properties of volume and transfer rates for a particular drug. One-, two- and three-compartment models are routinely used, but note that these compartments do not correspond precisely to anatomical structures. Consistent solubilities are assumed throughout, so the volumes are calculated based on partition coefficients = 1. The models are used mathematically to describe the changes in plasma concentration with time, and so predict and compare pharmacokinetic profiles. Figures 27.6 to 27.8 illustrate one-, two- and three-compartment models. The small 'k' in these diagrams denotes the rate constants for those intercompartmental equilibria.

One-compartment model

The simplest model is a one-compartment model. In this, all tissues are represented as a composite single compartment (1). A drug of dose D is administered to the compartment and is considered evenly distributed throughout. The plasma concentration (C) of the drug is measured to calculate the volume (V) of this hypothetical compartment, the plasma being the 'window' through which the compartment can be 'viewed'. By definition:

$$C = \frac{D}{V}$$

The elimination rate constant (k_{el}) defines the overall rate of removal of drug from this single compartment, and is a combination of all the modes of elimination for that drug.

Two-compartment model

The one-compartment model is too simple to describe accurately the behaviour of most drugs, and the single compartment is therefore divided into central (1) and peripheral (2) compartments. Again the plasma is the 'window' to the compartments and is not necessarily equivalent to the central compartment. The central compartment is the intermediary compartment through which the peripheral compartment is accessed. Many drugs, including thiopental, show a good approximation to this model.

Three-compartment model

Some drugs, such as propofol, require further compartments to be added to allow accurate pharmacokinetic predictions. In this model, a third, deep peripheral compartment is added, and this communicates with the central compartment, but at a much slower rate.

Any model is an approximation, but by increasing the number of compartments, the correlation with the real situation can be improved. However, the size of the improvements diminishes as the number of compartments increases.

Water analogue model

Mapleson described a model for the pharmacokinetic behaviour of inhaled anaesthetic agents using a series of interconnected cylinders of water (Figure 27.9). In this model, the height of the water determines the pressure and is analogous to the agent partial pressure. The cross-sectional area of each cylinder is analogous to the solubility of the agent in that tissue and its apparent physical volume, and the amount of agent in the tissue is represented by the volume of water in the cylinder. The resistance of the connecting pipes represents the transfer characteristics, a small-bore (high-resistance) tube representing a slow transfer. The model will proceed towards the equilibrium state in which all the cylinders will have an equal volume of water.

Volume of distribution

Volume of distribution may be explained using the models above. These model compartments are defined as having a consistent concentration throughout. Therefore, if the amount of drug in the compartment is known,

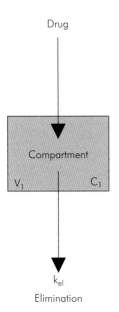

Figure 27.6 A one-compartment model

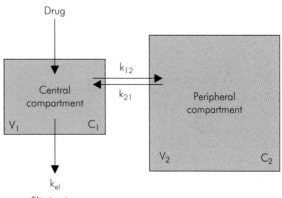

Figure 27.7 A two-compartment model

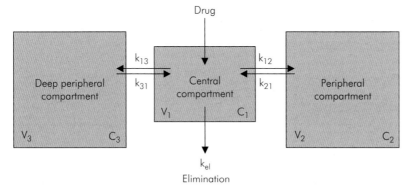

Figure 27.8 A three-compartment model

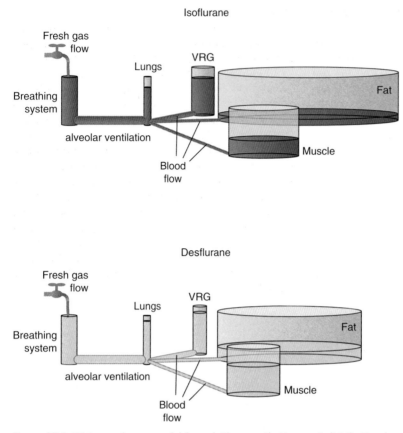

Figure 27.9 Water analogue model for volatile anaesthetic agent distribution based on Mapleson's description. Isoflurane and desflurane are used as examples, using the pharmacokinetic values in Chapter 29.

measuring the concentration of the drug will enable calculation of the apparent volume through which the drug is distributed. The model works on the basis that the drug is equally distributed throughout that calculated volume. Usually, the drug dose given is known and the plasma concentration that would exist if distribution occurred without elimination can be calculated. The apparent volume of distribution does not exist as an identifiable anatomical entity, but rather is a mathematical concept representing the composite result of multiple volumes with differing solubilities for a given drug.

The apparent volume of distribution is thus used as a tool to describe the way in which drugs are distributed. Drugs that are mainly confined to plasma have low volumes of distribution, while drugs that are highly tissue-bound have a high volume of distribution. The volume of distribution may easily exceed the total volume of the body. High tissue binding results in a low plasma

concentration. This low concentration spread evenly throughout the calculated volume for a given dose results in a very large value for volume of distribution.

Elimination kinetics

Zero- and first-order kinetics are used to describe the elimination characteristics of a drug. Most drugs are eliminated with first-order kinetics.

Zero-order kinetics

In zero-order kinetics the elimination system is saturated at clinical levels, and elimination is therefore constant and unrelated to drug concentration. A fixed mass of drug is eliminated in unit time irrespective of the blood concentration, and the concentration therefore declines at a constant rate. This is demonstrated in Figure 27.10, in which a constant amount of drug is removed in each time interval, resulting in a similar linear decline in drug concentration.

Ethanol provides an example of zero-order elimination, and high levels of phenytoin, thiopental and salicylates also show zero-order features. As the concentration falls so the elimination pathways may no longer be saturated, and first-order kinetics takes over. Kinetics may also be affected by saturation of other components such as protein binding, carrier-mediated active transport mechanisms and enzyme systems.

First-order kinetics

In the first-order model, the rate of drug elimination is proportional to the plasma drug concentration such that:

Elimination $= dC/dt \propto C$

where
dC = a small change in concentration
dt = a small change in time
C = concentration

The elimination pathways are not saturated, but are gradually recruited as the concentration of drug increases, and vice versa. The rate of change of drug concentration is therefore also proportional to the drug concentration. The change in concentration is a lowering of concentration, and so the formula has a minus sign. Thus, for first-order kinetics:

$$\frac{dC}{dt} = -kC$$

This can be calculated from the following derived formula:

$$C = C_0 e^{-k_{el}t}$$

where
k_{el} = elimination rate constant
C_0 = concentration (C) at time (t) = 0

Figure 27.11 demonstrates this process, in which a constant volume is cleared of drug in each time interval, resulting in an ever-declining rate of fall in drug and drug concentration. Although the drug concentration decreases with time, it approaches but never actually reaches zero. The rate of that decrease (the gradient of the slope) also falls with time. This is an exponential decay.

Half-lives and time constants

An important feature of the exponential function shown in first-order kinetics is the time taken for the concentration to halve (Figure 27.12). This is the half-life ($t_{\frac{1}{2}}$). Half-lives are hybrid constants that are dependent on primary constants. The time constant, another such feature, is based on the rate of change of concentration (the gradient of the plot). The time constant is the time that it would take for the drug concentration to reach zero if elimination continued at the rate of the chosen starting point. Time constants (τ) also apply to exponential functions of the form $y = 1 - e^{-x}$. Figure 27.13 shows the proportion of the initial concentration that exists after a given number of time constants. The initial concentration in this sense may be any point on the plot from which timing is started. As the time constant and half-life are constants for a given exponential function, they must have a constant relationship, which is described by the formula:

$$t_{\frac{1}{2}} = \tau \, \log_e 2 \qquad \text{and} \qquad \tau = \frac{1}{k_{el}}$$

Derivation of an expression relating the half-life and the elimination rate constant

Take the equation $C = C_0 e^{-k_{el}t}$.

By definition, at one half-life from time zero the concentration will be half that of the concentration at time zero (time zero can be chosen arbitrarily for this calculation):

$$\tfrac{1}{2}C_0 = C_0 e^{-k_{el}t_{\frac{1}{2}}}$$

⇓ Divide both sides by the common factor (C_0)

$$\tfrac{1}{2} = e^{-k_{el}t_{\frac{1}{2}}}$$

⇓ Take natural logarithm of both sides, $\log_e$

$$\log_e \tfrac{1}{2} = -k_{el}t_{\frac{1}{2}}$$

⇓ Rearrange

$$t_{\frac{1}{2}} = \frac{-\log_e \tfrac{1}{2}}{k_{el}}$$

as $-\log_e \tfrac{1}{2}$ equals $\log_e 2$, substitute to create the relationship between half-life and elimination rate constant:

$$t_{\frac{1}{2}} = \frac{\log_e 2}{k_{el}} = \frac{0.693}{k_{el}}$$

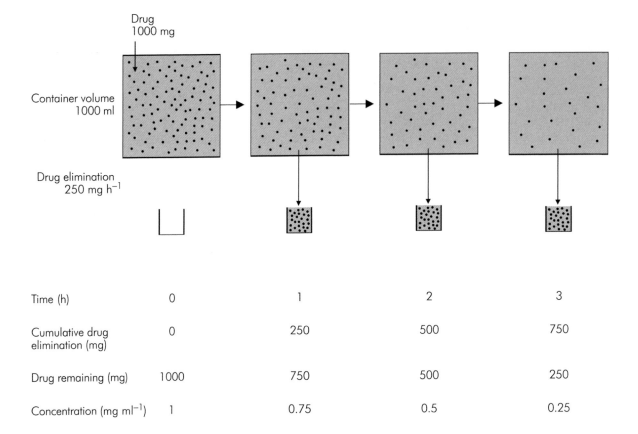

Time (h)	0	1	2	3
Cumulative drug elimination (mg)	0	250	500	750
Drug remaining (mg)	1000	750	500	250
Concentration (mg ml^{-1})	1	0.75	0.5	0.25

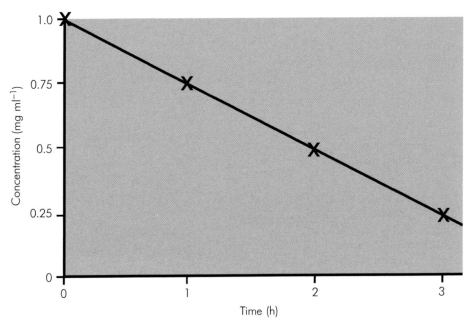

Figure 27.10 Effect of zero-order elimination on drug concentration

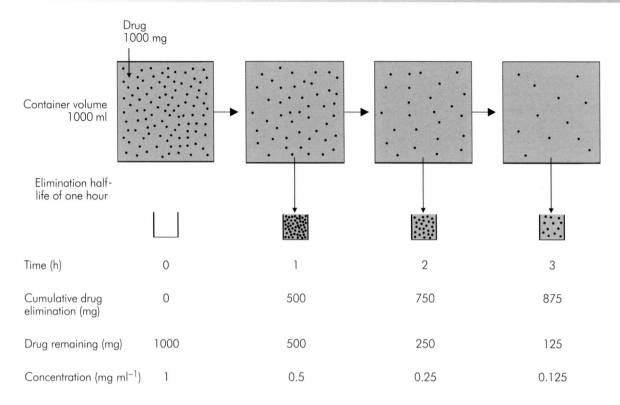

Time (h)	0	1	2	3
Cumulative drug elimination (mg)	0	500	750	875
Drug remaining (mg)	1000	500	250	125
Concentration (mg ml^{-1})	1	0.5	0.25	0.125

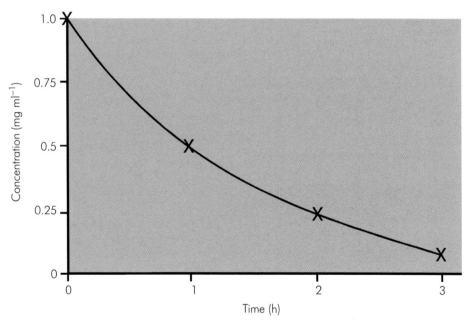

Figure 27.11 Effect of first-order elimination on drug concentration

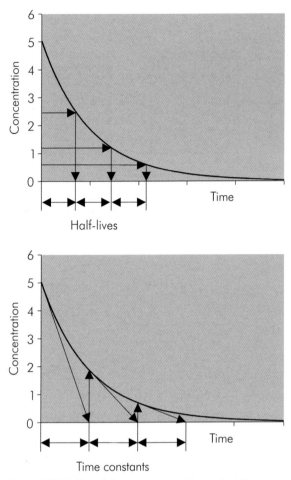

Figure 27.12 Plot of drug concentration against time showing half-lives and time constants (using linear scales)

Figure 27.13 Time constants and the concentration remaining

Number of time constants	Percentage of starting concentration remaining
N	e^{-N} (%)
0	100
1	37
2	13.5
3	5.0
4	1.8

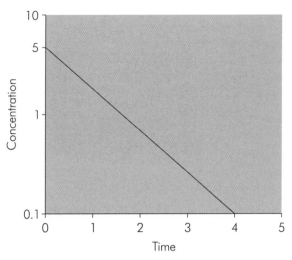

Figure 27.14 Semilogarithmic plot of concentration against time

The natural logarithm 'log$_e$' may also be written 'ln'. The concentration and rate of decline of concentration in Figure 27.12 fall exponentially with time. Mathematically and graphically, it is easier to work with linear relationships. Using a logarithmic scale for the concentration (or the natural logarithm of the concentration) against time on the original linear scale (Figure 27.12) produces a straight line (Figure 27.14).

The straight line can now be extrapolated to the y-axis (t = 0) to obtain a theoretical (or apparent) value for concentration at the time of injection (C_0). This is the predicted concentration if there was instantaneous uniform distribution of the drug of dose D throughout the compartment at the time of injection, before any elimination has occurred. This single-compartment model can then be used to calculate the volume of distribution (V_d) as follows:

$$C_0 = \frac{D}{V_d}$$

In practice, this simple exponential decline is masked in the clinical situation by the combined affects of absorption, distribution, redistribution and elimination. Most clinical data sets of plasma (or blood) levels of an intravenously injected drug have a pattern similar to Figure 27.15.

This two-compartment model can be seen to have two linear (graphical) components, which can be separated. The initial rapid decline is the result of rapid redistribution

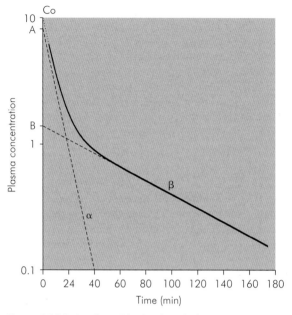

Figure 27.15 Semilogarithmic plot of plasma concentration against time

Step 3
Subtract B from C_0 to create concentration A.

Step 4
Subtract the β slope from the concentration plot to create a new straight line of slope α (the distribution element of the graph). Although it may seem unusual that a curve appears as the result of the addition of two straight lines in part of the graph, this is because of the logarithmic scale used for concentration. Observation of this scale shows that it does not reach zero at the x-axis.

Step 5
Use these values mathematically to calculate the following variables:

$$\alpha = \log_e 2/t_{\frac{1}{2}\,\alpha}$$

$$\beta = \log_e 2/t_{\frac{1}{2}\,\beta}$$

$$V_{dI} = dose/C_0$$

Area under the curve $(AUC) = A/\alpha + B/\beta$

throughout the central compartment being predominant. Later, redistribution to the peripheral compartments is predominant. Clearance is constant throughout, but elimination is proportional to concentration and is greatest earlier in the process. Each component has a half-life and volume of distribution. Elimination half-life $(t_{\frac{1}{2}\beta})$ is the usual value quoted. To calculate elimination half-life using the graph, the following steps may be followed.

Step 1
Extrapolate the straight line of the distribution phase to the y-axis (t = 0). Call this 'C_0' as before.

Step 2
The elimination phase has a slope of β. Extrapolate the straight line of the elimination phase to the y-axis (t = 0). Call this 'B'. This is the initial concentration that would have existed if there was instantaneous distribution to equilibrium on IV injection. This can be used to calculate a value for the volume of distribution following equilibration with the tissues. This is also an approximation of the volume of distribution at steady state (V_{dss}). However, this is calculated and defined as the volume of distribution when giving an infusion of a drug at exactly the same rate as total clearance of the drug.

Clearance
Clearance (Cl) represents the volume of blood completely cleared of drug in unit time. The amount of drug eliminated is therefore dependent upon the drug concentration, which is a first-order process. Typical units for clearance are mL of blood per kg body weight per minute (mL kg^{-1} min^{-1}). Total clearance is the sum of all the individual clearances, such as hepatic (Cl_H), renal (Cl_R) and others (Cl_X). Clearance can be calculated from a graph using AUC:

$$Cl = dose/AUC = \frac{dose}{A/\alpha + B/\beta}$$

In other words, clearance = volume of compartment × elimination rate constant.

Referring back to the two-compartment model, the volume of distribution at steady state (V_{dss}) is the usual volume quoted, as follows:

$$V_{dss} = V_{dI}(1 + k_{12}/k_{21})$$

where
k_{12}, k_{21} = intercompartment rate constants
V_{dI} = initial volume of distribution

As the plasma concentration is determined by the addition of the α and β profiles, $Cp = Ae^{-\alpha t} + Be^{-\beta t}$. Note that at t = 0, $e^0 = 1$, so $C_0 = A + B$.

Figure 27.16 Pharmacokinetic values for propofol

Compartment		$t_{1/2}$ (min)
Central (1)		2–3
Peripheral (2)		30–60
Deep peripheral (3)		180–480
V_{dl}	230 mL kg^{-1}	
V_{dss}	12 L kg^{-1}	

This is a 'best fit', and most drugs fit the two-compartment model. However, it should be remembered that this apparent mathematical model is derived from numerous distribution profiles and a range of tissue profiles. Some drugs, such as propofol, best approximate to a three-compartment model, that is a tri-exponential model. Values pertaining to this are shown in Figure 27.16.

Effective levels

Effective levels of volatile agents can be monitored by measurement of the end-tidal concentration. Blood levels of IV agents are not readily monitored, but desired concentrations can be targeted using pharmacokinetic models based on patient demographic data, and compared with plasma equivalents of MAC, which are:

MIR – minimum infusion rate that prevents response to surgical stimulus in 50% of patients

ED_{50} – a general term to describe the dose that is effective in 50% of subjects

EBC – effective blood concentration (sometimes called EC)

The strategy of a target concentration is one method of delivering the anaesthetic dose. A target concentration is chosen in a similar way to volatile agent concentration, and a computer-controlled pump calculates bolus and maintenance infusion rate based on patient details. The target concentration is altered according to clinical need and the pump adjusts accordingly. The concept of an effective blood concentration of the agent depends on the following conditions:

- Intensity of drug action (predictable from concentration at the receptor site)
- Concentration at the receptor site proportional to free plasma concentration

In total intravenous anaesthesia (TIVA) using propofol, the aim is to rapidly achieve a blood level of propofol that will induce anaesthesia, and then maintain this state until the procedure is complete. Discontinuing the infusion will then lead to a rapid recovery of consciousness as blood (and brain) concentrations of propofol fall. A constant infusion achieves a plateau level, but this is slow. A loading dose is therefore used, based on the volume of distribution (V_d) and the desired concentration (C_p) in the following way:

$$\text{Loading dose} = V_d \times C_p$$

This may be followed by a maintenance dose calculated from the total clearance and the desired plasma concentration (this being equal to the amount of drug being eliminated in unit time) in the following manner:

$$\text{Maintenance dose} = Cl \times C_p$$

Another method of maintaining a therapeutic level over a prolonged period is to administer intermittent doses, with each bolus given before the plasma level falls below the therapeutic threshold. For maximum interval, the dose used should raise the plasma level to the top of the therapeutic range without reaching toxic levels. Repetitive dosing results in a plateau once elimination (determined by concentration) equals administration rate. The dosing interval is usually approximately that of the terminal elimination half-life.

The various half-lives that are given for the decline in concentration of a given drug apply to specific circumstances. An initial redistribution component ($t_{1/2\alpha}$) and a slower terminal half-life ($t_{1/2\beta}$) describing what happens over a longer period of time, mainly due to elimination, are quoted for two-compartment models. In addition, if a drug is infused over a period of time, eventually a steady state occurs in which all tissues are in equilibrium, the plasma concentration is constant and elimination equals infusion rate. Stopping the infusion gives a decline with the longest possible half-life for that drug. However, usually infusions run for much shorter periods of time and so a steady state has yet to be reached. The half-life in this context (the context-sensitive half-life) is less than the half-life at steady state. The shorter the duration of the infusion the closer the half-life becomes to the redistribution half-life. Drugs with a low lipid solubility (such as alfentanil) are less affected by this than those with a high lipid solubility (such as fentanyl).

Context-sensitive half-life

The multicompartment models that are used to predict pharmacokinetic behaviour are more complex when infusions of drugs are used. The context is the duration of infusion. Drug boluses lead to decline in plasma concentration as a result of both redistribution and elimination. When infusions are given the aim is to maintain the plasma concentration, and this provides a sustained concentration difference between compartments leading to continuing redistribution into the peripheral compartments until eventually equilibrium may be reached. When the infusion is stopped elimination continues from the plasma (in proportion to plasma concentration), but once plasma concentration falls below that of the other compartments then diffusion back into the plasma occurs. The longer the infusion the greater the total amount of drug in the peripheral compartments, and so the more the plasma concentration will be maintained and the slower it will fall. So the terminal half-life does not adequately reflect the actual rate of fall in plasma concentration. The context-sensitive half-life is a concept to describe how the duration of infusion (the context) alters the effective elimination half-life of the drug. The same effect is seen with volatile anaesthetic agents, as described in Chapter 29, with the longer duration of inhalation leading to slower elimination by the lungs.

CHAPTER 28

Mechanisms of drug action

Sue Hill

Drugs exert their observed effects in a multitude of different ways. These may involve physicochemical, pharmacodynamic or pharmacokinetic interactions with biochemical and physiological systems of the body.

The main, intended action of a drug may not be the only effect that the substance has on the body, and there may be multiple modes of action. For example, many drugs interact with more than one type of receptor, and some may alter the pharmacokinetics of co-administered drugs by enzyme induction or inhibition.

Physicochemical mechanisms

These mechanisms are generally non-specific, and depend on the physicochemical properties of a drug including its molecular size, shape, whether it is a weak acid or weak base, the pK_a of its constituent groups and its lipid and water solubility.

Non-specific physicochemical mechanisms of action include:

- Charge neutralisation (pH effects)
- Osmotic effects
- Adsorption
- Chelation

Charge neutralisation

This mode of action is typified by the action of the antacid drugs. When sodium citrate is ingested, citric acid is produced. **Citric acid and sodium citrate act as a buffer-pair, reducing the concentration of hydrogen ions and increasing stomach pH.** Calcium bicarbonate is also an effective antacid, but the reaction produces carbon dioxide, which can cause abdominal distension and flatulence. To avoid this problem sodium citrate is preferred preoperatively to reduce the risk of aspiration-induced lung damage in high-risk patients requiring general anaesthesia. Sodium citrate should not be used long-term because of the high sodium load: antacid drugs for prolonged use should not be absorbed. Aluminium hydroxide preparations are relatively insoluble and longer-lasting, so come closest to ideal, although care should be taken in renal failure.

Another example of charge neutralisation is the use of protamine in reversing the effects of heparin (see Chapter 41). Protamine is a fish spermatozoal protein that is strongly basic due to a high arginine content, and carries a high density of positive charge; heparin is acidic and carries a negative charge. The combination of

Fundamentals of Anaesthesia, 4th edition, ed. Ted Lin, Tim Smith and Colin Pinnock. Published by Cambridge University Press. © Cambridge University Press 2017.

protamine and heparin produces a complex that has no anticoagulant effect.

Osmotic effects

Mannitol is an alcohol derivative of the sugar mannose. **Mannitol exerts an osmotic effect in the plasma**, like glucose, which leads to expansion of the extracellular volume and reduction of blood viscosity. It also has a diuretic effect, because it is freely filtered and minimally reabsorbed. Large volumes of mannitol must be avoided to prevent impaired tubular function as the result of the high plasma osmolality.

Adsorption

Non-specific adsorption of drugs to activated charcoal allows the latter to be used in the treatment of drug overdose by effectively removing free drug from the stomach. Charcoal is not always effective and is not useful in lithium, cyanide, iron, ethanol or methanol poisoning.

Chelation and inclusion complexes

Heavy metal ions such as lead, arsenic and copper can effectively be removed by using chelating agents. These agents have multiple oxygen, sulphur or nitrogen atoms that form coordinate bonds (where the ligand contributes both electrons) with the metal ion. **An ideal chelating agent will be water-soluble, not undergo biotransformation, have a low affinity for calcium and form non-toxic metal complexes that can readily be excreted.** Edetate calcium disodium ($Ca^{2+}Na_2^+EDTA$) and penicillamine are both used in lead poisoning; penicillamine is also of use in copper and mercury poisoning.

Cyclodextrins are bucket-shaped oligosaccharides produced from starch. α-Cyclodextrins are formed of six, β-cyclodextrins of seven and γ-cyclodextrins of eight sugar residues. They present a hydrophilic outer surface and an internal hydrophobic cavity that can trap other molecules by forming an inclusion complex. Modified cyclodextrins are used extensively for masking odours and as drug delivery systems for poorly water-soluble drugs. **Sugammadex is a γ-cyclodextrin reversal agent that selectively forms an inclusion complex with rocuronium** and less so with vecuronium but not with benzylisoquinolinium muscle relaxants. This produces effective reversal of rocuronium effects from any depth of neuromuscular blockade without the unwanted effects of widespread inhibition of acetylcholinesterase.

Pharmacodynamic mechanisms

Many drugs exert their effects through an interaction with specific and selective sites on receptors. Receptors are large proteins that are associated with cellular structures such as cell membranes, cytoplasm, intracellular membranes or nuclear material. The selectivity arises from the 3D chemical configuration of the drug, which matches a site on the relevant protein and allows binding to take place. The observed effect then results directly or indirectly from this interaction. This type of action is characterised by a lock-and-key mechanism involving different chemical forces that allow the drug first to approach its active site and then to fit into a selective binding area. Initial attraction may be by ionic forces, but stabilisation is due to van der Waals interactions once the drug is in close proximity to its selective binding site.

Interaction mechanisms include:

- Drug–cell membrane receptor
- Drug–voltage-gated ion channel
- Drug–intracellular membrane receptor
- Drug–cytosolic receptor mechanisms

Drug–cell membrane receptors

Many of the drugs we use in our anaesthetic practice act by interfering with the action of endogenous neurotransmitters at their receptors. **The most important neurotransmitter-associated receptors are ligand-gated ion channels and G-protein-coupled receptors.** Other membrane-dependent transduction mechanisms include tyrosine kinase and guanylyl cyclase-coupled receptors.

Ligand-gated ion channels

Ion channels that are opened as a result of binding of neurotransmitters are known as ligand-gated ion channels. They must be distinguished from ion channels that are opened as a result of a change in membrane potential (voltage-gated channels).

Many of the drugs we use interfere with ligand-gated ion channels that mediate very rapid transmission of information through the central and peripheral nervous systems. Neurotransmitters either depolarise the postsynaptic membrane, allowing forward transmission of electrical signals, or hyperpolarise the membrane, inhibiting such signals.

There are three distinct families of ligand-gated receptors, which can be distinguished by their subunit structure: pentameric, ionotropic glutamate and ionotropic purinergic receptors (Figure 28.1).

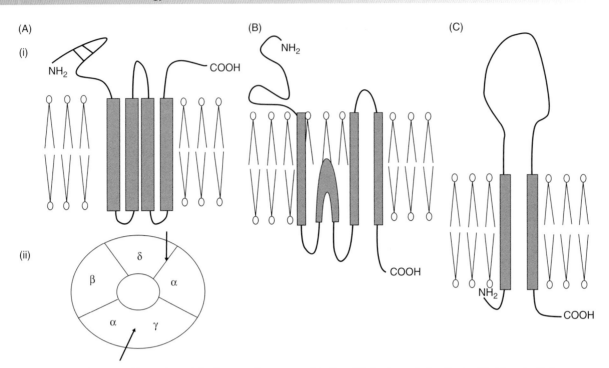

Figure 28.1 Schematic illustration of the ionotropic receptor families. (A) Pentameric family, typified by nicotinic acetylcholine receptor at the neuromuscular junction; (i) subunit configuration – note four transmembrane domains and two cysteine bridges near the NH₂ terminus; (ii) arrangement of subunits as seen from above – arrows show the two acetylcholine binding sites. (B) Ionotropic glutamate family, typified by NMDA receptor with three transmembrane domains and one re-entrant loop. (C) Purinergic ionotropic P2X receptors, with two transmembrane domains and a large extracellular loop.

Cys-loop pentameric receptors

Examples – the nicotinic acetylcholine receptor (nAChR), the γ-aminobutyric acid type A receptor (GABA$_A$), inhibitory glycine receptors (GlyR) and the 5-hydroxytryptamine (serotonin) type 3 receptor (5-HT$_3$).

Each subunit of this pentameric family has four helical transmembrane domains (TMDs). The name *cys-loop* comes from the fact that in the extracellular N-terminal region there are two disulphide cysteine bridges, forming a looped structure.

The pentameric family provides the most important sites of drug action for neuromuscular blocking agents, at the nAChR, and for many of our general anaesthetic agents, at the GABA$_A$ receptor; the action of general anaesthetic agents is discussed in greater detail below.

Subunit composition can vary for the nAChR. At the neuromuscular junction (NMJ), subunit composition is αεαβδ, but in the fetus it is αγαβδ; acetylcholine binds to the α–ε and α–δ subunit interfaces. Cooperative binding of two molecules of acetylcholine is required to produce the required conformational change and open the channel, which is then five times more selective for monovalent cations – Na$^+$ in particular – than for divalent cations such as Ca^{2+}. **Depolarising blockers, such as suxamethonium, bind to the same site as the natural transmitter acetylcholine and cause opening of the ion channel** by inducing similar conformational changes, although channel opening time is increased. Suxamethonium persists longer in the synaptic cleft than acetylcholine because it is not a substrate for acetylcholinesterase. As a result the receptor cannot return to its resting conformation but becomes desensitised: it no longer responds to the agonist, and neuromuscular blockade ensues. A similar picture is seen in the presence of irreversible inhibition of acetylcholinesterase by organophosphates: acetylcholine itself induces paralysis. In contrast, **the non-depolarising**

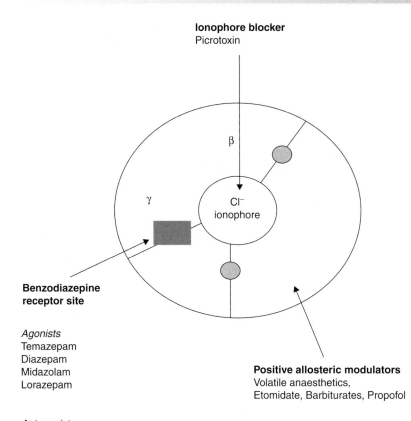

Ionophore blocker
Picrotoxin

β

γ

Cl⁻
ionophore

**Benzodiazepine
receptor site**

Agonists
Temazepam
Diazepam
Midazolam
Lorazepam

Positive allosteric modulators
Volatile anaesthetics,
Etomidate, Barbiturates, Propofol

Antagonist
Flumazenil

Figure 28.2 Active sites on the GABA$_A$/Cl⁻ ionophore/benzodiazepine receptor complex, looking from above. The grey circles show the two agonist sites for GABA, which are competitively inhibited by gabazine and bicuculline.

muscle relaxants compete for the same binding site as acetylcholine but the conformational change they induce prevents channel opening.

Nicotinic receptors are found at sites other than the NMJ, in particular at autonomic ganglia and in the CNS. In the CNS the subunit composition is very different from that at the NMJ, which accounts for the differing sensitivity of these receptors to cholinergic drugs. As discussed below, these neuronal nicotinic receptors are sensitive to the effects of certain general anaesthetic agents.

GABA and glycine are the major inhibitory neurotransmitters in the CNS, glycine predominantly in spinal cord and hindbrain, GABA supraspinally. Unlike the nAChR, **the GABA$_A$ channel is an anionic channel** favouring chloride passage through the synaptic membrane, resulting in hyperpolarisation and inhibition of forward signalling. Subunit stoichiometry depends on anatomical location, but 1α:2β:2γ and 2α:2β:1γ are most

common. **The benzodiazepine receptor (BDZR) site is associated with the GABA$_A$–chloride channel complex.** Activation of the BDZR is responsible for sedative and anticonvulsant effects due to positive allosteric modulation of GABA transmission, so increasing hyperpolarisation. The benzodiazepine binding site requires both α and γ subunits to be present, whereas etomidate binds with higher affinity to receptors with a β$_2$ or β$_3$ subunit. Important sites for drug binding on the GABA$_A$ receptor complex are shown in Figure 28.2.

Ondansetron inhibits 5-hydroxytryptamine type 3 (5-HT$_3$) ionotropic channels. Like nAChR, 5-HT$_3$ receptors are cation channels favouring monovalent over divalent cations. There are several types of serotoninergic receptors, but only type 3 are ionotropic; the others are all G-protein-coupled receptors. The centrally mediated antiemetic action is associated with vagolytic effects, as these receptors are also found on vagal afferents from the gastrointestinal (GI) tract. Ondansetron therefore has both central and peripheral effects.

Ionotropic glutamate receptors

There are three ionotropic glutamate receptor types, NMDA, AMPA and kainite. Other glutamate receptors are metabotropic G-protein-coupled receptors. NMDA receptors are formed from four subunits, two are pore-forming (NR1) and two regulatory (NR2). Glutamate binds to the NR1 subunit and its coactivator, glycine, to the regulatory subunit. All ionotropic glutamate receptors are equally permeable to Na^+ and K^+ but have a particularly high permeability to the divalent cation, Ca^{2+}, unlike the pentameric excitatory channels. **NMDA receptors are the site of action of ketamine, nitrous oxide and xenon**, all of which are non-competitive inhibitors of glutamate. There is a high density of NMDA receptors in the hippocampus and associated regions, which are important in the formation and recall of memories.

Ionotropic purinergic receptors: P2X subtypes

Receptors of this family form cation channels that are equally permeable to Na^+ and K^+ but also to Ca^{2+}. They are activated by ATP and its metabolites and are widely distributed in both central and peripheral neurones. The analgesic property of pentobarbital is thought to be due to inhibition of P2X receptors in the dorsal root ganglia. These ionotropic purinergic receptors are not to be confused with G-protein-coupled receptor forms of purinergic receptors: adenosine receptors (P1) and P2Y subtypes.

G-protein-coupled receptors (GPCRs)

Almost 1000 genes for GPCRs have been identified and all have a similar structure, although they can be divided into several distinct families. **GPCRs have seven helical TMDs, starting with the extracellular N-terminus and ending with the intracellular C-terminus.** The quaternary structure is such that these helices cluster together, held in the correct alignment by interactions with extracellular/intracellular domains. When a ligand binds, these helices twist in relation to each other, inducing a conformational change that is transmitted to the domain that is associated with G-protein coupling. The ligand binding site is determined by the composition of the second and third extracellular loops, whereas the second and third intracellular loops are associated with G-protein binding. **All adrenoceptors, muscarinic, cholinergic and opioid receptors work through a GPCR mechanism.**

G proteins are associated with the inner leaflet of the cell membrane and are not always associated with receptors. When the ligand binds, a conformational change occurs that increases the likelihood of the receptor becoming associated with its particular G protein. The kinetics of GPCR–G-protein interactions requires complex models to explain observed responses. Essentially the receptor can exist in a number of states, which differ in their affinity for agonist, antagonist or inverse agonist. Response is greatest when a full agonist is bound to the appropriate G protein. Once the GPCR–G-protein association takes place, there is a conformational change in the G-protein α subunit that allows dissociation of bound GDP in exchange for GTP and favours dissociation of the α subunit from the βγ dimer. The GTP-bound α subunit now has sufficient energy to interact with intracellular enzymes or cell-membrane-bound ion channels and either activate or inhibit these secondary mechanisms. The GTPase activity of the α subunit limits the duration of this activity and, once GTP is hydrolysed to GDP, further interaction is energetically unfavourable and the α subunit then re-associates with the βγ dimer, which has dissociated from the GPCR. In some situations the βγ dimer can also act as an intermediary by opening K^+ channels.

There are many different types of G protein, with subfamilies classified according to their α-subunit activity including Gs, Gi and Gq subfamilies: Gs and Gi proteins activate and inhibit adenylyl cyclase, respectively; Gq causes phospholipase C to hydrolyse phosphatidylinositol in the cell membrane, producing diacylglycerol (DAG) and inositol triphosphate (IP_3). All catecholamine action is mediated through GPCRs, although different adrenoceptor subtypes are associated with different subfamilies of G protein. Figure 28.3 lists some GPCRs and their G-protein associations that are of importance to the anaesthetist.

Other transmembrane messenger systems

Unlike GPCRs, tyrosine kinase receptors (Trk) do not rely on an intermediary protein for activity. The cytoplasmic portion of a Trk forms the catalytic site, which is activated by ligand binding to the extracellular portion of the receptor. The effects of many polypeptide growth factors, cytokines and hormones, including insulin, are through Trk activation.

The guanylyl-cyclase-coupled receptor (GCCR) is a single transmembrane protein responsible for the action of certain hormones, particularly atrial natriuretic peptide.

Figure 28.3 Some important GPCRs and their agonists and antagonists

Natural ligand/receptor type	G-protein α-subunit type	Agonist/antagonist drugs
Acetylcholine M_1, M_3 and M_5	Gq	Atropine, glycopyrrolate antagonists
Acetylcholine M_2 and M_4	Gi	Atropine, ipratropium, glycopyrrolate antagonists
Noradrenaline α_1	Gq	Phenylephrine agonist; phentolamine antagonist
Noradrenaline α_2	Gi	Clonidine agonist; yohimbine antagonist
Noradrenaline β_1 and β_2	Gs	Isoprenaline, salbutamol agonist (β_2); atenolol, propranolol, labetolol antagonist
Opioid receptors (all types)	Gi	Morphine, fentanyl, alfentanil, remifentanil (μ); pentazocine (κ)
$GABA_B$ receptors	Gi	Baclofen agonist
P1 adenosine receptors	Gi	Adenosine agonist
$P2Y_1$ and $P2Y_2$ receptors	Gi	ADP agonist; clopidogrel irreversible antagonist
Histamine H_1 receptors	Gq	Cetirizine antagonist
Histamine H_2 receptors	Gs	Ranitidine antagonist
Dopamine D_1 and D_5 receptors (postsynaptic)	Gs	Dopamine and dobutamine in kidney agonist
Dopamine D_2, D_3 and D_4 receptors (presynaptic)	Gi	Bromocriptine agonist; haloperidol, risperidone, chlorpromazine and clozapine (D_4 selective) antagonists
Serotonin $5-HT_{1A}$ receptors	Gi	Buspirone antagonist
Serotonin $5-HT_2$ receptors	Gs	Ketanserin antagonist
Angiotensin II AT_1 receptors	Gq	Losartan, valsartan antagonist

Voltage-gated ion channels

Voltage-gated ion channels are activated by a change in membrane potential. They are present in nerve axons, including presynaptically, and on smooth and skeletal muscle.

Local anaesthetics such as lidocaine and bupivacaine act by blocking voltage-gated sodium channels. They are usually administered in close proximity to peripheral neurones; activity requires access to the cytosolic side of the axon so lipid solubility is important, although the ionised form is active. Some anticonvulsants, such as phenytoin, lamotrigine and carbamazepine, act by blockade of central sodium channels, so reducing neuronal excitability. Voltage-gated calcium channel blockers such as nifedipine and verapamil act by blocking L-type calcium channels: antihypertensive and antianginal effects are associated with action on vascular smooth muscle, whereas myocardial effects produce their antiarrhythmic action.

Intracellular receptors

Receptors within the cell can be associated either with the cytosol or with any of the specialised intracellular membranes; of particular importance are receptors associated with the sarcoplasmic reticulum that regulate calcium release.

Intracellular hormone receptors

Lipid-soluble hormones interact with intracellular receptors. There is a superfamily of such receptors, including those for sex hormones, corticosteroids, thyroxine and vitamin D_3. **These receptors act as ligand-regulated** transcription factors that bind to DNA and influence the pattern of RNA production by either increasing or inhibiting specific protein production. Gene transcription is influenced by the recruitment of additional proteins that act as co-activators or co-repressors to remodel the quaternary structure of DNA. The oestrogen-receptor modulator tamoxifen inhibits transcription associated with tumour cells in certain cancers. In addition to hormone receptors, other nuclear receptors can also influence protein production: the antidiabetic drug rosiglitazone is a peroxisome proliferator-activated receptor type γ (PPAR-γ) agonist that stimulates protein transcription, leading to insulin sensitising activity within adipose tissue.

Adrenal steroid hormones
There are two types of corticosteroid receptor: MR (or type 1) is the mineralocorticoid receptor and GR (or type 2) the glucocorticoid receptor. **In the cytoplasm, GR is bound to an inhibitory protein, heat shock protein. Glucocorticoid binding displaces this inhibitor and triggers a conformational change that facilitates translocation and binding to specific regions on DNA.** GR is widespread in cells, whereas MR is restricted to epithelial tissue such as renal collecting tubules. Cortisol and aldosterone are equipotent at MR receptors: aldosterone-triggered activation is facilitated by the presence of 11β-hydroxysteroid dehydrogenase in epithelial cells, which metabolises cortisol to a compound that is inactive at the MR receptor.

Intracellular membrane-bound receptors
Intracellular membranes have GPCRs in addition to receptors that respond to secondary messengers produced by ligand–GPCR coupling at the cell membrane. Of particular importance is the control of intracellular calcium. **Endoplasmic reticulum contains IP$_3$ (inositol triphosphate) receptors and sarcoplasmic reticulum (SR) ryanodine receptors.** In skeletal muscle the ryanodine–L-type calcium channel complex triggers calcium release for excitation–contraction coupling. **Dantrolene acts at the ryanodine receptor to inhibit calcium release from the SR.** Several families with malignant hyperthermia have genetic abnormalities associated with the ryanodine receptor.

Pharmacokinetic actions
Drugs may exert their effects by interfering with the absorption, distribution and metabolism of endogenous substances involved in biochemical and physiological systems. In this section we consider drug–enzyme and drug–transporter mechanisms.

Drug interactions with enzymes
Enzymes of relevance to anaesthetists are those that metabolise neurotransmitters and those that inhibit non-neuronal homeostatic systems such as elements of the immune or coagulation cascades.

Interaction with neurotransmitter metabolism
Acetylcholine: acetylcholinesterase
The duration of acetylcholine activity at the NMJ is determined by acetylcholinesterase, which is found in the clefts of the postsynaptic membrane. Several enzyme molecules associate to form an oligomer that is anchored to the synaptic membrane with enzymatic sites facing into the cleft. The non-depolarising muscle relaxants, such as vecuronium and atracurium, competitively inhibit the association of acetylcholine with the nAChR; this inhibition can be overcome by the use of acetylcholinesterase inhibitors such as neostigmine, resulting in an increase in acetylcholine concentration in the synaptic cleft. The log-dose–response curve for acetylcholine is shifted to the right by the presence of vecuronium; in the presence of neostigmine the acetylcholine concentration increases, so producing a return of muscle contraction (Figure 28.4). It is important that some activity is present before neostigmine is given, or the relative increase in acetylcholine concentration is not sufficient to overcome the blockade completely.

There are two binding sites on acetylcholinesterase, the anionic and the esteratic sites. The anionic site attracts the positively charged quaternary nitrogen of acetylcholine, allowing the substrate to approach the esteratic site. This latter site contains a serine residue that is crucial for bond breakage and which is transiently acetylated. **Neostigmine binds to both anionic and esteratic sites**; it is a substrate for the enzyme, but instead of metabolism resulting in acetylation of the enzyme, carbamylation occurs. Although the carbamoyl group can dissociate from the esteratic site, the rate at which this occurs is very much slower than for an acetyl group; the enzyme remains inhibited sufficiently long for the synaptic concentration of neuromuscular blocking drug to fall to an insignificant level.

Catecholamine neurotransmission
Methyldopa is a substrate for the natural catecholamine synthetic pathway, and the metabolic product,

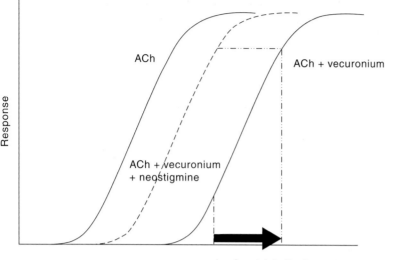

Figure 28.4 Addition of vecuronium shifts the log-dose–response curve to the right. Addition of neostigmine has the *apparent* effect of shifting the response back to the left (shown by the dashed curve), since the concentration of acetylcholine is increased (by an amount indicated by the solid arrow) in the presence of an acetylcholinesterase inhibitor.

methylnoradrenaline, is packaged into synaptic vesicles in the same way as the endogenous transmitter. However, methylnoradrenaline is less active than noradrenaline so autonomic control of blood pressure is impaired.

Endogenous catecholamines are metabolised by monoamine oxidase (MAO) and catechol-O-methyltransferase; inhibition of MAO is associated with antidepressant action. MAO is widespread, but is particularly associated with mitochondrial membranes in the synaptic terminal and hepatocytes. There are two forms of MAO, MAO-A and MAO-B. Non-selective MAO inhibitors (MAOIs) such as tranylcypromine and phenelzine are irreversible inhibitors. Selective MAO-A inhibitors (e.g. moclobemide) are reversible, shorter-acting inhibitors used in the treatment of depression, whereas the MAO-B inhibitor selegiline is used in the treatment of Parkinson's disease. The use of pethidine and indirectly acting synthetic catecholamines, such as ephedrine, is contraindicated in the presence of MAOIs. It is suggested that irreversible MAOIs are stopped for 2 weeks before surgery.

GABA metabolism

Enhancement of GABA transmission is a target for development of anticonvulsant drugs. Sodium valproate and vigabatrin both inhibit GABA-transaminase, which is responsible for breakdown of GABA.

Immunomodulatory action

NSAIDs, including aspirin, exert their effects by inhibiting cyclo-oxygenase, the enzyme responsible for the production of a variety of prostaglandins and related autocoids. These are derived from arachidonic acid, which is produced by activation of membrane-associated phospholipase C in response to inflammatory mediators. **There are two genetically determined forms of cyclo-oxygenase: cyclo-oxygenase 1 (COX-1), which is constitutively active, and cyclo-oxygenase 2 (COX-2), which is inducible.** It is this latter form that is produced in response to an inflammatory insult and is associated with the pain of inflammation. Aspirin and non-selective NSAIDs act by inhibiting both forms of the enzyme; reducing the action of the constitutive form is thought to be responsible for many of the unwanted actions of this group of drugs. The selective NSAIDs, such as etoricoxib, have a much higher affinity for the inducible form, COX-2, with an associated reduction in many unwanted effects such as gastric erosions and ulceration. A third type of cyclo-oxygenase exists, COX-3, which represents a post-transcriptional modification of the COX-1 gene product. It has been suggested that inhibition of COX-3 is the mechanism of paracetamol's antipyretic action, although this is disputed.

Drug interactions with transport proteins

The duration of action of many neurotransmitters is regulated by reuptake into neurones. Inhibition of pre-synaptic transport proteins will increase neurotransmitter availability at the postsynaptic membrane. Of particular interest are the selective serotonin reuptake inhibitors (SSRIs), such as paroxetine, which are effective anti-depressants with fewer unwanted effects than less selective drugs, such as imipramine.

In the renal tubule furosemide inhibits the $Na^+/K^+/2Cl^-$ symport mechanism in the thick ascending limb of the loop of Henle to produce its diuretic effect. Thiazide diuretics inhibit the Na^+/Cl^- symport in the distal tubule, a weak effect, since electrolyte concentrations in distal tubular fluid are relatively low.

Another transport mechanism of importance is the proton pump in the stomach, responsible for the secretion of hydrogen ions and maintenance of gastric pH. The $H^+K^+ATPase$ enzyme system at the secretory surface of gastric parietal cells is the target for proton pump inhibitors such as omeprazole.

The anticonvulsant tiagabine is an inhibitor of the GABA transport mechanism that is responsible for glial cell uptake of GABA from adjacent synapses.

Mechanisms of general anaesthetic action

Of the mechanisms of drug action described earlier in this chapter, those of particular relevance to anaesthesia involve neurotransmitter function. Figure 28.5 summarises ways in which neuronal traffic can be altered by drugs.

One of the most elusive mechanisms of drug action is that of general anaesthetics themselves. For many years this was thought to involve a non-specific physicochemical action, but now it is thought more likely that a specific receptor-based mechanism is responsible.

One of the main problems with investigating the mechanism underlying anaesthetic action is the lack of a clear definition of what constitutes general anaesthesia. The definition must include certain clinical observations: loss of conscious awareness, loss of response to noxious stimuli (antinociceptive effect). Importantly, the effect must be reversible. Animal models of anaesthesia can address antinociception and reversibility, but cannot measure conscious awareness.

It is likely that different general anaesthetic agents have differing profiles of pre- and postsynaptic activity at ligand-gated channels within the CNS. All these

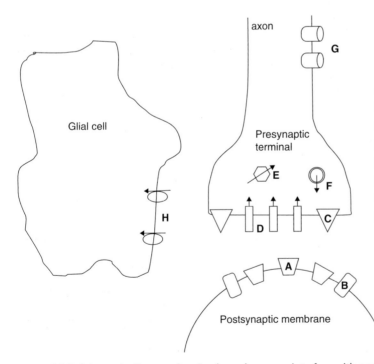

A. Inhibition/activation at postsynaptic receptors

B. Inhibition of membrane-bound enzymes

C. Inhibition/activation at presynaptic receptors

D. Inhibition of reuptake of neurotransmitter

E. Inhibition of intraneuronal metabolism

F. False transmitter formation

G. Inhibition axonal voltage-gated ion channels

H. Inhibition of transport into glial cells

Figure 28.5 Schematic diagram showing how drugs can interfere with neuronal traffic

effects result in depression of signals reaching the hippocampus and cortex so that explicit memory traces are not laid down, information processing is interrupted and unconsciousness ensues. The sedative effects seem to be mediated, at least in part, through the tuberomammillary nucleus, and the immobility induced by volatile anaesthetics is through spinal rather than supraspinal mechanisms. **The molecular sites of anaesthetic action are likely to be lipophilic sites on mainly ligand-gated ionic channels,** although we cannot entirely exclude effects on voltage-gated channels. As a result, an allosteric conformational change in the ion channel either enhances inhibitory or inhibits excitatory currents. At present, the best evidence is for enhancing the inhibitory effect of GABA at GABA$_A$ receptors and/or inhibition of excitatory currents at the NMDA receptor. The contribution made by action on glycine and neuronal nicotinic receptors has yet to be established. Whatever the effects of the anaesthetic agents, clinical anaesthesia is achieved by a balanced combination of agents contributing to the overall effect.

Anatomical sites of action

The anatomical sites of action of general anaesthetics are regions of the brain and spinal cord. Such sites must be involved both in physiological responses to nociception and in consciousness; certainly explicit but possibly also implicit memory mechanisms should be inhibited. Memory is associated with the limbic system, and the degree of awareness is related to depth of anaesthesia. Cortical afferent input and motor efferents must also be interrupted. It is likely that both spinal and supraspinal sites are involved in the action of anaesthetics.

Auditory and sensory evoked potential data support an anatomical site of action for volatile anaesthetic agents somewhere between brainstem and cortex, with the thalamus the most likely primary target. This fits with the integrative functions of the thalamus, but does not exclude the limbic system or certain cortical areas. Evidence suggests that several brain areas are affected by anaesthetics, each mediating different components of anaesthetic activity. The sedative effect of anaesthetics appears to be associated with the tuberomammillary nucleus. Inhibition of GABA receptors in this region, using the GABA antagonist gabazine, markedly reduces the sedative effects of propofol and pentobarbital, but not those of ketamine.

Molecular theories

At the beginning of the nineteenth century, when the anaesthetic effects of a number of agents were being investigated in animal models, Overton and Meyer independently described the linear correlation between the lipid (in particular olive oil) solubility of anaesthetic agents and their potency (Figure 28.6). This correlation was so impressive, given the great variation in structure of these agents, that it suggested a non-specific mechanism of action based on this physicochemical property. Later interpretation pointed out that any highly lipophilic area was a potential site of action, with cell membranes being the most likely contender, given the high concentration of lipids. Not all lipids give as good a correlation between solubility and potency. The best correlation occurs with lecithin, a constituent of cell membranes. However, there are problems with a unified theory based on lipid interactions: some general anaesthetics, such as ketamine, are extreme outliers. The stereoisomeric pair of steroidal agents alphaxalone and betaxalone have identical lipid solubility, but only alphaxalone has anaesthetic properties (perhaps explained by its GABA$_A$ agonism). Thus lipid solubility is likely to be relevant, but it does not in itself explain anaesthesia.

Membrane lipids

There are several potential lipophilic sites in cell membranes, including the lipid bilayer itself and the annular lipids surrounding ionic channels.

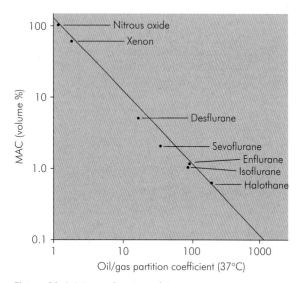

Figure 28.6 Meyer–Overton plot

Lipophilic anaesthetic agents can penetrate the bilayer and alter the molecular arrangement of the phospholipids in a manner described as 'fluidising' the membrane. The expansion of the membrane was thought to disrupt the function of membrane-spanning ionic channels. This theory explained why general anaesthetic agents could affect a number of ionic currents, as there was a generalised, non-specific change in membrane structure. However, many highly lipid-soluble molecules that can induce changes in lipid bilayers are not anaesthetic. Several halogenated hydrocarbons, including some with multiple fluorine substitutions, fail to elicit anaesthesia, and some actually induce seizures.

Rapid advances in receptor protein identification within the CNS, together with the observation that anaesthetic agents can alter enzyme function, led to theories based on interactions with specific proteins. It is now accepted that the relationship between potency and lipid solubility reflects the lipophilic nature of specific protein-based binding sites.

Protein site(s) of action
The evidence for a protein site of action

- General anaesthetic agents, at concentrations close to those producing anaesthesia, inhibit the firefly enzyme luciferase. The order of effective inhibition is the same as the order of potency for those anaesthetic agents.
- Saturable binding of halothane to rat brain synaptosomes suggested a limited number of binding sites. This would not be the case for a non-specific interaction.
- The enantiomers of certain general anaesthetic agents show stereoselective differences in the extent to which they alter ionic currents.

Anaesthetics may prevent afferent signals reaching the brain either by increasing inhibitory or by reducing excitatory pathways, or possibly by a combination of these two actions. Experimental work has therefore looked at both excitatory and inhibitory ionic channel function, including voltage-gated and ligand-gated channels, in the presence of anaesthetic agents.

We know that anaesthetic agents alter the conductance of voltage-gated sodium and calcium channels, although the concentrations at which such effects can be elicited are generally a little higher than found in vivo. The log-dose–response curve for anaesthesia shows a much steeper, left-shifted curve than that for depression of voltage-gated sodium channels. This suggests not only that anaesthesia occurs at a lower drug concentration, but probably that a different mechanism is responsible.

Several ligand-gated ionic channels are more sensitive to the action of general anaesthetics than are voltage-gated channels. The interactions at inhibitory ($GABA_A$ and glycine) and excitatory (neuronal nicotinic and NMDA) channels have all been studied. Figure 28.7 summarises the relative activity of a number of agents at these receptors.

$GABA_A$ receptor

The $GABA_A$ receptor has modulatory sites on the β subunit for benzodiazepines, barbiturates, propofol and volatile agents. In vitro investigation of the stereospecificity of the action of barbiturates and isoflurane support the notion of a specific binding site for each agent.

- Etomidate is clinically presented as an enantiopure preparation of the R(+) isomer; the S(−) form is inactive clinically. At the $GABA_A$ receptor there is a 30-fold difference in activity.

Figure 28.7 Effect of intravenous anaesthetic agents at ligand-gated ion channels

	Inhibitory transmitters		Excitatory transmitters	
	$GABA_A$	**Glycine**	**NMDA**	**Neuronal nicotinic cholinergic**
R-Etomidate	↑↑↑	–	–	–
S-Etomidate	–	–	–	–
Propofol	↑↑↑	↑	–	↓↓
Ketamine	–	–	↓↓↓	–

- Stereoisomers of the barbiturates pentobarbital and thiopental show a twofold difference in enhancing GABA activity at the $GABA_A$ receptor. There are no human studies with barbiturate stereoisomers, but animal studies suggest a twofold difference in potency, with S-barbiturates more potent than R-barbiturates.
- Stereoisomers of isoflurane have a 1.5-fold difference in efficacy at the $GABA_A$ receptor, although there is no clinical evidence for any difference in potency.

Anaesthetics increase channel opening time, so allowing for increased chloride entry resulting in hyperpolarisation. The effect is seen for etomidate, propofol, barbiturates and alphaxalone, as well as volatiles. Other pentameric receptors are influenced by some of these agents, but etomidate seems selective for the $GABA_A$ receptor. In contrast, propofol will also increase glycine channel opening time and is inhibitory at neuronal nicotinic and $5-HT_3$ receptors. Mutation studies suggest that each agent occupies a separate site, although all appear to be associated with the β subunit and are distinct from the benzodiazepine receptor site. There are at least 30 types of $GABA_A$ receptor, each with different stoichiometry of subunit composition. Different forms are likely to have varying sensitivities to anaesthetic agents. In vitro it has been shown that the $β_2$ and $β_3$ subunits are more sensitive to the effects of etomidate than is the $β_1$ subunit. A single amino acid substitution on the $β_2$ subunit can reduce the effect of etomidate on chloride conductance. However, animal experiments with genetically modified mice showed only a faster recovery from anaesthesia; EEG changes and loss of the righting reflex were the same as in wild-type mice. A mutation of $β_3$ subunits has been shown to prevent etomidate-induced suppression of hind-limb withdrawal and righting reflex. Animal models thus provide evidence for the importance of $GABA_A$ receptors in producing the state we call anaesthesia.

Glycine receptor

The major inhibitory transmitter in the spinal cord and brainstem is glycine. The glycine receptor is associated with a chloride channel similar to the $GABA_A$ receptor. Electrophysiological evidence suggests that although the spinal cord is not a major anatomical site for signal attenuation by intravenous anaesthetics, the volatile anaesthetics all markedly potentiate the action of glycine. The spinal cord is an important site for volatile agents, and activity correlates more with immobility than with awareness.

NMDA receptor

Neuronal signalling may also be reduced by inhibition of excitatory pathways. The excitatory amino acid glutamate has received a lot of attention, but interest has focused on the NMDA receptor as it is involved in long-term signal potentiation associated with learning and memory.

The NMDA receptor is activated by glutamate, modulated by magnesium, and is inhibited in a non-competitive manner by ketamine, nitrous oxide and xenon. It is therefore likely that this glutamate-mediated mechanism represents an additional pathway for the onset of the anaesthetic state. Some other anaesthetic agents, such as barbiturates, can reduce the effectiveness of glutamate but at a lower potency than for inhibition of $GABA_A$ receptor function. Any theory of anaesthesia should include both NMDA- and $GABA_A$-mediated pathways.

Adverse effects

Adverse effects of drugs may be either predictable or idiosyncratic, minor or life-threatening. Genetic factors may influence susceptibility. Predictable adverse effects are usually dose-dependent, and can potentially occur in anyone exposed to the drug in question. The higher the dose of drug, the more likely there will be associated adverse consequences. However, pharmacogenetic and environmental factors contribute to a wide inter-individual variability in the occurrence of such unwanted effects.

Physicochemical effects

Many drugs have a complex heterocyclic structure; some, such as sulphonamides, can be photoactivated to produce skin discoloration and dermatitis. This photosensitivity-induced dermatitis is seen in an extreme form in the porphyrias.

The chemical activity of certain drugs can alter the valency of metal ions that play an essential part in enzyme activity. Nitrous oxide changes cobalt from the monovalent to the inactive bivalent form in cyanocobalamin (vitamin B_{12}), which is a co-activator for methionine synthase. Prolonged exposure to nitrous oxide results in megaloblastic anaemia.

Pharmacodynamic effects

Pharmacodynamic effects usually arise from drug action at sites other than those responsible for the required effect. This may involve activity at the same receptor or enzyme but at a different anatomical location, or activity at a different receptor subtype, or it may happen because the drug can interact with more than one target. Such effects are dose-dependent and predictable, but there is a wide range of inter-individual variation depending on patient factors such as age, pathophysiology and genetic disposition.

The respiratory depressant effect of morphine typifies the first of these mechanisms: analgesia and respiratory depression are both associated with the μ opioid receptor, but at different central locations. A second example is of convulsions arising from toxic levels of local anaesthetic agents, such as lidocaine or bupivacaine, due to central inhibition of neuronal voltage-gated sodium channels: a dose-dependent phenomenon occurring at central rather than peripheral nerve axons.

The gastrointestinal effects of aspirin are secondary to its inhibition of the constitutive form of cyclo-oxygenase, COX-1, whereas its anti-inflammatory effect is due to acetylation of the inducible form, COX-2, so this characterises the second type of pharmacodynamic adverse effect. Another example is asthma triggered by the antihypertensive agent propranolol, which is due to actions at β_2-adrenoceptors, whereas the blood-pressure-lowering effect is a β_1-mediated action.

The third mechanism is demonstrated by the dry mouth and tachycardia associated with use of intravenous cyclizine, an H_1 antihistamine used as an antiemetic, which are a consequence of antimuscarinic effects at acetylcholine receptors.

Drugs used by infusion in the intensive care unit (ICU) often induce unwanted effects as duration of infusion increases. One is tachyphylaxis (the reduction in responsiveness of physiological systems to drugs due to continuous exposure), which requires escalating dose and eventually lost responsiveness. This is particularly evident with agonists and is related to receptor down-regulation. Conversely, receptor up-regulation can result in increased responsiveness that can produce adverse effects, such as exposure to suxamethonium several days after denervation injury. Receptor regulation is discussed further below. Other unwanted effects in the ICU are seen with non-depolarising muscle relaxants, which if given continuously can induce myelopathy, and with sodium nitroprusside, where excessive infusion rates can produce cyanide toxicity due to uncoupling of oxidative phosphorylation leading to tissue hypoxia.

Regulation of receptor activity and unwanted effects

Molecular mechanisms of receptor regulation for both GPCRs and ionotropic receptors underlie unwanted tachyphylaxis and tolerance to drugs. Interaction of a GPCR with an agonist increases the likelihood of receptor down-regulation and internalisation. The extent to which internalisation occurs depends upon the system in question. Agonist binding may activate GPCR-kinases (GRKs), which phosphorylate both the C-terminal and the domain associated with G-protein binding. Phosphorylation of the C-terminal then increases the affinity of the GPCR for β-arrestin, a protein that triggers receptor internalisation. This down-regulation of receptor activity is seen with β_1-adrenoceptor agonists such as dobutamine. Up- and down-regulation is also seen in ionotropic receptor populations. Of particular importance are the changes seen at the motor endplate following denervation injury, such as that seen following spinal injury. Under circumstances when acetylcholine availability is reduced, the homeostatic response is to increase the number of membrane receptors. Large numbers of receptors are inserted at extrajunctional sites; most importantly they are of the fetal ($\alpha\gamma\alpha\beta\delta$) rather than the adult type ($\alpha\epsilon\alpha\beta\delta$). Fetal-type receptors have a longer channel opening time, allowing a greater efflux of potassium, which may be sufficient to trigger arrhythmias. Similar effects are seen in burn injury and acute degenerative disorders. It takes time for a large number of new receptors to be made; suxamethonium can be used safely shortly after injury but is best avoided after 48–72 hours.

Pharmacokinetic effects

Adverse pharmacokinetic drug effects arise from alterations in distribution, metabolism or elimination of endogenous bioagents, or from biotransformation of the drug itself.

The bradycardia associated with neostigmine administration is due to increased acetylcholine concentrations at autonomic sites, particularly cardiac M_2-muscarinic receptors. In anaesthetic practice we anticipate this and co-administer an antimuscarinic agent, such as atropine or glycopyrrolate.

Drug metabolites can produce unwanted actions. Paracetamol is mostly converted to inactive compounds by conjugation with sulphate and glucuronide, but a small portion is metabolised via the cytochrome P450 (CYP) enzyme system. This is responsible for oxidation of paracetamol to a highly reactive intermediary metabolite, N-acetyl-p-benzo-quinone imine (NAPQI). Under normal conditions, NAPQI is detoxified by conjugation with glutathione. In overdose the conjugation pathways become saturated, and NAPQI production increases. When hepatocellular supplies of glutathione are reduced by more than 70%, NAPQI is free to react with elements of cellular membranes, resulting in acute hepatic necrosis and death.

Idiopathic adverse effects
Idiopathic adverse effects are generally unrelated to dose, and are usually unpredictable. Some involve well-understood hypersensitivity reactions that range from mild skin rashes to anaphylactic shock. Both pharmaco-genetic and environmental factors may contribute to an individual's response. Other idiosyncratic effects may result from inherited abnormalities.

Hypersensitivity reactions
These range from mild rashes through angioneurotic oedema to full-blown anaphylaxis. The mechanisms involve immune elements activated either with (anaphylactic) or without (anaphylactoid) previous exposure, and they are described in Chapter 2. **In anaesthetic practice, muscle relaxants account for about 80% of such hypersensitivity reactions**; the main culprits are suxamethonium and rocuronium. An immune-mediated mechanism is thought to underlie halothane hepatitis, where the oxidative metabolism of halothane produces a reactive intermediate, trifluoroacetylchloride, which leads to production of trifluoracetylated cellular proteins that act as haptens for immune-mediated fulminant hepatic necrosis on a second exposure. Fatality is high (50%) although the incidence is relatively low, about 1 in 10,000 exposures.

Pharmacogenetic influences
Pharmacogenetic abnormalities can account for several serious adverse effects with anaesthetic agents. **Malignant hyperthermia can be triggered by suxamethonium and the halogenated volatile agents.** The underlying defect in about 50% of families appears to be associated with an abnormal ryanodine receptor, which is intimately involved in the control of calcium release from sarcoplasmic reticulum in skeletal muscle. Inheritance is autosomal dominant and may also be associated with certain congenital myopathies.

Suxamethonium apnoea is an autosomal co-dominant response to abnormal plasma cholinesterase (pseudocholinesterase, butyrylcholinesterase) (see *Postoperative complications* in Chapter 4). Homozygotes show the most profound prolongation of neuromuscular blockade after suxamethonium use, but supportive ventilation is all that is required. In affected families, avoiding suxamethonium and mivacurium will prevent any problem.

Pharmacogenetics of other drug-metabolising enzymes, including the cytochrome P450 (CYP) system, can profoundly affect extent and duration of response. Although strictly not an adverse action, presence of an abnormal CYP2D6 isozyme can prevent conversion of codeine to morphine, with the unwanted consequence of inadequate analgesia. Slow acetylators will have prolonged effects of drugs such as hydralazine and isoniazid.

Mechanisms of drug interactions
We can describe the mechanism of interaction between drugs as physicochemical, pharmacokinetic or pharmacodynamic. **Some drug interactions can be exploited for therapeutic benefit.**

Clinically significant drug interactions commonly involve drugs with a low therapeutic index: anticoagulants, antiarrhythmics, anticonvulsants and hypoglycaemic agents. Furthermore, polypharmacy increases the risk of a significant drug interaction: patients on more than six drugs have an 80% chance of a drug interaction. Since the elderly are more likely to be on multiple therapies, and are often more sensitive to drug effects, they are more likely to experience such adverse interactions.

Physicochemical
The chemical interaction of two drugs may produce an insoluble or non-absorbable product. Of importance is the interaction between an acidic drug such as thiopental and a base such as sodium bicarbonate – when they are given intravenously through the same line an insoluble salt precipitates out. A similar problem occurs with thiopental (acidic) and suxamethonium (basic) during rapid sequence induction if a fluid flush is omitted between administration of the two drugs. For orally administered drugs, two drugs may interact in the stomach, reducing absorption and causing sub-therapeutic plasma levels of one or both. Antacids are notorious at reducing the absorption of antibiotics from the GI tract, particularly ciprofloxacin, rifampicin and tetracyclines. Ketoconazole is administered orally as a poorly soluble base that has to be changed to the more soluble hydrochloride salt by gastric acid. H_2-antagonists (such as ranitidine) and proton pump inhibitors (such as omeprazole) raise gastric pH, thus reducing the absorption of ketoconazole.

Pharmacokinetic
Drugs that alter the absorption, distribution, metabolism and excretion of other drugs are said to interact pharmacokinetically. Absorption is often affected through

physicochemical interactions, and delayed absorption may occur with drugs that produce stasis of the GI tract, such as opioids, but in general delayed absorption does not prevent drug entering the plasma, though it may reduce peak concentrations.

Distribution of drugs can be influenced by competition for plasma protein binding sites. This leads to an increased plasma level of free drug that could, theoretically, reach toxic levels. **Although many drugs are plasma-protein-bound, changes in the extent of protein binding due to drug displacement are rarely significant.** An increase in the free fraction may occur transiently, but increased elimination soon counteracts this effect. Significant interactions involving competition for binding sites occur only for drugs that are very highly protein-bound (in excess of 95%), and when the displaced drug is eliminated only in a dose-independent manner, i.e. zero-order kinetics (see *Elimination kinetics* in Chapter 27). Amiodarone and warfarin are highly protein-bound to albumin (99%); the increase in INR when they are used together was thought to be due to displacement of warfarin, but amiodarone also inhibits S-warfarin metabolism, which is

the more likely explanation. Small changes in free drug may also be of importance where the two drugs act on the same effector system but through different mechanisms. NSAIDs displace warfarin, but one affects blood clotting by reducing platelet adhesion while the other interferes with the coagulation cascade, and the combination results in an increased risk of bleeding.

The majority of clinically significant pharmacokinetic drug interactions involve induction or inhibition of metabolism. Many drugs are metabolised by the cytochrome P450 system of enzymes. These enzymes are subject to induction or inhibition by a wide range of agents, including tobacco, drugs and fruit juices (especially cranberry and grapefruit). Enzyme induction by one drug can increase the clearance of another, so reducing peak concentration and duration of activity. **The anticonvulsants phenytoin, phenobarbital and carbamazepine are cytochrome inducers that shorten the duration of aminosteroidal non-depolarising neuromuscular blockade**; bisbenzylisoquiloniums are not affected as their metabolism is different. Co-administration of drugs with cytochrome inhibitors such as ranitidine, fluconazole and

Figure 28.8 Drug interactions for the cytochrome P450 system. CYP2D6 is not inducible, unlike other isoforms. These interactions are considered clinically important according to the *British National Formulary*.

Drug combination	Drug affected	Result	Mechanism
Cimetidine + theophylline	Theophylline	CNS agitation, arrhythmias, nausea	Inhibition of CYP1A2
Tricyclic antidepressants (TCAs) + paroxetene	TCAs	Serotonin toxicity; agitation, hyperreflexia, arrhythmias	Inhibition of CYP2D6
Amiodarone + S-warfarin	S-warfarin	Increased INR; risk of bleeding	Inhibition of CYP2C9
Fluoxetine + phenytoin	Phenytoin	Phenytoin toxicity: ataxia, nystagmus, slurred speech, nausea & vomiting	Inhibition of CYP2C19
Clarithromycin + terfenidine	Terfenidine	Ventricular arrhythmias	Inhibition of CYP3A4
Carbamazepine + vecuronium	Vecuronium	Reduced duration neuromuscular blockade	Induction of CYP3A4
Rifampicin + S-warfarin	S-warfarin	Reduction in INR; risk of thrombotic events	Induction of CYP2C9
Chlorpropamide + rifampicin	Chlorpropamide	Poor diabetic control; reduced levels	Induction of CYP2C9

amiodarone may lead to toxic levels; the combination of fluconazole and terfenidine in particular leads to a high risk of ventricular arrhythmias. Figure 28.8 lists a number of important CYP interactions.

Plasma cholinesterase is responsible for suxamethonium metabolism, and there are several drugs that either inhibit or compete for this enzyme. Neostigmine inhibits plasma cholinesterase as well as acetylcholinesterase; suxamethonium-induced neuromuscular blockade is prolonged by neostigmine.

The interaction between probenecid and penicillin is used therapeutically. Both drugs compete for a transport protein for weak acids in the renal tubule so probenecid markedly reduces the rate of penicillin excretion.

Pharmacodynamic

Two drugs that act on a physiological system may either have the same effects (e.g. vecuronium and suxamethonium both produce neuromuscular blockade) or have opposing effects (e.g. phenylephrine vasoconstricts and nifedipine vasodilates). **Drugs that have similar physiological effects will, in combination, produce an overall response that is additive, synergistic or antagonistic. Additivity suggests a shared mechanism of action; synergism or antagonism is evidence for differing mechanisms of action.** Additivity is seen, for example, when vecuronium and rocuronium or isoflurane and sevoflurane are used together. Both tricyclic antidepressants (TCAs) and selective serotonin reuptake inhibitors (SSRIs) inhibit biogenic amine reuptake at central synapses. The combination of TCA and SSRI is additive, and can produce symptoms of serotonin toxicity such as agitation, hyperreflexia and hyperpyrexia. If a rise in synaptic serotonin concentration is produced by two different mechanisms, synergism can produce the life-threatening serotonin syndrome. The interaction between pethidine and monoamine oxidase inhibitors is now thought to be due to serotonin syndrome, since pethidine is a dose-dependent serotonin reuptake inhibitor.

Synergism is also seen when nifedipine and ACE inhibitors are used together for their antihypertensive effect; doses may need to be adjusted to prevent unwanted hypotension. Similarly, the hypotensive effect of volatile agents is significantly greater in the presence of ACE inhibitors. Synergism in antiplatelet activity is seen with aspirin and clopidogrel. Diuretics that increase potassium loss through different mechanisms, such as loop (furosamide) and thiazide (bendroflumethiazide) diuretics, when used together can rapidly precipitate severe hypokalaemia with the risk of arrhythmias in susceptible patients. In contrast, a combination of diuretics that have opposing effects on potassium loss can be used together safely, without the need for potassium supplements, such as bendroflumethiazide and amiloride, which is a clinically useful interaction.

Antagonism is seen with the combination of ACE inhibitors and angiotensin II receptor (AT_1) antagonists: receptor inhibition minimises the effectiveness of lowering angiotensin II concentration, and their combined antihypertensive effect is not as great as would be predicted from their individual activity.

CHAPTER 29

Anaesthetic gases and vapours

Tim Smith

Administration

Volatile anaesthetic agents are liquids with a low boiling point (BP) and high saturated vapour pressure (SVP) so that they evaporate easily. Volatile agents have higher saturated vapour pressures and lower boiling points than water. Most have a characteristic smell.

Volatile agents are administered via inhalation through the lungs and so enter the circulation via the pulmonary alveolar capillaries. Intravenously administered agents are injected into a small part of the venous system and are then diluted by mixing with other sources of the venous blood. The injected agent then passes through the right heart before reaching the pulmonary circulation. Inhaled agents bypass this venous phase and are fairly evenly spread through the ventilated alveoli. However, there is some delay in achieving sufficiently high alveolar concentrations for induction of anaesthesia.

Uptake of inhaled anaesthetic agents

Inhaled anaesthetics are administered so as to achieve levels in central neural tissue sufficient to produce anaesthesia without detrimental effects on other organs. At equilibrium, the partial pressures of the agents will be identical throughout the body, but the concentrations in different tissues will be determined by the partition coefficients (see Chapter 25, *Solubility and partition coefficients*). When a difference in partial

pressure exists between two compartments, there will be a movement down the pressure gradient until equilibrium is achieved.

Achievement of satisfactory brain levels of anaesthetic agent occurs in three stages:

- Delivery phase
- Pulmonary phase
- Circulatory phase

Delivery phase

The delivery phase involves the introduction of the anaesthetic agents into the gas to be inspired. The anaesthetic machine produces a fresh gas mixture which is passed into the anaesthetic breathing system. When a circle breathing system is used a vaporiser may be placed within this circuit. While the details of vaporiser and breathing systems are covered elsewhere (Chapter 46, *Breathing systems*), within this chapter it is important to appreciate that the settings dialled up on the anaesthetic machine do not guarantee the same levels in the inspired gas, because anaesthetic agent is lost in several ways:

- Dilution with existing gas in the breathing system
- Uptake by CO_2 absorbers
- Uptake by rubber and plastic components of the circuit

Inspired and expired concentrations of anaesthetic agents should ideally be monitored at the closest point to the patient.

Fundamentals of Anaesthesia, 4th edition, ed. Ted Lin, Tim Smith and Colin Pinnock. Published by Cambridge University Press. © Cambridge University Press 2017.

Pulmonary phase

The following factors influence the uptake of anaesthetic agents from inhaled gas to the blood:

- Inhaled concentration
- Alveolar ventilation
- Diffusion
- Blood/gas partition coefficient
- Partial pressure of agent in the pulmonary artery
- Pulmonary blood flow
- Ventilation/perfusion distribution
- Concentration effect
- Second gas effect

Inhaled concentration

The inhaled concentration directly affects the inhaled partial pressure or tension. The higher the tension the higher the levels achieved in the blood. Levels above the desired maintenance tension for the brain (over-pressure) are used to reach these maintenance levels more rapidly.

Alveolar ventilation

Ventilation of the lungs carries the volatile agent into the alveoli, and the pre-existing gas mixture is gradually replaced. At the same time, vapour is diffusing into the blood, so depleting its concentration in the alveoli. Increasing alveolar minute volume speeds up the approximation of alveolar to inspired levels. Increases in physiological dead space constitute wasted ventilation in terms of supplying vapour to the blood. In general, volatile anaesthetic agents depress respiration, so as anaesthetic depth increases alveolar ventilation falls. This is one reason for a reduction in the rate of uptake of volatile agents as anaesthesia progresses.

Diffusion

The small molecules of volatile agents pass easily through the pulmonary membrane, and in health diffusion is not a limiting factor. However, disease processes may reduce the surface area and increase the thickness of the alveolar membrane. For example, emphysema reduces the available area and pulmonary fibrosis increases the thickness of the membrane, so transfer of inhaled agents into the capillary blood may be delayed.

Blood/gas partition coefficient

The blood/gas partition coefficient (see Figure 25.14) determines the amount of agent that must be transferred to the blood to achieve equilibrium for a given tension,

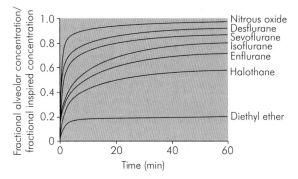

Figure 29.1 Wash-in curves for volatile anaesthetic agents

assuming that the blood volume is known and that there is no transfer to other tissues. This is an important point, because it is this tension that drives the agent into the brain and other tissues. A low blood/gas partition coefficient indicates low solubility in blood, so equilibrium will be reached with relatively small transfers of gas, and therefore equilibrium will be rapid. Conversely, a high coefficient indicates high solubility, and equilibrium will be slow. Nitrous oxide and desflurane, which have low blood/gas solubility coefficients, illustrate this point, and blood levels rapidly approximate to inspired levels. Agents such as halothane are much more soluble in blood and take considerably longer. Isoflurane is quicker. In practice, equilibration is affected by distribution to other tissues and the process is slower than the simple model above, and other factors influence the relationship between individual agents. Figure 29.1 shows wash-in characteristics for selected volatile agents obtained by plotting the fractional alveolar to inspired concentration as a ratio against time.

Partial pressure of volatile agent in the pulmonary artery

The rate of uptake of volatile agent from each alveolus is dependent on the tension difference between the alveolus and the capillary blood. As the concentration and tension in the blood rises the rate of uptake is reduced and so the rate of tension rise decreases.

Pulmonary blood flow

As blood passes through the pulmonary capillaries the tension of volatile agent in the capillary will increase and so reduce the rate of transfer in the latter part of the capillary. Therefore, increasing the blood flow will increase uptake.

Ventilation/perfusion distribution

Ventilation/perfusion mismatch will reduce perfusion of well-ventilated areas of lung and increase perfusion of alveoli poorly supplied with volatile agent.

Concentration effect

The uptake of volatile agent from the alveolus, during a small part of the respiratory cycle, reduces the amount left in the alveolus for subsequent parts of the cycle. Rate of uptake is proportional to the tension, which is the direct result of the concentration. Assuming that a smaller proportion of the other constituents of alveolar gas (e.g. nitrogen and oxygen) is absorbed, then the concentration of the anaesthetic agent will fall. The degree of fall will be influenced by its concentration, agents in low concentrations suffering a greater proportional loss than those in high concentrations. This means that the uptake of agents inhaled in high concentrations will be better maintained over the respiratory cycle than those administered at lower concentrations.

Second gas effect

The second gas effect embodies the same principles as the concentration effect. However, in this case the administration of a rapidly absorbed gas given in high concentration (typically nitrous oxide), together with a volatile agent of lower solubility, produces an increasing alveolar concentration of the second agent, thus promoting its absorption.

Circulatory phase

The following factors influence the transport of the dissolved volatile agent to the brain:

- Cardiac output
- Cerebral blood flow
- Distribution to other tissues

The distribution of blood to various tissues and compartments is described elsewhere (see Chapter 27, *Distribution*). While these principles apply to drugs that are intravenously administered, volatile agents behave in a similar fashion, with the driving force of partial pressure (tension) tending toward equilibrium. The uptake of agent by the tissues is proportional to tissue perfusion, solubility and arteriovenous tension difference. The formula is:

Uptake = tissue blood flow × tissue/blood solubility
× arteriovenous tension difference

The formula produces time constants for the exponential function of tissue anaesthetic tension against time. High cardiac output and low tissue solubility produce a low time constant.

Cardiac output

Of cardiac output, 70–80% is distributed to the vessel-rich organs (brain, heart, liver, kidney) that constitute about 9% of body mass. Of the total, 14% goes to the brain (2.2% of body mass). A large proportion of the absorbed anaesthetic is thus directed to the brain. By virtue of their high lipid solubility, the brain has a relatively high affinity for anaesthetic agents.

Cerebral blood flow (CBF)

Factors affecting the proportion of cardiac output going to the brain will influence cerebral uptake of volatile agents. In shock, CBF is relatively well preserved, and therefore more agent will go to the brain and equilibrium will be reached more rapidly. Increasing depth of anaesthesia during spontaneous ventilation increases CO_2 and secondarily CBF. Hyperventilation during induction of anaesthesia will reduce CO_2 and CBF and delay equilibrium.

Distribution to other tissues

Distribution of volatile agent to other tissues (dependent on the factors above) slows the initial rate of uptake by the brain. Later, these depots of anaesthetic agent act to maintain the blood and so brain levels, and they act as a damper to any changes in alveolar and blood levels. This is something of an advantage, but slows recovery as much as it does induction.

Minimum alveolar concentration (MAC)

Minimum alveolar concentration may be defined as the concentration of anaesthetic agent which at equilibrium will prevent a reflex response to skin incision in 50% of subjects. MAC acts as a guide to the concentration required for anaesthesia. Altitude reduces atmospheric pressure, and therefore reduces the concentration of anaesthetic agent for a given percentage, so minimum alveolar pressure might be a more useful concept. It is a form of ED_{50} (effective dose). Other measures of potency include AD_{95} (anaesthetic dose), which is the dose required to prevent response to surgical stimulus in 95% of subjects. Various factors affect MAC for a particular agent, e.g. species, age and concomitant drugs. In clinical practice, it is important to remember that the displayed MAC value on an anaesthetic monitor is calculated from a standard MAC for the identified volatile(s), and does not measure neuronal tissue levels.

The mechanism of action of anaesthetic agents is described in Chapter 28.

The ideal volatile agent

Although the ideal volatile agent does not exist, nonetheless it remains a useful concept. The characteristics of an ideal agent are given in Figure 29.2. A comparison of the physical properties of the major agents in clinical practice is given in Figure 29.3.

Specific pharmacology

The following agents will be considered in more detail: desflurane (D), halothane (H), isoflurane (I) and sevoflurane (S). Chemical structures of these four, as well as enflurane and nitrous oxide, are shown in Figure 29.4. In the comparative lists for each agent, molecular weight (MW) is given in daltons, boiling point (BP) in degrees Celsius, MAC in volumes %, and the coefficients are dimensionless.

General features
Physical

Physically, the volatile anaesthetic agents are relatively small, simple molecules, generally denser than water.

Figure 29.2 Characteristics of an ideal volatile agent

Physical
Liquid at room temperature
Low latent heat of vaporisation
Low specific heat capacity
SVP sufficiently high to allow for easy vaporisation
Stable in light
Stable at room temperature
Non-flammable
Inexpensive
Environmentally safe (locally and globally)

Pharmacological
Pleasant smell
Low blood/gas solubility
Potent enough to provide surgical anaesthesia without supplement (low MAC)
High oil/water solubility
Analgesic effect
Non-epileptogenic
No cardiac irritability
No cardiovascular depression
No respiratory depression
Non-irritant to airways
Muscle relaxation
No increase in intracranial pressure (ICP)
Unaffected by renal failure
Unaffected by hepatic failure
Minimal metabolism

Figure 29.3 Physical properties of volatile agents and anaesthetic gases

	MW (daltons)	BP at 1 atm (°C)	SVP at 20 °C (kPa)	MAC (% v/v)	Ostwald solubility coefficients (dimensionless) [a]					
					O/W	Bl/G	W/G	Br/G	O/G	Br/Bl
Desflurane	168	22.8	88.5	6.35	N/A	0.42	N/A	0.54	19	1.3
Enflurane	184.5	56.5	22.9	1.68	120	1.9	0.78	2.6	98	96
Halothane	197	50.2	32.5	0.75	220	2.3	0.8	4.8	224	1.9
Isoflurane	184.5	48.5	31.9	1.15	174	1.43	0.62	21	91	1.6
Sevoflurane	200	58.6	21.3	2.00	N/A	0.69	N/A	1.1	53	1.7
Nitrous oxide	44	− 88	5300	105	3.2	0.47	0.44	1.4	1.0	
Xenon	131.2	−108		71	19	0.12	0.075		1.8	0.17
Ethyl chloride[b]	64.5	13	132							

[a] O/W, oil/water; Bl/G, blood/gas; W/G, water/gas; Br/G, brain/gas; O/G, oil/gas; Br/Bl, brain/blood.
[b] Although no longer used as a volatile agent by inhalation, ethyl chloride remains in practice as a cutaneous analgesic when applied as a spray. It is included here for the sake of completeness.

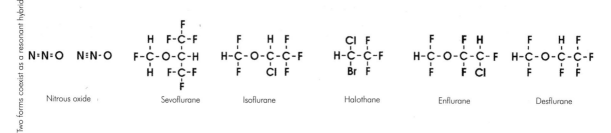

Two forms coexist as a resonant hybrid

Figure 29.4 Chemical structures of volatile agents

Figure 29.5 Ranking of clinical properties of volatile agents. D = desflurane, H = halothane, I = isoflurane, S = sevoflurane

	Worst	Worse	Better	Best
Induction	D	I	H	S
Cardiovascular stability	H	I	D	S
Respiratory irritation	D	I		H & S
Ease of titration	H	I	S	D
Emergence	H	I	S	D
Metabolism/toxicity	H	S	I	D

They rely on physical as well as pharmacological features to achieve their effect. For a particular carbon skeleton, changes in halogenation alter both physical and pharmacological properties. This is best demonstrated by the methyl ethyl ether skeleton common to desflurane and isoflurane.

Solubility is reduced with lowering of molecular weight. Fluoride ions are lighter than chloride and bromide ones, and thus desflurane, having fluoride ions in place of chloride, is comparatively less soluble than isoflurane. Potency increases with increasing molecular weight, and the lighter desflurane is less potent than isoflurane. This may be related to the strong correlation of oil/water solubility with pharmacological potency (see Chapter 28).

Increasing fluorination of a carbon skeleton increases saturated vapour pressure and stability but reduces boiling point, flammability and toxicity. Methyl ethyl ether is flammable, but desflurane, enflurane and isoflurane are not.

Clinical

The comparative clinical properties of the major volatile agents are summarised in Figures 29.5 and 29.6.

Central nervous system

Volatile agents cause a dose-dependent depression of cerebral activity on the EEG. Cerebral oxygen consumption reduces in line with this. Epileptiform spikes occur with enflurane. All the volatile agents increase CBF and thus ICP, and should be used with caution where raised ICP may be a problem. Apart from nitrous oxide, analgesia is not a feature of the volatile agents used in current practice.

Relative effects

Cerebral blood flow : $H > D, I, S$

ICP : $H > D > I, S$

Respiratory system

A dose-dependent depression of respiration occurs. This is manifest as reduced tidal volume with increased rate (except sevoflurane, which lowers rate), causing an overall reduction in alveolar minute volume. Arterial CO_2 levels rise. The responses to hypercarbia and hypoxia are reduced.

Halothane in particular, but also sevoflurane, causes bronchodilatation by reducing bronchial smooth muscle tone.

Desflurane and to a lesser extent isoflurane are irritant and stimulate bronchial and salivary secretion.

Figure 29.6 Grading of clinical properties of volatile agents. ○○○○ = least effect, ●●●● = maximum effect

	Halothane	Isoflurane	Desflurane	Sevoflurane
Pungency	●○○○	●●●○	●●○○	○○○○
Respiratory irritation	○○○○	●●○○	●●●○	○○○○
Respiratory depression	●●○○	●●●○	●●●●	●●○○
Cardiovascular depression	●●●○	●●○○	●○○○	●○○○
Coronary vasodilatation	●○○○	●●○○	●○○○	●●○○
Muscle relaxation	●●○○	●●●○	●●●○	●●●○
Intracranial pressure elevation	●●●●	●●○○	●●●○	●●○○

Relative effects

Respiratory depression : D > I > H, S

Cardiovascular system

Cardiovascular depression is usual, with varying effects on contractility, heart rate and vascular resistance. Contractility is reduced by all agents, by interference with calcium ion movement. In clinical practice, contractility is affected by other factors such as preload and sympathetic stimulation. Direct effects, and indirect effects such as hypercarbia from respiratory depression, also influence these factors. Desflurane in particular appears to maintain contractility initially, perhaps as a result of increased sympathetic stimulation. Baroreceptor reflexes are also depressed.

Heart rate is primarily affected by the balance between sympathetic and parasympathetic nervous systems. In general, heart rate increases in clinical usage. This is more marked with desflurane and isoflurane. However, halothane decreases heart rate, and sinus bradycardia, atrioventricular block and ventricular premature contractions are not uncommon, especially in the presence of hypercarbia and increased circulating catecholamine levels. Conduction velocity in the atrioventricular node, His–Purkinje system and ventricles is reduced.

Systemic vascular resistance (SVR) is reduced with isoflurane and sevoflurane. Desflurane and halothane have little effect.

Blood-pressure changes are the result of the above effects. In general, blood pressure is reduced by a combination of reduced contractility, preload and afterload.

Coronary vasodilatation alters coronary blood flow and may cause coronary 'steal'. This is more of a problem with isoflurane and sevoflurane than with the other agents.

Sensitisation of the myocardium to catecholamines, both endogenous and exogenous, may result in arrhythmias.

Relative effects

Conduction velocity slowing : H > I, S

Catecholamine sensitisation : H > D, I, S

Muscle relaxation

There is a dose-dependent depression of neuromuscular function, with potentiation of both depolarising and non-depolarising neuromuscular blocking agents. While this is probably mediated by the neuromuscular junction, there may also be a direct reduction in contractility.

Metabolic rate

A decrease in metabolic rate causes a secondary reduction in oxygen consumption and carbon dioxide production. Inhalation of 2 MAC of a volatile agent reduces basal metabolic rate of oxygen consumption ($BMRO_2$) by 30%.

Toxicity

Increasing fluorination of a carbon skeleton reduces both metabolism and toxicity. While 2.4% of enflurane is metabolised, the corresponding amount for desflurane is 0.02%. Higher levels of metabolism increase the amount of potentially toxic metabolites and so increase toxicity. Fluoride production is greater in the morbidly obese than in non-obese patients when using halothane or enflurane. There is no difference when using sevoflurane.

Soda lime

Formation of carbon monoxide can occur when dry (used) soda lime comes into contact with desflurane or isoflurane. Note that this is not a problem with halothane or sevoflurane. To avoid the problem, fresh soda lime should be used and prolonged periods of flushing the soda lime canister with dry oxygen and high gas flows should be avoided. At low flows, humidity will be high and the absorbent will function correctly.

Immune system

Volatile anaesthetic agents reduce the killing function of polymorphonuclear cells by interfering with calcium flux and superoxide generation.

Desflurane

Chemical name – 1,2,2,2-tetrafluoroethyl difluoromethyl ether (halogenated ether)

Properties

MW	BP	SVP	MAC	O/W	Bl/G	O/G	Br/Bl
168	22.8	88.5	6.35	N/A	0.42	19	1.3

Presentation – pure agent without preservative or stabilisers supplied in brown bottle with self-closing valve, which fits special vaporiser

Storage – at room temperature away from heat

Soda lime – compatible, but avoid exhausted, dry granules

CNS – anaesthesia, no analgesia; not epileptogenic

CVS – dose-dependent depression similar to isoflurane

RS – dose-dependent depression; respiratory irritant; increased secretions

Others – muscle relaxants potentiated; stimulation of salivary secretions

Elimination – predominantly via lungs; 0.02% metabolised in liver

Contraindications – risk of triggering malignant hyperthermia

Desflurane has a boiling point close to ambient temperature with a high saturated vapour pressure. This necessitates the use of a special heated pressurised vaporiser. Superficially, this looks similar to the usual plenum vaporisers, but closer examination reveals a sophisticated microprocessor-controlled unit. The desflurane is heated and the vapour kept under pressure. Pure desflurane is then injected into the incoming fresh gas, which is also heated. The system is very accurate. The vaporiser can be filled without switching off. The unit is mains-operated, and is locked until the operating temperature is reached.

The low blood/gas solubility coefficient is close to nitrous oxide, but desflurane is more potent. This produces a rapid response to changes in inhaled concentration, and rapid recovery. However, to the respiratory tract, it is the most irritant volatile agent and it increases bronchial and salivary secretions. This reduces the rate at which the inspired concentration may be increased during induction and offsets the benefit of its rapid approximation of inhaled and alveolar concentrations. Concentrations of above 6% during induction have a relatively high incidence of coughing, breath-holding and laryngospasm (especially in children under 12 years of age), and it is not recommended for inhalational induction in children.

Desflurane depresses cardiac contractility, but this is less pronounced than with the other agents, perhaps as a result of sympathetic stimulation. During prolonged anaesthesia, this depression is less prominent. Initially SVR does not change, but above 2.2 MAC it falls. As a result, the blood pressure falls and heart rate increases to compensate. Coronary vasodilatation and increased blood flow occur. There is a theoretical risk of coronary 'steal'. Desflurane does not sensitise the heart to catecholamines. There is a dose-dependent depression of the respiratory centre, with reduced tidal volume and increased rate. The response to carbon dioxide is reduced (shifted to the right). Desflurane potentiates the effects of muscle relaxants, benzodiazepines and opioids. As only 0.02% is metabolised, toxicity is likely to be very low.

Halothane

Chemical name – 1-bromo-1-chloro-2,2,2-trifluoroethane (halogenated alkane)

Properties

MW	BP	SVP	MAC	O/W	Bl/G	O/G	Br/Bl
197	50.2	32.5	0.75	220	2.3	224	1.9

Colour code – red

Presentation – clear, colourless liquid in brown glass bottle with keyed filling system collar; 0.1% thymol to protect against decomposition by light

Storage – at room temperature away from heat

Soda lime – compatible

CNS – anaesthesia, no analgesia; not epileptogenic

CVS – dose-dependent depression of contractility and heart rate; sensitisation to catecholamines

RS – dose-dependent depression (but may increase rate), reduced tidal and minute volumes; bronchodilatation; non-irritant

Other – postoperative shivering is common; muscle relaxants potentiated

Elimination – 60–80% unchanged via lungs, 20% metabolised in liver (metabolites are excreted in urine for several weeks)

Contraindications – risk of triggering malignant hyperthermia; contraindicated if previous pyrexia or jaundice following prior administration. For halothane hepatitis see Chapter 28, *Adverse effects*.

The thymol preservative does not readily evaporate, and therefore builds up in the vaporiser, which requires drainage and cleaning at regular intervals. Halothane may corrode aluminium, tin, lead, magnesium, brass and solder alloys in the presence of water. Halothane is usually administered via a specifically calibrated plenum vaporiser but draw-over vaporisers may also be used (e.g. Goldman).

Halothane produces anaesthesia without specific analgesia, and has a low propensity for causing nausea and vomiting. CBF and ICP are increased, and it should be used with caution if ICP is raised.

Halothane reduces myocardial contractility, and decreases heart rate by vagal stimulation. Phase 4 depolarisation and cardiac conduction velocity are slowed. The combination of this and increased irritability may allow ventricular premature beats, bigeminy and other rhythm disturbances to occur. There is no increase in circulating catecholamines, but administered adrenaline increases the risk of cardiac arrhythmias, especially in the presence of hypoxia and hypercarbia. The administration of adrenaline of greater than 1/100,000 concentration, more than 100 μg in 10 minutes, and more than 300 μg per hour should be avoided.

SVR is not affected. Blood pressure is reduced and left ventricular end-diastolic pressure is increased, leading to decreased coronary perfusion. This is offset by a reduction in cardiac oxygen utilisation.

Tidal volume is reduced and respiratory rate increased. The ventilatory response curve to carbon dioxide shifts to the right. Minute volume may fall or stay the same. Halothane is non-irritant to the respiratory tract and causes bronchodilatation; anatomical dead space is therefore increased. It reduces salivary and bronchial secretions and is still the agent of choice for inhalational induction where airways obstruction is a significant problem, e.g. epiglottitis.

Halothane reduces gastrointestinal motility and reduces uterine tone. Skeletal muscle tone is reduced and neuromuscular blockade is potentiated, but there may be postoperative shivering.

Increased depth of anaesthesia reduces renal blood flow, glomerular filtration rate and urine output.

The secretion of vasopressin, thyroxine, growth hormone and corticosteroids is increased. Insulin secretion is not affected but insulin sensitivity is increased; glucose levels do not change, however.

Halothane reduces metabolic rate, oxygen consumption and carbon dioxide production. Twenty per cent of halothane is metabolised and it takes 3 weeks to clear completely from the body. The main metabolites are trifluoroacetic acid, chloride and bromide, which appear in the urine. Of patients receiving halothane 50% show a temporary rise in glutathione S-transferase.

Isoflurane

Chemical name – 1-chloro-2,2,2-trifluoroethyl difluoromethyl ether (halogenated ether)

Properties

MW	BP	SVP	MAC	O/W	Bl/G	O/G	Br/Bl
184.5	48.5	31.9	1.15	174	1.43	91	1.6

Colour code – purple

Presentation – colourless liquid in brown glass bottle, with keyed filling system collar, without additive or preservative

Storage – at room temperature away from heat

Soda lime – compatible, but avoid exhausted dry granules

CNS – anaesthesia, no analgesia; not epileptogenic

CVS – decreased blood pressure and systemic vascular resistance; heart rate rises

RS – decreased volume, increased rate, decreased minute volume; moderate respiratory irritant; increases bronchial secretions

Other – muscle relaxants potentiated; stimulation of salivary secretions

Elimination – primarily via lungs; 0.2% metabolised in liver

Contraindications – risk of triggering malignant hyperthermia

Isoflurane is a potent volatile anaesthetic agent, with an average speed of equilibration between inspired and tissue levels. The physical properties of boiling point and saturated vapour pressure are very similar to halothane, so the vaporiser design is also closely related.

Isoflurane causes anaesthesia without specific analgesia. It is not epileptogenic. It causes cerebral vasodilatation and there is a risk of 'steal', where vasodilatation of healthy vessels diverts blood flow away from critically perfused areas supplied by non-compliant vessels, which cannot dilate further. This is compounded by the reduction in blood pressure. Total CBF is increased and ICP may rise.

Isoflurane acts directly on blood vessels, reducing blood pressure by reducing SVR. There is a compensatory increase in heart rate, but cardiac output changes little. Isoflurane has little effect on contractility (except at multiples of MAC, when contractility is adversely affected). The baroreceptor reflex is depressed. Myocardial work and oxygen consumption are reduced.

Isoflurane is pungent and causes some respiratory irritation, necessitating slower increases in inspired concentration than with halothane or sevoflurane, and making inhalational induction more difficult. Isoflurane reduces tidal and minute volumes with increased respiratory rate. It reduces the responses to hypercarbia and hypoxia and carbon dioxide rises. Bronchial smooth muscle tone is reduced with increasing depth, but during the initial stages of anaesthesia the respiratory irritancy may precipitate coughing and bronchospasm.

Isoflurane facilitates neuromuscular blockade.

Only 0.2% is metabolised, and toxicity from metabolites is therefore very low.

Sevoflurane

Chemical name – fluoromethyl-2,2,2-trifluoro-1-(trifluoromethyl) ethyl ether (halogenated ether)

Properties

MW	BP	SVP	MAC	O/W	Bl/G	O/G	Br/Bl
200	58.6	21.3	2.0	N/A	0.69	53	1.7

Colour code – yellow

Presentation – no preservative; supplied in brown bottle with keyed filling system collar

Storage – at room temperature away from heat

Soda lime – compatible, but may produce Compound A (see below)

CNS – anaesthesia, no analgesia; not epileptogenic

CVS – decreased heart rate, systemic vascular resistance and blood pressure but stable cardiac output; no myocardial sensitisation to catecholamines

RS – dose-dependent depression of respiratory rate and tidal volume; bronchodilatation

Other – muscle relaxants potentiated; uterine relaxation in pregnancy similar to isoflurane

Elimination – predominantly via the lungs; 5% metabolised by cytochrome P450

Contraindications – risk of triggering malignant hyperthermia

Sevoflurane has similar physicochemical characteristics to isoflurane, but is a little less volatile. It is administered using a plenum vaporiser. It differs from the other agents in having lower blood/gas and lower oil/gas solubilities. This produces a more rapid response to changes in inhaled concentration, and speedier induction and recovery. The higher MAC (2.0), indicating lower potency, is predictable from the oil/gas coefficient.

Sevoflurane produces anaesthesia without analgesia or epileptogenic spikes in a similar way to desflurane and isoflurane. ICP is raised, but this effect is minimal at less than 1 MAC.

Sevoflurane reduces blood pressure primarily by reducing SVR, with little effect on cardiac output until higher doses are used. It lowers heart rate, in contrast with isoflurane and desflurane. There is less coronary vasodilatation than with isoflurane, and coronary blood flow does not change. The reduced heart rate reduces myocardial oxygen consumption so the relationship between supply and demand may be improved.

Sevoflurane reduces tidal volume and respiratory rate. Hypoxic drive is reduced, as is sensitivity to carbon dioxide tension. Sevoflurane reduces bronchial smooth muscle tone and so increases anatomical dead space. It has low respiratory irritancy.

Uterine muscle is relaxed to a similar degree to isoflurane. The potentiation of neuromuscular blockade is similar to other agents. Malignant hyperthermia has occurred with sevoflurane so it should be avoided in at-risk patients.

Most sevoflurane is eliminated via the lungs. Five per cent is metabolised by cytochrome P450, producing hexafluoroisopropanol (CF_3-CHOH-CF_3) and inorganic fluoride ions. A plasma fluoride ion concentration of 50 μmol L^{-1} is quoted as the threshold for renal toxicity. Sevoflurane metabolism can produce levels above this threshold. The potentially hepatotoxic hexafluoroisopropanol is rapidly conjugated before it can cause damage.

Compound A

Sevoflurane is absorbed and degraded by CO_2 absorbers. At temperatures above 65 °C five breakdown products are formed (compounds A–E). In the lower temperatures encountered clinically, sevoflurane only produces compound A (CH_2F-O-C(CF_3)=CF_2) and a lesser amount of compound B (CHF_2-O-CH(CF_2-O-CH_3)-CF_3). The concentrations are higher with baralyme than with soda lime because baralyme attains a higher temperature and the breakdown is temperature-dependent. The concentrations of compounds A and B are substantially lower than the toxicity threshold in animal studies. Zeolite-coated soda lime may absorb these compounds. Possible toxicity effects are renal, hepatic and brain.

'Wet' and 'dry' formulations

In 1996 and 1997 specific batches of sevoflurane were found to contain hydrofluoric acid, which reacts with glass and can be toxic. This was because Lewis acids in the presence of some metals such as iron promote the breakdown of sevoflurane. However, the small amounts produced were unlikely to cause serious toxicity. Water inhibits Lewis acids. Two formulations of sevoflurane, 'wet' and 'dry', are now available, the 'wet' having had additional water added at the final stage of production. The 'wet' sevoflurane (330 ppm water) is supplied in a plastic bottle and the 'dry' (130 ppm) in a lacquer-lined aluminium bottle. Clinically there is no difference between the two products, and no convincing evidence of increased risk has yet been found. Stored according to manufacturers' instructions, there should be minimal degradation of either formulation of sevoflurane. Compound A production occurs in the soda lime canister, where water content will be considerably higher.

Nitric oxide

See Chapter 35, *Organic nitrates, nitrites and related drugs*.

Nitrous oxide

Structure – resonant hybrid of two forms, N=N=O and N≡N–O (anaesthetic gas)

Properties

MW	BP	SVP	MAC	O/W	Bl/G	O/G	Br/Bl
44	–88	5300	105	3.2	0.47	1.4	1.0

Critical temperature – +36.5 °C
Critical pressure – 72.6 bar
Presentation – supplied in cylinders as the pure liquid (no water vapour) under pressure (44 bar at 15 °C); filling ratio 0.75

Colour code – cylinders French blue; rotameter knob blue; pin index 3,5
Storage – at room temperature away from extremes of heat; non-explosive; not flammable but can support combustion because it decomposes to oxygen and nitrogen above 450 °C
Soda lime – compatible
CNS – analgesia, sedation; not epileptogenic
CVS – increased vascular tone, rise in blood pressure
RS – decreased tidal volume, increased rate; non-irritant
Other – increased skeletal muscle activity; emetogenic
Elimination – predominantly via lungs
Contraindications – diffuses into air-filled spaces causing expansion; prolonged use interferes with vitamin B_{12}

Nitrous oxide is a vapour rather than a gas (because it is usually met below its critical temperature). It is manufactured by heating ammonium nitrate (NH_4NO_3) to 240 °C. Toxic impurities (nitric oxide and nitrogen dioxide) and water vapour are removed. The gas is pumped into cylinders and the pressure causes it to liquefy. Any volatile liquid has a specific pressure for any given temperature (the saturated vapour pressure). In use, therefore, the pressure in the nitrous oxide cylinder is maintained until all the liquid nitrous oxide has been used; the pressure then falls rapidly. The pressure does in fact fall slightly during use because conversion of the liquid to vapour uses latent heat of vaporisation, which cools the remaining liquid. The amount of cooling is determined by the specific heat capacity of the liquid nitrous oxide.

As nitrous oxide has a low anaesthetic potency, it is usually administered using a needle control valve and a rotameter marked in litres per minute rather than a vaporiser marked in percentages. It may be administered via a Hudson mask, although scavenging is not then possible.

Rapid equilibration of the brain concentration with the inhaled concentration occurs, but the low anaesthetic potency necessitates the use of adjuncts to provide anaesthesia rather than dissociated sedation. Usually the adjunct is a volatile anaesthetic agent, but intravenous anaesthetic agents are also suitable. The importance of this agent in anaesthetic practice is that it reduces the concentration of volatile agent required so that induction and recovery can be more rapidly achieved than by using the volatile agent alone. This is of limited benefit with the newer agents (desflurane and sevoflurane). But isoflurane, and especially desflurane and sevoflurane, are relatively expensive, and concurrent use of nitrous oxide makes economic sense. The reduced concentration required is also advantageous when the volatile agent is irritant to the respiratory tract.

Nitrous oxide suppresses spinal impulses and may suppress supraspinal pathways in part by activation of inhibitory mechanisms. It has a moderate analgesic effect that may be effected through CNS endorphins and enkephalins. The analgesic effects are partly antagonised by naloxone.

Cerebral vasodilatation occurs, with increased CBF and raised ICP.

Myocardial contractility is reduced by a direct effect, but this is neutralised by an increased sympathetic tone (α and β stimulation). Vascular tone is increased generally, causing rises in central venous pressure, systemic vascular resistance and peripheral vascular resistance. Blood pressure is usually raised a little, but may decrease if cardiac output is compromised.

Nitrous oxide decreases tidal volume and increases respiratory rate. The overall effect is an increased minute volume. There is little effect on CO_2 tension, but the responses to hypercarbia and hypoxia are impaired. The gas is non-irritant to the respiratory tract, but ciliary activity is reduced.

Skeletal muscle activity is increased, probably because of supraspinal excitation. In contrast with the volatile agents, neuromuscular function is not affected and neuromuscular blocking agents are not facilitated. Neutrophil chemotaxis is impaired.

The oxyhaemoglobin dissociation curve (in vitro) is shifted to the left (affinity for oxygen increased).

Nitrous oxide interacts with vitamin B_{12} (cyanocobalamin), converting the monovalent cobalt to the bivalent form. This prevents it functioning as the coenzyme for methionine synthase and methyl malonyl CoA mutase. Methionine synthase catalyses conversion of homocysteine to methionine, and the demethylation of methyltetrahydrate. The latter is an essential step in the synthesis of thymidine for DNA synthesis. Bone-marrow DNA synthesis is impaired, resulting in megaloblastic changes with metabolic precursors appearing in the circulation. Eventually neutropenia and thrombocytopenia also occur. The initial changes are seen with exposure of 6–24 hours' duration, but in seriously ill patients as little as 2 hours will show effects. Chronic nitrous oxide abusers develop neurological damage similar to subacute combined degeneration of the cord secondary to a decrease in hepatic S-adenosyl methionine. Nitrous oxide may also have an inhibitory effect on methionine synthesis at very low concentrations (< 1000 ppm). COSHH regulations specify a time-weighted 8-hour exposure of less than 100 ppm.

Biotransformation occurs in minimal amounts. As nitrous oxide is relatively insoluble, it is excreted predominantly by the lungs. Anaerobic bacteria in the gut can also cause decomposition.

Nitrous oxide is more soluble in blood than nitrogen (34-fold). Nitrous oxide diffuses into air-filled spaces (containing oxygen, nitrogen, carbon dioxide and water vapour) quicker than nitrogen diffuses out, resulting in an increase in volume or an increase in pressure within a fixed volume space.

50% Nitrous oxide in oxygen (Entonox)

Presentation – supplied in cylinders as a gas under pressure (137 bar); liquefies at –6 °C; filling ratio 0.75

Colour code – cylinder body French blue, shoulder French blue and white quarters; pin index is a specific large single pin offset from centre

Storage – at room temperature away from extremes of heat; may separate if exposed to low temperatures (0 °C), in which case rewarm and invert to restore the mixture

Non-explosive – not flammable but supports combustion

CNS – broadly similar to nitrous oxide

CVS – broadly similar to nitrous oxide

RS – broadly similar to nitrous oxide

Other – mainly used as an inhaled analgesic (e.g. in labour)

Elimination – predominantly via lungs

Contraindications – as for nitrous oxide

Xenon (Xe)
Properties

MW	BP	MAC	O/W	Bl/G	O/G	Br/Bl
131.2	–108	71	19	0.12	1.8	0.17

Soda lime – compatible

CNS – anaesthesia, analgesia

CVS – very cardiostable, no reduction of contractility, increased CBF, no sensitisation to catecholamines

RS – non-irritant, increased tidal volume, reduced rate

Elimination – unchanged, via lungs

Xenon is a possible anaesthetic agent for the future. It is a rare or noble gas (like helium and argon) existing in monovalent form and present in atmospheric air in a concentration of 0.086 ppm (0.0000086%). It is obtained from fractional 'distillation' of liquefied air and is very expensive. At 20 °C xenon is above its critical temperature of 16 °C and so cannot be compressed to form a liquid, meaning that it is a gas rather than a vapour. Xenon is non-flammable and does not support combustion. As an anaesthetic agent it has a very low Bl/G solubility coefficient, giving rapid induction and emergence. It has a high MAC (low potency). It is highly cardiostable with no sensitisation of the myocardium to catecholamines and no reduction in contractility. It does not trigger malignant hyperthermia or cause respiratory irritation. At concentrations above 60% cerebral blood flow is increased. Xenon inhibits plasma membrane Ca^{2+} pumps and inhibits dorsal horn neurones by NMDA inhibition. Problems of expense and availability are the major obstacles to its use, as well as the difficulty of monitoring inspired and expired concentrations. Higher density and (to a lesser extent) higher viscosity than oxygen–nitrous oxide combinations result in the need for higher driving pressures during ventilation.

CHAPTER 30

Hypnotics and intravenous anaesthetic drugs

Tim Smith

General features

Anaesthetic drugs are usually administered by either the intravenous or the inhalational route, but they may also be given rectally or intramuscularly. The advantages of administering drugs intravenously rather than orally are listed in Figure 30.1.

Pharmacokinetics

The pharmacokinetic profiles of most IV anaesthetic drugs are similar to that of thiopental, which is shown in Figure 27.4. They result from a rapid transfer of drug from the blood to the brain tissue, followed by a rapid distribution to other tissues. This reduces the plasma level so that the drug diffuses back from the brain into the plasma, from where it is redistributed to other tissues. The result is a brief duration of anaesthesia with a rapid recovery. Elimination of the drugs subsequently occurs more slowly. Thiopental concentrations peak in the vessel-rich group of tissues (including the brain) within 1–2 minutes. Within a further 1 minute the brain level falls again because of redistribution to the muscle group, to reach near equilibrium in about 15–20 minutes. The redistribution to fat tissues is slow, peaking at 3 hours, owing to the relatively poor blood supply. However, the capacity of the fat tissues is large. The fat group contributes little to the immediate recovery but accounts for the prolonged elimination.

Fundamentals of Anaesthesia, 4th edition, ed. Ted Lin, Tim Smith and Colin Pinnock. Published by Cambridge University Press. © Cambridge University Press 2017.

Figure 30.1 Advantages of intravenous drug administration, compared with oral administration

Quick onset, as enteral absorption is bypassed
Dose not reduced by the first-pass effect (bioavailability 100%)
Lower total dose required
Quicker recovery with single dose due to redistribution, as gut does not act as reservoir
Greater control, therefore suitable for infusion

Adverse reactions

Adverse reactions to IV agents vary from the trivial (muscular movements) to the serious (anaphylactoid or anaphylactic reactions). The incidence of serious adverse reactions to common IV anaesthetic agents is shown in Figure 30.2.

Figure 30.2 Incidence of serious adverse reactions to intravenous drugs

Thiopental	1 in 14,000–20,000
Propofol	1 in 50,000–100,000
Etomidate	1 in 450,000

The ideal agent

No currently available IV drug fulfils the criteria of an 'ideal' anaesthetic agent. The concept remains useful, nonetheless, as a yardstick for assessing new drugs. Properties of an ideal agent are given in Figure 30.3.

Barbiturates

Examples – pentobarbital, phenobarbital, thiopental

Chemical structure

Barbiturates are based on barbituric acid, which contains the six-membered pyrimidine nucleus that is a building block of nucleosides. Oxypyrimidines may exist in two structural forms, enol and keto (Figure 30.4). Thiobarbiturates have a similar pair of structural forms. Chemically, barbituric acid is a condensation product (formation of the chemical bonds involves the removal of water molecules) of malonic acid and urea. Substitutions on atoms at positions 1, 2 and 5 confer and modulate hypnotic activity.

Figure 30.3 Properties of an ideal intravenous anaesthetic drug

Physical
Soluble in aqueous medium
Stable in solution
Stable in air within the container
Stable when diluted
Stable in light
Stable at room temperature
Inexpensive
Pharmacological
Potent enough to provide surgical anaesthesia without supplement
Induction in one arm–brain circulation time
High oil/water solubility
Analgesia
No pain on injection
Non-epileptogenic
No cardiac irritability
No cardiovascular depression
No respiratory depression
Muscle relaxation
No increase in intracranial pressure
Non-cumulative with infusion
Unaffected by renal and hepatic failure
Metabolites inactive and non-toxic
Non-teratogenic

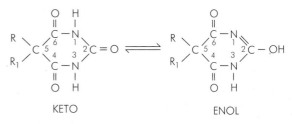

KETO   ENOL

Figure 30.4 Basic chemical structure of barbiturates, showing enol and keto forms

Structure–activity relationship

Barbituric acid has no hypnotic activity. Clinically active barbiturates are created by the addition of various alkyl groups to C-5. Barbiturates act at the $GABA_A$ receptor to increase the effect and duration of action of GABA and also block AMPA/kainite receptors and inhibit glutamate release via the P/Q type high-voltage-activated calcium channels. Oxybarbiturates (e.g. phenobarbital) are the basic form of barbiturate, which have a slow onset of

Figure 30.5 Structural classification of barbiturates

		Position 2	
		Oxygen	**Sulphur**
Position 1	**Hydrogen**	Oxybarbiturate (phenobarbital)	Thiobarbiturate (thiopental)
	Methyl group	Methylbarbiturate (methohexital)	Methylthiobarbiturate (no clinical use)

action and a long duration. They function well as basal hypnotics and sedatives but are too slow for use as anaesthetic agents. Replacing the oxygen on C-2 with sulphur produces a thiobarbiturate (e.g. thiopental), which has a rapid onset of action and a relatively short duration of action and recovery period. Replacing the hydrogen on N-1 of the basic oxybarbiturate with a methyl group produces a methylbarbiturate (e.g. methohexital). Methylbarbiturates also have a rapid onset and short duration of action plus a short recovery. However, they also produce some excitatory activity, which takes the form of sporadic uncoordinated movements during induction of anaesthesia. These may be mild or vigorous, but are usually distinguishable from the repetitive jerking of epileptiform convulsions, or the diffuse muscular shimmering (fasciculation) seen with suxamethonium. Modification of the alkyl groups on C-5 alters the potency of the drug. Oxy-, methyl-, and thio-barbiturates are all clinically useful, but the addition of both sulphur and a methyl group (methylthiobarbiturates) results in excessive excitatory activity, precluding the use of such a compound in the clinical setting.

The structural classification of barbiturates is shown in Figure 30.5.

Clinical effects

Phenobarbital and pentobarbital have a slow onset of action, and provide anxiolysis and anticonvulsant activity. The intravenously administered induction agent thiopental is the most relevant to anaesthetic practice: it is a water-soluble barbiturate agent that induces anaesthesia within one arm–brain circulation time of IV injection. It is highly lipophilic, and easily and rapidly crosses the blood–brain barrier to penetrate the brain.

Complications associated with barbiturate usage

Porphyria

The porphyrias are a group of diverse diseases of inborn or acquired errors of metabolism that result in the

Figure 30.6 Classification of porphyrias

Erythropoietic	Congenital erythropoietic porphyria
Hepatic	Acute intermittent porphyria Hereditary coproporphyria Variegate porphyria Porphyria cutanea tarda Toxic porphyria
Erythropoietic and hepatic	Protoporphyria

secretion of excessive amounts of porphyrins and precursors (Figure 30.6).

Porphyrins comprise four pyrrole rings linked together to form a larger ring. They are fundamental constituents of haemoglobin, myoglobin, cytochromes and catalases, and all contain iron. Porphyria is very rare in the UK. While still rare, **acute intermittent porphyria** is more common in South Africa, Sweden and Finland, and **variegate porphyria** is more common in Sweden and Finland. These are both inherited by autosomal dominance, and are the most relevant to anaesthesia. They affect the liver, where haem is produced as a component of the cytochrome P450 enzyme, and therefore affect drug metabolism. Many drugs increase porphyrin production, and administration may result in neurotoxic porphyrin levels. Drugs to avoid include barbiturates, benzodiazepines and steroids, but propofol is thought to be safe.

Subcutaneous extravasation

Extravasation of thiopental causes localised pain and tissue damage due to the highly alkaline medium in which it is mixed. It does not usually cause major sequelae, but injection in proximity to a nerve may cause damage. The pain and bruising can be reduced by dilution with a small dose (10 mL) of saline, or 10 mL 1% procaine, which vasodilates as well as diluting the thiopental. The damage is due to the high pH, and is immediate, so any damage limitation measures should be performed as quickly as possible.

Intra-arterial injection

Intra-arterial injection of thiopental is a potentially serious complication, causing endothelial damage. This is related to the change in pH of the solution as it is diluted in the blood, which results in a precipitation of insoluble microcrystals that block the narrowing arterial tree – whereas in veins any such crystals are carried away and diluted so that they dissolve before causing any problems. The precipitate causes arterial intimal damage, local release of noradrenaline and the release of ATP from damaged red cells and platelets, which initiates vascular thrombosis. Clinically there is pain, with delayed or absent onset of sleep. Blanching or cyanosis of the affected area, loss of the peripheral pulse of the injected limb and gangrene may occur. Arterial thrombosis may gradually develop, progressing for up to 15 days. The treatment is as follows:

Management of suspected intra-arterial injection of thiopental

- Stop the injection, but leave the needle or cannula in place.
- Dilute immediately by injecting normal saline into the artery.
- Administer local anaesthetic and/or vasodilator directly into the artery:
  - Lidocaine 50 mg (5 mL 1% solution)
  - Procaine hydrochloride 50–100 mg (10–20 mL 0.5% solution)
  - Phenoxybenzamine (α-adrenoceptor antagonist) 0.5 mg or infuse 50–200 µg min^{-1}
- Administer papaverine systemically 40–80 mg (10–20 mL 0.4% solution).
- Consider sympathetic neural blockade (stellate ganglion or brachial plexus block). This produces prolonged vasodilatation to improve circulation and tissue oxygenation while improving clearance of the crystals.
- Start IV heparin.
- Consider intra-arterial injection of hydrocortisone.
- Postpone non-urgent surgery.

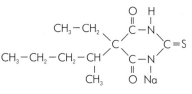

Figure 30.7 Structure of thiopental

Thiopental

Physical

Sodium thiopental is a thiobarbiturate. It is supplied in a rubber-topped bottle, as a pale yellow powder containing 6% anhydrous sodium carbonate (a base). The gaseous environment within the bottle is nitrogen. The sodium carbonate prevents CO_2 in the air from forming free acid that would react with the thiopental. The sodium ion replaces the hydrogen ion that associates with C-1 and C-2 of the base compound, as shown in Figure 30.7.

The powder is readily soluble in water, producing a 2.5% (2.5 g 100 mL^{-1}) solution with pH 11. At pH 11, having a pK_a = 7.6, it is almost entirely (99.9%) ionised. However, once in the blood the pH falls towards 7.4, at which 61% of the drug is non-ionised. This non-ionised portion is the more lipid-soluble and readily crosses the blood–brain barrier into the lipid-rich brain tissue. Of the drug, 60–80% is reversibly bound to protein (mainly to albumin) and is therefore non-diffusible and inactive.

Clinical

IV injection of thiopental rarely causes pain, and venous thrombosis occurs in only 3–4% of patients. Characteristically, the subject may be aware of a taste of onions or garlic before the onset of sleep. The redistribution half-life of 4 minutes leads to rapid recovery.

Central nervous system

Thiopental causes cortical depression, with a plasma level of 40 µg mL^{-1} being typical for sleep. Rapid and smooth induction of anaesthesia occurs within one arm–brain circulation time with a low incidence (4%) of minor excitatory movements. Thiopental has no analgesic activity and may be antanalgesic. It is an anticonvulsant agent. During induction, the EEG shows the onset of high-amplitude waves of 10–30 Hz, followed by depression of cortical activity with an isoelectric picture accompanied by occasional bursts of 10 Hz activity.

Cerebral metabolic rate of oxygen consumption ($CMRO_2$) is reduced, which leads to cerebral vasoconstriction with a concomitant fall in cerebral blood flow

(CBF) and ICP. The fall in blood pressure that also occurs leads to a fall in CBF, with an opposite effect on cerebrovascular resistance. The reduction in ICP and $CMRO_2$ are useful properties of thiopental for use in cerebral protection for situations such as cardiopulmonary bypass or standstill, and for the prevention of secondary brain damage in trauma.

A single large dose results in the return of wakefulness when the plasma level is higher than if smaller doses are used. This is termed acute tolerance. The technique of injecting a predetermined dose without slowly titrating it to effect allows the use of lower doses while still achieving satisfactory peak concentrations in the cerebral circulation and therefore the brain. A more rapid recovery results from a correspondingly more rapid fall in cerebral plasma thiopental concentration. Late recovery is also improved, as the total dose is lower.

Cardiovascular system

Thiopental causes a dose-dependent reduction in vascular tone with a reduction in SVR, CVP and PCWP. Preload and afterload are therefore both reduced, resulting in a decrease in mean arterial blood pressure and in left and right ventricular work. There is a slight compensatory increase in heart rate. High doses given rapidly can cause severe myocardial depression and hypotension, particularly in hypovolaemic patients or those receiving antihypertensive medication. Extreme caution should be exercised if thiopental is to be used in patients who cannot increase their cardiac output to compensate for a drop in vascular resistance, such as those with valvular stenosis or cardiac tamponade. Gradual administration can produce an isoelectric EEG without any significant effect on blood pressure or heart rate. Cardiac oxygen consumption is increased in normal individuals, but in ischaemic hearts the requirement is reduced.

Respiratory system

Thiopental causes a dose-dependent reduction in both respiratory rate and tidal volume. Manifestations of irritation such as cough and hiccup are uncommon, although it is less effective at depressing the laryngeal reflexes than propofol.

Other effects

Thiopental is not emetic. It has minimal effect on hepatic, renal or adrenal function. Uterine tone is unaffected, but it readily crosses the placenta, also diffusing back into the maternal circulation as plasma levels fall, so this is of little practical significance.

Metabolism

Metabolism occurs in the liver, with an extraction ratio of 0.1–0.4. Phase I mechanisms result in oxidation of the C-5 side chains, replacement of the sulphur with oxygen to produce pentobarbital and cleavage of the barbiturate ring into urea and a three-carbon portion. These actions are robust enough to cope with major liver dysfunction, so thiopental may still be suitable in hepatic failure. Clearance is insufficient to deal with repeated doses, and cumulation therefore occurs.

Complications

Extravasation causes local damage, and intra-arterial injection may cause serious damage distal to injection (see *Complications associated with barbiturate usage*, above). Avoid in porphyria.

Steroids

Examples – eltanolone, hydroxydione, minaxolone. At present there are no steroid anaesthetic agents available for clinical use.

Physical

The steroid anaesthetic agents are based on the familiar steroid nucleus. Note that oxy- and hydroxy- substitutions at 3 and 20 appear to be associated with anaesthetic activity.

Clinical
Central nervous system

Most of the steroid agents produce a rapid onset of action (within one arm–brain circulation time) with smooth induction of anaesthesia, and a rapid recovery.

Cardiovascular system

The steroids are less depressant to the cardiovascular system than barbiturates and propofol.

Respiratory system

The steroids are less depressant to tidal volume and respiratory rate than the barbiturates or propofol.

Other effects

Anaesthetic and endocrine activities appear to have no structural relationship. There is a low incidence of postoperative nausea and vomiting. Excitatory phenomena are frequently problematic.

Complications

Toxicity is generally low, with a high therapeutic index. Local irritation is a problem.

Eltanolone (pregnanolone)

Eltanolone produces rapid induction and recovery of anaesthesia, but this is slower than propofol and accumulation occurs. It is insoluble in water, so a soya bean emulsion is used. It has a terminal half-life of about 50–80 minutes. It has been abandoned because of cutaneous reactions.

Hydroxydione

Hydroxydione is a water-soluble steroid anaesthetic. It has little effect on cardiorespiratory physiology, some neuromuscular blockade with a low incidence of coughing and a very low incidence of nausea and vomiting. However, slow onset of action (several minutes), pain on injection and localised venous irritation have prevented its success.

Minaxolone

Minaxolone is a water-soluble steroid anaesthetic. It has a slow onset of action and its clinical usefulness has been limited by the excitatory activity, associated convulsions and abnormal liver function tests.

ORG 20599 and ORG 21465

These two water-soluble aminosteroid anaesthetic agents, which have a high therapeutic index (about 13) in animals, have been blighted by excessive excitatory movements and stability problems, which limit human application.

Butyrophenones

Examples – benperidol, droperidol, haloperidol
 Butyrophenones are covered in detail in Chapter 34.

Phencyclidine derivatives

Example – ketamine

Physical

Ketamine is a derivative of phencyclidine and cyclohexamine. It is supplied as an aqueous solution in several concentrations, formulated as a weak acid with a pH between 3.5 and 5.5. Ketamine has a single chiral carbon atom. It is supplied as a racemic mixture of the two stereoisomers.

Pharmacodynamics

Ketamine is a non-competitive antagonist of the calcium ion channel operated by the excitatory NMDA glutamate receptor that is likely to be responsible for anaesthesia, analgesia and neurotoxicity. Ketamine also inhibits the NMDA receptor by stereoselectively binding to the phencyclidine (PCP) binding site. Ketamine interacts with the δ, κ and μ opioid receptors. S(+)ketamine provides more potent analgesia than R(−)ketamine. There is stereoselectivity for κ and μ receptors but not δ receptors. Evidence suggests that ketamine may be an antagonist at the μ receptor and that analgesia is not μ-mediated. Ketamine, especially R(−)ketamine, also interacts weakly with the σ receptor (formerly classified as an opioid receptor). The potency of ketamine at the receptors is in the order $\mu > \kappa > \sigma > \delta$.

High doses of ketamine have a local anaesthetic action, and there is supportive evidence of fast sodium channel blockade.

Ketamine also acts stereoselectively at muscarinic acetylcholine receptors. This action is likely to be antagonist, as ketamine produces anticholinergic effects such as bronchodilatation, delirium and a sympathomimetic action. Ketamine anaesthesia is antagonised by anticholinesterases. It is thought that ketamine may also have an effect on voltage-sensitive Ca^{2+} channels.

Clinical

Ketamine has a slow onset of action, taking about 1 minute after IV injection to achieve an effect. Ketamine can be administered intramuscularly, with an onset of sleep in 2–5 minutes and duration of 12–25 minutes. The role of extradurally and intrathecally administered ketamine has yet to be established, but, in brief, it causes segmental blockade, and affects the receptors located in the spinal cord as described above.

Central nervous system

Ketamine produces sleep, analgesia and dissociation (a psychological detachment from the surrounding environment). The eyes frequently remain open, and eyelash, corneal and laryngeal reflexes are preserved to a variable extent. Muscle tone is increased and marked involuntary movements are common.

Unlike other typical induction agents, it affects the limbic system rather than the thalamocortical axis.

Analgesia is effected by inhibition of the affective, emotional component of pain mediated by the thalamic reticular system rather than the transmission of the nociceptive signals. As well as a slow onset time, the duration of action is much longer than that of the faster induction agents. The recovery may be associated with hallucinations, diplopia or temporary blindness. These effects are a particular problem with short procedures, but those lasting beyond an hour when anaesthesia has been maintained with other agents are less of a problem.

Dissociative side effects are less in males and children, and can be reduced by the concomitant use of opioids, benzodiazepine, droperidol or thiopental. There is no retrograde amnesia.

A significant rise (80%) in CBF, ICP, intraocular pressure (IOP) and $CMRO_2$ may persist for 30 minutes. The onset of effect is associated with a loss of α waves followed by a dominant θ wave on the EEG.

The (+) isomer is more potent than the (–) isomer for hypnosis, analgesia and dissociative effects, supporting the hypothesis that ketamine acts via receptor interaction.

Cardiovascular system

Ketamine increases heart rate, blood pressure and catecholamine levels by a generalised increase in CNS activity. These changes are marked, with 30–100% increases. Direct myocardial depression counteracts the increased sympathetic activity and may leave stroke volume unaffected. Arrhythmias are not common.

Respiratory system

Ketamine has the advantage that, in the absence of opioid, it does not depress respiration greatly. It is a bronchodilator, and protective reflexes are preserved to some extent. Preserved airway maintenance is particularly useful, but reflex protection of the airway from aspiration cannot be guaranteed. Because of the sparing of these reflexes and an increase in secretions, coughing, hiccup and laryngospasm are more prevalent than with thiopental.

Other effects

In both parturient and non-parturient patients, uterine tone is increased. This is a particular problem in the presence of placental abruption or umbilical cord prolapse.

Metabolism

The pharmacokinetic profiles of both stereoisomers are identical. Ketamine is metabolised in the liver by N-desmethylation to norketamine. Norketamine has a half to a third of the potency of ketamine and is subsequently hydroxylated. Hydroxylation of the ketamine ring plays a minor role in its metabolism.

Most appears in the bile, with 20% as metabolites in the urine, but some appears unchanged in urine and faeces.

Imidazoles

Example – etomidate

Physical

Etomidate is a carboxylated imidazole. It is soluble in water but is unstable so it is formulated either in a mixture of water and propylene glycol (pH 8.1) or in a lipid emulsion. Etomidate has two stereoisomers, with R(+) etomidate being the predominant enhancer of GABA binding to the $GABA_A$ receptor. Figure 30.8 shows the chiral carbon atom, and the ester linkage which is hydrolysed in its metabolism.

Clinical

Etomidate is a rapidly acting induction agent. It sometimes causes pain on injection, which is considerably lessened by using the lipid emulsion.

Central nervous system

There is rapid induction of anaesthesia within one arm–brain circulation time. Excitatory muscle movements are much more frequent than with thiopental. The EEG frequently shows epileptiform activity. Cerebral blood flow, ICP, $CMRO_2$ and IOP are reduced.

Cardiovascular system

Etomidate causes less cardiovascular depression than the barbiturates and is indicated when the cardiovascular status is delicate. It has relatively minor effects resulting in a fall in SVR, blood pressure and heart rate. There is a

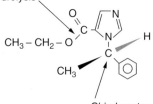

Figure 30.8 Chemical structure of etomidate

slight increase in contractility and cardiac output, but oxygen delivery and utilisation are preserved.

Respiratory system

Etomidate reduces both tidal volume and rate. Depression is much less than with the barbiturates.

Other effects

Histamine release is minimal. Etomidate has been used by infusion for ICU sedation. Unfortunately, it inhibits 11-β-hydroxylase and cholesterol cleavage, which results in inhibition of glucocorticoid and mineralocorticoid synthesis. The suppression of steroid synthesis (part of the stress response to surgery) lasts for 3–6 hours after a single dose, but it is only of clinical significance when infused. It is no longer licensed for use by infusion.

Metabolism

Etomidate is metabolised by esterases in the plasma and liver to produce inactive metabolites that are excreted in the urine and bile. A small amount is excreted unchanged.

Phenols

Example – propofol

Physical

Propofol is an alkyl phenol (2,6-di-isopropyl phenol), having minimal solubility in water. It is formulated as an isotonic 1% emulsion in a mixture of soya bean oil, purified egg phosphatide, glycerol and sodium hydroxide having pH 6–8.5. In this formulation, with a pK_a in water of 11, it is almost entirely ($>$ 99%) non-ionised. Of the drug, 98% is protein-bound.

Propofol may be diluted using 5% dextrose to a lower limit of 2 mg mL^{-1} (0.2%) for infusion. To reduce the incidence of injection pain, 1 mL of 0.5% or 1% preservative-free lidocaine may be added to 20 mL propofol.

It potentiates the activity of GABA at the GABA$_A$ receptor to prolong chloride channel opening, and also blocks voltage-operated sodium channels.

Clinical

Propofol provides a rapid and smooth induction of anaesthesia (within one arm–brain circulation time) and attenuates laryngeal reflexes better than the barbiturates.

Central nervous system

Propofol causes dose-dependent cortical depression. The EEG shows the development of α waves followed by slower δ waves as anaesthesia deepens. There is no epileptiform activity, although excitatory movements may be seen, particularly with larger doses. Propofol is an anticonvulsant, and reports of epileptic fits following prolonged propofol infusion are now thought to be due to the rapid clearance of the anticonvulsant propofol from the body with a rebound excitation. Arguably it may not be the first choice for electroconvulsive therapy (ECT), as recovery is no better than with other agents and it reduces convulsion duration (although the efficacy may be unaffected). It has some antiemetic activity.

The incidence of excitation, cough and hiccup are similar to those of thiopental. At equianaesthetic doses, laryngeal reflexes are attenuated more than with barbiturates, thus facilitating laryngeal mask insertion.

Cardiovascular system

Propofol causes a dose-dependent reduction in vascular tone that reduces SVR and CVP. The reduction in preload, together with a fall in contractility, contributes to the fall in cardiac output and subsequent hypotension. Heart rate remains relatively unchanged. The reductions in SVR, blood pressure and cardiac output are more pronounced than with thiopental. Propofol produces a variable but mild effect on heart rate.

Respiratory system

There is a fall in tidal volume with an increase in rate. The response to CO_2 is attenuated. Propofol is more depressant than thiopental. The response to intubation is suppressed more by propofol than by thiopental.

Other effects

The fat emulsion of propofol can produce hyperlipidaemia. It is routinely used for sedation of adults in critical care but is not suitable for such use in children under the age of 16 because of its association with hepatomegaly, metabolic acidosis and mortality.

Metabolism

Propofol is conjugated in the liver by glucuronidation to make it water-soluble, with 88% appearing in the urine and 2% in the faeces. Renal and hepatic failure have little effect on propofol metabolism.

Complications

Complications include excitation, and pain on injection, the incidence of which is affected by:

- Site of injection
- Speed of injection
- Concentration of propofol in the aqueous phase
- Buffering effect of blood
- Speed of IV carrier fluid
- Temperature of the propofol
- Concomitant use of adjunct drugs

Immediate pain is probably due to a direct irritant effect, while delayed pain occurring 10–20 seconds after the start of injection is probably the result of activation of the kinin system.

Pain on injection can be reduced by the following measures:

- Using large veins
- Slow administration so that dilution of the injectate occurs
- 1 mL of 0.5% or 1% preservative-free lidocaine added to 20 mL propofol
- Administration of 2 mL lidocaine 1% into the vein prior to propofol injection
- Using different lipid formulations

Extravasation causes no major damage. Intra-arterial injection results in some pain, loss of the pulse and some blanching, but long-term there is no damage. The solvent is non-irritant and there is a low incidence of hypersensitivity, but note that the solvent is a good bacterial culture medium.

Propofol occasionally results in green urine.

Benzodiazepines

Examples – diazepam, lorazepam, midazolam, temazepam

Chemical

The benzodiazepine skeleton is a set of two rings (benzene and diazepine: Figure 30.9), but most benzodiazepines also have a third ring at the R-5 position.

Structure–activity relationships are not clear, but modifications to the basic structure primarily affect the pharmacokinetic profile of the drug. Benzodiazepines may be classified as in Figure 30.10.

Pharmacokinetics

The benzodiazepines act on specific receptors, which are mainly in the grey matter of the CNS where the majority of synapses are located. The greatest number of receptors is in the cerebral cortex, followed by the cerebellar cortex, thalamus, hypothalamus and limbic system, with the

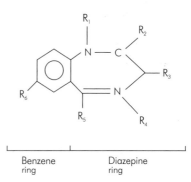

Figure 30.9 General structure of the benzodiazepine skeleton

Figure 30.10 Structural classification of benzodiazepines

Structure	Examples
1,4-Benzodiazepine	Diazepam Temazepam Lorazepam
Substituted 1,4-benzodiazepine	Triazolam
1,5-Benzodiazepine	Clobazepam
Imidazobenzodiazepine	Midazolam Flumazenil

lowest numbers in the brainstem and spinal cord. There are three subtypes of benzodiazepine receptor, represented by the abbreviation BDZ or ω. The properties of these are shown in Figure 30.11.

The clinical effects appear to be due to agonism at BDZ receptors attached to the $GABA_A$ receptor complex on the postsynaptic membrane. This facilitates the action of GABA, which opens the inhibitory chloride channel and hyperpolarises the membrane. Therefore, benzodiazepines do not act directly on the chloride channels, so the maximum effect is determined by the prevailing levels of GABA, which should ensure a high therapeutic index.

The search for endogenous ligands of the benzodiazepine receptors has not been conclusive. There are agonists at the benzodiazepine receptors (β-carbolines) which have the opposite effect by preventing the binding of GABA to its receptor site. This is called inverse agonism. It is different from antagonism because, rather than acting by preventing the binding of benzodiazepines with no intrinsic activity of its own, the inverse agonist causes a conformational change that is the opposite to that of the agonist. Efficacy is, in effect, negative.

Figure 30.11 Properties of benzodiazepine receptors

Receptor		Location	On GABA receptor	Postulated clinical effect
BDZ$_1$	ω_1	Central	yes	Sedation and hypnosis
BDZ$_2$	ω_2	Central	yes	Anticonvulsant
BDZ$_3$	ω_3	Central and peripheral	no	Not known

All the benzodiazepines are highly lipid-soluble and cross the blood–brain barrier readily. Used intravenously, the onset of effect usually takes longer than one arm–brain circulation time. Brain levels follow plasma levels closely. Orally administered benzodiazepines are readily absorbed as a result of the lipid solubility.

Drugs with a low lipophilicity have a lower transfer to brain and more drug is distributed peripherally (to vessel-rich tissues). This results in increased persistence of some drugs (although the elimination half-life is shorter) with a prolongation of recovery. For example, lorazepam has a short half-life compared with diazepam but is less lipophilic, so the effects may last less with the latter.

In rank order of lipid solubility: midazolam > diazepam > temazepam > lorazepam, but onset of action is much the same. The benzodiazepines are bound to albumin in the plasma.

Clinical
Central nervous system
The benzodiazepine family shares the following central effects:

- Anxiolysis
- Sedation
- Hypnosis
- Anterograde amnesia
- Anticonvulsant activity
- Skeletal muscle relaxation

Benzodiazepines reduce both rapid eye movement (REM) and slow-wave sleep, which in the short term may result in a deficit of REM sleep during treatment. Chronic administration results in tolerance, and withdrawal may result in rebound. The benzodiazepines are slow-acting induction agents with a prolonged recovery.

Cardiovascular system
Benzodiazepines administered intravenously have only minor depressant effects on the cardiovascular system in general. There is a slight reduction in SVR, preload,

Figure 30.12 Metabolism of benzodiazepines

Drug	Extraction ratio	Metabolism
Diazepam	Low	Oxidation
Lorazepam	Low	Conjugation
Midazolam	High	Oxidation
Nitrazepam	Low	Nitro-reduction
Temazepam	Low	Conjugation

cardiac output and blood pressure. However, elderly and hypovolaemic patients may be particularly sensitive to IV midazolam, and this should be used with caution.

Respiratory system
Oral benzodiazepines have minimal effects on respiration. However, IV benzodiazepines have a very variable although usually slight effect on breathing. Airway maintenance is impaired, and tidal volume is reduced, with reduced sensitivity to CO_2. Respiratory rate usually increases slightly. Depression is especially likely with the concomitant use of opioids and other central depressants.

Other effects
Benzodiazepines reduce skeletal muscle tone via an effect on the dorsal horn of the spinal cord.

Metabolism
A number of benzodiazepines have active metabolites, resulting in prolonged duration of action (Figure 30.12). These may have longer half-lives than the parent compound.

The metabolism of benzodiazepines produces metabolites that are also administered in their own right. Figure 30.13 shows the important interrelationships.

Diazepam
Diazepam is a 1,4-benzodiazepine that is insoluble in water. For IV administration it is therefore solubilised

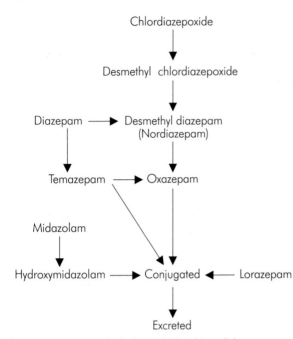

Figure 30.13 Metabolic interrelationships of the benzodiazepine family

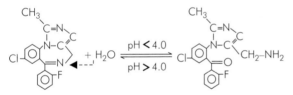

Figure 30.14 Structural equilibrium of midazolam

either in buffered propylene glycol and ethanol to a pH of 6.4–6.9 or in a soya bean lipid emulsion, to avoid causing thrombophlebitis and subsequent thrombosis.

It may be administered orally or intravenously. Diazepam is metabolised to N-desmethyldiazepam.

Midazolam

Midazolam is an imidazobenzodiazepine. This results in the ability of a water molecule to open the diazepine ring (Figure 30.14), thus encouraging aqueous solubility.

The equilibrium between the two forms of midazolam is determined by pH. The change from the one form to the other is relatively slow, having a half-life of 10 minutes. The pH in the ampoule containing midazolam hydrochloride is 3.0 and so the ring is open and it is soluble. Once subjected to body pH 7.4, the diazepine

Figure 30.15 Comparison of diazepam with midazolam

		Diazepam	Midazolam
Physical		No imidazole ring	Imidazole ring
		Insoluble in water	Soluble in water
		Lipid emulsion	Aqueous
Chemical		Consistent structure	Structural change
		High F/M ratio	Low F/M ratio
Clinical		Antiepileptic	Antiepileptic
		Longer duration	Shorter duration

ring closes and the midazolam becomes lipid-soluble, allowing it readily to cross the blood–brain barrier. In the plasma most of the midazolam (95%) is protein-bound. Midazolam is redistributed more rapidly than diazepam and so its duration of action is much shorter than that of diazepam.

Midazolam is hydroxylated in the liver to 4-hydroxy-midazolam, which has minimal clinical activity. In the elderly, the lower hepatic blood flow and metabolic activity result in a significantly higher elimination half-life.

Diazepam and midazolam are compared in Figure 30.15.

Lorazepam

Lorazepam is a 1,4-benzodiazepine used in the alleviation of anxiety and for sedation. It is used as a premedicant. It is available for oral, sublingual, IM and IV administration. The oral dose is 2–4 mg, and IV is 50 μg kg^{-1}. Oral bioavailability is 90%, with 90% protein-bound and a volume of distribution of 1 L kg^{-1}. It is predominantly eliminated by glucuronide conjugation followed by urinary excretion, with an elimination half-life of 10–20 hours.

Temazepam

Temazepam is an orally administered 1,4-benzodiazepine used in the alleviation of anxiety and for sedation. It is used as a premedicant, typically in doses of 10–40 mg (1 mg kg^{-1}, up to 30 mg syrup in children). Bioavailability is high, 76% is protein-bound and the volume of distribution is 0.8 L kg^{-1}. It is predominantly eliminated by glucuronide conjugation followed by urinary excretion, with an elimination half-life of 8 hours.

Flumazenil

Flumazenil is an imidazobenzodiazepine and a competitive benzodiazepine receptor antagonist, bearing the closest resemblance to the structure of midazolam. It is administered intravenously to antagonise the clinical effects of agonist benzodiazepines. It also antagonises inverse benzodiazepine receptor agonists.

Flumazenil is 40–50% protein-bound to albumin and rapidly redistributed, with a volume of distribution of 0.9 L kg^{-1}. Flumazenil has a high hepatic extraction ratio, with a total clearance of 15 mL kg^{-1} min^{-1}. Elimination half-life is about 50 minutes. Flumazenil is metabolised to a carboxylic acid derivative and a glucuronide, which are both inactive.

Cautions

Flumazenil has a short duration of action. It is important to realise that its effects may wear off before the benzodiazepine agonist has been cleared, with a re-emergence of the agonist effects. In addition, rapid antagonism of benzodiazepine sedation in a head-injured patient may precipitate an excessive rise in ICP. After chronic administration of benzodiazepines, flumazenil may provoke abrupt withdrawal effects.

Other hypnotic agents

Examples – buspirone, chloral hydrate, meprobamate, zolpidem, zopiclone

Buspirone

Buspirone is an azaspirodecanedione used for anxiolysis. It does not appear to act on benzodiazepine receptors, and the most likely mode of action is antagonism at 5-HT_{1A} receptors. It may also reduce acetylcholine activity and increase catecholamine activity. There is marked first-pass metabolism, with peak levels after 60 minutes. It is 95% protein-bound in the plasma. Buspirone is metabolised in the liver and has a half-life of 2–11 hours.

Chloral and related drugs

Chloral, chloral hydrate, triclofos and dichloraphenazone are interrelated metabolically. These drugs are administered orally as either tablets or elixir. Triclofos is said to cause less gastric irritation than chloral hydrate. Chloral hydrate is useful for premedication of small children. A dose of 50 mg kg^{-1} (up to 1 g) acts within 45 minutes. Doses from 6 mg kg^{-1} in adults will produce sedation.

Clinical effects
Central nervous system

The chloral derivatives cause central depression with a mild anticonvulsant activity. There is little interference with EEG sleep patterns. They have no analgesic activity.

Cardiovascular system

In normal dosage, there is minimal cardiovascular depression, but overdose causes profound depression, with supraventricular tachycardia a feature.

Respiratory system

In normal dosage, there is minimal respiratory depression, but overdose causes profound depression.

Metabolism

Alcohol dehydrogenase, present in the liver, red blood cells and other sites, plays a major role in the inactivation of these drugs. Trichlorethanol is conjugated with glucuronide.

Cautions

Problems include gastric irritation, hepatic enzyme induction or inhibition, and the displacement of drugs such as warfarin from plasma proteins.

Meprobamate

Meprobamate is a carbamate tranquiliser having anxiolytic, anticonvulsant and muscle-relaxant properties. It acts by inhibiting adenosine uptake. It is less effective than benzodiazepines and has a lower therapeutic index. Rapid absorption follows oral administration. Ninety per cent is excreted in the urine (mainly as the hydroxy metabolite and its glucuronide conjugate). It may precipitate convulsions in susceptible patients, particularly following withdrawal of the drug. Meprobamate is contraindicated in acute intermittent porphyria.

Zolpidem

Zolpidem is an imidazopyrine that acts at the benzodiazepine receptor complex of the $GABA_A$ receptor, to produce anxiolysis and sedation. It is selective for ω_1 receptor subtype, producing hypnosis without the ataxia or other ω_2 effects. The effects are reversed by flumazenil. Zolpidem is rapidly absorbed, with a bioavailability of 70%. Concentrations peak at about 1–3 hours, and it is 93% protein-bound. Zolpidem is metabolised to inactive metabolites in the liver, with a half-life of 2.4 hours.

Zopiclone

Zopiclone is a cyclopyrrolone with anxiolytic and sedative properties. It acts at the GABA–benzodiazepine receptor complex but appears to act at a different site from that affected by benzodiazepines. The overall effect is to enhance the action of GABA in promoting opening of the chloride channel. It does not reduce the amount of REM sleep. Zopiclone is well absorbed following oral administration and has a short elimination half-life of 5 hours.

Specific pharmacology

Units (unless stated otherwise) are:
Molecular weight (MW): daltons
Volume of distribution (V_d): L
Clearance (Cl): mL kg^{-1} min^{-1}
Terminal half-life ($t_{1/2}$): minutes

Diazepam

Structure – 1,4-benzodiazepine
Presentation

Oral – 2, 5, 10 mg tablets; 2 mg in 5 mL solution
IV – 5 mg mL^{-1} clear yellow solution of diazepam (osmolality 7775 mOsm kg^{-1}) in a mixture of solvents (propylene glycol (40%), ethanol (10%), benzoic acid/sodium benzoate (5%), benzyl alcohol (1.5%), pH 6.2–6.9); or white opaque oil-in-water emulsion (osmolality 349 mOsm kg^{-1}) using soya bean oil similar to intralipid (pH 6.0)
May also be administered rectally and intramuscularly
Storage – room temperature
Dose – IV bolus 0.1–0.3 mg kg^{-1}
Pharmacokinetics

MW	285
bioavailability	oral 86–100%
pH	6.2–6.9
protein binding	99%
V_d	1.2
Cl	0.4
$t_{1/2\alpha}$	70
$t_{1/2\beta}$	30 h

CNS – anxiolysis, hypnosis, sedation, anterograde amnesia; anticonvulsant; CBF, ICP and $CMRO_2$ reduced

CVS – blood pressure, cardiac output decreased; coronary vasodilatation increases coronary blood flow; myocardial oxygen consumption decreased
RS – respiratory depression; hypoxic drive reduced more than response to CO_2
Other – clearance reduced by concomitant cimetidine treatment
Elimination – hepatic metabolism to desmethyldiazepam (active $t_{1/2\alpha}$ at least 100 h), oxazepam and temazepam; oxidised and glucuronide derivatives excreted in urine; < 1% unchanged

Etomidate

Structure – imidazole
Presentation – clear colourless solution of 2 mg mL^{-1} etomidate in 10 mL 35% propylene glycol in water or 2 mg mL^{-1} in 10 mL lipid emulsion
Storage – room temperature
Dose – IV bolus 0.15–0.30 mg kg^{-1} (maximum 60 mg)
Pharmacokinetics

MW	342
pH	8.1
protein binding	76%
V_d	3.5
Cl	11.7
$t_{1/2\alpha 1}$	2.6
$t_{1/2\alpha 2}$	27
$t_{1/2\beta}$	75

CNS – rapid induction of anaesthesia (one arm–brain circulation time); excitatory phenomena common, reduced by opioids; recovery is dose-related; IOP, ICP, CBF and brain oxygen consumption ($CMRO_2$) reduced; epileptiform EEG features
CVS – systemic vascular resistance, mean arterial blood pressure fall; cardiac index and heart rate decrease slightly; atrial muscle function or contraction, ventricular dP/dt_{max}, mean aortic pressure, coronary blood flow are unchanged; myocardial oxygen delivery and consumption are preserved
RS – dose-dependent depression of tidal volume and rate; cough and hiccup common
Other – relatively high emesis rate (2–14%); pain on injection; venous thrombosis. There is no effect on renal or hepatic function. Steroid synthesis is inhibited, so infusions should not be used

Elimination – ester hydrolysis in plasma and liver, inactive metabolites; 87% in urine, 3% unchanged, rest in bile

Toxicity – adrenocortical suppression when infused over a long period; suppression direct and via ACTH

Contraindications – porphyria

Flumazenil

Structure – imidazobenzodiazepine, BDZ receptor antagonist

Presentation – clear colourless solution of 100 µg mL^{-1} flumazenil in 5 mL

Dose
  IV bolus – 100 µg increments up to 2 mg
  IV infusion – 100–400 µg per hour

Pharmacokinetics

protein binding	50%
V_d	0.9
Cl	15
$t_{\frac{1}{2}\alpha}$	7
$t_{\frac{1}{2}\beta}$	60

Clinical – antagonises the effects of central benzodiazepines; benzodiazepine withdrawal effects may occur

Elimination – almost entirely metabolised in the liver to the inactive carboxylate, which is excreted in the urine

Ketamine hydrochloride

Structure – phencyclidine derivative

Presentation – white crystalline powder for dilution with water, forming clear, colourless, aqueous solutions of 10, 50 and 100 mg mL^{-1}; 10 mg mL^{-1} isotonic with normal saline; 50 and 100 mg mL^{-1} contain 1:10,000 benzethonium chloride as preservative

Dose
  IV – 1–4.5 mg kg^{-1}
  IM – 4–13 mg kg^{-1}

Pharmacokinetics

MW	237.5
pH	3.5–5.5
protein binding	20–50%
V_d	3
Cl	17
$t_{\frac{1}{2}\alpha}$	10
$t_{\frac{1}{2}\beta}$	120–180

CNS – slow onset of dissociative anaesthesia, light sleep, analgesia, amnesia; the EEG shows θ activity; ICP, CBF and IOP are increased; analgesia is good for burns and fractures but poor for visceral pain

CVS – increases sympathetic tone, leading to increases in heart rate, cardiac output, blood pressure, central venous pressure; baroreceptor function is maintained; few arrhythmias

RS – protective respiratory reflexes are usually preserved, but cannot be relied upon; bronchodilatation

Other – nausea and vomiting are common; salivation is increased; uterine tone is increased; levels of adrenaline and noradrenaline are increased

Elimination – N-demethylation and hydroxylation to produce metabolites with reduced activity; metabolites then conjugated and excreted in the urine

Toxicity – rashes 15%; emergence delirium, hallucinations; pain on injection particularly with IM injection

Midazolam hydrochloride

Structure – imidazobenzodiazepine

Presentation – 1 mg mL^{-1} midazolam in 2, 5 and 50 mL; 2 mg mL^{-1} midazolam in 5 mL; 5 mg mL^{-1} midazolam in 2 and 10 mL; colourless aqueous solution of midazolam hydrochloride. Stable in water by virtue of opening of diazepine ring

Dose
  IV – 0.03–0.3 mg kg^{-1} depending on effect (sedation/anaesthesia) required; elderly are particularly sensitive
  IM – 0.07–0.1 mg kg^{-1} for premedication

Pharmacokinetics

MW	326
bioavailability	oral 44%; IM 80–100%
pH	3
protein binding	96%
V_d	1.1
Cl	7
$t_{\frac{1}{2}\beta}$	5 h

CNS – slow onset of action; anxiolysis, sedation, hypnosis, anterograde amnesia; anticonvulsant; CBF and $CMRO_2$ reduced

CVS – heart rate, systemic vascular resistance and blood pressure reduced

RS – tidal volume and minute volume reduced; rate increased but may cause apnoea; response to CO_2 impaired

Other – catecholamine levels reduced; renin, angiotensin and corticosteroid levels unaffected; skeletal muscle tone reduced; renal and hepatic blood flow reduced

Elimination – hydroxylated and conjugated with glucuronide in the liver, and is then excreted in urine

Toxicity – occasional pain on injection

Propofol

Structure – alkyl phenol derivative, 2,6-di-isopropyl phenol

Presentation – white, isotonic, neutral aqueous emulsion 10 mg mL^{-1}; also in 5 mg mL^{-1} and 20 mg mL^{-1}; 10% soya bean oil, 1.2% purified egg phosphatide, 2.25% glycerol, sodium hydroxide, water

Dose

Anaesthesia – IV bolus 2–2.5 mg kg^{-1}
Anaesthesia – IV infusion 4–12 mg kg^{-1} h^{-1}
Sedation – IV infusion 0.3–4 mg kg^{-1}

Pharmacokinetics

MW	178
pH	6–8.5
pK$_a$	11
protein binding 98%	98%
V$_d$	15
Cl	20
t$_{\frac{1}{2}\alpha1}$	2.5
t$_{\frac{1}{2}\alpha2}$	45
t$_{\frac{1}{2}\beta}$	3–8 h

CNS – rapid onset of anaesthesia (one arm–brain circulation); excitatory movements common; ICP, cerebral perfusion pressure and CMRO$_2$ reduced; anticonvulsant

CVS – systemic vascular resistance, cardiac output and blood pressure reduced; variable effect on heart rate, usually a slight increase

RS – tidal volume reduced, rate increased; response to CO_2 reduced; greater suppression of laryngeal reflexes than thiopental

Others – possible antiemetic effect; pain on injection; excitatory movements; renal and hepatic function unaffected

Elimination – liver and extrahepatic, unaffected by renal or hepatic disease; excreted in urine, 0.3% unchanged; non-cumulative when infused

Toxicity – a small risk of convulsions in epileptic patients; may cause bradycardia or asystole, possibly due to emulsion. Not licensed for use in pregnancy

Sodium thiopental

Structure – thiobarbiturate

Presentation – hygroscopic yellow powder of sodium thiopental with 6% sodium carbonate; reconstituted with water to 2.5% solution (2.5 mg mL^{-1}). Reconstituted solution must not be used after 24 hours

Dose – IV bolus 4–6 mg kg^{-1}

Pharmacokinetics

MW	264
pH	10.8
pK$_a$	7.6
protein binding	75%
V$_d$	1.96
Cl	3.4
t$_{\frac{1}{2}\alpha1}$	2–6
t$_{\frac{1}{2}\alpha2}$	30–60
t$_{\frac{1}{2}\beta}$	5–10 h

CNS – smooth, rapid induction of anaesthesia (one arm–brain circulation); CBF, ICP, IOP, CMRO$_2$ reduced; anticonvulsant, antanalgesic

CVS – negative inotropy; cardiac output, systemic vascular resistance and blood pressure reduced

RS – dose-dependent respiratory depression; response to CO_2 reduced; may cause laryngeal spasm or bronchoconstriction

Other – splanchnic vasoconstriction; no effect on pregnant uterus

Renal – vasopressin, renal plasma flow, urine output reduced

Hepatic – no effect, used in hepatic encephalopathy

Elimination – metabolised in the liver at 15% per hour; 30% remains by 24 hours; excreted in urine, 0.5% unchanged

Toxicity – tissue damage with extravasation; arterial constriction and thrombosis with intra-arterial injection

Contraindications – porphyria

CHAPTER 31

Analgesic drugs

Ian Power and Michael Paleologos

Opioids

The term *opioid* is defined as a natural, semisynthetic or synthetic compound that acts at opioid receptors. *Opiate* is a specific term to describe drugs derived from the opium poppy (*Papaver somniferum*).

Classification

Opioids may be classified in a number of ways according to chemical structure, production, receptor activity and specific receptor subtype affinity. A classification of opioids by origin and structure is shown in Figure 31.1. Naturally occurring opioids fall into two structural categories: those with a phenanthrene nucleus (morphine, codeine and thebaine) and benzylisoquinolines (papaverine and noscopine). Thebaine, despite being a relatively inactive opium derivative, is used as a precursor for the development of many semisynthetic opioid agonists and antagonists (buprenorphine, naloxone and oxycodone). Semisynthetic opioids are produced from chemical modification of naturally occurring opioids. Synthetic opioids may be further subdivided into four classes: anilinopiperidines (a type of phenylpiperidine), diphenylhaptanes, morphinans and phenylpiperidines.

Opioids may also be classified by their activity, affinity and efficacy at opioid receptors (Figure 31.2).

Partial agonists and mixed agonist–antagonists produce analgesia in opioid-naive patients, but may precipitate withdrawal in individuals who are dependent on full opioid agonists. They usually produce inadequate analgesia for treatment of severe pain, having a ceiling effect at less than the maximal effect of a full agonist. Hence they also produce less respiratory depression, constipation and

Fundamentals of Anaesthesia, 4th edition, ed. Ted Lin, Tim Smith and Colin Pinnock. Published by Cambridge University Press. © Cambridge University Press 2017.

Figure 31.1 Structural classification of opioid drugs

Classification	Structure	Examples
Naturally occurring	Morphine analogues	codeine, morphine
Semisynthetic	Morphine analogues	diamorphine, dihydrocodeine
	Thebaine derivatives	buprenorphine, oxycodone
Synthetic	Anilinopiperidines	alfentanil, fentanyl, phenoperidine, remifentanil, sufentanyl
	Diphenylheptanes	dextropropoxyphene, methadone
	Morphinans	levorphanol, butorphanol
	Phenylpiperidines	pethidine

Figure 31.2 Functional classification of opioid drugs

Classification	Example	Affinity	Efficacy
Pure agonists	Morphine	High	100%
Partial agonists	Buprenorphine	Medium	60–70%
Mixed agonist–antagonists	Pentazocine	Medium	Predominantly agonist
	Nalbuphine	Medium	Predominantly agonist
	Nalorphine	Medium	Predominantly antagonist
Pure antagonists	Naloxone	High	Zero
	Naltrexone	High	Zero

urinary side effects, and have a lower addiction potential. Mixed agonist–antagonists are associated with a much lower incidence of euphoria, but the production of psychotomimetic effects (hallucinations, depersonalisation) limits their clinical use.

Structure–activity relationships

Most opioids demonstrate optical activity, with the majority of the pharmacological effect being produced by one of the stereoisomers – usually the laevorotatory (S) isomer. Naturally occurring opioids are produced by stereospecific enzymes and are isolated as a single isomer, while synthetic opioids possessing a chiral carbon can only be synthesised as racemic mixtures. Some opioids require both stereoisomers for maximal efficacy (tramadol).

Phenylalanine and tyrosine are important structural elements of all opioid compounds, including the endogenous opioid peptides. Morphine is synthesised in the opium poppy from two molecules of tyrosine. All opioids

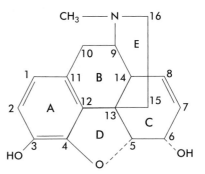

Figure 31.3 Chemical structure of opioids

have a tertiary positively charged (basic) nitrogen separated by an ethylene chain from a quaternary carbon, which is also attached to a phenyl group (Figure 31.3).

The presence of the tertiary nitrogen and its distance from the aromatic ring (4.55 Å for morphine and the related semisynthetic compounds) is considered to be essential for activity. The rigid pentacyclic (phenanthrene) frame of the morphine molecule has a three-dimensional structure in which rings A and B are coplanar and rings C and E are perpendicular to the AB plane. This configuration is common to many compounds with opioid activity. The flat benzene ring (A) lies against the flat part of the receptor, while the piperidine ring (E) fits into a groove in the receptor, to which it is attracted by virtue of its positively charged nitrogen atom.

Substitutions of functional groups on the rings or the core morphine molecule produce opioids with different pharmacological properties.

On the tertiary amine N-17, a short-chain alkyl substitution results in mixed agonist–antagonists such as buprenorphine and nalorphine. Hydroxylation of the C-14 in addition to this converts these into full antagonists. Naloxone is one such antagonist, produced by hydroxylation of nalorphine and modification of the C-6 hydroxyl group to double-bond oxygen. Removal of the methyl group (on the tertiary amine N-17) or replacing it with certain alkyl groups markedly reduces opioid agonist activity.

The phenolic group at C-3 probably interacts with the receptor, since the presence of a hydroxyl group maximises potency, while substituting it with a methyl to make codeine decreases potency 10 times. Longer alkyl side-chain substitutions produce even weaker agonists. Similar alkyl substitutions on C-1 also reduce potency.

C-6 substitutions with lipophilic groups increase activity. Oxidation of C-6 increases potency and the double acetyl substitution at C-3 and C-6 to produce diamorphine increases potency by increasing lipophilicity, despite the competing effects of the dual substitution.

Alterations to the pentacyclic structure of morphine produce the synthetic opioids. Removal of the oxide bridge between rings A and C produces the morphinans, which are generally more potent. Removal of the C ring from the morphinans creates the benzomorphan group. Removal of the methylene bridge from the benzomorphans produces the phenylpiperidine structure of which pethidine is the prototype. The molecule unfolds such that the tertiary nitrogen is now further from the aromatic ring. The phenylpiperidines are all developed from modifications to the structure of pethidine, with sufentanil being a thienyl derivative of fentanyl.

Opioid receptors

Opioid receptors are G-protein-coupled transmembrane receptors. These exist throughout the CNS, with particularly high concentrations in the periaqueductal grey area and the substantia gelatinosa of the spinal cord. They are also present outside the CNS, and this may account for some of the other opioid effects (gastrointestinal) and their postulated value in some peripheral anaesthetic techniques (such as intra-articular injection).

Classification

There have been a number of schemes used to define the various opioid receptor groups. These have in the main been merely new names for the same groups. Three main groups have been classified, to which a fourth (the nociceptin/orphanin receptor) has been added. The grouping has been defined by their response to different *prototype agonists*. The various classifications are shown in Figure 31.4. The current International Union of Basic and Clinical

Figure 31.4 Opioid receptor classification.

Classification	Receptors			
	MOP	**DOP**	**KOP**	**NOP**
	μ	δ	κ	
	OP_3	OP_1	OP_2	OP_4
Subtypes	$μ_1, μ_2$	$δ_1, δ_2$	$κ_1, κ_2, κ_3$	
Prototype agonist	morphine	Ala-leu-enkephalin	ketocyclazocine	
Endogenous ligand	Leu-enkephalin	Leu-enkephalin	dynorphin	nociceptin
	Met-enkephalin	Met-enkephalin	β-endorphin	orphanin FQ peptide
	β-endorphin	β-endorphin		

Pharmacology (IUPHAR) nomenclature for the opioid receptors is MOP (μ, OP_3), KOP (κ, OP_2), DOP (δ, OP_1) and NOP (OP_4). The OP_x type classification can lead to confusion once the receptors are subdivided. Separate genes for each class of opioid receptor have now been identified.

MOP

MOP receptors open potassium ion channels, causing hyperpolarisation and reduced neuronal firing. At the nerve terminal the action potential plateau shortens, thus reducing calcium ion influx and neurotransmitter release. MOP receptors are located in the:

- Primary afferent neurones (pre- and postsynaptic)
- Peripheral sensory neurones
- Periaqueductal grey matter
- Nucleus raphe magnus
- Rostral ventral medulla
- Thalamus
- Cerebral cortex

DOP

DOP receptors also open potassium ion channels, causing hyperpolarisation and reduced neuronal firing. At the nerve terminal the action potential plateau shortens, thus reducing calcium ion influx and neurotransmitter release. DOP receptors are located in the:

- Olfactory bulb
- Cerebral cortex
- Primary afferent neurones (presynaptic)
- Motor integration areas
- Nociception areas

KOP

KOP receptors, in contrast, directly close calcium channels, so that the end result is reduced neurotransmitter release. KOP receptors are found in the:

- Hypothalamus
- Nociception areas

NOP

NOP receptors directly close calcium channels, so that they too result in reduced neurotransmitter release. NOP receptors are located in the:

- Nucleus raphe magnus
- Primary afferent neurones

Sigma receptor

Following the original discovery of μ, δ and κ subtypes, a fourth variant, σ, was originally classified as an opioid receptor. The selective agonist N-allyl-normetazocine (SKF 10047) had been shown to produce mydriasis, tachypnoea, tachycardia and delirium after occupancy of this receptor. The σ receptor is no longer classified as an opioid receptor, as it does not meet the full criteria. Notably:

- It has a high-affinity binding for phencyclidine and related compounds.
- The σ-mediated effects are not reversed by naloxone.
- σ receptors are stereospecific for dextrorotatory isomers.

The σ receptor is not affected by opioids but is bound to by phencyclidine and haloperidol.

Pharmacodynamics

All opioid agonists share a similar pharmacodynamic profile, and demonstrate a sigmoidal dose–effect relationship. In addition to the variety of exogenous opioid agonists, there are a number of endogenous agonist ligands which act on opioid receptors. Many of these agonists lack specificity for a particular subtype of receptor, while the mixed agonist–antagonists exhibit agonist, partial agonist and antagonist actions on the various receptor subtypes (Figure 31.5).

Each of the opioid receptors arises from a separate gene. Opioid receptors belong to the superfamily of serpentine receptors, which contain seven membrane-spanning domains, with an extracellular N-terminus and an intracellular C-terminus. The transmembrane helices are arranged anticlockwise, forming a tight helical bundle. Importantly, the N-terminal and C-terminal tails, and the second and third extracellular loops, are responsible for ligand binding specificity, and for the differential regulation of and variation in coupling to effector systems. The four classes of opioid receptors all produce primary inhibitory effects following activation, via receptor coupling to inhibitory G proteins. This results in inhibition of adenylyl cyclase, with reduced formation of cyclic adenosine monophosphate (cAMP), closure of voltage-sensitive calcium channels, stimulation of inwardly rectifying K^+ channel opening causing membrane hyperpolarisation, and stimulation of phospholipase Cβ. Any excitatory or facilitatory effects of opioids can be explained by the inhibition of inhibitory pathways. Figure 31.6 summarises opioid receptor classification and molecular coupling mechanisms.

Stimulation of the NOP receptor may produce either a pro-nociceptive antanalgesic effect (supraspinal and spinal) or an antinociceptive effect (spinal – at high

Figure 31.5 Effects of opioid receptor activation

Actions	Receptors		
	MOP	DOP	KOP
	OP_3 (μ)	OP_1 (δ)	OP_2 (κ)
Analgesia: supraspinal	++	++	++
Analgesia: spinal	++	++	++
Respiratory depression	++	++	+
Miosis	++	++	++
Gastrointestinal motility decreased	++	++	0
Smooth muscle	++	++	0
Behaviour	Euphoria	Euphoria	Dysphoria
Sedation	++	++	+
Physical dependence	++	++	+
Other			Diuresis

concentrations). The function of this receptor is thought to be in setting pain thresholds and in the formation of tolerance to opioid therapy, although tolerance also develops to its antiopioid effects. Importantly, NOP receptor antagonists produce analgesia, prevent the development of tolerance to opioid analgesia, and may be useful for reducing some of the side effects associated with opioid therapy.

Clinical effects

Opioid agonists cause a range of mainly depressant and some stimulant actions on the CNS via specific receptors. They have little capacity to produce amnesia, have no intrinsic anticonvulsant activity and do not alter seizure threshold.

In anaesthesia, opioids are used for the production of analgesia and the maintenance of haemodynamic stability. Systemically administered opioids produce analgesia through actions at two anatomically distinct regions: supraspinal and spinal sites. They reduce the intensity of pain and the associated fear. This is achieved by raising the pain threshold, altering the reaction to pain, and inducing sleep and hypercapnia. Their efficacy is greater for continuous dull pain rather than sharp intermittent pain. They are less effective for the treatment of neuropathic pain.

CNS effects

Figure 31.7 lists the various effects of opioids on the CNS. Opioids cause a reduction in level of consciousness and eventually produce sleep, with the loss of responsiveness to verbal command. They produce a dose-related decrease in the MAC for volatile anaesthetics, with a ceiling of 60–70% reduction in MAC. They also increase cerebral vasoconstriction in the presence of vasodilating agents such as volatile anaesthetics. They do not cause a loss of cerebral autoregulation or reactivity to CO_2. A ceiling effect is reached on the EEG, with a slowing of EEG frequency and the production of high-voltage (δ) waves.

Cardiovascular effects

Opioids preserve cardiovascular stability to a greater extent than most other anaesthetic drugs. In normovolaemic patients they produce little perturbation in haemodynamic parameters, with minimal cardiac depression, no baroreceptor inhibition and a modest reduction in preload or afterload. Haemodynamic compromise may, however, be observed in individuals whose cardiovascular integrity is dependent on a high level of sympathetic tone, because opioids reduce central sympathetic outflow when even small doses can cause hypotension or cardiovascular collapse. Morphine has the greatest effect on the vascular system, owing to its propensity to cause histamine release

Figure 31.6 Opioid receptor molecular pharmacology

Receptor	Subtypes	Location	Endogenous ligand	Clinical effect
MOP (μ)	μ_1, μ_2	Pre- and postsynaptic on primary afferent neurones and peripheral sensory neurones Periaqueductal grey matter Nucleus raphe magnus Rostral ventral medulla Thalamus Cortex	β-endorphin Leu-enkephalin Met-enkephalin Dynorphin	Supraspinal analgesia (μ_1) Sedation (μ_1) Spinal analgesia (μ_2) Respiratory depression (μ_2) Bradycardia (μ_2) Hypothermia (μ_2) Miosis (μ_2) Euphoria (μ_2) Pruritis (μ_2) Nausea and vomiting (μ_2) Constipation (μ_2) Urinary retention (μ_2) Physical dependence
DOP (δ)	δ_1, δ_2	Olfactory bulb Cerebral cortex Pre-synaptic on primary afferent neurones, motor integration areas and nociception areas	Leu-enkephalin Met-enkephalin	Supraspinal analgesia (δ_1) Spinal analgesia (δ_1) Respiratory depression Constipation Physical dependence
KOP (κ)	κ_1, κ_2, κ_3	Hypothalamus Nociception areas	Dynorphin	Supraspinal analgesia (κ_3) Sedation Spinal analgesia (κ_1) Dysphoria Psychotomimetic effects ↓ vasopressin + diuresis
NOP		Nucleus raphe magnus Primary afferent neurones	Nociception/orphanin FQ peptide	Supraspinal anti-analgesia Spinal anti-analgesia and analgesia Urinary retention

and subsequent indirect effects on catecholamine release. This may result in a tachycardia with a reduction in systemic vascular resistance (SVR) and mean arterial pressure (MAP). The risk can be attenuated by pretreatment with histamine receptor antagonists and volume loading.

Opioids generally produce a negative chronotropic effect via central vagal excitation. Pethidine, however, has a homology with atropine and can produce a tachycardia, and it is the only opioid to produce significant direct myocardial depression when used at high doses. Myocardial depression is not observed unless extraordinarily high doses of morphine or the fentanyl congeners are administered. Morphine has indirect positive inotropic

effects at doses of 1–2 mg kg^{-1}, and blocks neurally and hormonally mediated venoconstriction to reduce preload, making it useful in the treatment of acute congestive heart failure.

Effects on other organ systems

The effects of opioids on the cardiovascular system and other organ systems are summarised in Figure 31.8.

Opioids are the most efficacious of all anaesthetic drugs for attenuating the stress response associated with pain, laryngoscopy and airway manipulation. The plasma concentrations of stress hormones (catecholamines, cortisol, vasopressin, aldosterone and growth hormone) increase during anaesthesia and surgery in proportion to

Figure 31.7 Opioid effects on the CNS

System		Effect
Musculoskeletal	Gait	↓ Physical performance Ataxia ↓ Spinal cord reflexes
	Rigidity	Rigidity occurs 60–90 seconds post-injection and abates spontaneously after 10–20 minutes Mainly thoracoabdominal and upper limb musculature, ↑ with ↑ age, ↑ speed of injection, ↑ dose, use of N_2O Mediated via nucleus raphe magnus
	Multifocal myoclonus	Non-seizure related, ↑ with pethidine
Neural	Central	Spectrum from abnormal eye movement, to contraction of extremities, to tonic–clonic movements Euphoria: especially for agents which cross the blood–brain barrier quickly Dysphoria in some individuals Subjective feelings of body warmth and heavy extremities Apathy ↓ Level of consciousness and eventually sleep ↓ Concentration and capacity for complex reasoning
	EEG	Effects vary between different opioids: slowing of frequency, production of high-voltage δ waves No capacity to produce EEG silence
Cerebrovascular	SSEPs	No effect on SSEPs
	ICP	No effect
	CBF	No effect, but ↑ vasoconstriction with vasodilators
		No loss of autoregulation or CO_2 reactivity $CMRO_2$ reduced by up to 10–25%
Vision	Edinger–Westphal nucleus	Miosis (via a ↓ in inhibition to the nucleus) except pethidine. Reversed by hypoxia and atropine
Thermoregulation	Peripheral effects	Promote hypothermia via ↓ BMR (10–20%), venodilatation, muscle relaxation
	Response	↓ Thermoregulatory responses (as for volatile agents)

the degree of operative trauma. This contributes to increased myocardial work, tissue catabolism and hyperglycaemia – responses associated with increased perioperative morbidity and mortality. Opioids reduce nociception, inhibiting the pituitary–adrenal axis, reducing central sympathetic outflow and influencing centrally mediated neuroendocrine responses. Fentanyl and its congeners (particularly sufentanil) are the most efficacious, but no opioid is completely effective.

Side effects

The organ-specific adverse effects of opioids observed in an individual depend on age, extent of disease, presence of organ dysfunction, concurrent administration of certain drugs, prior opioid exposure and the route of drug administration. Not all adverse effects are deleterious. A number of opioid-induced side effects are produced by activation of opioid receptors either centrally or peripherally, or in both areas. Serious allergic reactions

Figure 31.8 Opioid effects on major organ systems

System		Effect
Cardiovascular	Heart rate	Usually sinus bradycardia via central vagal excitation Occasionally sinus arrest Exacerbated by concomitant vagal stimuli (e.g. laryngoscopy) and β-blockers
	Mean arterial pressure	Usually no effect or a slight ↓ (unless significant bradycardia) Greater ↓ associated with histamine release
	Vascular tree	No effect on SVR (unless histamine release) Mild venodilatation with a ↓ in preload (due to ↓ central sympathetic outflow
	Myocardium	No effect on contractility (except for pethidine which is a depressant) No effect on metabolic rate Possible ischaemic preconditioning
	Excitability	↓ Myocardial conductivity, ↑ Refractory period, ↑ VF threshold
Respiratory	Mechanics	Equivalent ↓ in rate, tidal volume and minute ventilation at equianalgesic doses ↑ Pauses, irregular breathing and apnoeas
	Control	↑ Apnoeic threshold ↓ CO_2 sensitivity ↓ Carotid body chemoreception and hypoxic drive Voluntary control of respiration remains intact No effect on hypoxic pulmonary vasoconstriction
	Airway reflexes	↓ Airway reflexes with improved tolerance of ETT Antitussive via peripheral and central actions ↓ Mucociliary function Brief cough in up to 50% with bolus phenylpiperidines
Gastrointestinal	Stomach and intestines	↓ Peristalsis and secretions, and ↑ tone causing dry stool and constipation ↓ Gastric acid ↓ Gastric emptying with ↑ antral tone and ↓ LOS tone promoting ↑ aspiration risk ↑ Tone of pyloric, ileocaecal, and anal sphincters
	Biliary tree	↑ Bile duct pressure Sphincter of Oddi contraction (little clinical significance overall)
	Chemoreceptor trigger zone	Nausea and vomiting (worse with first dose and ↑ dose interval) Worse postprandial due to concomitant ↑ gastric antral tone
Genitourinary	Kidney	Antidiuresis as a result of ↓ RBF and ↓ GFR (predominates) ↓ Vasopressin release in response to osmotic stimuli
	Bladder	↑ Bladder and urethral tone Vesicular sphincter contraction
Immunity	Immune system	↓ Immunoglobulin production (uncertain significance) Reactivation of herpes simplex virus 2–5 days after neuraxial opioid

to opioids are exceedingly rare, although anaphylaxis has been reported.

At equianalgesic doses all opioids produce equivalent degrees of respiratory depression, with the elderly and neonates being at increased risk. Tolerance develops rapidly to this effect, and with chronic opioid exposure the risk of significant respiratory depression is reduced. Apnoea may occur in conscious patients, but is usually associated with other signs of CNS depression, and apnoeic patients can be instructed to breathe as voluntary control of ventilation remains intact. Sleep, or the concomitant use of other CNS depressants (except clonidine), potentiates the risk by further reducing sensitivity to CO_2.

Opioid-induced depression of airway reflexes is usually regarded as an advantageous side effect, although the impairment of mucociliary function is not. All opioids possess antitussive activity at less than analgesic doses, acting via central and peripheral mechanisms (opioids that do not cross the blood–brain barrier also depress coughing, e.g. pholcodine).

The incidence of nausea associated with opioid use is 10–60%, and this is markedly increased in pain-free and ambulatory patients (via opioid sensitisation of the vestibular nucleus). The ability to produce nausea and vomiting varies between opioids, and also between patients, but tolerance develops rapidly. Substituting one opioid for another may decrease the incidence, as may switching to oral administration.

Constipation remains the most common side effect of chronic opioid administration, and toxic megacolon may occur in patients with ulcerative colitis. Tolerance to this and other smooth muscle effects develops very slowly. Loperamide is a synthetic opioid which does not cross the blood–brain barrier, and it is used specifically as an antimotility agent. All opioids increase bile duct pressure and cause contraction of the sphincter of Oddi in a dose-dependent manner. Pethidine has been incorrectly reported to cause less smooth muscle spasm than the other full agonists, and is equally spasmogenic at equi-analgesic doses. Opioid effects on the biliary tree can be reversed by naloxone (except for pethidine, which produces any smooth muscle contraction via a direct action), nitroglycerine or glucagon.

Other smooth muscle effects involve the genitourinary system. Urinary retention and urgency occur frequently, and are more common in the elderly, and when opioids are administered neuraxially. This latter situation reflects a centrally mediated mechanism through receptors located in the sacral spinal cord.

There are a number of other centrally mediated opioid effects. The majority of these are of no clinical benefit and usually unpleasant. Opioids may cause pruritis with a spectrum of severity, and the mechanism and physiological significance are unknown. The pruritis predominantly affects the face and nose, and is independent of any histamine release. Substituting opioids may decrease the incidence, and it may be alleviated by low-dose naloxone therapy. Muscle rigidity begins at or just after the loss of consciousness, and may manifest as hoarseness in mild cases. Severe episodes can make ventilation almost impossible, even after intubation. It can be minimised by co-administration of induction agents and benzodiazepines, and may be prevented by pretreatment with muscle relaxants. It is aggravated by the use of nitrous oxide. It is seen more commonly with the potent phenylpiperidines than with morphine, the risk is increased with increased opioid dose, and it can be reversed by administration of naloxone.

Opioids decrease thermoregulatory thresholds to a similar degree to the potent volatile agents. Pethidine is unique in its ability to reduce shivering, probably via a KOP-mediated action, and has been effectively utilised for hypothermic, postoperative, blood transfusion-related and epidural-related shivering. Tramadol has also been demonstrated to be efficacious in this regard.

All alkaloids of opium cause a histamine weal when injected intradermally. Histamine release and associated hypotension are variable in incidence and severity, and are reduced by slow IV administration and ameliorated by intravascular fluid loading. The phenylpiperidines (except pethidine) are devoid of this side effect. The histamine release may be localised or generalised, and may cause subjective facial flushing and variable itch.

Opioid-specific effects

A number of important opioid-related therapeutic and adverse effects are specific to the individual opioid being used (e.g. codeine – antitussive and constipation). Pethidine is a unique opioid because of its non-opioid effects. It has a local anaesthetic effect of equivalent potency to cocaine, which gives it advantages when administered neuraxially, and it has a quinidine-like effect on cardiac muscle to reduce cardiac irritability and arrhythmias. Pethidine overdose produces the unique combination of cardiovascular collapse, mydriasis, hyperreflexia and convulsions in addition to respiratory depression.

The phenylpiperidine family (except remifentanil) has been associated with postoperative respiratory depression after high-dose administration, due to secondary peaks in plasma levels. This has been attributed to a number of possible aetiologies, but most probably results from the release of opioid from body stores, with increases in peripheral perfusion and shivering postoperatively.

Opioid metabolites

Some of the significant adverse effects of opioids relate to the production of toxic metabolites. Morphine-3-glucuronide (M3G) may be responsible for the neuroexcitatory effects observed with large-dose chronic morphine administration. Moreover, it may be an opioid antagonist and possibly associated with hyperalgesia (paradoxical pain) seen after morphine administration. Norpethidine has half the analgesic potency of pethidine, but 2–3 times the convulsant activity. Because of the long half-life of norpethidine, significant accumulation occurs within 48 hours and steady state is achieved within 3–6 days. Greater amounts of norpethidine are produced with oral administration. Norpethidine accumulation initially manifests as subtle mood alteration with anxiety, culminating in potentially fatal reactions at higher concentrations. Norpropoxyphene also has a weak opioid action, but causes central excitatory effects and cardiac conduction disturbances.

Not all opioid metabolites are inactive or toxic. In fact some are necessary for clinical efficacy. Examples include morphine and morphine-6-glucuronide (M6G), codeine and morphine, tramadol and its M_1 metabolite. The main metabolite of naltrexone, 6-β-naltrexone, is active with a longer half-life than its parent, and is necessary for the efficacy of naltrexone.

Pharmacokinetics

Figure 31.9 shows pharmacokinetic data for some commonly used opioids.

Administration

The choice of route of administration depends on the opioid being utilised, pain severity, the need for drug titration and any drug or patient contraindications to a particular route. The mode of administration may influence the onset of peak analgesia and side effects. For example, respiratory depression may occur 7 minutes after an IV dose of morphine, but not until ~30 minutes after IM or 6–10 hours after intrathecal dosing.

Certain routes confer advantages for specific opioids. Intrathecal administration may provide a greater quality and potentially a longer duration of pain relief, with a lower incidence of supraspinal effects. However, a higher incidence of specific side effects (nausea, urinary retention, pruritis) occurs. Hydrophilic opioids (morphine) and the active metabolites of diamorphine remain in the CSF for longer, where they produce prolonged analgesia. At higher doses they ascend to produce analgesia at higher segmental levels. An unfortunate and hazardous consequence of this migration is a dose-dependent risk of late respiratory depression (peak 6–10 hours after dose).

Figure 31.9 Pharmacokinetic data for commonly used opioids

Drug	Protein binding (%)	pK_a	Octanol/water partition coefficient	V_d (steady state) $L\ kg^{-1}$	$t_{1/2\beta}$ (min)	Cl (mL kg^{-1} min^{-1})	HER
Alfentanil	92	6.5	129	0.8	100	6	0.4
Buprenorphine	96	8.6		3.0	330	19	0.8
Codeine	10	8.2	0.6	5.4	180	11	0.4
Fentanyl	85	8.4	813	4.0	100	13	0.9
Morphine	35	7.9	1.4	3.5	180	15	0.8
Naloxone	45	7.9	34	2.0	70	25	0.9
Remifentanil	70	7.1	18	0.35	15	50	N/A
Tramadol	20	9.4	1.4	4.0	360	10	0.3

HER, hepatic extraction ratio; V_d, volume of distribution; $t_{1/2}$, half-life

The more lipophilic opioids bind rapidly to local sites, and from there are absorbed intravascularly before they can migrate cephalad.

In respect of epidural opioid pharmacokinetics, dural penetration is related to opioid molecular size and lipophilicity, with sufentanil, fentanyl, and morphine peak CSF concentrations occurring at 6, 20, and 60–240 minutes respectively. Only 3–5% of a morphine dose crosses the dura. Opioid lipophilicity is also important for uptake into peridural fat and epidural veins. Hence, plasma opioid concentrations of lipophilic opioids given epidurally are often equivalent to those levels achieved after IM administration.

No opioid agonist demonstrates dose-dependent pharmacokinetics. First-pass metabolism of orally administered opioids occurs in the liver and the intestinal wall (up to 50%). Opioids given IM or SC have 100% bioavailability, but peak plasma concentrations can vary up to fivefold depending on body temperature, site of administration and haemodynamic status. IV administration results in a much narrower range of plasma concentrations.

The lung exerts a significant first-pass effect on several highly lipid-soluble opioids. Prior administration of other lipophilic amines such as propranolol reduces pulmonary uptake, by saturating binding sites.

Distribution

Opioids undergo variable degrees of protein binding, primarily to α_1-acid glycoprotein, but also to albumin. Fentanyl, sufentanil, and alfentanil also bind to β-globulins, while morphine is bound mainly to albumin. Variability in plasma protein concentration only alters the free fraction for highly protein-bound opioids. Those opioids bound to the acute-phase reactant α_1-acid glycoprotein (especially alfentanil) can achieve variable free concentrations in states of inflammation, infection, malignancy and pregnancy. Dilution or states of low protein concentration increase the free fractions of all highly bound opioids, as does competition for binding sites from other drugs that are basic amines.

Due to their high lipid solubility, most opioids tend to be widely distributed throughout the body, resulting in a large volume of distribution (V_d). Redistribution thus has a significant effect on the decline in opioid plasma concentrations after bolus dosing and short-term infusions of certain opioids. Uptake by muscle, visceral organs and the lung contributes to this redistribution.

Receptor kinetics

The diffusion of an opioid to its site of action (biophase) is dependent on its lipid solubility, the driving concentration gradient and uptake into surrounding tissue. Opioid lipid solubility is usually quantified by a specific oil/water (usually octanol/water) partition coefficient. In addition, all opioids are weak bases that dissolve into solutions of protonated (ionised) and free base fractions. The relative proportions of these fractions are dependent on the pK_a of the specific opioid and the plasma pH. The un-ionised free base form is always more lipid-soluble than the ionised form, and thus the pK_a of any particular agonist is another determinant of its lipid solubility in vivo.

The concentration gradient driving diffusion is dependent on the dose and percentage protein binding. Only the unbound fraction of un-ionised drug constitutes the diffusible fraction, which provides the concentration gradient for diffusion into the biophase.

In the biophase the opioid receptor only recognises the protonated form of the opioid, and ion trapping in the context of an acidic CNS secondary to respiratory acidosis therefore amplifies opioid activity.

Binding to receptor sites depends on receptor affinity and on any non-receptor site binding (e.g. brain lipids). Hydrophilic morphine penetrates the blood–brain barrier slowly, but its low lipid solubility and little non-specific brain binding results in a large mass of drug eventually reaching the effect site, where it binds strongly to the MOP receptor. Moreover, morphine gets 'trapped' in the CNS, and this explains its longer duration of action than predicted by its elimination half-life. The onset and duration of action of an individual opioid therefore represents a complex interaction between its pK_a and the pH of plasma and the pH of the biophase, lipid solubility, and both protein and tissue binding.

Elimination

Opioids predominantly undergo liver metabolism (phase I and/or phase II reactions), with renal excretion of the more hydrophilic metabolites. Some of these metabolites also undergo biliary excretion. Small amounts of the more hydrophilic opioids may be excreted unchanged in the urine. Hepatic blood flow (HBF) is the primary determinant of plasma clearance (Cl) for most opioids, because of their high hepatic extraction ratios (HER).

Morphine

The biotransformation of morphine is unique among the opioids. In the liver 60–80% undergoes glucuronidation to morphine-3-glucuronide (M3G) and 10% to morphine-6-glucuronide (M6G). The remainder undergoes sulphation (significant in the neonate, where glucuronidation metabolism is immature), 5% is demethylated to normorphine, and a small amount is converted to codeine, with 10% being excreted unchanged in the urine. In healthy individuals up to 10% of glucuronidation occurs in extrahepatic sites (kidney and GI tract). The excretion of the morphine glucuronides is directly related to creatinine clearance. Ninety per cent of conjugated morphine is eventually excreted in the urine, and the remainder excreted in bile, sweat and breast milk. M6G is 2–4 times more potent than morphine, and has a much longer elimination half-life. Despite being more hydrophilic than morphine, M6G crosses the blood–brain barrier, from where its elimination is significantly slower. There is also some enterohepatic recirculation of morphine and its glucuronides, particularly in the setting of chronic oral therapy.

Diamorphine

Diamorphine is inactive and requires rapid deacetylation in the CSF, liver, and plasma to 6-monoacetylmorphine and morphine. These active metabolites are more hydrophilic, and their subsequent metabolism is as for morphine.

Codeine

Codeine is mainly metabolised in the liver to codeine conjugates and norcodeine, with some urinary excretion of free codeine. Up to 10% of a dose is also metabolised to morphine by the hepatic microsomal enzyme CYP2D6. This biotransformation is thought to be the major contributor to the analgesia produced by codeine. Due to genetic polymorphisms, 8% of western Europeans are deficient of this enzyme. These individuals require higher doses, and they may still not obtain effective analgesia. Additionally, the variability may lead to dangerously high morphine levels in breast milk.

Pethidine

The majority of pethidine metabolism involves hydrolysis to pethidinic acid, with little free urinary excretion (5%) of the parent drug – although this may be increased to 25% with urinary acidification (pH < 5). One-third of metabolism involves N-demethylation to norpethidine, which is then hydrolysed to norpethidinic acid. Enzyme induction resulting from chronic pethidine use (and carbamazepine therapy) increases the proportion transformed to norpethidine.

Fentanyl and sufentanil

The high lipid solubility of fentanyl and sufentanil contributes to their large volume of distribution, which causes rapid and continued peripheral tissue uptake, limiting initial hepatic metabolism. This results in greater variability in plasma concentrations (13-fold range for fentanyl) during the elimination phase, particularly with fluctuations in muscle blood flow that may contribute to secondary peaks in plasma concentration after large doses. Fentanyl, sufentanil and alfentanil undergo little unchanged renal excretion, being metabolised in the liver via similar pathways. These inactive metabolites are subsequently excreted in the urine. Alfentanil is mainly metabolised by CYP3A3/4 – the most abundantly expressed of the hepatic P450 enzyme isoforms. Variations in the activity of this enzyme are thought to explain the variability in the kinetics and dynamics of alfentanil infusions.

Remifentanil

Remifentanil is a structurally unique methyl ester that undergoes widespread and rapid extrahepatic metabolism by blood and tissue non-specific esterases. This process is non-saturable and results in a clearance that is several times hepatic blood flow. The primary metabolic pathway is de-esterification to a carboxylic acid metabolite, with 90% of the drug recovered from the urine in this form. This metabolite is also a full agonist at μ receptors, but has a potency 1/4600 that of the parent compound and is of no clinical significance even in renal failure. The high clearance and low volume of distribution of remifentanil mean that the offset of its effect is due to metabolism rather than redistribution; this explains its very short context-sensitive half-life irrespective of the duration of infusion. Hypothermia can reduce remifentanil clearance by up to 20%.

All highly lipid-soluble drugs are sequestered into fat stores after prolonged infusions. Even after large single boluses or sequential boluses there is likely to be a delayed clinical recovery because the fall in plasma drug concentration by elimination of drug from the central compartment is retarded by the return of opioid from the peripheral compartments. Hence, the time for the plasma drug concentration to fall by 50% after an infusion ceases is influenced by the duration of the infusion, representing the degree to which the peripheral compartment has become saturated – so-called 'context-sensitive'. The context-sensitive half-life for most opioids, except remifentanil, increases with increasing duration of infusion.

Figure 31.10 Factors influencing opioid pharmacokinetics and pharmacodynamics

Physiological state	Effect	Mechanism
Obesity	Overdosage	Central V_d is not reflected by actual body weight ↑ Total V_d prolongs elimination half-life
Elderly	↑ Sensitivity to opioid	↓ Neuronal cell mass ↓ Central V_d
	Prolonged effect of infusion	↓ Lean body mass with ↑ adipose tissue causes increase in total V_d ↓ HBF (by 40–50% by age 75)
Infant	Prolonged effect	↓ Conjugating capacity Immature renal function (both approach adult values by 1–3 months)
Renal failure	Morphine toxicity	Accumulation of M6G Possible hydrolysis of glucuronides back to parent compound Uraemia potentiates CNS depression and ↑ blood–brain barrier permeability
	Pethidine toxicity	Accumulation of norpethidine
Hepatic failure	↑ Sensitivity to opioids (in severe liver failure only)	Synergism if encephalopathic Altered integrity of blood–brain barrier ↑ Elimination half-life for pethidine and tramadol

For example, although fentanyl has an elimination half life of 3–5 hours, in the steady state its context-sensitive half-life is 7–12 hours.

Patient factors influencing opioid pharmacokinetics and pharmacodynamics

The pharmacokinetics and dynamics of opioids may be altered in a number of physiological states (Figure 31.10). The pharmacokinetic parameters of opioids are unrelated to absolute body weight except for distribution parameters. Rather, they correspond to lean body weight, and dosages should be on the basis of ideal (estimated lean) body weight. Caution in obese individuals is recommended when giving prolonged infusions of all opioids other than remifentanil, because their larger volume of distribution will prolong the elimination half-life.

Renal failure is only of clinical significance for the use of morphine and pethidine. The elimination half-life of morphine glucuronides increases from 4 to 14–119 hours in renal failure. Fatal and near-fatal CNS toxicities including convulsions and extreme tachycardia and hypertension have occurred with the use of pethidine from

norpethidine accumulation in individuals with renal failure. These CNS effects are not mediated by opioid receptors, and not reversible with naloxone. A similar accumulation occurs with norpropoxyphene. The clearance of the fentanyl congeners is not altered appreciably, although the reduction in plasma proteins may potentially alter the free fraction of the opioid.

Surprisingly, the pharmacokinetics of most opioids is unchanged in liver failure, except in the setting of liver transplantation. This demonstrates the substantial metabolic reserve of the liver, particularly in relation to conjugation reactions. Liver disease may be reflected by a variable reduction in metabolic capacity, hepatic blood flow (HBF) and hepatocellular mass. It also causes a reduction in plasma proteins and increases in total body water through the formation of oedema, which may alter distribution kinetics and unbound drug fractions. Synergistic and unpredictable CNS depression may occur in the setting of hepatic encephalopathy. The metabolism of morphine is the least likely to be altered by liver disease, mainly because of the preservation of glucuronidation in all but fulminant liver failure. Also, a significant contribution to metabolism (at least 30%) is by increased extrahepatic (kidney and GI tract) activity. Importantly, any reduction in liver clearance will increase the oral bioavailability of morphine. During liver transplantation the offset of the effect of morphine is due to redistribution. The metabolism and clearance of the fentanyl congeners is also relatively preserved in most stages of hepatic failure. Fentanyl and sufentanil disposition may be altered only if given in high doses in severe liver dysfunction. There is no change to the pharmacokinetic profile of remifentanil, even during the anhepatic phase of liver transplantation. Pethidine is the only opioid whose clearance is decreased in liver dysfunction. Similarly, considerable dosage reductions are necessary for tramadol, as the clearance is markedly reduced.

Acid–base changes have complex effects on opioid pharmacokinetics, with unpredictable consequences. Alterations in pH have competing effects on drug ionisation (with ion trapping), plasma protein binding and cerebral blood flow, which result in both respiratory acidosis and respiratory alkalosis prolonging the action of opioids.

The use of opioids is also cautioned in hypothyroid patients and those with adrenocortical insufficiency, because of the potential for significant effects on haemodynamics.

Opioid drug interactions

The opioids have limited but important interactions with other drugs. Predictably, they produce synergistic effects on the level of consciousness with other CNS depressants. Benzodiazepines, barbiturates and propofol act synergistically on loss of consciousness, but increase the risk of cardiovascular depression. In anaesthesia the use of opioids allows the concentrations of volatile anaesthetic agents to be reduced by up to 50% while ensuring amnesia and immobility, with the preservation of haemodynamic stability at low inhaled concentrations (≤ 1 MAC).

The use of opioids (particularly pethidine and tramadol) with monoamine oxidase inhibitors (MAOIs) may result in serious and potentially fatal sequelae. Morphine has been recommended as the preferred opioid for use in these patients. The interaction of pethidine with MAOI may produce excitatory (type I) or inhibitory (type II) reactions. Excitatory phenomena include agitation, headache, haemodynamic instability, fever, rigidity, convulsions and coma. This is attributed to excessive CNS serotonin activity, since both MAOI and pethidine block serotonin reuptake. The inhibitory syndrome consists of respiratory depression, coma and hypotension, and is the result of MAOI inhibition of hepatic microsomal enzymes with secondary pethidine accumulation. A similar excitatory ('serotonergic') syndrome is seen with the combination of tramadol and the selective serotonin–noradrenaline reuptake inhibitors (SNRIs). The risk is increased in individuals with CYP2D6 polymorphisms, which make them extensive metabolisers of tramadol.

Opioid antagonists

The only opioid antagonists currently used in clinical practice are naloxone and naltrexone.

Naloxone

Naloxone is an N-allyl derivative of oxymorphone. It is a pure opioid antagonist, having no intrinsic pharmacological activity. It has a high affinity for MOP but also blocks other opioid receptors. Naloxone reverses the respiratory depression and analgesia of opioids and precipitates withdrawal in opioid addicts. It may also block the actions of endogenous opioids. Intravenous administration of 200– 400 µg of naloxone will reverse the respiratory depressant effects of opioids, but incremental titration (1.5–3 µg kg^{-1}) is preferable in order to minimise the reversal of the analgesic effects of the opioids. Naloxone acts for approximately 30 minutes, so further doses or an infusion may be necessary to avoid the return of the respiratory-depressant effects of any agonist that outlasts the effects of naloxone. Naloxone is also effective in alleviating the pruritis and urinary retention of intrathecal and epidural opioids. Naloxone has an oral bioavailability of only 2% because of extensive first-pass metabolism.

Naltrexone

Naltrexone is an analogue of naloxone that has a longer duration of action (elimination half-life of 8 hours). Naltrexone is effective orally because it has a low first-pass effect. It is used as maintenance therapy in the management of dependency because it blocks the euphoria of high doses of opioids in relapsing cases.

Tramadol

Tramadol is a unique drug with a complex mode of action, only part of which is mediated through opioid receptors.

Tramadol is a phenylpiperidine analogue of codeine. Tramadol acts as a weak agonist at all types of opioid receptor, with some selectivity for the µ receptor. It has one-tenth the potency of morphine. Tramadol also blocks the reuptake of noradrenaline and 5-HT (serotonin) and facilitates release of the latter, to modify nociceptive transmission by activation of the descending inhibitory pathways in the CNS. Naloxone therefore only partially reverses the analgesic effects of tramadol. Tramadol is a racemic mixture of (+)tramadol and (–)tramadol and it appears that the two enantiomers have separate effects at opioid and non-opioid sites. (+)Tramadol affects μ receptors and 5-HT reuptake and release, while (–)tramadol inhibits noradrenaline release. Effects on α_2-adrenergic, NMDA and benzodiazepine receptors may be due to indirect effects secondary to noradrenergic effects.

Tramadol is used in the treatment of moderate to severe pain. It is well absorbed orally, with a bioavailability of 68%, and only 20% is protein-bound. Tramadol is extensively metabolised in the liver by N-desmethylation, O-desmethylation and conjugation, with 90% being excreted in the urine. The elimination half-life is 4–6 hours. The metabolite O-desmethyltramadol (half-life 9 hours) has 2–4 times greater analgesic potency than tramadol, and caution should be used in hepatic and renal impairment.

Tramadol exhibits little respiratory depression when compared to equianalgesic doses of morphine. Cardiovascular effects are minimal. Other reported side effects include dizziness, sedation, nausea, dry mouth, sweating and skin rashes. There is a low potential for abuse and physical dependence, although abuse has been reported. Tramadol is now a Schedule 3 Controlled Drug in the UK (does not require a register and signature).

Concomitant use of MAOIs is contraindicated. Co-administration with carbamazepine may decrease the concentration and effect of tramadol.

Non-steroidal anti-inflammatory drugs (NSAIDs)

Examples – diclofenac, ibuprofen, ketorolac, mefenamic acid, naproxen

The non-steroidal anti-inflammatory agents share several properties with aspirin and may be considered together. Injectable preparations of the 'aspirin-like' NSAIDs ketorolac, diclofenac, ketoprofen and tenoxicam provide perioperative analgesia free from opioid disadvantages of respiratory depression, sedation, nausea and vomiting, gastrointestinal stasis or abuse potential. NSAIDs have analgesic, anti-inflammatory and antipyretic effects, and those used for pain relief produce marked analgesia with less anti-inflammatory action.

NSAID absorption is rapid by all routes of administration, whether by mouth or by injection. The drugs are highly protein-bound, with low volumes of distribution, and the unbound fraction is active. Consequently, NSAIDs can potentiate the effects of other highly protein-bound drugs by displacing them from protein binding sites (oral anticoagulants, oral hypoglycaemics, sulphonamides and anticonvulsants).

Mechanism of action
Prostaglandin synthesis inhibition
Many NSAID and aspirin effects are mediated by inhibition of prostaglandin synthesis in peripheral tissues, nerves and the CNS (Figure 31.11). Aspirin acetylates and irreversibly inhibits cyclo-oxygenase, while NSAIDs act by competitive inhibition. However, the NSAIDs and aspirin may have other mechanisms of action independent of any effect on prostaglandins, including effects on basic cellular and neuronal processes. Prostaglandins (PG) were initially described as locally active substances from the prostate gland that produced smooth muscle contraction. Many are now recognised, based on a 20-carbon chain molecule, being one family of the eicosanoids (from Greek *eicosi*, twenty), oxygenated metabolites of arachidonic acid and other polyunsaturated fatty acids that include leukotrienes.

The rate of prostaglandin synthesis is normally low, being regulated by tissue stimuli or trauma, which activates phospholipases to free arachidonic acid, from which prostaglandins are produced by prostaglandin endoperoxide (PGH) synthase, which has both cyclo-oxygenase and hydroperoxidase enzymatic sites. Prostaglandins have many physiological functions including gastric mucosal protection, maintenance of renal tubular function and renal vasodilatation and bronchodilatation. Endothelial prostacyclin produces vasodilatation and prevents platelet adhesion, and platelet thromboxane produces aggregation and vessel spasm.

Cyclo-oxygenase isoenzymes
Two subtypes of cyclo-oxygenase enzyme (*constitutional* COX-1 and *inducible* COX-2) have been identified. NSAIDs, like aspirin, are non-selective cyclo-oxygenase inhibitors that inhibit both COX-1 and COX-2. Non-selective COX-1 and COX-2 inhibition confers both the analgesic and the adverse-effect profile of NSAIDs.

The two isolated COX isoenzymes have 75% amino acid homology, with complete preservation of the

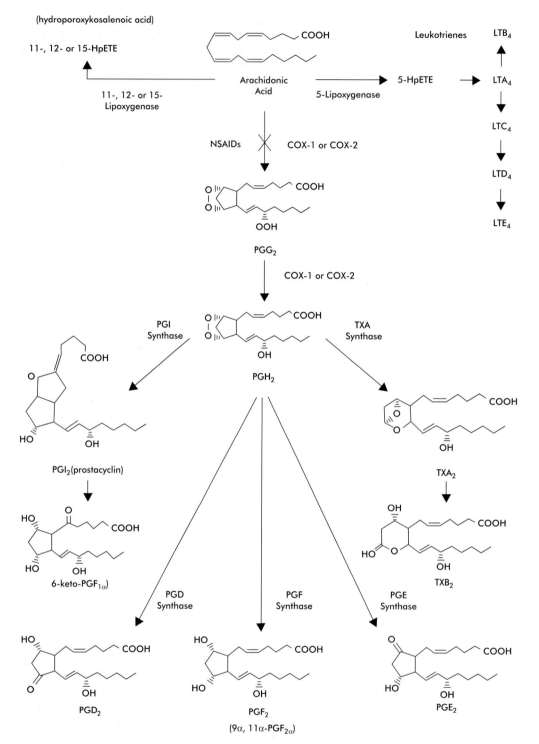

Figure 31.11 Prostaglandin synthesis pathways

catalytic sites for cyclo-oxygenase and peroxidase activity, with almost identical enzyme kinetics.

COX-1

COX-1 is a membrane-bound haemoglycoprotein with a molecular weight of 71,000 daltons found in the endoplasmic reticulum of prostaglandin-producing cells. The enzyme cyclises arachidonic acid and then adds a 15-hydroperoxy group to form the endoperoxide PGG_2, which is then reduced to the hydroxy form of PGH_2 by a peroxidase in the same COX enzyme protein. The COX-1 isoenzyme integrates into only a single leaflet of the lipid bilayer, and this is described as a monotopic arrangement. The enzyme has three independent folding units: an epidermal growth-factor-like domain, a membrane binding domain and an enzymatic domain. The helices of the membrane binding domains form a channel entrance to the active site, are inserted into the membrane, and thereby allow arachidonic acid to gain access into the interior of the lipid bilayer. The sites for cyclo-oxygenase and peroxidase activity are spatially distinct but adjacent to each other. The COX active site is a long hydrophobic channel. NSAIDs block COX-1 halfway down the channel by hydrogen bonding (reversible). Aspirin acetylates serine, irreversibly preventing access for arachidonic acid.

COX-2

COX-2 has a molecular weight of 70,000 daltons, with similar sites to COX-1 for the attachment of arachidonic acid, and a similar three-dimensional structure to COX-1. However, its active site has a greater volume, because it has a larger central channel with a wider entrance and a secondary internal pocket, and therefore COX-2 can accommodate larger drugs than COX-1. A single amino acid difference at position 523 is critical for the COX-1 and COX-2 selectivity of the NSAIDs. In COX-2 a valine molecule replaces the isoleucine molecule present at position 523 in COX-1. This valine molecule is smaller and produces a gap in the wall of the channel, giving access to a side pocket, which is the binding site of the COX-2 selective inhibitors. The larger isoleucine at position 523 in COX-1 blocks access of drug molecules to the side pocket.

The genes for the two isoenzymes are found on different chromosomes. Under physiological conditions COX-1 activity predominates, to produce prostaglandins that regulate rapid physiological responses such as vascular homeostasis, gastric function, platelet activity and renal function. The concentration of the COX-1 isoenzyme is low, but it may increase two- to fourfold in response to stimulation by hormones or growth factors. Low concentrations of COX-2 can normally be detected in the brain, kidney and the gravid uterus. COX-2 mRNA expression by monocytes, synovial cells and fibroblasts may be increased 10–80-fold when stimulated by growth factors, cytokines, bacterial lipopolysaccharides or phorbol esters. These factors increase COX-2 production and tissue PGE_2 concentrations, resulting in pain and inflammation.

Efficacy of NSAIDs

NSAIDs are effective as postoperative analgesics. The *number needed to treat* (NNT, essentially the number of patients in a study to whom the drug must be given to show a benefit) for ketorolac 10 mg is 2.6, diclofenac 50 mg 2.3, and ibuprofen 400 mg 2.4. For comparison, the NNT of morphine 10 mg (intramuscularly) is 2.9, and codeine 60 mg (orally) 16.7. When given in combination with opioids, NSAIDs produce better analgesia and reduce opioid consumption by 25–50%. NSAIDs are insufficient for sole use for the relief of very severe pain immediately after major surgery, although they are very useful analgesic adjuncts, improving pain relief while reducing opioid requirements.

Adverse effects

Prostaglandins are local tissue hormones regulating function, and interference with their synthesis can produce specific problems. With acute use the main concerns are the potential of producing peptic ulceration, interference with platelets, renal impairment and bronchospasm in individuals who have 'aspirin-induced asthma'. In general, the risk and severity of NSAID-associated side effects increases with age.

The gastric and duodenal epithelia have protective mechanisms against acid and enzyme attack involving prostaglandin production, and chronic NSAID use is associated with peptic ulceration and bleeding. Unfortunately, acute gastroduodenal damage and bleeding can occur even with short-term NSAID use.

Platelet cyclo-oxygenase is essential for the production of the cyclic endoperoxides and thromboxane A_2, which mediate vasoconstriction and platelet aggregation, the primary haemostatic response to vessel injury. Aspirin acetylates cyclo-oxygenase irreversibly, but NSAIDs inhibit platelet cyclo-oxygenase in a reversible fashion. Single doses of NSAIDs such as ketorolac and diclofenac inhibit platelet function (prolong skin bleeding time and inhibit platelet function in vitro), but do not tend to increase surgical blood loss in normal patients. However, the presence of a subclinical bleeding diathesis or administration of anticoagulants may increase the risk of significant surgical blood loss when NSAIDs are given.

Conversely, NSAIDs and COX-2 inhibitors have a small prothrombotic effect, which has led to guidance (European and UK) on their usage. The risk appears to be greatest with prolonged usage and higher doses, and for the more selective agents (COX-2 inhibitors and diclofenac). Diclofenac 150 mg has a similar risk to etoricoxib, and ibuprofen in doses of 2400 mg a day also increases risk. Naproxen 1 g daily and ibuprofen 1.2 g daily have not shown any increased risk.

Renal prostaglandins have important physiological roles, including the maintenance of blood flow and glomerular filtration, regulation of tubular electrolyte handling and modulation of the actions of renal hormones. The adverse renal effects of chronic NSAID use are well recognised. In certain clinical settings where there are high plasma concentrations of the vasoconstrictors renin, angiotensin, noradrenaline and vasopressin, intrarenal vasodilators including prostacyclin are produced and renal function can then be impaired by NSAID administration. The co-administration of other potential nephrotoxins, such as gentamicin, may increase the renal effect of NSAIDs. Nevertheless, with careful patient selection and monitoring the incidence of NSAID-induced renal impairment is low in the perioperative period.

Precipitation of bronchospasm is a recognised phenomenon in individuals with asthma, chronic rhinitis and nasal polyps. Such 'aspirin-induced asthma' affects 10–15% of asthmatics, can be severe, and features cross-sensitivity with NSAIDs. A history of aspirin-induced asthma is a contraindication to NSAID use after surgery. The mechanism is unclear, but the reaction increases with cyclo-oxygenase inhibitor potency. Cyclo-oxygenase inhibition may increase the arachidonic acid availability for production of inflammatory leukotrienes by lipooxygenase pathways. Aspirin-induced asthma is less common in children, and the susceptibility may be precipitated in adult life by viral illness.

Selective cyclo-oxygenase-2 inhibitors

Examples – celecoxib, etoricoxib, meloxicam, parecoxib

New drugs have been developed that selectively inhibit the inducible cyclo-oxygenase enzyme, COX-2, and spare the constitutive enzyme, COX-1. The COX-2 inhibitors include meloxicam, nimesulide and parecoxib – the injectable valdecoxib precursor. By sparing physiological-tissue prostaglandin production while inhibiting inflammatory prostaglandin release, COX-2 inhibitors offer the potential of effective analgesia but with fewer side effects than the NSAIDs. Unfortunately, associated cardiovascular prothrombotic toxicity has minimised their role in clinical practice. Valdecoxib has been withdrawn because of concerns about thrombotic events.

COX-2 inhibitors can produce effective analgesia for moderate to severe acute pain, such as after surgery, similar to that of the NSAIDs. Quoted NNTs are comparable to those for conventional NSAIDs: parecoxib 20 mg IV 3.0; parecoxib 40 mg IV 2.2.

COX-2 inhibitors produce less clinically significant peptic ulceration than other NSAIDs. However, peptic ulceration remains a significant adverse effect of the COX-2 inhibitors, and there is continuing debate on the role of COX-2 inhibitors in patients who have other risk factors for complicated ulcer disease: the elderly, those on aspirin or corticosteroids, those with a previous ulcer or *H. pylori* infection.

Platelets do not produce COX-2 (only COX-1), and so COX-2 selective inhibitors do not impair platelet function. Studies have confirmed the lack of an antiplatelet effect of COX-2 inhibitors, and a reduction in surgical blood loss in comparison to NSAIDs. Unfortunately, because they inhibit endothelial prostacyclin production while sparing platelet function, it is now apparent that COX-2 inhibitors can produce a tendency to thrombosis, increasing the risk of thrombotic adverse events.

COX-2 is resident (constitutive) in some tissues, including the kidneys, and COX-2 inhibitors have similar adverse effects on renal function to conventional NSAIDs.

Paracetamol

Paracetamol is the active metabolite of the earlier (more toxic) drugs acetanilide and phenacetin. It can be given orally, rectally or parenterally, has little anti-inflammatory activity, and is an effective analgesic and antipyretic. It is absorbed rapidly from the small intestine after oral administration Paracetamol has lower protein binding than NSAIDs (and hence fewer potential drug interactions) and a higher volume of distribution. The recommended dose in adults is 0.5–1 g oral or rectal, every 4–6 hours when necessary, and a maximum of 6 g a day in divided doses for acute use and 4 g a day for chronic use.

Paracetamol inhibits prostaglandin synthesis in the CNS. In clinical doses it has insignificant peripheral anti-inflammatory action. Unlike morphine, paracetamol has no apparent binding sites, and unlike NSAIDs it does not inhibit peripheral cyclo-oxygenase activity. There is some evidence of a central antinociceptive effect of paracetamol. Postulated mechanisms include central COX-2 inhibition, inhibition of a central cyclo-oxygenase, COX-3, that is selectively susceptible to paracetamol, and modulation of descending serotonergic pathways that suppress spinal cord nociceptive transmission. There is also evidence of agonism at the CB_1 cannabinoid receptor. Paracetamol may also inhibit prostaglandin production at the cellular transcriptional level, independent of cyclo-oxygenase activity.

Nitroxyparacetamol (nitroacetaminophen) is a novel potent nitric-oxide-releasing version with anti-inflammatory and analgesic properties that has a described mechanism of action in the spinal cord that differs from paracetamol, and has less hepatotoxicity.

The NNT of paracetamol is 3.8 (compared with morphine 10 mg IM 2.9, ibuprofen 400 mg 2.4, codeine 60 mg 16.7). The combination of paracetamol 1000 mg plus codeine 60 mg has an NNT of 2.2. Paracetamol is therefore an effective analgesic, with potency somewhat less than a standard dose of morphine. Paracetamol is an effective adjunct to opioid analgesia, and regular administration after surgery can reduce opioid requirements by 20–30%; the addition of NSAIDs to paracetamol also improves efficacy. Paracetamol is thus an integral component of multimodal analgesia in combination with NSAIDs and opioids. Paracetamol has fewer side effects than the NSAIDs, and can be used when the latter are contraindicated (asthma, peptic ulcers, bleeding diathesis). However, paracetamol overdose can produce severe liver damage. A small amount of paracetamol undergoes cytochrome P450-mediated hydroxylation, producing a toxic metabolite that is normally rendered harmless by liver glutathione conjugation. With excessive doses the rate of reactive metabolite formation exceeds that of glutathione conjugation, and the result is centrilobular hepatocellular necrosis. Doses of more than 150 mg kg^{-1} taken within 24 hours may result in severe liver damage, hypoglycaemia and acute tubular necrosis. Individuals taking enzyme-inducing agents are more susceptible. Early signs include nausea and vomiting, with right subcostal pain and tenderness. Damage is maximal 3–4 days after ingestion, and may lead to death. Treatment includes gastric emptying, and administration of methionine or acetylcysteine. Plasma paracetamol concentration versus time from ingestion indicates liver damage risk after overdose (acetylcysteine should be given if the plasma paracetamol concentration is greater than 200 mg L^{-1} at 4 hours and 6.25 mg L^{-1} at 24 hours after ingestion). Nitroxyparacetamol may have less hepatic toxicity than its parent drug.

Other analgesic drugs

α_2-Agonists

Examples – clonidine, dexmedetomidine

The α_2-agonists clonidine and dexmedetomidine have been shown to provide effective analgesia after a variety of surgical procedures. Attention has concentrated on spinal or epidural administration of clonidine to take advantage of the known attenuating effect of stimulating spinal α_2-receptors on pain perception. In general, α_2-agonists are useful only as adjuncts to conventional opioid analgesics because of the side effects of sedation, hypotension and bradycardia, which can be marked. Epidural administration has been shown to be more effective than the systemic route, supporting the theory that clonidine acts via spinal α_2-receptors. High-dose epidural clonidine has been successfully used as a sole analgesic following major abdominal surgery, but with a significant incidence of sedation and hypotension. There is some evidence that systemic clonidine administration may have some analgesic effect. Clonidine, when given orally as a premedication, reduces both the requirement for postoperative morphine and the incidence of nausea and vomiting. Clonidine is useful in the treatment of neuropathic pain, and can also be used to modify opioid withdrawal states. In addition, spinal infusions of clonidine with opioids and local anaesthetic agents may be of considerable benefit in the treatment of complex regional pain syndromes (CRPS).

Dexmedetomidine may be infused for ICU sedation as an alternative to propofol or midazolam. It has a distribution half-life of 8 minutes, a terminal half-life of 3 hours, a volume of distribution of 170 L and clearance of 50 L h^{-1}.

Anticonvulsants

Examples – carbamazepine, gabapentin, lamotrigine, phenytoin, sodium valproate, vigabatrin

Anticonvulsants are useful for the alleviation of neuropathic pain. Drugs used include carbamazepine, phenytoin, sodium valproate and the newer agents gabapentin, pregabalin, lamotrigine and vigabatrin. Suggested mechanisms of action include frequency-dependent block of sodium channels, calcium channel blockade and potentiation of GABA inhibition of spinal nociceptive pathways via increased release or reduced breakdown. Meta-analyses have demonstrated that anticonvulsants are effective for neuropathic pain, but with frequent adverse effects. For example the NNT for carbamazepine for trigeminal neuralgia is 2.6, while the *number needed to harm* (NNH) is only 3.4 patients. Therefore the effectiveness of anticonvulsants for neuropathic pain must be balanced against adverse effects, which may be serious. Common side effects include sedation, rashes, nausea, anorexia, dizziness, confusion and ataxia. Serious side effects are blood dyscrasias, subacute hepatic impairment, renal failure and Stevens–Johnson syndrome. Gabapentin (and pregabalin) offer the potential of similar efficacy with an improved safety profile, but gabapentin can produce the significant adverse effects of pancreatitis, altered liver function tests and Stevens–Johnson syndrome.

Antidepressants

Example – amitriptyline

The tricyclic antidepressants used to relieve neuropathic pain all have noradrenergic activity by inhibition of adrenaline reuptake from nerve endings, probably in descending modulatory inhibitory pain pathways. The antidepressants have similar NNT and NNH to the anticonvulsants and are again effective for the relief of neuropathic pain, but with the cost of common side effects, many related to a vagolytic effect. Some tricyclic side effects are transitory, such as dry mouth and sedation, but others are serious, including postural hypotension, urinary retention, narrow angle glaucoma, paralytic ileus and cardiac arrhythmias. The elderly are particularly susceptible to side effects when given tricyclic antidepressants. Unfortunately newer antidepressants with a better side-effect profile have not been shown to be as effective for the treatment of neuropathic pain.

Cannabinoids

Delta-9-tetrahydrocannabinol (Δ^9-THC) is the main active constituent of the cannabis plant (*Cannabis sativa*). It is used as a recreational drug but it has value as an analgesic and antiemetic in cancer treatment.

Two cannabinoid receptors have been identified, CB_1 and CB_2. These are both G-protein-coupled receptor complexes. CB_1 is the neuronal receptor found in the brain and spinal cord. Relatively few receptors are in the brainstem. CB_2 is predominantly found peripherally.

Δ^9-THC is highly lipophilic but has a low potency. Nabilone is a non-selective cannabinoid receptor agonist that is less lipophilic and a more potent agonist. Anandamide, a derivative of phospholipase D, has been identified as an endogenous ligand for CB_1. The breakdown pathway for this is inhibited by NSAIDs. The precise role of this in vivo is yet unclear.

Δ^9-THC causes:

- Antiemesis
- Analgesia
- Increased pulse rate
- Decreased blood pressure
- Muscle weakness
- Increased appetite
- Euphoria then drowsiness
- Psychological interference

The main use of cannabinoids at present is in antiemesis. Nabilone is a synthetic dibenzopyran cannabinol that acts on the vomiting centre. It is licensed for use for the antagonism of resistant cytotoxic-induced nausea, but has largely been superseded by ondansetron. Δ^9-THC has analgesic properties and causes less dysphoria and drowsiness than nabilone. The route of administration may also affect the spectrum of effects.

Lidocaine

The amide local anaesthetic lidocaine can be a very useful diagnostic test and treatment for neuropathic pain. The dose is 0.5–1.5 mg kg^{-1} h^{-1} by subcutaneous or intravenous infusion, and it may be continued for a number of days to control neuropathic pain quickly before long-term oral therapy is instituted if required.

NMDA antagonists

Examples – dextromethorphan, ketamine

The activation by excitatory amino acids (glutamate) of spinal cord dorsal horn N-methyl-D-aspartate (NMDA) receptors is essential for the development of central sensitisation after tissue damage. The anaesthetic agent ketamine is a potent NMDA receptor antagonist, and relatively low-dose ketamine given by subcutaneous or intravenous continuous infusion produces significant pain relief. When combined with opioids, ketamine improves analgesia and reduces side effects. Unfortunately the side effects of ketamine, including hallucinations, limit the use of this agent. A notable advantage of ketamine is that it is effective both for nociceptive and for neuropathic pain, which presents as burning stinging pain with allodynia and dysaesthesias. Ketamine can be of particular benefit in clinical situations where the pain may be of a mixed nociceptive and neuropathic nature (e.g. severe burns or cancer pain with nerve involvement). Dextromethorphan, a component of cough mixtures, is an alternative, although less potent, NMDA receptor antagonist that has been shown to reduce opioid requirements following abdominal surgery.

Steroids

The role of corticosteroids as analgesics is limited to short-term relief of neuropathic pain where nerve compression is a feature.

Future developments

Nicotinic acetylcholine receptor agonists

Epibatidine, from the skin of an Ecuadorian frog (*Epipedobates tricolor*) and used as an arrow poison, has potent analgesic properties, and is an agonist of nicotinic acetylcholine receptors (nAChR). There are two enantiomers of epibatidine, R(+)epibatidine being the naturally occurring substance. Pharmacologically their activity is similar. Nicotinic acetylcholine receptors have five subunits, but it is now known that there is considerable diversity in the amino acid composition of a particular subunit. For example, there are at least nine variants of α and four variants of β subunit, and this may explain the differing affinities for various agonists in different locations. In the CNS, nAChR has a higher affinity for epibatidine than for acetylcholine or nicotine. Epibatidine has numerous nicotinic agonist effects that make it unsuitable as a pure analgesic. If drugs with a high affinity for specific central nAChR groups involved in nociception can be developed without the multitude of other effects then this may be a future method of analgesia.

Tachykinins

Tachykinins are a group of neuropeptides including substance P and neurokinins A and B. Substance P and neurokinin A (NKA) are released in the spinal cord in response to peripheral noxious stimuli. Three tachykinin receptors (NK-1, NK-2, NK-3) have been identified. They enhance neurotransmission in the pain pathways. In acute nociception NKA is the main mediator acting on NK-2 receptors. In pathological pain such as inflammatory hyperalgesia NK-1 receptors are more important. Substance P is more active at NK-1, and in addition stimulates the release of peripheral inflammatory mediators such as bradykinin. NK-1 receptor antagonists inhibit pain transmission and appear to reduce inflammatory vasodilatation and plasma protein leakage.

Other centrally mediated contenders

Agonists and antagonists of a number of neurological systems may provide future advances in analgesia:

- Calcitonin gene-related peptide (CGRP) is released in the dorsal horn by afferent fibres in response to noxious stimuli. The neuropeptides somatostatin and galanin cause analgesia, while cholecystokinin inhibits opioid-mediated analgesia.
- Galanin is another neuropeptide released from afferent nociceptive neurones. It appears to inhibit nociceptive dorsal horn transmission.
- The amino acid glutamine, released by C fibres, is an agonist at NMDA receptors and may be responsible (in conjunction with substance P) for 'wind-up'. Ketamine blocks the NMDA ion channel, and this probably affects analgesia.
- Adenosine acts on A_1 (inhibitory) and A_2 (excitatory) receptors to influence synaptic transmission. Both receptor types are found within the CNS, including the dorsal horn. Intrathecal administration of adenosine analogues produces antinociception.

Specific pharmacology

In this section bioavailability applies to oral administration. Units (unless stated otherwise) are:
Volume of distribution at steady state (V_d): L kg^{-1}
Clearance (Cl): mL kg^{-1} min^{-1}
Terminal half-life ($t_{1/2}$): minutes

Alfentanil

Structure – anilinopiperidine opioid analogue of fentanyl

Presentation – colourless aqueous solution (500 μg mL^{-1} in 2 and 10 mL ampoules; 5 μg mL^{-1} ampoules also available)

Dose
IV bolus 10–50 μg kg^{-1}
IV infusion 0.5–1 μg kg^{-1} min^{-1}

Pharmacokinetics

Protein binding	92%
pK$_a$	6.5
V$_d$	0.8
Cl	6
t$_{1/2}$	100
Peak effect within 90 s, duration 5–10 min	

CNS – potent μ opioid receptor agonist, 10–20 times more potent analgesic than morphine

CVS – bradycardia, hypotension may occur. Obtunds cardiovascular responses to laryngoscopy and intubation in doses of 30–50 μg kg^{-1}

RS – potent respiratory depressant; chest wall rigidity may occur

Other – nausea and vomiting; no histamine release

Elimination – predominantly hepatic metabolism by N-dealkylation to noralfentanil, < 1% excreted unchanged via kidneys

Contraindications – concurrent administration with monoamine oxidase inhibitors

Codeine

Structure – a morphine analogue (3-methyl morphine); a principal alkaloid of opium

Presentation

Oral – tablets 15, 30 and 60 mg; syrup 5 μg mL^{-1}

IV – colourless aqueous solution, 60 μg mL^{-1} (1 mL ampoules). Often combined with non-opioid analgesics such as paracetamol as tablets (cocodamol, containing 8 or 30 mg of codeine)

Dose – oral/IM 30–60 mg, 4–6-hourly

Pharmacokinetics

Protein binding	10%
Bioavailability	60–70%
V_d	5.4
Cl	11
$t_{1/2}$	180

CNS – <20% analgesic potency of morphine, low affinity for opioid receptors, low euphoria, rarely addictive, low abuse potential

RS – produces some respiratory depression but not severe even in high doses; antitussive

Other – constipation (used as antidiarrhoeal), mild nausea and vomiting

Elimination – 10% metabolised to morphine in liver by demethylation, remainder metabolised to norcodeine or conjugated to glucuronides. Excretion in urine as free and conjugated codeine, norcodeine and morphine. Less than 17% excreted unchanged

Diclofenac

Structure – phenylacetic acid derivative, NSAID; potent inhibitor of cyclo-oxygenase enzyme (COX-1 and COX-2)

Presentation

Oral – enteric-coated tablets 25, 50 mg; sustained-release tablets 75, 100 mg; dispersible tablets 46.5 mg; suppositories 12.5, 25, 50, 100 mg

IM/IV – aqueous solution in 3 mL ampoules containing 75 mg diclofenac sodium, sodium metabisulphate, benzyl alcohol, propylene glycol and mannitol

Dose

Oral – 75–150 mg day^{-1} in 2–3 divided doses, children 1–3 mg kg^{-1} day^{-1}

Rectal – 100 mg 18-hourly; maximum daily dose 150 mg

Deep IM – 75 mg once or twice daily

IV infusion – 75 mg 6-hourly

Pharmacokinetics

Protein binding	99.5%
Bioavailability	60%
V_d	0.17
Cl	4.2
$t_{1/2}$	90

CNS – analgesic and anti-inflammatory; dizziness; vertigo

RS – bronchospasm in atopic and asthmatic individuals

GI tract – gastric irritation, dyspepsia, peptic ulceration; nausea and vomiting; diarrhoea; local irritation from suppositories

Other – renal impairment or failure; decreased renin activity and aldosterone concentrations by 60–70%; platelet aggregation inhibited; pain and local induration with IM injection; rashes and skin eruptions; transaminases raised and hepatic function impaired; blood dyscrasias; increases plasma concentrations of co-administered digoxin, lithium, anticoagulants and sulphonylureas

Elimination – significant first-pass metabolism in liver by hydroxylation then conjugation with glucuronide and sulphate; followed by excretion in the urine (60%) and bile (40%); < 1% unchanged in urine

Contraindications – asthma, gastrointestinal ulceration, hepatic and renal insufficiency, bleeding diathesis, haematological abnormalities, pregnancy and porphyria

Fentanyl
Structure – synthetic anilinopiperidine opioid
Presentation – colourless aqueous solution of citrate salt (preservative-free), 50 μg mL^{-1} (2 and 10 mL ampoules)
Dose
  IV – 0.5–3 μg kg^{-1} for spontaneous ventilation, 1–50 μg kg^{-1} for assisted ventilation.
  Epidural – 50–100 μg bolus, infusion 1 μg kg^{-1} h^{-1}
Pharmacokinetics

Protein binding	85%
pK$_a$	8.4
V$_d$	4
Cl	13
t$_{1/2}$	180
Peak effects in 5 min, duration of 30 min for smaller doses	

CNS – potent μ opioid receptor agonist, 60–80 times more potent analgesia than morphine; sedation
CVS – minimal effects even in higher doses, use in cardiac anaesthesia well established. Hypotension and bradycardia may occur particularly in hypovolaemic patients because of reduced sympathetic tone
RS – respiratory depression and reports of delayed respiratory depression probably as a result of enterohepatic circulation; high doses may increase chest and abdominal muscle tone so impairing ventilation
Other – nausea and vomiting, decreased gastrointestinal motility, negligible histamine release
Elimination – predominantly metabolised in liver by dealkylation to norfentanyl, an inactive metabolite; norfentanyl and fentanyl then hydroxylated and excreted in the urine (elimination half-life increased in liver disease and elderly)
Contraindications – concurrent administration with monoamine oxidase inhibitors

Ibuprofen
Structure – propionic acid derivative, NSAID; potent inhibitor of cyclo-oxygenase enzyme (COX-1 and COX-2)
Presentation – coated tablets 200, 400, 600 mg; slow-release tablets 800 mg; capsules 300 mg; syrup 100 mg 5 mL^{-1}; compound preparations with codeine (8 mg codeine/300 mg ibuprofen)
Dose – oral – 1.2–1.8 g day^{-1} in 3–4 divided doses (maximum 2.4 g day^{-1}); children 20 mg kg^{-1} in divided doses (maximum 40 mg kg^{-1} day^{-1}); not recommended in children < 7 kg
Pharmacokinetics

Protein binding	99%
Bioavailability	78%
V$_d$	0.15
Cl	0.75
t$_{1/2}$	120

CNS – mild analgesic and anti-inflammatory properties; malaise; dizziness; vertigo; tinnitus
RS – bronchospasm in asthmatics
GI tract – dyspepsia; gastic irritation; nausea and vomiting; diarrhoea
GUS – renal insufficiency and acute reversible renal failure
Other – rashes and hypersensitivity reactions; a few reports of toxic amblyopia
Excretion – metabolised in liver to two inactive metabolites and excreted in urine; < 1% excreted unchanged
Contraindications – asthma; history of peptic ulceration; renal insufficiency; haemorrhagic tendencies

Ketorolac
Structure – a pyrroleacetic acid, NSAID; potent inhibitor of cyclo-oxygenase enzyme (COX-1 and COX-2)
Presentation
  Tablets – 10 mg ketorolac trometamol
  IV/IM – clear, slightly yellow solution, 1 mL ampoules containing 10 and 30 mg ketorolac trometamol
Dose
  Oral – 10 mg 4–6-hourly (6–8-hourly in elderly), maximum 40 mg day^{-1} for 2 days
  IV/IM – 10–30 mg 4–6-hourly, maximum daily dose 90 mg in non-elderly, 60 mg in elderly,

renally impaired and patients < 50 kg, for a maximum of 2 days

Pharmacokinetics

Protein binding	99%
Bioavailability	85%
V_d	0.15
Cl	0.35
$t_{1/2}$	300

CNS – dizziness; tinnitus

RS – dyspnoea; asthma; pulmonary oedema

GI tract – dyspepsia; gastrointestinal irritation; peptic ulceration; nausea, vomiting and diarrhoea

Other – minimal anti-inflammatory effect at its analgesic dose; renal insufficiency; acute renal failure; hyponatraemia; hyperkalaemia; interstitial nephritis; thrombocytopenia and platelet dysfunction; rashes; pruritis and hypersensitivity reactions; flushing; pain at site of injection; increased risk of renal impairment with ACE inhibitors; reduced clearance of methotrexate and lithium; increased levels of ketorolac with probenecid

Elimination – mainly metabolised to inactive metabolite acyl glucuronide, about 25% metabolised to para-hydroxyketorolac, which has 20% of the anti-inflammatory and 1% of the analgesic activity of the parent drug. Excretion is primarily renal (92%), the remainder in bile (6%), and < 1% is unchanged

Contraindications – history of peptic ulcer disease; asthma and atopic tendencies; haemorrhagic diatheses; renal insufficiency; hypovolaemia and dehydration; pregnancy; children < 16 years

Morphine

Structure – a phenanthrene; a principal alkaloid of opium

Presentation

Oral – tablets 10, 20 mg; modified release tablets, 5, 10, 15, 30, 60, 100, 200 mg, solution of 10 mg 5 mL^{-1}, 30 mg 5 mL^{-1}; suppositories 10, 15, 20, 30 mg

IV – clear, colourless, aqueous solution of morphine sulphate, 10, 15, 20, 30 mg mL^{-1} (1 and 2 mL ampoules containing preservative 0.1% sodium metabisulphate)

Dose

SC/IM – 0.1–0.3 mg kg^{-1}, peak effect after 30 min, duration 3–4 h

Rectal – 15–30 mg 4-hourly

Intrathecal – 0.2–1 mg

IV – 0.05–0.1 mg kg^{-1}

Epidural – 2.5–10 mg

Pharmacokinetics

Protein binding	35%
Bioavailability	15–50%
pK_a	7.9
V_d	3.5
Cl	15
$t_{1/2}$	180

CNS – potent analgesic, agonist at μ, κ and δ receptors; sedation, drowsiness, euphoria, dysphoria, miosis (stimulation of Edinger–Westphal nucleus); tolerance and dependence

CVS – heart rate, systemic vascular resistance and blood pressure reduced

RS – respiratory rate and volume reduced, response to hypercarbia reduced; bronchoconstriction, antitussive, muscle rigidity

GI tract – nausea and vomiting, delayed gastric emptying, constipation, contraction of gallbladder and constriction of sphincter of Oddi causing reflux into pancreatic duct and an increase in serum amylase or lipase

Other – histamine release, itching, urticaria, increased tone of ureters, bladder and sphincter leading to urinary retention, increased vasopressin secretion, transient decrease in adrenal steroid secretion

Elimination – extensive first-pass metabolism: therefore oral dose 50% higher than IM dose. Conjugated in liver to morphine-3-glucuronide (70%) and morphine-6-glucuronide (5–10%), active metabolites more potent than morphine, the remainder demethylated to normorphine. Excreted predominantly in urine as conjugated metabolites; < 10% excreted unchanged. Accumulation of morphine-6-glucuronide may occur in renal failure

Naloxone

Structure – N-allyl oxymorphone opioid antagonist

Presentation – clear, colourless, aqueous solution containing 400 μg in 1 mL, or 20 μg in 2 mL naloxone hydrochloride

Dose – IV – increments 1.5–3 $\mu g\ kg^{-1}$, peak effect in 2 min; bolus 0.4–2 mg for suspected overdose repeated up to 10 mg lasts 20 min; may need to follow with infusion. Also administered SC and IM

Pharmacokinetics

Protein binding	45%
V_d	2
Cl	25
$t_{1/2}$	70

Clinical effects – pure opioid receptor antagonist acting at all opioid receptors; effects are related to withdrawal of the effects of any opioids and antagonism of endogenous opioids

Elimination – primarily by hepatic glucuronide conjugation followed by urinary excretion

Paracetamol

Structure – acetaminophen, a hydroxyphenylacetamide

Presentation

Tablets in various forms – 500 mg paracetamol

Suspension – 60 mg 5 mL^{-1}, 120 mg 5 mL^{-1}, 250 mg 5 mL^{-1}

Suppository – 60 mg, 125 mg, 250 mg, 500 mg

IV – clear colourless solution in 50 mL & 100 mL bottles containing 500 mg or 1 g paracetamol in low-pressure atmosphere of argon; also in plastic bottles

Dose

Oral – 500 mg to 1 g, 4–6-hourly, maximum 1 g day^{-1}

IV/IM – over 50 kg: 1 g 4–6-hourly, maximum 1 g day^{-1}; child 10–50 kg: 15 mg kg^{-1} 4–6-hourly, maximum 60 mg kg^{-1} day^{-1}; child < 10 kg: 7.5 mg kg^{-1} 4–6-hourly, maximum 30 mg kg^{-1} day^{-1}; infuse over 15 minutes

Pharmacokinetics

Protein binding	3%
Bioavailability	80%
V_d	1
Cl	5
$t_{1/2}$	150

CNS – analgesia

GUS – potentiation of vasopressin on water retention

Elimination – 80% metabolised by conjugation in the liver to glucuronide or sulphate. 10% hydroxylated by cytochrome P450 to the highly reactive and toxic N-acetyl-p-benzoquinone imine (NAPQI), which is rapidly inactivated by conjugation with glutathione. 4% excreted unchanged in urine

Overdosage – (10 g or 150 mg kg^{-1} in 24 hours) saturates the glutathione leading to free NAPQI, which damages the hepatic cell membrane. Early intervention by providing an alternative source of glutathione (N-acetylcysteine or methionine) can prevent this damage

Caution – Effervescent and soluble paracetamol preparations contain high levels of sodium, a 4 g daily dose typically containing 120–150 mmol of sodium

Remifentanil

Structure – synthetic anilinopiperidine opioid with a methyl ester linkage

Presentation – lyophilised white powder as 1, 2 or 5 mg vials for reconstitution, which forms a clear colourless solution containing 1 mg mL^{-1} remifentanil hydrochloride. Further dilution to a concentration of 50 μg mL^{-1} recommended for general anaesthesia. Reconstituted solution is stable for 24 hours at room temperature

Dose – IV – bolus at induction 1 μg kg^{-1} over not less than 30 s, maintenance infusion 0.05–2 μg kg^{-1} min^{-1} titrated to desired level. For spontaneous ventilation, starting dose 0.04 μg kg^{-1} min^{-1}, with range of 0.025–0.1 mg kg^{-1} min^{-1} titrated to effect

Pharmacokinetics

Protein binding	70%
V_d	0.35
Cl	50
$t_{1/2}$	15

CNS – potent μ opioid receptor agonist; analgesic potency comparable to fentanyl; rapid onset and recovery even after several hours' infusion

CVS – haemodynamically very stable; rarely bradycardia and hypotension

RS – respiratory rate and volume reduced, response to hypercarbia reduced; muscle rigidity, related to dose and rate of administration

Other – nausea and vomiting, no histamine release

Elimination – independent of hepatic and renal function, metabolised by de-esterification by non-specific plasma and tissue esterases to inactive metabolites that are excreted in urine. Unlike suxamethonium it is not a substrate for plasma cholinesterase and clearance is unaffected by cholinesterase deficiency or the administration of anticholinesterases. Not recommended for intrathecal or epidural use

Contraindications – concurrent administration with monoamine oxidase inhibitors

Tramadol

Structure – synthetic phenylpiperidine opioid analogue of codeine

Presentation

Capsules 50 mg (also modified-release preparations up to 200 mg available)

IV – clear colourless solution in 2 mL ampoules containing racemic mixture of 50 mg mL^{-1} tramadol hydrochloride

Dose

Oral – 50 mg to 100 mg, 4–6-hourly, maximum 400 mg day^{-1}

IV – 50 mg to 100 mg 4–6-hourly, maximum 400 mg day^{-1}; for postoperative pain up to 250 mg in first hour, maximum 600 mg day^{-1}

Pharmacokinetics

Protein binding	20%
Bioavailability	68%
V_d	2.7
Cl	5.9
$t_{1/2}$	400

CNS – weak, non-specific opioid receptor agonist, noradrenaline and 5-HT reuptake inhibitor and facilitator of 5-HT release

CVS – minimal

RS – minimal

Other – nausea and vomiting, no histamine release

Elimination – Metabolised in the liver (CYP2D6 and CYP3A4) to N-desmethyl-tramadol and O-desmethyl-tramadol (potent active metabolite with 9H half-life

Contraindications – concurrent administration with monoamine oxidase inhibitors

References and further reading

Rang HP, Ritter JM, Flower RJ, Henderson G. *Rang and Dale's Pharmacology*, 8th edn. Edinburgh: Churchill Livingstone, 2016.

CHAPTER 32

Neuromuscular blocking agents

Tim Smith

Mechanisms of neuromuscular blockade

The transmission of neuronal impulses to skeletal muscle can be prevented in many ways. These are summarised in Figure 32.1.

Drugs acting on the postjunctional nicotinic acetylcholine receptors (nAChR) of the skeletal muscle neuromuscular junction (NMJ) are generally used in clinical practice. These may be either depolarising or non-depolarising. The features of an ideal neuromuscular blocking agent are shown in Figure 32.2.

Depolarising blockade

Examples – decamethonium, suxamethonium

Suxamethonium is the only current therapeutic example of a depolarising blocking drug. However, any agonist of nicotinic acetylcholine receptors can also cause blockade if not rapidly cleared from the neuromuscular junction. Examples include nicotine and acetylcholine in the presence of excess anticholinesterase.

Mechanism of action

A depolarising block occurs when the agent stimulates the acetylcholine receptor and causes depolarisation. Persistence of the agonist at the receptor prevents repolarisation of the endplate and so it is refractory to further stimulation. As the agent diffuses away from the junctional cleft, repolarisation occurs and muscle action potentials are once more possible. The block is reversible, and attachment to the receptors is competitive. The block may be enhanced by a local increase in acetylcholine, as produced by anticholinesterases.

Clinical features

Depolarising blockade is characterised by rapid onset with muscle fasciculation, as groups of muscle fibres are depolarised. This is followed by a prolonged refractory period, which constitutes the blockade.

Neuromuscular test stimulation results in:

- Reduced single-twitch height
- Reduced train of four, all of equal amplitude
- No tetanic fade
- No post-tetanic facilitation

After suxamethonium administration there may be widespread muscular pains, which are worse on movement. They are particularly common in muscular young males after early ambulation. Muscle pains may persist for

Fundamentals of Anaesthesia, 4th edition, ed. Ted Lin, Tim Smith and Colin Pinnock. Published by Cambridge University Press. © Cambridge University Press 2017.

Figure 32.1 Mechanisms of neuromuscular blockade

Type of blockade

1. Prevention of acetylcholine synthesis
   Hemicholiniums

2. Prevention of acetylcholine release
   Botulinum toxin
   Local anaesthetic agents
   Magnesium ions

3. Depletion of acetylcholine stores
   Tetanus toxin

4. Blockade of the acetylcholine receptor
   (a) Depolarising blockade
       Suxamethonium
       Acetylcholine excess secondary to
       anticholinesterases
       Neostigmine
       Organophosphorus compounds
       Nicotine
   (b) Non-depolarising blockade
       Aminosteroids
           ORG 9487
           Pancuronium
           Pipecuronium
           Rocuronium
           Vecuronium
       Benzylisoquinolinium esters
           Atracurium
           Cis-atracurium
           Doxacurium
           Mivacurium

Figure 32.2 Features of an ideal neuromuscular blocking agent

Non-depolarising mode of action

Rapid onset of action

Short duration of action

Non-cumulative

No cardiovascular side effects

No histamine release

Spontaneous predictable reversal

High potency

Pharmacologically inactive metabolites

Unaffected by renal or hepatic failure

Figure 32.3 Causes of plasma cholinesterase deficiency

Pregnancy, third trimester

Collagen disorders

Carcinomatosis

Myocardial infarction

Liver disease

Hypothyroidism

Blood dyscrasias

Amethocaine

Ketamine

Pancuronium

Anticholinesterases

Oral contraceptives

Propranolol

Cytotoxic agents

Ecothiopate eye drops

several days. Pretreatment with benzodiazepines, lidocaine or small doses of non-depolarising agents may help. Dantrolene has also been used with some success.

Plasma cholinesterase abnormalities

Plasma cholinesterase (also known as butyrylcholinesterase or pseudocholinesterase) is a lipoprotein enzyme comprising four polypetide chains responsible for hydrolysing esters in many tissues. It is synthesised in the liver and is present in the liver, kidneys, pancreas, brain and plasma but not in erythrocytes. The normal range in plasma is $4000–12,000$ IU L^{-1}, and a fall of 700 IU L^{-1} or more is significant. Plasma cholinesterase is responsible for the metabolism of suxamethonium by hydrolysis of the two ester links of choline to succinic acid (see Figure 32.8).

Suxamethonium is also metabolised, slowly, by acetylcholinesterase.

A reduction in cholinesterase activity may be due either to a deficiency of cholinesterase molecules or to an abnormality of the enzyme. The causes of cholinesterase deficiency are listed in Figure 32.3. Levels fall to 75% of normal during pregnancy and to 67% of normal during

Figure 32.4 Inheritance of abnormal plasma cholinesterase

Type	Genotype		Dibucaine number	Fluoride number	Typical apnoea	Incidence
Normal	$E_1^u E_1^u$	homozygous	80	50	1–5 min	94%
Atypical	$E_1^u E_1^a$	heterozygous	60	50	10 min	1 : 25
Atypical	$E_1^a E_1^a$	homozygous	20	20	2 hours	1 : 3000
Silent	$E_1^u E_1^s$	heterozygous	80	50	10 min	1 : 25
Silent	$E_1^s E_1^s$	homozygous	minimal activity		2 hours	1 : 100,000
Fluoride-resistant	$E_1^u E_1^f$	heterozygous	75	50	10 min	1 : 300,000
Fluoride-resistant	$E_1^f E_1^f$	homozygous	65	40	2 hours	1 : 150,000

u, a, s and f are the four commonest of 25 possible gene variants for plasma cholinesterase

the first 7 days post partum. Patients with pre-existing genetic deficiencies are more prone to problems (e.g. suxamethonium apnoea – see *Postoperative complications* in Chapter 4) if acquired forms of deficiency coexist.

Plasma cholinesterase synthesis is controlled by a pair of autosomal recessive genes. Figure 32.4 shows possible genetic configurations, their incidence and dibucaine numbers. Assessment of plasma cholinesterase activity includes global plasma cholinesterase activity levels, and dibucaine and fluoride numbers. The dibucaine number quantifies the inhibition, by a 10^{-5} molar solution of dibucaine (a local anaesthetic previously available as cinchocaine), of the activity of plasma cholinesterase in the sample on benzoyl choline. It is expressed as a percentage. The fluoride number is similar but uses 5×10^{-5} molar sodium fluoride.

Plasma cholinesterase may also exist in excess, as a genetic variant or particularly in the presence of obesity or alcoholism. The result is a shortened duration of action of suxamethonium.

Plasma cholinesterase is also responsible for the metabolism of mivacurium, and the concomitant use of these drugs in susceptible patients may exaggerate problems.

Phase I and phase II blockade

Two distinct types of neuromuscular blockade (termed phase I and II blockade respectively) may result after the administration of suxamethonium. Figure 32.5 lists the features of each type.

Figure 32.5 Phase I and II blockade after suxamethonium administration

Phase I blockade
- Well-sustained response to tetanic stimulation
- No post-tetanic facilitation
- Train-of-four ratio > 0.7
- Potentiated by the effect of anticholinesterases

Phase II blockade
- Tetanic fade
- Post-tetanic facilitation
- Train-of-four ratio < 0.3
- Antagonised by the effect of anticholinesterases
- Tachyphylaxis

Non-depolarising blockade

Examples – atracurium, mivacurium, pancuronium, rocuronium, vecuronium

Mechanism of action

Non-depolarising neuromuscular blockade is the result of competitive occupancy of the postjunctional receptors preventing acetylcholine from reaching one or both α subunits of the receptor. This is probably a dynamic process, with both acetylcholine and the blocking agent in equilibrium with the receptors. At least 75% of receptors must be blocked before contraction fails. The process is competitive and reversible. The block can be antagonised by a local increase in acetylcholine, as produced by anticholinesterases. These muscle relaxants have no intrinsic activity at the neuromuscular endplate. Each has one or more quaternary ammonium groups. In the bisquaternary agents, these are usually 140 nm apart.

A graphic illustration of the process by which depolarising and non-depolarising drugs have their effects is shown in Figure 32.6.

Clinical features

The predominant effect of neuromuscular blocking agents is a reversible paralysis of skeletal muscle. This reduction in skeletal muscle activity reduces venous return and therefore reduces cardiac output and blood pressure.

Neuromuscular test stimulation results in:

- Reduced single-twitch height
- Reduced train of four, with twitch amplitude 1 > 2 > 3 > 4
- Tetanic fade
- Post-tetanic facilitation

The neuromuscular blocking agents also have anticholinesterase activity (Figure 32.7).

Aminosteroids

The acetylcholine-type fragment associated with the D ring of the steroid nucleus is probably responsible for most of the neuromuscular antagonism. The acetylcholine-type fragment associated with the A ring is probably responsible for the cardiovascular effects, especially the vagolytic aspects. Histamine release is not expected with the aminosteroid structure. In general, the aminosteroids are more slowly metabolised than the benzylisoquiniliniums.

Benzylisoquinolinium compounds

The chemical structure of benzylisoquinolinium is associated with histamine release. In general, the presence of an ester link promotes rapid degradation and metabolism, leading to a short half-life and rapid transition to complete recovery.

Elimination

The non-depolarising agents are usually metabolised in the liver. Other pathways exist, including spontaneous degradation and enzymatic hydrolysis within the plasma. These pathways are covered under *Specific pharmacology*, below.

The non-depolarising blocking agents may be potentiated by suxamethonium, intravenous and volatile anaesthetic drugs, opioids, aminoglycosides, tetracyclines, metronidazole, lincosamides, polymyxins, magnesium, verapamil and nifedipine, protamine, diuretics and catecholamine antagonists. The blockade is prolonged by hypothermia.

Anticholinesterases

Mechanism of action

The anticholinesterases inhibit the breakdown of acetylcholine by binding to the acetylcholinesterase enzyme in a competitive manner. This raises the background concentration of acetylcholine near the neuromuscular junction, which in turn overcomes the reduced number of functional nicotinic receptors on the muscle endplate, whether due to a reduced number of receptors (myasthenia gravis) or due to blockade of existing receptors (non-depolarising muscle relaxants). The anticholinesterases can be classified as either reversible anticholinesterases or organophosphorus compounds. While they all act on acetyl and plasma cholinesterase, the specific interaction with the enzyme varies between individual drugs.

Reversible anticholinesterases

Examples – distigmine, edrophonium, neostigmine, pyridostigmine

Acetylcholinesterase has an esteratic site and an anionic site in close proximity. Physiologically, the positively charged quaternary amine of acetylcholine binds to the anionic site. The acetyl ester combines with the esteratic site and the acetylcholine is hydrolysed. The anticholinesterases competitively occupy these sites and prevent acetylcholine access. The anticholinesterases have a quaternary amine group that is attracted to the anionic site and a carbamyl ester that binds covalently to the serine amino acid of the esteratic site. The quaternary amine group is not essential for activity, but when present it conveys enhanced potency and stability. The quaternary group also results in poor absorption following oral administration and a minimal transfer of the drug across the blood–brain barrier. Neostigmine is absorbed poorly from the gut as compared with the IV route. When neostigmine is used orally for the treatment of myasthenia gravis larger doses are therefore necessary. Equivalent doses of neostigmine are as follows: IV 0.5 mg; IM 1–1.5 mg; oral 15 mg.

Anticholinesterases also have some direct cholinergic agonist activity.

Physostigmine (no longer available) is an example of an anticholinesterase with several tertiary amine groups

Sequence 1: Normal depolarisation

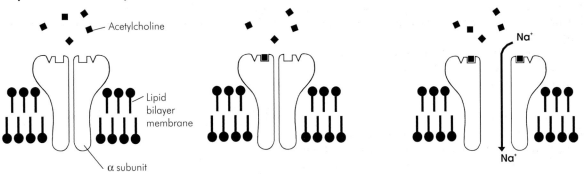

Acetylcholine released into the junctional cleft binds reversibly to receptor sites on the alpha subunits of the sodium ionophore. When the alpha site on each of the two subunits is occupied, the channel opens and allows depolarisation. Rapid metabolism enables rapid dissociation of receptor and agonist and the channel closes.

Sequence 2: Depolarising blockade

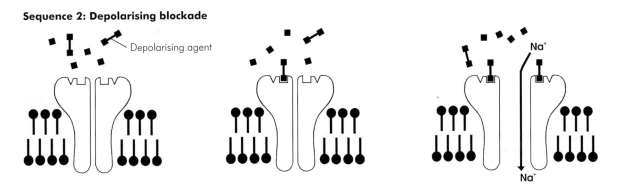

Suxamethonium and the released acetylcholine are both agonists of the receptor. When both receptors are occupied by any combination of these molecules the channel opens. However, the persistence of suxamethonium causes the channel to remain open long after the acetylcholine has been destroyed, maintaining a depolarised refractory endplate.

Sequence 3: Non-depolarising blockade

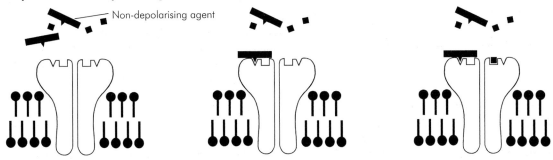

Non-depolarising drugs are antagonists and bind to the receptor without opening the channel. They subsequently prevent acetylcholine from binding and as two acetyl choline molecules are required for depolarisation only one receptor needs to be occupied by the antagonist to be effective.

Figure 32.6 Action of depolarising and non-depolarising muscle relaxants

Figure 32.7 Anticholinesterase activity of neuromuscular blocking agents

Drug	Concentration to produce 50% inhibition of enzymatic acetylcholine breakdown (μmol L^{-1}) in the presence of various neuromuscular blocking drugs	
	Acetylcholinesterase	Plasma cholinesterase
Suxamethonium	1300	640
Atracurium	340	420
Vecuronium	66	0.62

rather than the quaternary amine of the others. Consequently it is readily absorbed topically and orally and crosses the blood–brain barrier, but has no cholinergic agonist activity.

Edrophonium is only clinically effective for 5 minutes, and is used in the diagnosis of myasthenia gravis. Longer-acting agents are needed for treatment of the disease. Neostigmine is the only anticholinesterase routinely used to reverse planned neuromuscular blockade in clinical practice. Anticholinesterases have widespread effects subsequent to the stimulation of increased cholinergic muscarinic and nicotinic activity. Heart rate, vasomotor tone and blood pressure are reduced. At high dose levels sympathetic ganglion stimulation may predominate. Excess acetylcholine causes bronchoconstriction and increased bronchial secretion. Increased gastrointestinal tone and secretion occurs. Secretions of saliva, sweat and tears are also stimulated. These problems are prevented by the concomitant use of muscarinic anticholinergic drugs such as atropine or glycopyrrolate. Anticholinesterases can also cause a depolarising neuromuscular blockade when used in excess, or in the absence of non-depolarising blockade.

Neuromuscular blockade is terminated either by endogenous elimination of the drug and diffusion of the blocking agent away from the neuromuscular junction, or, in the case of non-depolarising agents, the effects can be overcome, in part, by inhibiting the metabolism of acetylcholine. If a long-acting muscle relaxant is used, it is possible for the blockade to re-establish if the effects of the anticholinesterase wear off before the neuromuscular blocking agent has left the receptors.

Organophosphorus compounds
Example – ecothiopate

These are primarily used as nerve gases and pesticides, and may feature in cases of poisoning. In general, they have no ionic binding component but bind covalently and irreversibly to the esteratic site of the cholinesterase enzyme by the release of a relatively weakly bound component of the drug. Consequently, the enzyme is not readily reactivated. Organophosphates tend to be highly lipid-soluble and readily cross the blood–brain barrier, causing central nervous system toxicity.

Ecothiopate differs from the other organophosphates in a number of ways. It is the only organophosphate in clinical use, and is used in the treatment of glaucoma. It too binds covalently to the esteratic site of the enzyme, but it also has a positively charged quaternary ammonium group that helps binding. This positive charge means that ecothiopate does not readily cross the blood–brain barrier, in contrast with other organophosphorous compounds. Although it is slowly hydrolysed it may nonetheless prolong the action of suxamethonium and mivacurium.

Selective binding agent
Example – sugammadex

Sugammadex is a selective relaxant binding agent specifically designed to target rocuronium (de Boer *et al.* 2006). It is a synthetic γ-cyclodextrin derivative (an oligosaccharide) devoid of intrinsic activity. In effect, each molecule forms a tube into which a single relatively small aminosteroid molecule of rocuronium or vecuronium fits. This binding is specific for rocuronium and vecuronium, effectively encapsulating it to rapidly reduce its unbound plasma concentration and also that at the neuromuscular endplate. Cyclodextrins are highly water-soluble, and sugammadex is excreted rapidly in the urine. The half-life is relatively short, and so further administration of rocuronium soon afterwards may be an option. An alternative benzylisoquinolinium non-depolariser could also be used, as these larger molecules will not fit within the cyclodextrin cavity.

Figure 32.8 Pharmacokinetic data for non-depolarising neuromuscular blocking agents

	ED$_{95}$ (mg kg^{-1})	Dose (mg kg^{-1})	V$_d$ (mL kg^{-1})	Clearance (mL kg^{-1} min^{-1})	Elimination t$_{1/2}$ (min)
Atracurium	0.2	0.3–0.6	170	5.5	20
Doxacurium	0.025	0.05	220	2.7	99
Mivacurium	0.08	0.07–0.25			
trans–trans isomer			150–267	51–63	1.9–3.6
cis–trans isomer			290–382	93–106	1.8–2.9
cis-cis isomer			175–340	3.7–4.6	34.7–52.9
ORG 9487	1.15^a	1.5–2.0	293	8.5	74
Pancuronium	0.06	0.05–0.1	200	1.8	115
Pipecuronium	0.049	0.07	309	2.4	137
Rocuronium	0.3	0.6	270	4.0	131
Vecuronium	0.046	0.05–0.1	260	4.6	62

^{a} Value quoted for ED$_{90}$

In contrast with anticholinesterase reversal, sugammadex:

- Is effective regardless of the state of neuromuscular blockade.
- Is devoid of intrinsic activity.
- Allows subsequent re-paralysis.

Specific pharmacology

Units (unless stated otherwise) are:
Volume of distribution at steady state (V$_d$): mL kg^{-1}
Clearance (Cl): mL kg^{-1} min^{-1}
Terminal half-life (t$_{1/2}$): minutes

Pharmacokinetic data for specific non-depolarising drugs are summarised in Figure 32.8, and the chemical structures of atracurium, rocuronium, suxamethonium and neostigmine are shown in Figure 32.9.

Atracurium dibesylate

Structure – bisquaternary benzylisoquinolinium diester. A plant derivative
Presentation – clear, colourless, aqueous solution of pH 3.5 (10 mg mL^{-1}, 2.5, 5, 25 mL ampoules). Storage in fridge at 2–8 °C, protect from light
Dose – IV bolus 0.3–0.6 mg kg^{-1}, infusion 0.3–0.6 mg kg^{-1} h^{-1}. Initial dose lasts 30 min. ED$_{95}$ = 0.2 mg kg^{-1}

Pharmacokinetics

Protein binding	82%
V$_d$	170
Cl	5.5
t$_{1/2}$	20

CNS – no increase in intraocular pressure (IOP) or intracranial pressure (ICP). Laudanosine, a metabolite and stimulant, crosses the blood–brain barrier and can cause convulsions if plasma concentration > 20 pg mL^{-1}
CVS – the small amount of histamine release may lower systemic vascular resistance, central venous pressure and pulmonary capillary wedge pressure
RS – paralysis of respiratory muscles; small risk of bronchospasm due to histamine release
Other – no effect on lower oesophageal sphincter pressure; placental transfer insufficient to cause an effect in the fetus
Elimination – non-cumulative. Hofmann elimination is the spontaneous fragmentation of atracurium at the bond between the quaternary nitrogen and the central chain. This occurs at body

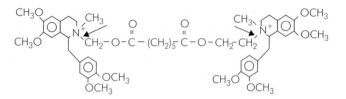

Atracurium

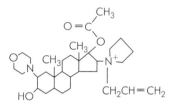

Rocuronium

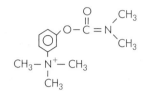

Neostigmine

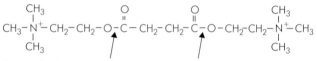

Suxamethonium

Figure 32.9 Chemical structures of commonly used neuromuscular drugs. The arrows indicate sites of cleavage (atracurium – Hofmann degradation; suxamethonium – ester hydrolysis)

temperature and pH, producing inactive products – laudanosine ($t_{1/2}$ = 234 min) and a quaternary monoacrylate ($t_{1/2}$ = 39 min). Atracurium is also metabolised by ester hydrolysis, producing a quaternary alcohol and a quaternary acid. These two mechanisms account for 40% of the elimination of atracurium, the remainder being by a variety of other mechanisms

Metabolites – 55% excreted in the bile within 7 h, 35% excreted in the urine within 7 h

Side effects – histamine release may cause bronchospasm, hypotension, and erythema and weals, generally or along the vein of injection

Cis-atracurium dibesylate

Atracurium contains a mixture of 10 geometric isomers. One of these, cis-cis-atracurium, is marketed as Cisatracurium. The features are as for atracurium except:

Presentation – clear, colourless, aqueous solution of pH 3.5 (2 mg mL^{-1} in 2.5, 5, 10, 25 mL ampoules, and 5 mg mL^{-1} in 30 mL vial). Store in fridge at 2–8 °C, protect from light

Dose – IV bolus 0.15 mg kg^{-1}; infusion 0.18 mg kg^{-1} h^{-1}. ED$_{95}$ = 0.05 mg kg^{-1}

This single isomer of atracurium avoids the histamine release but is similar to atracurium in other respects.

Mivacurium chloride

Structure – bisquaternary benzylisoquinolinium diester

Presentation – clear, colourless, aqueous solution of pH 4.5 (2 mg mL^{-1}, 5 and 10 mL ampoules) containing three stereoisomers – trans–trans (57%), cis–trans (36%), cis–cis (6%)

Dose – IV bolus 0.07–0.25 mg kg^{-1}; children 0.1–0.2 mg kg^{-1}; infusion 0.06 mg kg^{-1} h^{-1}. ED$_{95}$ = 0.08 mg kg^{-1} (children 0.1 mg kg^{-1})

Pharmacokinetics

Isomer	V_d	Cl	$t_{1/2}$
trans–trans	150–267	51–63	1.9–3.6
cis–trans	290–382	93–106	1.8–2.9
cis–cis	175–340	3.7–4.6	34.7–52.9

CNS – no effect
CVS – no effect
RS – respiratory muscle paralysis
Other – minimal placental transfer
Elimination – *trans–trans* and *cis–trans* isomers hydrolysed by plasma cholinesterase. The *cis–cis* isomer may be metabolised in part by the liver. Lasts twice as long as suxamethonium (24 min)
Toxicity – block antagonised by neostigmine. Block prolonged by reduced or atypical plasma cholinesterase as with suxamethonium. Block also prolonged if factors interfering with plasma cholinesterase are present. Heterozygotes for atypical plasma cholinesterase show a prolongation of effect of about 10 min

Neostigmine bromide
Structure – quaternary amine, alkylcarbamic acid ester
Presentation – clear, very pale yellow, aqueous solution in brown ampoule (2.5 mg in 1 mL)
Storage – protect from light
Dose – IV bolus 0.05–0.08 mg kg^{-1}. Peak effect 7–11 min; duration 40 min
Pharmacokinetics

V_d	700
Cl	8
$t_{1/2}$	40
Bioavailability after oral administration < 1%	

CNS – central hypotensive effect at high dose; miosis, blurred vision
CVS – causes bradycardia and decreases cardiac output
RS – bronchconstriction and reduces anatomical dead space
Other – increases in all the following: ureteric peristalsis, gastrointestinal peristalsis, sweating, lacrimation, gastric tone and lower oesophageal sphincter pressure
Elimination – hydrolysed by the acetylcholinesterase that it antagonises and by plasma cholinesterase to a quaternary alcohol. Some hepatic metabolism occurs with biliary excretion. 50–67% is excreted in the urine
Side effects – concomitant administration of anticholinergics is essential when used for reversal of neuromuscular blockade. The increased

gastrointestinal tone may promote anastomotic breakdown. Neostigmine inhibits the hydrolysis of suxamethonium and mivacurium and other drugs metabolised by plasma cholinesterase. High levels of neostigmine at the neuromuscular junction cause a direct blockade of the acetylcholine receptor, and the raised levels of acetylcholine have a depolarising blocking effect

Pancuronium bromide
Structure – bisquaternary aminosteroid
Presentation – clear, colourless, aqueous solution (4 mg in 2 mL)
Dose – IV bolus 0.05–0.1 mg kg^{-1}. Initial dose lasts 45–60 min. ED$_{95}$ = 0.06 mg kg^{-1}
Pharmacokinetics

Protein binding (albumin, γ-globulin)	15–87%
V_d	200
Cl	1.8
$t_{1/2}$	115

CNS – does not cross blood–brain barrier. No increase in IOP and ICP
CVS – increase in heart rate, cardiac output and blood pressure due to vagolytic action. Systemic vascular resistance unchanged
RS – respiratory muscle paralysis; some bronchodilatation
Other – increase in lower oesophageal sphincter pressure; may increase prothrombin time and partial thromboplastin time; small amount of placental transfer but no clinical effect on fetus
Elimination – 50% excreted unchanged, of which 80% appears in the urine. 40% is deacetylated in the liver to 3-hydroxy, 17-hydroxy and 3,17-dihydroxy derivatives which are eliminated in the bile. The 3-hydroxy compound has some neuromuscular antagonist activity
Note that pancuronium has some prejunctional activity.

Rocuronium bromide
Structure – monoquaternary aminosteroid
Presentation – aqueous solution (10 mg mL^{-1}, 5 and 10 mL ampoules)
Storage – in fridge at 2–8 °C; protect from light
Dose – IV bolus 0.6 mg kg^{-1}, infusion 0.3–0.6 mg kg^{-1} h^{-1}, initial dose lasts 38–150 min. ED$_{95}$ = 0.3 mg kg^{-1}. Onset

time of 1.5 min using $2 \times ED_{95}$, which may be shortened to 55 s using $4 \times ED_{95}$

Pharmacokinetics

V_d	270
Cl	4.0
$t_{1/2}$	131

CNS – no effect
CVS – increases heart rate, cardiac output and blood pressure slightly due to vagal blockade
RS – respiratory muscle paralysis
Other – no histamine release
Elimination – predominantly hepatic but also some renal elimination. Hepatic or renal failure can cause prolongation of effect

Sugammadex

Structure – synthetic oligosaccharide, γ-cyclodextrin derivative
Presentation – clear aqueous solution of sodium sugammadex containing hydrochloric acid (pH 7–8) and (100 mg mL^{-1}, 2 and 5 mL ampoules)
Storage – room temperature
Dose – IV bolus $2–4 \text{ mg kg}^{-1}$ up to 16 mg kg^{-1}

Pharmacokinetics

Protein binding	None
V_d	180
Cl	1.2
$t_{1/2}$	120

Elimination – renal

Suxamethonium chloride (succinylcholine)

Structure – dicholine ester of acetylcholine
Presentation – clear, colourless, aqueous solution of pH 3.0–5.0 with a shelf life of 2 years (50 mg mL^{-1} in 2 mL)
Storage – in fridge at 4 °C; spontaneous hydrolysis occurs in warm or alkaline conditions
Dose – IV bolus $0.3–1.1 \text{ mg kg}^{-1}$; children $1–2 \text{ mg kg}^{-1}$. Infusion 0.1% solution at $2–15 \text{ mg min}^{-1}$. It is effective within 30 s and lasts for several minutes

Pharmacokinetics

$t_{1/2}$	3.5

Protein binding occurs but the extent is not known because of the transient nature of the drug

CNS – small increase in ICP which may be of relevance in the head-injured patient
CVS – increased blood pressure, bradycardia
RS – paralysis of respiratory muscles
Other – increases IOP and intragastric pressure, and lowers oesophageal sphincter pressure (barrier pressure is increased). Increases gastric secretion and salivary production
Elimination – metabolised by plasma cholinesterase – complete recovery in 10–12 min. 2–20% is unchanged in urine. The elimination pathway is shown in Figure 32.10
Side effects – muscle pains, especially in muscular young males and after early ambulation, malignant hyperthermia trigger. May result in trismus, histamine release and hyperkalaemia – especially if denervation, burns, trauma or renal failure coexist
Contraindications – malignant hyperthermia susceptibility, burns, myotonia

Suxamethonium is a short-acting depolarising neuromuscular blocking agent. It is rapidly acting by virtue of rapid distribution to the neuromuscular junction and its depolarising mode of action. Its effect is terminated by diffusion away from the neuromuscular junction followed by rapid redistribution and hydrolysis. Hydrolysis occurs in two stages each removing choline. 80% is metabolised before reaching the neuromuscular junction.

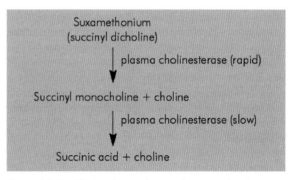

Figure 32.10 Elimination pathway of suxamethonium

Vecuronium bromide

Structure – monoquaternary aminosteroid, becomes bis-quaternary at pH 7.4

Presentation – freeze-dried, buffered, lyophilised cake for reconstitution, containing vecuronium bromide, citric acid monohydrate, disodium hydrogen phosphate dihydrate and mannitol

Storage – avoid light and temperatures in excess of 45 °C. Reconstitution with water for injections produces clear, colourless solution of pH 4.0

Dose – IV bolus 0.05–0.1 mg kg^{-1}, infusion 0.05–0.1 mg kg^{-1} h^{-1}. ED$_{95}$ = 0.046 mg kg^{-1}. Initial dose lasts 30 min

Pharmacokinetics

V_d	260
Cl	4.6
$t_{1/2}$	62

CNS – no increase in ICP
CVS – no effect

RS – respiratory muscle paralysis

Other – no increase in IOP; minimal placental transfer; no histamine release

Elimination – spontaneous deacetylation and hepatic metabolism. Of total dose, 10–25% is excreted in urine; the rest in the bile. Most excreted unchanged. Suitable in patients with absent renal function. Hepatic failure may prolong clinical effect, whereas chronic phenytoin therapy reduces the efficacy of vecuronium. There are three potential metabolites, 3-hydroxy, 17-hydroxy and 3,17-dihydroxy. These have minimal neuromuscular and vagolytic activity; only 3-hydroxy is found in any significant quantity and it has 50% of the neuromuscular blocking potency of vecuronium. Vecuronium is more stable in acidic solutions, and is therefore potentiated by respiratory acidosis

References and further reading

de Boer HD, van Egmond J, van de Pol F, Bom A, Booij LH. Sugammadex, a new reversal agent for neuromuscular block induced by rocuronium in the anaesthetized Rhesus monkey. *Br J Anaesth* 2006; **96**: 473–9.

CHAPTER 33

Local anaesthetic agents

Tim Smith

Local anaesthetic agents are used directly to block neuronal transmission. They also stabilise other electrically excitable membranes, and some examples, such as lidocaine, have clinically useful antiarrhythmic activity.

Structure

Local anaesthetic agents comprise a hydrophilic tertiary amine group linked to a lipophilic aromatic group. They are divided into esters and amides, based on the linking group. Figure 33.1 shows examples of these two types of local anaesthetic agent. Protonation of the highlighted amine nitrogen atom confers activity on the molecule once it is inside the cell.

Local anaesthetic agents exist in two states, acid (protonated) and basic (non-ionised) in equilibrium according to their pK$_a$ and ambient pH, as determined by the Henderson–Hasselbalch equation:

$$pH = pK_a + \log_{10} \frac{LA \text{ (base)}}{LA \text{ H}^+ \text{ (acid)}}$$

Local anaesthetic agents are weak bases. At physiological pH, there exists a mixture of non-ionised and ionised drug. This is important, as only the non-ionised drug passes through the membrane, yet it is only the ionised drug that is active. Small changes in pH have marked effects on the proportion of drug that is ionised, and therefore markedly influence the effect.

Mechanism of action

Injectable local anaesthetics must be soluble and stable in water. This is achieved by creating hydrochlorides of the drug. Hydrochlorides are soluble in water and produce an acid environment with a high degree of ionisation.

Local anaesthetic agents act by blocking the fast sodium channel in neuronal membranes. To do so the

Fundamentals of Anaesthesia, 4th edition, ed. Ted Lin, Tim Smith and Colin Pinnock. Published by Cambridge University Press. © Cambridge University Press 2017.

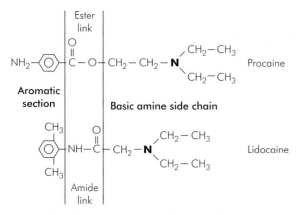

Figure 33.1 Chemical structure of an ester (procaine) and an amide (lidocaine)

drug must be in the protonated form and the ion channel must be in the open state. The drug enters the ion channel from the intracellular direction, but is administered extracellularly. Blockade by this route is use-dependent, because ionophores are only blocked while open.

The process by which local anaesthetic agents reach the sodium channel is illustrated in Figure 33.2, using lidocaine as an example:

1. The pK_a of lidocaine is 7.9, so extracellularly (at pH 7.4) 24% is in the non-ionised state and 76% in the ionised state.
2. The non-ionised drug is therefore relatively lipophilic, and it passes passively down the concentration gradient through the membrane into the cell.

Mechanism of action of LA action agents using lidocaine as an example

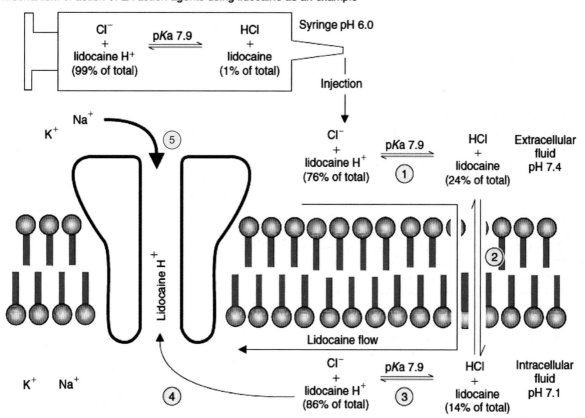

Figure 33.2 Mechanism of action of local anaesthetic agents, using lidocaine as an example. The stages indicated by circled numbers are described in more detail in the text.

3. Intracellularly, pH is about 7.1, and this shifts the balance of ionisation of the intracellular portion of drug towards the ionised state (86%).
4. The ionised drug, attracted by the negative charge of membrane protein, then passes into the open ion channel.
5. The channel remains open but is blocked to further transmission of sodium.

Another mechanism of action may contribute to the anaesthetic activity. This involves the passage of non-ionised drug through the membrane directly blocking the sodium channel, an effect that does not rely on the sodium channel being open.

The opening of the fast sodium channels in neuronal membranes and the passage of sodium through them are essential for the development and propagation of the action potential. The sharp upstroke of the action potential is gradually attenuated as more sodium channels become blocked. When the depolarisation is insufficient to generate the currents required to depolarise neighbouring membrane, then action-potential propagation and neuronal transmission cease.

Factors influencing activity

Figure 33.3 shows the pharmacological properties of important local anaesthetic agents.

Molecular weight

Molecular weight itself does not affect the pharmacological properties. However, increases in molecular weight tend to be indicative of increased side-chain size and therefore increased lipid solubility.

Lipid solubility

The higher the lipid solubility, the greater the penetration of the nerve membrane by the drug, so that higher lipid solubility results in greater potency. It also results in more toxicity and local irritancy. High lipid solubility also increases the rate of onset and duration of action of local anaesthetic agents.

pK_a

The lower the pK_a, the lower the degree of ionisation for any given pH and so the more rapid the speed of onset of the block. Increasing pK_a increases the ionised proportion of the drug so that intracellularly a higher proportion is in the active state. However, this also means that less is in the non-ionised, diffusible state, so the onset and offset of action are also slower. Figure 33.4 shows the effect of differences in pH and pK_a on the proportion of ionised and non-ionised local anaesthetic agents.

pH

Acidosis (low pH) increases the proportion of ionised drug in the interstitium, and therefore reduces the amount of drug able to cross the neuronal membrane. The local anaesthetic is therefore reduced in potency. Manipulation of the pH of the local anaesthetic solution by addition of alkali, buffers or carbonation may be used to alter the proportion of non-ionised drug.

Figure 33.3 Physicochemical and pharmacokinetic properties of local anaesthetic agents

	Molecular weight (Da)	pK_a (25 °C)	Partition coefficient (heptane buffer)	Protein binding (%)	Onset	Potency (relative to lidocaine)	Duration
Esters							
Amethocaine	264	8.5	4.1	76	Slow	4	Long
Procaine	236	8.9	0.02	6	Slow	½	Short
Amides							
Bupivacaine	288	8.1	27.5	96	Medium	4	Long
Lidocaine	234	7.9	2.9	64	Rapid	1	Medium
Prilocaine	220	7.9	0.9	55	Rapid	1	Medium
Ropivacaine	274	8.1	6.1	95	Medium	4	Long

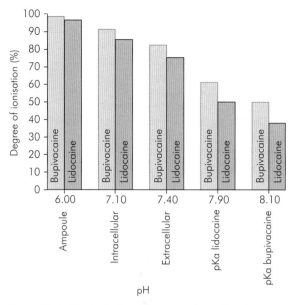

Figure 33.4 Effect of pH on the ionisation of local anaesthetic agents

Protein binding

The degree of protein binding reflects the ability of the drug to bind to membrane proteins: the greater the binding, the longer the duration of action. Increased binding to tissue protein correlates with an increase in the duration of action and probably indicates a higher affinity for membrane proteins (for example, the fast sodium ionophore).

Clinical effects and toxicity

See *Local anaesthetic toxicity* in Chapter 7.

Ester-linked agents

Amethocaine

Amethocaine (tetracaine) is an ester local anaesthetic agent used for topical anaesthesia. It is available as a gel (4%) for local anaesthesia of the skin before intravascular cannulation. Applied to the skin, it is effective within 45 minutes. It can then be removed, and remains active for 4–6 hours. The preparation should not be applied to inflamed or damaged skin or highly vascular tissues, as it is rapidly absorbed through mucosal surfaces. More dilute solutions (0.5% and 1%) are available for topical anaesthesia of the conjunctiva. Amethocaine is potent and readily absorbed, but in common with other ester local anaesthetics it may cause hypersensitivity.

Benzocaine

Benzocaine is an unusual ester local anaesthetic agent in that the side chain is an ethyl group with no amine component, and therefore remains un-ionised. Benzocaine has a low potency but it may cause methaemoglobinaemia. It is a component of some throat lozenges, and may be applied directly to painful skin ulcers.

Cocaine

Cocaine is a naturally occurring ester derived from benzoic acid, and extracted from the leaves of *Erythroxylum coca*. It is available in solution and pastes in concentrations ranging from 1% to 10%. It is mainly used for topical anaesthesia and to reduce bleeding during nasal surgery. Cocaine is rapidly taken up into mucous membranes to provide anaesthesia and intense vasoconstriction. This vasoconstriction limits systemic absorption, resulting in a bioavailability by this route of 0.5%. It is well known as a drug of abuse with high addictive potential, and in this role is taken by chewing, inhaling nasally, smoking or intravenously. It causes marked sympathomimetic activity, and arrhythmias are a definite risk. Systemic injection must be avoided. Systemically absorbed cocaine has a volume of distribution of 2 L kg^{-1}, with 98% being protein-bound. It is eliminated by plasma and liver esterases, having a clearance of 35 mL kg^{-1} min^{-1} and a half-life of 45 minutes.

Cocaine shares the same mechanism of action as the other local anaesthetic agents (pK_a = 8.7), and also inhibits catecholamine neuronal uptake-1. Synaptic levels of dopamine and noradrenaline increase, resulting in the central stimulation and euphoria, and vasoconstriction. Cocaine initially blocks the inhibitory pathways, resulting in euphoria, hyperthermia, altered vision and hearing, nausea and eventually convulsions. Higher levels of cocaine also block the excitatory pathways, resulting in central nervous depression leading to sedation and unconsciousness, with respiratory depression. Cocaine causes mydriasis and raised intraocular pressure. It is no longer used for local anaesthesia of the eye. The central stimulation increases respiratory rate and volume. A rise in sympathetic tone leads to tachycardia and hypertension, the latter being exacerbated by peripherally mediated vasoconstriction. High doses depress the myocardium. The general excitation also increases metabolic rate, which contributes to the hyperthermia and raises oxygen consumption and CO_2 production. The recommended maximum dose is 1.5 mg kg^{-1}. Cocaine should be avoided in porphyria.

Amide-linked agents

Bupivacaine

Bupivacaine is a long-acting local anaesthetic agent with a slow onset of action. Blockade of a large peripheral nerve such as the sciatic nerve may take 60 minutes, depending on the approach, but may last up to 48 hours. Intrathecal injection in contrast produces an acceptable block within a few minutes. Bupivacaine is particularly prone to causing myocardial depression and, once cardiac function is compromised, reversal may be slow and difficult. In part this is due to the relatively high pK_a, but an affinity for cardiac proteins is probably more important. Recommendations to minimise systemic toxicity specific to bupivacaine include:

- Avoid bupivacaine for IVRA.
- Avoid 0.75% bupivacaine in obstetric practice.
- Limit dose to 2 mg kg^{-1}.

Bupivacaine is predominantly metabolised by N-dealkylation to pipecolylxylidine (N-desbutylbupivacaine). Hydroxybupivacaine is also produced. The metabolites are excreted in the urine.

Levobupivacaine

Levobupivacaine is the S(–)enantiomer of racemic bupivacaine. It is clinically similar to racemic bupivacaine. The important differences are dose terminology and toxicity. Levobupivacaine is expressed as milligrams of base rather than of hydrochloride salt, so for a given (mg) dose there is 13% more activity. Animal studies demonstrate lower cardiotoxicity, but at present the maximum recommended dose remains at 2 mg kg^{-1}, and it is contraindicated for IVRA (Bier's block). Lower CNS toxicity is also apparent.

Lidocaine

Lidocaine (lignocaine) is primarily classified as a local anaesthetic agent but is also a class IB antiarrhythmic. It has a relatively rapid onset of action and intermediate duration. Combination with a longer-acting agent such as bupivacaine may produce a balance of onset and duration between the two component agents alone. The cardiotoxic potential of lidocaine at equivalent levels of CNS toxicity is about one-ninth that of bupivacaine.

Lidocaine is metabolised in the liver by microsomal oxidases and amidases. N-dealkylation followed by hydrolysis produces ethylglycine, xylidide and other derivatives that are excreted in the urine.

Prilocaine

Prilocaine is closely related to lidocaine in terms of pharmacological activity. It has the same pK_a (7.9) but is less lipid-soluble. Speed of onset and duration are similar. It is less toxic than lidocaine, due to high tissue fixation and rapid metabolism of systemically absorbed drug. Prilocaine is the drug of choice for IVRA.

Prilocaine is metabolised in the liver, lungs and kidney to O-toluidine, and then hydroxytoluidine, leaving less than 1% unchanged. O-toluidine is responsible for methaemoglobinaemia.

Methaemoglobinaemia

Metabolism of prilocaine following significant absorption (e.g. after 600 mg) to O-toluidine results in the oxidation of the ferrous ion (Fe^{2+}) of the haem in haemoglobin to ferric (Fe^{3+}) to produce methaemoglobinaemia. This results in cyanosis, and the abnormal haemoglobin shifts pulse oximeter readings towards 85% regardless of the true saturation. Methaemoglobinaemia is not usually clinically detrimental, but when the patient becomes compromised methylene blue (1–2 mg kg^{-1}) may be used as a treatment. Excess methylene blue (> 7 mg kg^{-1}) may also cause methaemoglobinaemia, and as the dye has a distinctive spectral absorption it also affects pulse oximeter accuracy.

Children (especially infants) are more susceptible to methaemoglobinaemia, because they have underdeveloped metabolic processes and fetal haemoglobin is more easily oxidised. Methaemoglobinaemia also occurs occasionally after application of EMLA cream.

Ropivacaine

Ropivacaine is closely related to bupivacaine in terms of pharmacological activity, as both drugs are pipecoloxylidides. Ropivacaine is produced as a single enantiomer with an enantiomeric purity of 99.5% for S-ropivacaine. As ropivacaine is less lipid-soluble than bupivacaine and less readily penetrates the neuronal myelin sheaths, C fibres are blocked more readily than A fibres. At high concentrations the blocking effect is similar for both drugs, but at lower concentrations ropivacaine preferentially blocks C fibres over the faster A fibres. Ropivacaine has a potential advantage that motor function can be spared (or show earlier recovery) while still achieving sensory blockade, if a suitable concentration of drug is used. Complete motor and sensory blockade can still be achieved if desired. In summary, ropivacaine provides sensory blockade similar to that of bupivacaine but motor blockade is slower in onset, less pronounced and shorter in duration. Ropivacaine is half as cardiotoxic as bupivacaine. It is mainly bound to α_1-acid glycoprotein in plasma.

EMLA

Eutectic mixture of local anaesthetic (EMLA) is a mixture of 2.5% prilocaine and 2.5% lidocaine used for topical anaesthesia of undamaged skin before intravascular cannulation and minor, superficial dermal and aural surgery. A eutectic mixture is one in which the constituents are in such proportions that the freezing (or melting) point is as low as possible, with the constituents freezing (or melting) simultaneously. The preparation is therefore unusual, as the local anaesthetics are not in aqueous solution, and both agents are in their pure form rather than the hydrochloride preparations used in the solutions. In theory, this means that both drugs are in the non-ionised state in EMLA. Once absorbed into the tissues, ionisation will occur. The commercial preparation (EMLA cream 5%) contains carboxypolymethylene and sodium hydroxide, resulting in an oil–water emulsion.

Lidocaine cream

4% lidocaine cream can be used topically as an alternative to EMLA or amethocaine. It avoids the higher allergenic properties of the ester local anaesthetics. It takes 30 minutes to work and can be left on for up to 5 hours.

Additives

Glucose

Standard solutions of local anaesthetic agents are slightly hypobaric at body temperature and pH, and therefore tend to move upwards in the cerebrospinal fluid away from the gravitational pull. Dextrose (glucose) is added to bupivacaine to increase the density of the solution. The specific gravity of hyperbaric (or 'heavy') bupivacaine is 1.026 at 20 °C. The specific gravity of cerebrospinal fluid is 1.005 at 37 °C, so the injected bupivacaine solution will sink due to gravity. Combined with knowledge of the spinal curves and manipulating the position of the patient, this helps to control the distribution of the local anaesthetic. Note that the specific gravity of a substance or solution is the density of that solution relative to the maximum density of water, which occurs at a temperature of 4 °C.

Vasoconstrictors

Adrenaline

Adrenaline is added to local anaesthetic solutions to reduce vascularity of the area by direct vasoconstriction, and in turn to reduce the systemic uptake of the drug. This has the following effects:

- Increased duration of nerve blockade
- Greater margin of safety for systemic toxicity
- Reduced surgical bleeding

Care must be taken to avoid the systemic effects of adrenaline due to systemic uptake. For example, combination with halothane anaesthesia may result in cardiac arrhythmias, especially ventricular excitation and fibrillation. Adrenaline-containing solutions should not be injected in the proximity of end-arteries such as the penile, ophthalmic (central artery of the retina) or digital arteries, as there is no collateral circulation to supplement the supply if vasoconstriction is severe. To minimise the risk of serious systemic actions consider the following:

- Avoid hypoxia and hypercarbia.
- Use dilute solutions (< 1:200,000).
- Limit of 100 µg per 10 minutes.
- Limit of 300 µg per hour.

Felypressin

Felypressin is an octapeptide derived from vasopressin (ADH). In common with vasopressin, felypressin is a powerful direct-acting vasopressor, but it is safe to use with halothane and has no antidiuretic or oxytocic activity. It may, however, cause coronary vasoconstriction.

Hyaluronidase

Hyaluronidase, supplied as a white fluffy powder, is used to facilitate the spread of a drug through connective tissues following subcutaneous or intramuscular injection. In addition to promoting the spread of local anaesthetics and other injections, it is also used to promote reabsorption of fluids and blood from extravascular tissues. Its effect is dependent on the temporary depolymerisation of hyaluronic acid. Hyaluronidase is stable in solution for 24 hours at room temperature.

pH manipulation

Alkalination of solutions by addition of bicarbonate increases tissue pH. This results in a higher proportion of non-ionised drug, which diffuses into the neurone

Figure 33.5 Local anaesthetic additives used for receptor-mediated analgesic effect

Drug	Receptor	Uses
Opioids	μ/κ	Central and peripheral
Clonidine	α_2-Adrenoceptor	Central and peripheral
Ketamine	NMDA	Central

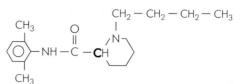

Bupivacaine

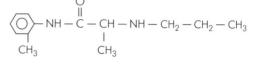

Prilocaine

Ropivacaine

Figure 33.6 Structures of common local anaesthetic drugs. The chiral carbon of bupivacaine (levobupivacaine) is shown in bold (C)

more rapidly. Preparation and storage are awkward, and the preparations are not widely available.

Additives with analgesic activity

Other agents developing roles in central and peripheral nerve blockade are shown in Figure 33.5. These additives are used to provide a synergistic effect on pain perception by interaction with specific receptors in the afferent pathways.

Specific pharmacology

n-Heptane/aqueous phosphate buffer partition coefficient indicates lipid solubility. Note that the use of octanol as lipid results in different figures. Units (unless stated otherwise) are:

Molecular weight (MW): daltons
Volume of distribution at steady state (V_d): L kg^{-1}
Clearance (Cl): mL kg^{-1} min^{-1}
Terminal half-life ($t_{1/2}$): minutes

Figure 33.6 shows the chemical formulae of the commonly used local anaesthetic agents.

Bupivacaine hydrochloride

Structure – amide local anaesthetic agent, pipecoloxylidide
Presentation – clear, colourless, aqueous solutions include:
Plain solutions (0.25%, 0.5%)
Solutions with 1:200,000 (5 µg mL^{-1}) adrenaline (0.25%, 0.5%)
Solutions for infusion – plain and opioid-containing
'Heavy' 0.5% with 80 mg mL^{-1} dextrose (specific gravity 1.026) for spinal anaesthesia
Recommended maximum dose – 2 mg kg^{-1} (150 mg plus up to 50 mg 2-hourly subsequently).

Pharmacokinetics

MW	288
pK$_a$	8.1
partition coefficient	27.5
protein binding	96%
V_d	1
Cl	7
$t_{1/2}$	30

Clinical – intermediate speed of onset, long action, four times as potent as lidocaine; propensity to cardiotoxicity
Elimination – 5% excreted as pipecoloxylidine after dealkylation in the liver, 16% excreted unchanged in urine

Levobupivacaine hydrochloride

As for bupivacaine hydrochloride except:
Structure – Laevorotatory enantiomer of racemic bupivacaine
Presentation – Plain solutions (2.5 mg mL^{-1}, 5.0 mg mL^{-1}, 7.5 mg mL^{-1})

Recommended maximum dose – 150 mg (2 mg kg^{-1}), total 400 mg in 24 h. 7.5 mg mL^{-1} contraindicated in obstetric practice

Pharmacokinetics

MW	288
pK$_a$	8.1
partition coefficient	27.5
protein binding	97%
V$_d$	1
Cl	9
t$_{1/2}$	80

Clinical – Levobupivacaine doses are expressed as milligrams of base compound, whereas racemic bupivacaine is expressed as the hydrochloride salt. Levobupivacaine therefore has 13% more activity than the same dose of racemic bupivacaine. Animal studies indicate lower CNS toxicity than bupivacaine

Elimination – Extensive metabolism with no unchanged levobupivacaine in urine or faeces. The major metabolite is 3-hydroxylevobupivacaine excreted in urine as sulphate and glucuronate conjugates (71% of dose in urine and 24% in faeces by 48 h)

Lidocaine hydrochloride

Structure – amide local anaesthetic agent, derivative of diethylaminoacetic acid

Presentation – clear, aqueous solutions include:
Plain solutions (0.5%, 1%, 2%)
Solutions with 1:200,000 (5 µg mL^{-1}) adrenaline (0.5%, 1%, 2%)
Gel (1%, 2%) with chlorhexidine for urethral instillation
Cream (4%) for topical anaesthesia (e.g. LMX 4)
Solutions for surface application to pharynx, larynx and trachea (4%) (coloured pink)
Spray for anaesthesia of the oral cavity and upper respiratory tract (10%)

Dose – topical, infiltration, nerve blocks, epidural and spinal; 0.5–10% available; 100 mg bolus then 1–4 mg min^{-1} for ventricular arrhythmias. Recommended maximum dose 200 mg (3 mg kg^{-1}); with adrenaline 500 mg (7 mg kg^{-1})

Pharmacokinetics

MW	234
pK$_a$	7.9
partition coefficient	2.9
protein binding	64%
V$_d$	1
Cl	9
t$_{1/2}$	100

Clinical – rapid speed of onset, intermediate action; class IB antiarrhythmic

Elimination – 70% by dealkylation in liver, < 10% excreted unchanged in urine

Prilocaine hydrochloride

Structure – amide local anaesthetic agent, secondary amine derived from toluidine

Presentation – clear, colourless, aqueous solutions include:
Plain solutions (1%, 4%)
Solutions with 0.03 unit mL^{-1} felypressin (3%)

Recommended maximum dose – 400 mg (6 mg kg^{-1}); with felypressin 600 mg (8.5 mg kg^{-1})

Pharmacokinetics

MW	220
pK$_a$	7.9
partition coefficient	0.9
protein binding	55%
V$_d$	3.7
Cl	40
t$_{1/2}$	261

Clinical – rapid speed of onset, duration of action intermediate between lidocaine and bupivacaine, potency similar to lidocaine; may result in methaemoglobinaemia

Elimination – rapidly metabolised to O-toluidine by liver, < 1% excreted unchanged

Ropivacaine hydrochloride

Structure – amide local anaesthetic agent, pipecoloxylidide

Presentation – clear, colourless, aqueous solutions of S-ropivacaine enantiomer include:
Plain solutions in 10 mL ampoules (2, 7.5, 10 mg mL^{-1})

Plain solution in 100 and 200 mL bags (2 mg mL^{-1}) for
epidural infusion

Recommended maximum dose – 250 mg (150 mg for
Caesarean section under epidural); cumulative dose of
675 mg over 24 h

Pharmacokinetics

MW	274
pK$_a$	8.1
partition coefficient	6.1
protein binding	94%
V$_d$	0.8
Cl	10
t$_{1/2}$	110

Clinical – intermediate onset, long duration of action
between lidocaine and bupivacaine, potency similar to
lidocaine; greater separation of sensory and motor
blockade, and lower cardiotoxicity than bupivacaine
may be advantages

Elimination – aromatic hydroxylation to 3- (and 4-)
hydroxy-ropivacaine, and N-dealkylation. 86% (mostly
conjugated) excreted in the urine, of which 1%
unchanged. 3- and 4-hydroxy-ropivacaine have
reduced local anaesthetic activity

Contraindication – IVRA

CHAPTER 34

Central nervous system pharmacology

Tim Smith

Many drugs act on the central nervous system (CNS), with various specific aims in mind. While certain categories of drugs are considered elsewhere (anaesthetic gases and vapours in Chapter 29, hypnotics and intravenous agents in Chapter 30), other drugs acting on the CNS have been grouped here. Antiemetic drugs are considered in detail, with specific pharmacology of individual agents to reflect their direct relevance to the practice of anaesthesia.

Antiemetic drugs

The causes of nausea and vomiting (NV) are legion, as illustrated by Figure 34.1, and antiemetic therapy is most effective when directed at the likely origin.

Postoperative nausea and vomiting (PONV) is a specific entity, and its treatment is more appropriately directed when other risk factors are considered. See Chapter 4 for the management of PONV.

Two distinct sites in the CNS, the vomiting centre and the chemoreceptor trigger zone, are implicated in the causes of NV (see Chapter 20). The chemoreceptor trigger zone lies in the area postrema outside the blood–brain barrier and possesses dopaminergic (D$_2$) and serotonergic (5-hydroxytryptamine, 5-HT$_3$) receptors. In contrast, the vomiting centre is a complex entity of interconnected areas located in the dorsolateral reticular formation of

Fundamentals of Anaesthesia, 4th edition, ed. Ted Lin, Tim Smith and Colin Pinnock. Published by Cambridge University Press. © Cambridge University Press 2017.

Figure 34.1 Causes of nausea and vomiting

Drug-induced
- Central effect – opioids, nitrous oxide
- Local effect – poisons, copper, sodium chloride
- Systemic effect – cytotoxic drugs

Pregnancy

Radiotherapy

Psychogenic

Vestibular
- Labyrinthitis
- Ménière's disease
- Motion sickness

Stimulation of vagal afferents in the pharynx

Hypotension

Migraine

Abdominal pathology

Raised intracranial pressure

the brainstem that possesses $5\text{-}HT_3$, D_2 and muscarinic (M_3) receptors. Histaminic (H_1) and neurokinin (NK_1) receptors are located in the nucleus of the tractus solitarius, which integrates afferent signals associated with emesis. The interaction of various drugs with these sites is shown in Figure 34.2.

The major classes of drug used to combat NV possess receptor antagonism at D_2, M_3, H_1 and $5\text{-}HT_3$ receptors. The more common agents and their receptor specificity are shown in Figure 34.3.

Antiemetic activity is ascribed to the following categories of drug:
- Anticholinergic drugs
- Phenothiazines
- Butyrophenones
- Antihistamines
- $5\text{-}HT_3$ receptor antagonists
- Cannabinoids
- Neurokinin receptor antagonists
- Steroids

Additionally, metoclopramide and domperidone are two peripherally acting antiemetic drugs of importance.

Anticholinergic drugs
Examples – atropine, hyoscine

Atropine and hyoscine cross the blood–brain barrier (unlike glycopyrrolate) and act on muscarinic cholinergic receptors in the vomiting centre and in the gastrointestinal tract. Anticholinergic drugs are antispasmodic, reducing intestinal tone and inhibiting sphincter relaxation. They also reduce salivary and gastric secretions and so reduce gastric distension. These are the drugs of choice for the treatment of motion sickness and opioid-induced nausea. Hyoscine has been popular for premedication in conjunction with opioids for this reason, and because it possesses a sedative effect. The side effects of anticholinergic drugs are predictable from the known effects of muscarinic cholinergic receptors. In particular, dry mouth and blurred vision can be a problem, and drowsiness is not uncommon. Bronchial secretions become more viscid, but a degree of bronchodilatation is seen (increasing anatomical dead space). Pupillary constriction may be abolished, which removes a useful indicator of depth of anaesthesia. Anticholinergic agents that cross the blood–brain barrier are implicated in the development of the central anticholinergic syndrome, which is detailed in Figure 34.4.

Treatment of the central anticholinergic syndrome is accomplished by the use of an anticholinesterase that can cross the blood–brain barrier. In practice, this requires a tertiary amine structure, and thus physostigmine would be the drug of choice, but it is no longer available.

Phenothiazines
Examples – perphenazine, prochlorperazine, promethazine

Phenothiazines have a variety of effects, including antiemesis. Trifluoperazine is a potent antiemetic, but its antipsychotic effects preclude its routine use for this purpose. Phenothiazines act on the D_2 receptors in the chemoreceptor trigger zone in the area postrema, and on M_3 receptors in the same way as anticholinergic agents. The major effect of promethazine is antihistaminic, although it has antidopaminergic and antimuscarinic activity that contribute to the antiemetic effect. Sedation may limit the usefulness of promethazine as an antiemetic drug. 6 mg of buccal prochlorperazine may be a useful alternative to IM injection.

Butyrophenones
Examples – benperidol, droperidol, haloperidol

Droperidol is an antagonist of D_2 receptors in the chemoreceptor trigger zone. It has potent antiemetic activity but can cause a dissociative phenomenon even in relatively small doses, when the patient appears outwardly content but experiences an unpleasant feeling of

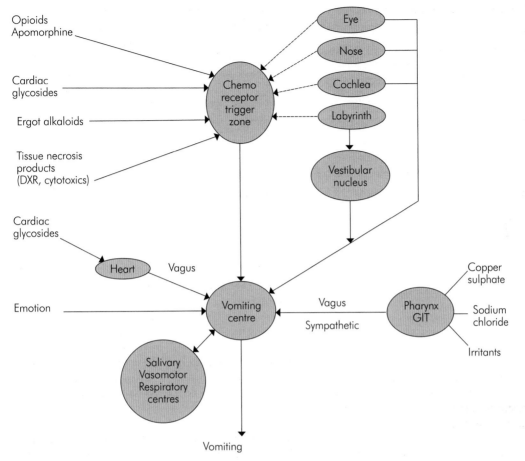

Figure 34.2 Causes of NV and sites of drug action

Figure 34.3 Receptor antagonism of antiemetic drugs

	D₂	M₃	H₁	5-HT₃
Hyoscine	0	++++	+	0
Promethazine	+	++	+++	0
Chlorpromazine	++	+	++	+
Metoclopramide	+	0	+	++
Droperidol	+++	0	+	+
Ondansetron	0	0	0	++++
Prochlorperazine	++++	+	+	0

Figure 34.4 The central anticholinergic syndrome

Causes
- Muscarinic anticholinergic drugs which cross the blood–brain barrier (typically atropine and hyoscine)

Risk factors
- Elderly patients most at risk

Features
- Excitement
- Drowsiness
- Ataxia
- Coma

Figure 34.5 Antiemetic drugs with antihistamine activity

Ethanolamines	Diphenhydramine Dimenhydrinate
Piperazines	Cyclizine Buclizine Cinnarizine
Phenothiazines	Promethazine

helplessness and vulnerability. It can prolong the QT interval of the ECG and is contraindicated in hypokalaemia and hypomagnesaemia.

Haloperidol and benperidol are primarily used as antipsychotic agents, but haloperidol possesses substantial anticonvulsant activity. It causes α_1-adrenoceptor blockade, which may result in postural hypotension.

Butyrophenones are metabolised in the liver. Side effects include extrapyramidal phenomena, neuroleptic malignant syndrome and hyperprolactinaemia with gynaecomastia.

Antihistamines
Examples – buclizine, cinnarizine, cyclizine, diphenhydramine

Several categories of drug may show antihistaminic activity. Figure 34.5 lists the main categories.

There are a number of chemically different agents that are antagonists at histaminergic receptors. The general term *antihistamine* tends to be used to describe anti-H_1 drugs alone. These are particularly effective in the treatment and prevention of motion sickness. The antiemetic action is centrally mediated, but H_1 antagonism may not be the sole mechanism of antiemesis. The sedative effects of antihistamines contribute to the treatment of nausea.

Ethanolamines (such as diphenhydramine) are potent antihistamines with some anticholinergic activity, which are thought to work at the labyrinth and the neural interface between the labyrinth and the vomiting centre.

Cyclizine is used for motion sickness and for PONV. It has anticholinergic activity, resulting in dry mouth, and can cause tachycardia if given intravenously. Cinnarizine is almost insoluble in water and only available in the tablet form. Buclizine has a long duration of action but is only available in combined formulation with other drugs.

5-Hydroxytryptamine (5-HT$_3$) receptor antagonists
Examples – granisetron, ondansetron, tropisetron

There are four basic types of serotonergic (5-HT) receptors (5-HT$_{1-4}$). 5-HT$_1$ receptors are subdivided further (5-HT$_{1A}$, etc.). An especially high density of 5-HT$_3$ receptors is found in the area postrema and nucleus tractus solitarius, where they are probably on the vagus nerve terminals. Receptors have also been identified on peripheral sections of the vagus nerve in the gastrointestinal tract, and the emetogenic effect of 5-HT release can also be blocked here.

Cannabinoids
Example – nabilone

Cannabis is derived from the plant *Cannabis sativa*. The active constituents of cannabis are called cannabinoids. Delta-9-tetrahydrocannabinol (Δ^9-THC) is the major active cannabinoid. A specific cannabinoid receptor has been identified in the CNS, and it is thought that cannabinoids act at the chemoreceptor trigger zone. Naloxone may be used to overcome their effects. Nabilone is a synthetic derivative of the naturally occurring tetrahydrocannabinol. It is effective against NV induced by opioids, cytotoxic therapy and radiotherapy. Taken orally, it is well absorbed and has a half-life of 120 minutes. Indications for cannabinoid therapy are limited by the side effects of hallucinations, psychosis, dizziness and dry mouth.

Neurokinin receptor antagonists
Example – aprepitant

Selective neurokinin (NK$_1$) receptor antagonists have been shown to have antiemetic activity via the nucleus of the tractus solitarius and dorsal motor nucleus of the vagus nerve. Aprepitant has a broader spectrum of antiemetic activity than 5-HT$_3$ antagonists. It has a half-life of 11 hours. Aprepitant is only available as oral capsules. Fosaprepitant is a prodrug of aprepitant and provides an intravenous alternative with rapid conversion in hepatic microsomes (97% conversion within 15 minutes) by dephosphorylation. Although fosaprepitant has some affinity for NK$_1$ receptors, the rapid conversion means that its clinical effect is produced by the resultant prepitant.

Steroids
Example – dexamethasone

Dexamethasone is a synthetic steroid that has found many diverse clinical uses. It appears to be effective in the prevention of PONV. Postulated mechanisms of action include prostaglandin inhibition (reducing the effect of surgically mediated tissue damage), inhibition of gut 5-HT release, inhibition of neuronal 5-HT and reduced release of endorphins. There may be a small risk of increased postoperative infection and of postoperative bleeding in high-risk patients on concomitant NSAIDs.

Posology of dexamethasone

Dexamethasone is supplied in ampoules containing 3.3 mg of dexamethasone per mL of solution. It also contains sodium and phosphate such that it combines two forms of dexamethasone. The molar masses are as follows: dexamethasone 392, phosphate 94, sodium 23. So the solutions contain 3.3 mg dexamethasone, which is equivalent to 4 mg dexamethasone phosphate or 4.3 mg dexamethasone sodium phosphate.

Peripherally acting antiemetic drugs
Examples – domperidone, metoclopramide

Metoclopramide and domperidone are chemically unrelated yet functionally similar. Metoclopramide hydrochloride is a white crystalline salt that is chemically related to procaine. It is readily soluble and stable in water. It has antidopaminergic (D_2) activity in the chemoreceptor trigger zone and also inhibits the emetic effects of gastric irritants. It also antagonises H_1 and $5-HT_3$ receptors and promotes gastric emptying through the pylorus. Extrapyramidal effects (such as oculogyric crisis) are the major potential side effects. Metoclopramide is indicated for PONV, opioid-induced nausea and NV related to cytotoxic drug treatment and radiotherapy.

Domperidone is a benzimidazole derivative that has both centrally and peripherally mediated effects. Peripherally, domperidone promotes gastric emptying and increases lower oesophageal sphincter tone. It crosses the blood–brain barrier (but only slowly) and then acts on dopamine receptors in the chemoreceptor trigger zone. This impaired transit across the blood–brain barrier reduces the incidence of extrapyramidal side effects. Domperidone is indicated for the treatment of PONV and opioid-induced NV but it is limited in its application as it cannot be given parenterally. The major application of the drug is in the treatment of cytotoxic and radiotherapy-induced NV. These agents may also be useful in promoting gastric transit when this is impaired by diabetic autonomic neuropathy.

Domperidone can also cause QT-interval prolongation and ventricular tachydysrhythmias, and sudden death has been reported.

Miscellaneous antiemetics
- Sedatives and anxiolytics often have an antiemetic effect by reducing the psychological component of the nausea. Propofol appears to reduce PONV.
- Betahistine is a histamine analogue used for the treatment of Ménière's disease and its associated NV.

Specific pharmacology of antiemetic drugs
Units (unless stated otherwise) are:
Volume of distribution at steady state (V_d): L kg^{-1}
Clearance (Cl): mL kg^{-1} min^{-1}
Terminal half-life ($t_{1/2}$): hours

Cyclizine hydrochloride and lactate
Structure – piperazine
Presentation
Oral – tablets 50 mg
IV/IM – 50 mg in 1 mL
Pharmacokinetics

Bioavailability	80%
$t_{1/2}$	10

Blood–brain barrier – crossed
CNS – antiemetic, with some sedation
CVS – slight tachycardia
RS – minimal effect
Other – increase in lower oesophageal sphincter pressure
Elimination – N-demethylation to norcyclizine (half-life 20 h, minimal activity), and also some to the oxide
Side effects – anticholinergic; dry mouth, blurred vision, drowsiness

Dexamethasone
Structure – glucocorticoid steroid
Presentation – IV, clear colourless solution; 8 mg dexamethasone in 2 mL; 3.3 mg dexamethasone in 1 mL (see box above)
CNS – may cause convulsions and increase ICP (but indicated for treatment of cerebral oedema)
CVS – minimal effect
RS – may be used for asthma and aspiration pneumonitis

Other – mineralocorticoid effects may be present to a limited extent
Elimination – liver metabolised
Side effects – as for hydrocortisone

Droperidol
Structure – butyrophenone
Presentation – clear colourless solution, 2.5 mg mL^{-1} in 1 mL for IV administration
Pharmacokinetics

Protein binding	90%
V_d	2
$t_{1/2}$	12

Blood–brain barrier – crossed
CNS – anxiolysis, placid state, indifference to environment, may be unpleasant feelings of helplessness not outwardly expressed; antiemesis via central D_2 antagonism in the chemoreceptor trigger zone
CVS – vasodilatation and decreased arterial pressure due to α-adrenergic blockade may occur when given intravenously
RS – minute volume, functional residual capacity and airway resistance all slightly decreased
Elimination – oxidative N-dealkylation in the liver
Side effects – extrapyramidal effects, gastrointestinal dysfunction, QT-interval prolongation

Metoclopramide hydrochloride
Structure – chlorinated procainamide derivative
Presentation
   Oral – tablets 10 mg, syrup 1 mg mL^{-1}
   IV – 10 mg in 2 mL
Pharmacokinetics

Protein binding	18%
V_d	2.8
Cl	10
$t_{1/2}$	4

CNS – antiemetic via chemoreceptor trigger zone, and by decreasing afferent activity from viscera to vomiting centre

CVS – some reports of hypotension, dysrhythmias and cardiac arrest
RS – minimal effects
Others – lower oesophageal sphincter pressure increased, gastric contractility and emptying increased, small intestine transport time accelerated; prolactin and aldosterone secretion increased; may increase ureteric peristalsis
Elimination – 80% in urine within 24 h, of which 20% unchanged, the rest conjugated or as sulphated metabolite
Side effects – drowsiness, dizziness, extrapyramidal effects

Ondansetron hydrochloride
Structure – 5-HT$_3$ receptor antagonist
Presentation
   Oral – tablets 4 mg
   IV – 4 mg in 2 mL (protect from light)
Pharmacokinetics

Bioavailability	60%
V_d	1.8
Cl	6
$t_{1/2}$	3

CNS – antiemetic
CVS – no effect with therapeutic doses
RS – no effect on respiratory regulation
Others – antagonises 5-HT$_3$ receptors on vagal afferents in small intestine, no effect on platelet function or prolactin secretion
Elimination – extensively metabolised in liver, main metabolite 8-hydroxyondansetron; metabolites conjugated; < 5% unchanged via urine
Side effects – constipation, headache, flushing

Prochlorperazine
Structure – piperazine phenothiazine
Presentation
   Oral – tablets 5 or 25 mg, buccal tablets 3 mg
   Suppositories 5 or 25 mg
   IM – clear colourless solution 12.5 mg in 1 mL
Pharmacokinetics

V_d	20
$t_{1/2}$	6

Figure 34.6 Modes of action of anticonvulsants

GABA facilitation	Benzodiazepines Barbiturates
GABA agonism	Progabide
GABA transaminase inactivation	Valproate Vigabatrin
Fast sodium channel blockade	Phenytoin
Presynaptic sodium channel stabilisation	Lamotrigine Valproate

Blood–brain barrier – crossed

CNS – antiemetic with neuroleptic effects, acting via dopaminergic (D_2) receptors

CVS – α-blockade occasionally causes postural hypotension; QT increased, ST depressed, T and U wave changes on ECG

RS – mild respiratory depressant effect

Other – lower oesophageal sphincter tone increased, antiadrenergic activity, antihistaminic and anticholinergic effects

Elimination – S-oxidation to a sulphoxide by the liver

Side effects – extrapyramidal effects

Anticonvulsant drugs

Epileptic events are the result of repetitive neuronal discharges in the CNS involving many neurones. Anticonvulsant drugs act by breaking these propagating and recycling currents, either by increasing inhibitory neurotransmitter levels or by facilitating their action by modulating the γ-aminobutyric acid (GABA) receptor function. There is the potential for new drugs to be developed that would inhibit excitatory neurotransmitters and their receptors (the N-methyl-D-aspartate agonist–receptor interaction is a likely target). The modes of action of anticonvulsants are listed in Figure 34.6.

The drug chosen for treatment of epilepsy depends greatly on the type of fits. Figure 34.7 shows treatment guidelines for different types of epilepsy.

In pregnancy, most anticonvulsant drugs carry a risk of neural tube defects, teratogenicity and coagulation disorders in the newborn. Counselling, antenatal screening, folate supplements and pre-delivery vitamin K should be considered. The greatest risk to mother and baby, however, is that of the re-emergence of convulsions. Fears about the drugs may lead to poor compliance in the

Figure 34.7 Types of epilepsy and drug choice

Status epilepticus	First line	IV Diazepam
	Subsequently	Phenytoin or Phenobarbital or Chlormethiazole or Paraldehyde
Prevention	Absences (petit mal)	Ethosuximide or Valproate
	Tonic–clonic	Carbamazepine or Lamotrigine or Phenytoin or Valproate or Phenobarbital
	Myoclonic	Valproate or Clonazepam or Lamotrigine or Ethosuximide
	Atypical (usually childhood, especially if any cerebral damage)	Clonazepam or Ethosuximide or Lamotrigine or Phenobarbital or Phenytoin or Valproate

complacent patient. In addition, the increase in body water during pregnancy will dilute the concentration of the anticonvulsant agent, thereby reducing its clinical effect.

Benzodiazepines

Examples – clobazam, clonazepam, diazepam

Benzodiazepines act by attaching to a specific area of the GABA–receptor complex. The benzodiazepine has an agonist activity at this site that facilitates the opening of the chloride channel by GABA. Chloride ions then flow down the concentration gradient into the cell, making it hyperpolarised (more negative) and so less excitable.

Diazepam is primarily used for the acute treatment of convulsions. It has the disadvantage of pronounced sedation, long half-life and active metabolite. Other benzodiazepines may be used prophylactically.

Barbiturates

Examples – phenobarbital, primidone

All barbiturates possess anticonvulsant activity, but phenobarbital is less sedative for a given anticonvulsant activity. It binds to the GABA receptor at a site distinct from the benzodiazepine receptor area, and facilitates the chloride channel opening. It is inhibitory at some excitatory synapses. The barbiturate primidone acts by being converted to phenobarbital.

Phenytoin

Phenytoin is a hydantoin that also has local anaesthetic and antiarrhythmic properties. It has structural similarities with the barbiturates. The site of action of phenytoin is the fast sodium channel responsible for depolarisation during an action potential. It binds to the channel when it is refractory following opening, and is therefore most effective when repetitive discharges occur. It may also interfere with calcium entry and with calmodulin protein kinases. Phenytoin can cause hirsutism, gum hyperplasia, megaloblastic anaemia and fetal malformations.

There is the potential for interaction with other drugs, including other anticonvulsants. The high degree of protein binding (85% bound to albumin) results in competition for the binding site with salicylates, phenylbutazone and valproate. Phenytoin metabolism is competitively inhibited by phenobarbital because of enzyme induction in the liver. The same hepatic microsomal enzymes are induced by phenytoin, phenobarbital, steroids, oestrogens and coumarins. As with ethanol, the enzyme system is readily saturated, so that as doses increase the metabolism changes from first-order kinetics (metabolism proportional to concentration) to zero-order kinetics (metabolism constant and maximal), and thus 'half-life' increases with dose.

Carbamazepine

Carbamazepine is structurally similar to the tricyclic antidepressants and has pharmacological similarities with phenytoin. It acts at voltage-gated sodium channels producing frequency-dependent depression of neuronal activity. It is also an agonist at the postsynaptic GABA receptor but it is unclear if this has significant effect in clinical use. With chronic usage, the half-life decreases from 30 to 15 hours due to enzyme induction.

Gabapentin and pregabalin

Gabapentin is an amino acid. The postulated mechanisms of action are listed in Figure 34.8. Gabapentin is used as adjunct treatment for partial seizures. It is also used to

Figure 34.8 Postulated mechanisms of action for gabapentin

Competes with Leu, Ile, Val, Phe for specific amino acid transmembrane transporter
Increases concentration and synthesis of brain GABA
Binds to $\alpha_2\delta$ subunit of voltage-sensitive Ca^{2+} channels
Reduces release of monoamine transmitter (noradrenaline, dopamine and 5-HT)
Inhibits voltage-sensitive Na channels
Increases 5-HT
Prevents neuronal death by inhibition of glutamate synthesis

treat neuropathic pain, trigeminal neuralgia and post-herpetic neuralgia. Pregabalin has the same mechanism of action but it is claimed to have more specificity for the target receptors, leading to a higher therapeutic index.

Valproate

Sodium valproate is a monocarboxylic acid that increases brain levels of GABA by inhibiting GABA transaminase and inactive presynaptic Na^+ channels. It is used for petit mal, myoclonic epilepsy and infantile spasms. It also has a role in the management of chronic pain, especially trigeminal neuralgia. It interferes with platelet numbers and function, and can cause neural tube defects.

Lamotrigine

Lamotrigine stabilises inactive presynaptic sodium channels and so reduces neurotransmitter release. It is used to treat partial seizures, tonic–clonic and myoclonic seizures. Concentrations are increased by carbamazepine and phenytoin (enzyme inducers) and reduced by valproate.

Vigabactrin

Vigabactrin binds to and inhibits GABA transaminase, resulting in increased GABA levels. It is used for partial epilepsy in combination therapy and as a sole agent for the treatment of the brief infantile spasms of West syndrome. Particular concerns are that a third of patients develop visual field defects, and that it may cause behavioural problems.

Figure 34.9 Classes of antidepressants

Tricyclic antidepressants (TCA)	Dibenzazepines Dibenzocycloheptenes
Monoamine oxidase inhibitors (MAOI)	Hydrazines Propargylamines Cyclopropylamines Reversible MAOI (RIMA)
Selective serotonin reuptake inhibitors (SSRI)	
Serotonin–noradrenaline reuptake inhibitor (SNRI)	
Selective noradrenaline reuptake inhibitor	
Noradrenergic and specific serotonergic antidepressants (NaSSA)	
Other antidepressants	Lithium

Tiagabine

Tiagabine is an adjunct antiepileptic used for treating partial seizures. It is a selective inhibitor of the GABA uptake carrier. A Cochrane review which found insufficient evidence of benefit in bipolar disorders noted that a significant proportion of patients had episodes of seizure or syncope (Vasudev *et al.* 2006). It is 96% protein-bound. It should be avoided in porphyria.

Levetiracetam

For use alone or as an adjunct for partial seizures and myoclonic seizures. No binding to the usual neurotransmitter agonist sites has yet been found, but it may work at a specific neuronal binding site, resulting in a selective action on epileptogenic neuronal tissue only. Non-epileptic neuronal tissue may therefore be unaffected.

Antidepressant agents

There are several different classes of antidepressant agents. The major categories of antidepressant drugs are listed in Figure 34.9.

Miscellaneous agents unrelated either structurally or functionally may also show antidepressant activity. Among these are nomifensine, maprotiline, venlafaxine, nefazodone, flupenthixol and L-tryptophan.

Tricyclic antidepressants

Examples – dibenzazepines (clomipramine, imipramine), dibenzocycloheptenes (amitriptyline, nortriptyline)

Tricyclic antidepressants are chemically related to the phenothiazines, but differ in that the central ring has an additional carbon atom. This changes the shape of the molecule from the planar phenothiazine molecule to a three-dimensional skeleton. Tricyclic antidepressants act by preventing reuptake of neurotransmitter (primarily noradrenaline) into the nerve terminal of monoaminergic neurones. This action is stronger at noradrenergic and serotinergic sites than at dopaminergic sites. Some drugs also act on presynaptic α_2-receptors to increase neurotransmitter release. Tricyclic agents also antagonise muscarinic cholinergic (amitriptyline is used in the treatment of nocturnal enuresis), H_1-histaminergic and α_1-adrenoceptors. In addition to the antidepressant effects, they cause sedation, weakness and fatigue. Cardiac effects include postural hypotension, sinus tachycardia and cardiac arrhythmias. Amitriptyline prolongs the PR and QT intervals on the ECG. In the plasma tricyclic antidepressants are 90–95% bound to albumin, and may become displaced by drugs such as aspirin which compete for the same binding sites.

While reuptake blockade occurs soon after administration, the onset of antidepressant action takes several weeks to develop. It is not clear why this is so, but it may be due to down-regulation of adrenergic and 5-HT receptors.

Tricyclic agents are metabolised by hepatic microsomal enzymes, and are therefore competitively antagonised by some neuroleptic drugs which share the same route of excretion. There are two main methods of metabolism: either N-demethylation, converting the tertiary amine to a secondary amine, or ring hydroxylation.

Monoamine oxidase inhibitors (MAOIs)

Examples – cyclopropylamines (tranylcypromine), hydrazines (iproniazid, phenelzine), propargylamines (pargyline, selegiline)

Two variants of monoamine oxidase have been described, MAO-A and MAO-B. MAO-A is more effective at oxidising noradrenaline and 5-HT than MAO-B, but types A and B are equally effective in the metabolism of dopamine and tyramine. Antidepressant activity is conferred by inhibition of MAO-A. MAOIs act by antagonising the breakdown of monoamine neurotransmitters after uptake into the nerve terminal. In most cases inhibition is irreversible.

Pargyline, phenelzine, tranylcypromine and iproniazid non-selectively inhibit both MAO-A and MAO-B, while clorygyline is selective for MAO-A. Selegiline is selective for MAO-B and is therefore not antidepressant but is used in Parkinsonism, acting by inhibition of dopamine oxidation. Reuptake blockade occurs soon after administration, but the onset of antidepressant action takes several weeks to develop. In a similar fashion to the tricyclic antidepressants, this may be due to down-regulation of adrenergic and 5-HT receptors. Patients being treated with MAOI drugs also become compromised in their ability to metabolise exogenously administered amines. The pressor effect of tyramine (which is found in cheese, broad beans, red wine and Marmite) is greatly enhanced. Indirect sympathomimetic drugs such as those found in cough medicines will show enhanced effects. A specific interaction with pethidine may result in profound coma.

Reversible MAOIs
Example – moclobemide

These drugs reversibly inhibit MAO-A, and are also called RIMAs (reversible inhibition of MAO-A). Caution should still be exercised with foods rich in tyramine and sympathomimetic agents, but the problem is likely to be less marked. The advantage of RIMAs is that they can be stopped and another antidepressant started without the need to wait several weeks for MAO enzyme regeneration.

Selective serotonin reuptake inhibitors (SSRIs)
Examples – fluoxetine, paroxetine, sertraline

SSRIs act by increasing the level of 5-HT at the neuronal receptors. The specificity for 5-HT results in fewer antimuscarinic and cardiac side effects than with other antidepressants. Sedation is less marked than with the tricyclic antidepressants. Diarrhoea and NV are more common, and headache, restlessness and anxiety may occur. Withdrawal should be slow, over several weeks, and MAOI therapy should not be started until 2–5 weeks after stopping the SSRI treatment (dependent on which drug was being taken). SSRI should not be started until 2 weeks after stopping MAOI therapy.

Serotonin–noradrenaline reuptake inhibitors (SNRIs)
Example – venlafaxine

Serotonin–noradrenaline reuptake inhibitors inhibit both noradrenaline and serotonin (5-HT) neuronal reuptake. Venlafaxine is a bicyclic phenylethylamine antidepressant that inhibits presynaptic reuptake of 5-HT, noradrenaline and to a much lesser extent dopamine. There is no effect on adrenergic, cholinergic or histaminergic **receptors**. The specificity results in lower adverse effects than with the tricyclic antidepressants.

Selective noradrenaline reuptake inhibitors
Example – reboxetine

Reboxetine is a selective inhibitor of noradrenaline reuptake. Again the specificity results in lower adverse effects than with the tricyclic antidepressants.

Noradrenergic and specific serotonergic antidepressants
Example – mirtazapine

Mirtazapine increases noradrenaline and 5-HT neurotransmission by blockade of α_2-adrenoceptors, and also blocks $5\text{-}HT_2$ and $5\text{-}HT_3$ receptors. The $5\text{-}HT_3$ blockade reduces the incidence of nausea. The specificity results in lower adverse effects than with the tricyclic antidepressants.

Lithium
Lithium is used prophylactically to suppress the manic element of bipolar depression (manic–depressive psychosis). It is unclear how the pharmacological activity of lithium produces the clinical effect. The active component of lithium carbonate is the lithium cation (Li^+). Chemically, lithium is the first element in group IA of the periodic table (the same group as sodium and potassium). It has atomic number 3 and a molecular weight of 7. It mimics cations, especially sodium. It passes through the fast sodium channels easily, being smaller, but the $Na^+K^+ATPase$ pump does not readily extract lithium from the cells, and it therefore tends to accumulate intracellularly, which in turn displaces potassium and reduces the outward leakage of potassium responsible for maintaining the negative intracellular potential. In this way, the transmembrane potential becomes reduced and neuronal depolarisation is facilitated. Lithium also reduces brain levels of noradrenaline and 5-HT acutely, reduces cAMP production, and reduces inositol triphosphate.

Lithium has a low therapeutic index, and plasma levels should therefore be maintained between 0.4 and 1.0 mmol per litre. Toxicity occurs with levels of over 2.0 mmol per litre. The half-life of the extracellular ion is about 12 hours, and lithium should be stopped 2–3 days before using a muscle-relaxant drug. This is particularly important for non-depolarising relaxants that are potentiated. It may also delay the onset and prolong relaxation with suxamethonium. The intracellular lithium takes a further 1–2 weeks to excrete. Lithium inhibits vasopressin activity in the kidney via cAMP and increases aldosterone secretion, which can result in renal tubular damage. Lithium inhibits thyroid hormone release and thyroid hypertrophy, and hypothyroidism may occur. Neurological effects include thirst, tremor, muscle weakness, confusion and seizures. Cardiac arrhythmias may be induced, and all toxic effects are enhanced if dehydration occurs. Close monitoring of clinical state, lithium levels and renal function is essential to minimise toxicity.

Antipsychotic drugs

A wide variety of drugs have antipsychotic activity. These have been variously referred to as neuroleptics, major tranquillisers and anti-schizophrenia drugs. Specific categories of drug that have antipsychotic activity include:

- Phenothiazines
- Butyrophenones
- Thioxanthines
- Benzamide
- Diphenylbutylpiperidine
- Dibenzodiazepines

The mode of action of these drugs in the treatment of psychosis is not precisely known. Various receptor systems have been implicated, including dopaminergic, noradrenergic and 5-hydroxytryptaminergic (serotonergic). It is likely that many different receptors are affected, but D_2-dopaminergic receptors are currently thought to be the most important. While D_1 receptors increase adenylyl cyclase activity generally, D_2 receptors are found both pre- and postsynaptically, and blocking potency at these receptors correlates closely with clinical potency. The delay in onset of a therapeutic effect from these drugs may in part be explained by a slow increase in the numbers of D_2 receptors over several weeks. Some antipsychotic drugs are formulated so that they may be administered by deep IM injection given at intervals of 1–4 weeks.

As antipsychotic agents affect so many receptors, a wide diversity of adverse effects results. These are listed in Figure 34.10.

Phenothiazines

Phenothiazines may be classified chemically by the side chain on the nitrogen atom of the phenothiazine base as follows:

- Aliphatic – chlorpromazine
- Piperidine – thioridazine
- Piperazine – fluphenazine

Figure 34.10 Adverse effects of antipsychotic drugs

Antidopaminergic
Antiemesis
Extrapyramidal features
• Facial grimacing
• Involuntary movements of tongue and limbs
• Oculogyric crises
• Torsion spasms
• Tasikinesia
• Akithisia
• Parkinsonism
• Tardive dyskinesia
• Increased prolactin secretion
Antimuscarinic
• Dry mouth
• Constipation
• Urinary retention
• Blurred vision
• Precipitation of glaucoma
Anti-α-adrenergic
• Postural hypotension
Antihistaminergic
• Sedation

The side chains alter the potency and specificity for the receptor types and in turn alter the clinical features (Figure 34.11).

Thioxanthines

Examples – flupenthixol, zuclopenthixol

Thioxanthines are similar in structure and function to the aliphatic phenothiazines, and therefore block D_2 receptors more than D_1. Flupenthixol is also employed clinically as an antidepressant agent.

Other antipsychotic drugs

Other miscellaneous antipsychotic drugs include sulpiride, which has a greater affinity for D_2 than D_1 receptors;

Figure 34.11 Receptor sensitivity of phenothiazines

Chain	Receptor blockade		Clinical effect		
	D$_2$	α-Adrenergic	Muscarinic	Extrapyramidal	Sedation
Aliphatic	+	+++	++	++	+++
Piperidine	++	++	+++	+	++
Piperazine	+++	+	+	+++	+

pimozide, which may prolong QT interval on the ECG; and clozapine, which has been associated with agranulocytosis.

Anti-Parkinsonian drugs

Parkinson's disease is caused by a dysfunction within the basal ganglia. The predominant change is a deficit of dopamine with an increase in dopamine D$_2$ receptors, but other neurotransmitters are also implicated in the pathology of the disease. Drugs that affect Parkinson's disease may act in any of the following ways:

- Increased dopamine synthesis (levodopa)
- Decreased peripheral conversion of levodopa (carbidopa)
- Decreased dopamine breakdown (selegiline)
- Dopamine receptor agonists (bromocriptine)
- Dopamine receptor facilitators (amantadine)
- Acetylcholine antagonists (benztropine)

Levodopa

Levodopa (L-DOPA) is used to increase brain levels of dopamine. Dopamine does not cross the blood–brain barrier, and racemic DOPA produces numerous systemic side effects without being effective. DOPA is well absorbed orally and 95% is converted into dopamine by DOPA-decarboxylase. This is then metabolised by mono-amine oxidase and catechol-O-methyl transferase (COMT). About 1% of the drug enters the brain, where it is converted into its active form, dopamine. Levodopa causes an increase in the number of dopamine (D$_2$) receptors in the brain.

Carbidopa

Used in conjunction with levodopa, carbidopa increases the proportion of the oral dose of levodopa entering the brain by inhibiting its peripheral conversion to dopamine. Carbidopa itself does not cross the blood–brain barrier, and therefore does not interfere with subsequent conversion in the brain.

Domperidone

Used in conjunction with levodopa, this dopamine antagonist only crosses the blood–brain barrier slowly, and it is used to reduce the peripheral effects of dopamine. It has important antiemetic activity peripherally and also at the chemoreceptor trigger zone. Domperidone permits the use of larger doses of levodopa than would otherwise be possible without gross unwanted effects. Domperidone is covered in more detail earlier in this chapter (see *Antiemetic drugs*).

Selegiline

Selegiline is a selective MAO-B inhibitor. This selectivity reduces the peripheral effects of conventional MAO inhibitors, which are largely due to MAO-A inhibition. There is no effect from tyramine-containing foods, and drug interactions are less severe and less common.

Dopaminergic drugs

Examples – bromocriptine, cabergoline, quinagolide

Dopaminergic drugs act by direct stimulation of central dopamine (D$_2$) receptors. They are reserved for patients in whom levodopa is ineffective. Predictably, these drugs inhibit prolactin secretion. They are sometimes referred to as 'dopamine facilitators'. Cabergoline lasts longer than bromocriptine and has fewer side effects. Bromocriptine and cabergoline are chemically related to the ergot alkaloids and may be associated with retroperitoneal, pulmonary and pericardial fibrosis. Quinagolide is not derived from ergot and may avoid this risk.

Amantadine

The mode of action of amantadine remains obscure. Possibilities include facilitation of dopamine release, inhibition of dopamine metabolism and direct D$_2$ agonist activity.

Acetylcholine antagonists

Examples – benzhexol, benztropine, orphenadrine, procyclidine

Certain muscarinic antagonists can cross the blood–brain barrier, having a preferential action on central muscarinic receptors, thus minimising their peripheral side effects. The central excitatory effects of acetylcholine are inhibited, and this may restore the imbalance between cholinergic and dopaminergic activity that occurs in Parkinson's disease. Cholinergic antagonists also antagonise presynaptic inhibition of dopaminergic neurones, so increasing dopamine release, which may prove therapeutic.

References and further reading

Diemunsch P, Schoeffler P, Bryssine B, *et al.* Antiemetic activity of the NK1 receptor antagonist GR205171 in the treatment of postoperative nausea and vomiting after major gynaecological surgery. *Br J Anaesth* 1999; **82**: 274–6.

Gan TJ. Risk factors for postoperative nausea and vomiting. *Anesth Analg* 2006; **102**: 1884–98.

Taylor CP, Gee NS, Su T, *et al.* A summary of mechanistic hypotheses of gabapentin pharmacology. *Epilepsy Res* 1998; **29**: 233–49.

Vasudev A, MacRitchie K, Rao SNK, Geddes JR, Young AH. Tiagabine in the treatment of acute affective episodes in bipolar disorder: efficacy and acceptability. *Cochrane Database Syst Rev* 2006; (3): CD004694.

Williams PI, Smith M. An assessment of prochlorperazine buccal for the prevention of nausea and vomiting during intravenous patient-controlled analgesia with morphine following abdominal hysterectomy. *Eur J Anaesthesiol* 1999; **16**: 638–45.

CHAPTER 35

Autonomic nervous system pharmacology

Tim Smith

The autonomic nervous system (ANS) comprises the sympathetic and parasympathetic nervous systems. Ganglionic synaptic transmission in the ANS is mediated by the release of acetylcholine from the preganglionic neurone. Both muscarinic and nicotinic receptors are involved in mediation of the postganglionic response, as are inhibitory dopaminergic interneurones. In general, sympathetic postganglionic neurones are noradrenergic, and parasympathetic postganglionic neurones are muscarinic (cholinergic). The two systems tend to have opposite actions. Deliberate pharmacological manipulation of the ANS is therefore aimed at sites where physiological or anatomical differences exist between the two systems.

Cholinergic system

The important structural features of the neurotransmitter acetylcholine are the strongly positive quaternary amine in the choline part of the molecule and the ester component with its partial negative charge. Choline receptor antagonists have either a tertiary or a quaternary amine (or both). Acetylcholine receptors are classified as either muscarinic or nicotinic. Nicotinic receptors are widespread in the body, and are found in both sympathetic and parasympathetic nervous systems. Drug actions at the nicotinic receptors of the neuromuscular junction, which is not part of the ANS, are covered in Chapter 32.

Muscarinic receptors

The muscarinic receptors are G-protein-coupled receptors. Five subtypes have been identified (M_{1-5}), but the most important ones are M_1, M_2 and M_3, which are all antagonised by atropine. M_1 receptors are found in the central nervous system (CNS), autonomic ganglia and gastric parietal cells, M_2 receptors are found in the heart and at presynaptic sites, and M_3 receptors are found in

Fundamentals of Anaesthesia, 4th edition, ed. Ted Lin, Tim Smith and Colin Pinnock. Published by Cambridge University Press. © Cambridge University Press 2017.

smooth muscle, vascular endothelium (causing vasodilatation) and exocrine glands.

Muscarinic agonists

Examples – carbachol, pilocarpine

Pharmacological features

In common with other agonists, these drugs bear a structural relationship to the relevant endogenous agonist (acetylcholine). Pharmacological activity is reduced by changing the nitrogen unit from quaternary to tertiary, by removing the ester and by increasing the length of the aliphatic component on the quaternary nitrogen. Such changes also reduce hydrolysis and increase the half-life. This is essential to enable the drug to be given by conventional intermittent doses.

Carbachol has a quaternary amino group with the acetyl component changed to a carbamyl group so that it produces both nicotinic and muscarinic effects. Pilocarpine has a tertiary amino group and possesses muscarinic effects only.

Clinical effects

Muscarinic agonists are used to constrict the pupil to reduce intraocular pressure in glaucoma, and to improve micturition by increasing detrusor muscle contraction.

The muscarinic agonists are often referred to as parasympathomimetics, because the peripheral muscarinic receptors are predominantly located in the parasympathetic system. Their effects are predictable from this knowledge, and are summarised in Figure 35.1.

Muscarinic antagonists

Examples – atropine, glycopyrrolate, hyoscine

Pharmacological features

Muscarinic antagonists compete with acetylcholine in the end effector organs of the parasympathetic system, and in the sweat glands, which are also muscarinic yet innervated by the sympathetic system. Atropine and hyoscine are naturally occurring agents formed from esters of tropic acid and either tropine or scopine. The tertiary amines such as atropine and hyoscine cross the blood–brain barrier, whereas quaternary amines such as glycopyrrolate and ipratropium do not.

Clinical effects

Muscarinic antagonists increase cardiac activity by increasing heart rate (blood pressure often rises as a result). They inhibit most secretions and sweating. In the gastrointestinal

Figure 35.1 Clinical effects of muscarinic agonists

Cardiovascular system
- Atrial contractility decreased
- Heart rate decreased
- Blood pressure decreased
- Systemic vascular resistance decreased

Respiratory system
- Mucous secretion stimulated
- Bronchoconstriction, with increased resistance and decreased dead space

Gastrointestinal system
- Propulsive activity increased
- Salivary, exocrine pancreatic, gastric and intestinal secretions stimulated

Urogenital system
- Sphincter tone decreased
- Detrusor tone increased

Eye
- Miosis
- Ciliary muscle stimulated (poor focusing on far objects)
- Lacrimation increased

and urinary systems there is increased sphincter tone and reduced motility. The pupils are dilated and accommodation is blocked, causing blurred vision. The clinical effects of the muscarinic antagonists are the opposite of those of the agonists, and are shown in Figure 35.2.

Atropine

Atropine is initially synthesised in the S(–) form by plants, but it spontaneously racemes, so the commercial preparation of atropine contains a mixture of both enantiomers, which are frequently referred to as hyoscyamine, in particular the R(+) enantiomer. There is an aromatic group in place of the acetyl group of acetylcholine, and there is a tertiary amino group in place of the quaternary one. The muscarinic effects are mainly due to the L form. Atropine is chemically related to cocaine, and consequently it has a weak local anaesthetic effect. Atropine readily crosses the blood–brain barrier and the placenta. Initially the drug causes CNS excitation, followed by depression.

Glycopyrrolate

Glycopyrrolate has a quaternary ammonium group and does not readily cross the blood–brain barrier, and

Figure 35.2 Clinical effects of muscarinic antagonists

Peripheral

Cardiovascular system
- SA node and atria hypopolarised
- Refractory period of SA node and atria increased
- Refractory period of AV node decreased
- Conduction velocity in SA node, atria and AV node increased
- Atrial contractility increased
- Heart rate increased
- Systemic vascular resistance increased (vascular receptors not innervated)
- Salivary gland arterioles vasoconstricted

Respiratory system
- Mucous secretion inhibited
- Bronchodilatation

Gastrointestinal system
- Sphincter activity increased
- Propulsion reduced
- Biliary tree constricted
- Salivary, exocrine pancreatic, gastric and intestinal secretions inhibited

Urogenital system
- Sphincter tone increased
- Detrusor tone reduced
- Erectile tissue vasoconstricts

Eye
- Mydriasis
- Ciliary muscle relaxed
- Lacrimal secretions reduced

Central
- Sedation
- Antiemesis
- Anti-Parkinsonian

therefore central anticholinergic effects are minimal. It also has the advantage that its duration of effect is similar to that of neostigmine, with which it is given concomitantly for the reversal of neuromuscular blockade.

Hyoscine

The muscarinic effects of hyoscine are due mainly to the L form. Hyoscine causes CNS depression, and as the hydrobromide has a useful role as a sedative and antiemetic in premedication. As the butylbromide it is a useful smooth muscle relaxant for treating gastrointestinal and genitourinary spasm. It is notable that the parenteral doses of these two preparations are 100-fold different.

Nicotinic receptors

The nicotinic acetylcholine receptors are part of a transmembrane protein ion channel. In the ANS, they are located in the ganglia. The pharmacology of the nicotinic receptors at the neuromuscular junction is discussed in detail in Chapter 32.

Nicotinic agonists

Nicotine is the most prevalent exogenous agent active at the nicotinic receptors. It preferentially affects autonomic ganglia rather than the neuromuscular junction, and causes central stimulation. When an excess of acetylcholine occurs, such as when acetylcholinesterase is blocked by an anticholinesterase (for example, neostigmine or an organophosphorus compound), there will be nicotinic stimulation of the ganglia. Stimulation of autonomic ganglia has no clinical application, but the following effects will be seen: vasoconstriction, hypertension, sweating and salivation. Gut motility may increase or decrease.

Nicotinic antagonists

Nicotinic antagonists cause blockade of autonomic ganglia. They have been superseded by drugs targeting more specific parts of the autonomic system. The neuromuscular blocking agent D-tubocurarine caused ganglion blockade as a side effect and has also been superseded by drugs with more specificity for the nicotinic receptors of the muscle endplate. This is made possible by the different subchain types (specifically the α subunit) and subtypes that make up the pentameric nicotinic receptor (see *Drug–cell membrane receptors* in Chapter 28).

Clinical effects

Drugs causing ganglion blockade reduce blood pressure by a combination of vasodilatation and inhibition of compensatory effects such as tachycardia. The vasodilatation affects both arterioles (afterload) and venules (preload). The effect on the capacitance vessels reduces venous pressure and consequently intraoperative venous oozing. In general use, ganglion blockade causes postural hypotension, as the venous tone does not increase to compensate for the upright position.

Drugs interfering with synthesis, release and metabolism of acetylcholine

Magnesium ions and aminoglycosides inhibit calcium entry into the synaptic terminal, and so prevent neuro-transmitter release. Botulinum toxin and β-bungarotoxin bind irreversibly to nicotinic nerve terminals and prevent neurotransmitter release (α-bungarotoxin blocks post-synaptic acetylcholine receptors). The main effect of these compounds is that of muscle paralysis. However, if venti-lation support is instituted then the excessive parasympa-thetic blockade is still a serious problem.

Metabolism of acetylcholine is inhibited by anticholin-esterases and organophosphorus compounds, resulting in excess levels of acetylcholine. Initially, these cause increasing levels of stimulation of the parasympathetic system, but further rises cause depolarising blockade of the postsynaptic membrane with muscle paralysis.

Adrenergic system

The postganglionic neurones of the sympathetic nervous system provide the adrenergic component of the ANS. The adrenoceptors (adrenergic receptors) are located on the postsynaptic membrane of the end organ. Catechol-amines are the agonists at these receptors, which are readily affected by circulating catecholamines and adren-ergic drugs. The ubiquity of the sympathetic nervous system results in diverse effects when drugs interfering with adrenergic neurotransmission are used.

Adrenoceptors

The adrenoceptors are structurally similar. They are G-protein-coupled receptors with seven transmembrane α-helical segments (see *Drug–cell membrane receptors* in Chapter 28). Drugs affecting the adrenergic system work either by being structurally similar to the neurotransmit-ter, or by interfering with storage, release or metabolism. Drugs with a structural similarity take the place of the endogenous agonist and either mimic (agonism) or block (antagonism) the effect on the receptor. The endogenous neurotransmitters and hormones noradrenaline, adrena-line and dopamine are used pharmacologically. The two basic divisions of adrenoceptors (α and β) are affected to different degrees by various drugs. They were originally defined by their responses to noradrenaline, adrenaline and isoprenaline in the following manner:

Agonist responses of adrenoceptors
- α-adrenoceptor: noradrenaline $\geq$ adrenaline $>$ isoprenaline

Figure 35.3 Characteristics of the adrenoceptor subtypes

Receptor	Location	Effect on neurotransmission
α_1	Postsynaptic	Excitatory
α_2	Presynaptic	Inhibitory
β_1	Postsynaptic	Excitatory
β_2	Postsynaptic	Inhibitory
β_3	Postsynaptic	–

- β-adrenoceptor: isoprenaline $\geq$ adrenaline $\geq$ noradrenaline

The subclassifications are now performed using selective antagonists. α- and β- receptors are further subdivided into α_1 and α_2, and β_1, β_2 and β_3. They may be located at different sites or at the same synapses, and drugs may have specificity for one subtype over another, although this is not usually exclusive. Figure 35.3 details the recep-tor subtypes and their characteristics.

Clinical effects
The clinical effects of the adrenoceptors are as follows:
- α_1 – vasoconstriction, gut smooth muscle relaxation, increased saliva secretion, hepatic glycogenolysis
- α_2 – inhibition of autonomic neurotransmitter (noradrenaline and acetylcholine) release, stimulation of platelet aggregation
- β_1 – increased heart rate, increased myocardial contractility, gut smooth muscle relaxation, lipolysis
- β_2 – vasodilatation, bronchiole dilatation, visceral smooth muscle relaxation, hepatic glycogenolysis, muscle tremor
- β_3 – lipolysis, thermogenesis

Drugs acting on the adrenoceptors may cause agonism, antagonism or partial agonism, and often have a mixture of effects at different receptor types. Figure 35.4 shows the relative agonism and antagonism of various drugs on the adrenoceptor subtypes.

Adrenergic drugs will be considered further according to their primary effect in the clinical setting.

Pharmacological features
The structure–activity relationship of adrenergic drugs is marked. The basic catecholamine structure consists of an

Figure 35.4 Drug–receptor interactions at adrenoceptors

	α_1	α_2	β_1	β_2
Agonists				
Noradrenaline	+++	+++	++	+
Phenylephrine	++	0	0	0
Clonidine	0	+++	0	0
Dopamine	+	0	++	++
Adrenaline	++	++	+++	+++
Dobutamine	0	0	+++	+
Salbutamol	0	0	+	+++
Isoprenaline	0	0	+++	+++
Antagonists				
Phentolamine	—	—	0	0
Phenoxybenzamine	—	—	0	0
Prazocin	—	–	0	0
Indoramin	—	–	0	0
Ergotamine	pa	—	0	0
Labetalol	—	–	–	–
Propranolol	0	0	—	—
Atenolol	0	0	—	–

$^+$, agonist activity; $^-$, antagonist activity; pa, partial agonist activity

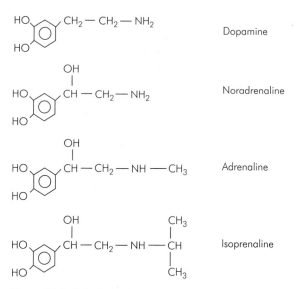

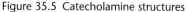

Figure 35.5 Catecholamine structures

Note that β-adrenoceptor agonists are covered in more detail in Chapter 37.

Clinical uses

Adrenoceptor agonists are administered systemically for myocardial failure (inotropic), sepsis (vasoconstriction and inotropy), anaphylaxis, nasal congestion and broncho-spasm. They may be administered peripherally to cause local vasoconstriction and so prolong the effects of local anaesthetics and reduce bleeding in the operative field. β_2-Agonists are effective in the treatment of asthma when inhaled, which reduces systemic effects.

Adrenaline

Adrenaline has both α- and β-agonist effects and many applications. It is an inotrope and chronotrope but sensitises the myocardium to arrhythmias. The ventricles in particular become hyperexcitable. There is generalised vasoconstriction, but dilatation of skeletal muscle arterioles.

Dobutamine

Dobutamine is a non-selective β-agonist with both chronotropic and inotropic effects. It is usually used for its inotropic effect, but tachycardia may limit the dose. It causes some vasodilatation, and this may require concurrent treatment with an α-agonist such as noradrenaline.

organic ring and side chain. Increasing the size of the attachment to the amino group of the side chain increases the affinity for β-receptors, which increases the effect of both agonists and antagonists, and reduces the effect of monoamine oxidase and the uptake 1 mechanism (U1) which removes catecholamines from the synaptic cleft. The β-hydroxy group is important for α-agonist activity and β-antagonism, while removal reduces receptor affinity. Substitution or repositioning of the catechol hydroxyl groups results in resistance to catechol-O-methyl transferase (COMT) and uptake 1. Removal of one or both catechol hydroxyl groups reduces or obliterates receptor affinity but leaves uptake 1 intact. The structure of the more common catecholamines is shown in Figure 35.5.

Adrenoceptor agonists

Examples – adrenaline, clonidine, dobutamine, dopamine, dopexamine, isoprenaline, noradrenaline

Dopamine

Dopamine is an agonist at α_1-, β- and dopamine receptors. The balance of these effects is dose-related. Initially only dopamine receptors are affected, but with increasing doses β-receptors and then α-receptors are also affected. Peripheral dopamine receptors are located in the renal arterioles and are responsible for vasodilatation. Dopamine is often used to maintain renal perfusion when this may be compromised. Increasing the dose recruits the β-receptors with their positive inotropic effect. This is limited by the onset of a tachycardia. Vasoconstriction (α_1) may become a problem as the drug dose increases.

Dopexamine

Dopexamine is an agonist of β_2-adrenergic and D_1 and D_2 dopamine receptors in the periphery. It also inhibits neuronal noradrenaline reuptake (uptake 1), so enhancing the β effects. It is a positive inotrope but has the principal effect of peripheral vasodilatation, especially of the splanchnic and renal arterioles. The resulting reduction in afterload improves cardiac output.

Isoprenaline

Isoprenaline is used in the treatment of bronchospasm, bradycardia and heart block. It is used to increase heart rate in complete heart block while electrical pacing is instituted. It is agonist at β_1- and β_2-receptors.

Noradrenaline

Noradrenaline is primarily an α_1-agonist and causes vasoconstriction (although it does have some β-agonist effects). It is particularly useful in patients with septicaemic shock, as they have a pathological reduction in systemic vascular resistance resulting in hypotension and hypoperfusion due to diversion of blood away from essential organs. The inotropic effect, although small, may also help. It may cause a reflex bradycardia if hypotension is overcorrected.

Salbutamol

Salbutamol is an effective bronchodilator, used in both the treatment and prophylaxis of obstructive airway disease. It is a selective β_2-agonist, and this minimises the undesirable effects such as tachycardia, although this β_1 effect does still occur with higher doses. It also has a role as a uterine relaxant for the treatment of premature labour and before delivery during Caesarean section.

Clonidine

Clonidine is an α_2-agonist used as a centrally acting antihypertensive agent that works by reducing noradrenaline release. Its role in preventing migraine is controversial. α_2-receptors are located on the presynaptic membrane of noradrenergic neurones, and have also been found in the spinal cord and at peripheral nerve endings. Clonidine may prolong the effect of epidurally administered local anaesthetic agents, although it is not licensed for this route.

Metaraminol

Metaraminol tartrate has both α- and β-agonist effects, with the α effect predominating. It increases systemic and pulmonary vascular resistance and causes increased systolic and diastolic blood pressures. Heart rate decreases in response and some inotropy occurs, although overall cardiac output may fall or may not change. Cerebral and renal blood flow are reduced by the vasoconstriction, and during pregnancy uterine tone is increased. β effects increase blood glucose levels.

α-Adrenoceptor antagonists

Examples – alfuzosin, doxazocin, phenoxybenzamine, phentolamine, tamsulosin

Uses

α_1-Adrenoceptor antagonists are used as antihypertensives and in benign prostatic hyperplasia.

Clinical effects

α-Blockade causes vasodilatation with reduced systemic vascular resistance and lowered blood pressure. There is a reflex increase in heart rate and cardiac output.

Phenoxybenzamine

Phenoxybenzamine is a haloalkylamine. The N-chloroethyl group binds covalently to part of the receptor. It therefore detaches from the receptor very slowly and behaves like a competitive irreversible antagonist. The recovery half-life is about 24 hours. Phenoxybenzamine is also an antagonist of acetylcholinergic, 5-hydroxytryptaminergic and histaminic receptors. Its primary effect is that of vasodilatation.

Phentolamine

Phentolamine affects both α_1 and α_2. It does not bind covalently and so is reversible.

Labetalol

Labetalol is an antagonist at both α_1- and β-receptors. The reflex tachycardia from the α-blockade is antagonised by the β-blockade. α-Blockade is more prominent when it is used intravenously, whereas β-blockade is the main effect when it is used orally.

Tamsulosin and alfuzosin

Tamsulosin and alfuzosin have specificity for the α_{1A}-adrenoceptor, giving targeted treatment of benign prostatic hypertrophy by smooth muscle relaxation.

β-Adrenoceptor antagonists

Examples: acebutolol, atenolol, metoprolol, nadolol, oxprenolol, pindolol, propranolol, sotalol

Mode of action

β-Adrenoceptors activate adenylyl cyclase. There are two subtypes of β-receptor (β_1 and β_2). In general, β_1-receptors tend to be excitatory and β_2-inhibitory. β-Adrenoceptor antagonists with a specific affinity for β_1-receptors alone are called selective, and those also affecting β_2-receptors are called non-selective. Even those classified as selective still have some β_2-antagonism. Some β-blockers are partial agonists (intrinsic sympathomimetic activity), so that at low dose there is increasing agonism as the dose increases, but a plateau is reached and there is antagonism of circulating catecholamines. They may have an advantage over the others in minimising bradycardia, reducing heart failure and maintaining perfusion to the extremities. The membrane-stabilising effect that some β-blockers have is, however, of little clinical importance. Figure 35.6 shows the selectivity and partial agonist properties of the β-blockers.

Figure 35.6 Partial agonism and selectivity of β-blockers

	Antagonist	Partial agonist
Selective	Atenolol Betaxolol Bisoprolol Esmolol Metoprolol Nadolol	Acebutalol Alprenolol
Non-selective	Propranolol Sotalol Timolol	Celiprolol Oxprenolol Pindolol

Uses

β-Blockers are used in the treatment of angina, hypertension, tachyarrhythmias, anxiety, glaucoma, migraine, phaeochromocytoma and thyrotoxicosis.

Clinical effects

The clinical effects (Figure 35.7) are predictable from knowledge of receptor locations. The important effects for clinical use are those of negative inotropy and negative chronotropy, which reduce blood pressure and myocardial work. Coronary blood flow is reduced, but this

Figure 35.7 Clinical effects of β-blockade

Peripheral

Cardiovascular system
- Conduction velocity in SA node, atria, AV node and ventricles reduced (β_1)
- Atrial contractility reduced (β_1)
- Heart rate reduced (β_1)
- Blood pressure reduced (β_1)
- Class II antiarrhythmic activity (β_1)
- Skeletal muscle (β_2) and coronary vasomotor tone increased
- Coronary blood flow reduced
- Cardiac oxygen demand reduced

Respiratory system
- Bronchoconstriction with increased resistance and reduced dead space (β_2)

Renal system
- Renin secretion inhibited (β_1)

Metabolic
- Less free fatty acid release (β_1)
- Glycogenolysis reduced (β_2)
- Insulin release reduced (β_2)
- Lipolysis (β_3)
- Thermogenesis (β_3)

Eye
- Reduced production of aqueous humour
- Constriction of ciliary muscle (β_2)

Central

- Reduced sympathetic tone
- Anxiolysis
- Tiredness
- Nightmares
- Sleep disturbance

effect is less than the reduction in myocardial work. These drugs are particularly effective when sympathetic tone is increased, for example following myocardial infarction, but care must be taken not to block a protective inotropic effect in incipient heart failure. The undesirable effects include bradycardia, bronchoconstriction, sleep disturbance, hypoglycaemia (especially with exercise) and cold extremities.

β-Blockers (whether selective or not) should be avoided in asthmatic patients. They should be used with caution in diabetes, peripheral vascular disease and heart failure. Calcium antagonists with negative inotropic effects (verapamil and diltiazem) act synergistically with β-blockers to cause hypotension, bradycardia and conduction defects, and they should not be administered contemporaneously.

Atenolol, celiprolol, nadolol and sotalol are very water-soluble and therefore penetrate the brain poorly and are primarily excreted in the urine. In general, the β-blockers are well absorbed orally, but the first-pass effect is particularly high with alprenolol, propranolol, metoprolol, oxprenolol and timolol. Bisoprolol and sotalol have a high bioavailability.

Atenolol

Atenolol is a popular selective β-blocker for the control of essential hypertension. In the clinical setting, patient compliance with the treatment is often apparent from a relatively slow heart rate. Bioavailability is 50% and protein binding is low. Atenolol is highly water-soluble and is largely excreted unchanged in the urine.

Esmolol

Esmolol hydrochloride is a short-acting β_1-adrenoceptor antagonist, and class II antiarrhythmic. This aryloxypropanolamine is rapidly hydrolysed to a low-activity acid by red cell esterases and has a half-life of only 9 minutes. It is used in the acute management of supraventricular tachycardias, hypertension and myocardial infarction, and is an option for suppression of the hypertensive response to laryngoscopy and intubation.

Propranolol

Propranolol is a non-selective β-blocker with no intrinsic sympathomimetic activity. It has been largely superseded by selective antagonists but still has a role in the management of phaeochromocytoma (in conjunction with α-blockade), thyrotoxicosis and crisis, acute hypertension and tachyarrhythmias. Propranolol has a high first pass

with a bioavailability of only 10–30%. It is lipid-soluble and highly protein-bound (90–95%).

Drugs interfering with synthesis, storage, release and metabolism of catecholamines

Examples – bretylium, carbidopa, guanethidine, methyldopa, reserpine

A few drugs act by interfering with the metabolic elements of the catecholamines rather than with receptor interactions. While not widely used now, as they lack specificity, these agents merit brief consideration.

Synthesis

Carbidopa inhibits dopa decarboxylase and so prevents the formation of dopamine, the first catecholamine in the chain of synthesis. Carbidopa does not cross the blood–brain barrier and is therefore used to minimise the peripheral effects of levodopa (L-DOPA) used in the treatment of Parkinsonism. The antihypertensive agent methyldopa is a false substrate for dopa decarboxylase and dopamine hydroxylase and results in the synthesis of a false transmitter – methyl noradrenaline. This is ineffective, and as it is not metabolised by monoamine oxidase it accumulates within the nerve terminal and displaces the true neurotransmitter, which becomes depleted.

Storage

Reserpine blocks the uptake and reuptake of noradrenaline, dopamine and 5-hydroxytryptamine in the neuronal terminals. The neurotransmitter accumulates within the cytoplasm where MAO inactivates it and transmitter levels fall. It affects both the sympathetic and central nervous systems but has been superseded by drugs that are more specific.

Release

Guanethidine was originally used as an antihypertensive but is now used in the management of chronic pain. It is transported by the uptake 1 mechanism and accumulates in the nerve terminals. Initially it causes release of noradrenaline from the vesicles and then inhibits release of the diminishing levels of noradrenaline. Bretylium has a similar mode of action. Guanethidine is used to treat reflex sympathetic dystrophy by IV regional sympathetic block (chemical sympathectomy), in which guanethidine is injected intravenously into an isolated limb.

Direct-acting vasodilating agents

Calcium channel antagonists

Examples – amlodipine, felodipine, nicardipine, nifedipine, nimodipine, nisoldipine

The calcium channel antagonists are covered in detail in Chapter 36. This is a mixed group of drugs having in common the blockade of various calcium ionophores in cell and intracellular membranes. These vasodilators relax vascular smooth muscle preferentially and dilate coronary and other arterial smooth muscle. They can be used in conjunction with β-blockers. Amlodipine, felodipine, nicardipine and nifedipine are used to treat both hypertension and angina. Isradipine and lacidipine are only useful in the treatment of hypertension. Nimodipine has a specificity for cerebral arterioles and is used to treat vascular spasm following subarachnoid haemorrhage or neuroradiological instrumentation.

Organic nitrates, nitrites and related drugs

Examples – glyceryl trinitrate, isosorbide di- and mononitrate, nitric oxide, nitroprusside

Uses

These are direct-acting vascular smooth muscle relaxants that are used to control and reduce blood pressure and to alleviate angina.

Mode of action

Both organic nitrates (NO_3^-) and sodium nitroprusside act in a similar way. Having diffused from the vascular lumen through to the smooth muscle they are converted to nitrites (NO_2^-) by reacting with –SH groups (thiols) in the tissues. Hydrogen ions within the cells then react with the nitrite to produce nitric oxide (NO). This in turn reacts with more thiols in the muscle cell to produce nitrosothiols. These stimulate guanylyl cyclase to convert guanosine triphosphate (GTP) to cyclic guanosine monophosphate (cGMP) in a comparable way to adenylyl cyclase. The cGMP then relaxes the smooth muscle. Nitric oxide may be administered by inhalation to selectively dilate pulmonary arterioles. It mimics the physiological mediation by the vascular endothelial cells of a number of circulating autacoids such as bradykinin, which stimulate nitric oxide synthase to convert arginine to citrulline and nitric oxide. This nitric oxide (formerly identified as endothelium-derived relaxing factor, EDRF) diffuses into the muscle cell, where it has its effect.

Clinical effects

The predominant effect is that of vasodilatation, affecting the venous system (preload) in particular. The reduction in preload reduces cardiac output, cardiac work and myocardial oxygen demand, and so these drugs are used to treat angina. Higher or more prolonged doses also dilate arterioles, including the coronary vessels, and therefore reduce afterload. In the ischaemic heart, these drugs may increase the blood flow to ischaemic myocardium by dilating collaterals that bypass partial vessel occlusions.

Flushing and headaches are common, and a reflex tachycardia develops, putting a practical upper limit on the degree of vasodilatation. All smooth muscle is affected somewhat, but the clinically important effect is confined to the cardiovascular system.

Patients using isosorbide dinitrate and other longer-acting nitrates may develop tolerance, perhaps because of depletion of the tissue thiols. Excessive levels of nitrates convert haemoglobin to methaemoglobin.

Glyceryl trinitrate

Glyceryl trinitrate (GTN) reduces blood pressure and coronary vascular resistance and increases subendocardial coronary blood flow by decreasing left ventricular end-diastolic pressure (LVEDP). It may be administered by infusion, by transdermal absorption using a skin patch, or by sublingual absorption using a spray or a tablet. Gastric acid rapidly inactivates glyceryl trinitrate, and once the desired effect is achieved it may be swallowed. Within the body it is rapidly hydrolysed in the liver, producing inorganic nitrite. Some is also converted to glyceryl dinitrate, which has a small amount of activity and a half-life of 2 hours.

Isosorbide dinitrate

Isosorbide dinitrate is usually given orally by a slow-release preparation, and so its effect is delayed compared with glyceryl trinitrate. It may also be given sublingually for rapid onset, and by infusion for precision control of symptoms or blood pressure. The effects are similar. It is converted to isosorbide mononitrate in the liver, with a half-life of 4 hours.

Isosorbide mononitrate

Isosorbide mononitrate, the active metabolite of isosorbide dinitrate, is given orally and is similar to its precursor.

Nitric oxide

Inhaled nitric oxide (in concentrations of about 40 ppm) is used to treat pulmonary hypertension in the intensive care setting. It diffuses through to the pulmonary vascular smooth muscle, where it interacts to cause cGMP-mediated relaxation. Further diffusion to the vascular lumen results in rapid inactivation, as it combines with haemoglobin to form methaemoglobin.

Nitroprusside

Sodium nitroprusside is used in the control of hypertension, and for induced hypotension during surgery. It affects both arterial and venous systems to cause a reduction in systemic vascular resistance followed by a compensatory tachycardia. It is administered by infusion in systems protected from light (brown syringes and yellow infusion lines are available). Nitroprusside metabolism produces the highly toxic cyanide ion (CN^-), some of which combines with haemoglobin to produce methaemoglobin, and the rest is converted to thiocyanate by rhodonase in the liver and subsequently excreted in the urine. Thiocyanate levels can be measured to monitor toxicity. A small amount combines with vitamin B_{12} to form cyanocobalamin. In excess the cyanide ion saturates these elimination processes and damages the cytochrome oxidase chain (fundamental for aerobic cellular energy production).

Potassium channel activators

Examples – minoxidil, nicorandil

Potassium channel activators act by opening potassium channels, resulting in hyperpolarisation of the cell membrane with a reduction in electrical activity. ATP has the opposite effect, closing the channels and depolarising the membrane. Nicorandil relaxes arterial smooth muscle and reduces systemic vascular resistance. The nitrate component of the drug causes venous smooth muscle relaxation with a fall in preload. It also has a direct dilating affect on coronary arterioles, to improve perfusion of ischaemic myocardium. Nicorandil is used to treat angina.

Minoxidil is also a potassium channel activator, and is reserved for resistant severe hypertension. The resulting vasodilatation causes a tachycardia and increased cardiac output, and fluid retention is also a problem. Concomitant use of a β-blocker and diuretic are essential. It causes hypertrychosis, and is used as a treatment for baldness.

I$_f$ current inhibitor

Example – ivabradine

Ivabradine inhibits the I$_f$ current in the sinoatrial node produced by sodium channel opening. This reduces the slow depolarisation phase in the pacemaker and so slows heart rate. It is used to treat angina in patients in sinus rhythm.

Endothelin receptor antagonists

Examples – bosentan, sitaxsentan

Endothelin receptors ET_A, ET_{B1} and ET_{B2} are G-protein-coupled receptors located in the endothelium and vascular smooth muscle. The endogenous agonist endothelin causes an increase in free intracellular calcium ions. Bosentan is a competitive antagonist at both ET_A and ET_B receptors, causing vasodilatation. It is licensed for some types of pulmonary hypertension. Sitaxsentan is a sulphonamide that is very selective for ET_A. It is also used as a pulmonary antihypertensive.

Prostacyclins

Examples – epoprostenol, iloprost

Epoprostenol (synthetic prostacyclin, PGI_2) and iloprost (a synthetic analogue of prostacyclin) are both potent vasodilators. Epoprostenol is used for inhibition of platelet aggregation, for example during haemodialysis. Iloprost is presented as a solution for nebulised inhalation, and so targets pulmonary vessels for the treatment of pulmonary hypertension.

cGMP phosphodiesterase inhibitor

Example – sildenafil

Sildenafil inhibits PDE5 (phosphodiesterase 5) to inhibit the nitric oxide stimulation of guanylyl cyclase to produce cGMP, causing vascular smooth muscle relaxation. Its specificity leads to its use as a pulmonary vasodilator, but it is perhaps better known for its use in treating erectile dysfunction.

Other agents of importance

Diazoxide

Diazoxide is a thiazide, but unlike its diuretic counterparts it causes sodium and water retention. Diazoxide antagonises the effect of ATP on potassium channels. It has a direct effect on arteriolar smooth muscle, and given intravenously causes marked hypotension and a reflex increase in heart rate and cardiac output. The increased sympathetic outflow also increases free fatty acids and blood glucose.

Hydralazine

Hydralazine acts both centrally and peripherally. The peripheral effect causes direct vascular smooth muscle relaxation. There is also a mild α-blocking action. The drop in blood pressure causes a reflex increase in sympathetic tone. Renal blood flow is increased. Headache, dizziness, nausea and vomiting are common side effects.

Specific pharmacology

Units (unless stated otherwise) are:
Volume of distribution at steady state (V_d): L kg^{-1}
Clearance (Cl): mL kg^{-1} min^{-1}
Terminal half-life ($t_{1/2}$): minutes

Adrenaline

Structure – catecholamine; α and β agonist

Presentation – IV/subcutaneous – 1 mg in 1 mL (1:1000) and 1 mg in 10 mL (1:10,000); also added to local anaesthetics 1:200,000 (1 mg in 200 mL)

Dose – highly variable, depending on indication and route

CNS – limited crossing of the blood–brain barrier but does cause excitation. Neuromuscular transmission facilitated

CVS – heart rate increased (may be reflexly reduced); contractility, stroke volume and cardiac oxygen consumption increased; systemic vasoconstriction, but vasodilatation in skeletal muscle; mean arterial pressure, systolic and pulse pressure increased, diastolic decreased; coronary blood flow increased

RS – bronchodilatation; respiratory rate and tidal volume increased; secretions more tenacious

Other – gastrointestinal tract tone and secretions decreased, splanchnic blood flow decreased; renal blood flow increased; bladder tone reduced but sphincter tone increased; clotting factor V increased, leading to enhanced platelet aggregation and coagulation; metabolic effects to increase gluconeogenesis and increase metabolic rate

Metabolism – by catechol-O-methyl transferase (COMT) in the liver and monoamine oxidase (MAO) in adrenergic neurones to inactive metabolites 3-methoxy-4-hydroxy phenylethylene and 3-methoxy-4-hydroxy mandelic acid

Contraindications – beware arrhythmias with halothane; caution with MAO inhibitors

Toxicity – there are many adverse effects, but the major ones are cardiac; increases cardiac sensitivity and irritability, so arrhythmias including VF and asystole are likely if given too quickly

Atropine sulphate

Structure – tertiary amine; muscarinic, anticholinergic antagonist

Presentation

Oral – tablets 600 µg

IV/IM – clear, colourless, aqueous solution containing a racemic mixture of 600 µg atropine in 1 mL

Dose – 10–20 µg kg^{-1}

Pharmacokinetics

Bioavailability	10–25%
Protein binding	50%
pK_a	9.8
V_d	3
Cl	17
$t_{1/2}$	150

CNS – variable stimulation or depression, antiemetic, anti-Parkinsonian; competitive antagonism of muscarinic receptors causes blockade of parasympathetic system and sweating

CVS – heart rate, AV nodal transmission and cardiac output increase (initial temporary bradycardia with low doses due to centrally mediated increase in vagal tone); blood pressure may increase; tachyarrhythmias

RS – bronchodilator with increased anatomical dead space; respiratory rate increased; secretions reduced

Other – gastrointestinal motility and secretions reduced; biliary antispasmodic effect; lower oesophageal sphincter pressure reduced; urinary tract tone and peristalsis reduced, bladder sphincter tone increased and retention may result; pupillary dilatation, inability to accommodate for near objects (may persist for several days) and raised intraocular pressure occur; metabolic rate increased

Metabolism – atropine ester hydrolysed into its component parts tropine and tropic acid by the liver, 94% of the dose appearing in the urine in 24 hours

Contraindications – beware glaucoma, hyperpyrexia especially in children; central anticholinergic syndrome

Clonidine hydrochloride

Structure – imidazoline-aniline derivative

Presentation

Oral – tablets/capsules 25, 100, 250 and 300 µg

IV – clear, colourless, aqueous solution containing 150 µg in 1 mL

Dose

Oral migraine/flushing – 50–75 µg twice daily

Oral antihypertensive – 50–600 µg 3 times daily

Slow IV – 150–300 µg for control of hypertensive crisis

Pharmacokinetics (IV dose)

onset	10 min
peak	30–60 min
duration	3–7 h
V_d	2
Cl	3
$t_{1/2}$	6–23 h

CNS – analgesia

CVS – transient α_1 effect causes increased SVR and blood pressure; α_2-agonism produces presynaptic inhibition of sympathetic noradrenaline release with reductions in SVR, blood pressure, venous return and heart rate; cardiac contractility and output are preserved; coronary blood flow increased; renal blood flow increased; rebound tachycardia and hypertension can result from sudden withdrawal

RS – no effect

Other – plasma catecholamine and renin reduced; blood glucose increased; reduction of MAC; may cause dizziness, drowsiness, headache, dry mouth and impotence

Metabolism – 65% unchanged in urine, 20% in faeces, 15% inactivated in liver

Dopamine hydrochloride

Structure – catecholamine; β and α agonist

Presentation – 400 mg (1600 μg mL^{-1}) and 800 mg (3200 μg mL^{-1}) in 250 mL 5% dextrose (other mixtures available)

Dose – IV infusion:
1–20 μg kg^{-1} min^{-1}
1–5 μg kg^{-1} min^{-1} increases renal blood flow
5–15 μg kg^{-1} min^{-1} inotropic
15–20 μg kg^{-1} min^{-1} vasoconstricts

CVS – contractility, stroke volume increased; little effect on heart rate; systemic vascular resistance, systolic, mean and diastolic blood pressures decreased; coronary blood flow increased

RS – carotid bodies stimulated, leading to reduced respiratory response to hypoxia

Other – splanchnic (including renal) vasodilatation; renal blood flow, glomerular filtration rate (GFR), urine (volume and sodium content) increased; prolactin secretion inhibited (also known as prolactin inhibiting hormone (PIH) secreted by the posterior pituitary)

Metabolism – by COMT and MAO to homovanillic acid and 3,4-dihydroxyphenylacetic acid. Predominantly excreted in urine, conjugated and unconjugated; 25% of the dopamine is taken up into adrenergic nerve endings and is converted to noradrenaline

Contraindications – nausea, tachycardia and arrhythmias; caution with MAO inhibitors

Dopexamine hydrochloride

Structure – catecholamine; dopamine (D_1 and D_2) and β_2 agonist

Presentation – colourless aqueous solution adjusted to a pH of 2.5, containing 50 mg dopexamine hydrochloride in 5 mL, and 0.01% disodium edetate; requires dilution prior to use

Dose – IV infusion – 0.5–6 μg kg^{-1} min^{-1} (start at 0.5 and increase by 0.5–1 μg kg^{-1} min^{-1} increments with at least 15-min intervals according to need

CNS – cerebral blood flow increased; dopexamine causes nausea by its action on D_2 receptors in the chemoreceptor trigger zone

CVS – stroke volume, heart rate and cardiac output increased; systolic blood pressure increased; systemic and pulmonary vascular resistance, diastolic blood pressure, LVEDP, pulmonary artery pressure reduced; coronary blood flow increased

RS – bronchodilatation

Other – mesenteric and renal vasodilatation with increased blood flow, diuresis and natriuresis; hyperglycaemia, hypokalaemia; splenic platelet sequestration; 40% of dose is bound to red cells

Metabolism – rapid tissue uptake, methylation and conjugation eliminate the drug

Contraindications – caution with MAO inhibitors

Dobutamine hydrochloride

Structure – catecholamine; β_1 and β_2 (and α_1) agonist

Presentation – 250 mg dobutamine and 4.8 mg sodium metabisulphite in 20 mL for further dilution prior to administration

Dose – infusion 0.5–40 μg kg^{-1} min^{-1}

CNS – stimulant at high dose

CVS – heart rate, stroke volume, cardiac output increased, atrioventricular node conduction enhanced; vasodilatation; systemic vascular resistance and left ventricular end-diastolic pressure (LVEDP) reduced; coronary perfusion may increase

RS – no effect

Other – β_1 effect increases renin output; urine output increases secondary to increased cardiac output

Metabolism – converted to 3-O-methyldobutamine by COMT; this is conjugated and excreted in urine (80%) and faeces (20%)

Contraindications – increasing doses cause tachycardia, hypertension and arrhythmias; angina may occur in susceptible patients; allergic reactions to the metabisulphite preservative have occurred

Ephedrine

Structure – sympathomimetic amine; α and β agonist

Presentation

Oral – tablets 15, 30 and 60 mg; elixir 15 mg in 5 mL
IV – clear, colourless, aqueous solution containing 30 mg ephedrine in 1 mL

Dose – IV – 3, 6 or 9 mg increments at minimal interval of 3–4 min. Maximum of 30 mg as tachyphylaxis ensues

CNS – stimulant effect (drug of abuse)

CVS – heart rate, stroke volume, cardiac output, myocardial oxygen consumption increased; SVR, diastolic, systolic and pulmonary pressures increased; coronary blood flow increased; splanchnic and renal vasoconstriction

RS – bronchodilator; respiratory rate and tidal volume increased; irritant to mucous membranes

Other – uterine, bladder and gastrointestinal smooth muscle relaxation; bladder sphincter tone increased; gluconeogenesis, metabolic rate and oxygen consumption increased; irritant to mucous membranes

Metabolism – up to 99% eliminated in urine unchanged; the rest by oxidation, demethylation, and hydroxylation of the aromatic part plus conjugation

Contraindications – tachyarrhythmias (especially with halothane), nausea and central stimulation

Esmolol hydrochloride

See Chapter 36

Glyceryl trinitrate

Structure – organic nitrate ester of nitric acid and glycerol (glycerine)

Presentation

Sublingual tablets and oral spray
Transdermal patches (5 and 10 mg)
IV – clear, colourless, aqueous solution containing 1 mg glyceryl trinitrate per mL with polyethylene glycol and dextrose; stored in amber ampoules with 5 and 50 mL solution

Dose

SL – 300 µg
TD – 5 or 10 mg per 24 h
IV – 0.2–3 µg kg^{-1} min^{-1}

Pharmacokinetics

V_d	0.04–2.9
Cl	600
$t_{1/2}$	2

CNS – intracranial pressure increased as a result of vasodilatation, and headache ensues if sublingual dose continues beyond desired antianginal effect

CVS – venodilator with arterial dilatation as dose increases; SVR, systolic, diastolic, venous and pulmonary artery pressures reduced, myocardial oxygen demand reduced; subendocardial coronary blood flow improved; heart rate is unchanged in failure but increased reflexly in normal state

RS – bronchodilatation, and may increase shunt

Other – relaxes other smooth muscle such as biliary and gut

Metabolism – hydrolysis of the ester bonds by red cells and the liver, and 80% of the dose is excreted in the urine

Contraindications – substantial amount of intravenously administered GTN binds to the plastic of giving sets and syringes, therefore reduced availability

Glycopyrrolate

Structure – quaternary amine; muscarinic anticholinergic antagonist

Presentation – IV – clear, colourless, aqueous solution containing 200 µg mL^{-1} in 1 and 3 mL ampoules

Dose

IV – 4–5 µg kg^{-1} (10–15 µg kg^{-1} in conjunction with neostigmine)
Children – 4–8 µg kg^{-1} (10 µg kg^{-1} in conjunction with neostigmine 50 µg kg^{-1})

Pharmacokinetics

Bioavailability	5%
V_d	0.4
Cl	13
$t_{1/2}$	50

CNS – does not cross the blood–brain barrier, so there is no effect on the eye; competitive antagonism of muscarinic receptors causes blockade of parasympathetic system and sweating

CVS – heart rate, AV nodal transmission and cardiac output increase, blood pressure may increase; tachyarrhythmias less common than with atropine

RS – bronchodilatation with increased anatomical dead space; secretions reduced

Other – gastrointestinal motility and secretions reduced; lower oesophageal sphincter pressure reduced; urinary tract tone and peristalsis reduced, bladder sphincter tone increased and retention may result; metabolic rate increased

Metabolism – excreted unchanged in the urine (85%) and faeces (15%)

Contraindications – in high doses the quaternary ammonium has a nicotinic antagonist effect of significance in myasthenia gravis; limited crossing of the placenta but can still cause fetal tachycardia

Hyoscine hydrobromide or butylbromide

Structure – tertiary amine, muscarinic anticholinergic antagonist; S-hyoscine (scopolamine) used

Presentation

  Oral – hyoscine butylbromide tablets 10 mg, hyoscine hydrobromide tablets 150 µg and 300 µg

  IV – hyoscine butylbromide clear colourless solution 20 mg in 1 mL, hyoscine hydrobromide 20 mg in 5 mL

Dose

  Oral – 150–300 µg hydrobromide for motion sickness
  IM – 200–600 µg hydrobromide for premedication
  Slow IV – 20 mg butylbromide for GI or GU spasm

Pharmacokinetics

Bioavailability	10%
Protein binding	11%
V_d	2
Cl	10
$t_{1/2}$	150

CNS – sedation, antiemesis, anti-Parkinsonian

CVS – initial tachycardia when given IV, but may later cause bradycardia due to central effect

RS – decreases secretions, bronchodilatation, slight ventilatory stimulation

Others – antisialagogue, antispasmodic for biliary tree and uterus; marked decrease in tear and sweat formation; decreases bladder and ureteric tone

Elimination – metabolised in the liver to scopine and scopic acid; unchanged, urine 2%, bile 5%

Toxicity – potential problem in patients with porphyria

Isoprenaline

Structure – catecholamine; β agonist

Presentation

  Oral – tablets 30 mg

  IV – colourless, aqueous solution adjusted to a pH of 2.5–2.8, containing 2 mg isoprenaline hydrochloride in 2 mL, with ascorbic acid and disodium edetate; requires dilution prior to use

Dose – IV infusion – 0.02–0.4 µg kg^{-1} min^{-1}

CNS – stimulant

CVS – heart rate, stroke volume and cardiac output increased; SA node automaticity and AV nodal conduction increased; SVR and diastolic blood pressure reduced; coronary blood flow increased; splanchnic and renal vasoconstriction, but flow may improve if treating low cardiac output

RS – bronchodilatation

Other – uterine and gastrointestinal smooth muscle relaxation; gluconeogenesis increased; antigen-induced histamine release inhibited

Metabolism – extensive first-pass effect if taken orally. 15–75% unchanged in the urine; the rest by COMT, then conjugated

Labetalol hydrochloride

Structure – 2-hydroxy-5-[1-hydroxy-2-(1-methyl-3-phenyl-propylamino) ethyl] benzamide hydrochloride; combined α_1-, β_1- and β_2-adrenoceptor antagonist

Presentation

  Oral – tablets 50, 100, 200, 400 mg

  IV – clear, colourless, aqueous solution containing 100 mg in 20 mL

Dose

  Oral – 100–1200 mg twice daily

  IV – slow bolus of 50 mg at 5-min intervals until blood pressure is controlled (duration 6–18 h, maximum dose 200 mg); IV infusion 15–160 mg h^{-1}

Pharmacokinetics

V_d	10
Cl	23
$t_{1/2}$	6 h

CNS – fatigue, confusion

CVS – heart rate, contractility, stroke volume, cardiac output, SVR, systolic and diastolic blood pressure decreased; coronary and renal blood flow increased

RS – potential risk of bronchoconstriction in asthmatic patients

Other – with IV use there is a compensatory increase in endogenous catecholamines; renin and angiotensin II reduced; platelet aggregation may be reduced

Metabolism – hepatic

Contraindications – as for other β-blockers; may interact with antiarrhythmics of class I and IV; crosses the placenta and causes clinical effects in the fetus, including bradycardia, hypotension, respiratory depression, hypoglycaemia and hypothermia in the neonate

Noradrenaline acid tartrate

Structure – catecholamine; α (and β) agonist

Presentation – clear, colourless, aqueous solution containing 0.2 mg mL^{-1} (in 2, 4 and 20 mL ampoules) or 2 mg mL^{-1} (2 mL ampoule) with sodium metabisulphite and sodium chloride. 1 mg noradrenaline acid tartrate (1 mL) contains 0.5 mg noradrenaline base, so the preparations contain 0.1 and 1 mg noradrenaline base per mL respectively

Dose – IV infusion 0.05–0.2 µg kg^{-1} min^{-1}

CNS – cerebral oxygen consumption reduced

CVS – generalised peripheral vasoconstriction, systolic and diastolic blood pressure increased; a reflex fall in heart rate occurs; cardiac output may fall slightly; coronary vasodilatation causes coronary blood flow to increase; ventricular rhythm disturbances may occur

RS – mild bronchodilatation, minute volume increases

Other – hepatic, renal and splanchnic blood flow reduced; pregnant uterus contractility increased, and this may compromise fetal oxygen supply; insulin secretion reduced; renin secretion increased; mydriasis; plasma water reduced by contraction of vascular space, and this increases haematocrit and plasma protein concentration

Metabolism – by MAO and COMT, which in combination produce 3-methoxy-4-hydroxy vanillylmandelic acid (VMA) in the urine. 5% excreted unchanged

Contraindications – caution with MAO inhibitors

Sodium nitroprusside

Structure – inorganic complex

Presentation – red-brown powder containing 50 mg sodium nitroprusside in a brown glass ampoule which is reconstituted in 2 mL 5% dextrose before further dilution. It should be protected from light, and yellow and brown giving sets and syringes are available for this purpose

Dose – IV infusion 0.1–1.5 µg kg^{-1} min^{-1} (maximum of up to 8 µg kg^{-1} min^{-1}). Maximum dose 1.5 mg kg^{-1}; starts to accumulate once rate > 2 µg kg^{-1} min^{-1}

Pharmacokinetics

V_d	0.2
Elimination	1 µg kg^{-1} min^{-1}
nitroprusside $t_{1/2}$	very short
thiocyanate $t_{1/2}$	2.7 days

CNS – cerebral vasodilatation increases intracranial pressure

CVS – dilates arterioles and venules with reduced blood pressure, reduced LVEDP, reduced myocardial oxygen demand; heart rate increases but contractility is unaffected

RS – hypoxic pulmonary vasoconstriction is impaired and arterial oxygen tension may fall

Other – gastrointestinal motility and lower oesophageal sphincter pressure are reduced; metabolic acidosis may occur

Metabolism – reacts with sulphydryl groups of plasma amino acids; higher concentrations cause non-enzymatic hydrolysis in red blood cells to produce five cyanide ions from each nitroprusside molecule. One of these combines with haemoglobin (iron in ferrous state) to form methaemoglobin (iron in ferric state); most of the rest is converted to thiocyanate by rhodonase in the liver and is then excreted in the urine; small amount of thiocyanate combines with vitamin B$_{12}$ to form cyanocobalamin

Toxicity – cyanide ions inhibit the cytochrome oxidase chain; plasma levels of > 80 µg L^{-1} produce tachycardia, sweating, hyperventilation, cardiac arrhythmias and retrosternal pain

CHAPTER 36
Cardiovascular pharmacology

Tim Smith

Antiarrhythmic drugs

Antiarrhythmic drugs are usually classified according to their effect on the electrophysiology of cardiac myofibrils. Figure 36.1 shows the different sites in the heart on which these drugs act. There are four basic classes of antiarrhythmic, with considerable variation in the chemical structure of the drugs within each functional class (Vaughan Williams 1970). Examples of the drugs by class are shown in Figure 36.2.

Class I

Class I drugs work in a similar way to local anaesthetic agents (lidocaine is used for both roles). They act by slowing sodium entry into cells through the fast voltage-gated sodium channels that primarily affect the non-nodal areas characterised by a fast depolarisation action potential. They reduce the maximum rate of rise of phase 0 depolarisation. The rate of phase 4 sinoatrial node

depolarisation may also be reduced, and with it spontaneous automaticity.

Fast voltage-gated sodium channels may exist in three states – resting, open and refractory. In normal myocardium their state switches between resting and open, but ischaemia results in prolonged depolarisation and the channel becomes refractory. The class I antiarrhythmics block open channels so that the more frequent the action potentials the more ionophores become blocked. The first action potential shows a slight reduction in phase 0 depolarisation. Subsequent action potentials show a progressive reduction in the rate of depolarisation as more channels are blocked. The block is therefore use-dependent.

Class I has three subdivisions, based on the effect on the action potential duration. The effect on action potential duration is related to the type of sodium channel affected, as follows:

Fundamentals of Anaesthesia, 4th edition, ed. Ted Lin, Tim Smith and Colin Pinnock. Published by Cambridge University Press. © Cambridge University Press 2017.

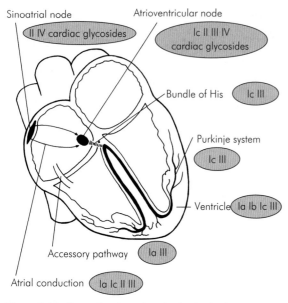

Figure 36.1 Sites of action of antiarrhythmic drugs

- Class IA (e.g. quinidine) – action potential duration increased
- Class IB (e.g. lidocaine) – action potential duration decreased
- Class IC (e.g. flecainide) – action potential duration unaffected

The key features of the subdivisions of class I antiarrhythmics are listed in Figure 36.3, and their ECG effects are shown in Figure 36.4.

Class IB antiarrhythmics have a receptor association/ dissociation cycle shorter than the cardiac cycle. The initial drug effect causes gradual blockade of the ionophores to develop during the action potential depolarisation. By the time the next action potential occurs, however, the drug will have dissociated from its receptor again. If a premature depolarisation (e.g. a ventricular premature beat) occurs then the myofibril will still be blocked. Class IB antiarrhythmics bind preferentially to refractory channels, and are therefore selective for ischaemic myocardium. Class IB drugs also elevate the fibrillation threshold. Lidocaine is discussed in Chapter 33. Mexiletine is similar but also has anticonvulsant properties, possibly due to GABA reuptake inhibition.

Class IC drugs have a much slower association/ dissociation cycle, lasting longer than the cardiac

Figure 36.2 Antiarrhythmic drugs by class

Class I
IA
• Quinidine
• Procainamide
• Disopyramide
• Cibenzoline
IB
• Lidocaine
• Phenytoin
• Mexiletine
• Tocainide
• Ethmozine
IC
• Flecainide
• Lorcainide
• Propafenone
• Indecainide
• Encainide

Class II
• Propranolol
• Esmolol
• Sotalol

Class III
• Amiodarone
• Bretylium
• Sotalol
• N-acetylprocainamide

Class IV
• Verapamil
• Diltiazem

cycle, so the block is relatively constant from cycle to cycle. The overall effect is a general reduction in excitability, and this is therefore more suitable for re-entrant-type rhythms. There is little selectivity for the refractory channels of ischaemic myocardium.

Class IA drugs have features midway between those of IB and IC.

Class IA antiarrhythmics are primarily used for supraventricular tachycardias, and class IB and C for ventricular tachycardias.

Figure 36.3 Features of the subdivisions of class I antiarrhythmic drugs

Class	Example	dV/dt of phase 0	Repolarisation	PR	QRS	QT
IA	Quinidine	Slowed	Prolonged	↑	↑	↑
IB	Lidocaine	Little effect	Shortened	0	0	↓
IC	Flecainide	Marked slowing	Little effect	↑↑	↑↑	0

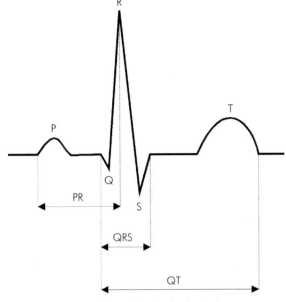

	Anti-arrhythmic group		
	I A	I B	I C
PR Interval	↑	—	↑
QRS Duration	↑	—	↑
QT Interval	↑	↓	—

Figure 36.4 ECG effects of antiarrhythmic drugs

Class II

Class II antiarrhythmics (β-blockers) competitively block the effects of circulating and neurotransmitter catecholamines, reducing arrhythmogenicity, heart rate and contractility. This slows and so lengthens phase 4 depolarisation, the phase which is shortened by catecholamines. The action potential is shortened and the refractory period of the atrioventricular (AV) node is prolonged. These Gs-coupled effects are mediated by a slow L-type Ca channel influx that may be particularly useful in preventing post-myocardial infarction ventricular arrhythmias, when catecholamine levels may be high. Some potassium, chloride and even sodium channel modulation may also be involved. β-blockers are covered in detail in Chapter 35.

Class III

Class III drugs (e.g. amiodarone, bretylium, sotalol) prolong repolarisation and therefore the action potential, and

increase the effective refractory period. Their principal uses are for the following arrhythmias:

- Atrial tachycardia
- Atrial flutter and fibrillation
- Re-entrant junctional tachycardia
- Ventricular tachycardia

Amiodarone is particularly effective for the treatment of atrial tachyarrhythmias when Wolff–Parkinson–White syndrome is also present. At higher doses, the effect may be similar to β-blockade and there is a quinidine-like action. Marked hypotension may result from IV administration.

Bretylium tosylate is reserved for use in resuscitation. It is given intravenously or intramuscularly in the treatment of ventricular fibrillation after DC shock and lidocaine have been tried. It accumulates in sympathetic ganglia and reduces noradrenaline release. There is an initial postganglionic discharge. It may cause hypotension, nausea and vomiting, and should be used with caution when a cardiac glycoside has been previously administered.

Sotalol is a β-adrenoceptor antagonist and is classified as both a class II and a class III antiarrhythmic. Sotalol causes both β_1 and β_2 antagonism (mainly by the L isomer). Its place amongst the class III antiarrhythmics is due to K^+ channel inhibition, which is equally attributable to both stereoisomers. It is indicated for the treatment of paroxysmal supraventricular tachycardia, ventricular premature beats and ventricular tachycardia. It is more suitable than lidocaine for the treatment of spontaneous sustained ventricular tachycardia secondary to coronary disease or cardiomyopathy. The usual precautions for β-blocker therapy apply. Use with caution when there is hypokalaemia and when other agents that prolong the QT interval are concurrently administered.

Class IV

There are numerous calcium antagonists (see below), having different sites of action. Verapamil and diltiazem have antiarrhythmic activity, but nifedipine does not. Slowing of calcium influx reduces the duration of phases 2 and 3 of the action potential. At the AV node, this action is particularly beneficial in preventing re-entry rhythm problems.

Adenosine

Adenosine is used for rapid conversion of paroxysmal supraventricular tachycardias back to sinus rhythm (including Wolff–Parkinson–White syndrome). It may also be used in the diagnosis of conduction defects. Adenosine is ubiquitous in the body, in combination with phosphate (e.g. cAMP) and has predominantly inhibitory effects. There are four specific types of adenosine receptor, A_1, A_{2A}, A_{2B} and A_3, the effects of which are detailed in Figure 36.5.

The effect of adenosine in causing transient slowing of AV nodal conduction allows normal sinus nodal discharge to initiate a normal pattern of electrical depolarisation throughout the heart, and so normal sinus rhythm resumes, before the drug has been eliminated. This appears to be mediated by increasing myocardial K^+ flux. The A_1 purinoceptors are linked by a stimulatory G protein to the same transmembrane K^+ channels that are opened by M_2-muscarinic acetylcholine receptors. It is an unusual drug in that a key to successful use is that its IV injection must be rapid. This is because it is

Figure 36.5 Receptor effects of adenosine

A_1
- Inhibition of AV nodal conduction
- Reduced heart rate
- Reduction of atrial contractility
- Decreased cardiac excitability in response to adrenaline
- Antihypertensive
- Inhibition of excitatory amino acid release in CNS and PNS
- Decreased cerebral excitability during hypoxia and epilepsy
- Renal vasoconstriction leading to reduced diuresis
- Bronchoconstriction
- Enhanced response to insulin
- Antilipolytic

A_{2A}
- Vasodilatation (increasing coronary and cerebral blood flow)
- Inhibition of platelet aggregation
- Stimulation of nociceptive neurones

A_{2B}
- Anti-inflammatory
- Inhibition of GI tract tone

A_3
- Cardioprotection

metabolised rapidly, with a half-life of only 8–10 seconds. Unlike verapamil, it can be used safely in conjunction with β-blockers, but is contraindicated in asthma, sick sinus syndrome, and second- and third-degree AV heart block.

Cardiac glycosides

The cardiac glycosides are a group of naturally occurring compounds used to improve myocardial contractility and reduce cardiac conductivity. Cardiac glycosides are found mainly in three botanical species, white foxglove (*Digitalis lanata*), purple foxglove (*D. purpurea*) and climbing oleander (*Strophanthus gratus*).

Chemistry

The cardiac glycosides share the same basic structure:
- Steroid nucleus (cyclopentanophenanthrene)
- Lactone ring (five- or six-membered) – the aglycone
- Carbohydrate (up to four monosaccharide units)

The carbohydrate moiety is responsible for solubility, and the lactone ring confers pharmacological activity. Saturation of the lactone rings reduces potency, and opening of the ring abolishes the pharmacological activity. Only rings A and D of the steroid nucleus are coplanar, whereas in adrenal steroids rings A and C, and B and D are coplanar.

Pharmacological effects
Cardiac glycosides increase myocardial contractility and slow conduction at the AV node. Isometric and isotonic contraction of both atrial and ventricular muscle is improved. Cardiac glycosides cause directly mediated vasoconstriction.

Clinical uses
Cardiac glycosides are used to improve contractility in hypervolaemic myocardial failure. In chronic atrial fibrillation ventricular rate becomes slower because of a direct reduction in AV nodal conduction and by a secondary reduction in vagal tone.

Mechanisms of action
Sodium–potassium adenosine triphosphatase ($Na^+K^+ATPase$)
Cardiac glycosides specifically and reversibly bind to cardiac cell membrane $Na^+K^+ATPase$, which alters the electrolyte balance inside the myocardial fibres with more sodium and less potassium intracellularly. This results in a reduction of the transport of sodium into the cell using the Na^+Ca^{2+} ion exchange system, and intracellular calcium is better maintained and increased. The increased calcium may be responsible for the positive inotropy. However, at higher doses this interference with an essential membrane pump may be responsible for toxicity.

Interference with neuronal catecholamine reuptake
At low biophase concentrations, there is an increase in local catecholamine levels due to interference with neuronal catecholamine reuptake. This has positive inotropic and chronotropic effects, and may in fact increase overall $Na^+K^+ATPase$ activity. There is also an increase in local acetylcholine levels, resulting in negative inotropic and chronotropic effects.

Elimination
The glycosides are highly bound to cardiac muscle, and therefore have very high volumes of distribution. This slows elimination considerably, as most are excreted

Figure 36.6 Side effects of cardiac glycosides

Heart block
Cardiac arrhythmias
Fatigue
Nausea
Anorexia
Xanthopsia
Confusion
Neuralgia
Gynaecomastia

unchanged in the urine, both by simple filtration and also by tubular secretion. Digitoxin is the exception, being primarily metabolised by hepatic microsomal enzymes.

Toxicity
The cardiac glycosides have a very low therapeutic index. Most of the toxic effects are due to potassium loss. It is therefore particularly important to consider potassium-sparing diuretics when diuretics are needed in conjunction with cardiac glycosides. Side effects of the cardiac glycosides are listed in Figure 36.6.

Contraindications
Digoxin is contraindicated in hypertrophic cardiomyopathy as it may increase outflow obstruction and cause sudden failure. It is also contraindicated in cardiac amyloidosis.

Magnesium
Magnesium is the fourth most prevalent cation in the body, and the second intracellularly. Of total body magnesium, 53% is in bone, with 27% in muscle and only 0.3% in plasma. Its physiological roles include incorporation as a cofactor in over 300 enzyme systems, inhibition of IP_3-gated calcium channels, muscle contraction, neuronal activity, neurotransmitter release and adenylyl cyclase regulation.

Pharmacologically, magnesium is used as replacement therapy. Magnesium deficiency is not uncommon in hospital patients, and in particular two-thirds of intensive care patients may be magnesium-depleted. Magnesium is effective in the treatment of eclampsia and pre-eclampsia and in preventing the hypertensive response to intubation. The treatment of cardiac dysrhythmias is particularly indicated if hypokalaemia coexists. A list of possible uses is given in Figure 36.7.

Calcium antagonists

Calcium is involved not only in muscle contraction but also in neurotransmitter release, hormone secretion, platelet aggregation and enzyme function. There are numerous calcium channels across cell and other membranes. These may be active or passive, triggered by chemical mediators or voltage changes, and may be coupled with other ionic exchange. The term *calcium channel blocker* is generally used to describe those agents with a role in cardiovascular manipulation. These act primarily on the voltage-gated (L-type) calcium channels, preventing opening of the ionophore. There are three main groups (papaverines, benzothiazepines, dihydropyridines), each having characteristic actions. However, even within these groups, there is considerable difference between the individual chemical structures of the drugs, and in their calcium-channel specificity. The myocardial depression caused by the volatile anaesthetic agents halothane, enflurane and isoflurane is also the result of an alteration in calcium flux. Figure 36.8 shows the relative potencies of the three representative calcium antagonists.

All three groups of calcium antagonist reduce systemic vascular resistance and central venous pressure by vasodilatation. This vasodilatation is more pronounced in the arterial system, and as it is combined with a slight negative inotropic effect blood pressure falls. The reduction in afterload and contractility reduces myocardial workload and oxygen requirement. All calcium antagonists cause coronary vasodilatation, but this is only of clinical relevance in coronary artery spasm.

Calcium antagonists may also interfere with noncardiac calcium channels, affecting, for example, neuromuscular blockade and insulin secretion.

Papaverines

Examples – methoxyverapamil, teapamil, verapamil

Papaverines predominantly act on cardiac muscle, inhibiting the slow calcium entry during phases 2 and 3 of the cardiac-muscle action potential. This lengthening of the action potential makes them appropriate for tachyarrhythmias, especially re-entry supraventricular tachycardias and others of atrial origin. They also slow AV conduction, giving them a role in the management of

Figure 36.7 Possible pharmacological uses of magnesium therapy

Correction of magnesium deficiency
Control of eclampsia and pre-eclampsia
Inhibition of premature labour
Improvement of cardiac contractility
Limitation of myocardial infarct size
Component of cardioplegia (a mixture to arrest the heart during cardiac surgery)
Correction of cardiac dysrhythmias: emergency treatment of torsades de pointes, digoxin toxicity, life-threatening atrial and ventricular dysrhythmias
Prevention of hypertensive response to intubation
Reduction of catecholamine release in phaeochromocytoma surgery
Treatment of asthma

Figure 36.8 Relative clinical effects of calcium antagonists

	Verapamil (papaverine)	Diltiazem (benzothiazepine)	Nifedipine (dihydropyridine)
Reduction in SVR	++	+	+++
Coronary vasodilatation	++	++	++
Reduction in contractility	++	0	+
Reduction in blood pressure	+	0	++
Reflex increase in sympathetic tone	+	0	++
Slowing of AV nodal conduction	+++	++	0

atrial flutter and tachycardia. Papaverines have relatively little effect on vasomotor tone, but the reduction in contractility is more marked than with the other calcium channel blockers.

Benzothiazepines
Example – diltiazem

Diltiazem affects both cardiac and smooth muscle, causing relatively mild reductions in systemic vascular resistance, blood pressure and cardiac output. It is used as an antiarrhythmic drug and for the treatment of angina and hypertension.

Dihydropyridines
Examples – amlodipine, nicardipine, nifedipine, nimodipine

The dihydropyridines predominantly act on smooth muscle. Clinically this mainly affects vascular tone, causing peripheral vasodilatation primarily on the arterial side, and so reduces afterload. This reduces cardiac workload and may improve peripheral perfusion. The resultant drop in blood pressure results in a partial compensatory increase in heart rate and cardiac output. They also cause coronary vasodilatation, but this is not generally of clinical benefit. Dihydropyridines are used to treat hypertension, angina and heart failure. Nimodipine acts preferentially on cerebral arteries and is used to prevent vascular spasm after subarachnoid haemorrhage.

Phosphodiesterase inhibitors
Selective phosphodiesterase inhibitors are used for their inotropic and vasodilator properties. They selectively inhibit the phosphodiesterase 3 isoenzyme (PDE3) responsible for the breakdown of cAMP in myocardial muscle and vascular smooth muscle. This is in contrast to the methylxanthines such as theophylline (see Chapter 37), which non-specifically inhibit all five PDE isoenzymes. There are two chemical types of PDE3 inhibitor, bipyridines and imidazolines.

Mode of action
Inhibition of PDE3 causes an increase in intracellular cAMP, and to a lesser extent cGMP, in myocardial and vascular smooth muscle cells. The cAMP is responsible for phosphorylation of protein kinases in the cell. In the myocardium, this increases the influx of calcium through the slow calcium channels of the sarcolemma by increasing both the number of channels open and the duration of the open state. The sarcoplasmic reticulum is also affected, facilitating faster calcium release. The net effect is an increase in calcium ion availability in the cell for contraction. The raised level of cAMP is also responsible for improved reuptake of calcium into the sarcoplasmic reticulum, so that active myocardial relaxation is also improved, leading to an overall improvement in myocardial function.

In smooth muscle, the cAMP causes phosphorylation of the myosin light chain kinase, which reduces the affinity for the calmodulin complex and dephosphorylates the myosin light chains. This results in relaxation and secondary vasodilatation. The increase in cGMP also mediates smooth muscle relaxation.

Clinical effects
PDE3 inhibitors improve contractility in the failing heart without increasing the myocardial oxygen utilisation. The positive inotropic effect is greater than that of the cardiac glycosides and there is little chronotropic activity. Conduction in the atrium and AV node is increased, with little effect on the His–Purkinje system. PDE inhibitors cause vasodilatation, and therefore reduce preload and afterload. Coronary vascular resistance is also reduced, but this does not appear to cause coronary steal. PDE3 inhibitors also cause some bronchodilatation, but this is not a major feature. These agents are used in the short-term treatment of severe congestive cardiac failure when other measures have failed. They work synergistically with β-adrenoceptor agonists, and can work when the latter used alone have failed.

Bipyridines
Example – milrinone

Milrinone is supplied as a pale yellow solution of the lactate salt. It is administered as a loading dose followed by infusion. It may potentially cause hypotension because of vasodilatation, necessitating close monitoring. Eighty per cent is eliminated unchanged in the urine, and it is therefore greatly influenced by decreases in renal function. In severe myocardial failure, glomerular filtration rate is often reduced and so half-life is increased from the normal 1 hour to several hours.

Imidazolines
Example – enoximone

Enoximone is supplied as a pale yellow solution in ethanol, propylene glycol and sodium hydroxide and has a pH of 12. It is administered as a loading dose followed by infusion. Enoximone reduces the refractoriness of the atrium and AV node and shortens the ventricular refractory period. Ventricular tachycardias and ectopic beats have been observed in some patients who have received enoximone. The propensity to cause hypotension (due to vasodilatation) necessitates monitoring of blood pressure. Enoximone is metabolised in the liver, producing a mixture of active and inactive metabolites, and has a half-life of about 4 hours.

Selective imidazoline receptor agonists (SIRAs)

Example – moxonidine

Selective imidazoline receptor agonists are used for antihypertensive therapy. These drugs act by selective agonism at the imidazoline subtype 1 receptor (I_1) in the rostral ventrolateral pressor area and ventromedial depressor areas of the medulla oblongata. This area is responsible for sympathetic activity, and an agonist effect at I_1 receptors results in a reduction of general sympathetic nervous system activity which produces the desired effect. SIRAs have a minor effect at the α_2-receptor which might potentially result in sedation, but in practice this is not seen, and the commonest side effect is dry mouth.

An example from this group is moxonidine, a centrally acting antihypertensive agent for mild to moderate hypertension. Moxonidine is also an α_2-adrenoceptor agonist acting similarly to clonidine. Moxonidine improves insulin release in response to glucose. It may exacerbate cardiac conduction defects and should be withdrawn slowly over a 2-week period. Caution is necessary when administering moxonidine with benzodiazepines, as the sedative effects of the latter become enhanced.

Renin–angiotensin system

Antagonism of the renin–angiotensin system at various levels is used to control hypertension by reducing vasomotor tone and by reducing salt and fluid retention. The first site of interference in this cascade is by antagonism of the β-adrenoceptors responsible for renin secretion. Next in line are the angiotensin-converting enzyme (ACE) inhibitors, then the angiotensin II receptor antagonists.

Angiotensin-converting enzyme inhibitors

Examples – captopril, enalapril, lisinopril, perindropril, ramipril

Mechanism of action

ACE inhibitors block the action of angiotensin-converting enzyme (ACE), a carboxypeptidase in the lungs that converts the inactive angiotensin I (Ang I) into the active angiotensin II (Ang II, an octapeptide). Angiotensin II causes profound vasoconstriction and release of aldosterone, resulting in sodium and water conservation. ACE is relatively non-specific, and it also inactivates bradykinin (a vasodilator) and other kinins. These three activities produce a rise in intravascular volume and vasomotor tone with the resultant increase in blood pressure. ACE inhibitors antagonise these effects. ACE inhibitors may also cause specific renal vasodilatation, and so further enhance sodium and water excretion. The reduced breakdown of bradykinin is responsible for the side effect of dry cough experienced with ACE inhibitors. The effects of ACE inhibitors include a reduction in:

- Sodium and water retention
- Vasomotor tone
- Preload
- Afterload
- Myocardial work

ACE inhibitors are indicated in hypertension, congestive cardiac failure, myocardial infarction and diabetic nephropathy. They are particularly effective when renin levels are raised, such as when sympathetic tone is increased. Myocardial infarction and congestive cardiac failure may show such increases. In antihypertensive therapy the ACE inhibitors may be used alone or in conjunction with other agents using different systems, such as diuretics and calcium antagonists. β-Blockers reduce renin secretion, so the benefit of adding an ACE inhibitor will be limited.

Angiotensin-II receptor antagonists

Examples – irbesartan, losartan, valsartan

Mechanism of action

The classification of the AT-II receptor deserves further clarification. ACE converts angiotensin I to angiotensin II. Angiotensin I is inactive and does not have identified receptors, whereas angiotensin II is highly active. There are two receptor subtypes for angiotensin II (roman numerals) which have been numbered (with arabic numerals) AT_1 and AT_2. AT_1 receptors are G-protein-coupled receptors responsible for vasoconstricton and aldosterone secretion. The role of the AT_2 receptors is less clear, but they are thought to be antiproliferative for endothelial cells and to be involved in smooth muscle proliferation and differentiation. The angiotensin II receptor antagonists block the AT_1 receptor.

Figure 36.9 Clinical effects of AT-II inhibitors

Reduced sodium and water retention
Reduced vasomotor tone
Reduced preload
Reduced afterload
Reduced blood pressure, especially if sodium depletion
Reduced myocardial work
Variable reduction in aldosterone levels
Blockade of negative feedback produces a rise in renin, Ang I and Ang II
Increased insulin sensitivity
Reduced catecholamines and atrial natriuretic peptide (ANP)
Increased plasma potassium concentration

Uses

The AT-II inhibitors are used as antihypertensive agents and have clinical effects similar to the ACE inhibitors. Their main advantage is the absence of an effect on kinins, so the persistent dry cough of ACE inhibitors is not seen.

Features

The clinical features of AT-II inhibitors are very varied. The main effects are shown in Figure 36.9.

Diuretics

Diuretics promote the loss of water and sodium via the urine. Interference with sodium reabsorption in the renal tubule causes increased sodium loss, and the sodium takes water with it. Their precise effect is determined by which part of the renal tubule they affect. Other drugs may also indirectly increase renal water loss. The sites of action of the various diuretics are shown in Figure 36.10.

Loop diuretics

Example – frusemide

These act on the thick (upper) part of the ascending loop of Henle by reducing sodium and chloride reabsorption. This interferes with the generation of the interstitial hypertonicity which is used by the collecting duct to reabsorb water. A smaller effect is due to the increased delivery of filtrate to the distal tubule. These are the most efficacious diuretics, causing up to 25% of sodium and water in the filtrate to be excreted. Loop diuretics also cause vasodilatation either directly or indirectly. This increases renal blood flow without affecting the glomerular filtration rate. The protein left in the efferent capillaries supplying the remainder of the nephron is therefore more dilute and has a lower oncotic pressure, which reduces reabsorption from the nephron. Subsequently more filtrate enters the loop of Henle, which is the primary site of action of the loop diuretics. In congestive cardiac failure, the venodilatation reduces preload before any diuretic effect is seen.

Loop diuretics work as antihypertensives by reducing both blood volume and vascular tone. The vascular effects may be mediated by interference with prostaglandin E_2 and I_2 degradation.

Loop diuretics present more filtrate to the distal convoluted tubule. The sodium–potassium exchange pump reabsorbs more sodium, and therefore more potassium is excreted. Hydrogen ions are also excreted in exchange for some of the potassium, and bicarbonate concentration increases. Patients on loop diuretics are therefore at risk of hypokalaemia and metabolic alkalosis. Calcium and magnesium loss also occurs. Uric acid secretion is reduced.

Loop diuretics are highly protein-bound, and therefore do not readily pass through the glomerular membrane. They are actively secreted into the proximal convoluted tubule (via the organic acid transport system) and then travel along the tubule to the luminal membrane of the loop of Henle. Excretion occurs via the urine, and they are non-cumulative.

Thiazide diuretics

Example – bendrofluazide

Thiazides act on the luminal membrane pump of the distal convoluted tubule by inhibiting active sodium and chloride reabsorption. They are medium-efficacy diuretics, causing up to 10% of sodium and water in the filtrate to be excreted. More sodium reaches the distal tubules, and this results in high potassium loss in the same way as with the loop diuretics, but because this is the main mode of thiazide action potassium loss is a much greater problem. Magnesium excretion is increased, but calcium and uric acid excretion are reduced.

Thiazides also cause direct vasodilatation. Owing to the ability to cause hyperglycaemia they are best avoided in diabetics. Excretion is by glomerular filtration and by

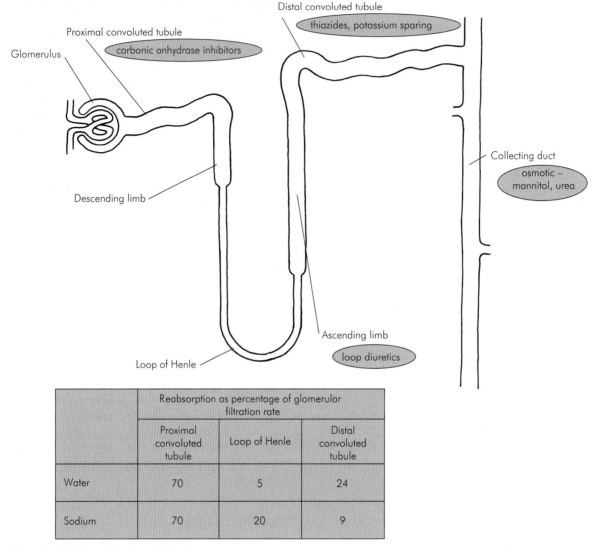

Figure 36.10 Sites of action of diuretics

	Reabsorption as percentage of glomerular filtration rate		
	Proximal convoluted tubule	Loop of Henle	Distal convoluted tubule
Water	70	5	24
Sodium	70	20	9

tubular secretion using the uric acid secretion mechanism, which reduces uric acid excretion.

Potassium-sparing diuretics
Examples – amiloride, spironolactone

Potassium-sparing diuretics act on the distal convoluted tubule and collecting duct. They are low-efficacy diuretics, causing only 5% of sodium and water in the filtrate to be excreted, but have the advantage that they conserve potassium and are mainly used to minimise potassium loss caused by more effective diuretics. The decrease in potassium secretion increases the hydrogen ion secretion and thus reduces bicarbonate excretion. They also reduce uric acid excretion. Spironolactone inhibits the sodium–potassium exchange pump of the extraluminal membrane of collecting duct cells. Triamterene and amiloride interfere with the sodium channels through which the effects of aldosterone are mediated. Amiloride also inhibits sodium–potassium exchange in the proximal tubule.

Osmotic diuretics

Examples – mannitol, glucose, urea

Osmotic diuretics (such as mannitol and glucose) act by passing freely through the glomerular basement membrane, but being non-reabsorbable once in the tubule. The resultant effect is dependent directly upon the number of molecules, and so a large number of molecules is required to produce a clinical effect. They must usually be given intravenously. Urea is classified as an osmotic diuretic but is actively secreted into the tubule as well.

Carbonic anhydrase inhibitors

Example – acetazolamide

Carbonic anhydrase inhibitors inhibit the enzymatic breakdown of carbonic acid, and so interfere with the reabsorption of sodium in exchange for hydrogen ion secretion, especially in the proximal tubule. Their diuretic effect is mild. Their use is now mainly reserved for treatment of glaucoma and epilepsy. Other examples of carbonic anhydrase inhibitors are methazolamide and dichlorphenamide.

Specific pharmacology

Here, bioavailability applies to oral administration. Units (unless stated otherwise) are:

Volume of distribution at steady state (V_d): L kg^{-1}
Clearance (Cl): mL kg^{-1} min^{-1}
Terminal half-life ($t_{1/2}$): hours

Adenosine

Structure – a nucleoside comprising adenine (6-amino purine) and D-ribofuranose (pentose sugar)

Presentation – IV – clear aqueous solution of adenosine 6 mg in 2 mL 0.9% sodium chloride

Dose – IV – bolus 3 mg over 2 s, then bolus 6 mg after 1–2 min if necessary, then bolus 12 mg after 1–2 min if necessary; stop if high nodal block develops

Pharmacokinetics

$t_{1/2}$	8–10 s

CNS – rare occurrence of blurred vision, headache, dizziness

CVS – inhibits AV nodal conduction, reduces contractility, vasodilatation; palpitations, flushing, hypotension, severe bradycardia may occur

RS – dyspnoea, bronchospasm may occur

Other effects – nausea

Elimination – rapid cellular uptake, adenosine deaminase, phosphorylation to nucleotide

Contraindications – second- and third-degree heart block and sick sinus syndrome unless artificial pacemaker functioning; asthma

Interactions – dipyridamole inhibits adenosine uptake (if essential, use 0.5–1 mg dose); xanthines (caffeine, aminophylline) are potent inhibitors of adenosine; drugs slowing AV nodal conduction

Amiodarone hydrochloride

Structure – iodinated benzofuran derivative, class III antiarrhythmic

Presentation
Oral – tablets 200 mg, 100 mg
IV – clear, pale yellow solution, 150 mg in 3 mL

Dose
Oral – loading regimen, then 200 mg per day; onset of action by oral route is 6 days
IV – 5 mg kg^{-1} over 20 min to 2 h

Pharmacokinetics

Bioavailability	22–86%
Protein binding	97%
$t_{1/2}$	54 days

CNS – peripheral neuropathy rare; nightmares, tremor, ataxia; corneal microdeposits (benign and reversible)

CVS – slows heart rate and may cause bradycardia and AV block

RS – may rarely cause diffuse pulmonary alveolitis and fibrosis

Other effects – metabolite blocks conversion of T_3 to thyroxine and may therefore cause hypo- or hyperthyroidism. Thyroid function should be monitored. It may cause chronic liver disease, and transaminases often rise, especially at start of treatment

Elimination – it is de-iodinated and has a very long half-life because it is highly lipid-soluble and highly tissue-bound, which may result in cumulation; toxic effects may still be present months after treatment stopped

Digoxin

Structure – sterol lactone with sugar moiety, cardiac glycoside

Presentation

Oral – tablets 62.5, 125 and 250 µg, elixir

IV – clear, colourless, aqueous solution, 125 µg mL^{-1}

Dose

IV – up to 1 mg loading dose by slow (25 µg min^{-1}) injection

Typically 10 µg kg^{-1} once daily oral or IV; monitor levels, plasma concentrations (nmol L^{-1}) – therapeutic 1.3–1.5; toxic 3.5

Pharmacokinetics

Bioavailability	75%
Protein binding	25%
V_d	8
$t_{1/2}$	35

Clearance – $0.88 \times$ creatinine clearance + 0.33

CNS – nausea, vomiting, dizziness, anorexia, fatigue, apathy, malaise, visual disturbance, depression and psychosis

CVS – positive inotropy, especially in hypervolaemic failure; negative chronotropy; slowing of AV conduction; in excess may cause complete heart block, and most rhythm disturbances, especially bradycardias

Other effects – mild intrinsic diuretic affect; abdominal pain, diarrhoea; gynaecomastia (steroid-related); intestinal necrosis (oral route); skin rashes; thrombocytopoenia

Elimination – 10% metabolised in the liver by progressive removal of the sugar moieties; 60% excreted unchanged in the urine by glomerular filtration and active tubular secretion

Toxicity increased by low potassium, low magnesium, high sodium, high calcium, acid–base disturbance and hypoxaemia. Poorly removed by dialysis as highly tissue-bound; digoxin-specific antibody fragments available for treatment of poisoning.

Diltiazem

Structure – benzothiapine calcium antagonist, class IV antiarrhythmic

Presentation – tablets 60 mg; slow-release 90, 120, 180, 200, 240 mg

Dose – 60–120 mg, 6–8 hourly

Pharmacokinetics

Bioavailability	35%
Protein binding	80%
V_d	5.3
Cl	15
$t_{1/2}$	5

CNS – no effect

CVS – causes peripheral and coronary arterial vasodilatation; decreases systemic and peripheral resistance; slows AV nodal conduction; exacerbates the negative inotropic effects of volatile agents

RS – antihistamine effect

Other effects – renal artery dilatation increases renal plasma flow; local anaesthetic effect; reduced lower oesophageal sphincter pressure in achalasia; may inhibit platelet aggregation

Elimination – 2% is excreted unchanged in the urine; deacetylation and demethylation produce active metabolites which are conjugated with glucuronides and sulphates; renal failure has no effect on elimination

Esmolol hydrochloride

Structure – aryloxypropanolamine, β-blocker, class II antiarrhythmic

Presentation – IV – clear aqueous solution 10 mL of 250 mg mL^{-1} for dilution and infusion; 10 mL of 100 mg mL^{-1} for undiluted boluses; 250 mL of 100 mg mL^{-1} for infusion

Dose – 50–200 µg kg^{-1} min^{-1}; a loading dose may be used

Pharmacokinetics

Protein binding	56%
V_d	3.43
Cl	285
$t_{1/2}$	9.2 min

CVS – mainly β_1; used for acute supraventricular tachycardia, acute control of hypertension and myocardial infarction; negative chronotrope and inotrope, cardiac output falls by 20%

RS – selectivity minimises increases in airway resistance

Elimination – metabolised by red cell esterases producing methanol and a primary acid (70–80% as this in urine) which has weak β-antagonism and a half-life of 3.5 hours; < 1% is excreted unchanged in the urine. Use with caution in renal failure; hepatic failure has no effect

Nifedipine

Structure – dihydropyridine calcium antagonist, class IV antiarrhythmic

Presentation – tablets 10 and 20 mg and capsules 5 and 10 mg; the yellow, viscous liquid in the capsules has been used sublingually for speedy control of blood pressure; a solution is available for direct intracoronary injection

Dose – oral – 10–20 mg 8 hourly, 20–40 mg 12 hourly slow-release formulation

Pharmacokinetics

Bioavailability	65%
Protein binding	95%
V_d	0.8
Cl	10
$t_{1/2}$	5

CNS – marginal increase in cerebral blood flow; headache, flushing, dizziness

CVS – decreases systemic and peripheral vascular resistance, decreases pulmonary artery pressure, reflex increase in heart rate and cardiac output; increases epicardial and coronary blood flow, negative inotrope

RS – no effect

Other effects – increases red cell deformability, decreases platelet aggregation, decreases thromboxane synthesis; reduces lower oesophageal sphincter pressure; increases renin, increases catecholamines; increases hepatic blood flow; oedema of legs; eye pain; gum hyperplasia

Elimination – 85% in urine; 15% in bile; non-cumulative

Verapamil

Structure – synthetic papaverine derivative, class IV antiarrhythmic

Presentation – tablets 40, 80 and 120 mg; IV 5 mg in 2 mL

Dose – oral – 40–120 mg 8 hourly; IV 10 mg (0.075–0.20 mg kg^{-1})

Pharmacokinetics

Bioavailability	20%
Protein binding	90%
V_d	4.5
$t_{1/2}$	5

CNS – dizziness, headache

CVS – slows cardiac action potential; slows AV nodal conduction; decreases systemic vascular resistance; decreases blood pressure, heart rate and cardiac output; increases coronary blood flow

RS – no effect

Other effects – local anaesthetic effect; constipation

Elimination – 70% excreted in urine as conjugated metabolites, 5% unchanged; non-cumulative; half-life is increased in hepatic disease

Interactions – avoid concurrent use with β-blocker as it may cause asystole or hypotension

References and further reading

Small R. Anti-arrhythmic drugs. *Anaesth Intensive Care Med* 2006; 7: 294–7.

Vaughan Williams EM. Classification of anti-dysrhythmic drugs. In Sande E, Flensted-Jensen E, Oleson KH, eds., *Symposium on Cardiac Dysrhythmias*. Södertälje: Astra, 1970, pp. 449–72.

CHAPTER 37
Respiratory pharmacology

Tim Smith

Administration and modes of action

Drugs acting on the airways may be administered systemically or by inhalation. The inhaled mode allows a higher concentration of agent to be delivered directly to the bronchial tree, which minimises absorption and accompanying systemic effects. Some drugs are metabolised in the lungs, resulting in a non-hepatic first-pass effect.

Typically, only 10% of an inhalationally administered bronchodilator reaches the lungs. Most of this is deposited in the upper airways with little benefit, with about 3% reaching the alveoli. Distribution is little affected by the presence of obstructive airways disease, or by particle size.

Bronchial calibre is fundamentally affected by two opposing systems. Factors that cause an increase of intracellular cAMP (such as sympathetic stimulation) result in bronchodilatation. The reverse situation involves factors that raise the intracellular concentration of cGMP (such as parasympathetic stimulation) to cause bronchoconstriction. The physiological and pharmacological influences on bronchial calibre are summarised in Figure 37.1.

Leukotrienes are involved in the development of bronchospasm. They are so named because of their presence in white blood cells (the *leuko* component) and their chemical bonds (a *triene* system of double bonds). They are a group of eicosanoids (bioactive lipid derivatives of arachidonic acid). Leukotrienes are produced by the action of the enzyme 5-lipoxygenase, which is found in white blood cells (particularly eosinophils) and mast cells, among other tissues. When activated, 5-lipoxygenase binds to the cell membrane and associates with five-lipoxygenase-activating protein (FLAP), the resulting complex causing change in arachidonic acid to produce leukotriene A_4 (LTA_4). This is a precursor of a whole family of leukotrienes, LTA_4 to LTF_4. LTC_4, D_4 and E_4 are spasmogenic, and comprise the substance formerly termed 'sRS-A'.

Control of bronchial calibre
Adrenoceptor agonists
β_2-agonists

Examples – bambuterol, formoterol, salbutamol, salmeterol, terbutaline

Selective β_2-adrenoceptor agonists are used in the treatment of bronchospasm and for prophylaxis. This selectivity is not absolute, and high doses of these drugs will cause β_1 effects (tachycardia, tremor, hyperglycaemia, increased insulin secretion and hypokalaemia).

β_2-agonists reverse bronchospasm caused by histamine release, platelet-activating factor and members of the leukotriene family, particularly C_4, D_4 and E_4.

Fundamentals of Anaesthesia, 4th edition, ed. Ted Lin, Tim Smith and Colin Pinnock. Published by Cambridge University Press. © Cambridge University Press 2017.

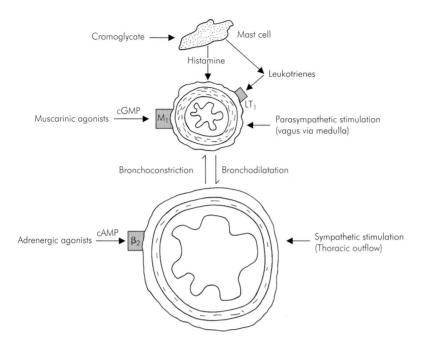

Figure 37.1 Causes of changes in bronchial calibre

The β_2-agonist salbutamol is the most widely used agent in the treatment of asthma. It is conjugated in the liver and excreted in both conjugated and unchanged forms in urine and faeces. Terbutaline is a similar drug that may have advantages in some patients because it has fewer sympathomimetic side effects. Terbutaline may be used antenatally to stimulate fetal lung surfactant production. Bambuterol is a prodrug of terbutaline.

β_2-agonists (in particular ritodrine, salbutamol and terbutaline) may be used as uterine relaxants for the management of premature labour or excessive contractions, or during Caesarean section to facilitate delivery. Administration for this purpose may be inhalational.

Other adrenoceptor agonists
Examples – adrenaline, ephedrine, isoprenaline, orciprenaline

Ephedrine, isoprenaline, orciprenaline and adrenaline are non-selective sympathetic agonists with bronchodilator (β_2) actions, which are infrequently used. Adrenaline has re-emerged as an effective inhaled agent for the treatment of acute tracheolaryngobronchitis (croup) and laryngeal oedema. A dose of 0.5 mL kg^{-1} 1:1000

adrenaline up to a maximum of 5 mL may be nebulised, and given according to effect.

Anticholinergic agents
Examples – ipratropium bromide, tiotropium bromide

Anticholinergic agents are given inhalationally and, as with other inhaled bronchodilators, only 10% of the dose reaches the lungs. These drugs act at muscarinic acetylcholine receptors and so inhibit bronchoconstriction. Systemically administered anticholinergic drugs also affect these receptors. Anticholinergic agents have the following respiratory effects:

- Bronchodilatation
- Reduced airways resistance
- Increased anatomical dead space
- Increased physiological dead space

Ipratropium bromide (N-isopropylatropine) is a non-selective muscarinic antagonist at M_1, M_2 and M_3. It has a rapid onset of action, but takes 2 hours to peak, lasting for 4–6 hours. Of the orally deposited drug, 70% passes unprocessed into the faeces. A small amount of drug is absorbed systemically from the oral mucosa, and this is metabolised by the liver. Antagonism at the (negative feedback) M_2 receptor increases acetylcholine release, which may limit the effectiveness of its M_1-mediated bronchodilatation. Ipratropium also blocks the M_1-muscarinic acetylcholine receptors on mast cells, limiting degranulation. It is primarily used for prophylaxis of bronchospasm, frequently in combination with other inhaled agents.

Tiotropium has a longer half-life, allowing once-daily administration, and remains preferentially bound to M_1 and M_3 compared with M_2, so improving efficacy.

Methylxanthines
Examples – caffeine, theophylline

The methylxanthines are stimulant bronchodilators derived from plant alkaloids which have both a local effect on the bronchial tree and a general central stimulating effect which increases respiratory drive. They have a multimodal mechanism of action that includes:

- Phosphodiesterase inhibition
- Facilitation of β_2 action
- Enhanced Ca^{2+} release from sarcoplasmic reticulum in striated muscle
- Adenosine receptor antagonism

Inhibition of phosphodiesterase directly and via β_2 effects causes bronchodilatation similar to that of β_2-agonists. The enhanced release of calcium within the sarcoplasmic reticulum improves the function of the respiratory muscles. Methylxanthines are potent inhibitors of adenosine receptors and inhibit smooth muscle contraction by increasing cAMP and by direct interference with calcium entry.

Clinical effects
Respiratory system
Methylxanthines cause bronchodilatation, with increased anatomical dead space. They are effective against bronchospasm owing to the release of histamine, platelet-activating factor and leukotrienes. The force of respiratory skeletal muscle contraction is increased, as is respiratory rate. Respiratory work is increased with relatively less fatigue. Methylxanthines are effective prophylactically, and are also indicated for the treatment of acute attacks of bronchospasm.

Cardiovascular system
Heart rate and cardiac contractility are increased and peripheral vascular resistance is markedly reduced due to smooth muscle relaxation. This combination of effects may be helpful in the treatment of left ventricular failure.

Central nervous system
There is general stimulation, which increases respiratory rate. Although CNS excitation is relatively non-specific, both vasomotor and respiratory centres are markedly affected. Convulsions are a potential hazard.

Other effects
These include the stimulation of gastric acid and pepsin secretion, diuresis (by dilatation of afferent glomerular arterioles) and inhibition of uterine contraction.

The methylxanthines can be considered as a family of agents with theophylline as the parent compound. Although theophylline is well absorbed orally, its rapid elimination in the liver by cytochrome P450, and variable protein binding of about 40%, leads to unpredictable clinical effects. Theophylline levels are measured in the plasma during chronic administration to ensure adequate therapeutic concentrations. Aminophylline, the ethylene diamine salt of theophylline, is more water-soluble (but highly alkaline in solution). This improved water solubility is required for intravenous administration.

Steroids
Examples – beclomethasone, budesonide, fluticasone

Inhaled and systemic steroids may be used in the treatment and prevention of bronchospasm secondary to obstructive airways disease. Steroids act directly on intracellular receptor sites, have an anti-inflammatory action that reduces mucosal oedema and swelling, and also interfere with many mediators of airways resistance. Chemical mediators suppressed by steroid treatment include prostaglandins, thromboxanes, prostacyclin, leukotrienes, platelet-activating factor and histamine. There are multiple other effects of steroids, including reductions in inflammation, smooth muscle tone, vascular permeability and pulmonary vascular resistance, all of which are useful in the treatment of bronchospasm.

The effects of inhaled steroids can be summarised as follows:

- Inhibition of arachidonic acid metabolites
- Inhibition of inflammatory response
- Stabilisation of mast cells
- Catecholamine synergism

Although inhaled steroids are used for prophylaxis, acute attacks require systemic steroids – but their action by this route is slow in onset.

Beclomethasone is an inhaled steroid given in typical doses of 100–400 μg, 2–4 times a day. Budesonide may have advantages in reaching the bronchioles in a more reliable manner, with less systemic effects.

Cromoglicate

Cromoglicate, an inhaled membrane-stabilising agent, is only effective in the **prevention** of bronchospasm. It inhibits the action of platelet-activating factor on eosinophils, mast cells and platelets, suppresses axonal reflexes caused by irritants and acts as a mild mast-cell stabiliser. This may be mediated by inhibition of calcium entry into the mast cell.

Bioavailability by the inhaled route is 10% (1% orally). Of the drug, 70% is protein-bound and it is excreted unchanged (50% in urine, 50% in bile). It has a half-life of 90 minutes, but its duration of action is several hours.

Leukotriene receptor antagonists

Examples – montelukast, zafirlukast

The release of cysteinyl leukotrienes C_4, D_4, and E_4 from eosinophils, basophils and mast cells is involved in the genesis of asthma. Leukotrienes increase mucus production, cause airway wall oedema, eosinophil migration, airway smooth muscle proliferation, bronchoconstriction and airway hyper-responsiveness. The leukotriene receptor antagonists are highly selective, and competitive. They block the effects of leukotrienes on the LT_1 receptor on bronchial smooth muscle and so antagonise the bronchoconstriction. They also reduce leukotriene production.

Montelukast and zafirlukast are indicated for the **prevention** of mild to moderate asthma as an adjunct to inhaled steroids, cromoglicate and intermittent β_2-agonists, but not in the treatment of acute attacks. Exercise-induced and aspirin-induced asthma may be particularly suitable for treatment. They are administered orally with a bioavailability of 60–80%, although with food this drops substantially. They achieve peak plasma levels at 2–3 hours. Metabolism is hepatic.

Respiratory centre stimulants

Example – doxapram

Respiratory centre stimulants act by increasing respiratory drive. As their site of action is not purely the respiratory centre, increasing doses produce the effects of generalised CNS stimulation such as restlessness, anxiety and convulsions. Doxapram is useful in the management of central respiratory depression either as a result of chronic lung disease or from drug therapy, but should not be used in patients with respiratory obstruction in whom the normal central drive is preserved, as this may lead to further exhaustion and precipitation of respiratory collapse.

Doxapram acts via the carotid sinus chemoreceptors (and also centrally, causing stimulation of the respiratory centre) to cause increased respiratory rate and tidal volume. Clinical effects last only 5–10 minutes, and further boluses or infusion may be required for longer duration of effect. Doxapram has a higher therapeutic index than the other respiratory stimulants, and because of this it has found a limited niche in the recovery area.

Other general analeptics also cause respiratory centre stimulation, but the more generalised CNS excitation precludes their use as specific respiratory stimulants.

Mucolytics

Examples – carbocisteine, methylcysteine

Carbocisteine and methylcysteine (given orally) may be used to reduce the viscosity of sputum as an aid to expectoration. Dornase alpha is a specific mucolytic agent that is a genetically synthesised enzyme acting by cleavage of extracellular DNA. The specific use of dornase alpha is administration by inhalation in selected cystic fibrosis patients.

Surfactant

Surfactant is a physiologically occurring lipid–protein complex produced in the lung by type II alveolar cells. It lines the alveolar lung surface and has its effect by reducing surface tension, which increases pulmonary compliance. Surfactant mainly comprises dipalmitoylphosphatidylcholine. Synthetic, porcine and bovine forms of surfactant have been used to treat respiratory distress in neonates, the route of administration being by direct instillation into the lungs.

Specific pharmacology

Units (unless stated otherwise) are:
Volume of distribution at steady state (V_d): L kg^{-1}
Clearance (Cl): mL kg^{-1} min^{-1}
Terminal half-life ($t_{1/2}$): hours

Aminophylline

Structure – ethylene diamine salt of the methylxanthine theophylline

Presentation

Oral – modified-release tablets 225 mg

IV – clear solution 25 mg mL^{-1}

Dose

Oral – up to 300 mg three times daily

IV – cautious slow infusion 500 µg kg^{-1} h^{-1} adjusted by serum theophylline concentrations

CNS – direct respiratory stimulant, may cause convulsions

CVS – myocardial contractility and heart rate rise, cardiac output increased; marked peripheral vasodilatation (offset slightly by vasomotor centre stimulation)

RS – bronchodilatation by β_2 action, direct respiratory centre stimulation; rise in respiratory rate

Other – general smooth muscle relaxation; renal blood flow increased

Elimination – demethylation and oxidation in the liver followed by urinary excretion

Caution – rapid IV administration may result in convulsions, tachycardia and collapse

Beclomethasone

Structure – synthetic corticosteroid

Presentation – metered inhaler, 50, 100 or 200 µg per puff

Dose – up to maximum of 800 µg daily (adult)

CNS - steroid psychosis rare but possible in high dosage

CVS - hypertension and fluid retention possible in high dosage

RS - reduction in airway sensitivity, reduction of bronchospasm; risk of *Candida albicans* infection

Other - adrenal suppression possible; osteoporosis is a risk in chronic therapy

Budesonide

Structure – synthetic corticosteroid

Presentation – metered inhaler, 50 or 200 µg per puff

Dose – 200–400 µg twice daily

CNS - steroid psychosis rare but possible in high dosage

CVS - hypertension and fluid retention possible in high dosage

RS - reduction in airway sensitivity, reduction of bronchospasm; risk of *Candida albicans* infection

Other - adrenal suppression possible; osteoporosis a risk in chronic therapy

Doxapram

Structure – monohydrated pyrrolidinone

Presentation – clear colourless solution, 100 mg in 5 mL, or 2 mg mL^{-1} in 500 mL 5% dextrose

Dose – IV – 1–1.5 mg kg^{-1}, onset 30 s, peak 2 min, lasts 10 min

Pharmacokinetics

V_d	1.5
Cl	5
$t_{1/2}$	3

CNS – carotid body chemoreceptors and respiratory centre stimulation; higher doses cause restlessness, dizziness, headache, hallucinations, convulsions

CVS – stroke volume and cardiac output increased; heart rate and blood pressure may increase

RS – tidal volume increased; rate increased with higher doses or if slow; minute volume increased. CO_2 response curve shifted to left

Others – may increase urine output, salivation, and motility of GI and urinary tracts

Elimination – 95% metabolised primarily by liver, 5% unchanged in urine

Side effects – potentiates sympathomimetic amines; increased effect if on MAOI; may cause agitation and increased skeletal muscle activity when concurrent with aminophylline therapy

Caution – if respiratory failure not due to inadequate respiratory drive, will cause agitation and convulsions

Ipratropium bromide

Structure – quaternary derivative of N-isopropyl atropine

Presentation – metered inhaler 20 µg per puff, nebuliser solution 250 µg mL^{-1} also available; maximum effect 30 min after administration, duration 6 h

Dose – up to 40 µg three times daily

CNS – no effect

CVS – no effect

RS – bronchodilatation, occasional irritation and cough; paradoxical bronchospasm possible but rare

Other – may produce glaucoma and urinary retention (anticholinergic effects)

Salbutamol

Structure – synthetic amine

Presentation – clear solution 5 mg in 5 mL, tablets 4 and 8 mg, syrup 2 mg in 5 mL, inhalation powder 200 and 400 µg, nebuliser solution 5 mg mL^{-1}

Dose – IV – 250 µg bolus; 3–20 µg min^{-1} by infusion
Pharmacokinetics

Protein binding	8–64%
V_d	2.2
Cl	6.7
$t_{1/2}$	4

CNS – may cause excitation, anxiety, tremor
CVS – β_2 effects cause vasodilatation with decreased blood pressure; higher doses cause β_1 effects with tachycardia
RS – bronchodilator for prophylactic and therapeutic use
Other – crosses placenta and may cause fetal tachycardia
Elimination – 30% unchanged in urine; the rest unchanged in faeces, small amount of conjugated form also appears in urine and faeces

Sodium cromoglicate
Origin – derivative of khellin, found in the oil of a Middle Eastern herb, *Ammi visnaga*
Presentation – metered inhaler, 5 mg per puff, Spincap 20 mg, nebuliser solution 10 mg mL^{-1} (also available as eye drops)
Dose – up to 20 mg four times daily; duration of single dose 6 h
Pharmacokinetics

Bioavailability	10%
Protein binding	70%
$t_{1/2}$	90 min

CNS – no effect
CVS – no effect
RS – prophylactic against bronchospasm; may produce coughing and throat irritation
Other – used in food allergy and inflammatory eye conditions

Zafirlukast
Structure – a complex cyclopentyl carbamate; a leuko-triene receptor antagonist
Presentation – film-coated tablet 20 mg
Dose – oral – 20 mg twice daily, peak 3 h
Pharmacokinetics

Bioavailability	73%
Protein binding	99%
Cl	5
$t_{1/2}$	7

RS – bronchodilator by inhibition of leukotriene-mediated smooth muscle contraction
Elimination – hepatic by cytochrome P450
Side effects – Churge–Strauss syndrome has been reported. Look out for eosinophilia, vasculitis, rhinitis and sinusitis
Caution – it inhibits cytochrome P450, so caution should be exercised with concomitant use of warfarin, phenytoin or phenobarbital
Contraindications – moderate to severe renal or hepatic impairment

CHAPTER 38
Endocrine pharmacology

Tim Smith

Blood sugar control

The physiological control of blood glucose is complex. While the major role belongs to insulin, a multitude of other hormonal influences apply. It should also be remembered that insulin has other actions beyond the regulation of blood glucose.

Pharmacological control of blood glucose becomes necessary in situations of elevation and depression of blood glucose beyond the homeostatic limits, in other words due to hyperglycaemia or hypoglycaemia. The causes of failure in regulation of blood glucose are given in Figure 38.1.

Treatment of hypoglycaemia is directed towards administration of glucose and removal of the root cause. Treatment of hyperglycaemia includes removal of the cause, administration of insulin in the acute phase and at a later stage augmentation of both the secretion and effect of endogenous insulin.

Insulin receptor

The insulin receptor is a complex of four glycoprotein subunits ($\alpha\alpha\beta\beta$) linked by disulphide bridges to form a cylinder. The α subunits are entirely extracellular and contain the insulin binding site. The β subunit spans the

Figure 38.1 Failure of glucose control

Hypoglycaemia	
Deficiency of glucose intake and failure of compensatory mechanisms	
Excess insulin	insulinoma
	iatrogenic
Hyperglycaemia	
Deficiency of insulin	
Decreased end-organ sensitivity to insulin	
Excess administration of glucose solutions	

cell membrane, and the intracellular part has tyrosine kinase activity. The α subunit has a repressive effect on this activity that is removed by the conformational change resulting from insulin binding. The tyrosine kinase acts on insulin receptor substrate 1 (IRS-1), triggering a chain of action culminating in the activation of glycogen synthetase, phosphorylase kinase and glycogen phosphorylase. IRS-1 is also a substrate for insulin-like growth factor 1

Fundamentals of Anaesthesia, 4th edition, ed. Ted Lin, Tim Smith and Colin Pinnock. Published by Cambridge University Press. © Cambridge University Press 2017.

(IGF-1) receptors. The binding of insulin to the α subunit changes the insulin receptor formation to form a trans-membrane tunnel allowing glucose (and other molecules) to pass through the membrane. The activated β subunit autophosphorylates at six or more tyrosine residues and these phosphorylate intracellular proteins, resulting in second-messenger effects on fat, protein and glycogen synthesis. Insulin has a very high affinity for the insulin receptor. This may be due to subsequent binding to the second α subunit. The interaction does not conform to the law of mass action. The insulin–receptor complex is internalised and the receptors recycled, while the insulin itself is degraded in lysosomes.

Glucose

Ideally, glucose should be administered by mouth. Its rapid absorption ensures rapid correction of limited hypoglycaemia. In more severe situations, the unconscious patient requires IV administration. Dextrose 5% has little calorific value (840 kJ L^{-1}). The treatment of hypoglycaemia usually requires a 20% dextrose solution (3.36 MJ L^{-1}) or alternatively a 50% solution (8.4 MJ L^{-1}). Glucose (20%) requires a large vein but can be administered peripherally, but 50% glucose should always be given via a central venous line. Both 20% and 50% solutions can cause damage to the blood vessels and are viscous. Extravasation of concentrated glucose solutions will cause local necrosis.

Glucagon

Glucagon is a polypeptide (smaller than insulin) formed in the A cells of the pancreas and also in the upper gastrointestinal tract. Glucagon has a large number of roles in the regulation of metabolism, all of which are directed to the raising of blood glucose. Although the majority of effects are physiological, glucagon has been used therapeutically in two main areas, for the rapid restoration of blood glucose in severe hypoglycaemia and in cardiogenic shock, due to its positive inotropic effect.

Insulin

Soluble (otherwise known as unmodified) insulin may be given subcutaneously or intravenously. It is short-acting and has a half-life in the circulation of 5 minutes. Subcutaneous administration results in more gradual absorption. Administration of IV insulin allows rapid control in ketoacidotic hyperglycaemia.

Long-term control of diabetes requires a variety of preparations of insulin with differing absorption characteristics

Figure 38.2 Temporal characteristics of subcutaneous insulin preparations

	Onset (hours)	Peak (hours)	Duration (hours)
Short-acting	0.5–1	2–4	8
Intermediate-acting	1–2	4–12	12–24
Long-acting	2–4	24–40	36

for precise control. Longer-acting insulin may be obtained by the formation of insulin complexes using either zinc or protamine or both. The addition of zinc produces a crystalline insulin of intermediate action. The addition of protamine produces isophane insulin, which also has an intermediate duration of action. These insulin preparations may be mixed with soluble insulin (to make *biphasic* insulins), which will lessen temporal fluctuations in plasma insulin.

Long-acting insulin is produced by combination with both protamine and zinc (protamine zinc insulin). This preparation should not be mixed with soluble insulin because the soluble insulin will combine with any free protamine in the solution. Figure 38.2 gives a guide to the time-related effects of the different categories of insulin.

Insulin may be bovine, porcine or human, the animal products being purified by crystallisation. Bovine insulin has three differences from human in its amino acid sequence, and porcine one. These foreign sequences in the insulin or in impurities may be antigenic, leading to insulin resistance and immunoreactivity. To overcome this the insulin is highly purified, but alternatively human insulin may be used. This is the preferred choice in modern therapy. Human insulin is either synthesised by bacteria or created by enzymatic modification of porcine insulin.

Insulin is mainly used in the treatment of diabetes mellitus, but it may also be indicated in parenteral feeding to aid glucose utilisation.

Oral hypoglycaemic agents
Sulphonylureas

Examples – chlorpropamide, glibenclamide, gliclazide, glipizide, tolbutamide

Sulphonylurea drugs act by augmenting endogenous insulin secretion from existing B cells within the islets of

Figure 38.3 Effect of sulphonylureas

Augmented by	Phenylbutazone
	Salicylates
	Alcohol
	Monoamine oxidase inhibitors
Diminished by	Thiazides
	Corticosteroids
	Oestrogens
	Frusemide

Langerhans. Sulphonylureas bind to receptors on the pancreatic B cells and increase the sensitivity of the cells to glucose. The potassium permeability of B cells is reduced by blockade of the ATP-dependent potassium channel. The membrane becomes depolarised, leading to calcium influx and subsequent secretion of insulin.

In excess, sulphonylureas have the propensity to cause hypoglycaemia. Most are metabolised in the liver, resulting in the formation of active metabolites. The sulphonylureas and metabolites are excreted in the urine. They cross the placenta and can cause hypoglycaemia in the newborn. There is competition for albumin binding sites with sulphonamides, aspirin and other highly protein-bound drugs. Factors affecting the action of the sulphonylurea family are given in Figure 38.3.

Chlorpropamide is active for 1–3 days, inactivated in the liver and excreted in the urine. It has a vasopressin-mimicking action on renal tubules and a disulfiram-like effect in the presence of alcohol. Glibenclamide has a duration of about 24 hours. Tolbutamide has a short half-life of about 5 hours, and may decrease thyroid iodide uptake. The third-generation sulphonylureas (such as gliclazide) have a biphasic effect and are metabolised in the liver.

Biguanides
Example – metformin

Biguanides decrease hepatic gluconeogenesis and increase insulin-mediated peripheral glucose uptake. They act by increasing the sensitivity of target tissues (skeletal muscle, adipose tissue and hepatocytes) to insulin. They have no effect on insulin secretion and do not require functioning B cells in the islets of Langerhans. Metformin also lowers low-density lipoproteins (LDL) and very-low-density lipoproteins (VLDL) in the plasma.

Metformin does not bind to plasma protein and is excreted unchanged in the urine, with a half-life of 3 hours. All biguanides carry a risk of lactic acidosis, possibly due to inhibition of oxidative phosphorylation.

Thiazolidinediones
Examples – pioglitazone, rosiglitazone

Thiazolidinediones are new agents intended for the treatment of type 2 diabetes mellitus. Like the biguanides, they sensitise target tissues to insulin. The thiazolidinediones activate nuclear peroxisome proliferator-activated receptor γ (PPAR-γ), predominantly in adipose tissue. This increases transcription of genes in adipocyte differentiation and lipid and glucose metabolism, resulting in reduced blood glucose and a corresponding fall in insulin secretion. Thiazolidinediones increase high-density lipoprotein (HDL) cholesterol and may prove to reduce cardiovascular risk. They are to be used in conjunction with sulphonylureas or metformin. Disadvantages include weight gain and possible risks of hepatotoxicity.

Meglitinide analogues
Examples – nateglinide, repaglinide

Nateglinide and repaglinide belong to a class of oral hypoglycaemic agents structurally related to meglitinide (the non-sulphonylurea moiety of glibenclamide). They inhibit ATP-dependent potassium channels in pancreatic B cells in the presence of glucose. They bind to a receptor site distinct from that of the sulphonylureas and stimulate prandial insulin release. They act synergistically with metformin and thiazolidinediones by specifically targeting postprandial hyperglycaemia. Nateglinide is a phenylalanine derivative and repaglinide is a carbamoylmethyl benzoate.

Thyroid hormones and antithyroid drugs

Hypothyroidism
Deficiency of thyroid hormones is treated with replacement therapy, usually with L-thyroxine (T_4). If a rapid onset of action is required (e.g. hypothyroid coma) then tri-iodothyronine (T_3, liothyronine) is used. This is effective within a few hours and lasts up to 48 hours.

Hyperthyroidism
Excess of thyroid secretions may be treated in several ways: surgical reduction of the thyroid gland, inhibition

of the peripheral actions (β-adrenoceptor antagonists) or specific targeting of thyroid hormone synthesis and secretion.

Specific antithyroid drugs have a variety of effects; the thioureylenes (such as carbimazole) block organification of iodine, potassium iodide inhibits secretion of thyroid hormones, and radio-iodine causes destruction of thyroid follicle cells.

Thioureylenes

Examples – carbimazole, propylthiouracil

Thioureylenes may take 3–4 weeks to take effect. Their major action is the inhibition of iodination of thyroglobulin-bound tyrosine by opposing thyroperoxidases. There is also evidence of inhibition of iodinated tyrosine coupling, and suppression of antibody synthesis in Grave's disease. The thiocarbamide group is essential for the therapeutic activity of carbimazole. Carbimazole is rapidly converted to another, active, thioureylene called methimazole. A rare but serious side effect of carbimazole therapy is the development of agranulocytosis.

Iodine/iodide mixtures

These inhibit iodine substitution on the tyrosine moieties, resulting in a decreased output of thyroid hormone by the gland.

Radio-iodine

Radio-iodine (^{131}I radioisotope) emits β rays. These cause cellular destruction but are rapidly attenuated and have an effective penetration of only 2 mm. Iodine-131 also emits γ rays that enable imaging.

Adrenocortical steroids

Examples – betamethasone, cortisone, dexamethasone, fludrocortisone, hydrocortisone, prednisolone, prednisone, triamcinolone

Hydrocortisone (cortisol) is naturally occurring, whereas the other examples are synthetically derived. Cortisone has minimal activity and must be converted to hydrocortisone in the liver first. Corticosteroids are used as replacement therapy in Addison's disease and similar conditions, and in higher doses for suppression of various inflammatory processes. Steroid choice is determined in part by the relative glucocorticoid and mineralocorticoid effects. Hydrocortisone is suitable for replacement therapy and short-term use. Long-term use causes excessive fluid retention compared with alternatives such as prednisolone. The relative glucocorticoid and mineralocorticoid

Figure 38.4 Relative potencies of the effects of corticosteroids

Drug	Gluco-corticoid	Mineralo-corticoid
Hydrocortisone	1	1
Cortisone	0.8	0.8
Prednisone	4	0.25
Prednisolone	4	0.25
Methylprednisolone	5	minimal
Dexamethasone	25	minimal
Aldosterone	0.3	400
Fludrocortisone	10	300

potencies are given in Figure 38.4. The pharmacological effects of steroids are manifold, including:

- Inhibition of inflammation
- Improved transport of cellular oxygen
- Preservation of lysosome membrane integrity
- Inhibition of complement C5 activation
- Inhibition of plasminogen activator
- Negative feedback on hypothalamus, and pituitary and adrenal cortex atrophy
- Inhibition of neutrophil and macrophage recruitment
- Red cell and neutrophil counts selectively increased

Corticosteroids diffuse into cells and act on specific intracellular receptors. The complex subsequently produced then moves to the nucleus and increases synthesis of certain enzymes. Glucocorticoids are lipid-soluble and are transported in the plasma by corticosteroid-binding globulin (CBG) and albumin. CBG is relatively specific for endogenous steroids and does not bind synthetic steroids readily. Because of its low capacity, it may become saturated when therapeutic doses of steroids are used.

The therapeutic effects of steroids are primarily a feature of the glucocorticoid effects. The side effects may be caused by either glucocorticoid or mineralocorticoid components. Mineralocorticoid side effects are seen early and mimic those of hyperaldosteronism – sodium and water retention, and increased renal potassium and calcium excretion. Glomerular filtration rate is increased. In the gut there is increased calcium absorption, but this is insufficient to offset the renal loss. The glucocorticoid side effects tend to be seen with chronic administration and

Figure 38.5 Side effects of steroids

Mineralocorticoid
- Sodium retention
- Potassium loss
- Water retention
- Renal calcium loss
- Hypertension

Glucocorticoid
- Muscle wasting
- Fat deposition
- Liver glycogen deposition
- Thin, friable skin
- Poor wound healing
- Reduced immunity
- Cataracts
- Raised intraocular pressure
- Osteoporosis
- Hyperglycaemia

are seen relatively late on, mimicking Cushing's syndrome. The side effects of steroid therapy are listed in Figure 38.5.

Oxytocic drugs

Oxytocin

Oxytocin is an octapeptide similar to vasopressin. The pharmacological preparation is synthetic, hence the trade name Syntocinon. It binds to specific sites in the myometrium, causing uterine contraction. This is probably mediated by increases in potassium permeability which reduce the membrane potential, making it more excitable. Uterine sensitivity to oxytocin increases from minimal in the non-pregnant to maximum at term. Oxytocin also causes contraction of breast-duct smooth muscle with milk ejection.

Oxytocin causes direct vasodilatation, and a mild vasopressin-like antidiuretic effect, which may become significant if it is used for prolonged infusion. There is metabolism by both renal and hepatic routes.

Ergometrine

Ergometrine stimulates uterine contraction (possibly via 5-HT receptors), and also causes vascular smooth muscle contraction although the effect is slight. It has a very mild α-adrenergic blocking action. These effects are mediated via dopaminergic and 5-HT receptors. Ergometrine is a potent emetic, acting on the chemoreceptor trigger zone

and vomiting centre (via D_2 receptors). After treatment with ergometrine there may occasionally be a clinical picture of hypertension with headache and blurred vision which lasts several days. Ergometrine acts within 30–60 seconds of IV administration (IM 2–4 minutes, orally 4–8 minutes), and lasts 3–6 hours. The drug is metabolised by the liver and excreted in the bile.

Carboprost

Carboprost tromethamine is a prostaglandin used in the management of severe obstetric haemorrhage secondary to uterine atony that is unresponsive to oxytocin and ergometrine. It may be administered by deep intramuscular injection. Side effects include nausea and vomiting, diarrhoea, flushing and bronchospasm. There have been very rare reports of cardiovascular collapse with prostaglandin use.

Renal hormones

Vasopressin and analogues

Vasopressin

Vasopressin (antidiuretic hormone, ADH) is an octapeptide similar to oxytocin. It may be used pharmacologically but its short half-life (10 minutes) is a disadvantage. Vasopressin acts on the vasopressin 2 (V_2) receptor to permit water reabsorption from the renal collecting duct and is a very potent direct-acting vasoconstrictor (V_{1a} receptor). Vasopressin also increases hepatic glycogenolysis, increases factor VIII activity and encourages platelet aggregation and degranulation. It is also involved in the release of ACTH-RH in the hypothalamus (V_{1b}/V_3). The vasopressin receptors are all G proteins. An intravenous preparation of vasopressin is available, but synthetic analogues last longer and are more useful.

Desmopressin (1-deamino-8-D-arginine vasopressin or DDAVP)

Desmopressin is used for the diagnosis and treatment of diabetes insipidus. It has an antidiuretic potency about 12 times that of vasopressin, but it has only 0.4% the vasoconstrictor activity. Desmopressin increases factor VIII activity in the same manner as vasopressin and is used to cover minor surgical procedures in mild haemophilia. It may be given by oral, intravenous, intramuscular, subcutaneous or nasal administration. Desmopressin is metabolised by proteases and then excreted in the urine. It has a half-life of 75 minutes.

Other vasopressin analogues include felypressin, which has a predominantly vasoconstrictor action and is used as an adjunct for local anaesthetics in place of adrenaline, and lypressin, which is similar but shorter in duration (10 minutes).

The nasal route of administration is used for these agents. Terlipressin, a prodrug for vasopressin, is used to control bleeding from oesophageal varices. Terlipressin requires IV administration.

Vasopressin antagonists
Demeclocycline

Demeclocycline is a tetracycline derivative which opposes the effect of vasopressin. It has been used in cases of inappropriate vasopressin secretion.

Vasopressin receptor antagonists

Examples – conivaptan, lixivaptan, tolvaptan

Figure 38.6 shows the relative potencies of lixivaptan, conivaptan and tolvaptan. Tolvaptan is therefore a combined V_{1a}/V_2 receptor antagonist.

These drugs are used in chronic heart failure with high levels of circulating vasopressin, and in hyponatraemia when water loss can be specifically facilitated. Tolvaptan is used in the latter. The drugs also inhibit cytochrome P450 CYP3A4, a potential problem with concurrent use of drugs such as clarithromycin and simvastatin.

Renin–angiotensin system

Inhibition of the renin–angiotensin system (see Chapters 16 and 36) may be effective in the control of hypertension. Renin secretion is increased by catecholamines (β_1 effect) and reduced by β-blockers. Angiotensin-converting enzyme (ACE) inhibitors inhibit the conversion of angiotensin I to angiotensin II. Angiotensin II receptor inhibiting drugs inhibit the vascular receptor for this pathway, thus preventing vasoconstriction.

Figure 38.6 Relative potency of vasopressin antagonists

Drug	$V_2 : V_{1a}$ relative potency
Lixivaptan	100
Conivaptan	30
Tolvaptan	10

Specific pharmacology

Dexamethasone
See Chapter 34

Hydrocortisone

Structure – glucocorticoid steroid

Presentation – IV/IM – white powder as sodium succinate for reconstitution with water for injection (many other preparations are available)

Dose – IV – 100–500 mg 6–8 hourly, onset 2–4 h, lasts 8 h

CNS – mood changes

CVS – restores vasomotor tone of small blood vessels, reduces vascular permeability and resultant tissue swelling

RS – reduces bronchial wall swelling caused by asthma or anaphylaxis

Other – anti-inflammatory agent with multiple uses

Elimination – hepatic conversion to tetrahydrocortisone

Side effects – anaphylactoid reactions have occurred

Cautions – congestive cardiac failure, hypertension, peptic ulceration, glaucoma, epilepsy, diabetes mellitus, history of tuberculosis, effect of anticholinesterases antagonised

Insulin (soluble)

Structure – glycopeptide; formed as pro-insulin with a connecting peptide, the C fragment

Presentation – clear colourless solution of human insulin pH 6.6–8.0 (containing glycerol and m-cresol)

Dose – SC/IM/IV – typically up to 8 IU per hour, based on intermittent blood glucose monitoring; used as replacement for low endogenous insulin, may be necessary in total parenteral nutrition to facilitate glucose uptake into cells

Oxytocin

Structure – synthetic octapeptide identical to human oxytocin

Presentation – IV/IM – clear colourless solution, 5 or 10 IU in 1 mL (available in combination with ergometrine 500 µg in 1 mL, as syntometrine)

Dose – IV to augment labour by infusion of variable magnitude; following Caesarean delivery slow bolus of 5 or 10 IU

CNS – no effect

CVS – bolus administration causes transient hypotension with reflex tachycardia. Following term delivery usually offset by placental autotransfusion

RS – no effect

Other – breast duct smooth muscle contraction, promoting milk ejection

Elimination – rapid metabolism by plasma oxytocinase (use separate line if transfusing blood or plasma)

Side effects – uterine spasm or rupture, hypotension, water intoxication (secondary to the vasopressin-like effect)

References and further reading

Mitchell SLM, Hunter JM. Vasopressin and its antagonists: what are their roles in acute medical care? *Br J Anaesth* 2007; **99**: 154–8.

CHAPTER 39

Gastrointestinal pharmacology

Tim Smith

Reduction of gastric acidity

Although gastric acidity is extremely variable, in health gastric pH may be as low as 1.0 (hydrogen ion concentration 100 mmol L^{-1}). In anaesthetic practice a pH > 3.5 (hydrogen ion concentration 300 mmol L^{-1}) is sought, to minimise the risk of acid aspiration syndrome. Many drugs may be used to reduce gastric acidity, acting in a variety of ways (Figure 39.1).

H$_2$ receptor antagonists

Examples – cimetidine, famotidine, nizatidine, ranitidine

Histamine has two primary effects on the gastrointestinal tract, mediated by H$_1$ and H$_2$ receptors. H$_1$ agonism causes contraction of gut smooth muscle, whereas H$_2$ agonism causes secretion of gastric acid. The H$_2$ antagonists typically resemble the imidazole-ring end of histamine and are hydrophilic. The H$_2$ antagonists are reversible competitive antagonists which each feature a five-membered ring similar to the imidazole of histamine, with a specific structure as follows:

- Cimetidine – imidazole ring
- Famotidine – guanidinothiazole ring
- Nizatidine – thiazole ring
- Ranitidine – furan ring

H$_2$ antagonism inhibits both basal levels and stimulated release of gastric acid. Pepsin secretion is reduced in line with the decrease in gastric volume even though secretion of pepsin is mediated by acetylcholine. As pepsin is usually secreted in excess of requirements, this does not present a problem. H$_2$ receptors are also present in the uterus, heart, blood vessels, ductus arteriosus and the lower oesophageal sphincter. Clinically, the H$_2$ antagonists have little effect on these other tissues, and there are no clinical applications related to these sites.

Cimetidine

Cimetidine is an H$_2$ antagonist with slight antiandrogenic effect that may cause gynaecomastia and impotence. Peak effect is achieved 80 minutes after oral administration, and the terminal half-life is 2 hours. It is given twice daily, is metabolised in the liver and binds to cytochrome P450, causing inhibition. It also reduces hepatic blood flow. Seventy per cent of cimetidine is excreted unchanged in the urine. T lymphocytes have H$_2$ receptors, and blockade of these may inhibit suppressor T-cell function, resulting in enhanced immune system activity. This effect may be harmful in the presence of autoimmune conditions or after organ transplantation. H$_2$ receptors in the atria are

Fundamentals of Anaesthesia, 4th edition, ed. Ted Lin, Tim Smith and Colin Pinnock. Published by Cambridge University Press. © Cambridge University Press 2017.

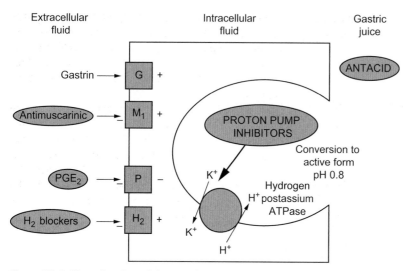

Figure 39.1 Sites of action of drugs reducing gastric acidity

responsible for atrial rhythmicity, and cimetidine may cause bradydysrhythmias, especially when given intravenously.

Famotidine

Famotidine is an H_2 antagonist that may be intravenously administered twice daily. It reduces acid and pepsin content, reduces gastric volume, and is about 50 times more potent than cimetidine. It is excreted in the urine, having a half-life of 3 hours and a duration of action of 10 hours. Cytochrome P450 is unaffected.

Nizatidine

Nizatidine is currently the H_2 antagonist with the shortest half-life (1.3 hours). It may be given orally or intravenously. It does not affect cytochrome P450. In high doses, nizatidine may increase salicylate absorption. Nizatidine also causes non-competitive inhibition of acetylcholinesterase similar to that caused by neostigmine, and so possesses prokinetic activity too.

Ranitidine

Ranitidine has a peak effect 100 minutes after oral administration, and the terminal half-life is 2.5 hours. There is a substantial first-pass effect that is avoided by use of the intravenous preparation. It is metabolised in the liver and binds to cytochrome P450, causing inhibition, but this effect is only about one-tenth that of cimetidine and thus rarely achieves clinical significance.

Proton pump inhibitors

Examples – esomeprazole, lansoprazole, omeprazole, pantoprazole, tenatoprazole

The proton pump inhibitors (PPIs) directly affect the acid-secreting pump of the gastric parietal cells, in effect bypassing the muscarinic, gastrin and H_2 receptors. Available proton pump inhibitors are substituted benzimidazoles (imidazole and benzene ring together) joined to a pyridine ring by a sulphenyl group. PPIs are weak bases (high pK_a) and are administered orally in buffered capsules to minimise the effects of gastric acid before arrival at the site of action. This allows slow release and gradual absorption of the dose. They are readily absorbed in this non-ionised form. They are prodrugs and are activated by exposure to acid conditions (pH 0.8–1.0) in the gastric parietal-cell canaliculi on the luminal surface of the stomach. This causes protonation of one nitrogen atom of the imidazole ring and that of the pyridine ring, which are therefore ionised. The two additional hydrogen ions (protons) then join with the oxygen on the sulphur atom to release water, and in doing so another ring is formed. The end result is a planar tetracyclic sulphonamide which is the active form of the PPI. The active form accumulates within the parietal canaliculi near the luminal surface and binds to the target enzyme. The sulphur of the PPI combines covalently with sulphydryl groups of cysteine amino acid residues in the H^+K^+-ATPase pump and so prevents hydrogen ion passage. These inhibitors are therefore very selective. The PPIs are strongly bound to the pump enzyme, and so the effect of these drugs is much longer than the elimination half-lives would suggest.

Omeprazole

The structure of omeprazole constitutes substituted benzimidazole and pyridine rings joined by a sulphox-ide link. It is a prodrug, converted within the parietal cell to sulphenamide, the active form. It has a highly selective effect that increases over several days to a plateau, probably because the reduced gastric acid reduces its degradation and increases bioavailability. Plasma distribution half-life is only 3 minutes, but gradual absorption and accumulation in the parietal cells results in a prolonged therapeutic effect. There is minimal crossing of the blood–brain barrier but free crossing of the placenta. Omeprazole undergoes hepatic metabolism. Untoward effects are limited, although long-term use may result in hypergastrinaemia, thought to be of little consequence. Cytochrome P450 is inhibited, leading to a prolonged half-life of benzodi-azepines and phenytoin as well as other agents sharing this elimination pathway.

Lansoprazole and pantoprazole, second-generation agents, are similar in structure to omeprazole. Both achieve higher bioavailability (lansoprazole 85% and pantoprazole 75%). Gradual absorption and accumulation in the parietal cells results in a prolonged therapeutic effect. The drug is conjugated in the liver and excreted in the urine (80%) and faeces.

Lansoprazole has a still higher bioavailability (85%), elimination half-life 0.9 hours (clearance 31 L h^{-1}, volume of distribution 29 litres, 50% excreted in urine). Unchanged drug is eliminated by the biliary route.

Rabeprazole binds more rapidly to the proton pump than the other PPIs, and also dissociates more easily.

Tenatoprazole

This proton pump inhibitor is distinct from the others in that it is an imidazopyridine (imidazole and pyridine ring together) rather than having a benzimidazole skeleton. This gives it a longer plasma half-life (7 hours), which may prove to reduce tolerance in the future.

Prostaglandins
Example – misoprostol

Prostaglandins E_2 and I_2 (PGE_2, PGI_2) inhibit gastric acid secretion and stimulate the production of mucus and bicarbonate, and therefore have a protective effect on the gastric mucosa. Natural prostaglandins are rapidly elim-inated, and synthetic analogues have therefore been developed.

Misoprostol is a synthetic prostaglandin E_2 analogue that reduces gastric acid secretion and antagonises the antiprostaglandin effects of the NSAIDs. It is most useful when these are a factor in the causation of ulcer forma-tion, and it can be used in conjunction with NSAIDs (to prevent further ulceration) when alternatives to NSAIDs are unacceptable. The only untoward effect of note is the occurrence of diarrhoea.

Antacids
Examples – aluminium hydroxide, sodium citrate

Antacids act in a simple chemical manner by neutral-ising acid in the stomach in the following manner:

$$acid + base \rightarrow salt + water$$

It is important that the by-products of this reaction are not toxic and cause minimal side effects. The commonest problem encountered is the production of CO_2 causing gastric distension with discomfort, nausea and belching. Antacids are given to alleviate symptoms of dyspepsia and reflux oesophagitis, or to neutralise acid preoperatively when a significant risk of acid aspiration exists. In the awake patient laryngeal reflexes protect the lungs from damage. In the anaesthetised patient the antacid may be aspirated and cause damage, a factor which influences antacid choice. Sodium citrate (0.3 molar) is the common-est antacid used in anaesthetic practice, because it is non-particulate.

The simplest antacids are those containing the following bases, either alone or in combination: magne-sium carbonate, hydroxide or trisilicate; aluminium hydroxide or glycinate. Sodium bicarbonate may also be used. Solubility and speed of reaction are important in antacids suitable for clinical use; sodium and potassium hydroxide are very soluble and are therefore very basic. These readily neutralise the acid, but any excess would render the stomach contents alkaline, causing potentially more damage than gastric acid. A solution is to use agents that either dissolve slowly or are less soluble. Magnesium carbonate has a crystalline structure that slows its reaction with the acid even though it is highly soluble, and the hydroxides of aluminium and magnesium have a low

Figure 39.2 Problems of antacid therapy

Salt and water retention
Alkalosis
Belching and regurgitation
Constipation or laxative effect
Lung damage from aspiration

solubility but react rapidly. The problems of antacid therapy are summarised in Figure 39.2.

A relatively large number of molecules is required for a chemical effect compared with receptor-based pharmacological methods. This can lead to excess salt and water absorption, with predictable consequences. Sodium bicarbonate is so readily absorbed that it may cause iatrogenic non-respiratory alkalosis. Bicarbonate and carbonate compounds release CO_2 within the stomach, resulting in belching and the risk of regurgitation. Calcium compounds cause constipation, and magnesium compounds have a laxative effect. Most of the antacids are suspensions and are therefore particulate in nature. Such particles, if aspirated, may lead to lung damage similar to acid aspiration syndrome.

Mucoprotective drugs

Mucoprotective drugs achieve their principal effects either through cytoprotective activity or by enhancing endogenous defence mechanisms. A mechanically protective barrier against acid damage to the gastric mucosa may be formed, and some agents stimulate endogenous secretion of mucus from the gastric mucosa.

Chelates and complexes

Examples – sucralfate, tripotassium dicitratobismuthate

Sucralfate

Sucralfate is a complex of sulphated sucrose and aluminium hydroxide that, although possessing little antacid activity, has a profound cytoprotective effect. It may be used, with caution, in critically ill patients unable to tolerate enteral feeding, to protect the gastric mucosa, and it is also used in ulcer treatment to promote healing in conjunction with acid-lowering drugs. It adheres to damaged gastric mucosa perhaps by virtue of its negatively charged component and forms a protective layer. It also stimulates the production of prostaglandins (particularly E_2), bicarbonate and mucus. Thromboxane release is inhibited, and the production of natural sulphydryl compound is increased. Sucralfate stays in the stomach for many hours, and only small amounts are absorbed. Aspiration of the drug may lead to pneumonitis, and the absorption of digoxin and warfarin is inhibited.

Tripotassium dicitratobismuthate

The bismuth chelate tripotassium dicitratobismuthate promotes the healing of peptic ulcers. Its mechanism of action is unclear but may be related to its binding to glycoproteins at the base of the ulcer.

Carbenoxolone

Carbenoxolone is used to promote peptic ulcer healing. It is a synthetic derivative of glycyrrhisinic acid which is found in liquorice. It probably enhances mucous secretion from the gastric mucosa and so provides protection from the hydrochloric acid and pepsin in the stomach. Carbenoxolone has mineralocorticoid effects, and patients may develop sodium and water retention with hypertension, signs of fluid overload and potassium depletion.

Antispasmodics

Antispasmodic agents mostly comprise muscarinic anticholinergic drugs, but include direct-acting smooth muscle relaxants. They are used for irritable bowel syndrome and diverticular disease.

Anticholinergics

Examples – atropine, dicycloverine, hyoscine, propantheline

Muscarinic anticholinergic agents reduce acid secretion and reduce gastrointestinal tone, including lower oesophageal sphincter tone. The dose required usefully to reduce gastric acid secretion causes numerous side effects related to inhibition of other muscarinic receptors. At lower doses they function as antispasmodics and are used in irritable bowel syndrome and diverticular disease. Selectivity is improved by using quaternary amino agents that do not cross the blood–brain barrier (poldine methylsulphate and propantheline bromide) and by using anticholinergics specific for the M_1 receptor (dicycloverine, formerly known as dicyclomine). The muscarinic M_1 receptors are present in parasympathetic ganglia supplying parietal gastric cells. The muscarinic receptors affecting the heart, eyes and bladder are primarily M_2 receptors.

Pirenzipine is a tricyclic antimuscarinic agent which inhibits oesophageal motility and reduces gastric volume and acidity. Pirenzipine is a relatively selective antagonist at the M_1 receptor that is found on the postganglionic fibres in the gastric mucosal plexus. In contrast, it is the M_3 receptor subtype that is located on the parietal cell. The reduction of lower oesophageal sphincter pressure caused by pirenzipine renders the drug unsuitable in anaesthetic practice.

Direct-acting smooth muscle relaxants
Examples – alverine, mebeverine, peppermint oil

Drugs of this mixed group all cause direct relaxation of gastric mucosal smooth muscle.

Prokinetic agents
Examples – domperidone, erythromycin, metoclopramide

Prokinetic agents are drugs used to stimulate enteral propulsion. Most are drugs known for other uses. The final common pathway seems to be via acetylcholine, but many other neurotransmitters are involved in the production of activity.

Domperidone and metoclopramide act via peripheral dopaminergic (D_2) antagonism. These are detailed in Chapter 34 (see *Peripherally acting antiemetic drugs*).

Erythromycin is an agonist of the motilin receptor. Motilin is a powerful prokinetic acting on the G-protein-coupled motilin receptor in the mucosa. Motilin and erythromycin release nitric oxide. Erythromycin is covered in more detail in Chapter 42.

The H_2 antagonist nizatidine (see *H_2 receptor antagonists*, above) also has an anticholinesterase effect similar to that of neostigmine and thus has prokinetic properties.

Laxatives
Constipation may result from a variety of causes. Within the hospital population, it is commonly iatrogenic. Drugs that cause constipation are listed in Figure 39.3.

There are four main categories of laxative: bulking agents, faecal softeners, osmotic laxatives and stimulants.

Bulking agents
Bulking agents are usually derived from bran, and increase the bulk of stools by absorbing and retaining water. These agents are usually administered as a dietary supplement. The only minor untoward effect is that of a minor reduction in the absorption of some drugs.

Figure 39.3 Drugs causing constipation

Opioids
Phenothiazines
MAOIs
Antacids
NSAIDs
Ganglion blockers

Faecal softeners
Faecal softeners are oily compounds that soften the consistency of stools. Liquid paraffin is the most common agent given by mouth. It is unpleasant tasting and potentially dangerous if aspirated. There may be a minor reduction in the absorption of fat-soluble vitamins.

Osmotic laxatives
Osmotic laxatives include magnesium salts (usually sulphate), phosphates and lactulose. These agents act by drawing water into the large bowel by an osmotic effect. Their major use is in the preparation of bowel before surgery.

Stimulants
Stimulants are poorly understood drugs that can have profound effects. It is thought that mucosal permeability is increased, although other effects may be mediated via the prostaglandin system. This group includes danthron derivatives (senna), diphenylmethane derivatives (bisacodyl) and anthraquinones. Absorption may occur, and there is a risk of hepatotoxicity. Some of these agents may be abused by patients.

Specific pharmacology
Here, bioavailability applies to oral administration. Units (unless stated otherwise) are:

Volume of distribution (V_d): L kg^{-1}
Clearance (Cl): mL kg^{-1} min^{-1}
Terminal half-life ($t_{1/2}$): hours

Lansoprazole
Structure – substituted benzimidazole
Presentation – capsules 15, 30 mg
Dose – 15–30 mg daily

Pharmacokinetics

Bioavailability	85%
Protein binding	97%
pK$_a$	8.5
t$_{1/2}$	1.7

CNS – headache, dizziness
CVS – no effect
RS – no effect
Other effects – rash; pruritus; eosinophilia; gynaecomastia; liver dysfunction; hyponatraemia; hypomagnesaemia

Omeprazole
Structure – substituted benzimidazole
Presentation – tablets 10, 20, 40 mg; IV 40 mg
Dose – 20 mg daily, increasing to 40 mg daily
Pharmacokinetics

Bioavailability	35%
Protein binding	95%
pK$_a$	3.97
t$_{1/2}$	1

CNS – headache, dizziness
CVS – no effect
RS – no effect

Other effects – rash; pruritus; eosinophilia; gynaecomastia; liver dysfunction; hyponatraemia; hypomagnesaemia

Ranitidine
Structure – furan derivative, five-membered oxygen-containing ring with three tertiary amine groups in the side chains
Presentation
  Oral – tablets 150 and 300 mg
  Clear aqueous solution (50 mg in 2 mL) for IV/IM use
Dose
  Oral – 150 mg twice daily
  Slow IV/IM – bolus 50 mg 6–8-hourly
Pharmacokinetics

Bioavailability	50–60%
Protein binding	15
V$_d$	1.5
Cl	10
t$_{1/2}$	2

CNS – no effect
CVS – no effect
RS – no effect
Other effects – placenta is readily crossed
Interactions – the increase in gastric pH increases the non-ionised proportion of some drugs (such as benzodiazepines) and so increases their absorption

CHAPTER 40
Intravenous fluids

Tim Smith

Intravenous fluids are characterised by being given in relatively large volumes compared with other drugs. This is in part a feature of their non-receptor mode of action, and often there are multiple functional components in the fluid administered. The uses of IV fluids are summarised in Figure 40.1.

Crystalloids

Crystalloids are relatively small molecules that dissociate into ions and form true solutions. In clinical terms, crystalloids pass through the capillary and glomerular membranes easily, but do not readily pass through cell membranes. This situation only applies immediately after administration, as metabolism and membrane pumps soon alter the distribution. The constituents of the commonly used IV crystalloid fluids are shown in Figure 40.2.

Water

Water is the essential solvent of all the IV fluids. 1.5 mL $kg^{-1} h^{-1}$ is a typical requirement for IV maintenance, and this will be the primary determinant of the volume given. The solutes determine how widely the water will be distributed in the body.

Electrolytes
Cations

Sodium is primarily an extracellular ion. Typical sodium requirement is 1 mmol $kg^{-1} day^{-1}$. In contrast, **potassium** is primarily an intracellular ion. In concentrations similar to plasma levels, potassium solutions can be given rapidly, but this will have little effect on total body potassium. Replacement of potassium by the IV route should be done slowly and requires careful monitoring when more concentrated solutions are used, to avoid cardiac arrhythmias and cardiac arrest. The addition of potassium to crystalloid solutions such as Ringer's lactate (Hartmann's) is an attempt to mimic the electrolyte composition of plasma.

Calcium may be used to improve myocardial contractility when plasma levels are depleted. It is available as calcium chloride 10% ($CaCl_2$, which contains 0.68 mmol mL^{-1} = 680 mmol L^{-1} calcium ions). Note that using the combined atomic weight of calcium and two chlorine atoms (MW 111) does not provide the actual molarity of calcium. This is because calcium chloride (dihydrate) has two water molecules closely associated with it in the crystalline form in which it is weighed ($CaCl_2.2H_2O$). Calcium is also available as the gluconate 10% (0.22 mmol mL^{-1}). However, this preparation may be negatively inotropic, and can cause coronary vasoconstriction. Calcium may be useful when large amounts of blood and fresh frozen plasma have been rapidly transfused.

Magnesium is important in enzyme systems, and in muscle and neuronal function. Magnesium can be used therapeutically for arrhythmias (especially torsades de pointes), myocardial infarction, eclampsia and pre-eclampsia.

Fundamentals of Anaesthesia, 4th edition, ed. Ted Lin, Tim Smith and Colin Pinnock. Published by Cambridge University Press. © Cambridge University Press 2017.

Anions

Chloride is the predominant anion in the body, and is a constituent to maintain the cationic/anionic balance of most IV fluids. **Bicarbonate** may be used to manipulate the pH of IV fluids. As heat sterilisation destroys the ion and thus produces CO_2, these solutions are sterilised by filtration and are relatively expensive. Phosphorus in the form of **phosphate** is the main intracellular anion. It is not routinely required in IV fluids but is important in long-term nutrition. Phosphate buffers are an important constituent of blood cell storage solutions.

Solutions

Sodium chloride 0.9% is the correct generic term for the solution isotonic with body fluids. It is also referred to as *normal saline*. 'Normal' in this sense is used to mean that it has the same tonicity as physiological fluids, and *twice normal saline* refers to sodium chloride 1.8%, which is used in cases of hyponatraemia. Unfortunately, 'normal' is an imprecise term that could also be interpreted in this case as 1 molar sodium chloride.

Compound sodium lactate (Hartmann's) solution uses lactate (another base present in the body) in place of bicarbonate so it can be heat-sterilised. Lactate is readily metabolised in the liver.

Sodium bicarbonate 8.4% solution is used for the immediate correction of metabolic acidosis. Its alkalinity and high osmolality can easily cause tissue damage if small veins are used or if extravasation occurs. It contains 1000 mmol of sodium ions per litre, and this carries a risk of fluid retention, which may be a particular problem if the acidosis is the result of renal failure.

Bags of IV fluid may contain more volume than stated on the packaging. A litre bag of Hartmann's solution, for example, may contain 1050 mL. This is to offset the priming volume of the giving set, but this clearly only applies to the first bag.

Colloids

Colloids tend to be larger molecules than crystalloids, and are dispersed throughout the solvent rather than forming true solutions. The component particles tend to arrange as groups of molecules and so do not readily pass through

Figure 40.1 Uses of IV fluids

Volume replacement	Total body water Extracellular water Intravascular (blood) volume
Provision of metabolic substrates	Electrolytes Carbohydrate Amino acids and protein Fatty acids
Manipulation of acid–base balance	Forced acid or alkaline diuresis
Coagulopathy correction	Platelets Clotting factors
Improving oxygen carriage	
Diluent for drugs	If caustic If low solubility
Osmotic effects	
Manipulation of blood viscosity	

Figure 40.2 Constituents and physicochemical properties of crystalloids

	Na^+	K^+	Ca^{2+}	Cl^-	HCO_3^-	Osmolality	pH
Sodium chloride 0.9%	150	0	0	150	0	300	5
Dextrose 5%	0	0	0	0	0	280	4
Dextrose 10%	0	0	0	0	0	560	4
Dextrose 4% saline 0.18%	30	0	0	0	30	255	4.5
Hartmann's solution	131	5	2	111	29	278	6
Sodium bicarbonate 8.4%	1000	0	0	0	1000	2000	8

Ionic concentrations in mmol L^{-1}, osmolality in mOsm kg^{-1}

Figure 40.3 Constituents and physicochemical properties of colloids

	Na$^+$	K$^+$	Ca^{2+}	Mg^{2+}	Cl$^-$	Osmolality	pH
Gelofusine	154	0.4	0.4	0.4	125	279	7.4
Haemaccel	145	5.1	6.25	0	145	301	7.3
Dextran 70 (dextrose 5%)	0	0	0	0	0	287	3.5–7
HAS 4.5%	100–160	< 2	0	0	100–160	270–300	6.4–7.4
HAS 20%	50–120	< 10	0	0	< 40	135–138	6.4–7.4

Ionic concentrations in mmol L^{-1}, osmolality in mOsm kg^{-1}

Figure 40.4 Serious adverse reactions following the use of intravenous colloids

Solution	Frequency
Succinylated gelatin	1 : 13,000
Polygeline	1 : 2000
Dextran 70	1 : 4500
Hetastarch	1 : 16,000
Human albumin	1 : 30,000

clinical semipermeable membranes. They therefore have an oncotic potential that is usually measured as colloid osmotic pressure (COP). As the number of molecules per volume of solution is usually lower than in crystalloid solutions, boiling point and freezing point are less affected for a given mass of solute. Increasing the amount of colloid has little effect on osmotic pressure, so electrolytes are used to achieve iso-osmolality with blood. The constituents of common colloids are shown in Figure 40.3. The frequency of serious adverse reactions varies between solutions, and a comparison is given in Figure 40.4.

Gelatins

Examples – Gelofusine, Haemaccel

Gelatins are proteins derived from hydrolysing collagen. These are succinylated (succinyl groups are added to the lysine amino residues which comprise approximately 5% of the total). Cross-linking with urea is an alternative to succinylation. Gelatins are prescribed by their proprietary names, as the generic term gelatin does not indicate the various component differences of the solutions. They all contain gelatin with an average molecular weight of 30,000 daltons. The main differences between preparations are in the electrolyte composition. Particular changes include using magnesium instead of calcium, using acetate rather than bicarbonate, and manipulating pH and chloride content. The merits of these strategies are controversial.

Gelofusine (Braun)

Gelofusine is a 4% solution of succinylated gelatin in saline in which the gelatin is prepared by hydroxylation and succinylation of bovine collagen. Other ions are present in negligible amounts because of the manufacturing process. The calcium present does not warrant line flushing before giving citrated blood.

Characteristics

Relative viscosity	1.9
Gel point	0 °C
t$_{1/2}$	2–4 h
COP	35 mmHg

The majority of renal excretion occurs within 24 hours, and the incidence of severe anaphylaxis is about 1 in 13,000 (Figure 40.4).

Haemaccel (Hoechst)

Haemaccel is a 3.5% solution of polygeline in a mixed salt solution. Polygeline is a degraded and modified gelatin with 6.3 g nitrogen equivalent per litre containing traces of phosphate and sulphate. The gelatine is cross-linked with urea, which may be released after hydrolysis, a potential problem in patients with renal failure.

Characteristics

Relative viscosity	1.7
Gel point	< 3 °C
$t_{1/2}$	6 h
COP	28 mmHg

Dextran 70

The dextrans are glucose polymers, solutions of which are classified according to the average molecular weight of the dextran molecules contained: Dextran 70 (average MW 70,000 daltons) is used as a volume expander. It also reduces thromboembolism by blood volume expansion, reduction of blood viscosity and lowering of erythrocyte and platelet aggregation. Dextran 70 is supplied in a solution of sodium chloride 0.9%.

Hydroxyethyl starches (HES)

These are composed of at least 90% amylopectin that is etherified with hydroxyethyl groups to slow down its metabolism. The degree of substitution is indicated by the prefix – hetastarch (0.6), pentastarch (0.5), tetrastarch (0.4) – which reflects the number of hydroxyethyl groups per glucose unit. The tetrastarches are the latest generation. The starch solutions have a large range of molecular weights. The polymerised glucose units are primarily joined by 1–4 linkages and the hydroxyethyl groups are attached to the 2 carbon of the glucose moiety, making the resultant polymer similar to glycogen.

Hydroxyethyl starches are referred to in the form 6% HES 130/0.4. This means a 6% solution of HES with an average molecular weight of 130,000 and a molar substitution ratio of 0.4 (a tetrastarch). 6% has the same oncotic potential as plasma, with 10% being higher. The higher the molecular weight the greater the persistence of the molecules, but there will in turn be fewer of them to contribute to the oncotic potential (this being based on the *number* of molecules). The higher the substitution ratio the more slowly the drug is eliminated.

Hetastarch is 6% hetastarch in sodium chloride 0.9% with pH modification by sodium hydroxide. It is almost entirely derived from amylopectin. It has an average molecular weight of 450,000. Molecules with a molecular weight below 50,000 daltons readily pass through the glomerular membrane, and 40% is excreted by this route within 24 hours. The hydroxyethyl–glucose bond remains intact, and usually < 1% of the total dose remains in the body after 2 weeks. Hetastarch has a colloid osmotic pressure of 20 mmHg.

Pentastarches have an average molecular weight of 200,000, all suspended in sodium chloride solution.

Tetrastarches have an average molecular weight of 130,000, and alternative electrolyte solutions to sodium chloride are also available. They are the latest generation, with the aim of improving safety.

Hydroxyethyl starches can interfere with coagulation, they can migrate to and persist outside the vascular compartment, and anaphylaxis can occur. Renal impairment is a particular risk in the critically ill. In 2013 the Commission on Human Medicines (CHM) suspended the use of HES infusions in critically ill patients and those undergoing surgery.

Human albumin solutions (HAS)

Derived from human plasma by fractionation (the old term is plasma protein fraction), human albumin is heat-sterilised, and thus the risk of infective transmission is very low. HAS may be supplied as 4.5% (40–50 g L^{-1}), to reflect normal plasma, or 20% (150–250 g L^{-1}), in which water is removed together with the dissolved salts. It is sometimes called 'salt-poor albumin', as the sodium concentration is also lowered. At least 95% of the protein in HAS is albumin, and this has been stabilised using sodium n-octanoate. HAS is used as a colloid especially if high albumin loss has been a problem (e.g. in burns patients). The 20% albumin solution will oncotically draw water from tissues and may be useful in the treatment of hypoalbuminaemia. A simple formula for calculating the amount of albumin needed in hypoalbuminaemia is:

$$Albumin\ required\ (g) = [desired\ total\ protein\ (g\ l^{-1})$$
$$- actual\ total\ protein\ (g\ l^{-1})]$$
$$\times plasma\ volume(1) \times 2$$

The use of HAS is still controversial. In addition to its colloid properties, it is involved in plasma molecular carriage, coagulation and membrane integrity. It is also a free radical scavenger. Low serum albumin is associated with poor outcome. Large volume resuscitation depletes albumin, probably because of redistribution. Theoretical benefits of albumin replacement are yet to be proven in practice.

Haemoglobin solutions (experimental)

Stroma-free haemoglobin (SFH)

Stroma-free haemoglobin has shown some promise experimentally as a blood substitute. The advantages and disadvantages of SFH are outlined in Figure 40.5.

Figure 40.5 Stroma-free haemoglobin

Advantages
- Effective oxygen carrier
- Passes easily into smallest capillaries
- No need for cross-match
- Infection risk minimal
- Storage and transport at ambient temperature
- Long shelf life

Disadvantages
- Low P_{50}
- Poor intravascular persistence
- Nephrotoxicity
- Immunological effects
- Free radical production
- Increased nitric oxide scavenging

Oxygen affinity

The P_{50} of intracellular haemoglobin is 3.6 kPa, but this drops to 1.6 kPa when free in the plasma, due to loss of 2,3-DPG from the haemoglobin molecule. This very high affinity for oxygen severely reduces its release to the tissues. In the clinical setting extra-erythrocytic haemoglobin coexists with intra-erythrocytic haemoglobin, and it has been shown that intracellular haemoglobin supplies most oxygen to the tissues until very low haematocrits (< 0.2) are reached. Pyridoxylation of haemoglobin reduces the high oxygen affinity.

Intravascular persistence

Free haemoglobin dissociates to monomers and dimers with molecular weights well below the renal threshold (69,000 daltons) and is rapidly excreted. The dimer binds to haptoglobin in plasma, but within 4 hours 25–40% of unmodified haemoglobin will have passed into the urine. Polymerisation of the haemoglobin produces a molecule of MW 600,000 daltons ($t_{\frac{1}{2}}$ 38 hours). Other methods include intramolecular cross-linking of haemoglobin, and conjugation of haemoglobin with large molecules (e.g. dextran).

Nephrotoxicity

Red cell lysis releases haemoglobin and stroma. Minute amounts of stroma can cause renal damage, so the haemoglobin solution must be washed thoroughly following lysis to produce stroma-free haemoglobin. Haemoglobin is not nephrotoxic, but severe hypovolaemia itself can cause clogging of the distal tubule.

Nitric oxide scavenging

This is increased by permeation of haemoglobin into the tissues. It results in vasoconstriction and possible neurotoxicity.

Microencapsulated haemoglobin

The physiological carriage of haemoglobin in erythrocytes avoids the problems of high oncotic pressure, prevents loss in the urine, and provides the most efficient micro-environment for the haemoglobin. Microencapsulated haemoglobin (non-capsule) is like an artificial red blood cell. A membrane of synthetic polymers, cross-linked protein, lipid protein and lipid polymer is created with a solution of haemoglobin and enzyme inside. The haemoglobin cannot leak out and therefore remains as a tetramer. There is no membrane antigen. Ideally the membrane is permeable to hydrophilic material but does not allow leakage of 2,3-DPG. These artificial cells are about 1 μm in diameter (compared with 7 μm for a red blood cell), which results in rapid clearance from the circulation. A less sophisticated alternative is to use a phospholipid and sterol bilayer liposome to encapsulate the haemoglobin.

Synthetic oxygen carriers

Normally only 4% of the oxygen delivered is carried in solution (0.0225 mL O_2 100 mL^{-1} blood kPa^{-1}), the rest being carried as oxyhaemoglobin. To rely entirely on dissolved oxygen (if this could all be extracted) would require either an increased cardiac output to 13 litres per minute or an inspired oxygen pressure of 2–2.5 bar. The latter is the principle behind the treatment of carbon monoxide poisoning, but it requires hyperbaric equipment and risks oxygen toxicity. Therefore an oxygen carrier is required that will carry oxygen more efficiently than plasma or plasma substitutes, and that will release it to the tissues. There are two options: and chelating agents and perfluorocarbons.

Chelating agents (experimental)

These are synthetic compounds based on porphyrin. They can contain iron or another metal. They need modification to avoid oxidation of the ferrous ion, a function normally carried out by the globulin, after which they may be incorporated into a membrane.

Perfluorocarbons

Perfluorocarbons (PFCs) are based on a carbon skeleton with fluorine atoms, but they may also have oxygen and nitrogen atoms as part of this skeleton. PFCs absorb oxygen without having a specific binding site. This produces a linear increase in oxygen content proportional to the oxygen partial pressure. They also absorb other low-polarity gases (carbon dioxide, carbon monoxide, nitrogen) and volatile anaesthetic agents in proportion to the individual partial pressures. Fluosol-DA is a mixture of F-decalin (FDC) and F-tripropylamine (FTPA) in a ratio of 7 FDC : 3 FTPA. The only clinical use was for distal coronary perfusion during angioplasty, because the maximum concentration possible did not carry sufficient oxygen. Sufficient oxygen transport is only achieved by hyperbaric partial pressures of oxygen. Second-generation PFCs using egg-yolk lecithin emulsions allow much higher concentrations of PFC to be used, thus raising the oxygen-carrying capacity to clinically useful levels for whole-body perfusion at atmospheric pressure.

References and further reading

Moral V, Aldecoa C, Asuero MS. Tetrastarch solutions: are they definitely dead? *Br J Anaesth* 2013; **111**: 324–7.

CHAPTER 41
Pharmacology of haemostasis

Tim Smith

The ways that haemostatic processes may be altered pharmacologically are classified in Figure 41.1, while Figure 41.2 shows the effects of the commoner drugs on the coagulation system.

Anticoagulants

Anticoagulants are drugs that interfere with the process of fibrin plug formation, to reduce or prevent coagulation. This effect is used to reduce the risk of thrombus formation within normal vessels and vascular grafts. The injectable anticoagulants are also used to prevent coagulation in extracorporeal circuits and in blood product storage. There are two main types of anticoagulants: oral anticoagulants and injectable anticoagulants (heparins).

Oral anticoagulants

Oral anticoagulants inhibit the reduction of vitamin K. Reduced vitamin K is required as a cofactor in γ-carboxylation of the glutamate residues of the glycoprotein clotting factors II, VII, IX and X, which are synthesised in the liver. During this γ-carboxylation process, vitamin K is oxidised to vitamin K 2,3-epoxide. The oral anticoagulants prevent the reduction of this compound back to vitamin K in the liver, and they do this by virtue of their structural similarity to vitamin K. Their action depends on the depletion of these factors, which decline according to their individual half-lives (Figure 41.3).

There are two groups of oral anticoagulants:
- Coumarins (warfarin and nicoumalone)
- Inandiones (phenindione)

Warfarin has the most widespread use. Phenindione is more likely to cause hypersensitivity, but is useful when there is intolerance to warfarin.

Warfarin sodium

Warfarin is administered orally as a racemic mixture. It is rapidly absorbed, reaching a peak plasma concentration within 1 hour with a bioavailability of 100%. However, a clinical effect is not apparent until the clotting factors become depleted after 12–16 hours, reaching a peak at 36–48 hours. Warfarin is 99% protein-bound (to albumin) in the plasma, resulting in a small volume of distribution. Warfarin is metabolised in the liver by oxidation (L-form) and reduction (D-form), followed by glucuronide conjugation, with a half-life of about 40 hours.

Warfarin crosses the placenta and is teratogenic during pregnancy. In the postpartum period it passes into breast milk, which is a particular problem as the gut flora responsible for producing vitamin K_2 and hepatic function in the newborn are not fully developed.

Warfarin has a low therapeutic index and is particularly prone to interactions with other drugs. Interactions increasing the effect of warfarin occur in several ways:

Figure 41.1 Mode of action of pharmacological alteration of haemostasis

Mechanism	Class	Examples
Coagulation (fibrin clot formation)	Procoagulants	Desmopressin
		Vitamin K
	Anticoagulants	Coumarins
		Inandiones
		Heparin
		Calcium chelating agents
Fibrinolysis	Fibrinolytic drugs	Streptokinase
		Urokinase
	Antifibrinolytics	Aprotinin
		Tranexamic acid
Platelet function	Antiplatelet drugs	Aspirin
		Prostacyclin
	Platelet enhancers	Ethamsylate

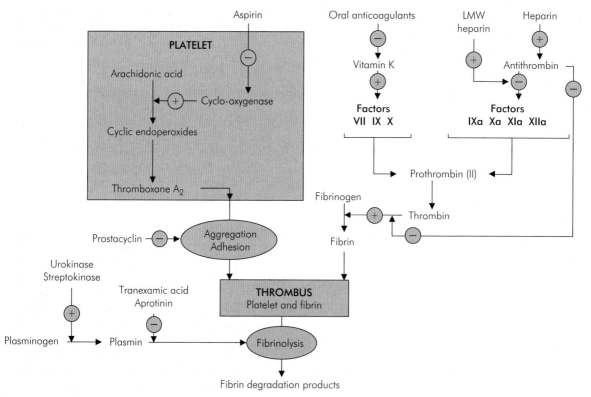

Figure 41.2 Effect of drugs on the coagulation pathway

Figure 41.3 Half-lives of vitamin-K-dependent clotting factors

Factor	Half-life (hours)
II	60
VII	6
IX	24
X	40

- Competition for protein binding sites
- Increased hepatic binding
- Inhibition of hepatic microsomal enzymes
- Reduced vitamin K synthesis
- Synergistic antihaemostatic actions

Drugs such as NSAIDs, chloral hydrate, oral hypoglycaemic agents, diuretics and amiodarone displace warfarin from albumin binding sites, resulting in higher free plasma levels and greater effect. This effect is made more significant because normally only 1% of warfarin is free and a small change in protein binding has a dramatic effect on free warfarin levels. D-Thyroxine increases the potency of warfarin by increasing hepatic binding. Ethanol ingestion may inhibit liver enzymes responsible for warfarin elimination. The effect of warfarin may also be increased by acute illness, low vitamin K intake and drugs such as cimetidine, aminoglycosides and paracetamol. Broad-spectrum antibiotics reduce the level of gut bacteria responsible for vitamin K_2 synthesis, and may enhance the effect of warfarin where the diet is deficient in vitamin K. Other anticoagulants, and particularly antiplatelet drugs, increase the clinical effects of warfarin.

Interactions decreasing the effect of warfarin can occur in several ways, notably:

- Induction of hepatic microsomal enzymes
- Drugs that increase levels of clotting factors
- Binding of warfarin
- Increased vitamin K intake

The effect of warfarin may be reduced by induction of hepatic enzymes by barbiturates and phenytoin. Oestrogens increase the production of vitamin-K-dependent clotting factors (II, VII, IX, X). Cholestyramine binds warfarin, reducing its effect. Carbamazepine and rifampicin reduce the effect of warfarin, but the mechanism of this effect is not clear.

Heparins

Heparins are injectable anticoagulants that act by binding to antithrombin, resulting in a profound increase in antithrombin activity.

Structure

Heparins are a group of sulphated acid glycosaminoglycans (or mucopolysaccharides) comprising alternate monosaccharide residues of N-acetylglucosamine and glucuronic acid and their derivatives. The glucuronic acid residues are mostly in the iduronic acid form and some are ester-sulphated. The N-acetylglucosamine residues may be deacylated, N-sulphated and ester-sulphated in a random manner. This results in a chain of 45–50 sugar residues of variable composition based on the above units. The molecules are attached by the sulphated components to a protein skeleton consisting entirely of glycine and serine amino acid residues. The molecular weight of heparin ranges from 3000 to 40,000 daltons, with a mean of 12,000–15,000. Endogenous heparin is located in the lungs, in arterial walls and in mast cells as large polymers of molecular weight 750,000. It is present in the plasma at a concentration of 1.5 mg per litre.

Heparin has a strong negative charge and is a large molecule, so there is minimal absorption following oral administration. It is supplied as heparin sodium and heparin calcium.

Mechanism of action

Heparin has the following effects:

- Inhibition of coagulation by enhancing the action of antithrombin on the serine protease coagulation factors (IIa, Xa, XIIa, XIa and IXa)
- Reduced platelet aggregation
- Increased vascular permeability
- Release of lipoprotein lipases into plasma

The negatively charged heparin binds to the lysine residue in antithrombin, an α_2-globulin, which in turns increases the affinity of the arginine site of antithrombin for the serine site of thrombin (factor II). This increases inhibitory activity of antithrombin 2300-fold. This reversible bond is the feature of a specific antithrombin binding site comprising five particular residues. This particular pentasaccharide sequence is present randomly in about one-third of the heparin molecules. For full activity of heparin on thrombin (IIa), a heparin molecule must have at least 13 extra sugar residues in addition to the pentasaccharide antithrombin binding site sequence. The covalently bonded thrombin–antithrombin complex is inactive, but once it is formed the heparin is released and the complex is rapidly destroyed by the liver. The active heparin section is then free to act on more antithrombin. Heparin acts in a similar way on the other activated serine protease coagulation factors (XIIa, Xa and IXa). The binding of heparin to both the clotting factor and antithrombin is important in the above enhancement of antithrombin. The activity of heparin on factor Xa is also mediated by increasing the affinity of antithrombin for the clotting factor, but heparin does not bind to factor Xa. Factor Xa inhibition is enhanced with lower levels of heparin than those required for thrombin inhibition. Heparin reduces platelet aggregation secondary to the reduction in thrombin (a potent platelet aggregator). The increase in plasma lipase results in an increase in free fatty acid levels.

Low-molecular-weight heparins
Examples – dalteparin, enoxaparin, tinzaparin

The low-molecular-weight (LMW) heparins are fragments of depolymerised heparin purified to contain the antithrombin-specific binding site. Therefore they all inhibit factor Xa. The molecular weight of LMW heparins ranges from 3000 to 8000, with a mean of 4000–6500. They comprise 13–22 sugar residues. The LMW heparins have a full anti-Xa activity but much reduced antithrombin activity, and require the presence of antithrombin for their effect. The reduction in interference with thrombin gives LMW heparins the following advantages:
- Minimal alteration of platelet function
- Better intraoperative haemostasis
- Possible better venous thromboembolic prophylaxis in orthopaedic practice

Administration
Heparin is administered intravenously and subcutaneously. A typical adult dose for thrombosis prophylaxis is 5000 IU subcutaneously 8–12-hourly. For full anticoagulation, as used during cardiopulmonary bypass, a dose of 3 mg kg^{-1} (300 IU kg^{-1}) is used to achieve 3–4 IU heparin mL^{-1} blood. Heparin has an immediate action within the plasma. It has a volume of distribution of $40–100 \text{ mg kg}^{-1}$ and is bound to antithrombin, albumin, fibrinogen and proteases. Increase in acute-phase proteins (during acute illness) can significantly alter the clinical effect. Heparin also binds to platelet and endothelial protein, reducing

bioavailability and effect. The drug is metabolised in the liver, kidney and reticuloendothelial system by heparinases that desulphate the mucopolysaccharide residues and hydrolyse the links between them. Heparin has a half-life of 40–90 minutes.

LMW heparins are also administered subcutaneously, and have the advantage of once-daily administration. They may be used in extracorporeal dialysis circuits, and have been used in cardiopulmonary bypass. LMW heparins are much less bound to proteins in the plasma, platelets and vascular walls, and bioavailability after subcutaneous administration is at least 90%. The levels of free LMW heparin are therefore much more predictable and require less monitoring. Peak anti-Xa activity is achieved within 3–4 hours after subcutaneous injection and activity has halved after 12 hours. Elimination is predominantly renal, and half-life may be raised in renal failure.

Effects on coagulation studies
Heparin increases activated partial thromboplastin time (APTT), thrombin time (TT) and activated clotting time (ACT) but does not affect bleeding time. Heparin therapy is routinely checked using the APTT and, on cardiopulmonary bypass, using ACT.

Heparin relies on the presence of antithrombin for its activity. Prolonged heparin therapy may lead to osteoporosis by an unknown mechanism.

Protamine
Protamines are a group of basic, cationic (positively charged) proteins of relatively low molecular weight. Protamine is used to neutralise the effects of heparin and LMW heparins. This occurs because the negative charge of the heparin is attracted to the positive charges of the protamine. 1 mg of protamine sulphate neutralises 1 mg (100 IU) heparin. Protamine (in excess) has anticoagulant activity, although this effect is not as powerful as that of heparin.

Activated factor X inhibitors
Examples – apixaban, fondaparinux, rivaroxaban

Apixaban, fondaparinux and rivaroxaban act by inhibiting factor Xa.

Fondaparinux is a synthetic pentasaccharide based on a sequence of sugars found in heparin that forms a highly specific binding site for antithrombin III. This binding substantially increases the anticoagulant effect of heparins and is likely to be the mechanism of action of fondaparinux. It may be of particular use when heparin-induced thrombocytopenia is a risk. It is contraindicated in the presence of bacterial endocarditis.

These drugs share the potential for causing active bleeding and are not easily monitored by laboratory tests. Achieving the right balance between prevention of dangerous excess clotting and causing of problematic bleeding has led to a number of NICE guidelines and a scene that is continually changing.

Thrombin (factor II) inhibitors

Examples –argatroban, bivalirudin, dabigatran

Argatroban, bilvalirudin and dabigatran inhibit thrombin (factor II) in the final common pathway of the classic clotting cascade directly.

Like the factor Xa inhibitors, these drugs may cause active bleeding and are not easily monitored. Again, it is important to follow NICE guidelines.

Calcium chelating agents

Calcium is an essential cofactor in the coagulation system. Agents that bind calcium will therefore inhibit coagulation. Citrate is used to bind calcium in stored blood to prevent its coagulation. In vivo, the citrate is metabolised by the liver, reversing this inhibition. However, massive transfusion may temporarily overload the liver's capacity to metabolise citrate, particularly if metabolic rate is reduced by the cooling effect of the transfusion or by deliberate hypothermia, as used in cardiac surgery. To some extent this may be overcome by administering calcium ions.

Fibrinolytic agents

Fibrinolysis may be **activated** or **inhibited** pharmacologically.

Plasminogen activators

Examples – alteplase, reteplase, streptokinase

The plasminogen activators act by catalysing the conversion of plasminogen to plasmin, the enzyme responsible for the enzymatic degradation of fibrin clot. Plasminogen activators are used to destroy clots in the following situations:

- Venous thrombosis
- Pulmonary embolus
- Retinal thrombosis
- Myocardial infarction

The drugs may also remove clot formed in response to haemorrhage, so bleeding from other sites is a risk. In some cases this can be minimised by administering the activator directly to the desired site of thrombus by catheter. However, this is technically difficult and the delay in doing so may remove any benefit. Some of these agents require heparin and/or aspirin to prevent reformation of thrombus. They may reduce levels of plasminogen, α_2-antiplasmin, α_2-macroglobulin and C_1-esterase inhibitor.

Alteplase (rt-PA) is a synthetic form of tissue-type plasminogen activator (a glycoprotein). Anistreplase is a ready-combined complex of plasminogen and streptokinase that is blocked by an anisoyl group. Once in the body the anisoyl group leaves the complex, which produces plasmin and so activates fibrinolysis. Reteplase is another recombinant plasminogen activator. These three agents act on fibrin-bound plasminogen.

Streptokinase is obtained from group C **haemolytic streptococci** cultures. Streptokinase induces an immune response that produces antibodies to the drug, limiting its useful duration to 6 days. Allergy is common. Patients frequently have antibodies to protein from previous exposure to the *Streptococcus*.

Fibrinolytic inhibitors

Examples – aprotinin, tranexamic acid

The fibrinolytic inhibitors act by inhibiting the enzymatic activity of plasmin on fibrin. They are used to prevent the breakdown of fibrin clot when excessive bleeding during surgery is a risk. Uses include the reduction of blood loss during surgery in haemophiliacs, in cardiac surgery, and in thrombolytic overdose.

Aprotinin is a polypeptide and inhibitor of proteolytic enzymes in general, but specifically it is used for its action on plasmin and kallikrein. It has also been tried in the treatment of acute pancreatitis. Tranexamic acid inhibits the fibrinolytic activity of both plasmin and pepsin. It is useful in upper gastrointestinal haemorrhage and in surgery in haemophiliacs, and it can be administered orally or intravenously.

Antiplatelet drugs

Aspirin

Aspirin irreversibly inactivates platelet cyclo-oxygenase (COX-2) by acetylation of the terminal serine amino acid. This inhibits endoperoxide and so thromboxane (TXA_2) production within the platelets. More importantly, endothelial cells generate new cyclo-oxygenase, whereas platelets are unable to do so. As it is an irreversible process, the effect on an individual platelet is permanent for the 4–6-day lifespan of the platelet. Aspirin is not specific for platelet cyclo-oxygenase, but this is more readily inactivated than the endothelial cyclo-oxygenase responsible for prostacyclin production. Aspirin should be stopped 7–10 days before surgery to allow regeneration of normally functioning platelets. It may be restarted 6 hours postoperatively. Prolonged aspirin usage may reduce circulating levels of factors II, VII, IX and X.

Other NSAIDs also inhibit COX, but are generally less potent, and the inhibition is reversible, so that the overall effect on platelet function is small.

Prostacyclin

Synthetic prostacyclin (epoprostenol) inhibits platelet aggregation and dissipates platelet aggregates. It can be used in haemodialysis, but must be given as an infusion because of a short half-life (about 3 minutes). Prostacyclin is also a potent vasodilator, so patients should be observed for hypotension, flushing and headaches.

P2Y$_{12}$ inhibitors

Examples – cangrelor, clopidogrel, prasugrel, ticagrelor, ticlopidine

Thrombin, TXA$_2$ and ADP among other agents act on platelet surface receptors to stimulate platelet aggregation (Wallentin 2009). To stimulate aggregation, two receptor types must be activated: the P2Y$_1$ ADP receptor that releases calcium and the P2Y$_{12}$ ADP receptor, a G-protein-coupled transmembrane receptor that activates cAMP. There are two sets of P2Y$_{12}$ inhibitors. The thienopyridines clopidogrel, prasugrel and ticlopidine are prodrugs and their active metabolites bind covalently, irreversibly to the P2Y$_{12}$ ADP receptor for the lifespan of the platelet. Cangrelor and ticagrelor are reversible anatgonists competing at the ADP binding site on the P2Y$_{12}$ ADP receptor.

Glycoprotein IIb/IIIa inhibitors

Examples – abciximab, eptifibatide, tirofiban

Platelet aggregation is mediated by glycoprotein IIb/IIIa receptors on the platelet surface which bind to fibrinogen. Glycoprotein IIb/IIIa inhibitors block these binding sites.

Other haemostatic modifiers

Viscosity

Dextrans reduce the viscosity of blood and may reduce the incidence of venous thrombus formation by improving the flow characteristics of the relatively slow-flowing venous circulation.

Coagulation factors

Coagulation factors may be administered as extracts (antithrombin III and factors VIIa, VIII, IX and XIII) or as fresh frozen plasma (FFP). Vitamin K may be used to increase levels of factors II, VII and IX when there is a deficiency of vitamin K or excess of oral anticoagulant therapy. Vitamin K$_2$ is produced by gut bacteria. These are reduced by broad-spectrum antibiotics and are deficient in the newborn (haemorrhagic disease of the newborn). Desmopressin increases levels of factor VIII. This may be useful to decrease surgical oozing in mild haemophilia, and in cases of massive transfusion, when clotting factors are reduced.

Platelet action

Ethamsylate reduces capillary bleeding, probably by correcting abnormal platelet adhesion. It also inhibits the antiplatelet action of some NSAIDs, in addition to a weak arteriolar constricting action. It is contraindicated in porphyria.

References and further reading

Wallentin L. P2Y$_{12}$ inhibitors: differences in properties and mechanisms of action and potential consequences for clinical use. *Eur Heart J* 2009; **30**: 1964–77.

CHAPTER 42
Antimicrobial therapy

Jim Stone

Principles of antimicrobial therapy

The factors that must be assessed before choosing antimicrobial therapy are shown in Figure 42.1.

After treatment has commenced, the duration of therapy must be determined and regularly reassessed, together with the need to modify the antibiotic(s) in terms of both type and dose, depending on the clinical condition of the patient and laboratory results, e.g. sensitivity tests, plasma drug levels, white blood count and inflammatory markers such as C-reactive protein (CRP) and procalcitonin.

Fundamentals of Anaesthesia, 4th edition, ed. Ted Lin, Tim Smith and Colin Pinnock. Published by Cambridge University Press. © Cambridge University Press 2017.

Figure 42.1 Factors influencing antimicrobial therapy

Patient factors
- Age
- Weight
- Renal function
- Hepatic function
- Antimicrobial allergy
- Immune deficiency or suppression
- Pregnancy
- Significant medical conditions
- Site of infection
- Severity of infection
- Prophylaxis or treatment required

Organism factors
- Virulence
- Predicted microbe population
- Predicted antimicrobial susceptibility

Drug factors
- Spectrum of antimicrobial activity
- Route of administration
- Pharmacokinetics
- Synergy or antagonism with other antimicrobial agents
- Toxicity profile
- Interactions with non-antimicrobial compounds
- Local antibiotic prescribing policies

Antimicrobial therapy in renal failure

Most antibiotics or their metabolites are renally excreted. Accumulation of potentially toxic compounds may therefore arise unless careful monitoring and dose adjustments are performed. Some antimicrobials (e.g. aminoglycosides) are nephrotoxic, while others should be avoided if there is pre-existing renal disease, and different methods of dialysis have differing abilities to clear certain compounds.

Mechanisms of action

Antimicrobials work by interfering with bacterial or fungal cellular functions. They target structures and functions specific to the target microbe or those that have an alternative metabolic pathway in human cells. These mechanisms target four groups of microbial sites:
- Cell wall
- Cell membrane
- Protein synthesis
- Nucleic acid synthesis

Cell wall synthesis

Bacteria have a cell wall to prevent swelling and lysis in hypotonic environments. The cell wall comprises N-acetyl glucosamine, acetyl muramic acid and a polypeptide, which form multiple cross-links. This maintains the three-dimensional integrity of the structure. The cell wall can range from several molecular layers thick in Gram-negative bacteria to 100 layers in the Gram-positive organisms. Antimicrobials that inhibit cell wall synthesis cause the growing cell to burst, and so are normally bactericidal. Antibacterial drugs targeting the cell wall cannot affect eukaryotic cells by this mechanism.

Cell membrane permeability

Drugs that selectively interfere with cell membrane permeability are active against bacterial and fungal cells. Selectivity is conferred by targeting components of bacterial or fungal cell membranes that are not found in the host. Negatively charged lipids are abundant in the cell membranes of Gram-negative bacteria and are the target of polymyxins such as colistin and polymyxin B. Sterols are present in both fungal and human cell membranes. Imidazoles and triazoles interfere with sterol synthesis, and toxicity occurs with higher doses. Polyenes such as amphotericin and nystatin bind to the fungal sterols and open pores in the membrane, leading to destruction of the molecular composition of the cytoplasm.

Protein synthesis

Where bacterial and human ribosomes differ, they can be targeted by antibiotics. Those agents that reversibly inhibit protein synthesis are bacteriostatic. Those that bind to the 30S subunit of the bacterial ribosome are bactericidal.

Nucleic acid synthesis

Rifampicin inhibits DNA-dependent RNA polymerase. The quinolones inhibit DNA synthesis and disrupt the final coiling of the DNA helix essential for its transcription. Nucleic acid analogues such as aciclovir attach to the active site of the enzymes of DNA synthesis and so block DNA synthesis.

Mechanisms of resistance

Bacteria, viruses and fungi can all mutate, and indeed do so frequently. Antimicrobial agents exert a selective pressure on microbial populations favouring resistant mutants. Because of the speed at which microorganisms multiply (every 20 minutes in the case of *Escherichia coli* in optimal growth conditions), it can be seen that the opportunity for the development and spread of resistance is considerable.

As well as spontaneous mutation within a bacterium, organisms may acquire resistance genes in a number of ways. This genetic material may be transmitted either on the bacterial chromosome or via extra-chromosomal DNA or plasmids. Bacterial genes can be transferred at the time of bacterial conjugation or via bacterial viruses (bacteriophages). Once a resistance gene has emerged it may therefore be readily transmitted between bacteria of the same species. However, interspecies transmission can also occur.

Bacterial plasmids are autonomously replicating genetic elements consisting of circular double-stranded DNA. They vary in size, and some may contain a number of different resistance genes as well as genes coding for a range of virulence and bacterial survival factors.

Transposons are genes which allow movement of genetic material attached to them from one bacterial chromosome to another or between bacterial chromosomes and plasmids. Hence a resistance gene that originally arose in a bacterial chromosome could move to a more mobile bacterial plasmid. Similarly, genes on plasmids (which may be less stable than chromosomal DNA) can be integrated into the bacterial chromosome of new species or strains.

There are about eight distinct mechanisms of resistance recognised, some of which may be combined within a single organism to increase the degree of resistance. Many of these resistance mechanisms can make the bacteria less 'fit' than sensitive strains, offering some hope that resistance could decline if antibiotic selective pressure is withdrawn.

Enzymic destruction. This is usually the most efficient mechanism, and it tends to have the least negative impact on the bacterium. Resistance to β-lactam antibiotics (see below) is largely a consequence of production of β-lactamase enzymes by bacteria. Aminoglycoside-modifying enzymes (of which there are more than 30) are the next most prolific group, conferring resistance to gentamicin, tobramycin and sometimes amikacin.

Altered target sites. Altered penicillin-binding proteins (PBPs) are the reason why strains of *Staphylococcus aureus* are resistant to meticillin, flucloxacillin and almost all of the cephalosporins (MRSA strains). In these strains the *mecA* gene codes for PBP2a, which has a low affinity for β-lactam antibiotics. A similar mechanism confers penicillin resistance in some *Streptococcus pneumoniae* and *Neisseria gonorrhoeae*. Resistance to the macrolides is often due to altered bacterial ribosomal binding sites. The glycopeptide (vancomycin and teicoplanin) resistance seen in vancomycin-resistant enterococci (VRE) is caused by alterations in bacterial peptidoglycan cell wall components. Quinolone (e.g. ciprofloxacin) resistance may be due to modified bacterial DNA-gyrase (the principal site of action of this class of antibiotics).

Protection of target sites. Recently described plasmid-mediated quinolone resistance works by protecting DNA-gyrase, and some tetracycline resistance is due to interference with the ability of the drug to bind to bacterial ribosomes without there being an obvious change to the ribosome.

Overproduction of target. Sulphonamides and trimethoprim resistance is a result of bacteria overproducing their target-site enzymes DHPS and DHFR respectively.

Bypass of metabolic pathway. Trimethoprim and sulphonamides are folic acid inhibitors. Some organisms, e.g. enterococci, can utilise folate from alternative sources.

Bind-up of antibiotic. Excess of binding sites in the bacterial cell wall is responsible for reduction in susceptibility to glycopeptides in *Staphylococcus aureus* (so-called vancomycin-intermediate *S. aureus* or VISA).

Decreased permeability. The movement of hydrophilic molecules through the outer bacterial lipid membrane is via porin proteins, which form channels through which they can pass. Mutations to the genes encoding for porin proteins or their expression may therefore confer a degree of resistance by preventing the antibiotic molecules passing through these channels. Aminoglycoside, quinolone and carbapenem resistance in certain Gram-negative bacteria, e.g. *Pseudomonas aeruginosa*, is a good example. Usually the resistance is low-level as molecules useful to the bacterium will also be blocked to some degree. However, when combined with active efflux (see below) the resistance will be greater.

Antibiotic efflux. Active efflux is a common mechanism of resistance, which, when it is present in conjunction with reduced antibiotic permeability, may confer high-level resistance. Essentially the antibiotic, on gaining access to the bacterium, is actively pumped out again before it can attach to its binding site. Quinolones, macrolides, β-lactams and tetracyclines may all be subject to this form of resistance.

Beta-lactams

This is the single largest group of antimicrobial agents presently available. It includes penicillins, cephalosporins, carbapenems and monobactams.

Mechanism of action

The β-lactam antibiotics target the penicillin-binding proteins (PBPs). These are cell-wall synthesising enzymes located in the cytoplasmic membrane. PBPs are not present in mammalian cells, which accounts for the low toxicity of these drugs. The bacterial cell wall is weakened and osmotic lysis occurs. Penicillins and cephalosporins show synergy with antibiotics acting on targets within the bacterial cell because the cell-wall changes increase the permeability of the cell to other compounds.

Acquired resistance

Bacteria exhibit resistance to β-lactams by four mechanisms:

- Enzymatic destruction of β-lactam (β-lactamases). These enzymes may be encoded for by genes present on either bacterial chromosomes or plasmids. There are many types of β-lactamase, and their classification is complex. First described in the 1940s, they are ubiquitous. In recent years, extended-spectrum β-lactamases (ESBLs) have been identified which attack most penicillins and cephalosporins, including the third-generation cephalosporins such as cefotaxime.

  Since 2010, there has been a rapid increase in metallo-β-lactamase enzymes, which are also often referred to as carbapenemases (although they also destroy other β-lactam antibiotics).
- Bacterial modification of PBP target (MRSA).
- Reduced permeability of the bacterial cell membrane to β-lactams (often referred to as porin-channel mutants).
- Active efflux pump (mainly in Gram-negative bacteria) – the bacterium excretes the drug.

Note that the last two mechanisms may act in synergy in some bacteria (such as *Pseudomonas*) to increase the degree of resistance.

Penicillins

Examples – amoxicillin, benzylpenicillin, flucloxacillin, piperacillin, temocillin

Adverse effects

These are few. Allergy is the most common problem and may occur in 1–10% of exposed individuals. True anaphylaxis is rare (0.05%) but has a potential mortality rate of 10%. It is important to obtain a good allergy history, including the type of allergy. Individuals with a history of anaphylaxis, urticaria or rash immediately after penicillin administration should not receive a penicillin or other β-lactam, as there is a small risk of cross-hypersensitivity with cephalosporins and carbapenems.

In very high doses with meningitis and renal impairment, penicillins and other β-lactams may cause convulsions.

Benzylpenicillin

Benzylpenicillin is active against Gram-positive bacteria, most anaerobes and certain Gram-negative cocci (*Neisseria* spp.). Most strains of *Staphylococcus aureus* produce β-lactamase and are resistant.

Benzylpenicillin is unstable in acid and must be given parenterally. It is distributed widely, penetrating pleural, pericardial, peritoneal and synovial spaces, but not cerebrospinal fluid in the absence of meningeal inflammation. Low levels are found in saliva. It is excreted mainly by tubular secretion in the kidney, with an elimination half-life of 30 minutes. This process is blocked by probenecid. Aspirin and sulphonamides also prolong the half-life.

Amoxicillin

Amoxicillin has a relatively broad spectrum of activity. It is active against bacteria covered by benzylpenicillin and several Gram-negative species, *Haemophilus influenzae* and most faecal streptococci (enterococci). Resistance is common and is usually due to β-lactamase production by the bacterium.

Amoxicillin is stable in gastric acid, and achieves good bioavailability after oral administration. It is otherwise very similar to benzylpenicillin. It has a half-life of 1–1.5 hours. Skin rashes are more common with amoxicillin than with benzylpenicillin.

Amoxicillin is the drug of choice for most acute lower respiratory tract infections acquired in the community, for sensitive strains of *Neisseria gonorrhoeae*, and for faecal streptococcal (enterococcal) infections.

Flucloxacillin

Flucloxacillin and related compounds (meticillin, cloxacillin) are unaffected by staphylococcal β-lactamase but have a narrower spectrum of activity than benzylpenicillin. Resistance to them is conferred by an altered target site (the PBP). These are the meticillin-resistant *Staphylococcus aureus* (MRSA) – meticillin sensitivity being the basis of the laboratory method of typing the bacterial subspecies.

Flucloxacillin is well absorbed orally but high protein binding (95%) limits its diffusion into some compartments, notably cerebrospinal fluid. It has a half-life of 45 minutes. Flucloxacillin remains the drug of choice for non-MRSA staphylococcal infections.

Flucloxacillin may rarely cause cholestatic jaundice and hepatitis, and it must be used with caution in patients with hepatic impairment.

Piperacillin and Tazocin

Piperacillin is distinguished from amoxicillin mainly by its activity against *Pseudomonas aeruginosa* and related species. It is however destroyed by bacterial β-lactamase. It is therefore now combined with a β-lactamase inhibitor (tazobactam) to produce Tazocin. This compound has a significantly improved spectrum of activity.

Poor absorption necessitates parenteral administration. These drugs are sodium salts, and the high doses required to treat severe sepsis may cause sodium overload. They are mainly used for known or suspected *Pseudomonas* infections and, usually in combination with aminoglycosides, for the treatment of febrile neutropenic patients.

Most β-lactam antibiotics exhibit antibacterial synergy when given with aminoglycosides, and there is some evidence that they may also be synergistic against Gram-negative bacteria when given with quinolones.

Clavulanic acid

Clavulanic acid is not an antibiotic but is an inhibitor of most β-lactamases (like tazobactam). In combination with amoxicillin it improves the spectrum of activity.

Co-amoxiclav (a combination of clavulanic acid and amoxicillin) has been a particularly successful compound. Pharmacokinetically the combination closely mimics that of amoxicillin alone. In addition to the side effects of amoxicillin, there is a small risk of cholestatic jaundice. Co-amoxiclav is used in the treatment of soft tissue infections (including bites), lower respiratory tract infections and urinary tract infections, and for surgical prophylaxis.

Because of the risk of cholestatic jaundice and hepatitis it must be used with caution (if at all) in patients with hepatic impairment.

Temocillin

Temocillin is an injectable penicillin. It lacks activity against Gram-positive organisms and *Pseudomonas*. However, it has a high degree of stability to β-lactamases, including extended-spectrum β-lactamases (ESBLs). It therefore may be an alternative to carbapenems (e.g. meropenem) in some situations, which is important if the use of the latter compounds is to be controlled.

Cephalosporins

Examples – cefixime, cefotaxime, cefpirome, ceftaroline, ceftazidime, ceftriaxone, cefuroxime, cephalexin

These compounds are based on cephalosporin C, a fermentation product of *Cephalosporium acremonium* cultivated from a Sardinian sewage outfall in 1948. They may be classified into seven groups (Figure 42.2).

Cephalexin

Cephalexin is active against most Gram-positive cocci, except fecal streptococci and MRSA. It is also moderately active against some enterobacteria (including *Escherichia coli*). It has negligible activity against *Haemophilus influenzae*.

Cephalexin is stable to gastric acid and almost completely absorbed when given by mouth, and 10% is protein-bound. There is reasonable penetration into bone and purulent sputum. It is almost entirely excreted in the urine, with a half-life of 50 minutes.

Cephalexin occasionally causes hypersensitivity, diarrhoea and abdominal discomfort, and rarely Stevens–Johnson syndrome.

Cefuroxime

Cefuroxime is more active than cephalexin against most of the Enterobacteriaceae, and has useful activity against *Haemophilus influenzae*. It is similar to cephalexin against Gram-positive cocci. It is not absorbed from the intestinal tract and is usually administered intravenously. It is well distributed, but cerebrospinal fluid levels are not sufficient to treat bacterial meningitis. It is excreted unchanged in the urine, one-half being the result of tubular secretion, with a half-life of 80 minutes.

Cefuroxime is used in the treatment of urinary, soft-tissue, bone, intra-abdominal and pulmonary infections and septicaemia. It is ineffective against faecal streptococci

Figure 42.2 A classification of cephalosporins

Group	Generation	Examples	Effect of β-lactamase	Antibacterial activity
1	1st	Cephazolin	Stable	Moderate
2	2nd	Cephalexin Cefaclor	Moderately stable	Moderate
3	2nd	Cefuroxime Cephamandole	Resistance	Moderate
4	3rd	Cefotaxime Ceftriaxone	Stable	Potent: especially Gram-negatives
5	3rd	Cefixime Cefpodoxime	Stable	Potent: especially Gram-negatives
6	3rd	Ceftazidime Cefsulodin	Stable	Potent: especially Gram-negatives and *Pseudomonas*
7	4th	Cefpirome	Stable	Enterobacteriaceae

and most anaerobes. Its use in surgical prophylaxis has been discouraged in recent years because of the association between cephalosporins and *C. difficile*-associated diarrhoea.

Cefotaxime

Cefotaxime is similar to cefuroxime but with much greater activity against many Gram-negative bacteria (e.g. coliforms and Gram-negative cocci including β-lactamase-producing strains). It is usually active against penicillin-resistant strains of *Streptococcus pneumoniae*. It has only moderate activity against *Listeria monocytogenes* (amoxicillin must be added if meningitis or septicaemia with this organism is suspected) and limited efficacy against anaerobes (requiring the addition of metronidazole if polymicrobial sepsis is considered likely). It has minimal activity against *Pseudomonas aeruginosa*.

Cefotaxime is administered intravenously. Unlike other cephalosporins, it is metabolised in the body to desacetyl-cefotaxime, and both the parent compound and metabolite are renally excreted. It has an elimination half-life of 80 minutes.

Cefotaxime has a very wide range of indications, including lower respiratory infections, septicaemia, meningitis, intra-abdominal sepsis, osteomyelitis, pyelonephritis, neonatal sepsis and gonorrhoea.

Ceftriaxone

Ceftriaxone is almost identical to cefotaxime in terms of its spectrum of activity and is prescribed for similar infections. However, it has a much longer serum half-life, allowing for once- or twice-daily dosing schedules. Because of this it is often used in the outpatient and home intravenous therapy setting for the management of difficult skin/soft-tissue infections.

Cefixime

Cefixime is an oral third-generation cephalosporin. Intestinal absorption remains relatively poor and it has a limited role in the hospital setting.

Ceftazidime

Ceftazidime is similar to cefotaxime but much more active against *Pseudomonas aeruginosa*. It is less active against Gram-positive cocci than other cephalosporins.

It is 17% protein-bound. Distribution of the drug around the body is similar to cefotaxime. It is mainly excreted renally, with a half-life of 2 hours.

It tends to be reserved for use as an anti-pseudomonal agent.

Cefpirome

Cefpirome is a fourth-generation cephalosporin similar to ceftazidime utilised for Gram-negative bacteria including

Pseudomonas aeruginosa. 10% is protein bound and 80% is renally excreted with a half-life of 2 hours.

Ceftaroline

Ceftaroline is a fifth-generation cephalosporin active against MRSA and Gram-positive bacteria.

Carbapenems

Examples – ertapenem, imipenem, meropenem

Carbapenems are bicyclic β-lactam compounds with a carbapenem nucleus. Their mechanism of action is similar to that of other β-lactam antibiotics but they seem to have a greater affinity for penicillin-binding protein 2 (PBP-2). This results in faster bacterial death and, in theory, less endotoxin release. They are extremely broad-spectrum antibiotics, because they are resistant to most β-lactamases (including the newer ESBLs). They are, however, susceptible to the recently described metallo-β-lactamases, which are beginning to threaten their efficacy in several parts of the world including India and the Middle East.

Pharmacokinetics

Carbapenems are administered intravenously. Excretion is predominantly by glomerular filtration. Carbapenems exhibit a phenomenon known as the *post-antibiotic effect*. This is a prolonged inhibition of bacterial growth for a period of time after the concentration of antibiotic has fallen below the accepted minimum inhibitory concentration (MIC). Therefore 6-, 8- and even 12-hourly dose regimes can be effective.

Adverse effects

Adverse effects are similar to those of other β-lactams. Neutropenia is a rare complication and is reversible on stopping the drug. Neurotoxicity appears to be more of a problem than with other β-lactam antibiotics but is primarily seen in patients with renal insufficiency and on high doses, particularly neonates and the elderly.

Imipenem

Imipenem is chemically unstable in its natural form and is supplied in crystalline form. It is highly active against virtually all Gram-positive and Gram-negative pathogenic bacteria, including anaerobes. Poor intracellular penetration of eukaryotic cells prevents its use against intracellular infections such as *Legionella*. It is rapidly bactericidal against a majority of organisms but is only bacteriostatic

against faecal streptococci. MRSA is not susceptible, and *Pseudomonas aeruginosa* can rapidly develop resistance.

Imipenem is rapidly destroyed by dehydropeptidase 1 in renal tubules. It is administered with cilastatin, a selective competitive inhibitor of this enzyme. Cilastatin has similar pharmacokinetic properties to imipenem, and inhibition of dehydropeptidase has no apparent adverse physiological consequences.

Meropenem

Meropenem is similar to imipenem but is stable to human renal dehydropeptidase, rendering the addition of cilastatin unnecessary. It is more active than imipenem against some Gram-negatives but less active against Gram-positives. The main benefit is that it is less neurotoxic than imipenem.

Monobactams

Example – aztreonam

Monobactams have only a single β-lactam ring, while penicillins, cephalosporins and carbapenems all have two. Note that only Gram-negative aerobic bacteria are sensitive. Aztreonam is highly active against most of the Enterobacteriaceae, *Haemophilus influenzae* and *Neisseria*, and has some activity against *Pseudomonas aeruginosa*.

Pharmacokinetics

Intestinal absorption is poor, so aztreonam is given by intravenous or intramuscular injection. Distribution in the body is similar to that of other β-lactams. Elimination is renal, by a combination of glomerular filtration and tubular secretion. Aztreonam has a half-life of 2 hours.

Adverse effects

Aztreonam is similar to other β-lactams. However, as a monobactam, there appears to be very little cross-hypersensitivity with penicillins or cephalosporins. Aztreonam should still be used with caution in patients with severe penicillin allergy. Aztreonam does not seem to interfere with platelet function, unlike some cephalosporins and penicillins.

Glycopeptides and lipopeptides

Examples – teicoplanin, vancomycin (glycopeptides); daptomycin (lipopeptide)

The glycopeptides are a group of complex, high-molecular-weight compounds that are usually slowly bactericidal and prevent bacterial cell wall synthesis at the substrate level. Glycopeptides are active against most

Gram-positive bacteria but they do not penetrate the outer membrane of Gram-negative organisms because they are large polar molecules.

Acquired resistance

Acquired resistance is uncommon. Gene mutations occur, which alter cell-wall precursors. These precursors are called Van-A (which produces resistance to both vancomycin and teicoplanin and is inducible and present on plasmids – allowing transfer between strains), Van-B and Van-C (which produce resistance to vancomycin only and are present on bacterial chromosomes – less easy to transfer to other species). Resistance has been reported principally in various *Enterococcus* species, which have been named vancomycin-resistant enterococci (VRE). The mechanism of resistance is not entirely clear.

The presence of mucopolysaccharide slime reduces the susceptibility of coagulase-negative staphylococci. This is often present when there are microcolonies on the surfaces of joint and heart valve prostheses or on intravenous and peritoneal dialysis cannulae.

Vancomycin

Vancomycin is used to treat difficult Gram-positive bacterial infections including MRSA, staphylococcal or streptococcal infective endocarditis, coagulase-negative staphylococci on indwelling materials and antibiotic-associated colitis (*Clostridium difficile*).

Spectrum of activity

Vancomycin is effective against Gram-positive cocci (including MRSA), coagulase-negative staphylococci (e.g. *Staphylococcus epidermidis*), streptococci, enterococci, bacilli, corynebacteria, *Listeria monocytogenes* (moderate), and Gram-positive anaerobes (*Clostridium perfringens* and other *Clostridia* spp. including *C. difficile*). Resistance is sometimes encountered in enterococci (VRE strains), which can cause line-associated bacteraemias.

Pharmacokinetics

Vancomycin is administered intravenously, because intestinal tract absorption is poor and intramuscular injection causes pain and necrosis. Protocols for continuous infusion are available but there seems to be little difference in efficacy between twice-daily short-duration infusions (1–2 hours depending on dose) and continued infusion therapy.

It is widely distributed, reaching most body compartments except the cerebrospinal fluid. It may also be administered into CSF shunts and into the peritoneum, and for antibiotic-associated colitis it is given orally. It is occasionally administered by intravitreal injection for difficult eye infections.

When given by the oral route it remains mainly in the intestinal tract. It is an effective oral treatment for *C. difficile*-associated colitis.

Vancomycin is 55% protein-bound. It is excreted, unchanged, mainly by glomerular filtration, with a half-life of 6–8 hours. Plasma monitoring is normally performed on pre-dose serum but is required mainly in those with renal impairment or on prolonged high-dose regimes. Note that it is not removed effectively by either haemodialysis or haemofiltration. When it is given orally for *C. difficile* infection, monitoring of blood levels is not normally required unless given in high doses for an extended period to patients with severe renal impairment.

Adverse effects

Adverse effects include hypersensitivity, nephrotoxicity, ototoxicity and occasionally neutropenia. Chemical thrombophlebitis is relatively common when vancomycin is administered via a peripheral vein. Vancomycin-induced histamine release with rapid infusion produces the 'red man syndrome'. This comprises itching, flushing, angio-oedema, hypotension and tachycardia. Bronchospasm does not occur. It normally resolves within 1 hour of the infusion stopping. It is prevented by antihistamines. The hypotensive effect may be severe. Nephrotoxicity and ototoxicity may be related to impurities in earlier preparations, and are now rare.

Teicoplanin

Teicoplanin has slightly greater activity against some streptococci and slightly less activity against staphylococci than vancomycin. It is distributed similarly to vancomycin but is more protein-bound (> 90%). The serum half-life is considerably longer (47 hours) than that of vancomycin, partly because of the protein binding. It may be given by rapid IV infusion or intramuscularly. It is less toxic than vancomycin but, for difficult-to-treat infections, periodic serum levels (pre-dose) are advised to ensure adequate concentrations are being achieved.

Daptomycin

Daptomycin is a cyclic lipopeptide. It is generally more active than glycopeptides against a range of Gram-positive bacteria, including some vancomycin-resistant entero-cocci (VRE). Most significantly, it is more rapidly bactericidal than either vancomycin or teicoplanin. It does not have activity against Gram-negative bacteria.

Aminoglycosides

Examples – amikacin, gentamicin, netilmycin, streptomycin, tobramycin

Aminoglycosides are naturally occurring or semisynthetic polycationic compounds with aminosugars glycosidically linked to aminocyclitols.

Mechanism of action

Aminoglycosides bind to the 30S subunit of the bacterial ribosome, causing inhibition of protein synthesis. It is not known why aminoglycosides are usually rapidly bactericidal, whereas other inhibitors of protein synthesis are bacteriostatic. Aminoglycosides cause cell-membrane leakiness and consequent cell death. In general, aminoglycosides are active against *Staphylococcus aureus*, a majority of the coagulase-negative staphylococci, the Enterobacteriaceae, and most are effective against *Pseudomonas aeruginosa* and other *Pseudomonas* spp.

Acquired resistance

There are three mechanisms of resistance to aminoglycosides:

- Altered binding site
- Reduced uptake/permeability
- Aminoglycoside-modifying enzymes

Resistance is increasing in the Enterobacteriaceae (e.g. *E. coli* and *Klebsiella* spp.) and is particularly common in ESBL and carbapenemase-producing strains.

Adverse effects

Aminoglycosides are nephrotoxic and ototoxic (vestibular and auditory). Toxicity is directly related to plasma levels, which should be monitored closely, particularly with impaired renal function. Slow IV injection will minimise the risk, but toxicity is principally associated with elevated trough levels. Ototoxicity is usually irreversible, but renal function often recovers. Once-daily dose regimes are associated with a lower risk of toxicity.

The ototoxicity is put to use in chemical vestibular labyrinthectomy, with gentamicin delivered to the middle ear to treat Ménière's disease.

Gentamicin

Gentamicin is active against the Enterobacteriaceae, some *Pseudomonas* spp. (e.g. *Ps. aeruginosa*) and staphylococci. It has limited activity against streptococci and *Listeria* spp. Gentamicin is used for serious Gram-negative bacterial infections. It is rapidly bactericidal and has a strong synergistic effect with β-lactams. Poor tissue penetration limits its usefulness in the treatment of deep soft-tissue infections and abscesses. Similarly, typhoid and other intracellular infections are relatively resistant. Selective decontamination of the intestine by oral administration may be useful, but can increase bacterial resistance.

Gentamicin is administered parenterally, because oral bioavailability is low (1%), typically in a dose of 3–5 mg kg^{-1} day^{-1}, once-daily. Divided doses (total daily dose 2–3 mg kg^{-1}) are used in patients with infective endocarditis. Tissue and cell penetration is poor but it crosses the placenta. Excretion is renal, mainly by glomerular filtration, with an elimination half-life of 2 hours.

Amikacin

Amikacin has a similar antibacterial spectrum to gentamicin, but is less susceptible to most of the aminoglycoside-modifying enzymes. It is reserved for specific sensitive strains. It is also active against *Mycobacterium tuberculosis* and other 'atypical' mycobacteria, including strains resistant to streptomycin. Any nephrotoxicity and ototoxicity that occurs is usually reversible.

Streptomycin

Streptomycin is particularly effective against *Mycobacterium tuberculosis*, but is also active against many Gram-negative aerobic bacteria and staphylococci. Resistance can develop as a single-step mutation that changes the structure of the ribosomal target site.

Macrolides

Examples – clarithromycin, erythromycin

Macrolides are naturally occurring antibiotics produced mainly by streptomycetes. They comprise a macrocyclic lactone ring with two sugars attached, one being an amino sugar. They are grouped according to the number of atoms in the lactone ring, e.g. 14 for erythromycin and clarithromycin.

Mechanism of action

Macrolides bind to the 50S ribosome of bacteria to inhibit protein synthesis, probably by preventing the first translocation. Macrolides appear to have a therapeutic effect below their in-vitro minimum inhibitory concentration. This may be achieved by inhibiting attachment and adherence by bacterial protein adhesions and by suppressing bacterial toxin and coenzyme production. Macrolides are active against most Gram-positive bacteria, Gram-negative organisms, some strains of *Haemophilus*, *Legionella*, *Campylobacter jejuni* and *Helicobacter pylori*. Some anaerobes are sensitive, including most Gram-positive streptococci and some species of *Bacteroides*.

Acquired resistance

Acquired resistance is relatively common. There are three mechanisms of resistance to macrolides:

- Altered binding site (the ribosome)
- Drug inactivation
- Active efflux of the drug from the bacterial cell

Changing the target site results in resistance to all the macrolides and also to lincosamides and streptogramins. The resistance genes can be on either the bacterial chromosome or the plasmid.

Erythromycin

Erythromycin is bitter, insoluble in water and inactivated by acid. The estolate and ascitrate are the most stable in gastric acid. Enteric and film-coated tablets of the base are available, but incomplete absorption occurs, with considerable inter-patient variation. Erythromycin is distributed widely throughout the body. It tends to be retained longer in liver and spleen. Very low levels are obtained in the cerebrospinal fluid, even in the presence of meningeal inflammation. The normal serum half-life is 1.4 hours, increased to 5 hours in anuric patients, so that only slight dose adjustment is required in renal failure. It accumulates with liver disease. It is eliminated primarily by hepatic inactivation and excretion in the bile, with active intestinal reabsorption. Less than 15% of active drug is excreted in the urine. It is usually given 6-hourly.

Erythromycin causes gastrointestinal upset, hepatotoxicity, ototoxicity and cardiotoxicity. Erythromycin is a gastric irritant, and a stimulant of intestinal motility (prokinetic). Nausea, vomiting and diarrhoea are common. Erythromycin may cause intrahepatic cholestasis, particularly during pregnancy. Ototoxicity is usually due to high-dose erythromycin lactobionate administration in patients with renal or severe liver dysfunction.

Cardiotoxicity is very rare but potentially fatal. Allergic reactions are rare (< 0.5%). Thrombophlebitis is a major problem with IV administration. Drug interactions include increased serum levels of prednisolone, theophylline, carbamazepine, ciclosporin, warfarin and terfenadine.

Clarithromycin, a derivative of erythromycin, has slightly greater activity and higher tissue levels. It requires only twice-daily administration.

Tetracyclines

Examples – doxycycline, minocycline, tetracycline

Mechanism of action

Tetracyclines bind to the 30S subunit of the bacterial ribosome and prevent the binding of aminoacyl-tRNA. Protein synthesis is prevented, resulting in a bacteriostatic effect. Tetracyclines have a very broad spectrum, including Gram-positive and Gram-negative bacteria, spirochaetes, some mycobacteria, *Mycoplasma*, *Chlamydia*, *Rickettsia*, *Coxiella* and protozoa. Minocycline even shows some activity against the fungus *Candida albicans*.

Acquired resistance

Acquired resistance is very common. This is plasmid-mediated and so is easily spread between different bacterial species, and is associated with multiple resistance genes. There are four mechanisms of resistance:

- Decreased cell entry
- Increased drug efflux
- Ribosomal protection by the formation of a cytoplasmic protein
- Chemical modification requiring nicotinamide adenine dinucleotide phosphate (NADPH) and oxygen

Resistance and newer, more effective antibiotics have limited the use of tetracyclines, but they remain the preferred treatment for chlamydial and rickettsial infections, Q-fever, anthrax and plague (*Yersinia pestis*).

Tetracycline

Tetracycline is particularly active against *Vibrio cholerae*, *Aeromonas hydrophila* and *Plesiomonas shigelloides*.

Tetracycline is less protein-bound (24%) and less lipophilic than doxycycline and minocycline. Penetration is quite good into most body tissues, although levels in tears and saliva are low. The serum half-life is about 7 hours. Excretion is mainly renal (by glomerular filtration) and biliary. The bioavailability of tetracycline following oral administration is less than for minocycline and doxycycline and declines proportionally with increasing doses. Absorption is better in the fasting state but impaired by ferrous ions.

Adverse effects

Adverse effects include gastrointestinal (nausea, epigastric pain, vomiting and diarrhoea), superinfections, hyperpigmentation, photosensitivity, dental discolouration in children, hepatotoxicity, nephrotoxicity, haematological (leucopenia and thrombocytopenia) and benign intracranial hypertension.

Bacterial and fungal superinfections are particularly frequent with tetracycline treatment. There are four types of nephrotoxicity:

- Aggravation of pre-existing renal disease
- Association with acute fatty liver
- Interstitial nephritis
- Nephrogenic diabetes insipidus and renal failure

Weak neuromuscular blockade and potentiation of non-depolarising neuromuscular blockade is seen, and this is not reversed by calcium or anticholinesterases.

Doxycycline

Doxycycline is semisynthetic. It is active against some tetracycline-resistant strains of *S. aureus*. It is more active than most other tetracyclines against *Streptococcus pyogenes* and *Nocardia* spp. It is strongly lipophilic, allowing widespread tissue distribution. 80–90% is protein-bound, the highest of any tetracycline. It has a long half-life of 15–25 hours. Specific uses include chlamydial infection of the eye and genital tract. It is also a treatment of choice for patients with Lyme disease (causative agent *Borrelia burgdorferi*).

Chloramphenicol
Mechanism of action

Chloramphenicol reversibly binds to the 50S subunit of the bacterial ribosome to inhibit bacterial protein synthesis. It is therefore bacteriostatic against most organisms, but at high concentrations it is bactericidal against *Haemophilus influenzae* and *Neisseria meningitidis* and some streptococci.

Chloramphenicol is a broad-spectrum antibiotic, active against most Gram-positive bacteria, anaerobic streptococci, Gram-negative bacteria, branching bacteria (*Actinomyces israelii*) and some mycobacteria.

Acquired resistance

Resistance is widespread, largely plasmid-mediated, and readily transferred between species.

Pharmacokinetics

Chloramphenicol is well absorbed from the intestinal tract, and intravenous and topical ophthalmic preparations are available. It is well distributed throughout the body, including the cerebrospinal fluid and the eye. The serum half-life is 1–3 hours. It is inactivated by hepatic glucuronide conjugation, then excreted by glomerular filtration with some active tubular secretion.

Adverse effects

Chloramphenicol causes the following adverse effects:

- Bone marrow suppression
- Grey baby syndrome
- Optic neuritis
- Ototoxicity

Bone marrow suppression is the most important toxic effect of chloramphenicol. There are two types: an idiopathic aplastic anaemia with pancytopenia (incidence 1 in 24,500 to 1 in 40,800) with a high mortality rate, and more commonly a dose-related and reversible marrow depression.

Grey baby syndrome results from reversible myocardial dysfunction causing circulatory collapse. This is seen in premature neonates who have very high serum levels of chloramphenicol. It has a mortality rate of 50%, but survivors recover 24–48 hours after chloramphenicol is stopped.

Chloramphenicol inhibits the activity of several liver enzymes, and concomitant administration may result in elevated levels of tolbutamide and phenytoin.

Chloramphenicol is rarely used systemically except in patients with meningitis and with severe proven penicillin allergy. Mostly it is administered as a topical preparation for eye infections.

Fusidanes
Example – fusidic acid

Mechanism of action

Fusidanes are a group of naturally occurring antibiotics that inhibit bacterial cell protein synthesis. They are active against most Gram-positive bacteria (including MRSA) and Gram-negative cocci. Tolerance rapidly develops if they are used as monotherapy.

Pharmacokinetics

Fusidic acid is well absorbed following oral administration. 95% is protein-bound. It penetrates pus and wound exudates well and achieves high concentrations in brain abscess cavities, although it does not enter the cerebrospinal fluid. Levels in bone and joint are high following either IV or oral administration. It is eliminated by liver metabolism and biliary excretion, with a half-life of 9 hours. Fusidic acid is reserved for severe staphylococcal sepsis, in combination with a second anti-staphylococcal agent.

Adverse effects

Fusidic acid may cause abnormal liver function, jaundice and thrombophlebitis.

Quinolones

Examples – ciprofloxacin, levofloxacin, ofloxacin, moxifloxacin

The quinolones are synthetic antimicrobials having a dual ring structure based on the 4-quinolone nucleus, and are closely related to nalidixic acid.

Mechanism of action

Quinolones inhibit bacterial DNA-gyrase, which promotes the supercoiling of double-stranded DNA. Quinolones are particularly potent against Gram-negative bacteria, including the Enterobacteriaceae (*E. coli, Klebsiella aerogenes, Salmonella typhimurium* etc.), *Haemophilus influenzae* and *Neisseria* spp. Quinolones are also active against *Pseudomonas aeruginosa* (not moxifloxacin) and related species, *Legionella pneumophila* and *Chlamydia* spp.

Acquired resistance

Acquired resistance is uncommon but increasing. Four mechanisms are known:
- Altered target site (DNA-gyrase enzyme)
- Protection of target site (this is a plasmid-mediated resistance mechanism and is therefore potentially readily transmissible)
- Reduced permeability of bacterial cell
- Active efflux of the quinolones from the bacterium

Reduced bacterial permeability to the quinolones also reduces susceptibility to β-lactams. Resistance is common in *S. aureus* (including MRSA) and is also seen in *Pseudomonas aeruginosa* and some Enterobacteriaceae (including ESBL and carbapenemase-producing strains).

Ciprofloxacin

Ciprofloxacin is active against the vast majority of Gram-negative aerobic bacteria, including *Pseudomonas* and *Legionella* species. Aerobic Gram-positive bacteria and mycobacteria are generally moderately susceptible. Ciprofloxacin is active against *Chlamydia* spp., *Rickettsia* spp., *Coxiella* spp. and *Plasmodium falciparum*. There is little activity against most spirochaetes.

Most quinolones have a similar pharmacokinetic profile. Ciprofloxacin is readily absorbed, with a bioavailability of 80%. Tissue penetration is generally good except for cerebrospinal fluid, even with inflamed meninges. Prostatic tissue levels are approximately twice those in the plasma. Ciprofloxacin is inactivated in the liver and excreted in the urine and faeces, but 70% is excreted unchanged. There is active tubular secretion. The elimination half-life is about 4–5 hours. 11% is also excreted by direct transepithelial elimination into the intestinal tract.

Adverse effects include gastrointestinal symptoms; headache, dizziness, insomnia; arthralgia, acute interstitial nephritis; leucopenia, eosinophilia, thrombocytosis and thrombocytopenia; and hypersensitivity reactions. Ciprofloxacin inhibits cytochrome P450, resulting in increased serum concentrations of some drugs, including theophylline and caffeine. There is a strong association between quinolone use and *C. difficile* infection.

Ofloxacin and levofloxacin

Ofloxacin has a similar activity to ciprofloxacin but the longer half-life allows once-daily administration. It is mainly excreted in the urine. Levofloxacin is an isomer of ofloxacin. The main benefit is slightly superior activity against *Streptococcus* pneumonia.

Nitroimidazoles

Example – metronidazole

Mechanism of action

Nitroimidazoles are synthetic antimicrobials that act by destroying DNA. They are only active when the nitro group is in the reduced form induced by the very low redox values achieved by anaerobic bacteria and some protozoa. Nitroimidazoles are only active against anaerobes, some micro-aerophilic bacteria (*Helicobacter pylori*) and certain protozoa.

Acquired resistance

Resistance in *Helicobacter pylori* is thought to be due to the redox potential internally not being low enough. Resistance in anaerobic bacteria is very rare. Some strains of *C. difficile* have shown reduced susceptibility to metronidazole in recent years.

Metronidazole

Metronidazole is active against anaerobes (*Peptococcus* spp., *Clostridium* spp., *Bacteroides* spp., fusobacteria), micro-aerophilic organisms (*Helicobacter pylori, Gardnerella vaginalis*), protozoa (*Entamoeba histolytica, Giardia intestinalis, Trichomonas vaginalis*) and a few helminths.

Oral metronidazole is rapidly absorbed, almost completely. Bioavailability is 60–80% when given rectally. Only 20% is protein-bound. It is widely distributed in body tissues, including cerebrospinal fluid, pleural fluid, breast milk, saliva, vaginal secretions, abscess cavities and the prostate. The elimination half-life is 6–10 hours, and 60–80% is excreted in the urine.

The adverse effects of metronidazole include central nervous (headache, dizziness, confusion, depression, incoordination and peripheral neuropathy); gastrointestinal (nausea, vomiting, abdominal discomfort and diarrhoea); haematological (neutropenia and thrombocytopenia). It has a metallic taste, and may cause intrauterine mutation. Metronidazole gives a disulfiram-type reaction with alcohol, enhances warfarin anticoagulation, and impairs phenytoin and lithium clearance. Concomitant administration of cimetidine increases plasma metronidazole.

Metronidazole elevates lithium and digoxin levels and interferes with the effectiveness of the contraceptive pill.

Rifamycins

Example – rifampicin

Mechanism of action

Rifamycins specifically inhibit bacterial DNA-dependent RNA polymerase, preventing the transcription of RNA from the DNA template. Eukaryotic RNA polymerase is unaffected. They have indications beyond antituberculous therapy due to their wider spectrum of action than other antimycobacterial agents.

Rifamycins are particularly active against Gram-positive bacteria, Gram-negative cocci and mycobacteria. Resistance is rapid, so combination therapy is essential. Penetration of rifampicin into soft tissue and bone has made it an excellent compound for the treatment of difficult orthopaedic infections caused by staphylococci, including prosthetic joint infections. Intracellular penetration makes it a useful adjunct in treatment of patients with *Legionella* infection and Q fever (*Coxiella burnetti*).

Pharmacokinetics

Rifampicin is well absorbed following oral administration. 80% is protein-bound. Rifampicin is distributed throughout the body, including cerebrospinal fluid, bone, tears, saliva, abscesses and ascitic fluid. The plasma half-life is 4 hours. Elimination is mainly by liver metabolism, producing an active metabolite. The urine turns an orange-red colour.

Adverse effects

Rifampicin is well tolerated but may cause:

- Hypersensitivity reactions
- Gastrointestinal effects
- Hepatotoxicity
- Thrombocytopenia
- Acute renal failure
- Influenza syndrome

Rifampicin induces liver microsomal enzymes, increasing the rate of metabolism of the contraceptive pill, corticosteroids, anticoagulants, digoxin, quinidine and tolbutamide.

Trimethoprim
Mechanism of action

Trimethoprim inhibits dihydrofolate reductase, the enzyme catalysing the conversion of folinic acid to folic acid. It therefore indirectly inhibits DNA synthesis. Trimethoprim is active against many Gram-negative bacteria, including most enterobacteria, *Haemophilus influenzae* and *Bordetella*. It has moderate activity against Gram-positives, including MRSA and streptococci. *Enterococcus faecalis* can utilise preformed folinic acid and becomes relatively resistant if the patient receives supplements containing folinic acid. Anaerobes are intrinsically resistant. Trimethoprim is active against some non-bacterial pathogens.

Acquired resistance

Resistance is increasingly common. The mechanisms are:
- Modification of target enzyme
- Altered metabolic pathway
- Reduced cell-membrane permeability

Plasmid-coded synthesis of a mutant enzyme is probably the most important mechanism, and enables easy inter-species transfer.

Pharmacokinetics

Trimethoprim is almost insoluble in water, and is rapidly absorbed from the gastrointestinal tract. 42% of the drug is protein-bound. Trimethoprim is extensively distributed in the body, and reaches cerebrospinal fluid and prostatic tissue. Excretion is almost entirely renal, with about 70% excreted in the first 24 hours. Trimethoprim is a weak base, so elimination is facilitated by acidic urine.

Adverse effects

Adverse effects are due to folate deficiency. This can be offset by giving a folate supplement, which the bacterium cannot use.

Sulphonamides

Examples – sulphadiazine, sulphadimidine

Mechanism of action

Sulphonamides inhibit folic acid synthesis (at an earlier stage than trimethoprim). Sulphonamides inhibit the incorporation of para-aminobenzoic acid (PABA) into folinic acid, and therefore indirectly inhibit DNA synthesis. Sulphonamides are broad-spectrum agents, active against Gram-positive and Gram-negative bacteria and some protozoa (*Toxoplasma gondii* and *Plasmodium* spp.). When combined with trimethoprim (co-trimoxazole) it is the treatment of choice for *Pneumocystis* pneumonia (PCP).

Acquired resistance

This is very common, with complete cross-resistance between sulphonamides. Of *Neisseria meningitidis* in the UK, 15% is resistant, and most species of Enterobacteriaceae are now resistant.

Pharmacokinetics

Sulphonamides are well absorbed from the intestine and are widely distributed around the body, including cerebrospinal fluid and the eye. Elimination is mainly by hepatic acetylation, but some oxidation and glucuronidation occurs. The parent compound and metabolites are excreted in the urine.

Adverse effects

Sulphonamides cause renal damage, rashes and bone marrow depression, and they interfere with fetal bilirubin transport. Older sulphonamides cause crystalluria. Newer sulphonamides produce a hypersensitivity reaction resulting in tubular necrosis or vasculitis. Rarely, they may cause Stevens–Johnson syndrome, which is often fatal. Sulphonamides cross the placenta, increase free plasma bilirubin and may cause kernicterus. Sulphonamides compete for plasma protein binding sites to affect oral anticoagulants and oral hypoglycaemic agents.

Antimycobacterials

Examples – ethambutol, isoniazid, pyrazinamide

These drugs are used specifically for their antimycobacterial action. Some aminoglycosides, quinolones and macrolides are also active against mycobacteria.

Ethambutol

Ethambutol inhibits the synthesis of arabinogalactan, a cell-wall polysaccharide. It is employed in combination with other agents when resistance is suspected. The most important side effect is optic neuritis, which can be irreversible.

Isoniazid

Isoniazid inhibits mycolic acid synthesis. Resistance is common but toxicity is unusual. The neurological effects can be minimised by using pyridoxine (vitamin B_6). Isoniazid forms part of all standard anti-tuberculous regimes.

Pyrazinamide

Pyrazinamide is bactericidal and resistance is uncommon. It is particularly active against intracellular bacilli. It is usually well tolerated, but uric acid excretion may be inhibited, resulting in gout. It is a component of all modern short-course anti-tuberculous regimes.

Antivirals

The main mechanisms of action of antiviral agents are:

- Direct inactivation of virus prior to cell attachment and entry
- Blocking viral attachment to host cell membranes
- Blocking virus uncoating
- Preventing integration of virus into the host cell membrane
- Blocking transcription or translation into viral messenger RNA

- Interfering with glycosylation steps, viral assembly and release

Currently most compounds in clinical use are nucleoside analogues that block nucleic acid metabolism. They include the anti-herpesvirus agents (e.g. aciclovir), the broad-spectrum antiviral ribavirin, and the anti-HIV agents zidovudine, stavudine and didanosine.

Two agents that are active against influenza virus are amantadine and rimantadine. They appear to prevent acidification of the virus interior, required to allow fusion of the viral envelope to the endosome, which normally leads to the release of viral RNA.

Human α-interferon is produced by recombinant DNA technology using *E. coli*. It renders cells resistant to infection by a wide range of viruses. Its main clinical use is the treatment of some cases of hepatitis B and hepatitis C.

Principles of antimicrobial stewardship

According to the Infectious Diseases Society of America (IDSA):

Antimicrobial stewardship refers to coordinated interventions designed to improve and measure the appropriate use of antimicrobials by promoting the selection of the optimal antimicrobial drug regimen, dose, duration of therapy, and route of administration.

Given the rise in antimicrobial resistance, good antimicrobial stewardship is a vital component in the battle to preserve the efficacy of existing antimicrobial agents. Strict adherence to departmental, hospital and national guidelines is required, and audit of compliance with guidelines is routinely performed by hospital pharmacists in conjunction with medical microbiologists.

Patients receiving antibiotic therapy should have their treatment reviewed regularly (on a daily basis if a hospital inpatient). As well as clinical parameters for measuring response to treatment there is an increasing trend for the use of biomarkers such as C-reactive protein and procalcitonin. The latter is particularly effective in the monitoring of the inflammatory response to bacterial infection and has led to reduced duration of antibacterial therapy in critical care and other hospital departments.

Antimicrobial prophylaxis in surgery

Most antibiotic prophylaxis is prescribed and administered by anaesthetists in line with a range of guidelines, usually locally produced but based on information provided by national or international bodies such as IDSA and the Scottish Intercollegiate Guidelines Network (SIGN), as well as by various UK colleges and societies covering specific areas including orthopaedics, obstetrics and gynaecology.

In the UK the SIGN guideline on *Antibiotic Prophylaxis in Surgery* is the principal reference, most recently updated in June 2014. It should be noted that this guideline does not cover anticipated infection in patients undergoing emergency surgery for contaminated or dirty operations or transplant surgery.

The principles governing antimicrobial prophylaxis are essentially the same for most procedures, namely: short duration (usually a single dose except in exceptional circumstances), given at a time and dose which allows for peak serum and tissue levels to be achieved for the duration of surgery. The choice of agent should ensure cover against the most likely bacterial pathogens to be encountered. Note that this latter consideration should also take into account the results of screening (e.g. for MRSA) and previous microbiology reports.

References and further reading

Infectious Diseases Society of America. Promoting antimicrobial stewardship in human medicine. www.idsociety.org/Stewardship_Policy (accessed 20 March 2016).

Scottish Intercollegiate Guidelines Network. *Antibiotic Prophylaxis in Surgery: a National Clinical Guideline.* SIGN Publication 104. Edinburgh: SIGN, 2008, updated 2014.

CHAPTER 43
Clinical trials and basic statistics

Leon Vries and Ted Lin

Clinical trials

> The World Health Organization defines a **clinical trial** as any research study that prospectively assigns human participants or groups of humans to one or more health-related interventions to evaluate the effects on health outcomes.

As the above definition states, this should be a prospective process in which the participants or subjects are identified and randomised at the start of the study and subsequently followed forward in time. Data are gathered, evaluated and analysed, and the results may then be published in a peer-reviewed journal.

Clinical trials can be used to compare diagnostic criteria or treatments for a specific disease. Alternatively they may also be used more generally to investigate the effects of preventive measures, behavioural patterns or lifestyle factors on health.

Types of trial
Phased clinical trials
Phase I trials
After drugs have been tested on animals, valuable information on safety and efficacy will have been obtained.

> In **phase I trials** a new drug is tested for the first time on humans. Therefore, they are often referred to as 'first in man studies'.

People who participate in phase I trials may be healthy volunteers or people who failed to respond to conventional treatments. The groups are typically small, and the dosing regime is often determined at this stage by looking at the side-effect profile and the metabolism of the new drug. A maximum tolerated dose (MTD) is usually ascertained. A substantial number of new drugs never make it past this stage and are not investigated further.

Fundamentals of Anaesthesia, 4th edition, ed. Ted Lin, Tim Smith and Colin Pinnock. Published by Cambridge University Press. © Cambridge University Press 2017.

Phase II trials

After the maximum dose and safety have been established in phase I trials, the investigators may move to a phase II trial.

> In **phase II trials** the main aim is to establish the efficacy of a treatment by starting small groups of patients on different dosing regimes. The patients may or may not be randomised at this point.

The feasibility and subsequent design of a larger phase III trial is determined at this stage if the results of the phase II trial are positive.

Phase III trials

This stage of trial is commonly known as a randomised controlled trial (RCT). It uses the information about dosing and efficacy obtained in the phase I and II trials.

> In a **phase III trial** the aim is to determine the effectiveness of the new intervention against a control group. The control-group patients may receive the conventional or standard treatment, a placebo, or no treatment at all.

The process of randomisation is designed to ensure that all participants have the same likelihood of ending in any of the groups.

Another difference is the size of patient groups in a phase III trial. They are much larger than the phase I and II trials and, generally speaking, the larger the groups, the more reliable the outcome of the study. Due to their size and complexity, these trials often take years to complete.

Quite often, the required number of patients is so large that a multicentre effort is necessary. If a study included a comparison of the complication rates between two techniques, and the rate of the complication in question was very low, a multicentre trial would be required to generate sufficient numbers in order to obtain a statistically significant result. Multicentre trials invariably carry a higher cost and require an increased organisational effort. Inter-centre differences in practice may result in protocol violation bias, and a robust universal study protocol must guard against this.

Following a phase III trial, a drug licence may be granted. The licence is time-limited and, additionally, new drugs are kept under heightened surveillance using the yellow card system as denoted by a black triangle in the BNF and via online reporting to the MHRA.

Phase IV trials

> **Phase IV trials** are also called post-marketing or surveillance studies. They are designed to monitor the long-term safety and efficacy of the new intervention.

Uncommon side effects of a new drug are sometimes only discovered at this stage, because the number of studied patients in the phase III trial was not sufficient to reveal the low incidence of a particular side effect. These types of trials are usually carried out by the pharmaceutical industry (Figure 43.1).

Figure 43.1 Phased clinical trials

Phased clinical trials			
Phase	**Size**	**Aim**	**Characteristics**
I	Small (< 30)	Find maximum safe dose and metabolism details	First time a new treatment is used on humans. No randomisation
II	Small to medium (< 100)	Establish initial efficacy of new treatment	Results are used to design phase III trial. May or may not be randomised
III	Large (100–1000s)	Establish whether new treatment is better than control intervention	Randomised. Control group (conventional treatment, no treatment or placebo)
IV	Large	Monitor long-term safety and efficacy	Post-marketing or surveillance studies. No control group

Crossover studies

> A **crossover study** is a longitudinal (non-parallel) trial where the patient receives each of the study interventions.

Patients are typically randomised to receive a certain sequence of treatments. It is imperative that the treatment or intervention is of rapid offset and short duration, otherwise the effect of a treatment may be 'carried over' into the next treatment phase and interfere with that treatment. Also the order in which the treatments are delivered may have an influence on outcome. Despite these two limitations, crossover studies are not so much influenced by confounding variables because, in effect, each patient acts as his or her own control. Furthermore, statistical analysis of these paired data is relatively straightforward and powerful.

The most appropriate groups of patients for crossover studies are those with chronic conditions.

Cohort, cross-sectional and case–control studies

In simple terms, a cohort is a group of people who share some characteristic. These people can be followed, either prospectively or retrospectively, and a correlation between exposure or characteristic and the disorder can be established.

In cross-sectional studies the proportion of people with a disorder is compared to the proportion of people who are exposed to a risk factor or not at a specific point in time.

Case–control studies compare groups of patients with and without the disorder and look at the number in each group that were exposed to a certain factor.

Meta-analyses and systematic reviews

> The limitations of a small trial could include lack of power and showing no difference in treatment effect where one actually exists. This is addressed by a **meta-analysis**. The main aim of a meta-analysis is to maximise the statistical precision of the effect of a particular intervention. Meta-analyses often form the basis of a wider systematic review of a subject.

It is vitally important to ensure that only methodically sound and well-conducted trials are included in a meta-analysis. The results of the trials are typically expressed as odds ratios with 95% confidence intervals. All trials to be included should be 'weighted' for the standard error of the relative risk. Trials with small standard errors generally have narrow confidence intervals and as a result carry a heavy weight. Only when all this is in place should the quantitative results from the individual studies be combined into a single value.

Limitations from meta-analyses mainly come from the potential for bias. Investigators may include or exclude certain trials, and reviewers and editors, both of the source journals and those assessing the meta-analysis, may be more inclined to accept studies showing positive findings (publication bias).

For further discussion of this topic, see *Systematic reviews*, at the end of this chapter.

Trial design

There are fundamental differences between the designs of phase I, II and III trials. In the first two phases, dosing regimes, safety and efficacy have been established, and in phase III trials it is of pivotal importance that the trial starts with a clearly defined main objective and corresponding outcome measure, including the statistical analysis to be used. These issues, which should be addressed from the start, will now be considered in further detail.

Sample size

> The **sample size** for a phase III trial is usually established early on in the trial design and is based on a power analysis.

The sample size is calculated to maximise the chance of finding a statistical difference between treatment groups, where a real difference exists. The analysis is usually based on information obtained in phase I or II trials or in pilot studies, and it must therefore take account of the small sample sizes of those studies. Other considerations are the expected effects in the new treatment and in the conventional or placebo group. Estimates derived from these small initial studies are frequently too optimistic, due to the fact that they are not randomised and have a huge potential for bias.

The power of a study is the likelihood of the null hypothesis being rejected correctly. This is given as $1 - \beta$, where β is the probability of making a type II error, or accepting a false negative hypothesis. A power of 0.9 for a study is good, giving a 90% chance of demonstrating a difference when it is present ($\beta = 0.1$, giving a 10% chance of accepting a false negative or making a type II error). A minimally acceptable level of power is 0.8, as this equates to an 80% chance of detecting a statistical difference, where such a difference truly exists. When designing a study, its power is selected according to other factors in the trial (see *Types of error*, below).

Variability

Variability in the interpretation of the outcome measures can reduce the chance of finding a statistically significant difference. Both inter- and intra-observer variability are well-recognised sources of error. Taking repeated measurements could produce a pooled value for the variable, which might be a better reflection of the true value.

Another source of variability arises from the selection criteria of the groups. When strict and highly selective criteria are used, it will produce a group with little variability, whereas if the group is selected with few and wide criteria, variability will be high. It could be more difficult to find a statistically significant result in the latter group. On the other hand, a highly selective group will make it easier to find a difference, but the result may apply only to this specific group of patients, and it may not be possible to extrapolate to a wider population.

Bias

The validity of the results of a trial depends heavily on its ability to eliminate bias. Bias is inherent in human nature and is often difficult to eliminate entirely. With the correct application of appropriate techniques, the study groups can be kept as similar as possible. If bias has been eliminated it is more likely that a true result will be obtained. If not, the result might reflect either over- or under-reporting of the difference between the groups. Bias may be outside the investigators' instigation. Researchers may inadvertently favour particular observations or changes. One source of bias is the analysis of ongoing cumulative data, which may cause a study to be terminated once a statistically significant result has been obtained. The most common types of bias are summarised in Figure 43.2.

Randomisation

> Meticulous **randomisation** ensures that every participant in the trial has exactly the same chance of ending up in any of the groups. Acceptable methods of achieving this include computer-generated random numbers, flipping a coin or rolling dice.

Allocation on the basis of year of birth, hospital number, day of admission or alternating allocation can all lead to selection bias.

Figure 43.2 Examples of bias in clinical trials

Type of bias	Description
Selection bias	Systematic difference in acceptance or rejection for inclusion in trial. Systematic difference in assignment of treatment
Ascertainment bias	Patient or investigator knows which treatment is administered
Allocation bias	The investigator allocates a patient to the group that he feels might benefit the patient most
Dropout/withdrawal bias	Dropout may be more frequent in one group
Protocol violation bias	Failure to follow protocol (for example on missing data)
Inappropriate crossover design bias	Curable or lethal conditions are inappropriate for this type of trial
Publication bias	Tendency to submit and publish trials with positive findings
Time-lag bias	Studies with positive findings are published more quickly
Potential breakthrough bias	Overemphasis of a positive finding while ignoring a previous negative finding

Despite the use of acceptable randomisation techniques, groups may become different during the course of the trial, and the use of block or stratified randomisation can minimise this phenomenon.

- The number of patients in each group is kept closely together by allocation of patients in 'blocks' of equal numbers. In any block the same number of patients will be allocated to each group.
- To minimise the differences in age, sex and other characteristics, stratified randomisation will put patients in blocks for each variable, thus ensuring equal distribution of these characteristics across all groups.

Blinding

Ascertainment bias may occur if the patients and/or the investigators know which arm of the study they are in. The process of blinding tries to eliminate this source of bias. In a single-blind trial only the investigator knows which group the patient is allocated to. Ideally, neither the patients nor the investigators are aware of the treatment identity (double-blind trial).

Despite the fact that many trials claim to be double-blinded, some of them are not truly so. For example, the effect or the side effect of the treatment may be apparent to the investigator, or even to the patient, thus resulting in ascertainment bias.

Trial implementation

Ethical approval

All clinical trials require prior review and approval by an ethics committee. The most important function of this committee is to ensure protection of the potential subjects of medical research. The committee can be at national, regional or local level, and it consists of medical and lay members.

An application for approval should consist of a thorough explanation of the trial. This should include a demonstration of the potential benefits, a trial protocol, previously published relevant papers and a description of the trial that is to be handed to patients. The explanation should detail the possible benefits and side effects and/or complications. This information forms the basis for the consent form to the trial, which is to be signed by the investigator and the patient.

The committee might either reject or approve the application, or it might request changes to be made to the trial design prior to approval.

Data collection

Included in the study protocol should be the method of data collection and interpretation to be used. The data could be in various formats, such as answers to questionnaires, physiological variables, laboratory results or pain scores. Ideally, these should be entered into an electronic database. For small trials with relatively few data, a spreadsheet could be used. For larger, multicentre trials, commercially available databases are more appropriate.

There are several ways to minimise the potential errors in data collection:

- Firstly, there should be clear guidelines regarding the variables to be measured, and investigators should be able to access a study protocol manual for reference.
- Secondly, a brief synopsis of the guidelines printed on the forms to be used could avoid errors. Closed questions with yes or no answers are preferable to open questions, which could be open to interpretation.
- Thirdly, the data collectors should have had adequate training in the data collection process.

A brief test period prior to the start of the clinical trial could highlight any pitfalls or mistakes in the protocol.

All machines, monitors and laboratory equipment to be used in the trial should be checked and calibrated regularly in accordance with the manufacturers' instructions.

Data analysis

Again, the method of data analysis to be used should be set out in the trial design. Investigators should ensure that the statistical tests to be used are appropriate for the type of data. It is sensible to seek expert statistical help at the time of the trial design.

There are sometimes a number of patients who at some point may be excluded from the trial. They may develop morbidity or complications, which may preclude them from further participation. Non-compliance of the patient may also lead to exclusion. It is important that the number of patients eliminated from the trial is mentioned and explained in the publication of data.

End of trial

The trial can end by stopping the recruitment of new patients or by ending follow-up. It should be detailed in the study protocol when and how a trial will end. Sometimes, the ethics committee that granted approval for the trial requires notification when a study finishes. At times, trials are temporarily stopped or even closed early because of unacceptable side effects or when it is plainly obvious that a real benefit exists.

Presentation of results

When results are obtained from the processed data, these can be presented at a local level or at national or international meetings, or they can be published in peer-reviewed scientific journals. Investigators should review their data critically and truthfully and adhere to the manuscript guidelines of the relevant journal. The manuscript should contain a detailed description of the trial design, so that readers can validate the procedures and statistical analysis used.

The authorship is an important issue. An author should have been involved with the trial design, implementation, data analysis and drawing of conclusions. The conclusions and implications of the study should be discussed, and this should be related to previously published relevant articles. Also, social and financial implications must be discussed, and whether the patients and circumstances in the study are widely applicable to the general population.

Basic statistics

A knowledge of statistics is required in designing studies for research, analysing the data collected in studies, and writing for publication – as well as for the critical assessment of published research work. Statistical techniques are also a key component of evidence-based medicine, used in systematic reviews and meta-analysis. The remainder of this chapter reviews the application of statistical methods in:

- Describing data
- Collecting data
- Testing and interpreting data

Data description

Types of data

Data are obtained by recording measurements or observations, and can be classified into different types.

> Data may consist of numbers (**numerical data**) or group names/labels (**categorical data**). It is important to choose the appropriate statistical test to suit the type of data.

Numerical data

Obtained from measurements (e.g. height, weight) or counts (e.g. number of operations, number of children). Numerical data can be divided into continuous and discrete data:

- *Continuous data* – can take any value over the range measured, depending only on the accuracy of the measurement device.
- *Discrete data* – can only take whole-number or integer values.

Categorical data

Consists of group names or labels. Categorical data can be further divided into unordered and ordered data.

- *Unordered* – the data come from groups which are mutually exclusive and not ordered in any way, e.g. blood group (A, B, O), sex (M, F, other).
- *Ordered* – the data groups are mutually exclusive and also ordered or ranked, e.g. socioeconomic class, staging of a disease.

Displaying data

Raw data usually consist of a collection of numbers and labels (Figures 43.3 and 43.4).

Graphical display gives a visual summary of the data. Graphs and charts are useful in characterising data because:

Figure 43.3 Numerical data for noradrenaline infusion in a patient

Noradrenaline infusion rate (mL h^{-1})	1.1	2.3	3.0	4.5	5.2	6.7
Mean BP (mmHg)		56	78	80	88	87	90

Figure 43.4 Categorical data for two postoperative analgesics

Postoperative pain at 4 hours	none	mild	moderate	severe
Group 1	23	11	9	2
Group 2	31	6	6	0

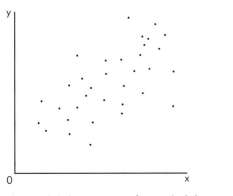

Figure 43.5 Scattergram of numerical data

Occurrence of ABO blood groups in the UK

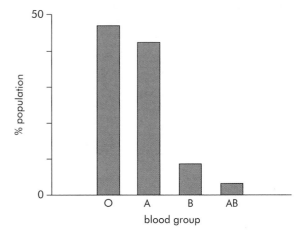

Figure 43.7 Bar chart of categorical data

Use of anaesthetic agents 2015 – 2016 St Elsewhere Hospital

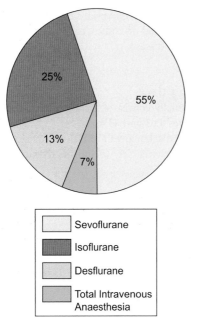

Figure 43.6 Pie chart of categorical data

Frequency distribution for body weight in a sample of 120 people

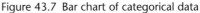

Figure 43.8 Histogram – frequency distribution of continuous numerical data

- With a small number of points a relationship can be sought between the independent (x) and dependent (y) variable.
- With a large number of data points, grouping the data points into categories or ranges enables the distribution to be visualised.

Figures 43.5 to 43.8 illustrate some common types of graph. Small numbers of numerical data, plotting y against x, can be displayed as a *scattergram* (Figure 43.5). Larger numbers of categorical data can be plotted as a *pie chart* (Figure 43.6). A *bar chart* can also be used to represent categorical data. Figure 43.7

illustrates the occurrence of blood groups in the UK, by plotting the percentage of population for each blood group. Sometimes continuous numerical data can be plotted as a *histogram* (a form of bar chart in which the area of each bar is proportional to the number of observations) in order to produce a frequency distribution (Figure 43.8).

Frequency distributions

Plotting numbers of data points in each category for categorical data produces a histogram showing the *frequency distribution*. Continuous numerical data may also be represented in this way by dividing the variable into ranges and plotting the frequency of data points occurring in each range. Figure 43.8 shows body weights for a sample of people. In this sample the number of people in each range (vertical axis) is plotted against body weight (horizontal axis). The following points can be made about frequency distributions:

- The area under a frequency distribution is proportional to the total number of data points (total number of people) in a sample.
- For large samples or whole populations the frequency distribution tends towards a smooth curve.
- A frequency distribution can be normalised by converting frequencies to relative frequencies, dividing each frequency by the total number of points in the sample. This makes comparisons between samples easier.

> When sample sizes are large the normalised frequency distribution approximates to the *probability density* function for the population.

Probability

Statistical methods are required because of biological variation between individuals. We cannot obtain black and white answers from our interpretation of data, we can only obtain a probability of a value being representative for a population, or for a hypothesis being true or false.

> **Probability** is usually expressed as a number from 0 to 1. If the probability of an event occurring is 0 it will not occur, and if the probability is 1 the event is certain to occur.

- In any individual, the probability of death occurring in their lifetime is 1 ($P = 1$).
- The probability of 'heads' occurring when a coin is tossed is 0.5 ($P = 0.5$).
- The probability of being blood group B in the UK is 0.08 ($P = 0.08$).

It is often useful to plot the probabilities for a variable having a specific value or falling into a particular category, as this gives an overall view of how the variable is distributed throughout the population. This curve is called a *probability density curve*.

Probability density curves

A probability density curve plots the probability of occurrence (probability density) against the value of variable for a population. Frequency distribution curves for samples from a whole population approximate to the probability density curve if the frequencies are converted to relative frequencies and the sample numbers are large.

Probability density curves are useful in describing the distribution of data values in populations. Naturally occurring data tend to follow recognised probability density curves, which can be defined by characteristic equations. These equations represent families of curves which depend on the values of parameters in the equations.

Probability density curves can also be derived for statistical parameters such as t and χ^2. These parameters are sometimes simply referred to as statistics, and are calculated from the data obtained in research studies. Such curves enable probabilities to be derived for specific values of the parameters. These probabilities (or P-numbers) are the end product, when data are statistically tested for the null hypothesis (see below).

A probability density curve has the following properties:

- The height of the curve at any point equals the probability of that value of x occurring.
- The maximum height of the curve cannot be greater than 1.
- The area under the curve between any two values of x equals the probability of x occurring in that range of values.
- The total area under the curve equals 1, since the curve covers all probabilities for the variable x.

Recognised probability density curves
Normal distribution

> The **normal distribution** is the most common probability density curve in biological data. It is based on the idea of a representative or average value for a population, and is a symmetrical bell-shaped curve.

The normal distribution describes many numerical variables – e.g. blood pressure, body temperature, body weight, haemoglobin level – and it is central to many statistical methods. The curve is defined by its mean value (μ) and its standard deviation (σ). Figure 43.9 shows two normal distributions with different mean values μ_1 and μ_2 ($\mu_2 > \mu_1$), and different standard deviations σ_1 and σ_2 ($\sigma_2 < \sigma_1$).

For example, consider plotting a probability density curve for systolic BP, over the whole population in the UK (this can only be approximated to by taking a very large sample). If the probability density is plotted against systolic BP, a normal distribution curve is obtained (Figure 43.10). The mean, mode and median are 120 mmHg. There are much lower probabilities for pressures 180 mmHg or

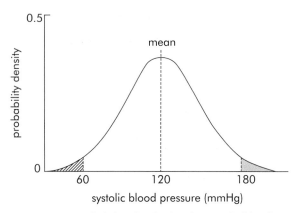

Figure 43.10 Probability distribution for systolic blood pressure

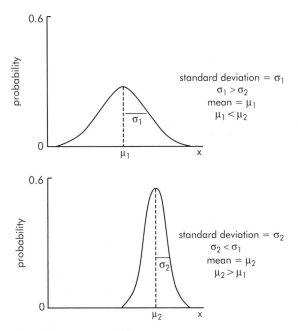

Figure 43.9 Normal distribution

Binomial distribution

These curves describe the probability distribution of proportions. Proportions occur in a sample in which a binary variable is recorded. Binary variables only have two possible values or states, e.g. 0 or 1, dead or alive, diseased or disease-free, ventilated or spontaneously breathing. Consider recording deaths in a sample (n) of ICU admissions. A number (r) will have died and a number ($n - r$) survive. These curves plot probability against the number of individuals (r) with the chosen outcome. The binomial distribution curves alter shape according to the total number (n) of individuals in the sample, and the probability (π) of the chosen outcome occurring. Figure 43.11 shows a binomial distribution plotting probability against r. It is skewed for $\pi < 0.5$ or $\pi > 0.5$ and becomes symmetrical at $\pi = 0.5$. The shape of the distribution curve also varies with n and tends towards a normal distribution as n increases (> 40).

Poisson distribution

This is used to describe the probability distribution of rates of occurrence, e.g. the respiratory rate of a patient (breaths per minute), the number of ICU admissions per week, the incidence of prostatic cancer per year. The Poisson distribution plots probability against the rate of events occurring. These probability density curves only depend on the average rate of events recorded over a period of time (μ). The distribution is skewed for low values of μ (< 10), but tends towards a normal distribution when μ is high (> 20) (Figure 43.12).

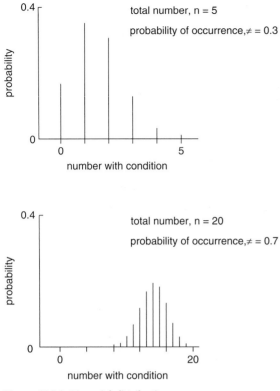

Figure 43.11 Binomial distribution

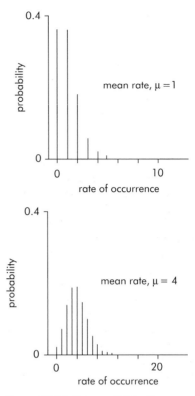

Figure 43.12 Poisson distribution

60 mmHg occurring. These occur in the outermost portions of the curve, called the *tails*. The shaded area equals the probability of systolic blood pressures > 180 mmHg occurring. The hatched area equals the probability of systolic blood pressures < 60 mmHg occurring.

Describing numerical data

Consider a set of values for a variable x. The values are $x_1 + x_2 + x_3 \ldots x_n$ and have been divided into ranges and plotted as a frequency distribution in Figure 43.13. These data can then be described by two main characteristics:

- An **average** or representative value
- A measure of the **spread** of values

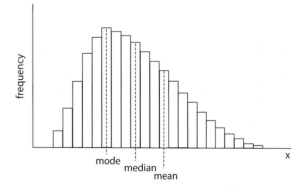

Figure 43.13 Mean, mode, median – skewed distribution

The average value

There are three choices for an average or representative value:

- *Mode* – This is the most commonly occurring value in the set of data values.

- *Median* – This is the value in the data set which has an equal number of data points above it and below it. It is sometimes called the geometrical mean, as the area above the median equals the area below.

- *Mean* – This is short for the arithmetical mean value, and is the most useful of these choices.

Calculation of mean value for a sample of n values of x

First sum all the values:

$$\text{Sum of values} = x_1 + x_2 + x_3 \ldots x_0$$

Using mathematical notation $= \sum_{i=0}^{i=n} x_i$ (abbreviated to Σx_i)

Then the mean, $m = \Sigma x_{xi}/n$

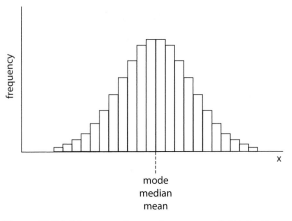

Figure 43.14 Mean, mode, median – normal distribution

In Figure 43.13 it can be seen that the frequency distribution is not symmetrical but is *skewed*. The mode, median and mean are all given by different values of x. Medical variables usually have a normal-shaped frequency distribution, which is symmetrical and has mean, mode and median values all coinciding (Figure 43.14).

The spread of values

The spread of a set of data can be calculated numerically in the case of a normal distribution, and is given by the standard deviation (s), which is derived from the variance (s^2).

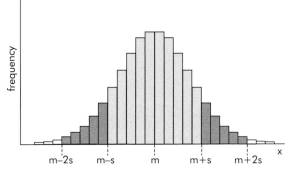

Figure 43.15 Normal distribution – m, s and $2s$

Calculation of variance (s^2)

Consider the above set of data, consisting of n values for a variable x. Then, using the above calculation, the mean, m, can be calculated. The variance is calculated from the deviations of each value from the mean and the number of degrees of freedom (DF), where DF $= n - 1$.

The deviation of each value from the mean is given by

$$\text{Deviation} = x_i - m$$
$$\text{Squared deviation} = (x_i - m)^2$$
$$\text{Sum of squared deviations} = \Sigma(x_i - m)^2$$
$$\text{Variance}(s^2) = \frac{\Sigma(x_i - m)^2}{\text{DF}} = \frac{\Sigma(x_i - m)^2}{n - 1}$$
$$\text{Standard deviation}(s) = \text{square root of variance}$$
$$= \sqrt{\frac{\Sigma(x_i - m)^2}{n - 1}}$$

In a normal distribution the **standard deviation** gives a measure of the spread of values. Figure 43.15 shows the frequency distribution for a normally distributed variable x, in which the mean value is m and the standard deviation is s. Then 68% of the values lie within the area $m \pm s$ (light shaded area), and 96% lie within $m \pm 2s$ (light and dark shaded areas). The smaller the standard deviation the more the data points cluster around the mean value, and the narrower the frequency distribution.

Sampling

Recording a number of numerical values from a whole population is known as sampling. The larger the number of data points recorded the closer the information

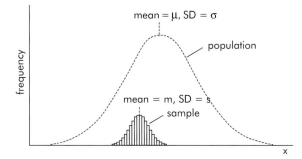

Figure 43.16 Population frequency distribution and sample frequency distribution

obtained from the sample is to the true situation for the whole population. In a population of a million people, taking a sample from 10 individuals is not likely to be as accurate in representing the whole population as sampling 1000 individuals.

In descriptive statistics a convention exists of representing sample parameters with Roman (normal) letters, but using Greek letters to represent true parameters for the whole population.

Figure 43.16 shows how a sample with mean m and standard deviation s is related to a normally distributed population with mean μ and standard deviation σ. The population frequency distribution is represented by the broken line, while the sample is represented by the smaller histogram. Note the following:

- The population distribution is shown as a smooth curve because it usually covers a very large number of individuals.
- The area of the sample histogram is small compared to the area of the population distribution curve, because the number of individuals in the sample is small compared to the population.
- The sample mean, m, is only an estimate of the true population mean, μ. It is unlikely that the sample mean will coincide with the population mean. Therefore there will be an error (error $= \mu - m$) in the estimated mean. A *standard error of the mean* (SEM) can be calculated for samples.

Standard error of the mean (SEM)

When a mean value is calculated from a sample set of data, the value obtained (m) is only an estimate of the true mean (μ). The true mean can only be calculated by measuring every value in the population. However a standard error of the mean can be calculated using the standard deviation (s) of the sample, and the number of data points in the sample (n):

$$SEM = \frac{s}{\sqrt{n}}$$

If a number of samples were to be taken from a population, each sample would provide its own estimate (m_1, m_2, ...) of the true mean (μ). These estimates (m_1, m_2, ...) would form a normal distribution centred about μ.

> The **standard error of the mean** (SEM) is the standard deviation of the distribution of sample means, and gives an idea of how close the estimated mean value is likely to be to the true mean value. In order to quantify this 'closeness', the *confidence limits* have to be calculated.

Confidence limits

When reporting a calculated mean value, it is sometimes quoted as $m \pm$ SEM. This only gives an idea of the ratio between mean value and SEM. Consider a calculated mean value

$$= m \pm SEM$$

$$= 10 \pm 2$$

It is not immediately apparent where the real mean (μ) lies in relation to the estimate (m). In order to clarify this, a *confidence interval* (CI) is determined around m, within which a reader can be confident the true mean (μ) lies. The wider the CI, the poorer the estimate. The CI is defined by two values, the *confidence limits* (CL). There is a 95% probability of the CI containing the true mean (μ). In a normally distributed sample, the confidence limits are calculated from the SEM by

Confidence limits (CL) $= \pm 1.96$ (SEM)

Thus in the above example the mean value can now be quoted as

$$m = 10(6.08, 13.92)$$

A reader then knows that the estimated mean is 10 and there is a 95% chance of the true mean lying within the range 6.08 to 13.92 (Figure 43.17).

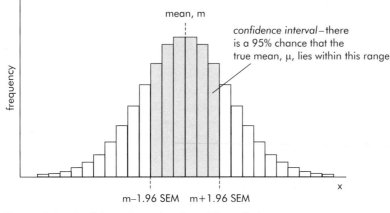

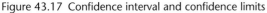

Figure 43.17 Confidence interval and confidence limits

> The **confidence interval** (CI) gives an idea of the reliability of a mean value estimated for a population from a sample. The wider the CI, the poorer the estimate.

Describing categorical data

As discussed above, categorical data take the form of variables which are labelled rather than measured. A common situation, referred to previously, is to sample a group of individuals in whom there are only two possible outcomes (categories) of interest. In such cases the data are described as binary, and the sample is considered in terms of proportions.

Proportions

Consider a group of n individuals, in whom there exist two possible categories. Let the number of individuals in one category be r, out of the total number n. This can be expressed as a proportion r/n.

For example, 10 (r) deaths occurred out of a sample of 100 (n) admissions to ICU. The proportion of deaths (p) is given by

$$p = r/n$$
Proportion of deaths $= 0.1$

Confidence limits for a proportion (p) can be obtained from

$$CL = p \pm 1.96\sqrt{p(1-p)n}$$

> ### Confidence limits and confidence interval for a proportion
>
> The concepts of *confidence limits* and *a confidence interval* can still be applied to a proportion, since proportions are obtained by sampling and follow a binomial distribution curve (see above).

Thus in the above example the confidence limits can be quoted as

$$CL = 0.1 \pm 0.0588$$

Proportion of deaths $= 0.1(0.041, 0.16)$

Contingency tables

Studies are often designed to look for differences in outcome between two or more groups of patients who have been exposed to different treatments or risk factors. The results can be conveniently displayed in a contingency table. In a contingency table the *column variable* labels each column with an outcome, while the *row variable* assigns each group to a row. In its simplest form it appears as a 2×2 table.

Consider a study examining the incidence of influenza in two groups of patients, one treated with a vaccine and the other not vaccinated. There are only two outcomes for the patients, either they catch influenza or they do not. The contingency table thus appears as in Figure 43.18.

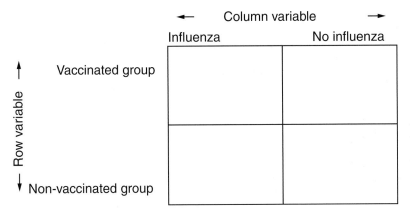

Figure 43.18 2 × 2 contingency table for influenza vaccinated and non-vaccinated groups

Larger contingency tables occur in studies examining multiple outcomes (increased number of columns) or more than two groups (increased number of rows). Contingency tables are important in the analysis of categorical data because of the use of the chi-squared test when testing non-parametric data. It should be noted, however, that many studies comparing proportions in two groups result in a 2 × 2 contingency table, which can be tested more effectively using parametric tests as described below. (see *Parametric and non-parametric tests*).

Data collection

Several different types of study can be designed. These can be broadly divided into:

- *Observational studies* – In these the investigator simply observes events occurring. Observational studies may be either cross-sectional (observations at one instant of time) or longitudinal (observations following the time course of events, e.g. plasma concentrations of a drug to determine pharmacokinetic parameters).
- *Experimental studies* – In these an investigator influences the outcome, e.g. administering a drug to observe its effect on blood pressure.

Experimental studies

Experimental studies in general may seek to relate 'cause' and 'effect' in an area of medicine, and may have been initiated by the results of a simple observational study. Many experimental studies in medicine are clinical trials which seek a specific answer by comparison, as in the comparison of the effects of two drugs, or the comparison of a drug against placebo. The results of a clinical trial may ultimately be applied in clinical practice. As discussed earlier in this chapter (see *Types of trial*), clinical trials vary in design and may be described as parallel, crossover, cohort or case–control studies.

The design of an experimental study must take account of a number of issues, which may confound its results. These include:

- *Randomisation* – This refers to the method of selecting individuals for each of the groups in a study, and it is one of the important ways of reducing bias. Randomisation is usually performed by tossing a coin, using a random number generator program in a computer, or by using random number tables.
- *Bias* – This is any systematic departure of results from the real situation, and may arise for different reasons. *Observer bias* occurs when an observer consistently under-records or over-records specific data values. *Selection bias* occurs when patients are not randomised into their study groups, or they are not representative of the population the results are to be applied to. *Publication bias* occurs when either favourable or unfavourable results are preferentially selected for publication. *Patient bias* may be introduced by patients who are trying to 'help' the investigators by only reporting positive results.
- *Sample numbers* – This is an important feature when designing a study because the size of sample groups will affect the SEMs obtained on statistical testing and can therefore determine the significance of the results. Appropriate selection of sample numbers is aided by power calculation (see below).
- *Blinding* – In a study comparing treatments and controls, observer and patient biases can be reduced by

Figure 43.19 Type I and Type II errors (H_0 = null hypothesis)

Error	Definition	Probability	Comment
Type I	False rejection of H_0	α – also significance level	Detects false difference/effect
Type II	False acceptance of H_0	β – related to power	Misses true difference/effect
		Power = $1 - \beta$	

'blinding' both patients and observers to the status of the individual patient under study. *Double blinding* means that neither the patient nor the observer knows whether the patient is a control or is receiving treatment; where only the patient can be blinded this is called *single blinding*.

- *Replication* – Measurements can be made more precise if they are repeated when made and an average taken.

Types of hypothesis

Studies often compare data collected from two groups. The question asked by such studies can be reduced to proving or rejecting a simple hypothesis. There are two types of hypothesis:

- **Null hypothesis** (H_0) – there is no difference between the two groups studied.
- **Alternative hypothesis** (H_1) – there is a difference between the groups studied.

Consider a study of two groups of subjects, one treated with a new medication and the other treated with placebo. The question to be answered is, 'Is the new medication effective?'

By convention the hypothesis to be proved or rejected is taken to be the null hypothesis. The null hypothesis states there is no difference between the groups. Thus if the null hypothesis is proved no significant difference exists between groups and the treatment is therefore ineffective. However, if the null hypothesis is rejected, then a difference exists between groups, and the treatment is effective. This leads to the definition of two types of error.

Types of error

Testing the null hypothesis leads to the definition of two types of error (Figure 43.19):

- **Type I error** – rejecting the null hypothesis when it is true (i.e. finding a false difference between groups). This is equivalent to finding a positive effect of treatment when there is none. The probability of making a type I error is also equal to α, which is used as a label for the level of significance (see below).
- **Type II error** – accepting the null hypothesis when it is untrue (i.e. missing a true difference between groups). This is equivalent to overlooking a therapeutic effect of treatment. The probability of making a type II error is called β.

Power of a study

The ability of a study to detect a difference between groups is referred to as the *power* of the study.

The **power of a study** is defined as its ability to detect a difference between groups or an effect of treatment. Since a type II error is a false detection of no difference between groups, power can be defined mathematically as the probability of not obtaining a type II error (i.e. missing a true difference):

Power of a study = $1 - \beta$

β is the probability of making a type II error. Therefore power increases as β decreases. A level of power commonly chosen for a study is 0.9 (i.e. $\beta = 0.1$).

The power of a study depends on various factors:
- *Sample size* – larger sample sizes increase study power.
- *Treatment effect* – the more effective the treatment the greater will be the difference (d) between groups, and study power will increase.

Calculating numbers of patients required in a study

Consider the common example of comparing the efficacy of two analgesics in two groups of patients using visual analogue scores (VAS). The number of patients (n) in each group required can be estimated as follows:

- Select power required, usually $1 - \beta = 0.9$ (90%). The probability of a type II error is then $\beta = 10\%$. Find percentage point (b) in normal distribution corresponding to $\beta = 10\%$ ($b = 1.28$).
- Select level of significance, usually $\alpha = 0.05$. Find percentage point (a) in normal distribution corresponding to α (e.g. for $\alpha = 0.05$, $a = 1.96$).
- Estimate variances of measurements by pilot study or from previous work (s_1^2 and s_2^2), e.g. let variance of VAS measurements in pilot study be 14, thus assume $s_1{}^2 = s_2{}^2 = 14$.
- Estimate anticipated difference in effect (d) between mean VAS scores of the two groups, using pilot study or review of literature. Alternatively select a minimum difference in mean VAS values to be detected by the study. Here let $d = 3$.

Then the number of patients in each group to be studied is given by

$$n = \frac{(a+b)^2(s_1{}^2 + s_2{}^2)}{d^2}$$

$$= \frac{(1.96 + 1.28)^2(14 + 14)}{9}$$

$$= \frac{10.5 \times 28}{9}$$

$$= 32.6$$

Therefore a minimum of 33 patients in each group is required to produce a study power of 90% with the estimated parameters and treatment effect difference suggested above. This calculation will vary according to the study design, since different values may be chosen for power, level of significance and outcome measure difference.

- *Variability of measurements* – less variability in measurements increases study power. Variability is represented by the variance of the measurements (s^2).
- *Level of significance* – a greater value for the significance level (α) increases the power of a study. Thus setting $\alpha = 0.05$ produces a more powerful study than setting $\alpha = 0.001$ (see *Level of significance*, below).

Data interpretation

P-number

However convincing data obtained by research studies may appear to be in demonstrating differences between sample groups, there is always a possibility that apparent differences are not meaningful, having arisen simply by chance. In a study, the probability of there being no difference between two groups is referred to as the *P*-number. If treatment is applied to one group and not to another group, then the lower the *P*-number the more likely that the treatment is effective.

Definition of *P*-number

By convention, statistical testing is performed to determine the probability of the null hypothesis (H_0) being true. This probability is referred to as the *P*-number or simply *P*.

If the *P*-number is less than a chosen value, called the level of significance (α), then H_0 is rejected and the differences found are accepted as being statistically significant. If the *P*-number is greater than the level of significance (α), then H_0 is accepted and there are no significant differences between groups.

In clinical research α is usually chosen as $\alpha = 0.05$, i.e. H_0 is only rejected when the probability for it being true is $\leq 5\%$.

Obtaining P-numbers

The choice of an appropriate statistical test depends on the type and form of data recorded. Statistical tests usually involve complex or repetitive arithmetic, readily performed by computers, and result in a value for a specific parameter or *statistic* depending on the test applied (e.g. a *t*-test will give a value for *t*, a χ^2 test will give a value for χ^2).

These statistics have known probability density curves. Figure 43.20 shows probability density curves for *t*. Different curves are produced by differing *degrees of freedom* (DF). The DF relates to the number of data points in each

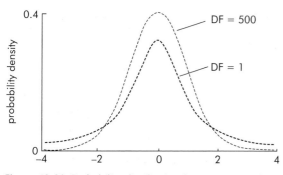

Figure 43.20 Probability distribution for t, DF = 1 and DF = 500

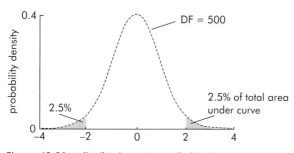

Figure 43.21 t distribution – two-tailed testing

group and the number of groups tested. In the case of a t-test, using the value of t obtained by testing the data, a corresponding P-number (probability for H_0 being true) can be looked up in numerical tables representing the probability density curves for t.

For example, consider a comparison between two groups, drug and placebo, involving 501 patients (DF = 500). If H_0 is true there is no difference between groups and the drug is ineffective. If H_0 is rejected, there is a difference between groups and the drug is effective. Applying a t-test to the data gives a value of t = 2, and the appropriate section in the t table may show:

t	P
1	0.03
2	0.04
3	0.05

Looking at the distribution curve in Figure 43.21, it can be seen that t = 2 is at the upper end (tail) of the distribution curve, where probabilities for the null hypothesis being

Figure 43.22 Summary for P-number (P) and level of significance (α)

P	The probability that H_0 is true
α	The level of significance. Usually α = 0.05
$P \leq \alpha$	H_0 is rejected – differences between groups are statistically significant
$P \geq \alpha$	H_0 is accepted – differences between groups are not statistically significant

true are low. From the t table, P = 0.04, so the null hypothesis can be rejected and the drug can be considered to be effective.

Level of significance (α)

Consider the probability density curve for t in the above example (Figure 43.21). The shaded area in the upper tail equals the probability of H_0 being true for all values of $t \geq 2$. Similarly t = –2 defines a small area at the lower tail of the curve which equals the probability of H_0 being true for $t \leq -2$. Because the probability levels are very low for values of t in these tail areas, it is unlikely that H_0 is true, and H_0 can be safely rejected. These areas therefore represent rejection areas for H_0.

In clinical research 95% probability (P = 0.95) is usually accepted as 'proving the case', so if $P \geq 0.95$ H_0 is accepted. Another way of expressing this is to say that if P < 0.05, H_0 is rejected. Therefore the total area for rejection of H_0 is the sum of the two shaded tail areas, which is equal to 5%. This is called the level of significance (α). Usually

$$\alpha = 0.05$$

Note that if H_0 is rejected falsely due to poor-quality or inaccurate data, a type I error has occurred. Thus the probability of making a type I error must also be equal to α (see *Types of error*, above).

Consider data demonstrating a difference in mean blood pressure between two groups of patients, one group treated with an antihypertensive and the other group treated with placebo. Statistical testing of the data may give P = 0.03 for the difference between the groups. This result means that there is only a 3% probability of H_0 being true. For α = 0.05, H_0 is rejected, the difference is significant, and the antihypertensive is effective.

The relationship between P and α is summarised in Figure 43.22.

Single-tailed and two-tailed testing

This refers to the setting of the significance level (α). In the above discussion α is shown to be equal to the area of rejection of H_0 in the probability density curve for t. This area consists of the two 'tails' in the distribution. This is the usual situation, and is referred to as *two-tailed testing* or two-sided testing (Figure 43.21).

> **Two-tailed testing** is the usual practice in setting the level of significance in a study. In this case α is set to an area (usually 0.05) consisting of the upper and lower 'tails' in the probability density curve for t.

Under some circumstances it may be valid to assume that t cannot assume negative values, in which case the upper tail rejection area can be increased from 2.5% to 5%, still maintaining the level of significance at $\alpha = 0.05$. This is *single-tailed testing*, and it can only be used under certain circumstances.

In a study investigating the difference between a treatment group and a control group, the results may demonstrate one of three outcomes:

- Treatment is the same as control and H_0 accepted. This means the treatment is ineffective.
- Treatment produces better outcomes. The treatment is effective and H_0 is rejected (upper tail).
- Treatment produces worse outcomes. The treatment is harmful and H_0 is rejected (lower tail).

Usually clinical studies are subjected to two-tailed testing, allowing for better or worse outcomes. Occasionally, however, a single-tailed test is used, because it can be assumed that the treatment can only affect the patient one way, i.e. make them better.

For example, consider testing a placebo treatment against no treatment. This assumes that the placebo can only make a patient feel better or the same, but not worse. This comparison can only reject the null hypothesis on the basis of the 'treatment' being better, and only one tail of the statistic probability distribution is used.

Single-tailed testing increases the rejection area at the single tail, compared to two-tailed testing (Figure 43.23). This can sometimes bring borderline P-numbers, which fail to demonstrate a significant difference, into significance. However, the assumptions made to justify single-tailed testing have to be valid.

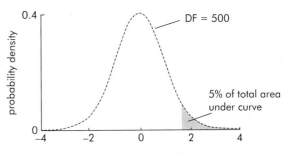

Figure 43.23 t distribution – one-tailed testing

Parametric and non-parametric tests

When tests are applied to data that fit a known probability density curve (i.e. one represented by a characteristic equation with defined parameters) these tests are referred to as *parametric tests*. Several defined probability density curves are well known. The most familiar is the *normal distribution* (bell-shaped curve, assumed in many biological and physiological data sets). Others include the *binomial distribution* and the *Poisson distribution* (see Figures 43.11 and 43.12).

In medical studies the data often follow a normal distribution, and parametric testing is often associated with normally distributed data. Parametric tests include the Student's t-test. However, binomially distributed data occur in a significant number of clinical studies, and appropriate parametric tests can be applied to these data.

When testing data in which the probability density curve cannot be assumed, *non-parametric tests* are used. These include ranking tests and the chi-squared test.

The chi-squared test is applied to data in the form of contingency tables. It is therefore usually used for non-parametric data presented in this form. Chi-squared testing may also be used for parametric data fitted to a contingency table, but it is less specific than the appropriate parametric tests and is therefore not usually used in this context.

> **Parametric tests** are applied to data which fit a known probability density curve (usually a normal distribution).
> **Non-parametric tests** are applied to data which do not fit a known probability distribution (such as a normal distribution).

Statistical tests

The type of testing used depends on the data collected. As noted above, the first consideration is whether data are parametric or non-parametric. Next the number of groups from which the data are collected must be considered. In practice comparisons between two groups form a large portion of medical studies. In this section the main emphasis will be on these types of data.

Comparing numerical data from two groups

Groups of patients are often compared to detect differences between the groups. The data collected may be normally distributed or of unknown probability density distribution.

> When normally distributed numerical data are collected from two groups of patients, the mean values for each group are usually compared, and this is commonly done with the *Student's t-test*. For data that do not fit a known probability density curve the most commonly used non-parametric test is the *Wilcoxon rank sum test*.

Student's *t*-test

This test compares the means of two small samples of numerical data, and determines whether the difference between the means is significant. The test obtains a value for the statistic *t*, which can be used to obtain a *P*-number from tables. The null hypothesis states that there is no difference between the groups, and the *P*-number represents

---

the probability that this hypothesis is true. Thus if $P > 0.05$, the difference between the means is not significant.

If the two samples of data come from the same individuals, such as in a crossover study, then the samples are said to be *paired* and the SEM is reduced. There is therefore an advantage in using paired data.

Consider comparing blood pressure measurements to find the effect of a new antihypertensive in one group of patients ($n_1 = 12$) against placebo in another group ($n_2 = 10$). If analysis of the results produced a statistic $t = 2.2$, looking up this value in the *t* tables for degrees of freedom (DF) $= n_1 + n_2 - 2 = 20$ gives the following:

t	*P*
1.7	0.1
2.1	0.05
2.8	0.01

This gives a probability $P < 0.05$ for the null hypothesis, and therefore makes the difference between groups significant and the antihypertensive effective.

Ranking tests

When non-parametric numerical data are recorded, the data cannot be assumed to fit a known probability density curve. Comparison between two groups then requires a non-parametric test such as the *Wilcoxon rank sum test*. Ranking combines the two groups to be compared into one single large group, and assigns each individual a rank according to the magnitude of the data measurement. The ranks are then summed for each group, and the rank sums are compared.

Testing categorical data from two groups

Categorical data do not fit any recognised probability density distribution, and are usually presented in the form of a contingency table (see Figure 43.18).

Chi-squared test

> The **chi-squared (χ^2) test** is a non-parametric test for the differences between group data as they appear in the contingency table. No assumptions need to be made about the probability distributions of the recorded data.

> ### Calculation of the *t* statistic
>
> The *t* statistic is calculated from the difference between the means and the standard error for this difference as
>
> $$t = \frac{\text{difference in means}}{\text{standard error of difference in means}}$$
>
> Given two independent sample groups of n_1 individuals and n_2 individuals, with means m_1 and m_2 and standard deviations s_1 and s_2:
>
> $$\text{Difference in means} = m_1 - m_2$$
> $$\text{SEM of difference in means} = \text{SEM}_1 + \text{SEM}_2$$
> $$t = \frac{m_1 - m_2}{\sqrt{s_1^2/n_1 + s_2^2/n_2}}$$

Calculation for Wilcoxon rank sum test

Consider recording the average weekly alcohol consumption of 12 individuals, five females (n_1) and seven males (n_2) (Figure 43.24). Is there a significant difference in alcohol consumption between males and females?

Rank sum for females $= 3+4.5+7+9.5+11.5 = 35.5$
Rank sum for males $= 1+2+4.5+6+8+9.5+11.5$
$= 42.5$

For samples of $n \leq 15$, the statistic for the test (z) is taken as the rank sum of the smaller group (n_1). Thus here $z = 35.5$.

Referring to the Wilcoxon two-sample rank sum table, the relevant line (for $n_1 = 5$ and $n_2 = 7$) shows the ranges for z:

		Two-tailed P value		
n_1	n_2	0.05	0.01	0.001
5	7	17,38	15,40	

At $P = 0.05$, this table shows a range of values for z between 17 and 38. Here $z = 35.5$, and the null hypothesis is accepted. There is no difference in alcohol consumption between males and females.

If the results were different and $z < 17$, then $P < 0.05$ and the null hypothesis would be rejected – i.e. female alcohol consumption is less than that of males. Similarly, for $z > 38$, the results would have demonstrated that females consume more alcohol than males.

Figure 43.24 Average weekly alcohol consumption of five women and seven men

Sex	Consumption (units)	Rank
F	0	11.5
M	10	8
M	15	6
F	16	4.5
F	18	3
M	22	1
M	0	11.5
M	16	4.5
M	20	2
F	8	9.5
M	8	9.5
F	14	7

This test is used to test the relationship between the row and column variables in a contingency table. It does not provide a specific answer to a question such as 'what are the odds of catching a particular disease if vaccinated or not vaccinated' as in the proportion testing below. It provides an estimate of how significant the differences observed between column and row variables in the contingency table are. As with other tests, the null hypothesis (H_0) is tested for. In this case H_0 is that there is no difference between groups, and therefore both rows are samples from the same population.

Comparison of two proportions

A proportion is obtained from a group of patients who can be divided into either of two outcomes (outcome X or outcome Y), e.g. dead or alive, disease-positive or disease-free. Such outcomes are referred to as *binary* outcomes, since there are only two possibilities.

Comparing proportions

In simple studies, proportions are compared between two groups, one of which (Group A) has been treated, tested, or exposed to a risk factor, while the other group (Group B) is a control. The results of such a comparison may be expressed in three different ways, as a *risk difference*, a *relative risk* or an *odds ratio*.

Some examples of such studies (with the basic question to be asked of the results in brackets) might be:
- Incidence of prostatic cancer in two groups: smokers and non-smokers (is smoking a risk factor for prostatic cancer?)

Calculation of χ^2

A χ^2 value is determined by comparing the observed values in the table with expected values. The expected values are calculated as if there was no difference between the groups (rows).

Consider a simple 2×2 contingency table for two groups of patients (Figure 43.25). The *observed* numbers in each category for each group are shown outside the brackets.

If there were no difference between groups, all of the patients could be considered as one big group of 30 patients. In such a case equal numbers would be expected in each of the outcome columns for each group. The *expected* values would then be those bracketed in the contingency table, and using these the χ^2 value can be calculated. Using the χ^2 value, a P-number can be obtained by looking it up in the appropriate table for χ^2. The value for χ^2 is calculated by

$$\chi^2 = \Sigma \frac{(\text{observed} - \text{expected})^2}{\text{expected}}$$

In the example shown in Figure 43.25:

$$\chi^2 = \frac{(2-5)^2}{5} + \frac{(8-5)^2}{5} + \frac{(13-10)^2}{10} + \frac{(7-10)^2}{10}$$
$$\chi^2 = 5.4$$

In order to obtain a value for the P-number the degrees of freedom (DF) for the contingency table must be identified. For a 2×2 table DF = 1. The P-number is then obtained by looking up its value in the section of the χ^2 table for DF = 1, which is shown below:

χ^2	P
3.84	0.5
5.02	0.025
6.63	0.01

Thus for $\chi^2 = 5.4$, $P < 0.025$. This means that the differences between the groups shown in the contingency table are significant.

Figure 43.25 Example contingency table for χ^2 test

	Outcome 1	Outcome 2
Group A ($n = 10$)	2 (5)	8 (5)
Group B ($n = 20$)	13 (10)	7 (10)
Totals	15	15

- Incidence of influenza in two groups: vaccinated and non-vaccinated (is vaccination effective against influenza?)
- Incidence of primary hepatoma in two groups: Hep B Ag positive and Hep B Ag negative (is Hep B Ag a risk factor for primary hepatoma?)

Such data will present as a 2×2 contingency table. Consider the example in Figure 43.26, showing influenza rates in two groups, one vaccinated and the other not vaccinated. The basic question to be answered with these data is 'How effective is the vaccine?' This table can be interpreted in different ways, by calculating:

- The difference in risk (probability of contracting influenza) between vaccinated and non-vaccinated groups. This is the **risk difference**.
- The ratio of the risk in the vaccinated group to that in the non-vaccinated group. This is the **relative risk**.
- The odds of contracting influenza in the vaccinated group, compared with the odds in the non-vaccinated group. This is the **odds ratio**.

Figure 43.26 Example 2×2 table for comparison of proportions – influenza vaccination

	Influenza	No influenza	Total
Vaccinated	30	300	330
Not vaccinated	80	270	350

Risk

> **Risk** can be defined as the probability of a condition occurring in a sample group.

If 30 patients out of the vaccinated sample of 330 (shown in Figure 43.26) contracted influenza, the risk (probability) of contracting influenza in that group is calculated as 30/330 = 0.09.

Risk difference (absolute risk reduction, ARR)

> **Risk difference** is the difference in risk of contracting a condition between treated and untreated groups.

Normally treatment would be expected to reduce the risk of a disease occurring, and this difference is sometimes referred to as the *absolute risk reduction* (ARR), which is usually expressed as a percentage.

> Risk in the vaccinated group, $r_1 = 30/330$
> $= 0.09$
> Risk in the non-vaccinated group, $r_2 = 80/350$
> $= 0.23$
> Risk difference, $r_1 - r_2 = 0.09 - 0.23$
> $= -0.14$
> $ARR = 14\%$
>
> This means that vaccination decreases the risk of contracting influenza by 0.14 (14%).

Number needed to treat (NNT)

> **NNT** is defined as the number of patients that need to be treated in order to save one disease event.

If ARR is expressed as a percentage (i.e. the number of disease events saved per 100 patients), then

$NNT = 100/ARR$

In the example from Figure 43.26:

$NNT = 100/14$
$= 7.14$

Number needed to harm (NNH)

> **NNH** is defined as the number of patients that need to be treated in order to produce one harmful side effect

A treatment may cause an increase in a disease condition as an unwanted side effect, e.g. increased incidence of peptic ulceration with the use of NSAIDs. In such a case there may be a positive risk difference between the control group ($r_2 = 0.1$) and the treated group ($r_1 = 0.2$).

Risk difference, $r_1 - r_2 = 0.2 - 0.1$
$= 0.1$
$ARR = 10\%$
$NNH = 100/10$
$= 10$

Relative risk

> **Relative risk** is the ratio of the risk in the treated group to the risk in the untreated group. Sometimes this ratio is presented in terms of the *relative risk reduction* (RRR), often quoted as a percentage.

Risk in the vaccinated group, $r_1 = 0.09$
Risk in the non-vaccinated group, $r_1 = 0.23$
Relative risk, $r_1/r_2 = 0.09/0.23$
$= 0.39$

This means that the risk of contracting influenza in the vaccinated group is only 39% of the risk in the unvaccinated group. Alternatively, this can be stated by saying that vaccination reduces the number of influenza cases by 100% – 39%: a relative risk reduction (RRR) of 61%. RRR can also be obtained by ARR divided by control event rate (or control-group risk, r_2). In this case ARR/CER = 0.14/0.23 = 0.61.

Odds ratio

When an event (e.g. disease) occurs in a group, rather than calculating risk in a group (probability) the proportion of event to non-event occurring can be expressed as *odds*.

The odds of an event occurring are defined as the ratio:

$$\text{Odds} = \frac{\text{Probability of event occurring}}{\text{Probability of event not occurring}}$$

Referring again to Figure 43.26, the odds of contracting influenza in the vaccinated group are given by:

$$\text{Odds}_1 = 30/300$$
$$= 0.1$$

The odds of contracting influenza in the non-vaccinated group are given by:

$$\text{Odds}_2 = 80/270$$
$$= 0.29$$

The *odds ratio* (OR) is then calculated as $\text{Odds}_1/\text{Odds}_2$:

$$\text{OR} = 0.1/0.29$$
$$= 0.34$$

This means that the odds of contracting influenza in the vaccinated group are only 34% of those in the non-vaccinated group.

> **Odds ratio** is the most commonly used method of comparing two proportions. It has the following properties:
> - Odds ratio (OR) approximates to relative risk (RR) when the outcome is rare.
> - When the outcome is common, RR does not discriminate well, because in such a situation it tends to a value of 1. This is not so with OR.
> - OR is the measure of choice in case–control studies.

Diagnostic or screening tests

A study may be performed to assess the value of a diagnostic or screening test, such as PSA for prostatic cancer, BIS score > 35 for awareness, Mallampati score for difficult airway. Such tests do not perform perfectly, and in some cases the condition may be missed (*false negatives*) while in others the test may give a *false positive* result.

Testing a group of patients will result in a 2 × 2 contingency table.

Consider the example shown in Figure 43.27, in which 100 people are screened for diabetes with a single fasting blood sugar. Subsequent glucose tolerance testing reveals those who truly have diabetes. Out of the 100 subjects, 20 test positive and 80 test negative, but only 16 are subsequently proved to have the condition.

Sensitivity

> **Sensitivity** is a measure of how good a test is at correctly identifying patients who *have* a condition, since the test will not detect all cases with the condition, but will produce a number of false-negative results.

In the above example (Figure 43.27) how good is the test at detecting the presence of diabetes?

$$\text{Sensitivity} = \frac{\text{Number of positive test results}}{\text{True number with condition}}$$
$$= 12/16$$
$$= 0.75$$

A high blood sugar result will pick up 75% of diabetics.

Specificity

> **Specificity** describes how good a test is at confirming the absence of a condition in patients who *do not have* the condition, since the test will not be negative in all patients without the condition, but will produce a number of false-positive results.

Figure 43.27 Example 2 × 2 table for a diabetes screening test

Proven diagnosis	Test positive	Test negative	
16 diabetic	12	4 (false negatives)	sensitivity = 12/16
84 non-diabetic	8 (false positives)	76	specificity = 76/84
	20	80	
	PPV = 12/20	NPV = 76/80	

How good is the test at confirming the absence of the condition?

$$\text{Specificity} = \frac{\text{Number of negative test results}}{\text{True number without condition}}$$
$$= 76/84$$
$$= 0.9$$

A low blood sugar result will pick out 90% of people without diabetes. 10% of patients who do not have diabetes will have a false-positive blood sugar.

Positive predictive value (PPV)

> **PPV** indicates how reliable a test is at detecting the presence of a condition, since some patients may produce false-negative results.

How good is the test at predicting the condition when the result is positive?

$$\text{PPV} = \frac{\text{Number of true positive test results}}{\text{Total number of positive results}}$$
$$= 12/20$$
$$= 0.6$$

A positive blood sugar result gives a 60% chance of diabetes being present.

Negative predictive value (NPV)

> **NPV** indicates how effective a test is at confirming the absence of a condition, since some patients may produce false-positive results.

How good is the test at predicting absence of the condition when the result is negative?

$$\text{NPV} = \frac{\text{Number of true negative test results}}{\text{Total number of negative results}}$$
$$= 76/80$$
$$= 0.95$$

A negative blood sugar result gives a 95% chance of diabetes being absent.

Likelihood ratio (LR)

> **Likelihood ratio** gives an idea of how likely it is that a positive test result means that the condition is truly present.

Given a positive result in the test, what is the likelihood that a person has the condition compared to the likelihood of obtaining a positive result in somebody free from the condition?

$$\text{LR} = \frac{\text{sensitivity}}{1 - \text{specificity}}$$
$$= 0.75/1 - 0.95$$
$$= 15$$

Given a positive result, a person is 15 times as likely to have diabetes as to be free from the condition.

Multiple groups
Parametric data

When more than two groups are studied, data may be analysed by **analysis of variance** (ANOVA). Consider investigating the postoperative analgesic requirements for patients from k different cities, with n patients in each group. The data obtained would give k different mean values $(m_1 \ldots m_k)$.

Is there a true difference between the means? Or is the variation in the mean values simply due to individual variation rather than geographical variation? The null hypothesis is that no difference exists and the groups are all from the same population.

ANOVA compares the variance across the mean values $(m_1 \ldots m_k)$ to the variance within each group of n patients. This statistic is called F, and it has a known F distribution that can be used to give P-numbers for values obtained from ANOVA testing. The number of degrees of freedom (DF) in this test is specified for the number of groups $(k - 1)$ and the number of patients in each group $(n - 1)$.

This test is known as *one-way analysis of variance* because a single factor is being tested for. It is equivalent to repeated t-testing between pairs of groups. The calculation is complex, but it is commonly available on computer software.

Non-parametric data

The Kruskal–Wallis test can be used to analyse non-parametric data from more than two groups. This test is an extension of the Wilcoxon rank sum test, and is not described further here.

Testing relationships

Data may be collected in order to try and define a relationship between two variables. If a relationship is found this is used as a model, and predictions can be made using this model. The simplest relationship mathematically is a linear one, and plotting a graph of one variable against the other will produce a straight-line graph.

Correlation

> **Correlation** describes the strength of relationship between two numerical variables, such as height and body weight, age and systolic blood pressure. This is quantified by measuring these variables in a sample of the population and calculating their correlation coefficient, r. (The full name for r is the Pearson product moment correlation coefficient.)

If two variables x and y are measured in a group of individuals they can be plotted against each other to produce a scatter plot. The shape of this scatter plot will be determined by their degree of association (Figure 43.28):

- If all of the points lie perfectly on a straight line the variables are said to be linearly correlated, and $r = +1$ or -1, depending on whether the gradient of the straight line is positive or negative.
- If the points form a shapeless cloud with no apparent axis or direction the variables are uncorrelated and $r = 0$.
- For intermediate degrees of correlation a best-fit straight line can be drawn through the data points, and r will assume values between 0 and ± 1.

Correlation describes a purely mathematical relationship and does not imply any causal relationship. For example, random fasting blood sugar levels may show some degree of correlation with shoe size. This does not mean that wearing

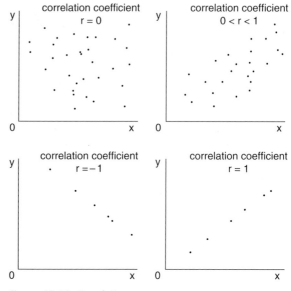

Figure 43.28 Correlation

big shoes causes high blood sugars, but simply implies an associative relationship rather than a causal one.

Testing for correlation between two variables

As in other statistical tests, when testing for correlation between two variables the null hypothesis ($r = 0$) is tested for and a P-number is determined from statistical tables. If $P < 0.05$ for the value of r and the given sample, then the null hypothesis is rejected and the variables are considered to be linearly correlated.

Calculation of the value of r is laborious and is commonly available in commercial software packages. Manually, r is calculated by first determining the mean values for x and y. Let these mean values be x_m and y_m.

Then find the differences between the coordinates of each data point (x, y) and the mean point (x_m, y_m). The arithmetic is given in the following formula:

$$ r = \frac{\Sigma(x - x_m)(y - y_m)}{\Sigma(x - x_m)^2(y - y_m)^2} $$

A value for r on its own is not enough to assess the degree of correlation in the data. This is because r is dependent on the size of the sample. If there are only two points in the sample $r = 1$ by definition. The greater the number of points the lower the value of r that is significant. With normally distributed data, five points in a sample might give $r = 0.8$, which is not significant. However, a sample of 150 points may yield a value of $r = 0.2$, which is significant.

Points to note about correlation:

- The Pearson correlation coefficient is calculated for normally distributed variables. For non-parametric data use Spearman's rank correlation coefficient.
- A value for r^2 is sometimes calculated, and this is useful as a measure of the fraction of the variability in one variable that is due to the linear relationship with the other variable.
- The correlation found in a sample of data only exists within the boundaries of the range of data points examined.

Linear regression

Linear regression takes the process of investigating the relationship between two variables a step further than correlation analysis.

> **Linear correlation** enables an observer to assess the degree of linear association between two variables but provides no further information upon which predictions can be made.
>
> **Linear regression** is used to mathematically model the relationship between two continuous variables by identifying the gradient and intercept of the best-fit line.

Consider the measurement of two continuous variables x and y from a sample of a population (Figure 43.29). These data can be plotted as a scatter diagram. Linear regression is used to define the best straight line fitting the points of the scatter diagram. Here it is assumed that one variable, x, is independent, and that the other variable, y, is dependent on x. In this case the equation for the best-fit straight line (or regression line) is given by

$$y = bx + a$$

where b is the gradient of the regression line and a is the intercept.

The coefficients b and a are also called the *regression coefficients*.

The regression line is thus a mathematical model for the relationship between y and x, and it is sometimes referred

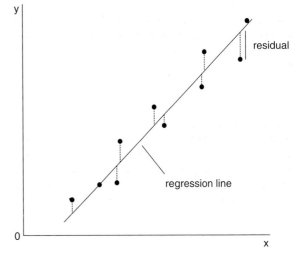

Figure 43.29 Linear regression

to as the regression of y on x. By knowing the coefficients a and b, any value of y can be calculated for a given value of x using the regression line.

Performing linear regression analysis

In order to calculate the regression coefficients a and b, a method of *least squares* is used. This method selects the best straight line, which minimises the sum of the vertical distance of each point from the regression line (the sum of the residuals). Figure 43.29 shows a regression line for a set of data points. The residuals are shown as dotted lines. The regression line is chosen so as to minimise the sum of these residuals. Certain assumptions are made when using this method:

- There is a linear relationship between x and y.
- The observations in the sample are independent.
- The variables y and x are normally distributed.
- The variance of the y values at all values of x is the same.

Calculation of the gradient (b) and the intercept (a) is usually performed on readily available software. Manual calculation is reasonably straightforward but laborious. Initially mean values x_m ($= \Sigma\, x/n$) and y_m ($= \Sigma\, y/n$) are calculated:

$$\text{gradient,}\quad b = \frac{\Sigma(x - x_m)(y - y_m)}{\Sigma(x - x_m)^2}$$

$$\text{intercept,}\quad a = y_m - bx_m$$

The null hypothesis in linear regression is that the gradient is zero, in which case there is no linear relationship between *x* and *y*. A probability can thus be calculated, which if $P < 0.05$ will reject the null hypothesis and indicate significance for the regression coefficients.

Goodness of fit for the regression line to the data is assessed by calculating a value for correlation coefficient squared (r^2). This is the proportion of the variability in *y* due to the linear relationship with *x*. If this is high (> 0.7) the line is a 'good' fit.

Systematic reviews

Many research studies may be performed over a period of decades before a particular treatment becomes employed routinely in clinical practice. Part of the process that may eventually result in a change in practice consists of reviewing the results from the different studies in order to reach a conclusion as to the efficacy of the intervention.

A conventional review is a 'narrative' or 'expert' review by an author, who gives a subjective opinion based on selected literature. Such a review can be misleading due to bias introduced by the selection of literature and differing methods of assessing results across studies.

A **systematic review** attempts to reduce this bias by using systematically assembled collections of literature and a standardised method of analysing the collected results.

Systematic reviews of appropriate collections of medical literature are provided by the Cochrane Collaboration. This is an independent international organisation, dating from 1993, which provides continually updated literature reviews covering a wide range of medical interventions and other topics.

Meta-analysis

The collective analysis of results from different studies is known as **meta-analysis**. In order to combine the results from different studies there must be criteria for selecting the studies to be included in the meta-analysis:

- The studies must be of the same type, producing the same format of results. The most common type of study included is a randomised controlled trial (RCT) comparing two groups.
- The studies should have the same type of outcome. This can be a *fixed effect* or *binary outcome*, e.g. dead or alive. Such studies produce a 2×2 contingency table, which is usually analysed to give an odds ratio (OR) or absolute risk reduction (ARR). This is the most common type of study in meta-analyses.

- Alternatively the studies can have a variable outcome, or *random effect*. These studies require a more complex analysis to combine their results.
- The studies must be statistically *homogeneous*. This means there should not be considerable variation between the outcome measures. Statistical homogeneity can be tested for, and may be quoted as a *Q* number.

Although systematic reviews and meta-analyses can be more powerful than individual studies they are still subject to their own sources of bias. These include:

- *Publication bias* – Trials that demonstrate a positive effect are more likely to be published than those that show a negative or non-significant effect.
- *Variable trial quality* – Differences in methodology can exaggerate outcome results, e.g. inadequate randomisation of allocation, small samples, poor blinding.
- *Heterogeneity* – Statistical heterogeneity can be tested for, but clinical heterogeneity may cause incompatibility due to population differences or differences in definition of variables.

Meta-analysis for a fixed effect most commonly results in a *forest plot*, which combines the results from a number of

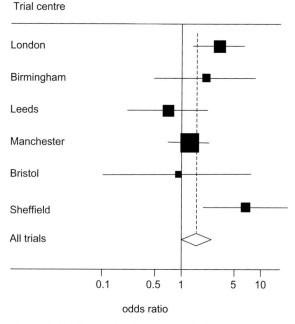

Figure 43.30 Forest plot for meta-analysis

studies. For example, consider a systematic review and meta-analysis for a new thromboprophylactic drug. This has been tested on hip-replacement patients, and six studies from different centres have met the inclusion criteria and been selected for review. The results are presented as odds ratios (OR) for positive venograms with confidence intervals (CI). The results of the meta-analysis are shown in Figure 43.30. This shows the study labels (trial centres) with the corresponding OR and CI on the axes. The horizontal axis is the OR and CI, while the vertical axis is the line for no effect (OR = 1). At the bottom of the diagram is the summary result for the meta-analysis, showing the resultant OR (open diamond), with the width of the diamond representing the resultant CI. The results from the individual trials are weighted before combination to allow for differences in quality of data. Different methods of weighting are used. One method is inverse variance weighting, while another is Mantel–Haenszel weighting. Degree of weighting is indicated by the width of the solid square representing the OR for each trial.

CHAPTER **44**

Applied physics

Ted Lin and Rajani Annamaneni

Fundamentals of Anaesthesia, 4th edition, ed. Ted Lin, Tim Smith and Colin Pinnock. Published by Cambridge University Press. © Cambridge University Press 2017.

Units and derived units

Quantifying physical dimensions and properties requires the definition of units of measurement. Many traditional and varied systems of measurement have evolved, but progress towards standardisation of units continues. The system adopted in 1960 was the International System of Units (Système International d'Unités, SI units).

SI units

The **SI system** is a coherent system based on the use of seven fundamental units, two supplementary units and an unlimited number of derived units.

'Coherent' in this context refers to the fact that there is a single unit for each fundamental quantity in the SI system, and all derived units are formed by simple multiplication of fundamental units. This means that consistent use of SI units in all equations and calculations produces an answer in the appropriate SI unit automatically without scaling or conversion. Unfortunately in medical sciences traditional units still persist, and it is necessary to be aware of some conversions between units.

Fundamental units

The seven fundamental units and two supplementary units in the SI system are shown in Figure 44.1.

Derived units

Most units that are derived from the fundamental units have a name (e.g. joule, watt). However, in the SI system, some of the derived units have not been named. These are shown in Figure 44.2.

Named derived units

Some commonly used named derived units are shown in Figure 44.3. These have been named after famous scientists who originally investigated the physical laws.

Unit multiplication factors

Basic or derived units may be prefixed by a letter that denotes a multiplying factor. The more common multiplying factors are shown in Figure 44.4. These letters increase or decrease the value of the unit by powers of 10.

Figure 44.1 Fundamental units and supplementary units in the SI system

Quantity	Unit	Symbol
Fundamental		
• Length	metre	m
• Mass	kilogram	kg
• Time	second	s
• Electric current	ampere	A
• Temperature	kelvin	K
• Amount of substance (specify particles, e.g. atoms, molecules, ions)	mole	mol
• Light intensity	candela	cd
Supplementary		
• Angle	radian	rad
• Solid angle	steradian	sr

Figure 44.2 Derived SI units

Phenomenon	Derived unit	Symbol
Area	square metre	m^2
Volume	cubic metre	m^3
Density	kilogram per cubic metre	$kg \cdot m^{-3}$
Velocity	metre per second	$m \cdot s^{-1}$
Acceleration	metre per second per second	$m \cdot s^{-2}$

Conversion between pressure units

As noted above, many non-SI units are still commonly used in clinical practice, mainly because of tradition or context. This particularly applies to pressure measurements in anaesthesia, where pressures may range from airway pressures (measured in cmH_2O) through to gas cylinder pressures (measured in atmospheres). There are therefore many different units of pressure still in daily use.

It is useful to be familiar with the conversion between pressure units (Figure 44.5).

Figure 44.3 Named derived units

Phenomenon	Derived unit	Name (symbol)	Unit description
Force	$kg \cdot m \cdot s^{-2}$	newton (N)	Force required to accelerate a mass of 1 kg at 1 $m \cdot s^{-2}$
Pressure	$kg \cdot m^{-1} \cdot s^{-2}$	pascal (Pa)	Pressure which exerts a force of 1 newton per square metre of surface area
Frequency	$1 \cdot s^{-1}$	hertz (Hz)	Number of cycles of a periodic activity per second
Energy	$kg \cdot m^2 \cdot s^{-2}$	joule (J)	Energy expended in moving a resistive force of 1 newton a distance of 1 metre
Power	$kg \cdot m^2 \cdot s^{-3}$	watt (W)	Rate of energy expenditure of 1 joule per second
Electric charge	$A.s$	coulomb (C)	Electric charge passing a fixed point in a conductor when a current of 1 ampere flows for 1 second

Figure 44.4 Prefixes used to denote unit multiplication factors

Prefix	Letter	Multiplying factor
exa	E	10^{18}
peta	P	10^{15}
tera	T	10^{12}
giga	G	10^{9}
mega	M	10^{6}
kilo	k	10^{3}
hecto	h	10^{2}
deca	da	10
deci	d	10^{-1}
centi	h	10^{-2}
milli	m	10^{-3}
micro	m	10^{-6}
nano	n	10^{-9}
pico	p	10^{-12}
femto	f	10^{-15}
atto	a	10^{-18}

Figure 44.5 Conversion between pressure units

Basic unit	Converted equivalent	
1.0 kPa	1000	$N \cdot m^{-2}$
	0.01	bar
	0.01013	atmospheres
	104	$dyne.cm^{-2}$
	7.5	mmHg
	10.2	cmH_2O
	0.145	pounds force per square inch
	20.9	pounds force per square foot

Converting units

When converting physical values between one system of units and another, it is useful to treat the conversion as an equation. In this case each side of the equation must be multiplied or divided by the same factor in order to keep the equation valid.

Fundamental constants

These are basic constants which have internationally agreed values. An example is the speed of light in a vacuum, which is now given the value of 299,792,458 m s^{-1}. This enables the unit of length to be defined. The metre is now defined as the length of the path travelled by light in a vacuum during a time interval of 1/299,792,458 of a second.

Other fundamental constants include the elementary charge of an electron (1.602×10^{-19} C), the Faraday constant (9.648×10^4 C mol^{-1}), the Avogadro constant and the gas constant ($\mathbf{R}$).

Converting mmHg to kPa

If the partial pressure of oxygen is 158 mmHg, what is the partial pressure of oxygen in SI units?

7.5 mmHg = 1.0 kPa (see Figure 44.5)

so dividing both sides of the conversion factor equation by 7.5 gives:

$$1.0 \text{ mmHg} = \frac{1.0}{7.5} = 0.133 \text{ kPa}$$

and multiplying both sides by 158 gives:

158 mmHg = 158 × 0.133 = 21 kPa

Mechanics

Mechanics is the study of how objects around us move or remain at rest. This subject requires an understanding of the quantities listed in Figure 44.6.

Mass and weight

Mass is the amount of matter present and is a property of an object which remains constant no matter where the object is located.

Weight is the gravitational force acting on an object and is given by the product of mass (m) times the acceleration due to gravity (g):

Weight = $m\,g$

The weight of an object therefore varies according to its location. It will be less on the moon than on earth, and it will be greater at the North Pole than at the Equator.

Force and pressure

The relationship between force and pressure is

$$\textbf{Pressure} = \frac{\text{Force}}{\text{Area}}$$

Force required when injecting with a syringe

Consider the force used when when injecting with a large syringe compared to a small syringe. In order to eject fluid from either syringe the same pressure must be developed. However, the force required to depress the plunger of the syringe will depend on the cross-sectional area of the syringe barrel, since

Force = pressure × cross-sectional area

For example, let the pressure required in the syringe equal p, and consider a 2 mL syringe with a radius a. The force required is given by

Force = $p \times \pi\, a^2$

Compare this with a 20 mL syringe in which the radius is $2a$. Here the force required becomes

Force = $p \times \pi\, 4a^2$

Thus four times the force is needed to depress the plunger in a 20 mL syringe compared to that required in a 2 mL syringe (Figure 44.7).

Figure 44.6 Some basic quantities in mechanics

Quantity	Vector or scalar	Description	SI unit
Displacement	Vector	Distance measured in a given direction	m
Velocity	Vector	Change in displacement per second	$m \cdot s^{-1}$
Acceleration	Vector	Change in velocity per second	$m \cdot s^{-2}$
Mass	Scalar	Amount of matter present in an object	kg
Force	Vector	An external 'push' or 'pull' which when applied to an object can change its state or motion	N
Weight	Vector	Gravitational pull acting on an object	N
Pressure	Scalar	Force per unit area	Pa
Energy	Scalar	Capacity to do work (stored work)	J
Work	Scalar	Energy expended when a force moves its point of application	J
Power	Scalar	Work done per second	W

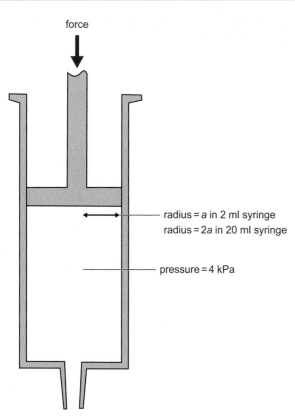

radius = a in 2 ml syringe
radius = $2a$ in 20 ml syringe

pressure = 4 kPa

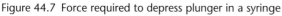

Figure 44.7 Force required to depress plunger in a syringe

Work done by a force

The work done by a force acting on an object can be calculated by the product of force and the distance moved through by its point of application.

> **Work done** = Force × distance moved

Consider the work done by a force F raising an object of mass m throught a height h (Figure 44.8). In order to lift the mass, the force must be at least equal to the weight of the object:

$F = m.g$

where g = acceleration due to gravity

Work done = $m.g.h$

The work done in raising the object has resulted in a gain in potential energy due to its increase in height (energy by virtue of position or state). This potential energy represents a capacity to do work, or may be converted to another form of energy such as kinetic energy, if the object were

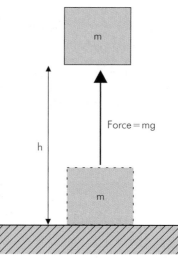

Figure 44.8 Work done by force raising a mass

allowed to fall. As the object falls it loses potential energy but gains kinetic energy (energy by virtue of its velocity).

Work, energy and power

Work and energy are closely related, since the expenditure of energy usually results in the performance of useful work, and similarly the performance of work often produces changes in energy levels. Energy is not destroyed but merely converted from one form to another. In a mechanical system, when energy is expended in doing work or converted from one form to another, there is usually an apparent 'loss' due to the inefficiencies of any real system (e.g. friction). This apparent 'loss' of energy often appears as a production of heat.

Power

Power is the rate of doing work or the energy expended per unit time. To calculate the power output of a machine or process, divide the total work done by the time taken.

> **Calculation for the power output of intermediate metabolism**
>
> Consider 24 hours given basal metabolic rate of 2400 kcal per day.
>
> Total energy expended = 2400×10^3 cal
> $\qquad\qquad\qquad\qquad = 9.98 \times 10^6$ J
> Total time taken $\quad = 24$ h
> $\qquad\qquad\qquad\qquad = 86,400$ s
> Average power output = 115 watts

Hydrostatics

This is the study of fluids and their pressure and volumes while they are at rest. An understanding of hydrostatics is useful when considering:

- Pressure measurement by a barometer or manometer
- How chest drains work
- Work done in compressing gases by a ventilator
- Work of breathing done by the body
- Work done by the myocardium in providing the cardiac output

Hydrostatic pressure

Manometers and barometers measure pressure using a column of fluid. This is done by balancing the unknown pressure against the pressure produced by the weight of a column of fluid.

- In a **barometer** the measuring column of fluid is mercury and closed to the atmosphere. The column of mercury is then balanced against the atmospheric pressure acting on the reservoir (Figure 44.9).
- In a **manometer** the measuring column is open to the atmosphere and an unknown pressure is applied to the base of this column via a closed limb as in the sphygmomanometer, in which the fluid is mercury. For measuring lower pressures the fluid may be water or alcohol.

Barometric pressure

A barometer balances atmospheric pressure (P_{atm}) acting on the surface of a reservoir against the pressure at the base of a column of mercury. The mercury column must therefore be in a sealed glass tube, since if it were open, as in the sphygmomanometer, no difference in mercury levels would exist.

Calculation of the pressure at the base of the mercury column in a barometer

$$\text{pressure} = \frac{\text{force}}{\text{area}}$$

$$= \frac{\text{weight of mercury column}}{\text{cross-sectional area}}$$

$$= h\rho g$$

where height of column (h) = 0.76 m, density of mercury (ρ) = 13.6×10^3 kg m^{-3}, and acceleration due to gravity (g) = 9.81 m s^{-2}.

Therefore the atmospheric pressure measured by a column of mercury 760 mm tall is given by:

$$\begin{aligned} \text{Atmospheric pressure} &= 0.76 \times 13.6 \times 10^3 \times 9.81 \\ &= 101,396 \text{ Pa} \\ &= 101.4 \text{ kPa} \end{aligned}$$

This can be used to convert between kPa and mmHg:

760 mmHg = 101.4 kPa

7.49 mmHg = 1 kPa

Gauge pressure

When an unknown pressure is measured relative to atmospheric pressure (as is usually the case in clinical practice) the value obtained is referred to as a 'gauge' pressure. This is the case in measurements such as blood pressure or airway pressure.

Absolute pressure

An absolute pressure measurement includes the effect of the atmosphere, and is therefore equal to the sum of atmospheric pressure plus the gauge pressure. Clearly barometric pressure is an absolute pressure measurement.

Work done by a ventilator in compressing inspiratory gases

When a volume of gas is compressed work is done, and potential energy is gained by the gas. This is analogous to the storage of potential energy in a spring when it is compressed. The work done in compressing a volume of gas from volume V_1 to V_2 with a pressure (p) can be found by plotting a pressure–volume curve and finding the area under the curve (Figure 44.10):

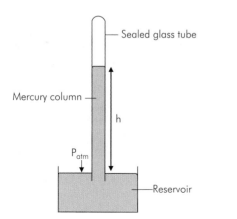

Figure 44.9 Calculation of pressure in a barometer

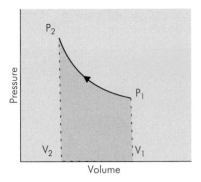

Figure 44.10 Pressure–volume curve during inspiration with variable pressure

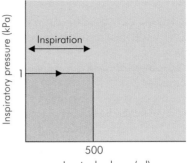

Figure 44.11 Pressure–volume curve with constant pressure showing work done

$$\text{Work} = \int_{V_2}^{V_1} p \, dV$$

Inspiratory work

In order to estimate the inspiratory work in delivering a breath of 500 mL, a simple example can be taken.

Consider a constant inspiratory pressure of 1.0 kPa applied to produce a tidal volume of 500 mL in a patient (Figure 44.11). The inspiratory work done per breath would then be $1000 \times 0.5 \times 10^{-3}$ J = 0.5 J.

When the complete inspiratory–expiratory cycle of a ventilator is plotted the pressure and volume axes are traditionally shown as in Figure 44.12. Note the arrangement of the axes, with pressure on the x-axis and volume on the y-axis: this is done to give the familiar inspiratory–expiratory loop. Work is performed in compressing the inspired gas and expanding the patient's lungs (inspiratory curve). This stores potential energy as elastic energy in the gases and tissues of the respiratory system, which then performs work in restoring the lungs to their original volume (expiratory curve). In an ideal system with 100% efficiency the inspiratory and expiratory curves would coincide, since no energy is wasted in frictional losses. The amount of energy put into the system during inspiration is thus returned in full during expiration. In practice when this cycle of events is plotted on a pressure–volume curve, as in Figure 44.12, the inspiratory and expiratory curves do not coincide, and a loop is formed. This phenomenon is known as *hysteresis*, and the area of the loop represents the inspiratory and expiratory work 'wasted' over the complete cycle.

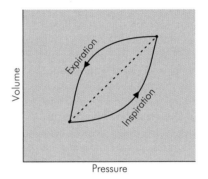

Figure 44.12 Pressure–volume loop for ventilator cycle, showing hysteresis

Work of breathing

Under resting conditions the work done in inspiration can be approximated by considering a simple model as described above.

Work of breathing, at an expenditure of 0.5 J per breath and a resting respiratory rate of 12 per minute, is given by

$$\text{Work done per minute} = 12 \times 0.5 \text{ J}$$
$$= 6 \text{ J}$$
$$\text{Power used} = 6/60 \text{ J s}^{-1}$$
$$= 0.1 \text{ W}$$

Allowing for the fact that respiratory muscles are only about 10% efficient, the total expenditure on work of breathing is approximately 1 W, which is equivalent to 1% of basal metabolic requirements. Under stressful or pathological conditions work of breathing may increase tenfold or more and represent a significant energy requirement.

The work of breathing during spontaneous respiration is considered in further detail in the section on 'Respiratory Physiology'.

Work done by the myocardium

The work performed by the myocardium of the left ventricle during each cycle of the heart can be derived from a pressure–volume loop plotted for the ventricle (Figure 44.13). This loop is described in detail in Chapter 14 (see Figure 14.18.). Calculation of the area of this loop gives the work done per cycle by the left or right ventricle, which can then be normalised for body surface area to give left or right ventricular stroke work index (LVSWI or RVSWI).

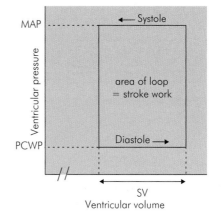

Figure 44.13 Pressure–volume loop for left ventricle

Calculation of myocardial power output

Figure 44.13 shows an example for the pressure–volume loop of a left ventricle. A gross simplification of the loop enables an estimate to be made. The work done per cycle is then given by

Stroke work done $= (MAP - PCWP) \times SV$

where
MAP = mean arterial pressure = 90 mmHg = 12 kPa
PCWP = mean pulmonary capillary wedge pressure
      = 7.5 mmHg = 1 kPa
SV = stroke volume = 80 mL $= 0.080 \times 10^{-3}$ m^3

Therefore, for a heart rate of 70 min^{-1}:

Stroke work done $= (12 \times 10^3 - 1 \times 10^3) \times 0.08 \times 10^{-3}$
                  $= 0.88$ J

Power output $= \dfrac{0.88 \times 70}{60}$
             $= 1$ W

Assuming a 10% efficiency for the myocardium, the total energy requirements to provide 5.6 L min^{-1} of cardiac output becomes approximately 10 W, i.e. approximately 10% of basal metabolic requirements.

Heat

Heat is a form of energy which can be transferred from hot objects to cooler objects. Temperature is a measure of how hot or cold an object is i.e. a measure of its thermal state. Therefore heat energy will tend to pass across a temperature gradient from high to low temperatures. When heat is transferred to an object its temperature will increase, similarly the loss of heat energy from an object will be accompanied by a fall in temperature.

Units of heat energy

Heat energy is measured in joules (J), but traditionally has also been measured in calories (cal) or kilocalories (kcal or Cal).

---

1 calorie is defined as the amount of heat required to raise the temperature of 1 g of water by 1 °C:

1 cal $= 4.16$ J
1 kcal (Cal) $= 1000$ cal

Temperature scales

Temperature scales have been defined in the past by using known fixed temperatures, such as the boiling and freezing points of water at one standard atmosphere pressure. Some temperature scales are compared in Figure 44.14 using these points.

The boiling and freezing points of water, however, vary according to ambient pressure, and nowadays a more invariant point called the *triple point of water* (see below) is used to define the two most commonly used temperature scales of kelvin and degrees Celsius. Practical

Figure 44.14 Commonly used temperature scales, showing freezing and boiling points of water

Scale	Freezing point H_2O	Boiling point H_2O
Kelvin	273.15 K	373.15 K
Celsius	0 °C	100 °C
Fahrenheit	32 °F	212 °F

methods of measuring temperature are discussed in Chapter 45.

Specific heat capacity and heat capacity
In an object the relationship between temperature change and amount of heat energy added or removed depends on the size of the object and the material it is composed of.

> **Specific heat capacity, s** ($kJ\ kg^{-1}\ °C^{-1}$) is the amount of heat required to raise the temperature of 1 kg of a substance by 1°C. For example, the specific heat capacity of water is 4.16 kJ $kg^{-1}\ °C^{-1}$. The average specific heat capacity of body tissues is between $3-4\ kJ\ kg^{-1}\ °C^{-1}$
> **Heat capacity, T** ($kJ\ °C^{-1}$) is the amount of heat required to raise the temperature of an object by 1°C. If the object has a mass = M, and is composed of material with a specific heat capacity = s, then it has a heat capacity given by
>
> $$T = M\ s\ (kJ\ °C^{-1})$$
>
> Thus the heat capacity of a 70 kg adult, assuming a specific heat capacity of 3.5 kJ $kg^{-1}\ °C^{-1}$, is given by
>
> $T = 70 \times 3.5$ kJ
> $= 245$ kJ ($= 58.9$ kcal)

Gases, liquids and solids
The addition or removal of heat energy to or from a substance will not only cause a variation in its temperature, but can also cause that substance to change its physical state. Any substance can exist in three states (phases) as a solid, liquid or gas. The conditions determining which state exists are temperature and pressure.

At any given pressure the transition between solid and liquid occurs at a fixed temperature, the 'freezing point', while the transition between liquid and gas occurs at the 'boiling point'. However, changes in ambient pressure cause boiling and freezing points to vary. At sea level water boils at 100 °C, but at 5500 m, where atmospheric pressure is approximately halved, the boiling point of water decreases to 80 °C.

Critical temperature
Both pressure and temperature can change the state of a substance. Thus gases can be liquefied either by cooling or by increasing the pressure. However, there is a temperature above which any gas cannot be liquefied by increasing pressure. This is the critical temperature (T_C).

> **Critical temperature** is defined as the maximum temperature at which a gas can be liquefied by increasing ambient pressure. Above critical temperature the gas cannot be liquefied by increasing ambient pressure.

The critical temperature for oxygen is –119 °C, and therefore oxygen in a cylinder at room temperature is always gaseous, no matter how much the pressure is increased. However, the critical temperature for nitrous oxide is 36.5 °C. This means that at normal room temperature (20–25 °C), a cylinder of nitrous oxide contains a mixture of liquid and gas. Should the ambient temperature exceed 36.5°C (as in a tropical country), the nitrous oxide in a cylinder will only exist in gaseous form.

Variation of physical state with pressure and temperature
The way in which temperature and pressure determine the physical state of a substance is illustrated in Figure 44.15. This figure shows curves plotting volume against pressure for a given mass of substance. Each curve is plotted at a given temperature and is called an isotherm. The middle curve is plotted at the critical temperature (T_C), while T_H is plotted at a temperature above T_C, and T_L is less than T_C.

T_H– at temperatures higher than the critical temperature, the substance exists only as a gas and the variation of volume with pressure, at constant temperature, follows a simple hyperbolic curve or inverse relationship, according to Boyle's law.

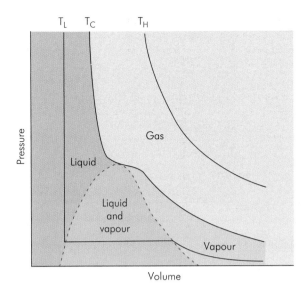

Figure 44.15 Isotherms for nitrous oxide

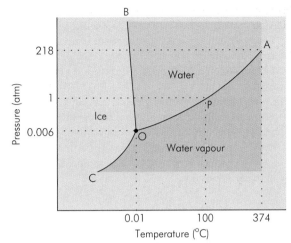

Figure 44.16 Triple point of water

T_C– at the critical temperature, the substance exists as a vapour at low pressures (i.e. below critical pressure). However, when pressure increases above critical pressure the vapour liquefies, producing an inflexion point in the curve. Further increases in pressure do not then decrease the volume, as the liquid state is effectively incompressible.

T_L– at temperatures lower than critical temperature, the substance exists as a liquid at high pressures. As the pressure decreases the volume remains constant until a point is reached when the liquid begins to boil (i.e. at the saturated vapour pressure, SVP) and a mixture of liquid and vapour is produced. The volume of this mixture at SVP varies according to the degree of vaporisation. When complete vaporisation has occurred, volume again follows an inverse relationship with pressure.

The isotherms map out areas which define the physical state of the substance. At temperatures above T_C (plain area) the substance exists only as a gas. At temperatures below T_C the substance may be in liquid form (darker shaded area); it may be a vapour (lighter shaded area); or it may exist as a mixture of both. This diagram is typical for a substance such as nitrous oxide, where T_C is equal to 36.5 °C.

> **Critical pressure** – the minimum pressure, at critical temperature, required to liquefy a gas
> **Critical volume** – the volume occupied by 1 mole of gas at critical temperature and critical pressure

Triple point of water

Water can exist in three phases, as water vapour, liquid water and ice. These phases will depend on temperature and pressure as shown in Figure 44.16. The transition between water and water vapour is demarcated by the boiling point of water (P), which is 100 °C at 1 atmosphere, but which increases with increasing pressure (OA).

Water vapour and water therefore coexist along OA. Similarly the freezing point of water (0 °C at 1 atmosphere) separates water and ice, but decreases with increasing pressure (OB). Ice and water thus coexist along OB. Finally, OC separates ice and water vapour, and these phases coexist along this line.

> **Triple point of water**
>
> There is a single point (O) at which the three phases of water coexist, at a pressure of 0.006 atmospheres and 0.01°C. This is the triple point of water (Figure 44.16).

Vapours and gases

The term **gas** is applied to a substance which is normally in its gaseous state at room temperature and atmospheric pressure. Its critical temperature is below room temperature and therefore it cannot exist as a liquid.

The term **vapour** refers to a gaseous substance which is normally in liquid form at room temperature and atmospheric pressure, since its critical temperature is above room temperature. Thus a vapour is a gaseous substance which is below its critical temperature under ambient conditions.

Saturated vapour pressure and its relationship to boiling point

A vapour is formed from a liquid by evaporation, or the escape of molecules from the liquid surface. This process also occurs from the surface of solids to a small extent by a process known as *sublimation*.

When evaporation takes place from the surface of a liquid the concentration of vapour above the liquid increases. This process continues until a state of equilibrium is reached when no further increase in vapour concentration occurs. At this stage the vapour is said to be saturated, and the vapour pressure is the *saturated vapour pressure* (SVP).

Saturated vapour pressure (SVP) can be defined as the pressure exerted by a vapour when in contact and equilibrium with its liquid phase. The SVP of a liquid increases with temperature (Figure 44.17). The temperature at which the SVP becomes equal to atmospheric pressure is the boiling point of the liquid.

Latent heat

When a substance changes phase, from liquid to gas or from solid to liquid, the molecular separation and bonding change. Water molecules in steam are about 12 times further apart than in liquid water. This increased separation of the molecules represents stored potential energy since the hydrogen bonds between water molecules in liquid water are very strong. Work is therefore required to achieve this molecular separation, which is provided by the latent heat absorbed.

If ice is heated from a sub-zero temperature (Figure 44.18), its temperature will rise steadily except

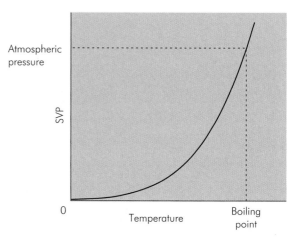

Figure 44.17 Variation of SVP with temperature

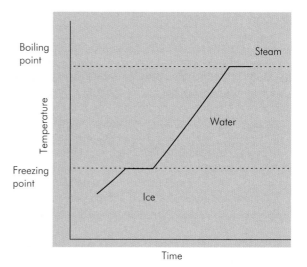

Figure 44.18 Variation of temperature of a block of ice being heated

when it passes through the two transitions in phase from solid to liquid (freezing point) and from liquid to gas (boiling point). At these transition points the temperature remains constant while latent heat is absorbed to increase molecular separation. The latent heat associated with these changes in state is known as *latent heat of fusion* and *latent heat of vaporisation*, respectively.

Liquids also evaporate at temperatures lower than their boiling point and will also require latent heat of vaporisation

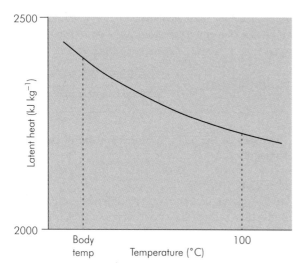

Figure 44.19 Variation of latent heat with temperature

to achieve this change in state. However, the cooler the liquid the greater the amount of latent heat required to increase the liquid molecular energy levels to those possessed by vapour molecules. Thus specific latent heat of vaporisation increases as temperature decreases (Figure 44.19), and is usually quoted at a given temperature.

> **Specific latent heat of fusion** is the energy required to change 1 kg of substance from solid to liquid, without change in temperature. The specific latent heat of fusion for water is 334 kJ kg^{-1}.
>
> **Specific latent heat of vaporisation** is the energy required to change 1 kg of substance from liquid to vapour, without change in temperature. The specific latent heat of vaporisation of water at 100 °C is 2260 kJ kg^{-1}. At 37 °C, the specific latent heat of water is 2420 kJ kg^{-1}.

Heat loss due to ventilation with cool dry gases

Poor preparation of inspired gases can cause a patient to lose body heat, because:

- The gases are not warmed and heat is lost in warming the gases to body temperature.
- The gases are not humidified and heat is lost due to evaporation in order to humidify the gases in the respiratory tract.

These losses can be calculated as follows:

> ### Calculation of heat loss in warming gases
>
> Consider ventilating with air at 20 °C (body temperature = 37 °C) with a minute volume of 6 L min^{-1}. The specific heat capacity (s) of air is 998 J kg^{-1} °C^{-1} and the density of dry air at normal temperature and pressure (NTP) is 1.29 kg m^{-3}.
>
> Mass (M) of air in the minute volume
> $$= \text{volume } (m^{-3}) \times \text{density}$$
> $$= 0.006 \times 1.29 = 7.74 \times 10^{-3} \text{ kg}$$
>
> Heat required to warm air to body temp
> $$= M\,s\,(37 - 20)$$
> $$= 7.74 \times 10^{-3} \times 998 \times 17$$
> $$= 131 \text{ J min}^{-1}$$
> $$= 2.2 \text{ W}$$
>
> If basal metabolic requirements are approximately 100 W this represents just over 2% of basal requirements.
>
> ### Calculation of heat loss in humidifying gases
>
> Fully saturated air at 37 °C contains approximately 43 g m^{-3} (0.043 kg m^{-3}) of water. Assume 6 L min^{-1} of ventilation with dry gases which become 100% humidified in the respiratory tract. If the specific latent heat of vaporisation of water at 37 °C is 2420 kJ kg^{-1}, then the amount of water vapour required to humidify the inspired minute volume is given by
>
> Mass of water evaporated min^{-1} = $6 \times 10^{-3} \times 0.043$
> $$= 2.58 \times 10^{-4} \text{ kg}$$
>
> Heat lost by evaporation min^{-1}
> $$= 2.58 \times 10^{-4} \times 2420 \times 10^{3}$$
> $$= 624 \text{ J}$$
> $$= 10.4 \text{ W}$$
>
> Thus the total heat losses due to using cool unhumidified gases are
> $$= 2.2 + 10.4$$
> $$= 12.6 \text{ W}$$

Humidity

Humidity is a measurement of the amount of water vapour present in the air. It may be presented in two ways, either as an *absolute humidity* value or as a *relative humidity* value.

> **Absolute humidity** – the mass of water vapour present in a given volume of air. The units of measurement are grams per cubic metre ($g\ m^{-3}$) or kilograms per cubic metre ($kg\ m^{-3}$). Absolute humidity value will not vary with the temperature of the air.
>
> **Relative humidity** – the ratio of the mass of water present in a given volume of air at a given temperature, to the mass of water required to saturate that given volume at the same temperature. Relative humidity is usually expressed as a percentage, and varies with temperature.

Figure 44.20 shows how the relative humidity (RH) of a sample of air which is saturated at 20 °C (RH = 100%) decreases as temperature increases. The amount of water vapour required to saturate air at 20 °C is approximately $17\ g\ m^{-3}$. However, at 37 °C, approximately $43\ g\ m^{-3}$ is required for saturation, so the RH of the given sample decreases to 39%. From this example it can be seen that humidifying inspired gases at room temperature results in only about 40% RH at body temperature.

Calculation of RH from water vapour pressure and SVP

Since the partial pressure exerted by a gas is proportional to the mass of gas present, the relative humidity can be

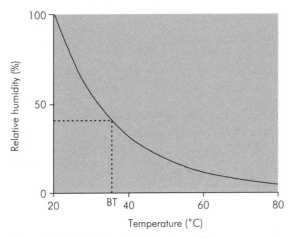

Figure 44.20 Variation of relative humidity with temperature

determined from the actual water vapour pressure and the saturated water vapour pressure at the given temperature:

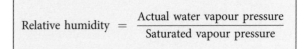

$$\text{Relative humidity} \ = \ \frac{\text{Actual water vapour pressure}}{\text{Saturated vapour pressure}}$$

Methods of humidity measurement are discussed in Chapter 45.

Heat transfer

Heat energy can be transferred by different mechanisms:

Conduction – When one end of a bar of metal is held in a fire the cool end gradually gets hotter as heat travels along the bar. This form of heat transfer is conduction. In the metal the atoms maintain a mean fixed position, unlike the case of a liquid or gas. The atoms, however, are free to vibrate about their mean position, the amplitude of this motion being dependent on the temperature of the solid. When this vibration is increased by raising the temperature in one region, the vibration is transmitted to neighbouring atoms, causing their temperature to increase and heat to be transferred. Clearly conduction requires physical continuity or contact. Net movement of the medium transferring heat does not occur in conduction. Conduction also occurs in liquids and gases, but the transfer of heat in these cases occurs mainly by convection.

Convection – This mechanism describes the transfer of heat in a liquid or gas when one region becomes heated. Increasing the temperature locally in a liquid or gas causes the density locally to decrease. This less dense fluid then rises to be replaced by cooler denser fluid. This results in a *convection current*, or the bulk movement of the fluid with an accompanying transfer of heat energy. Hot air currents in the atmosphere and the continuous movement of water in a kettle as it boils are examples of convection.

Radiation – Heat energy can also be transferred by electromagnetic radiation in the form of infrared radiation (see Figure 44.76). This enables heat transfer to occur across a vacuum in the absence of any physical continuity or surrounding medium. Radiation is the mechanism by which heat is transferred from the sun to earth. Any object is capable of both emitting and absorbing infrared radiation with a resultant loss or gain of heat energy.

The importance of these mechanisms in anaesthesia lies in heat losses suffered by a patient during prolonged periods of anaesthesia or sedation. These mechanisms are considered, together with additional factors such as losses due to evaporation from the respiratory tract and by sweating, in Chapter 21.

Gases

Gases, unlike solids and liquids, are compressible and change their volume when different pressures are applied to them. Therefore the physical behaviour of a gas can be described by three parameters, pressure (P), volume (V) and temperature (T). This is summarised by the **gas laws** for a fixed mass of gas:

The gas laws

The relationship between volume and pressure at constant temperature (**Boyle's law**):

Pressure is inversely proportional to volume

$$P \propto \frac{1}{V}$$

$$PV = \text{constant}$$

The relationship between volume and temperature at constant pressure (**Charles' law**):

Volume is proportional to temperature (kelvin)

$$V \propto T$$

$$\frac{V}{T} = \text{constant}$$

The relationship between pressure and temperature at constant volume (**Gay-Lussac's law**):

Pressure is proportional to temperature (kelvin)

$$P \propto T$$

$$\frac{P}{T} = \text{constant}$$

The ideal gas equation

The above three laws can be summarised into a single equation, the **ideal gas equation**:

$$\frac{PV}{T} = \text{constant}$$

This equation enables us to convert from one set of conditions to another when a fixed mass of gas undergoes changes in pressure, volume or temperature, since

$$\frac{P_1 V_1}{T_1} = \frac{P_2 V_2}{T_2}$$

The gas constant (R)

The ideal gas equation may be written as

$$PV = kT$$

where k is a constant dependent on the mass of gas present. If n = number of moles of gas present, the ideal gas equation becomes:

Ideal gas equation

$$PV = n\mathbf{R}T$$

where $\mathbf{R}$ is known as the **universal gas constant**, and can be evaluated by considering 1 mole of gas at 273 K (0 °C) at a pressure of 1 atmosphere. This gives a value of

$$\mathbf{R} = 8.32 \text{ joules per } °C$$

Gas contents in a cylinder

From the ideal gas equation, the pressure exerted by any gas is dependent on the number of moles present. Therefore, in a fixed volume such as a gas cylinder, the pressure in the cylinder is a measure of the amount of gas contained (e.g. in an oxygen cylinder). However this does not apply to a vapour (where liquid and gas phases are present, such as in a full nitrous oxide cylinder), since the pressure then reflects the saturated vapour pressure. However, it should be noted that the critical temperature (Tc) for nitrous oxide is only 36.5 °C, and if ambient temperature rises above this value nitrous oxide cannot exist in its liquid state.

Avogadro's hypothesis

The above gas laws apply to any gas as long as the 'given mass' of gas remains the same, since gas behaviour is determined by the number of molecules present rather than the absolute mass present. This idea is based on a hypothesis proposed by Amedeo Avogadro in 1811, which stated:

Avogadro's hypothesis

Equal volumes of gases, under the same conditions of temperature and pressure, contain equal numbers of molecules.

An important conclusion following from this hypothesis was that gaseous elements exist as molecules (O_2 and N_2) rather than as single atoms. This explained apparent anomalies in behaviour between gaseous elements and gaseous compounds.

The Avogadro constant

1 mole of gas or vapour contains the same number of molecules. This is the Avogadro constant:

Avogadro constant $= 6.022 \times 10^{23}$

Volume occupied by 1 mole of gas or vapour:

1 mole of any gas or vapour occupies 22.4 litres at NTP (0 °C or 273 K, and 1 atmosphere).

Dalton's law of partial pressures

Dalton's law of partial pressures states that if a mixture of gases is placed in a container then the pressure exerted by each gas (partial pressure) is equal to that which it would exert if it alone occupied the container.

Thus in any mixture of gases (e.g. alveolar gas, fresh inspired gases, air), the partial pressure exerted by each gas is proportional to its fractional concentration.

Calculation of partial pressures in a mixture of gases

Consider a mixture of 5% carbon dioxide, 15% oxygen and 80% nitrogen. If the mixture exerts a total pressure of 100 kPa, then the partial pressures exerted by each gas are $pCO_2 = 5$ kPa, $pO_2 = 15$ kPa and $pN_2 = 80$ kPa.

Similarly, if the total pressure exerted by the gas mixture is increased to 200 kPa, then the partial pressures become $pCO_2 = 10$ kPa, $pO_2 = 30$ kPa and $pN_2 = 160$ kPa.

Adiabatic compression or expansion of gases

Adiabatic, when applied to the expansion or compression of a gas, means that heat energy is not added or removed when the changes occur. Thus when compression of a volume of gas occurs, it is accompanied by a temperature rise, and similarly expansion of a volume of gas will produce a temperature fall. Practical consequences of this are that compression of gases will require added cooling to avoid unwanted heating of the system.

Alternatively, expansion of gases in the airway during jet ventilation can produce localised cooling, which in turn can reduce the humidity of injected gases. A practical application of the adiabatic expansion of gases lies in the cryoprobe. Here expansion of gas in the probe is used to produce low temperatures in the tip for cryotherapy.

Hydrodynamics

Gases, liquids and fluid behaviour

Although gases and liquids differ considerably in their physical properties, they display similar behaviour under flow conditions, and can both be described as being 'fluid'. The following points are similarities in behaviour between gases and liquids:

- Liquids and gases both fill the shape of their container, and are subject to constraints imposed by gravity. However, because of their lower density, gases are less affected by gravity than liquids.
- The flow behaviour of gases and liquids is largely determined by density and viscosity, although gases have much lower density and viscosity than liquids.
- In both gases and liquids, flow is produced by the application of a pressure gradient.

The similarity between gases and liquids in flow behaviour has led to the development of *fluid dynamics*, which is the study of fluids in motion, and applies equally to both gases and liquids.

Viscosity

Viscosity may be thought of as the 'stickiness' of a fluid. This property of a fluid can show itself in many ways. Imagine trying to pour treacle from a bottle compared to pouring water from the same bottle. Viscosity will affect the flow of fluids through a tube: the more viscous the fluid, the slower the flow through the tube. Gases are far less viscous than liquids, and viscous effects only become apparent at much higher flow velocities in gases compared to liquids.

The viscosity of a fluid can be quantified by its *coefficient of viscosity*. In order to understand how the coefficient of viscosity for a fluid is obtained, the concepts of *shear stress* and *shear rate* are required.

Shear stress and shear rate

A viscous force, or drag, is felt on any object if it moves through a fluid, or if the fluid moves past the stationary object. Figure 44.21 shows a thin, flat plate with a fluid flowing past it. Away from the plate, the fluid flow is faster, but closer in towards the plate the fluid is slowed down by the presence of the plate until at the surface the fluid is not moving. This happens at any surface because of adhesion between the fluid and the solid surface; it is known as the 'no-slip' condition. Near to the surface, the flow pattern is deformed from one of uniform flow velocity to one in which layers of fluid parallel to the direction of flow 'slip' against each other, giving rise to a drag effect or 'shearing' action. This shearing action at the surface gives a drag force per unit area of the plate, which is called the *shear stress*. This is illustrated in Figure 44.21. The lengths of the arrows represent the velocity of the fluid, which diminishes to zero next to the plate. The velocity of flow thus varies between these fluid layers, i.e. a velocity gradient perpendicular to the direction of flow, or *shear rate*, is produced.

Coefficient of viscosity

The coefficient of viscosity (or simply 'viscosity') of a fluid can be defined by considering laminar flow in which two parallel layers of fluid are slipping against each other. As described above this produces two effects, a shear stress between the layers, and a velocity gradient at right angles to the direction of flow (shear rate). The coefficient of viscosity (or viscosity) is defined by:

$$\text{viscosity, } \eta \;=\; \frac{\text{shear stress}}{\text{shear rate}}$$

The units of viscosity are poises, after Poiseuille, who discovered the laws governing the flow of fluids through tubes. Water has a viscosity of 0.0101 poises at 20 °C, while air has a viscosity of 0.00017 poises at 0 °C.

Viscosity varies with temperature. Liquids generally become less viscous with increasing temperature, while gases become more viscous as temperature rises.

Newtonian fluids

These are fluids in which viscosity, η, is constant, regardless of the velocity gradients produced during flow. Many fluids, including water, are Newtonian. Some fluids, however, do not behave in this way, such as the shear-thinning fluids whose viscosity falls as the shear rate between layers increases, and the rheotropic fluids, which become more viscous the longer the shearing persists. Blood is a well-known shear-thinning fluid.

Measurement of viscosity

Viscometers are used to obtain a measurement for the coefficient of viscosity. The simplest form of viscometer allows fluid to flow under the influence of gravity down a fine-bore calibrated tube. The rate of fall of the fluid meniscus is detected by photocells from which the viscosity can be calculated.

A more complicated device uses the viscous drag created by spinning a small drum containing a sample of fluid. A pointer is mounted on a float suspended in the sample and is displaced by the torque due to the viscous drag. This records the viscosity measurement on a scale.

Viscosity and the damping of fluid flow

The viscous shearing action in a fluid flow dissipates energy as heat and is analogous to frictional effects between two solid surfaces rubbing against each other. This dissipative effect dampens the motion of fluid in a system, and thus viscous effects form a major component of *damping* in any hydrodynamic system. As with mechanical or electrical systems, damping is an important factor in determining the behaviour of the system.

Viscous effects can also affect the pattern of flow, since fluid flow can occur with two different basic patterns,

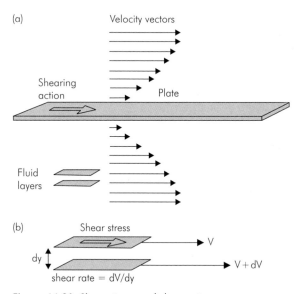

Figure 44.21 Shear stress and shear rate

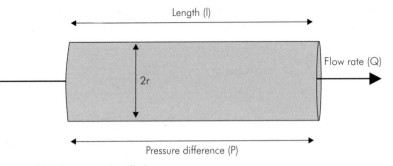

Figure 44.22 Hagen–Poiseuille law

laminar flow and turbulent flow. Laminar flow is smooth and streamlined while turbulent flow is rough, containing eddies of swirling fluid which disrupt the flow and create greater drag. The characteristics of these flow patterns are discussed in more detail below.

Flow through tubes

When a pressure difference is applied across the ends of a tube, fluid will flow from the high pressure to the low pressure. An analogy can be drawn with an electrical circuit. Fluid flow (electrical current) occurs along the tube (conductor) because of the driving pressure difference (voltage), and energy is dissipated by the viscous drag (shear stress) between the fluid and the tube (electrical resistance).

Hagen–Poiseuille law

Hagen (in 1839) and Poiseuille (in 1840) discovered the laws governing laminar flow through a tube. Consider a pressure P applied across the ends of a tube of length L and radius r (Figure 44.22). Then the flow rate, Q, produced is proportional to:

- the pressure gradient (P/L)
- the fourth power of the tube radius (r^4)
- the reciprocal of fluid viscosity (η^{-1})

This is often combined as the Hagen–Poiseuille equation and attributed to Poiseuille, a surgeon, who verified this relationship experimentally.

Hagen–Poiseuille equation

$$\text{Flow rate}, Q = \frac{\pi P r^4}{8 \eta L}$$

Kinematic viscosity

As noted above, the viscosity of a fluid influences its flow pattern by creating a damping effect. However, the inertial properties of the fluid (dependent on fluid density) also affect the flow pattern. Thus the relative effects of inertial and viscous forces can determine the nature of fluid flow in any given situation. This is taken into account by using the kinematic viscosity (μ), which is defined as the ratio of the viscosity to the density (ρ):

$$\text{Kinematic viscosity}, \mu = \frac{\eta}{\rho}$$

If the kinematic viscosity is high, rapid irregular flow patterns in a fluid will be well damped, but if it is low then disturbances such as swirling eddies may persist for a long time.

Reynolds number and turbulence

The Reynolds number (Re) is used to determine whether the flow will be laminar or turbulent in any given situation. It includes the kinematic viscosity and the ratio of the inertial forces to the viscous damping forces in the fluid, and is given by:

$$\textbf{Reynolds number, Re} = \frac{v L}{\mu}$$

Where v = the mean flow velocity for flow through a tube, or the velocity a long way from an object, and L = a characteristic length of the system, such as the diameter of a tube.

At low Reynolds numbers, the viscous forces dampen minor irregularities in the flow, resulting in a laminar pattern. A high Reynolds number means that the inertial forces dominate, and any eddies in the flow will be easily created and persist for a long time, creating turbulence. For flow though a tube, a Reynolds number of less than 2000 tends to give laminar flow, while between 2000 and 4000 the flow may be a mixture of laminar and turbulent depending on the smoothness of the fluid entering the tube. Above 4000, the flow will certainly be turbulent.

Velocity profiles for laminar and turbulent flow in a tube

If we looked at the velocities across a tube, the velocity profile, the shapes would be different for laminar and turbulent flow, as shown in Figure 44.23.

Laminar flow – Figure 44.23a shows the profile for laminar flow. This is much more pointed than the flat central portion of turbulent flow. The arrows are flow velocity vectors and are all parallel to the axis of the tube. There is a gradual decrease in flow velocity as the walls of the tube are approached. Laminar flow tends to occur when viscous effects predominate – i.e. with viscous fluids, in narrow tubes, or at low flow velocities.

Turbulent flow – If the flow velocity of the fluid in Figure 44.23a is increased, turbulent flow will be produced (Figure 44.23b). This contains irregular flow vectors and swirling eddies. The velocity vectors vary continuously in time, but a velocity profile (broken line) can still be drawn, by averaging the velocity vectors in time. In the turbulent case the velocity vectors are greater in magnitude but the profile is flatter across the centre of the tube. The velocity gradient at the walls is steeper because of an increased viscous drag associated with the turbulence. Flow resistance effects are relatively greater in turbulent flow than in laminar flow. Turbulence tends to occur at high flow velocities, when density

(inertial) effects predominate – i.e. with thin dense fluids and in wide-bore (orifices) or irregular tubes.

Transition between laminar flow and turbulence

When flow is slow it remains laminar, and both viscous drag and pressure drop along the tube increase in proportion with flow velocity. As flow velocity increases, there is an increased tendency for small eddies to disrupt the flow until at higher velocities the flow becomes turbulent. When flow is turbulent there is an abrupt change in the viscous forces, as reflected by an increased pressure drop along the tube. The slope of a graph plotting pressure drop against flow velocity becomes steeper at the laminar–turbulent transition. This transition is illustrated in Figure 44.24, and at this point the Reynolds number exceeds the threshold of approximately 2000.

A mixture of laminar and turbulent gas flow patterns is found in the airways of the lung during normal breathing. Turbulent flow occurs in the trachea and main bronchi at peak flow rates during quiet breathing, while flow in the small airways remains laminar under virtually all conditions.

Effect of varying cross-section on flow velocity

In many situations flow occurs through tubes with a varying cross-sectional area, as illustrated in Figure 44.25. The fluid is assumed to be incompressible, an assumption which is clearly valid for liquids, and which under normal circumstances remains surprisingly valid for gases. The volume flow rate is the product of the area of the tube and the average flow velocity, and since no fluid leaves or enters the tube, the volume flow rate must be the same at point 1 as it is at point 2. This statement can be written as:

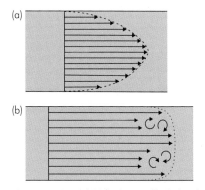

Figure 44.23 (a) Velocity profile in laminar flow; (b) velocity profile in turbulent flow

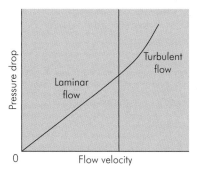

Figure 44.24 Velocity–pressure drop curve showing transition between laminar and turbulent flow

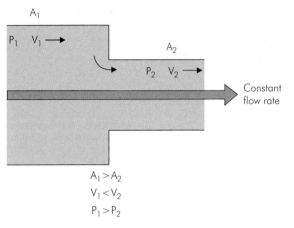

Figure 44.25 Constant volume rate flow through a tube with varying cross-section

$$A_1.v_1 = A_2.v_2$$

As the fluid moves from a larger cross-section (point 1), to a smaller cross-section (point 2), the velocity increases (from v_1 to v_2). Similarly, on moving from a smaller cross-section to a larger cross-section the velocity of flow will decrease.

Pressure and velocity: Bernoulli's equation

The pressure in the fluid can be related to its flow velocity by considering the balance between potential and kinetic energy for the fluid. The fluid has potential energy due to the pressure driving it in the direction of flow, and kinetic energy because it is moving. Since it is moving faster at point 2 than at point 1, its kinetic energy at point 2 is higher. For a gain in kinetic energy to occur, some potential energy must have been lost, i.e. a pressure drop occurs between point 1 and point 2. Thus the increased velocity at point 2 is accompanied by a reduced pressure. The relationship between pressure (P), and velocity (v) at any point in a fluid is given by:

Bernoulli's equation

$$\frac{1}{2}\rho v^2 \quad + \quad P \quad = \quad \text{constant}$$

$$\begin{bmatrix} \text{kinetic} \\ \text{energy} \end{bmatrix} \qquad \begin{bmatrix} \text{potential} \\ \text{energy} \end{bmatrix}$$

This equation applies to incompressible flow, assuming no change in potential energy due to gravity (i.e. flow does not occur uphill or downhill). This is a good approximation for gases, in which gravitational effects are usually negligible, or liquid flow in horizontal tubes.

Bernoulli's equation shows that as the velocity of a fluid increases, the pressure falls, or alternatively if the pressure of a gas flow falls, it gains velocity. This is illustrated by the example of gas escaping from a cylinder at high pressure through a nozzle to the atmosphere. The gas in the cylinder acquires a high speed as it exits through the nozzle to atmospheric pressure. The potential energy initially contained in the gas, due to it being compressed, has been converted to kinetic energy as the pressure falls to atmospheric pressure.

Venturi effect

The Venturi effect refers to the low pressure that is produced by a constriction in a duct with fluid flowing through it. As seen from the above discussion, this arises as a result of the Bernoulli principle. The Venturi effect is applied in devices such as the flow-driven nebuliser. The Venturi flow meter (Figure 44.26) also uses the Venturi effect to estimate flow velocity from the drop in pressure at a tube constriction. However, the pressure drop is not proportional to the flow velocity, and the device needs to be carefully calibrated.

Injection of gas through a jet

The use of gas injected through a narrow jet or cannula occurs in jet ventilation, the use of the Sanders injector and some types of fixed-performance oxygen masks. In these devices high-pressure gas is injected through a small orifice into a duct or airway open to the atmosphere. The injected gas forms a high-velocity stream which drags surrounding air behind it (entrainment) due to the viscosity of the gases. This is often erroneously referred to as

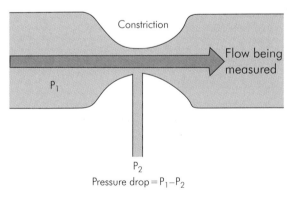

Figure 44.26 Venturi flow meter

a 'Venturi' effect but can more accurately be attributed to viscous drag.

Electricity

Basic quantities and units

Definitions of *charge*, *current*, *potential* and *potential difference* together with their units are given below.

Electric charge

An electric charge may be positive or negative, and is produced by the accumulation of an excess or deficit of electrons in an object. Charge is measured in coulombs. Like charges tend to repel each other and opposite charges attract each other.

Definition of the coulomb

The coulomb is defined as an electric charge equal in magnitude to the charge possessed by 6.24×10^{18} electrons.

1 coulomb can also be defined from the unit of current (the ampere: see below) as that charge which passes any point in a circuit in a second, when a steady current of 1 ampere is flowing.

Electric current

Most useful electrical effects are produced by the movement of charge. Any movement of electric charge forms an electric current. The current flowing in a conductor can be measured as the number of coulombs passing any given point per second. The unit of current is the ampere (A or amp), where

1 ampere (A) $= 1$ coulomb s^{-1}

1 milliampere (mA) $= 1 \times 10^{-3}$ amp

1 microampere (μA) $= 1 \times 10^{-6}$ amp

Definition of the ampere

If two conducting wires are close to each other they will produce a force between them due to their magnetic fields, which depends on the size of the current in the wires.

The ampere is defined as the current which, if flowing in two parallel wires of infinite length, placed 1 metre apart in a vacuum, will produce a force on each of the wires of 2×10^{-7} newtons per metre (Figure 44.27).

Magnetic effects of an electric current

When a current flows through a conductor it produces magnetic lines of force around the conductor (Figure 44.28). This effect was discovered by Oersted and later applied by Michael Faraday to give rise to the development of electric motors and generators. Currents flow easily in conductors, which commonly include

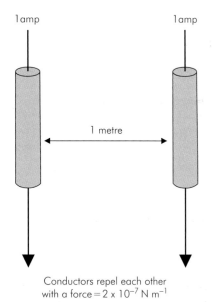

Conductors repel each other
with a force $= 2 \times 10^{-7}$ N m^{-1}

Figure 44.27 Definition of the ampere

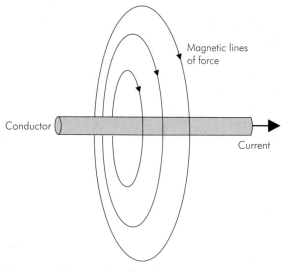

Figure 44.28 Magnetic effect of current

metals and electrolyte solutions. Materials which do not conduct current are insulators. There are some materials with intermediate conducting properties (semiconductors), e.g. silicon, which have revolutionised electronic technology.

Electrical potential

If a positive electrical potential exists at a point, any positive charge at that point will possess potential energy and will tend to move away from it to a point at lower potential. Electrical potential is analogous to height in a gravitational field where a mass possesses potential energy due to its height, and always tends to move downhill. The electrical potential of the earth is taken as a reference point for zero potential, and is usually referred to simply as 'earth'.

Potential is measured in volts. Charge will only move between points separated by a potential difference (also measured in volts).

Potential difference (voltage)

When a potential difference (often referred to as a 'voltage' – these terms have become interchangeable) is applied across a conductor it produces an electric current. A current is a flow of positive charge from a higher potential to a lower potential. (Note that this is a definition according to convention, and in reality only electrons, which are negatively charged, can move in a circuit).

Definition of the volt

1 volt is defined as a potential difference producing a change in energy of 1 joule when 1 coulomb is moved across it.

Electric circuits

An electric current is defined as a movement or flow of charge, and by convention the direction of the current is taken as the direction of flow of positive charge. In an electrolyte solution these charges may be positive or negative ions. In a wire the only mobile charges are the electrons, so the direction of current flow is opposite to the movement of the electrons. Consider a simple circuit, as in Figure 44.29. An electric current flows from positive to negative and lights the lamp. However, this current is actually formed by a movement of electrons in the opposite direction.

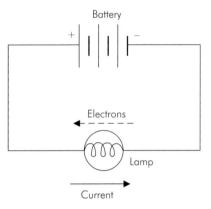

Figure 44.29 Simple circuit

Resistance

Electrical resistance is the electrical property of a conductor which opposes the flow of current through it. Electrical resistance is measured in ohms (Ω).

Ohm's law

Ohm's law states that the current flowing through a resistance is proportional to the potential difference across it. In Figure 44.30, the potential difference across the resistance = V volts, the current = I amps, and the resistance has a value of R Ω. Then

$V = I R$ volts

Example for Ohm's law

Find the current flowing when a resistance of 250 Ω is connected across a 12 volt battery

$$V = I R$$
$$I = \frac{V}{R} = \frac{12}{250}$$
$$= 0.048 \text{ A}$$
$$= 48 \quad \text{mA}$$

Power

Power is energy expended or work done per second, and has the units of joules per second or watts. In an electrical circuit the flow of current through a resistance requires the expenditure of energy, which appears as heat.

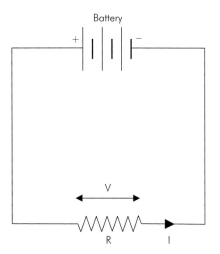

Battery

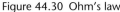

V

R   I

Figure 44.30 Ohm's law

Power

Dissipated in a resistance (R), by the passage of an electric current through it, power (P) is given by:

$P = V I$ watts

Substituting for I or V, this may become

$P = I^2 R$ watts

$\quad = \dfrac{V^2}{R}$ watts

Direct current (DC) and alternating current (AC)

The terms DC and AC are normally used to describe the electricity supply to a circuit or system, and are applied to either voltages or currents.

DC describes current which only flows in one direction, i.e. the polarity always remains the same. Generally DC is supplied by a battery (or power adaptor), and if the voltage supplied is plotted against time it will give a graph as shown in Figure 44.31a.

AC describes a supply in which the current reverses direction cyclically. If the voltage is plotted against time the sinusoidal curve shown in Figure 44.31b is produced. AC is the normal mains supply and has this form because of the way in which electricity is generated and distributed. An AC voltage is described by its amplitude (peak value) and frequency. The amplitude of mains voltage is 340 V and it has a frequency of 50 Hz.

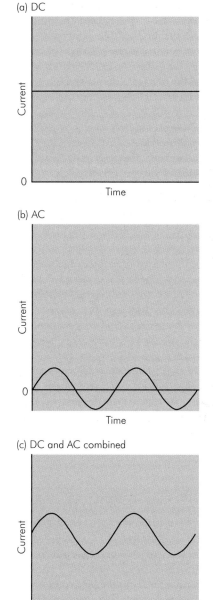

(a) DC

(b) AC

(c) DC and AC combined

Figure 44.31 (a) Direct current (DC); (b) alternating current (AC); (c) DC with AC superimposed

RMS value

Usually mains voltage is quoted as 240 V, which is the root mean square (RMS) value. The RMS value for an

AC voltage is the DC voltage or current which would have the same heating effect. This is used to compare AC and DC, because the heating and lighting effects (power dissipation) of a current are not dependent on the direction of flow. It is obtained mathematically by squaring the value of the voltage/current, averaging this squared value over time and then taking the square-root value.

AC currents and voltages are important because they can be used to carry information. In this case they are usually referred to as signals. The properties of signals measured and generated in the body, or *biopotentials*, are discussed in more detail in Chapter 45. Often electrical currents and signals are a combination of DC and AC (Figure 44.31c).

Phase angle

A simple AC voltage or current often takes the form of a sine wave, with successive identical cycles in voltage, as shown in Figure 44.32a. In this diagram voltage is plotted on the y-axis and time on the x-axis. The duration of a cycle is the period (T, in seconds), which is the time between successive positive or negative peaks.

The same electrical signal can also be shown as a sine wave by plotting voltage on the y-axis and phase angle (measured in degrees) on the x-axis (Figure 44.32b). The voltage cycles repeatedly with changes of phase angle, each cycle extending over an angle of 360°.

Thus any point in an electrical sine wave can be defined either as a point in time or as a phase angle.

Phase (angle) difference

It can be useful to compare the relative timing or phase (angle) difference between two sine waves in an electrical circuit (e.g. a comparison between an AC voltage across a resistance and the AC current flowing through the resistance). This comparison is made sometimes because it can give useful information about the behaviour of the circuit. The simplest case is when the two signals are perfectly 'in step' (Figure 44.33a), in which case the phase difference is zero (or it could also be considered to be 360°). If the two waves were out of step such that the positive peak of one wave coincided with the negative peak of the other, the phase difference would be 180° (Figure 44.33b).

The phase differences between two sine waves can take a value between 0° and 360°, and may sometimes

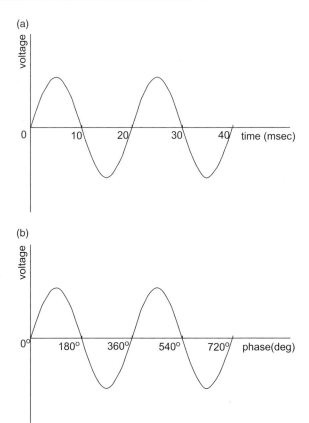

Figure 44.32 (a) AC voltage signal plotted in time; (b) AC voltage signal plotted against phase angle

be expressed as one wave either leading or 'lagging' the other. Figure 44.33c shows a case of current leading the voltage by 90°.

Impedance and reactance

The response of many circuit elements to DC and AC can be very different. Some devices may have a very low ability to resist the flow of AC, but offer a high resistance to DC, or vice versa (see below).

- **Resistance** is a measure of a device's ability to resist DC current. It is represented by R and measured in ohms.
- **Reactance** describes a device's ability to resist the flow of AC. The reactance of a device will be dependent on the frequency of AC applied. It is normally represented by X and is also measured in ohms.

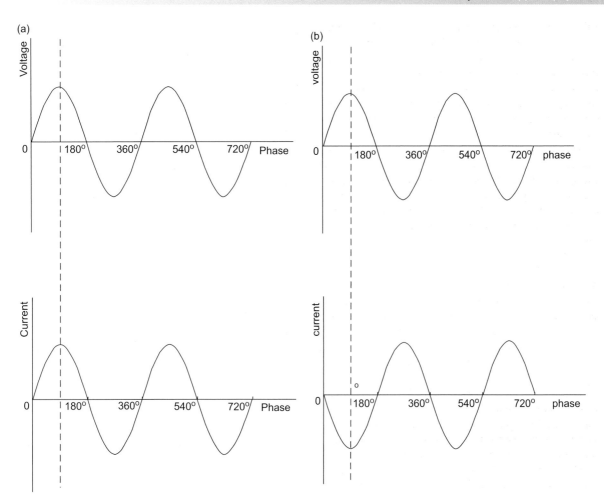

Figure 44.33 (a) AC voltage and current in phase (phase difference = 0°); (b) AC voltage and current 180° out of phase; (c) AC current leading voltage by 90°

Impedance

The electrical impedance of a device is obtained by mathematically combining its reactance and resistance. It is normally represented by Z and is measured in ohms.

$$Z = \sqrt{R^2 + X^2}$$

Impedance will vary with frequency because of the reactive component.

Circuit elements

Figure 44.34 shows some symbols representing circuit elements which are commonly encountered. The properties of some of them are outlined below.

Resistors

Resistance is the property of a conductor (a resistor) to oppose the flow of both AC and DC alike. A resistor in a circuit can be used to reduce currents or voltages. Often multiple resistors are used in a circuit. These can be combined in order to calculate the values of currents and voltages produced in different parts of the circuit.

> ### Series resistors
>
> A series arrangement (Figure 44.35) is 'end to end'. Combination of these values is by simple addition. The total for series resistance, R_T, where $R_1 = 5\ \Omega$ and $R_2 = 3\ \Omega$, is given by
>
> $$R_T = R_1 + R_2$$
> $$= 8\ \Omega$$
>
> ### Parallel resistors
>
> A parallel arrangement (Figure 44.36) is 'side by side'. The total for parallel resistances, R_T, where $R_1 = 5\ \Omega$ and $R_2 = 3\ \Omega$, is given by
>
> $$1/RT = 1/R1 + 1/R2$$
> $$= 1/5 + 1/3 = 8/15$$
> $$R_T = 1.9\ \Omega$$

Wheatstone bridge circuit

This circuit consists of a ring of four resistances supplied by a DC voltage across diagonally opposite corners of the ring A and C (Figure 44.37). The values of the resistances are balanced using a variable resistor R_1, such that points B and C are at exactly the same potential. This occurs when

$$\frac{R_1}{R_3} = \frac{R_2}{R_4}$$

When this condition is fulfilled, if a galvanometer, G, is connected between B and D no current will be detected and the bridge is 'balanced' or 'zeroed'. The bridge circuit is very sensitive to any variation in the value of the resistances, and if one of them changes a current will be detected on G.

The circuit is applied by using a strain gauge as one of the resistances (R_2) e.g. as in a piezoresistive pressure transducer. When the measured pressure varies the resistance of the strain gauge, the bridge circuit registers a current in G.

Capacitors

Capacitance describes the property of a circuit element (a capacitor) enabling it to store electric charge. A capacitor consists of two conducting plates separated by a thin layer of insulating material (or dielectric).

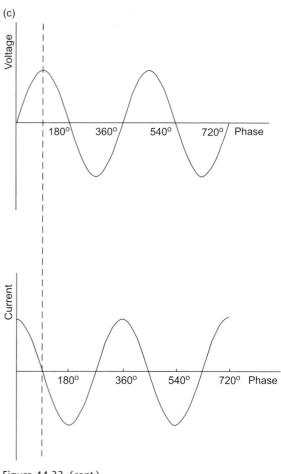

Figure 44.33 (*cont.*)

When a voltage is applied across the plates, there is an initial surge of current as charge moves onto the plates, but when the plates have become charged no more current flows. Figure 44.38 shows a capacitor charging circuit and the current (Figure 44.38b) and voltage (Figure 44.38c) changes occurring when the switch is closed. The amount of charge stored depends on the size of the capacitance, which is measured in farads (F). This in turn depends on the size of the capacitor plates, the separation of the plates and the dielectric material used. The physical size of a capacitor depends on the materials used and the working voltage, but one with a capacitance of 1 F would be impractical in most circuits, being the size of a shoebox, and thus more practical units of microfarads (μF) and picofarads (pF) are used.

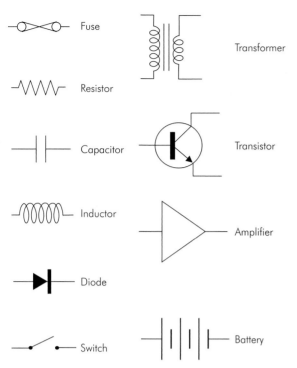

Figure 44.34 Circuit elements

Capacitance is given by

$$C = \frac{Q}{V}$$

In a circuit a capacitor has the useful property of being able to 'pass' AC signals, since electrostatic forces between the capacitor plates transmit AC current changes, but to 'block' DC, since there is no direct contact between the plates.

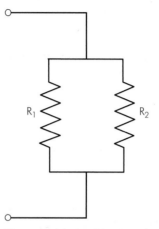

Figure 44.36 Combination of parallel resistors

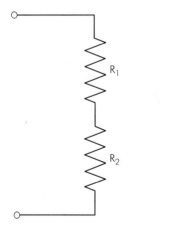

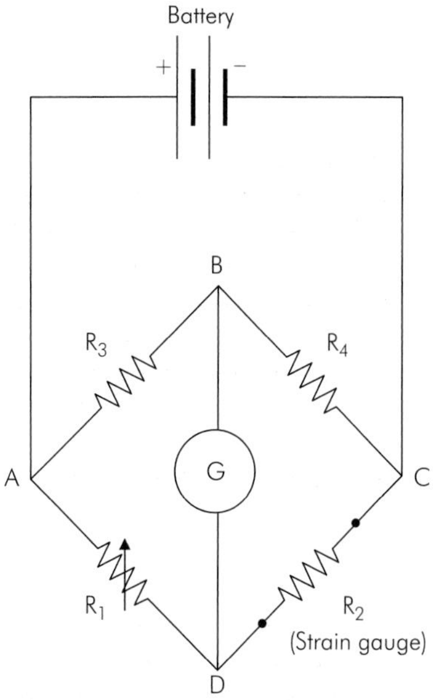

Figure 44.35 Combination of series resistors

The charge (Q) stored can be calculated given the value of the capacitance (C) and the voltage (V) applied across the capacitor plates:

$$Q = C\,V \text{ coulombs}$$

The resistance of a capacitor (to DC) is very high, since it is effectively an open circuit. However, the reactance of a

Figure 44.37 Wheatstone bridge circuit

capacitor (to AC) is low and decreases with frequency. This enables it to be used to bypass unwanted AC signals to earth in cases of electrical interference. The frequency dependence of capacitors also means that they are useful components in filters.

The values of two capacitors can be combined in a circuit, to give a total value depending on their configuration.

Parallel capacitors

Parallel capacitors are shown in Figure 44.39. Combination of these values is by simple addition. Calculation of total capacitance C_T for parallel capacitors where $C_1 = 16\ \mu F$ and $C_2 = 32\ \mu F$ is given by

$$C_T = C_1 + C_2$$
$$= 16 + 32$$
$$= 48\ \mu F$$

Series capacitors

Figure 44.40 shows series capacitors. Calculation of total capacitance C_T for series capacitors where $C_1 = 16\ \mu F$ and $C_2 = 32\ \mu F$ is given by

$$\frac{1}{C_T} = \frac{1}{C_1} + \frac{1}{C_2}$$
$$= \frac{1}{16} + \frac{1}{32} = \frac{3}{32}$$
$$C_T = 10.7\ \mu F$$

Inductors

Inductance describes the property of a circuit element (an inductor) to delay the passage of an electric current through it. An inductor is made by forming a conductor into coils, which are often wound around a core (or 'former') of ferrous material. This construction has the effect of producing a concentrated magnetic field through the axis of the inductor and around it, whenever a current flows (Figure 44.41).

When a voltage is applied across the terminals of an inductor (Figure 44.42a), current does not flow immediately but increases slowly in step with the build-up of the magnetic lines of force (Figure 44.42b.) Similarly, if the voltage is switched off, the current does not fall to zero immediately but dies down slowly, since as the magnetic field collapses it maintains the current flow for a while. This behaviour can be described as a 'lag' between the

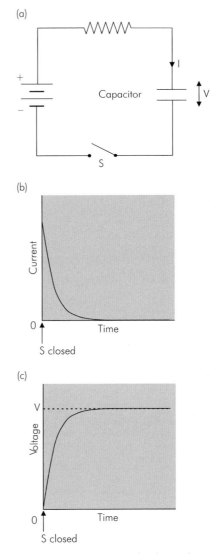

Figure 44.38 Current and voltage changes in a capacitor: (a) a capacitor charging circuit; (b) current changes when switch is closed; (c) voltage changes when switch is closed

current and voltage, giving a phase lag of 90° between current and voltage.

When a voltage is applied across the terminals of an inductor, as occurs when the switch, S, is closed in the circuit of Figure 44.42a, current does not flow immediately but increases slowly in step with the build-up of magnetic lines of force (Figure 44.42b). Similarly, when the voltage is switched off, the current does not fall to zero

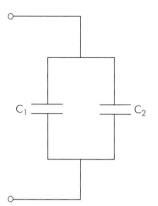

Figure 44.39 Combination of parallel capacitors

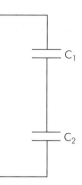

Figure 44.40 Combination of series capacitors

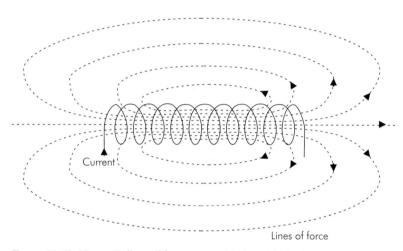

Figure 44.41 Magnetic lines of force generated by an inductor

immediately but dies down slowly (Figure 44.42c), since as the magnetic field collapses it maintains the current flow for a while. This behaviour can be described as a 'lag' between the current and voltage, giving a phase lag of 90° between current and voltage.

The build-up and collapse of the magnetic field around an inductor tends to slow down changes in current flow, whenever the applied potential difference varies. The behaviour of inductors in an electrical circuit is thus analogous to the inertial effect of masses in a mechanical system. The unit of inductance is the henry (H).

An inductor has a relatively low resistance to DC, simply equal to that of the coils of wire. However, when AC is applied to an inductor, the continually varying current meets a comparatively high reactance. The reactance of an inductor increases with frequency. Inductances therefore tend to 'block' AC but 'pass' DC.

Inductors are therefore used as components in filters and to 'smooth out' spikes and surges in power supplies.

Defibrillator circuit

A circuit using both capacitance and inductance is the defibrillator circuit (Figure 44.43). Its operation consists of two phases, charging and discharging. These phases are controlled by the switch S_1.

When charging (Figure 44.43a), S_1 connects the capacitor to the DC power supply, which charges it to deliver the required amount of energy or number of joules set by the operator.

(a)

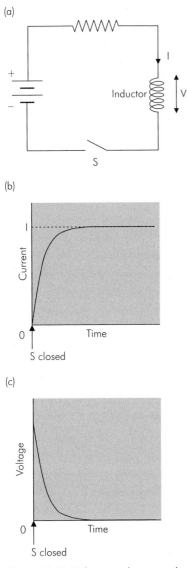

(b)

(c)

Figure 44.42 Voltage and current changes in an inductor: (a) circuit; (b) current and (c) voltage changes produced when the switch is closed

The energy stored by a charged capacitor depends on its capacitance (*C*) and the applied voltage (*V*), since

Energy stored $= 1/2\ CV^2$ joules

So if $C = 100\ \mu F$ and $V = 2000\ V$:

Energy stored $= 0.5(100 \times 10^{-6})(2000)^2$
$= 200\ J$

(a) Defibrillator charging

5000 volts DC

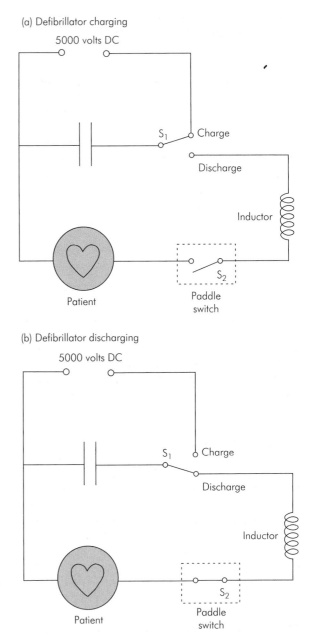

(b) Defibrillator discharging

5000 volts DC

Figure 44.43 Defibrillator circuit: (a) charging; (b) discharging through patient

On discharge (Figure 44.43b) S_1 connects the capacitor to the patient circuit, which enables the stored charge to be delivered to the patient via the switch (S_2) on the paddles. The inductor, L, in the discharge circuit has the effect of slowing down and spreading out the delivered pulse of energy to the myocardium, which makes it more effective than the shorter sharper spike waveform that would be delivered without the inductance.

Transformer

A transformer consists of two inductances wound around the same ferrous core (former). The close physical relationship between the two coils means that current changes in one circuit (the primary winding) will induce currents in the second coil (the secondary winding) via the coupling effect of the magnetic field (Figure 44.44).

> In a **transformer** the voltage produced across the secondary (V_2) will depend on the number of turns in the primary winding (N_1) and the secondary winding (N_2), and the voltage V_1 applied across the primary
>
> $$V_2 = V_1 . \frac{N_2}{N_1}$$

A transformer can thus be used to 'step up' or 'step down' voltages in circuits. Transformers are commonly used in distributing the electrical power supply from the national grid to domestic users. An alternative use for transformers is in transferring signals between circuits and devices such as microphones or loudspeakers.

Diode

A diode is a semiconductor (silicon or germanium) device which only enables current to flow through it in one direction. It is often used to convert AC to DC (Figure 44.45) in order to provide a DC power supply from the AC mains. This is commonly found in the 'mains adaptors' used as a charger or substitute for equipment batteries, or to provide the DC current to charge the capacitor in a defibrillator circuit. Diodes are also used in protective circuits and to process signals in measurement systems.

Transistor

Transistors are also semiconductor devices. These are used to amplify small current signals, enabling small electrical signals of a few microamps to be converted to much greater signals of tens of milliamps. The basic transistor consists of a tiny slice of semiconductor material with connections to three regions, the base (b), collector (c) and emitter (e). A common configuration allows a small signal fed into the base to produce an amplified signal in the collector circuit (Figure 44.46). In the early days of transistor electronics a circuit would be

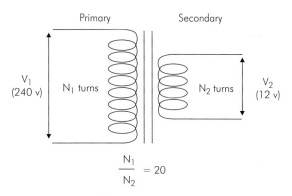

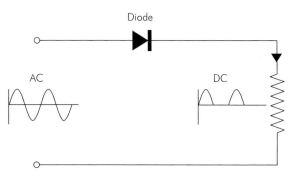

$$\frac{N_1}{N_2} = 20$$

Figure 44.44 Transformer

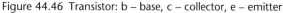

Figure 44.45 Diode circuit converting AC to DC

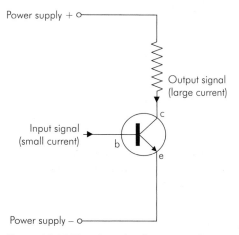

Figure 44.46 Transistor: b – base, c – collector, e – emitter

constructed using a few separate transistors. In modern electronics many thousands or even millions of transistors may be incorporated into a single semiconductor 'chip', which in turn is simply a single component in a more complex device such as a personal computer.

Electrical safety

The hazards associated with the use of electrical equipment are:

- Electric shock – macroshock
- Electric shock – microshock
- Diathermy hazards
- Electrical burns
- Fire and explosion

Electric shock (macroshock)

Electric shock (macroshock) occurs with the external application of a voltage to the skin, causing an electric current to pass through the body tissues. Commonly electric shock occurs from the AC mains supply.

The 'mains' supply

The mains supply in the UK consists of a 'live' line carrying the generated voltage (240 V RMS) and a 'neutral' line, which acts as a return for the current supplied. The 'neutral' line is earthed at the generator. In an intact mains circuit the current supplied in the 'live' line is equal to the return current in the 'neutral' line.

How electric shock occurs

Electric shock occurs from the mains supply when the body forms a circuit between the live mains line and a local earth connection or the neutral mains line.

Earthed circuit – The local earth connection may occur via the floor or ground (Figure 44.47). Alternatively, earthing may take place by inadvertent contact with earthed metalwork such as an anaesthetic machine or operating table (Figure 44.48).

Isolated circuit – In the absence of an earth connection, an individual or circuit is said to be electrically 'isolated' or 'floating'. However, current can still flow if contact with an alternative return path such as the neutral supply line is made (Figure 44.49).

Effects of electric shock

The effects of electric current flowing through body tissues depend on the following factors:

- Whether the current is AC or DC
- The magnitude of the current
- The tissues current passes through
- Current density
- Duration of current passage
- Pre-existing disease

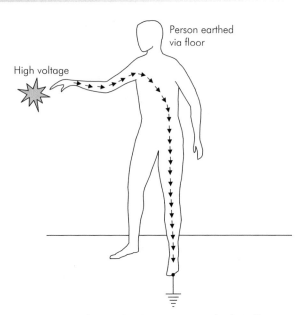

Figure 44.47 Electric shock in person earthed via floor

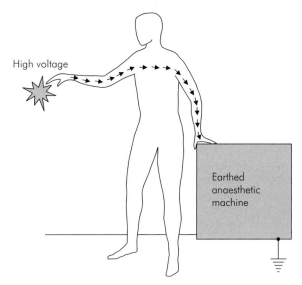

Figure 44.48 Electric shock in person earthed by touching metalwork

Whether the current is AC or DC DC produces a single muscle spasm on contact which often throws the victim clear. Arrhythmias can be precipitated, but DC shock is also used to cardiovert arrhythmias. Prolonged exposure to low DC currents can produce chemical burns.

AC will cause muscle spasm due to tetanic effects which are maximal at mains frequency (50 Hz). When contact is made through the hand, muscle spasm may

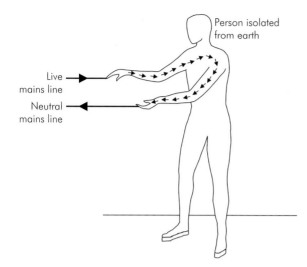

Live mains line →

Neutral mains line ←

Person isolated from earth

Figure 44.49 Electric shock in isolated person by return through neutral line

Current (mA)	Effects
0–5	Tingling sensation
5–10	Pain
10–50	Severe pain Muscle spasm
50–100	Respiratory muscle spasm Ventricular fibrillation Myocardial failure

- The tissue impedance – tissue impedance is usually low ($< 500\ \Omega$).

cause the individual to grip the contact uncontrollably, prolonging duration of the shock. AC at mains frequency is also more likely to cause arrhythmias than higher frequencies. The risk of arrhythmias decreases significantly at frequencies above 1 kHz, and at diathermy frequencies (> 1 MHz) this risk is negligible. AC currents also cause localised sweat release, which lowers skin resistance and increases tissue current (see below). AC shock is about three times as dangerous as DC for the same magnitude of current.

The magnitude of the current When an electric shock is received from the AC mains, different physiological effects are caused as the current increases in magnitude. These are summarised in Figure 44.50.

Currents above 100 mA may not only disturb normal function in conducting tissues, but can disrupt epithelium and cell membranes. There may also be a direct heating effect on tissues, depending on current density (see below), duration of application and local cooling.

The main factors determining the magnitude of a current during electrocution are:
- The voltage applied to the skin.
- The impedance (AC resistance) of the skin contact – location of the skin, thickness and sweating can all affect skin contact resistance significantly. Skin contact resistance can vary between 1000 and 200,000 Ω.
- The impedance of the earth connection – when the earth connection occurs via the floor the impedance of footwear becomes important.

Calculation of current in electric shock arm to ground (with insulating shoes)

Consider an electric shock received from the live mains wire (240 V) in a person (Figure 44.47) where the skin impedance is 2000 Ω, tissue impedance is 300 Ω and the earth contact resistance through shoes is 200,000 Ω.

If the current pathway lies through the right hand along the right arm, through the body and then via the feet to earth:

$$\text{Total resistance} = 2000 + 300 + 200{,}000$$
$$= 202.3\ \text{k}\Omega$$
$$\text{Current} = \frac{240}{202{,}300}$$
$$= 1.2\ \text{mA}$$

Normally this current would not have any harmful effects, although it might be discernible as a tingling sensation. However, if the earth contact resistance were reduced (low-resistance shoes or bare feet) this current could reach harmful levels.

Calculation of current in electric shock arm to ground (without shoes)

$$\text{Total resistance} = 2000 + 300 + 2000$$
$$\text{Current} = \frac{240}{4300}$$
$$= 55.8\ \text{mA}$$

This is a painful and potentially harmful current.

The **tissues or organs the current passes through** Currents passing through conducting tissues can disrupt normal physiological function. Consider an individual with one hand in contact with live mains terminal and the other hand earthed through an anaesthetic machine (Figure 44.48).

Calculation of current in electric shock arm to arm

The current pathway in this case is right hand and arm, chest, left arm and hand. The current flowing is given by

Total resistance $= 1000 + 300 + 1000$
$= 2.3\ \text{k}\Omega$

$$\text{Current} = \frac{240}{2300}$$
$$= 104\ \text{mA}$$

This current through the chest would not only deliver a painful shock but also carries a significant risk of inducing ventricular fibrillation or other arrhythmias, since it will pass through the heart.

Current density This is obtained by dividing the total current flowing by the cross-sectional area that the current flows through. The effect of electric currents on tissues will be more dependent on current density in the tissue than on the total current passing through the tissue. If a current passes through a diathermy probe tip the current density will be much higher than in the case of the diathermy pad (Figure 44.51). Thus tissue is burnt at the probe but not at the pad. If the pad is improperly applied, the contact surface area may be reduced and unwanted burns may occur. It is therefore important to

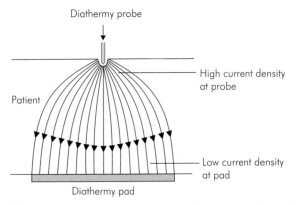

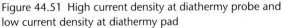

Figure 44.51 High current density at diathermy probe and low current density at diathermy pad

ensure that diathermy electrode plates are properly and uniformly applied to the patient in order to avoid accidental burns.

Duration of current passage The longer the duration of current flow, the more damage is caused to tissues in the current path, since the total amount of heat dissipated in the tissues depends on time:

$$\text{Power} = V\,I = I^2\,R\ \text{watts}$$

$$\text{Total heat} = I^2\,R\,T\ \text{joules}$$

where T = time in seconds

A small DC current, which may not produce excessive heating of tissues locally, can still produce 'chemical' burns by an electrolytic effect.

Pre-existing disease in a patient The presence of ischaemic heart disease increases the likelihood of problems such as arrhythmias.

Prevention of electric shock (macroshock)
Macroshock is prevented by the following measures:

Classification of equipment – Equipment should be designed to suitable specifications. Different classes of equipment are specified for the medical working environment, for use in different applications. The safety specifications refer to the risk of electric shock, as in the following classification:

Class I – earthed

Class II – double-insulated not earthed

Class III – low voltage (< 24 V) battery-powered

Earth circuits – These are integral to the design of equipment in order to:
- Reduce risk of electric shock
- Reduced interference
- Reduce leakage currents

Earth connections reduce the risk of electric shock by maintaining exposed metalwork at zero potential. Such metalwork cannot then deliver an electric shock current if inadvertently contacted.

However, unwanted earth connections may also increase the risks of macroshock if an individual is already in contact with a high voltage, since contact with earthed metalwork can then complete the circuit (Figure 44.48).

Earth connections can also provide a discharge pathway for static charges or leakage currents, which reduces the risk of microshock. Poor design of earth circuits, however, can actually generate *leakage currents*, which

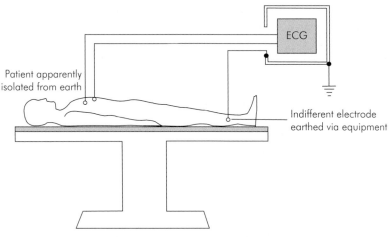

Figure 44.52 Unwanted earth connection via indifferent ECG electrode

can act as a source of microshock. This occurs where multiple earth connections are used, each connection being at a slightly different potential, causing small currents to flow through earth circuits or patients.

Poorly designed or faulty equipment can also act as a source of *microshock*. Unwanted earth connections can occur where a patient is attached to multiple electrodes (Figure 44.52) or intravascular monitoring equipment (e.g. pulmonary artery catheter, Figure 44.53). Should these connections to the patient include several earth connections, each at a slightly different potential, small leakage currents can be produced flowing through the patient.

Leakage currents

This term refers to small electric currents ($< 500\ \mu\text{A}$) which arise unintentionally. These currents may originate through faulty equipment, faulty components, faulty earth connections or the accumulation of static charges. Such currents can pass or 'leak' down to earth through a designed safety circuit (e.g. earth connection, antistatic shoes), or they may flow through an unintentional pathway, creating a risk of microshock.

The **optimum earth circuit** connects all earth circuits to earth at a single point via a good-quality contact (Figure 44.54).

Earthing casing or shielding around conductors carrying AC reduces both the transmission and pick-up of interference signals, particularly in the case of high frequencies. Coaxial cables are often used in sensitive circuits, with an earthed outer conductor surrounding and screening an inner wire.

Isolated patient circuit – An option most commonly used is the isolated patient circuit, in which there is no earth connection to the patient. This can be achieved by using an isolating transformer.

Isolating transformer – This system supplies all equipment attached to the patient via a transformer so that no equipment associated with the patient is directly connected to the mains.

Circuit breaker – This is a sensitive mains switch which operates to disconnect the mains whenever abnormal currents are detected, arising from dangerous equipment faults or the occurrence of electrocution.

Suitable footwear – Footwear impedance should be designed to isolate the wearers from earth. The impedance should be high enough to prevent large current passing to earth (avoiding electric shock) in case of contact with a high-voltage source, but low enough to allow a leakage current to earth to prevent the wearer and clothing from accumulating a static charge. Such shoes normally have an impedance of between 100 kΩ and 1 MΩ.

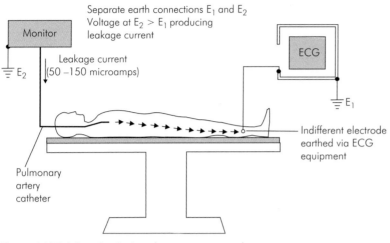

Figure 44.53 Microshock via pulmonary artery catheter

Microshock

> In **microshock**, current is delivered internally to the myocardium causing arrhythmias. The conducting pathway may be through an intravenous catheter or pulmonary artery catheter and its contained fluid.

Figure 44.53 shows a patient earthed via two circuits. One is via the pulmonary artery catheter monitor (E_2), and the other is via an indifferent ECG electrode (E_1). If the voltage at E_2 is greater than the voltage at E_1, even by 100 mV, then a leakage current may be generated, great enough to cause microshock. The magnitude of currents required to produce ventricular fibrillation in microshock is in the order of 100–150 µA. This is much smaller than in the case of macroshock.

Some potential sources of microshock
- Central venous catheter
- Pulmonary artery catheter
- Temporary external pacemaker
- Oesophageal temperature probe in lower third of oesophagus
- Statically charged staff touching any of the above

Prevention of microshock
- Appropriate equipment in good order. Equipment specifications may refer to leakage current generation and the risk of microshock:
  - CF (cardiac, floating) – leakage < 50 µA through cardiac connection
  - BF (non-cardiac, floating) – leakage < 500 µA through patient connection with single fault
- Suitable footwear impedance
- Antistatic flooring
- Isolated patient circuit – with no earth connection to patient
- Optimum design of earthing circuits for equipment (Figure 44.54)
- Correct humidity in theatre

Diathermy hazards
Diathermy uses high-frequency (0.4–1.5 MHz) currents to generate heat in the tissues during surgery. This is applied via a probe to produce coagulation and cutting effects. The most common risks in the use of diathermy are of unwanted diathermy burns, as well as the usual risks of electric shock associated with the use of any electrical equipment. In addition diathermy signals can cause interference in monitoring equipment and possibly indwelling pacemakers.

Prevention of diathermy hazards
- Use of isolated patient circuit
- Use of isolating capacitor – In diathermy an isolating capacitor is used which effectively 'short-circuits' high-frequency diathermy currents to earth (see *Capacitors*, above), reducing the risk of unintentional diathermy burns. However, at low frequencies (mains frequency and DC) the patient remains isolated, reducing the risk of macroshock and microshock (Figure 44.55).

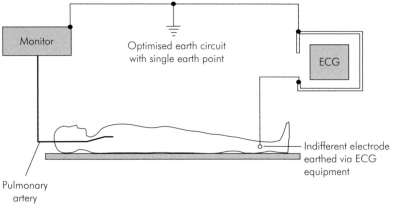

Figure 44.54 Optimised earth circuit with single earth connection

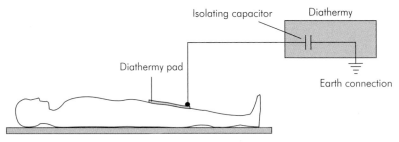

Figure 44.55 Isolating capacitor in diathermy equipment

- Proper application of diathermy pad.
- Avoiding inadvertent patient contact with earthed metalwork.
- Use of bipolar diathermy – This form of diathermy uses a pair of probes, one to deliver the diathermy signal and the other to act as a return circuit. They are arranged as the arms of forceps, which restricts the current field to a small area surrounding the forcep tips. In this way no diathermy pad is required and no electric field exists in the peripheral parts of the patient's body. This reduces the risk of unwanted peripheral diathermy burns, and also decreases possible inteference with monitoring equipment and pacemakers.

Electrical burns

Burns may occur during electrocution in different ways:
- Flash burns – This describes the effect of arcing around the individual in high-voltage (> 1000 V) shock, when electric arcing occurs to earth from the body or clothing.

- External burns – These may occur due to ignition of clothing or other inflammable materials around the individual, e.g. gases or vapours.
- Tissue burns – These may occur at the point of contact with the high-voltage source or earthing point. They are localised and are due to the passage of high-density electric currents, sometimes with accompanying arcing.

Fire and explosion

In an operating theatre there is a risk of fire or explosion due to the ignition of gas mixtures. The mixture usually consists of a fuel with oxygen or another oxidising agent such as nitrous oxide.

Inflammable gas mixtures may simply burn, generating temperatures of several hundred degrees Celsius at atmospheric pressure.

Explosions are a much more violent reaction generating a rapid rise in temperature to several thousand degrees Celsius, and a high-pressure shock wave which propagates outwards at speeds greater than the speed of sound.

For explosion or fire to occur the following are required:

- An inflammable agent – Examples include diethyl ether, cyclopropane, ethyl chloride and ethyl alcohol.
- An oxidising gas – These include oxygen, air, and nitrous oxide.
- Inflammable or explosive concentrations – Inflammable agents will only burn between flammability limits in different oxidising gases, e.g. the concentration flammability limits for cyclopropane in air are 2.4–10%, while in oxygen the limits for cyclopropane are 2.5–60%. Explosions occur when the mixture reaches stoichiometric proportions. Stoichiometric concentrations occur when the proportions of inflammable agent and oxidising gas are the same as the ratios required by the chemical reaction. An excess concentration of inflammable agent or oxidising gas reduces the likelihood of explosion.
  For example, the reaction for cyclopropane when it burns is

$$2C_3H_6 + 9O_2 \rightarrow 6CO_2 + 6H_2O$$

  Therefore a stoichiometric mixture consists of 2 parts cyclopropane to 9 parts oxygen, which is equivalent to an 18% concentration in oxygen or a 4.3% concentration in air.
- A source of ignition and activation energy – These include diathermy, electrostatic sparks and surgical lasers.

Prevention of fire and explosion

- Use of non-flammable agents
- Avoiding high-risk (5 cm radius) and low-risk (25 cm radius) zones with electrical equipment likely to generate sparks
- Use of appropriate antistatic equipment, footwear and clothing
- Awareness of equipment specifications (Figure 44.56):
  - The APG label refers to equipment which is safe to use within the high-risk zone, where oxygen and nitrous oxide may be the oxidising agents.
  - The AP label is used for the low-risk zone, where anaesthetic gases and air mixtures provide the risk.
- Adequate air conditioning, with 5–10 air changes per hour
- Appropriate scavenging system
- Use of specialised equipment in the surgical field during laser surgery

Ultrasound

Ultrasound scanning is increasingly used in anaesthesia and critical care. It is applied in:

- Acquiring vascular access
- Performing nerve blocks
- Estimating cardiac function, and detecting valve defects and pericardial collections
- Detecting pleural effusions
- Detecting collections in trauma
- Using Doppler to monitor adequacy of circulation (e.g. transcranial circulation during carotid surgery or limb circulation with the use of an intra-aortic balloon pump)

Sound

Sound travels as waves composed of alternating regions of compression and rarefaction. The particles of the medium in which the sound wave is travelling move backwards and forwards about a mean position, in the direction of propagation of the wave (Figure 44.57).

> **A sound wave** is a longitudinal compression wave (compare this with the transverse nature of light waves, or surface waves) and requires a medium to propagate in (compare this with electromagnetic waves, which can propagate through a vacuum).

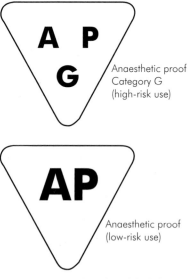

Figure 44.56 APG and AP labels for equipment suitable for use with inflammable gas mixtures

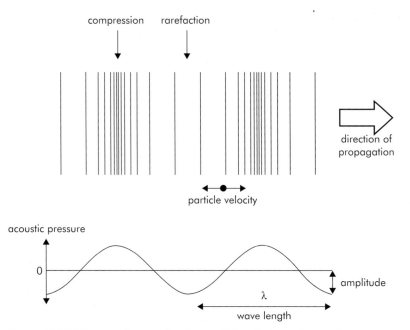

Figure 44.57 Ultrasound wave, showing particle velocity and acoustic pressure

The behaviour of sound waves is described by basic parameters and relationships that are common to all wave phenomena.

Frequency

The frequency (*f*) of a sound wave is the number of compression cycles which occur at any given point per second, and it is measured in hertz (Hz). The greater the frequency of a sound wave the higher its tone or pitch (e.g. in the musical scale middle C is 262 Hz, top C is 2093 Hz). The audible frequency range will vary according to age and species, and many examples of sound waves are generated outside the audible range for humans. *Ultrasound* is used to describe sound waves at frequencies above the audible range. The ultrasound frequencies used in medical scanning are usually between 2 and 20 MHz.

Some examples of frequency ranges for sound waves are shown in Figure 44.58.

Figure 44.58 Sound frequency ranges

Quantity	Frequency range
Adult hearing	15 Hz to 20 kHz
Child hearing	15 Hz to 40 kHz
Bat hearing	up to 200 kHz
Medical ultrasound	2 MHz to 20 MHz

Wavelength

Wavelength (λ) is the distance between two adjacent pressure peaks or troughs in a sound wave. It will vary with the medium that the wave is travelling in. The significance of the wavelength in ultrasound scanning is that detectable reflection of ultrasound waves will only occur from objects with dimensions much greater than the wavelength being used. Wavelength therefore becomes an important factor in determining the discriminative ability of an ultrasound scan. Detail in a scan will therefore be greatest at shorter wavelengths (and higher frequencies – see below).

Wavelength and discrimination

The discrimination of detail in an ultrasound scan is dependent on wavelength, and will thus be greatest at high frequencies. Using frequencies of 10 MHz in soft tissues (assuming velocity of propagation, $v = 1540$ m s^{-1}) will give a wavelength of:

$$\text{Wavelength}, \lambda = \frac{1540}{10,000,000}$$
$$= 1.5 \text{ mm}$$

Therefore objects with dimensions less than 1.5 mm will not be adequately visualised on the scan.

Velocity of propagation

Sound waves will travel through a given medium with a characteristic velocity of propagation (v). This will vary slightly with ambient conditions in the medium such as density, pressure and temperature. As with other wave phenomena, the velocity of propagation will be related to frequency (f) and wavelength (λ) by

velocity (v) = frequency (f) $\times$ wavelength (λ)

The velocity of sound in air is 330 m s^{-1}, while in water it travels much faster at 1500 m s^{-1}. The clinical use of ultrasound involves the use of ultrasound through various tissues with different velocities of propagation. Some examples are shown in Figure 44.59, below.

Acoustic impedance

As sound waves propagate through the particles (molecules) of a medium, the pressure peaks and troughs cause the particles to oscillate about their mean undisturbed position. These pressure changes and oscillations will gradually become attenuated as the wave progresses and its energy is dissipated. This process is analogous to the dissipation of electrical energy occurring when an electrical current passes through a resistance (or impedance) in a circuit. The local pressure increase produced in a sound wave is called the acoustic pressure (p) and is equivalent to electrical potential in a circuit, while the particle velocity (v) produced by the wave is equivalent to electrical current. These parameters (p and v) are dependent on the medium, and their ratio represents a property of the medium, its *acoustic impedance*.

Figure 44.59 Velocities of propagation and acoustic impedances of body tissues

Tissue	Velocity of sound (m s^{-1})	Density (kg m^{-3})	Acoustic impedance (kg m^{-2} s^{-1}) $\times 10^{-4}$
Gas	330	1.3	0.0004
Fat	1470	970	1.43
Blood	1570	1020	1.53
Muscle	1568	1040	1.63
Bone	4080	1700	6.12

$$\text{Acoustic impedance,}\, z = \frac{\text{acoustic pressure,}\, p}{\text{particle velocity,}\, v}$$

A material's acoustic impedance is also related to its characteristic speed of sound and its density. Thus:

Acoustic impedance, $z = \rho\, c$

where c = speed of sound and ρ = density of the material

Some acoustic impedances for common tissues are shown in Figure 44.59.

Reflection and acoustic impedance

Sound waves are reflected when they are incident on a smooth boundary between two media with different acoustic impedances (Figure 44.60). This type of reflection is called specular or mirror reflection since it is analogous to the reflection of light at a mirror. Specular reflection obeys the normal laws of reflection, as in the reflection of light from a mirror.

Angle of incidence = angle of reflection

Some sound is transmitted across the boundary, while some is reflected. The amount of sound transmitted depends on the acoustic impedances (z_1 and z_2). The percentage of sound reflected (R) at a boundary is given by:

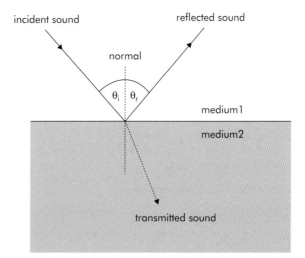

θ_i (angle of incidence) = θ_r (angle of reflection)

Figure 44.60 Reflection of ultrasound at a boundary

$$R = \frac{I_R}{I_i}$$

Where I_i = incident intensity, I_R = reflected intensity

$$R = \left[\frac{Z_1 - Z_2}{Z_1 + Z_2}\right]^2 \times 100\%$$

Consider the effect of differences in acoustic impedance on the reflected sound. If acoustic impedances differ by 10% where $z_1/z_2 = 1.1$, then the amount of sound reflected will be < 0.25%. However, when $z_1/z_2 = 10$, the amount of reflected sound is > 80%.

Acoustic impedances are important in ultrasound scanning because:

- In order to obtain efficient transmission of sound from the ultrasound probe to the tissues, 'matching' of acoustic impedances must be obtained by the use of appropriate gels, otherwise most of the sound energy is reflected from the boundary between probe and tissues.
- Since objects are only visualised by their reflected ultrasound, those objects with the greatest 'mismatch' in acoustic impedance at their boundaries will show up brightly. Thus boundaries between different soft tissues will not be as bright as those between soft tissue and air, or soft tissue and bone.
- When there is a significant mismatch in acoustic impedance at a boundary between tissues most of the incident ultrasound is reflected, leaving a 'shadow' behind the boundary or object. Common examples are bone surfaces or air spaces. Calculation of the reflected ultrasound shows that at a soft tissue to bone surface 30–40% of the incident ultrasound is reflected, while at a soft tissue to air boundary 99.99% reflection occurs. Thus the 'shadow' created by an air-filled target is denser than that distal to a bony target.

Scatter

When sound waves are incident on objects or surface irregularities with dimensions comparable to or less than the wavelength, the sound waves are not reflected wholesale as in specular reflection, but are scattered. This has the effect of reducing or attenuating the sound intensity

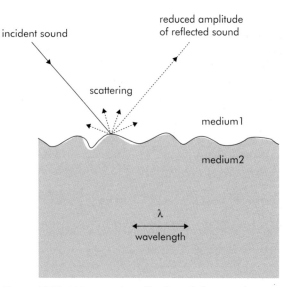

Figure 44.61 Non-specular reflection of ultrasound at a boundary

without producing an image of a boundary or object. This is sometimes referred to as non-specular reflection (Figure 44.61).

Refraction

When ultrasound is transmitted across a boundary between tissues, the transmitted ultrasound is deviated from its original course. This is due to refraction. The deviation can be measured by the angle of refraction, which is dependent on the ratio of velocities of propagation in the two media. This phenomenon is analogous to the refraction of light and obeys the same law, Snell's law:

$$\frac{\text{Sin } \theta_i}{\text{Sin } \theta_r} = \frac{\text{velocity of sound in medium}_1}{\text{velocity of sound in medium}_2}$$

Refraction effect in ultrasound scanning can lead to 'focusing' effects behind fluid-filled objects (Figure 44.62).

Power and acoustic intensity

The instantaneous energy content of a sound wave at any particular point in the wave is dependent on the kinetic energy and potential energy of the particles at that point. It is more meaningful to consider the power, P, generated by the sound wave, which is energy per second given to the medium particles (this is measured in joules s^{-1} = watts). By electrical analogy:

Acoustic power = acoustic pressure × particle velocity

$$P = p.v$$

A quantity used to compare effects of a sound wave on tissues is the acoustic intensity (I), which is the power passing through unit cross-sectional area of tissue. In practice acoustic intensity is measured in milliwatts per square millimetre (mW mm^{-2}). Ultrasound scanning is associated with acoustic intensities of < 1.0 mW mm^{-2}.

Acoustic intensities in an ultrasound field are compared using the logarithmic decibel (dB) scale:

$$\text{Change in acoustic intensity} = 10 \log_{10} \frac{I_1}{I_2} \text{ dB}$$

Thus a reduction in acoustic intensity by 50% is referred to as a 3 dB loss in intensity.

Attenuation of sound wave intensity in an ultrasound scan

The intensity of sound waves in a scan varies throughout the field and is generally reduced with increasing distance from the probe. The sound intensity is decreased by various mechanisms. These include:

- Absorption by tissues – which is dependent on frequency and accounts for most of the attenuation
- Reflection of the beam
- Scatter
- Divergence of the beam due to it not being perfectly parallel-sided

---

Averaged intensity units

When estimating the exposure of tissues to ultrasound energy it is useful to calculate an average value for acoustic intensity. Ultrasound fields produced when scanning patients are generated by pulses from the probe. The acoustic intensity in the tissues is therefore not constant in time, and neither is the acoustic pulse amplitude constant over the scanned field. Thus in order to obtain a practical value the peak acoustic intensity is averaged over both time and space (I_{SPTA}). The exposure of the tissues is then dependent on I_{SPTA} and the duration of exposure.

Harmful effects of ultrasound on tissues

The clinical use of ultrasound is generally a safe procedure, but ultrasound can damage tissues via its *heating effect*, *cavitation* and *mechanical effect*. The heating effect of ultrasound is the mechanism which has caused the

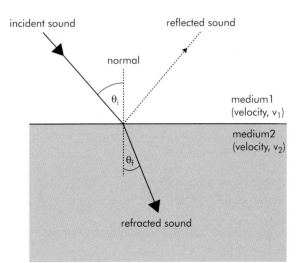

$$v_2 > v_1$$

$$\frac{\sin \theta_i}{\sin \theta_f} = \frac{v_1}{v_2}$$

Figure 44.62 Refraction of ultrasound

most concern, and this is thought to be most significant in the dividing tissues of the fetus during its first 8 weeks. Prolonged temperature rises of $> 1.5\,^{\circ}\text{C}$ are considered to be hazardous to fetal tissues.

Heating effect

Factors which determine temperature rise in tissues

- Total dose of ultrasound = mean intensity × duration
- Acoustic impedance
- Heat dissipation from the targeted area

The absorption of ultrasound energy determines the temperature rises produced in tissues exposed to ultrasound. Thus bone is likely to suffer much higher temperature rises than soft tissues in an ultrasound field.

It has been estimated that temperature rises in tissues $> 1\,^{\circ}\text{C}$ may be produced by B-mode scanning, and higher temperatures during Doppler mode because of the continuous wave nature of the ultrasound in Doppler mode.

Significant thermal effects due to ultrasound are not recorded as occurring at intensities below 1 mW mm^{-2} for unfocused ultrasound or < 10 mW mm^{-2} for focused ultrasound. Duration of exposure for unfocused ultrasound is considered safe up to 500 seconds, and up to 50 seconds with focused ultrasound.

Cavitation

Cavitation refers to the production and excitation of gas bubbles in tissues exposed to ultrasound. The negative pressures produced by ultrasound are mainly responsible for producing cavitation bubbles, but continuous-wave ultrasound (as in Doppler) is required, and it is not likely to occur during diagnostic scanning. Higher intensities, as during therapeutic ultrasound used by physiotherapists, may produce cavitation. Pre-existing gas bubbles or gas spaces in tissues (such as lung tissue) may also become excited by ultrasound waves and if violently excited may undergo collapse (collapse cavitation) with the generation of damaging effects and temperatures.

Mechanical effect

An object in a continuous-wave ultrasound field may experience a force due to incident sound waves on one surface which is not balanced by an equal force on the opposite surface. It will therefore experience a net mechanical force moving it in the direction of travel of the ultrasound waves. Small objects such as red blood cells can be agglomerated in this way by Doppler-mode exposure.

Ultrasound scanners

Ultrasound imaging is achieved by the transmission of pulses of sound waves, each pulse containing 2–3 compression cycles. These pulses are emitted by a transducer (ultrasound probe) into the tissue field, and reflected from objects in the field back to the transducer, which also acts as a receiver. Ultrasound scanning can be used in different modes.

Piezoelectric effect

Ultrasound transducers use the piezoelectric effect both for generating and for receiving signals. The piezoelectric effect refers to a property of certain crystalline materials (commonly ceramic lead zirconate titanate, PZT) in which application of a voltage across opposite faces of a crystal causes change in the width of the crystal. The crystal can thus be used as an emitting transducer to produce ultrasound from an electrical input signal (Figure 44.63a).

(a)
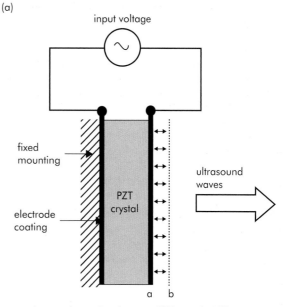

input voltage signal causes PZT crystal width to oscillate between a and b, generating ultrasound.

(b)
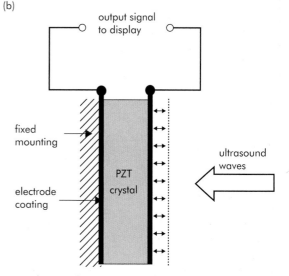

ultrasound waves cause PZT crystal width to oscillate between a and b, generating output signal.

Figure 44.63 (a) Piezoelectric effect: (a) transmitter; (b) receiver

The reciprocal effect can be applied to use the same crystal as a receiving transducer, since sound waves incident on the exposed surface of a crystal will cause a small change in its dimensions resulting in the production of a voltage across its width (Figure 44.63b).

A-mode

This scan mode is the most basic type and simply detects the range of a tissue boundary from the transducer. It displays the reflected ultrasound pulses from a single line scan on a time axis (Figure 44.64). Its main advantage is that it can accurately give the time delay between reflected pulses (hence distance between tissue boundaries/thickness of fluid layer). In addition, reflected pulse amplitudes can give an idea of the acoustic attenuation of tissue layers. This is not a particularly useful mode in clinical practice.

B-mode

This scan mode extends the A-mode to two dimensions to display the reflecting surfaces over a 'slice' of tissue. The reflected pulse amplitudes are displayed using a brightness scale. Thus surfaces producing high-amplitude reflections are outlined as 'bright' or 'white'. This is the most widely used mode in anaesthesia and can provide the most easily interpreted displays, which can be correlated with anatomical cross-sections (Figure 44.65).

M-mode

This mode is used to detect the movement of reflecting surfaces along a single scan line. It is the mode used in cardiac work to monitor the movement of valves. M-mode scanning is usually used in conjunction with B-mode scanning. The B-mode scan is used initially to select the best single line for the M-mode scan.

The M-mode scan plots distance from transducer on the vertical axis against time on the horizontal axis (Figure 44.66).

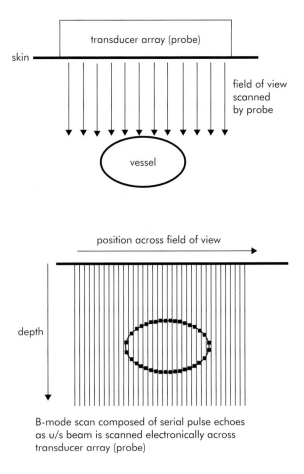

B-mode scan composed of serial pulse echoes as u/s beam is scanned electronically across transducer array (probe)

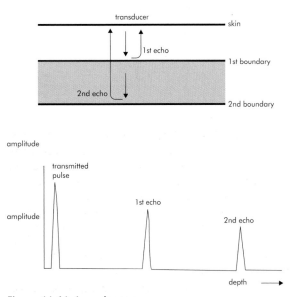

Figure 44.64 A-mode scan

Figure 44.65 B-mode scan

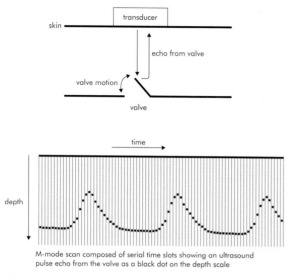

M-mode scan composed of serial time slots showing an ultrasound
pulse echo from the valve as a black dot on the depth scale

Figure 44.66 M-mode scan

Doppler mode

When scanning in Doppler mode the velocity of moving
targets, such as the red cells in blood vessels, can be
detected and displayed using a colour scale on an
M-mode scan. This mode depends on a mechanism
known as the Doppler effect.

Typically blood flow moving towards the transducer
is displayed with increasing velocity passing from a red
to yellow scale, while flow away from the transducer is
displayed on a dark blue to light blue scale. It should be
noted that these colours do not indicate arterial or
venous function of blood vessels. Usually venous flow
velocities are too low to produce a display in Doppler
mode.

Doppler effect

When ultrasound pulses are reflected from a moving
target the wavelength of the reflected waves will be different from the wavelength of the incident waves. This
occurs because the reflecting surface of the target is
moving relative to the medium.

Since the velocity of the ultrasound waves in the
medium is constant, the overall effect of a moving target
is to produce wavelength difference (and hence a frequency shift, the *Doppler shift*) between incident and
reflected waves. This frequency shift can be detected by
the receiver and is known as the *Doppler effect*.

Doppler shift

If a target is moving towards the receiver (observer) it
'bunches' the peaks and troughs of the reflected waves
closer together (Figure 44.67b).

If the frequency of the incident waves $= f$

the velocity of propagation $= u$

and the velocity of the target $= v$

Then

Wavelength of the incident waves, $\lambda_i = \dfrac{u}{f}$

And

Wavelength of the reflected waves, $\lambda_r = \dfrac{u - v}{f}$

$\lambda_r < \lambda_i$

and hence the frequency of the reflected waves
received is increased by the Doppler effect.

Similarly, if the target is moving away from the
receiver the peaks and troughs of the reflected wave
are spread further apart (Figure 44.67c):

$\lambda_r > \lambda_i$

and the frequency of the reflected waves is decreased
by the Doppler effect.

A classic and often-quoted example of the Doppler
effect is the rise in tone of a train whistle as it
approaches a static listener, and its fall in tone as the
train passes by and speeds away.

B-mode scanning for nerve blocks or vascular access

B-mode scanning irradiates a 'slice' of tissue with ultrasound using a probe. This probe consists of a linear array
of crystal transducers usually etched from a single block of
PZT. The use of such an array enables the ultrasound
beam to be swept electronically across the probe to produce the ultrasound field. Different types of probe can be
used, varying in size, shape of field and frequency range.
A common probe used in nerve blocks or vascular access
is 28 mm wide, producing a parallel-sided field 1 mm
thick. The depth of penetration can be adjusted depending
on the machine and the probe, but typically it may range

(a) Doppler effect – target stationary

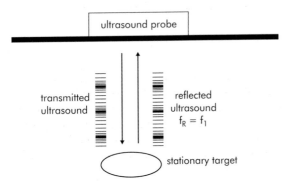

(b) Doppler effect – target moving towards ultrasound probe

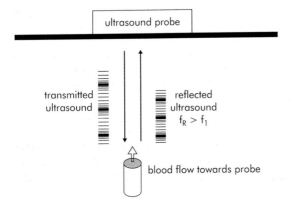

(c) Doppler effect – target moving away from ultrasound probe

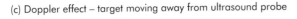

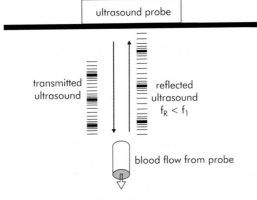

Figure 44.67 Doppler mode

from 2 to 6 cm. This can be visualised as a field with the approximate dimensions of a credit card.

The usefulness of a B-mode scan will depend on its resolution of detail, the width of the field covered and the depth of penetration. The pulses of ultrasound produced will have a mark/space ratio which, together with the ultrasound frequency (and wavelength), the design of the probe and the power of the scanner, will determine the performance. There is usually a trade-off between increasing frequency to obtain more detail in the scan and decreasing frequency to obtain more depth of penetration.

Interpretation of B-mode scans
When interpreting a B-mode scan, a knowledge of the underlying anatomy is essential and an awareness of limitations and artefacts is useful. A sample scan of the supraclavicular region is shown in Figure 44.68a, with a diagram of the corresponding anatomy in Figure 44.68b.

Limitations and artefacts of B-mode scans
- B-mode scans represent only a thin two-dimensional slice of tissue.
- Angle of incidence – maximal reflection occurs with reflection at angle of incidence = 0, i.e. when the ultrasound beam is at right angles to the target. Hence an injection needle will only be visualised if it lies within the 1 mm thickness of the ultrasound field and crosses the direction of the beam.
- Enhancement – occurs distal to fluid-containing cysts or blood vessels because of low attenuation within the target and refractive effects.
- Shadowing – occurs behind targets, due to either high reflection at the boundary (e.g. lung) or high attenuation (e.g. bone).

Special applications of ultrasound in anaesthesia, emergency medicine and critical care
FATE: focus assessed transthoracic echocardiography
This is a point-of-care test used to quickly assess ventricular function, pericardial and pleural collections and valve functions in the critical care unit or emergency

(a)

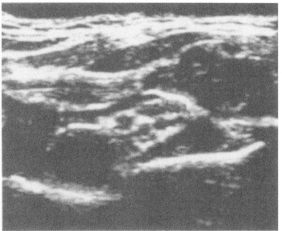

(b)

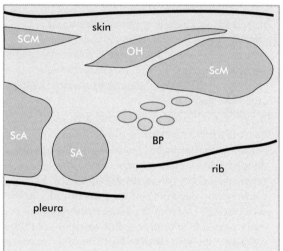

OH   = omohyoid

ScM = scalenus medius

BP   = brachial plexus

SA   = subclavian artery

SCM = sternocleidomastoid

ScA = scalenus anterior

Figure 44.68 (a) Ultrasound scan of brachial plexus; (b) diagram of anatomy seen in scan

department. Four transthoracic views are used. This tool is designed for use by non-echo-trained personnel and hence is not intended as a full examination.

FAST: focused assessment with sonography for trauma

This is a rapid bedside assessment of trauma patients to detect collections of blood. Pelvic, perihepatic, perisplenic and pericardial regions are examined for free fluid. An extended examination to include the pleural space is called eFAST. This technique is quick, non-invasive and as sensitive as diagnostic peritoneal lavage in an unstable trauma patient.

TOE: transoesophageal echocardiography

The echocardiography probe is placed in the oesophagus, which is close to the base of the heart (Figure 44.69). This means there is small attenuation of ultrasound and a higher-frequency transducer can be used. Hence resolution and image quality are better than with the transthoracic route. In addition, posterior structures such as the descending thoracic aorta and the atria are better visualised as they are nearer the probe in the oesophagus. The disadvantages of TOE are that it is more invasive, less tolerated by awake patients and contraindicated in oesophageal pathology. TOE is now routinely practised in the perioperative care of cardiac surgical patients.

Magnetic resonance imaging

Magnetic resonance imaging (MRI) was developed in the early 1970s and came into commercial use in the 1980s. It has the following advantages:

- Displays chemical differences between tissues
- Does not involve ionising radiation
- Can display blood flow
- Can display 3D slices from axial, coronal, sagittal and oblique views

MRI scanning uses the interaction between the hydrogen molecules in body tissues and a superimposed magnetic field to image the tissues under examination. This does not involve the use of ionising radiation (x-rays) or transmission of sound energy through the tissues.

Basic principles of MRI

> **The principle of MRI scanning** uses the normal stable spinning state of hydrogen nuclei in body tissues.
>
> The natural spin of the charged particles in a nucleus gives it magnetic properties causing it to behave as a microscopic bar magnet or magnetic dipole (Figure 44.70).
>
> Application of a high-intensity external magnetic field causes all these microscopic magnetic dipoles to align with this external field.
>
> These nuclei are then disturbed by electromagnetic radiofrequency (RF) pulses fired into the static high-intensity magnetic field. Each RF pulse causes the hydrogen nuclei to acquire an added 'wobble' or *precession* to their original spin (Figure 44.71a).

A gravitational analogy to this phenomenon is the spinning top which can be disturbed from its stable vertical position, causing it to wobble or precess. Once the precession has been initiated, it will naturally die away or 'decay', as the spinning top realigns itself in a vertical position (Figure 44.71b).

In MRI scanning, the precession of a nucleus has its own natural frequency, referred to as the Larmor frequency. This characteristic frequency depends on the structure of the nucleus and the magnitude of the magnetic field surrounding it. During precession the nucleus emits electromagnetic (radio) waves which are received by the MRI scanner and can be processed to construct the MRI image. The RF pulse frequency can be set to the characteristic value for hydrogen nuclei (protons), enabling these nuclei to be selectively stimulated and visualised in the image. This is usually the case in MRI scanning, as hydrogen is the most abundant nucleus in tissues. This sequence of events is summarised in Figure 44.72.

Changes in the magnetic field caused by the RF pulse

The response of different tissues to the RF pulse occurs because of changes in the high-intensity magnetic field set up by the MRI scanner. Consider reference axes which are labelled, according to convention, x, y, and z (Figure 44.73a). Initially all hydrogen nuclei are aligned with the high-intensity magnetic field along the z-axis (Figure 44.73b). When an RF pulse is fired the axes of the hydrogen nuclei are all shifted by an angle α (Figure 44.73c). This angle is the 'flip' angle or angle of precession. The effect of the RF pulse is to add a transverse magnetic component to the magnetic field in plane xy at right angles to the z-axis (Figure 44.73c). This produces a resultant magnetic field, M_r (Figure 44.73d) from the vector addition of the two components, a longitudinal component (M_z) and a transverse component (M_{xy}).

Relaxation phase after RF pulse excitation

After the RF pulse excites the hydrogen nuclei from their equilibrium state into precession, the hydrogen nuclei gradually 'relax' back into their equilibrium state.

As the nuclei relax they lose the energy gained from the RF pulse by transfer to the surrounding tissues and by emission of Larmor-frequency electromagnetic waves.

Individual tissues will produce different signals during the relaxation phase. Varying the sequence of RF pulses applied enhances differences between normal and abnormal tissues in the MRI image.

> **The relaxation phase** is important, because it is during this phase that information leading to construction of the MRI image is collected.
>
> Two time constants, T1 and T2, characterise the relaxation phase, and these can be used to enhance the MRI scan image.

Relaxation time constants (T1 and T2)

Relaxation of the *transverse component* is the decay of the precessional motion to zero. This process is an exponential decay process contributed to by the loss of coherence or 'dephasing' of the precessional spin of each nucleus. Decay of the precessional motion is characterised by a **time constant T2** (spin–spin time constant – the time taken to lose 37% of its maximum displacement value).

Relaxation of the *longitudinal component* or restoration of the longitudinal magnetic field is an inverse exponential process. Restoration of the longitudinal magnetic field is characterised by a **time constant T1** (spin–lattice time constant – the time taken to recover 63% of its original equilibrium value).

These T1 and T2 time constants vary for different tissues. Some sample times are shown in Figure 44.74.

T1- and T2-weighted images

Different effects in the MR image can be achieved by varying the sequence of RF pulses applied to 'weight' the image towards the T1 or T2 time constant.

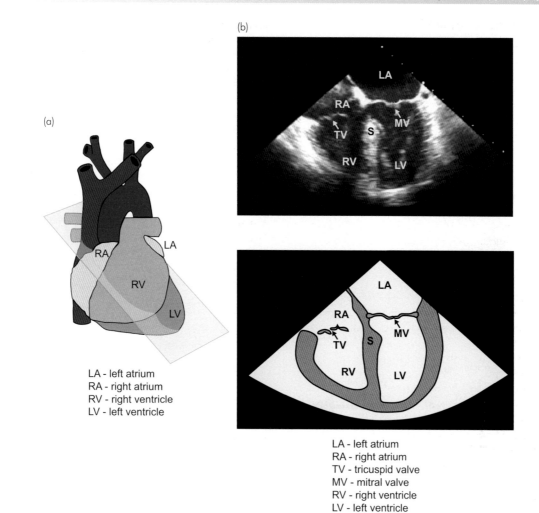

Figure 44.69 Transoesophageal echocardiography: (a) TOE scan plane; (b) example of TOE scan and diagram of anatomy

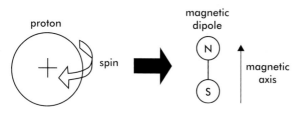

Figure 44.70 Magnetic equivalence of a spinning proton

- In a T1-weighted image, tissues with a long T1 time (e.g. CSF) will appear dark, while short T1 time tissues (e.g. fat) will appear bright.

- In T2-weighted images tissues with long T2 (e.g. CSF) will appear bright, while short T2 tissues (e.g. muscle) will appear dark.

TI-weighted images usually show good contrast between tissues, with clear boundaries. Fluids appear dark and fat appears bright, with other tissues intermediate greys. T1 weighting can enhance the contrast between grey and white matter compared to T2 weighting, because of the greater difference in T1 values as compared with similar T2 times for the tissues. The *shorter* the T1 time the brighter the tissue on MRI image.

(a)

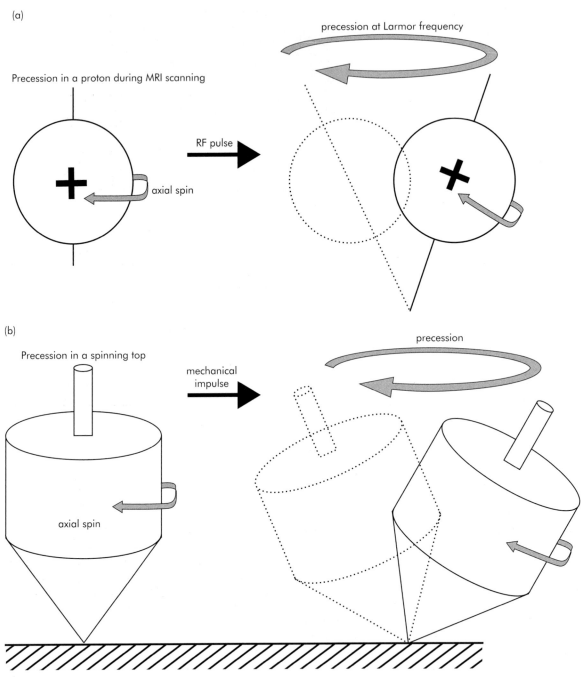

Figure 44.71 Precession: (a) in a proton excited by an RF pulse; (b) in a spinning top

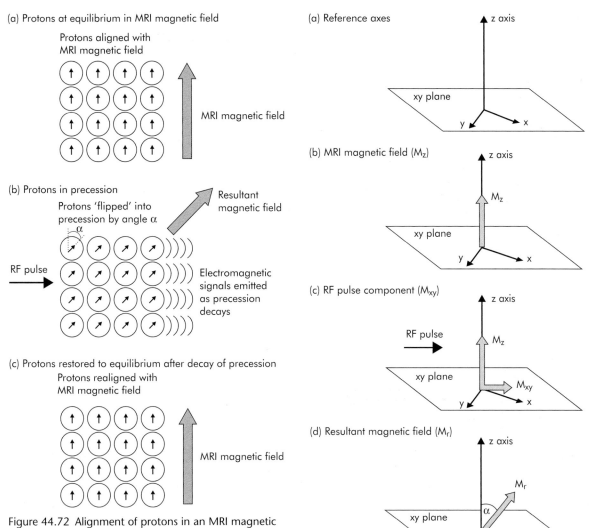

(a) Protons at equilibrium in MRI magnetic field

Protons aligned with MRI magnetic field

MRI magnetic field

(b) Protons in precession

Protons 'flipped' into precession by angle α

RF pulse

Resultant magnetic field

Electromagnetic signals emitted as precession decays

(c) Protons restored to equilibrium after decay of precession

Protons realigned with MRI magnetic field

MRI magnetic field

Figure 44.72 Alignment of protons in an MRI magnetic field: (a) at equilibrium; (b) precession of protons and 'flip' angle; (c) realignment following precession decay

(a) Reference axes

z axis

xy plane

y   x

(b) MRI magnetic field (M_z)

z axis

M_z

xy plane

y   x

(c) RF pulse component (M_{xy})

z axis

RF pulse

M_z

xy plane

M_{xy}

y   x

(d) Resultant magnetic field (M_r)

z axis

M_r

α

xy plane

y   x

Figure 44.73 (a) Reference axes in MRI magnetic field; (b) MRI magnetic intensity vector (M_z); (c) RF pulse transverse component vector (M_{xy}); (d) Resultant magnetic field producing precession and 'flip' angle

T2-weighted images show fluids as bright and other tissues as varying greys. Oedematous tissues appear brighter against normal tissues, and hence the appearance of pathological areas is often enhanced due to oedema. Abnormal collections of fluid can also be visualised more readily by using T2 weighted images. Note that, in contrast to T1 weighting, the *longer* the T2 time the brighter the tissue on MRI image.

Pulse sequences

The RF pulses used to excite the hydrogen nuclei or protons in the patient's tissues are a carefully selected and pre-adjusted sequence. There are two main types of pulse sequence used, spin echo (SE) and gradient echo (GE). Both sequences can weight an MR image towards T1 or T2 to achieve the image quality required. SE sequence pulses produce the best-quality images, but use a longer-duration pulse sequence, which may take several minutes to obtain an image. GE sequencing is much more rapid because of a shorter pulse sequence, but image quality may be impaired by inhomogeneities in the main magnetic field.

The MRI scanner

An MRI image is obtained by placing the patient in the high-intensity magnetic field generated by a large-bore circular magnet. This magnetic field is generated within the magnet (in a tunnel) but an outer or 'fringe' field exists which can cause interference with external apparatus or equipment. It is important that this magnetic field is free from inhomogeneities, which can impair the quality of the final image. Magnets used may be of the following types (Figure 44.75):

- Permanent – low field strength for their weight but non-uniform. No power consumption, but continual loss of field strength. Small fringe field.
- Resistive – good field strength and power-to-weight ratio. Power consumption and heat generation (> 30 kW).
- Superconducting – good power-to-weight ratio, with a high-quality field.

Magnetic field strength is measured as the density of magnetic lines of force or magnetic flux density. The units of magnetic flux density are gauss (G) or tesla (T). The tesla is the SI unit.

$$1\ T = 10,000\ G$$

The earth's magnetic field is approximately 50 µT (0.5 G). A simple bar magnet may produce a magnetic field of 50 G. An MRI magnet produces magnetic field intensities of between 0.2 T and 2 T, depending on clinical application.

MRI scanner coils

The tunnel inside an MRI scanner magnet is lined by systems of coils which perform the following functions:

- Gradient coils – these coils superimpose magnetic gradients on the static magnetic field. The gradients provide a spatial reference framework which enables the scanner to pick out a 'slice' on the z-axis and a point in the xy-plane.
- Transmitter coils – these coils transmit the RF pulse sequence.
- Receiver coils – these coils receive the Larmor-frequency radio waves emitted during the relaxation phase. In some machines the same set of coils may be used for receiving and transmitting.

In addition there may be active shield coils around the outside of the scanner – these coils generate an opposing field to reduce the 'fringe' magnetic field and radiation of RF signals from the scanner.

Biohazard effects of MRI exposure

Exposure to MRI scanning involves exposure to static and time-variant magnetic fields and radiofrequency (RF) electromagnetic waves. There are no known fatalities due to this type of radiation exposure. However, there are fatalities associated with MRI scanning caused by

Figure 44.74 Examples of T1 and T2 time constants for some different tissues in an equilibrium magnetic field of 1 T (tesla)

Tissue	T1 (milliseconds)	T2 (milliseconds)
CSF	2160	160
Grey matter	810	100
White matter	680	90
Muscle	730	45
Fat	240	80

Figure 44.75 Magnet types and properties

	Permanent	Resistive	Superconducting
Strength (tesla)	0.06–0.2 T	0.1–0.3 T	0.5–2.0 T
Fringe field	small	small	large
Weight	up to 80 tonnes	2 tonnes	6 tonnes

hazards such as projectile injury from metallic objects in the MRI field, displacement of an aneurysm clip and pacemaker displacement or dysfunction. Some biological effects of exposure to RF or magnetic fields include:

- RF exposure may produce heating of tissues or heating of conductors (monitoring cables) in contact with the patient. Safety recommendations are designed to limit temperature rises to below 1 °C.
- Exposure to time-variant magnetic fields may produce peripheral nerve stimulation with associated discomfort, by inducing currents in the body.
- High-intensity static magnetic field exposure can produce mild sensory discomfort, including vertigo, nausea and taste sensations. It is accepted that fields up to 2 T produce no harmful biological effects.
- There are no recorded effects on fetuses, pregnancies or fertility.

Although MRI scanning is considered to be a safe technique for patients and staff, the National Radiological Protection Board in the UK has issued guidelines for safety, which are usually complied with.

Light

Light is a type of electromagnetic (EM) wave and forms a narrow band of frequencies in the EM spectrum (Figure 44.76), defined as those frequencies detectable by the human retina. The EM spectrum covers many different forms of radiation ranging from low radio frequencies at the lower end of the spectrum, to γ rays at the high-frequency end of the spectrum. Wavelengths of low-frequency radio signals are hundreds of metres ($> 10^2$ m), while those of γ radiation are in the order of 10^{-12} m or less.

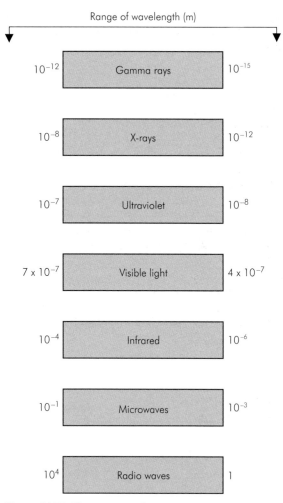

Figure 44.76 Electromagnetic spectrum

Dualistic nature of light

Light has a dualistic nature and not only behaves like electromagnetic waves but may also be considered as a stream of discrete particles or quanta of energy called photons.

The electromagnetic radiation of light is produced by the transverse vibration of photons emitted from the light source. This concept is useful when examining the action of light on photocells and photomultipliers as applied in oximetry and spectrophotometry.

Transverse waves, light waves and light rays

A light wave can be visualised as being analogous to a surface wave on water occurring when a stone is dropped into a pond. The surface wave is formed by water particles moving up and down, and the shape of a wave as it moves across the surface is called a wavefront. The wave moves across the surface in a plane at right angles to the particle motion. This is called a transverse wave (Figure 44.77). The direction that waves travel in is often represented by a single straight line at right angles to the plane of particle motion giving rise to the wave. This is referred to as a ray (Figure 44.78).

A stone dropped into water at X creates circular waves which travel outwards

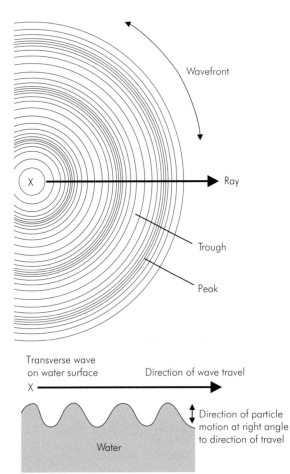

Figure 44.77 Particle motion, wavefront and ray in a transverse wave

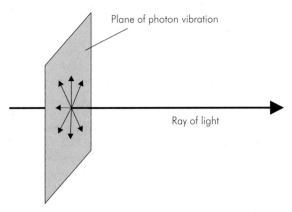

Figure 44.78 Light ray, showing plane of photon vibration

Wavelength of light

Wavelengths of light are normally quoted in nanometres (1 nm = 10^{-9} m), which have replaced the more traditional unit of the ångström (1 Å = 10^{-10} m). The lowest frequencies of visible light are dark red with wavelengths of around 700 nm, while the highest frequencies visible are violet with wavelengths of around 400 nm.

Speed of light

The speed of light in a vacuum is a fundamental constant in physics, with a defined value of 299,792,458 m s^{-1}. This value is now used to give the definition for the standard unit of length, the metre. The speed of light decreases with the density of the medium. Thus light travels more slowly in air and is even slower in glass.

Refraction of light

A consequence of the changes in the speed of light between different media is that the path of light is 'bent' when it travels across a boundary from one medium to another. Consider light travelling from air to glass, as shown in Figure 44.79. The light path is represented by a 'ray' or line drawn at right angles to the wave front. As the ray crosses the boundary from air to glass it 'bends' towards the normal. When light passes from a dense medium to a less dense medium, its path is deviated away from the normal.

The refraction of the light can be quantified using two angles, the angle of incidence (i) and the angle of refraction (r) (Figure 44.79). The deviation produced is dependent on the ratio of the speeds of light in the two media (c_1 and c_2), which will be a constant.

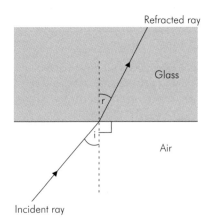

Figure 44.79 Refraction of light

Snell's law states that for light travelling between two given media

$$\frac{\sin i}{\sin r} = \frac{c_1}{c_2}$$

The refractive properties of a medium are measured by its absolute refractive index (n), which is defined by:

> **Refractive index** = $\dfrac{\text{speed of light in a vacuum}}{\text{speed of light in medium}}$
>
> $$n = \frac{c}{c_1}$$

When considering light passing from air to a medium, the value of the refractive index relative to air is virtually the same as its absolute value, because the refractive index of air is 1.0003 (i.e. the speed of light in air is almost the same as in a vacuum). Snell's law then becomes

$$\frac{\sin i}{\sin r} = \frac{1}{n}$$

Refraction results in the apparent distortion of images and distances, when viewing objects in one medium from another. This is why an object at the bottom of a pool of water appears closer to the surface than it actually is. Refraction is also responsible for the actions of lenses, including that in the eye. The refractive index for glass is typically 1.5, for water 1.33.

Reflection of light

When a light ray is reflected from a boundary between two media or from a surface (Figure 44.80), the geometry is again defined by the angles made with the normal to the surface. In this case the angle of incidence (i) is always equal to the angle of reflection (r). The use of reflection occurs in mirrors and the design of dish aerials or mirrors to focus light or other waves.

Total internal reflection

When light passes from a dense medium to a less dense medium (e.g. glass to air), Snell's law will only apply over a range of angles. This is because the angle of refraction is greater than the angle of incidence, the light being deviated away from the normal (Figure 44.81a). As the angle of incidence increases, a value is reached when the angle of refraction becomes 90° (Figure 44.81b). This value of the angle of incidence is called the critical angle (C). In this case, applying Snell's law:

$$\frac{\sin C}{\sin 90°} = \frac{1}{n}$$

When the angle of incidence exceeds C, total internal reflection occurs (Figure 44.81c). This is used in the construction of prisms to guide light in optical equipment, and also in the use of optical fibres to conduct light in fibreoptic equipment. The critical angle for glass is approximately 42°.

Polarised light

All electromagnetic waves, including light, are transverse waves. This means that the particle movement giving rise to the wave is in a plane at right angles to the direction the wave is travelling in (see Figure 44.78). Frequently the particle movement occurs in many different directions within the plane described. This is the case in light emitted by a high-temperature source such as a light filament or the sun, since it is emitted at random from the atoms in the source. This type of light is said to be *unpolarised*, and can be considered to be a mixture of vertical and horizontal components.

Unpolarised light may be filtered so that only light with particle oscillation in a single direction (vertical or horizontal) is allowed to pass. The light is then said to be *polarised*. Light can be polarised by passage through different crystals (e.g. quinine iodosulphate, toumaline). Vertically polarised light can only pass through a crystal with its optical axis aligned vertically (Figure 44.82). If such a crystal were then to be rotated through 90° (i.e. become horizontally aligned) it would only allow horizontally polarised light to pass.

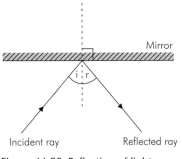

Figure 44.80 Reflection of light

(a) i < C

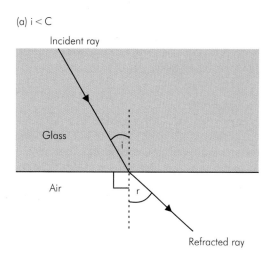

(b) i = C

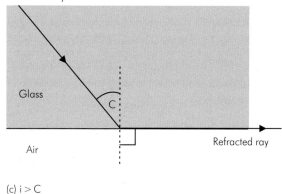

(c) i > C

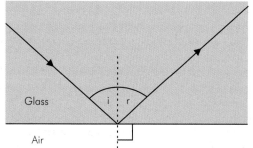

Figure 44.81 Refraction of light passing from a dense to a less dense medium, with (a) angle of incidence < critical angle; (b) angle of refraction = 90° at critical angle of incidence; (c) angle of incidence > critical angle

Dextro- (*d*) and laevo- (*l*) rotatory substances

Many pharmacological compounds are optically active, causing polarised light to rotate either to the right or to the left. The optical activity of such substances can be investigated by using a combination of a vertically aligned (polariser) and a horizontally aligned (analyser) crystal filter (Figure 44.83a). In combination, these two filters do not allow any light to pass. When an optically active substance is placed between the filters the vertically polarised light is rotated and some light then passes through the analyser (Figure 44.83b). The analyser is then rotated until the light passing through is once again extinguished (Figure 44.83c). The rotation of the analyser must then match the rotation caused by the substance under test. A dextrorotatory substance used is D-tubocurarine, while adrenaline, noradrenaline, L-atracurium and L-bupivacaine are examples of laevorotatory substances.

> Optical rotation (*d* and *l*) is determined by the physical 'handedness' of the molecule (D and L). However, physically right-handed molecules can be either dextro- or laevorotatory. This and newer terms (S, R, + and –) are explained in depth in Chapter 25.

Luminous intensity and the candela

It is required sometimes to quantify the luminous intensity or brightness of a source. This can be defined by the amount of light energy emitted per second (power) through unit solid angle (steradian) by the source, and is measured in candelas.

The candela is the luminous intensity of a source emitting light at 540×10^{12} Hz with an intensity of 1/630 watt per steradian.

Light transmission and absorbance (optical density)

When light passes through a substance some of the energy is absorbed. The absorption of light energy is dependent on the length of the path travelled and the absorptive properties of the substance. The absorption of monochromatic light (single wavelength) by a layer of solution or gas is used in absorption oximetry and spectrometry.

Consider the absorption of monochromatic radiation by a layer of substance. It is determined by a combination of two laws:

Lambert–Bouguer law – When a layer of solution of known thickness (*d*) is transilluminated by

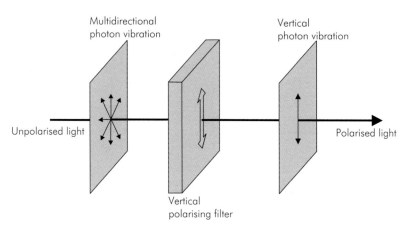

Figure 44.82 Non-polarised light filtered to give polarised light

monochromatic light, the transmitted light (I) is related to the incident light (I_O), by

$$I = I_O \, e^{-(ad)}$$

where (ad) is the 'absorbance' or 'optical density' of the layer of solution.

This in turn is the product of its thickness (d) and the quantity (a) known as the extinction coefficient of the solution (Figure 44.84).

Thus if the absorbance of the solution layer is 1.0, only 37% of the light is transmitted, but doubling the absorbance to 2.0 reduces the transmitted light to 13.5%.

Beer's law – This states that for a solution absorbance is a linear function of molar concentration.

Combining the above laws gives the Lambert–Beer law.

Lambert–Beer law

This relates the transmitted light to both molar concentration and thickness of the solution layer by expressing the absorbance as

Absorbance $= \varepsilon \, c \, d$

where ε = molar extinction coefficient, c = molar concentration, d = thickness.

To measure the concentration of a particular compound in a mixture, the mixture is transilluminated with monochromatic light at the wavelength where absorbance is maximal. The machine must be calibrated with a pure solution of the compound, and then the measured concentration can be calculated. Further details of this technique are given in Chapter 45.

Lasers

Laser is an acronym derived from Light Amplification by Stimulated Emission of Radiation, and it is applied to devices which emit a special form of light radiation. Laser light has the following characteristics:

- It is monochromatic.
- All radiated waves are in phase.
- The light waves emitted do not diverge but remain in a narrow beam.
- High light energy intensities can be produced with a relatively low-power source.

Stimulated emission

This describes the reaction when a high-energy atom is struck by an incoming photon. The high-energy-state atom is 'stimulated' to lose energy by giving out two light particles with the same phase and frequency. This process is called *stimulated emission* (Figure 44.85a). These emitted photons can then each stimulate the further emission of photons by striking two further high-energy atoms. In this way, provided that a suitable population of high-energy atoms can be maintained, a cascade amplification process is set up resulting in a high-energy light source emitting waves which are all in phase (Figure 44.85b).

Laser construction

All lasers consist of three basic parts:

- A source of energy to raise the electrons from the ground state to an excited one (a process known as pumping).

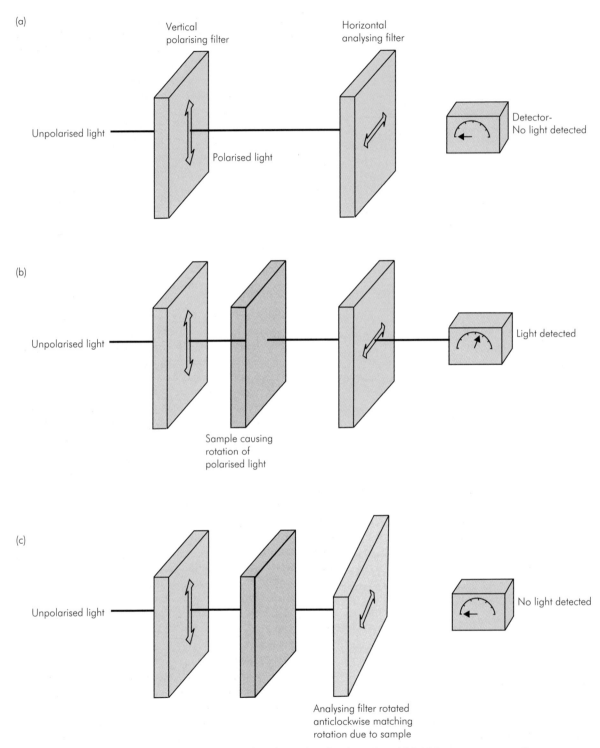

Figure 44.83 (a) Polariser and analyser filters used to determine *d* or *l* rotation: (a) initial setup – zero reading; (b) insertion of sample causing rotation of light – positive reading; (c) rotation of analysing filter to indicate *d* or *l* rotation – zero reading

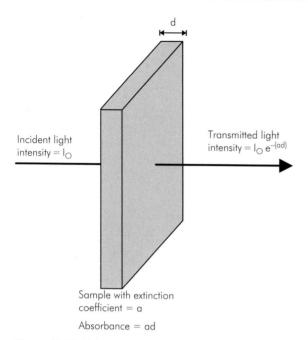

Figure 44.84 Light transmission and absorbance of a layer of material

- A suitable laser substance capable of stimulated emission.
- A system of mirrors to reflect light repeatedly back-wards and forwards through the laser substance. This process amplifies the light many times over.

Figure 44.85c shows a simplified diagram of a ruby laser. The pumping energy source is a flash tube, which feeds continuous or pulsed energy into the laser material to pro-duce high-energy-state atoms. These undergo stimulated emission, producing photons which are then reflected back-wards and forwards between the mirrored surfaces. The reflected photons in turn produce further stimulated emis-sion, and an amplifying cascade is built up. At one end the mirror is partially transparent, allowing light to escape as a highly parallel coherent beam. This beam can then be focused to produce extremely high light power intensities.

Many substances can act as laser materials. The prop-erties of some lasers commonly used in surgery are sum-marised in Figure 44.86.

Laser safety

Lasers are classified according to their degree of hazard from class 1 (the least dangerous) to class 4 (most danger-ous). Domestic lasers (e.g. DVD players, laser printers) are safe because of the wavelengths used and their low power. However, all surgical lasers are class 4, being inherently hazardous as they are specifically designed to damage tissue. Safety precautions when working with lasers include:

- Appropriate training for all staff.
- A designated suitably equipped area with all exposed surfaces matt finished.
- All instruments with matt finish.
- No inflammable material in the vicinity of the patient or in the operating field.
- All theatre staff must wear protective eye glasses, and protection for the patient's eyes and skin against stray laser light.
- The laser theatre must be well ventilated with a suitable smoke extraction system.
- Precautions against use of inflammable or explosive anaesthetic gases.

X-rays

X-rays are a form of EM radiation with wavelengths in the range 10^{-10} m to 10^{-13} m. The main properties of x-rays in medical applications are their ability to penetrate tissue and their ionising effect. The latter represents a hazard in their use but a property which is also used therapeutically in x-radiotherapy.

X-rays are generated in an x-ray tube, by bombarding a high-temperature anode with electrons generated by a cathode (Figure 44.87). The electrons are accelerated in the tube using a high-voltage electric field. X-ray machines are thus rated by the current and voltage that can be delivered. A portable x-ray set, for example, may deliver 100 mA at 90 kV.

Radioactive isotopes and radiation

An element may exist in different forms due to variations in its nuclear structure.

These different forms are called isotopes of the elem-ent. Each isotope will differ in atomic mass number but will possess the same atomic number. Some basic facts about the structure of an atom are as follows:

- The nucleus consists of neutrons and protons and is orbited by electrons.
- The atomic mass number is equal to the number of neutrons plus the number of protons in the nucleus. It is the nearest integer to the atomic weight.
- The atomic number is equal to the number of protons in the nucleus and determines which element is present.

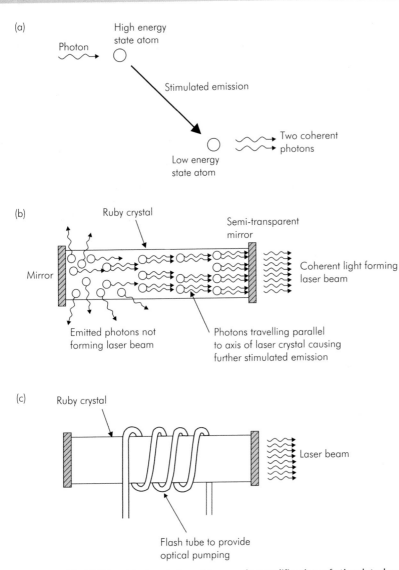

Figure 44.85 (a) Stimulated emission; (b) cascade amplification of stimulated emission; (c) components of a ruby laser

Notation used to identify isotopes is

atomic mass number
atomic number [element symbol]

For example, $^1_1$H is the symbol for hydrogen.

Some isotopes are stable and retain their nuclear structure indefinitely, while others are unstable and decay spontaneously. Unstable isotopes are said to be radioactive, and they decay by emitting radiation. Some examples of stable and unstable isotopes are shown in Figure 44.88.

Radioactive decay

Decay of a radioactive isotope involves the emission of nuclear particles from the substance resulting in the formation of another isotope or another element. An example is the uranium series, which occurs when uranium decays. This series of reactions finally results in the formation of lead, but involves a chain of intermediate decay reactions. Some of these are illustrated in Figure 44.89. Each of these reactions involves the emission of a specific type of particle with a characteristic mean

Figure 44.86 Properties of some surgical lasers

Laser material	Application	Properties
Synthetic ruby	Early use in eye surgery	
Argon	Replacement for ruby laser in eye surgery Retinal coagulation and repairing retinal detachment Removal of birthmarks	Passes through vitreous and aqueous humour Absorbed by haemoglobin Also absorbed by pigmented skin Can be transmitted by optical fibres for endoscopic application
Carbon dioxide	The most commonly used laser in surgery Superficial surgery, removing thin layers of tissue at a time	Absorbed by water, therefore low penetration to < 200 mm Cannot be used endoscopically
Nd-YAG (neodymium yttrium aluminium garnet)	Coagulation and cutting	Not absorbed by water, therefore good penetration of tissues Can be used endoscopically

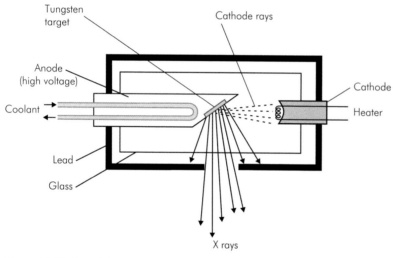

Figure 44.87 X-ray tube

energy level. Each reaction also has a particular half-life (see below).

The energy possessed by elementary particles (e.g. electrons or protons) is usually measured in electronvolts (eV). The electronvolt is defined as the change of kinetic energy occurring when a particle with a charge of e (the charge on an electron) moves through a potential difference of 1 volt.

$1 \text{ eV} = 1.602 \times 10^{-19}$ joules

$1 \text{ MeV} = 1.602 \times 10^{-13}$ joules

Radiation from radioactive isotopes
The types of radiation emitted from radioactive isotopes are:

α particles – a combination of 2 protons and 2 neutrons (equivalent to a helium nucleus). For example:

$$^{226}_{88}\text{Ra} \rightarrow {}^{222}_{86}\text{Rn} + {}^{4}_{2}\text{He}$$
radium   radon   helium (α particle)

β particles – an electron which is negatively charged, derived from a neutron splitting to give a proton and a high-energy electron. The creation of another proton

Figure 44.88 Some of the stable and unstable isotopes of hydrogen and carbon

Element		Atomic number	Neutrons	Atomic mass number	Stability
Hydrogen	^1_1H	1	0	1	stable
Deuterium	^2_1H	1	1	2	stable
Tritium	^3_1H	1	2	3	unstable
Carbon	$^{10}_6\text{C}$	6	4	10	unstable
Carbon	$^{12}_6\text{C}$	6	6	12	stable
Carbon	$^{14}_6\text{C}$	6	8	14	unstable

in the nucleus will increase the atomic number of the atom and thus change the element present:

$$^{14}_6\text{C} \quad \rightarrow \quad ^{14}_7\text{N} \quad + \quad e^-$$
$$\text{carbon 14} \qquad \text{nitrogen} \qquad \text{electron (β particle)}$$

Sometimes an electron may be emitted from the nucleus with a positive charge, in which case it is called a positron.

γ radiation – electromagnetic radiation with wavelengths $< 10^{-12}$ m, which is emitted during most nuclear reactions, usually following the emission of an α or β particle.

Decay half-life

The decay of a radioactive element from one isotopic form to the next form in its series follows an exponential decay curve, i.e.

$$N = N_0\, e^{(-\lambda t)}$$

where N is the number of atoms of the element present at time $= t$, N_0 is the number of atoms present at time $= 0$, and λ is the decay constant for the element.

λ is related to the decay time constant (K) for the element by

$$\lambda = \frac{1}{K}$$

The half-life for the element ($T_{1/2}$) is the time for the mass of element to decay to a half of its initial mass, and is related to the time constant, K, by

$$T_{1/2} = 0.693\, K$$

The half-life may have a value ranging from seconds to millions of years (Figure 44.89).

Units of radioactivity

The activity of a radioactive sample is measured by the number of disintegrations occurring per second. The SI unit of measurement used is the becquerel, which is defined as

1 becquerel (Bq) = 1 disintegration per second $\left(\text{s}^{-1}\right)$

The curie is a traditional unit referring to the activity of one gram of radium, where 1 curie $= 3.7 \times 10^{10}$ disintegrations per second $= 3.7 \times 10^{10}$ Bq.

Applications of radioactive isotopes

Radioactive isotopes are used in many applications clinically. These include:

- Measurements with labelled substances – use of chromium-51 to measure red cell volume
- Cancer therapy – use of yttrium-90 in pituitary tumours
- Diagnostic uses – imaging techniques with technetium-99, as in assessment of cardiac function

Measurement of exposure to ionising radiation

Exposure to ionising radiation can result in both short- and long-term sequelae.

The short-term effects of radiation exposure appear as the symptoms of acute radiation sickness. These are dose-dependent and include nausea, vomiting, anorexia, general lassitude and weakness, and can lead to death over a period of days or less. The long-term effects include an increased incidence of cancers and genetic defects in the population which occur after a period of years.

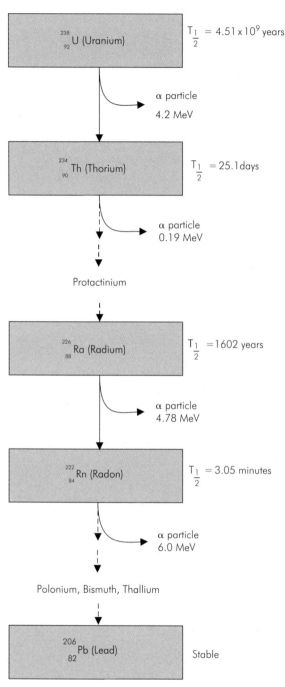

Figure 44.89 Uranium series

A dose of radiation can be measured by the effects it produces in a number of different ways.

Energy absorbed by air

A dose of radiation can be measured by the energy absorbed by the irradiated air.

> The röntgen is a unit used to measure x-radiation dosage.
>
> - **1 röntgen (R)** is the dose of x-radiation giving 83.3 ergs of energy to 1 gram of air.

Energy absorbed by body tissue

The röntgen does not provide a measure of the effects of radiation on the body, since the energy absorbed depends on the substance irradiated, and therefore the energy absorbed by body tissues will not be the same as that absorbed by air.

> The SI unit of absorbed radiation dose is the gray.
>
> - **1 gray (Gy)** is the dose of radiation giving an absorbed energy of 1 joule per kilogram of soft tissue.

Biological effect

Different types of ionising radiation provide different levels of biological hazard when absorbed. Thus even though the same amount of energy may be absorbed from different types of radiation, different sequelae may result. For instance, 200 kV x-rays are less damaging than γ rays or β particles; and α particles are even more damaging in their ionising effect, by a factor of 10 or more. Therefore, to assess risk in exposure to ionising radiation a unit of biological effect is used.

> The SI unit of biological effect is the sievert.
>
> - **1 sievert (Sv)** is the radiation dose equivalent to 1 Gy of absorbed radiation from 200 kV x-rays in terms of biological damage.

Thus if 1 Gy of radiation is absorbed from 200 kV x-rays, the biological dose equivalent will be 1 Sv by definition. However, an absorbed dose of 1 Gy from α particle radiation will have a dose equivalent to 10 Sv.

Biologically significant doses of radiation

Biologically significant levels of ionising radiation have been estimated in terms of their acute effects and their effect on the incidence of cancer and genetic defects in the population. These are at best an estimate, since the rate of delivery of a given dose can vary as well as individual response. An average dose of 1 mSv per individual over a population is believed to increase the incidence of cancer by 13 and genetic defects by 8 per million of population during the following years. A whole-life exposure of 1 Sv is thought to reduce lifespan by 1 year.

Some estimated doses of ionising radiation are shown in Figure 44.90.

Figure 44.90 Some estimated ionising radiation doses

Description	Dose/time
Maximum permitted dose	5 mSv per year
Natural background dose	1.25 mSv per year
Dose causing nausea	1 Sv per few hours
Dose causing death within days	10 Sv per few hours

CHAPTER 45

Clinical measurement

Ted Lin and Rajani Annamaneni

Clinical measurement in anaesthesia is usually concerned with the *direct* measurement of a physical quantity such as the pressure, flow or concentration of a gas. Alternatively, assessment of a physiological parameter such as neuromuscular blockade, depth of anaesthesia or pain levels may be required. In these instances measurement is made *indirectly*, using a related physical variable such as a stimulated muscle twitch, the electroencephalogram or a visual analogue scale.

The process of measurement is performed using apparatus which can be referred to as the *measurement system*. This may be as simple as a ruler with pencil and paper, or as sophisticated as the integrated electronic monitoring systems available in operating theatres and intensive care units.

Measurement systems

Measurement of a physical quantity is a process in which the quantity being measured provides an input signal to a measurement system, which processes this

> ### Interpreting measurements
>
> The data obtained by making measurements can only be interpreted correctly if:
>
> - The relationship between the data and the physical quantity or parameter being measured is understood.
> - The characteristics of the measurement system are known.

signal to give output in the form of a reading or display. This concept is illustrated in Figure 45.1, where a measurement system is represented as a 'black box' with an input and output.

The measurement system in turn consists of component 'black boxes' representing:
- A transducer – a detecting element which converts the quantity being measured (the input) into usable data or

Fundamentals of Anaesthesia, 4th edition, ed. Ted Lin, Tim Smith and Colin Pinnock. Published by Cambridge University Press. © Cambridge University Press 2017.

INPUT

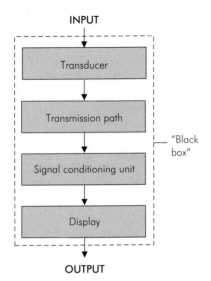

"Black box"

OUTPUT

Figure 45.1 The measurement system as a 'black box'

Figure 45.2 Analogue and digital methods of signal storage and display

Function	Analogue	Digital
Display	Oscilloscope Moving coil meter Chart recorder	Digital voltmeter Light-emitting diodes Liquid crystal display
Storage	Magnetic tape Chart	Computer hard disk Floppy disc Magnetic tape CD-ROM USB flash drive

a signal, usually an electrical signal. Examples of common transducers are:

o   a microphone, which converts sound to an electrical signal
o   a thermistor, which converts temperature variations into an electrical signal
o   a piezoelectric crystal, which converts pressure variations into an electrical signal

- A transmission path – this is the means by which the transducer signal is transferred to the signal conditioning unit or the display unit. Examples include electrical or optic cables, a length of tubing or an infrared link.
- A signal conditioning unit – this processes the transducer signal in order to make it suitable for display or storage. Signal processing includes functions such as amplification, filtering, and analogue to digital conversion. It may occur before or after the signal passes along the transmission path.
- A display and/or storage unit – this provides the output of the system as a display and also stores the signals or data. It may employ analogue or digital methods. Sometimes a distinction is drawn between a system displaying a signal (e.g. capnograph) as opposed to a numerical value (e.g. capnometer). Some examples are given in Figure 45.2.

Characteristics of a measurement system

> **The performance of a measurement system** is characterised by its *static* and *dynamic* characteristics. These determine the relationship between the quantity being measured (input) and the measurement (output).
>
> - **Static characteristics** define the performance of a measurement system when dealing with an input that is not changing or only changing slowly. Under these circumstances there is enough time for the system to reach a steady state before the measured quantity changes, so that the output follows changes in the input accurately.
> - The **dynamic characteristics** of a system reflect its ability to respond to rapidly changing inputs. Every system requires a certain time to settle to a steady state when presented with a change in its input. This response time may affect the accuracy of the measurement, since if the input is changing rapidly, the measuring system may not have adequate time to reach steady state and thus will not give an accurate reading.

Static characteristics

- **Accuracy** – This refers to the closeness between the measurement obtained and the 'true' value of the quantity being measured. For example, if a pressure has a 'true' value of 10 cmH_2O, an accurate system may read 10.01 cmH$_2$O and may be described as having an accuracy of 0.1%. In an inaccurate system reading 11 cmH$_2$O the accuracy may be quoted as 10% (Figure 45.3a).

- **Sensitivity** – This is the relationship between changes in the output reading of the system and changes in the measured quantity. The sensitivity of a pressure measurement system may be described as the change in output signal voltage for a given change in pressure, e.g. 1 volt per cmH$_2$O for a sensitive system or 100 millivolts per cmH$_2$O for a system 10 times less sensitive. Less sensitive systems will cover a wider range of pressure measurement than sensitive systems (Figure 45.3b).

- **Linearity** – In a linear measurement system the output reading varies in proportion to the measured quantity. Thus in a linear pressure measurement system, if the pressure doubles the output voltage will double. When the output voltage is plotted against the input pressure, a straight line is obtained. The gradient of this line gives the sensitivity of the system. It is usually desirable for a system to be linear, and any non-linearity is quoted as a percentage of the operating range of the instrument (Figure 45.3b). Some instruments may be intrinsically non-linear, reflecting their underlying mechanism – e.g. hot wire ammeter, rotameter.

- **Hysteresis** – This is a property of a measurement system which produces an error dependent on whether the measured value is decreasing or increasing. Hysteresis in a mechanical device is caused by elastic energy stored in the system, or frictional losses and slack movement of moving parts. Figure 45.3c shows how hysteresis in a measurement system produces errors in the measurement of increasing and decreasing pressures.

- **Drift** – This is variation in the reading from an instrument which is not caused by change in the measured quantity. It is usually caused by the effect of internal or external temperature changes on the measurement system, and unstable components in the system.

Dynamic characteristics
Step response
An important dynamic characteristic of any measurement system is its response to a rapid increase in input or a 'step' function (Figure 45.4). This can be simulated by dipping a thermometer at room temperature into boiling water, or rapidly opening a tap connecting a pressure

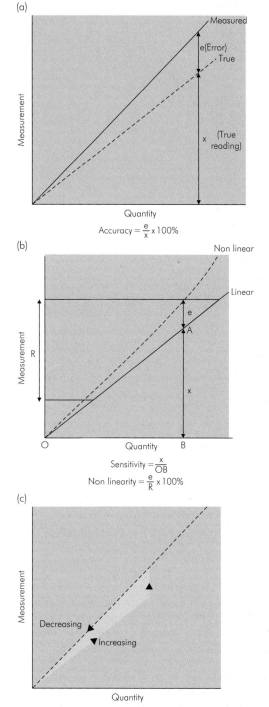

Figure 45.3 Static characteristics of a measurement system: (a) accuracy; (b) sensitivity and linearity; (c) hysteresis

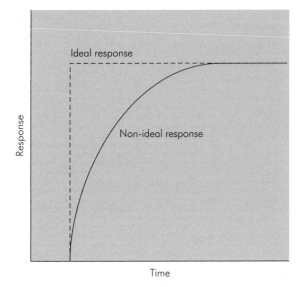

Figure 45.4 Ideal and non-ideal step responses of a measurement system

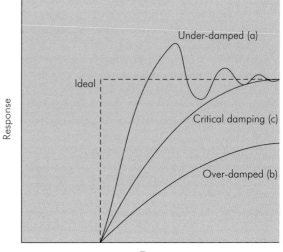

Figure 45.5 Effects of damping on the step response of a system

gauge to a pressurised container. In a perfect measuring instrument, the output or 'step response' produced by a step input should also be a step function, occurring instantaneously to give a reading of the measured quantity.

In practice, the step response differs from the ideal due to the properties of the system, and the output only reaches a 'true' steady state value after a finite time. The time lag for an instrument between a step input and the output reaching its final value is reflected by:

- Response time – the time taken from occurrence of the step input to the instrument output reaching 90% of its final value
- Rise time – the time taken for the output of the instrument to rise from 10% to 90% of its final value (Figure 45.4)

Damping

The step response of an instrument may also fall short of the ideal in the shape of the output signal produced. Some examples are shown in Figure 45.5. In response curve (a), *under-damped*, the output overshoots and oscillates about the true value; in curve (b), *over-damped*, the response does not reach the true value in the time plotted; and in curve (c), *critical damping*, the output reaches a steady reading of the true value within a short time with no overshoot. The property which determines the nature of the step response is called the *damping* of the system.

> ## Damping
>
> Damping is an important factor in the design of any system. In a measurement system it can lead to inaccuracy of the readings or display.
>
> - **Under-damping** can result in oscillation and overestimation of the measurement.
> - **Over-damping** can result in underestimation of the measurement.
> - **Critical damping** is usually an optimum compromise resulting in the fastest steady-state reading for a particular system, with no overshoot or oscillation.

All instruments will possess damping, which affects their dynamic response. This includes mechanical, hydraulic, pneumatic and electrical devices. In an electromechanical device such as a galvonometer there are mechanical moving parts such as the meter needle and bearings. Damping in these components arises from frictional effects on their movement. This may arise unintentionally or may be applied as part of the instrument design to control oscillation of the needle when it records a measurement. In a fluid (gas or liquid)-operated device damping occurs because of viscous forces which oppose the motion of the fluid, while in electrical systems damping is provided electronically by electrical resistance which opposes the passage of electrical currents.

Frequency response

Any measurement system in practice will only respond to a restricted range of frequencies, either by design or due to the limitations of its components. If the system were to be tested with input signals of the same amplitude but different frequencies it would only produce an output over a limited range of frequencies. Within this frequency range the system may respond more sensitively to some frequencies than others. When the system response is plotted against signal frequency the resultant curve is called the *frequency response* of the system (Figure 45.6).

Bandwidth

The highest frequency that a system responds to is the *high cutoff frequency*, above which input signals will produce no output. An example of such a cutoff is in the frequency response of the human auditory system, which at best may have a high cutoff frequency of 20 kHz. Similarly a system may possess a *low cutoff frequency*, the lowest frequency audible by the human ear being 15 Hz. The frequency range between low and high cutoff

frequencies, is referred to as the bandwidth, which in the human ear is 19.985 kHz.

Distortion due to poor frequency response

Any input signal can be characterised by its frequency spectrum (see below), which defines the different frequency components into which the signal can be resolved. Distortion may occur if the frequency response of a measurement system does not cover the spectrum of a signal, thus blocking part of the input signal. Alternatively, an instrument may be more sensitive to certain frequencies and enhance or attenuate them, causing it to give falsely high or low readings within its operating frequency range. This can occur at natural frequencies or resonances and anti-resonances (see below). Distortion due to poor frequency response of a system is illustrated in Figure 45.7.

It might initially be assumed that the ideal frequency response for a system would be one with equal sensitivity at all frequencies, from very low to very high (i.e. a flat response from 0 to ∞ Hz), but this would also enable 'noise' to pass through the system with the measurement signal, causing error and distortion.

The frequency response of a mechanical system is determined by its inertial and compliance elements (equivalent to masses and springs), while in an electrical circuit it is determined by the inductances and capacitances. There is often a design compromise between providing accuracy and reducing noise levels.

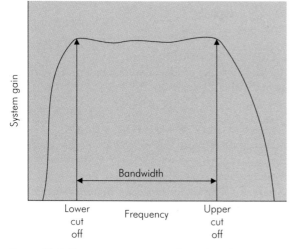

Figure 45.6 Frequency response of a system to an input signal with constant amplitude but at different frequencies

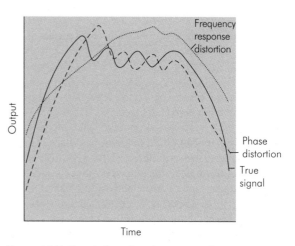

Figure 45.7 Signal distortion due to poor frequency response and phase response

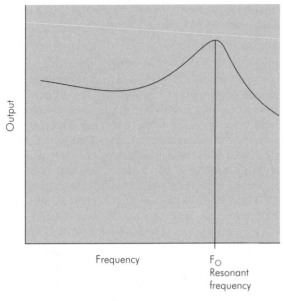

Figure 45.8 Resonant frequency response

Figure 45.9 Common biological potentials

Signal	Voltage range	Frequency range (Hz)
Electroencephalogram (EEG)	1–500 μV	0–60
Electrocardiogram (ECG)	0.1–50 mV	0–100
Electromyogram (EMG)	0.01–100 mV	0–1000

Natural frequencies or resonances

A measurement system may possess natural frequencies or resonances determined by inertial and compliance elements in a mechanical system (or inductances and capacitances in an electrical circuit). These resonances appear as peaks in the system's frequency response and can produce distortion in a signal display and errors in the readings (Figure 45.8). Good design practice can ensure that these resonances do not lie in the operating frequency range of the instrument, or can use appropriate levels of damping to smooth out these unwanted peaks in an instrument's frequency response.

Phase shift response

Fourier analysis demonstrates how a signal is composed of a series of component frequencies. In a signal being processed, each frequency component will undergo a different delay in time or phase shift as it passes through the measurement system (a phase shift is a time delay expressed as an angle, i.e. the units are degrees or radians – see *Phase angle*, under *Electric circuits* in Chapter 44). If the relative phases between frequency components of a signal are altered too much, distortion of the signal occurs and inaccuracy is introduced. Any measurement system will have a *phase shift response*, consisting of the phase shift occurring at different frequencies, which can be plotted against the frequency axis. In a simple system at resonant frequency the phase shift will be 90°. This phase shift response will be dependent on the components of the system, and can be responsible for distortion or errors in an instrument (Figure 45.7).

Electrical signals

In modern measuring instruments the transducer usually produces an electrical current or voltage, which varies according to the measured parameter. This voltage or current is a signal. Signals in clinical measurement are usually voltage signals or *biological potentials*. Most biological potentials vary in time, many in a repetitive or cyclical fashion – e.g. electrocardiogram, airway pressure during respiration. Some signals, such as the electroencephalogram and evoked potentials, are not cyclical but vary irregularly.

Biological potentials

The characteristics of some common biological potentials are outlined in Figure 45.9.

Characteristics of electrical signals

Electrical signals can be described in the following ways:

- *As a voltage (or current) varying in time* – The amplitude of a signal is the range of variation between maximum and minimum values (Figure 45.10).
- *As periodic or non-periodic* – A signal which varies with a repeating pattern in time, at regular intervals, is said to be periodic. The simplest type of periodic signal is a sine wave (Figure 45.10).

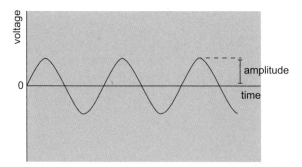

Figure 45.10 Periodic signal plotted against time – sine wave

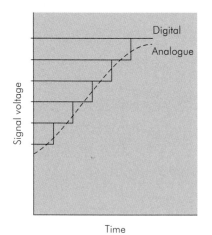

Figure 45.11 Analogue and digital signal

- *As analogue or digital* – An analogue signal is continuous in time and the magnitude of the signal varies smoothly without discernible increments. A digital signal is produced from an analogue signal by sampling the signal at regular intervals, and can be represented by a set of numbers. This adapts the signal for processing by digital systems and manipulation by computer (Figure 45.11).
- *As a series of frequency components* – A mathematical method of analysis was invented by Baron de Fourier in 1822. This has evolved both theoretically and practically to become one of the most powerful tools used in signal processing. Application of Fourier analysis to a signal enables it to be described by its *frequency spectrum*.

Frequency spectrum of a signal

> The description of a signal by its **frequency spectrum** can be summarised by:
> - Any signal varying continuously in time can be broken down into a collection of sine and cosine waves, which if added together yield the original signal.
> - The component waves exist as sine–cosine pairs at the same frequency.
> - Each pair of components has a combined amplitude and can be plotted as a point on the frequency axis, giving the frequency spectrum for the signal.

Conversion of a signal into its frequency components is referred to as spectral analysis or Fourier analysis. Fourier analysis is most suitable for *periodic wave forms*, but can still be used for *non-periodic wave forms* using an approximation (or mathematical 'trick') which treats the waveform as if it were a periodic signal with a very long period.

Figure 45.12a shows a square-wave signal plotted against the time axis as a time-variant periodic signal. It can also be plotted against the frequency axis as a series of frequency components or harmonics (Figure 45.12b). This gives an approximation to the frequency spectrum of the square wave. The frequency spectrum of a signal is related to the shape of its waveform. In general the more 'spiky' and 'pointed' the waveform, the higher the range of component frequencies contained.

Electrical 'noise'

A signal may be modified by any of the components of the measurement system. If the changes introduced are intentional, they represent *signal processing* or *signal conditioning*. Unwanted alteration of the signal by the system is distortion and introduces error.

Noise can change the amplitude of a signal and alter its appearance on display, causing inaccuracy. Noise signals may be generated by the components of the measurement system itself, or may be picked up as interference from external sources such as diathermy or fluorescent lighting.

Signal-to-noise ratio

In some cases the noise signals may be so large as to obscure the measurement signal altogether. An awareness

(a) Square wave plotted against time – 'time variant signal'

(b) Square wave plotted against frequency – 'frequency spectrum'

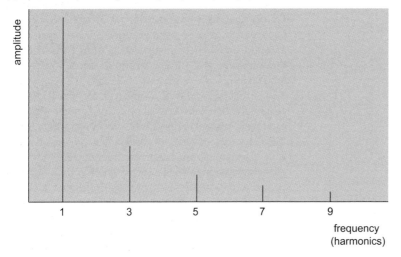

Figure 45.12 Square wave plotted against (a) time – time-variant signal; (b) frequency – frequency spectrum

of the magnitude of noise components in the signal is necessary in order to assess the accuracy of the measurements. This can be expressed by the signal-to-noise (S/N) ratio.

Signal processing

Signal processing improves a raw signal by:

- **Amplification** – Many biological signals are very small in amplitude (e.g. EEG signals may only be in microvolts, while ECG signals may only be in millivolts). Such signals are usually too small to drive display or storage units, and require amplification.

Electrical 'noise' is an unwanted component added to the signal by the signal processing system or due to outside electrical interference.

The **signal-to-noise (S/N) ratio** is the ratio of signal amplitude to noise amplitude expressed in decibels (Figure 45.13).

Low-amplitude signals are also unsuitable for transmission, since noise signals picked up may be of similar or greater amplitude, giving a low S/N ratio and obscuring the signal.

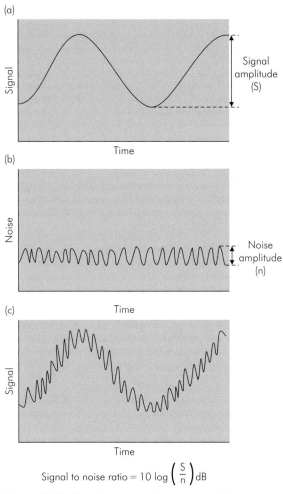

(a)

Signal

Time

Signal amplitude (S)

(b)

Noise

Time

Noise amplitude (n)

(c)

Signal

Time

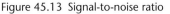

$$\text{Signal to noise ratio} = 10 \log \left(\frac{S}{n} \right) \text{dB}$$

Figure 45.13 Signal-to-noise ratio

- **Spectral analysis** – A signal is usually displayed as a time-varying voltage or currrent. In some cases (e.g. cerebral function monitoring) a display of the signal frequency spectrum is required, which can be achieved using electronic processing. A common method first converts the analogue signal to a digital signal, and then applies a mathematical algorithm called the Fast Fourier Transform (FFT). Transformation of a signal to its spectral components can also make some processing functions such as filtering easier and more accurate, and it also enables more complex analysis to be readily performed by computers.

- **Analogue to digital (A to D) conversion** – This conversion is often required before applying other processing functions, and is always necessary in order for the signal to be stored and analysed in a computer. This is because most electronic manipulation of signals uses digital electronics as opposed to analogue methods.

- **Averaging to remove noise** – In some cases the amplitude of the measurement signal may only be a fraction of the noise amplitude (i.e. the S/N ratio is very low). In such a case, the wanted signal may be completely obscured by noise. If the wanted signal is repetitive and the noise is random in time, multiple repetitions and summations of the noisy signal lead to an increase of the S/N ratio as the random noise cancels itself out. This is called averaging and is used in the extraction of evoked potentials, where the evoked signal is only a few millivolts in amplitude, hidden in background noise (EEG signals and neuromuscular activity). Averaging over 2000 or more repetitions may be required to obtain a clear signal.

- **Filtering to remove noise** – Often noise signals are in a different frequency range from the wanted measurement signal. In these cases the noise can be reduced by using filters to block out the unwanted frequencies:
  - *A low pass filter* rejects all frequencies above a given threshold. Such a filter would be used to avoid high frequency interference from a source like diathermy.
  - *A high pass filter* rejects low frequencies below a set threshold.
  - *A notch filter* rejects a specific frequency such as 50 Hz to avoid pick-up from mains cables.

Amplifiers

An amplifier is an electronic 'black box' which increases the amplitude of an electrical signal fed into its input. The purpose of an amplifier in measuring systems is to increase the power of a low-amplitude signal so that it can be used to drive a display or storage unit. The amplifier requires a power supply, and it channels power from this power supply into the input signal, increasing its voltage and current levels.

Characteristics of an amplifier include:

- **Gain** – this is the ratio of the amplitude of the output signal (A_O) to the input signal (A_I). It is usually expressed in decibels (dB – these units may be used to express any ratio by taking 10 times the $\log_{10}$ of the ratio).
- **Frequency response and phase response** – these are determined by the amplifier's circuit design.
- **Upper cutoff frequency** – this is the upper frequency limit above which signals are blocked or 'cut off'. It is measured in hertz (Hz).
- **Lower cutoff frequency** – this is the lower frequency limit below which signals are blocked or 'cut off'.
- **Bandwidth** – this is the extent of the frequency range passed by a system or amplifier: i.e. the amplifier only amplifies signals within this frequency range. It therefore lies between upper and lower cutoff frequencies and is also measured in frequency units (Hz).
- **Input impedance** – this is the electrical impedance 'seen' by the transducer signal at the input of the amplifier. Maximum power transfer takes place when the input impedance of the amplifier matches the output impedance of the trandsducer. It is measured in ohms.
- **Output impedance** – this is the electrical impedance seen 'looking' back into the output terminals of the amplifier. Maximum transfer of signal power from the amplifier requires matching of the output impedance to the input impedance of the transmission path or the display unit.

Calculation of gain

If the output amplitude produced by an amplifier, A_O, is 100 times the input amplitude, A_I:

$$\begin{aligned} \text{Amplifier gain} &= 10 \log (A_O/A_I) \\ &= 10 \log 100 \\ &= 20 \text{ dB} \end{aligned}$$

Pressure measurement

Pressure is defined as force per unit area and is measured in various units in the clinical setting, depending on the quantity being measured. Some examples are shown in Figure 45.14.

Figure 45.14 Units in the clinical measurement of pressure

Quantity measured	Unit
Blood pressure	mmHg
Airway pressure	cmH_2O
Partial pressure of blood gas	kPa
Gas cylinder pressure	bar, psi

In anaesthesia, pressure measurements are usually made in gases (gas cylinders, anaesthetic machines, breathing circuits) or liquids (intra-arterial pressure monitoring).

Pressures are not usually absolute measurements but are generally measured relative to atmospheric pressure. When interpreting pressure measurements various factors should be considered:

- **Transmission path** – Pressure transducers are often remote from the site at which pressure is sampled. The pressure is transmitted to the transducer by a length of tubing. The dynamic characteristics of this transmission path can significantly affect the final pressure measurements and signal displayed.
- **Sampling site** – Pressure may be sampled at a site remote from where the measurement is actually required, due to lack of access. Although static pressures may be equal throughout a closed system, pressures may differ significantly in a dynamic situation. A common example is the measurement of proximal airway pressures, which may not necessarily reflect distal airway pressures, particularly in the presence of bronchospasm.
- **Static or fluctuating** – If the pressure is not varying rapidly it can be considered as static, in which case the dynamic characteristics of the transmission path and measuring system may not affect the measurement significantly. This may not be the case when measuring a rapidly fluctuating pressure.

Common types of device used to measure pressure in gases or liquids include:

- Aneroid gauge
- Manometer
- Piezoresistive strain gauge

Aneroid gauge

This type of gauge is a mechanical device which uses the pressure being measured to operate a mechanism coupled to a pointer. It can be used to measure high or low pressures, but is usually employed when measuring pressures greater than 1 bar (1000 cmH$_2$O).

In the Bourdon gauge the measured pressure is connected to a spiral tube which uncoils as the pressure increases. This uncoiling movement is coupled to a pointer which indicates the pressure. Another form of aneroid mechanism relies on the expansion of a capsule produced by connection to the sampled pressure. This expansion again drives a pointer over a scale (Figure 45.15).

- *Advantages* – simple technology, mechanically robust and convenient to use. Operate in any position and do not require power supply. Suitable for high or low pressures.
- *Disadvantages* – not suitable for very low pressures (< 5 cmH$_2$O). Not easily recalibrated.

Manometer

This is the most basic device for measuring pressures, and because of its simplicity it represents a standard method of calibrating other devices. The unknown pressure is measured by balancing it against the pressure due to a column of a liquid (Figure 45.16). The liquids used most commonly are water for lower pressures and mercury for higher pressures. The manometer is so fundamental to pressure measurement that pressure units commonly employed are cmH$_2$O and mmHg. Accuracy and sensitivity can be increased by angling the manometer tubing and using a liquid with a lower density than water (e.g. alcohol). Surface tension between the liquid and the manometer tubing can cause an error, which causes the water manometer to read too high and the mercury manometer to under-read.

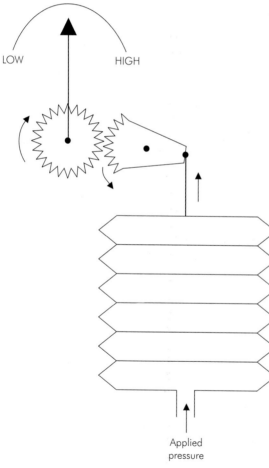

Figure 45.15 Aneroid gauge

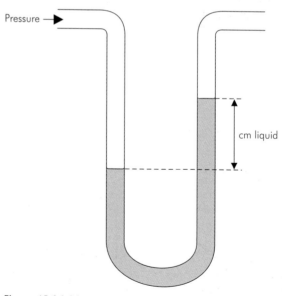

Figure 45.16 Manometer

- *Advantages* – simplicity of mechanism and no need for calibration. A standard method used to calibrate other techniques of pressure measurement.
- *Disadvantages* – bulkiness of the device and lack of a direct reading.

Piezoresistive strain gauge

This device is based on a semiconductor material with piezoresistive properties which cause it to vary in electrical resistance when subjected to a mechanical strain. The semiconductor is deposited onto the surface of a thin diaphragm which flexes when a pressure difference is applied across it. The distortion of the diaphragm produces a strain in the piezoresistive material which forms one arm of a bridge circuit (see *Wheatstone bridge circuit* in Chapter 44) etched onto the diaphragm. This results in a small signal current from the transducer which can then be amplified and processed (Figure 45.17).

- *Advantages* – versatility, since it can be used for measurement of high or low pressures. The electronic signal and display make it suitable for online display, automated data logging and linking to a computer. It is also easily adaptable for measuring differential pressures, since the diaphragm can be mounted with each face of the diaphragm enclosed in its own chamber and isolated from the other. Differential pressures can be used to measure gas flows, with the use of a suitable pneumotachograph head.
- *Disadvantages* – requires power supply and signal processing unit. Susceptible to electrical interference but has to be used in electronically hostile environments (operating theatres and intensive care units).

Blood pressure measurement

Blood pressure is an important determinant of tissue perfusion, oxygen delivery and cardiac work; it varies between individuals and is subject to a diurnal rhythm (lowest when the subject sleeps).

Recorded blood pressures reflect not only cardiovascular performance but also artefact (Figure 45.18).

Failure to recognise this can result in errors of interpretation and inappropriate action.

Variation due to the site of measurement

Changing the site of measurement, such as altering the level at which an arterial pressure transducer is positioned, will alter the blood pressure reading obtained because of the hydrostatic pressure difference between

Figure 45.18 Factors affecting blood pressure measurement

Cardiac output
The pulsatile nature of blood flow
Systemic vascular tone
Hydrostatic pressure variation in the circulatory system
The characteristics of the measurement system used

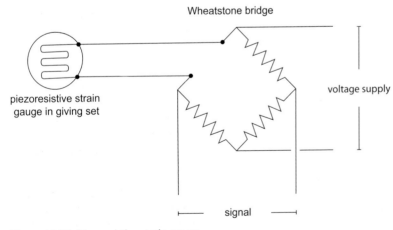

Figure 45.17 Piezoresistive strain gauge

the transducer positions. For this reason, a standard reference point is taken, usually the level of the heart (right atrium), so that all pressures measured are relative to that in the right atrium.

> ### Error in blood pressure due to height of measurement
>
> Changing the measurement site by 10 cm in height produces an error of 7.5 mmHg in the blood pressure measurement.

Since blood flow is pulsatile, the blood pressure varies according to the phase of the cardiac cycle. Thus peak (systolic), trough (diastolic) and mean pressures are defined individually, when discussing blood pressure measurements.

Methods of measuring blood pressure

The value of the displayed blood pressure is a function of the method used to measure it. The validity of any such measurements is strongly influenced by the observer's familiarity with the particular strengths/weaknesses of the technique employed. These can be divided into *indirect* and *direct* methods.

Indirect methods of measuring blood pressure

These methods are most commonly based on an occlusive cuff, which is inflated to a pressure above that of the artery and then slowly deflated. Once the cuff pressure falls below that of the artery peak pressures, pressure transients begin to pass beneath the cuff. These transients can be detected by a 'sensing' cuff, by manual palpation or by auscultation, and the pressure in the occluding cuff can then be recorded. In this way systolic and diastolic blood pressure values can be derived from these pressure transients, and can be measured manually or automatically.

Manual occlusive cuff methods

Manual methods rely on auscultation and palpation and are historically the earliest, but have become superseded by automated non-invasive techniques, which provide a continuous display of blood pressure. These manual methods, however, provide a historical perspective.

Riva-Rocci (1896) – described the use of an occlusive cuff to measure systolic pressure by palpation.

Korotkov (1905) – again using an occlusive cuff, Korotkov first described the measurement of blood pressure by auscultation. 'Korotkov sounds', heard over the artery

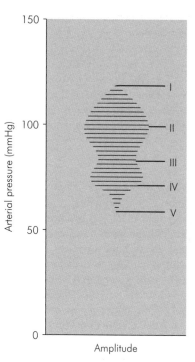

Figure 45.19 Korotkov sounds

as the cuff pressure falls, are the result of turbulent blood flow, vibration in the arterial wall, and pressure transients created as the extent of arterial occlusion decreases (Figure 45.19):

Phase I – a clear tapping synchronous with the pulse.

Phase II – sounds become softer approximately 5–10 mmHg below phase I.

Phase III – as the diastolic point approaches, sounds become more intense.

Phase IV – sounds suddenly become muffled, then, 5–10 mmHg later,

Phase V – sounds disappear.

Von Recklinhausen (1931) – described a dual cuff (occlusive and sensing) technique, employing aneroid valves in series within a sealed metal block, the oscillotonometer. This provided a visual measure of systolic, diastolic and mean arterial pressures displayed on a dial, connected by levers to an aneroid gauge.

- *Advantages* – these manual methods are simple and well established. They do not require sophisticated equipment or power supplies. They encourage patient contact.

- *Disadvantages* – dependent on operator technique and require manual intervention.

Flush method

This is an occlusive cuff method used for neonates. The arm is milked of blood before inflation of the occlusive cuff, which is then slowly deflated. The systolic point corresponds to the pressure at which flushing of the arm occurs (this point more closely reflects the mean arterial pressure).

Automated occlusive cuff methods (oscillometry)

Oscillometry is the most common method of automatic blood pressure measurement in clinical practice and is a development of Von Recklinhausen's oscillotonometer. The accuracy of blood pressure measurement has been improved by coupling the rate of cuff deflation to heart rate. A single occlusive cuff is employed using a dual sensing connection, which replaces the double cuff of the oscillotonometer. A pneumatic pump periodically inflates the cuff to a point 25–30 mm Hg above the systolic pressure and allows air to escape through a bleed valve, producing controlled deflation (approximately 2–3 mmHg s^{-1}). Vibrations of the arterial wall produce pressure transients which are transmitted via a sensing channel to an electrical transducer in the apparatus. The data is then analysed by a microprocessor which calculates systolic, diastolic and mean arterial pressures. The effects of electrical noise are reduced by comparing successive arterial pulsations as the cuff pressure decreases. If these do not correlate the data are rejected.

An example of pressure transients during cuff deflation is shown in Figure 45.19.

Systolic pressure corresponds to the point where the amplitude of pulsations is increasing, and is approximately 25–50% of maximum. Diastolic pressure corresponds to the point where the amplitude of pulsations has declined to 80% of the maximal pulse amplitude. Mean arterial pressure is the maximum amplitude point.

- *Advantages* – the principal advantages of these instruments is that they free the operator's hands, allowing measurements to be obtained conveniently when access to the patient is difficult, allow calculation of the mean arterial pressure, include alarm capabilities, and provide the capacity for data transfer.
- *Disadvantages* – while correlating fairly well with invasive measurements, they are less accurate at extremes of blood pressure (will over-read at low pressures and under-read at high pressures), and

should not be regarded as any more accurate than manual techniques. All these instruments assume the presence of a regular cardiac cycle; when this is absent, e.g. in atrial fibrillation, blood pressure measurements become inconsistent. The automatic cuff increases the risk of underlying tissue damage (in the elderly, particularly when the frequency of measurement is high, and the instrument is used for prolonged periods). Incorrect cuff placement may be responsible for nerve entrapment injuries (the ulnar nerve at the elbow).

Penaz technique

In oscillometry blood pressure measurement relies on gradual deflation of a cuff, which limits the frequency of measurement (maximum frequency of measurement is usually 1 min^{-1}). To overcome this limitation, a continuous non-invasive technique was first described by Penaz in 1973. This monitors the diameter of the digital artery using an infrared plethysmograph, which is mounted in a pneumatic cuff. The infrared signal responds to arterial dilatation and contraction during each cardiac cycle. This infrared signal is used to servocontrol a pump which maintains it at a constant level corresponding to mean arterial pressure, by inflating and deflating the cuff. Thus as the artery dilates in systole cuff pressure is increased, and as arterial diameter reduces during diastole, cuff pressure decreases. This duplicates the arterial pressure wave form in the cuff, which is then displayed on the machine.

- *Advantages* – this method provides a record of the changing trends in blood pressure, and in patients with normal or vasodilated fingers it correlates well with invasive methods.
- *Disadvantages* – results are less reliable in patients with peripheral vascular disease. Small differences in cuff positioning/tightness result in significant changes in the measured pressure. These measurements display a downward drift because of relocation of tissue fluid, necessitating repeated calibration. When used for periods in excess of 20–30 minutes, the cuff causes discomfort; where there is poor peripheral blood flow, there is the potential for vascular occlusive damage.

Continuous arterial wall tonometry

An alternative to the Penaz technique monitors changes in arterial wall elasticity/tonometry. A standard arm cuff is inflated to a constant low pressure (usually 30 mmHg), and the instantaneous changes in cuff pressure that result from arterial distension are interpreted by complex algorithms. Evaluation of response and accuracy of this device is mixed; the general impression is that at best it provides only a fair comparison with direct methods.

Doppler ultrasound

This method employs a transducer probe which transmits and receives ultrasound waves. These are coupled to the skin by a layer of gel, and positioned directly over the artery. Movements in the arterial wall caused by pressure transients as they pass beneath the cuff cause Doppler shifts in the frequency of the transmitted ultrasound waves. The amplitude of the shift provides a measure of the systolic and diastolic pressures. This technique should not be confused with the Doppler detection of blood flow in arteries, which analyses the reflection of ultrasound from the red blood cells in the vessel.

- *Advantages* – can be used for patients of all ages.
- *Disadvantages* – requires the accurate positioning of the transducers, and the use of the correct ultrasound coupling medium. The signals are prone to movement artefact, and are distorted by diathermy, dysrhythmias and atrial fibrillation.

Sources of error in indirect methods

In comparison with direct methods of blood pressure measurement (taken as the gold standard), indirect methods tend to slightly under-read, with the diastolic pressure showing the greatest degree of variability. The sources of error include:

- *Korotkov sounds* – these are complex sounds, with a large proportion of the sound energy being below the audible range. This reduces sound transmission to the observer. In addition, observer detection of the sounds will be dependent on aural acuity. The generated sounds are flow-dependent, and thus factors affecting flow can introduce inaccuracy (e.g. in high-output states, and after exercise, phase V may not occur)
- *Cuff size* – the width of the cuff affects the measured value of blood pressure. When too narrow, there is a tendency to overestimate; if too wide, underestimation occurs. As a consequence, there have been efforts to standardise the widths of blood pressure cuffs. The World Health Organization (WHO) recommends that adult cuffs should be 14 cm wide, and should cover two-thirds of the length of the upper arm, or its width

Figure 45.20 Recommended blood pressure cuff widths for different ages

Age (years)	Cuff width (cm)
Adult	12–14
4–8	9
1–4	6
Neonate	2–5

should be 20% greater than the diameter of the arm. Suggested widths are shown in Figure 45.20.

- *Zero/calibration errors* – particularly in aneroid devices.
- *Pneumatic leaks* – recommended working life for cuffs
- *Speed of deflation* – when too fast, then there is insufficient time to detect audible change.

Direct method: intra-arterial pressure monitoring

This provides an invasive, continuous measure of blood pressure by beat-to-beat reproduction of the arterial pressure waveform. It is particularly useful:

- In patients with cardiovascular instability
- Where blood pressure manipulation is required (inotropes or vasodilators)
- Where non-invasive blood pressure measurement is likely to be difficult and/or inaccurate (obesity)

The method requires the insertion of a short parallel-sided cannula into an artery. A continuous flow of either saline or heparinised saline (1 U mL^{-1}) at rates between 1 and 4 mL h^{-1} is used to reduce clot formation in the cannula. The cannula is connected by a short length of narrow-bore non-compliant plastic tubing containing saline to a pressure transducer, which is usually of the piezoresistive strain gauge type. More recently catheter tip pressure transducers have been developed but remain comparatively expensive. As noted above, the piezoresistive strain gauge produces a low-amplitude signal requiring signal processing before analysis and display.

The design of an intraarterial pressure monitoring system must take into account the following considerations:

- The frequency and phase shift responses of the system have to be adequate to allow good reproduction of the arterial signal. An approximate guide is that acceptable accuracy requires a frequency response extending to

8–10 times the maximum heart rate expected. In humans, the most important information is contained within the frequency range 0–20 Hz. The system can thus be designed to have an upper cutoff frequency > 20 Hz.

- The transducer and connecting tubing should be chosen to avoid natural frequencies or resonances occurring within the desired frequency response. Mechanical resonances due to the properties (compliances and inertial elements) of the transducer and column of saline in the connecting tubing can be shifted above the desired cutoff frequency by reducing the diameter of the connecting tubing.
- Components must also be chosen to provide the optimum degree of damping. Usually 'critical damping' is aimed for, but since frequency response, phase shift response and damping requirements may conflict a compromise may have to be arrived at. It is important to be able to recognise abnormal levels of damping in order to interpret the arterial waveforms appropriately. Figure 45.21 illustrates over-damping, under-damping and appropriate damping of arterial waveforms.

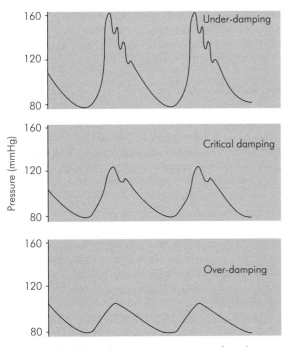

160
120
80
Under-damping

160
120
80
Critical damping

Pressure (mmHg)

160
120
80
Over-damping

Figure 45.21 Effect of measurement system damping on the arterial pressure waveform

- *Advantages* – this method provides a continuous display of the pressure wave form, providing an immediate assessment of blood pressure which is regarded as the gold standard.
- *Disadvantages* – as with any invasive technique, there are potential problems:
  - Cannulation – this can be difficult, particularly in low-output states, and may require consideration of multiple sites before success.
  - Disconnection – if unrecognised, this may result in serious blood loss and, in the extreme, exsanguination.
  - Infection is particularly relevant in cases of prolonged use (e.g. in the intensive care unit). Aseptic technique at the time of insertion, care of the catheter site (including appropriate dressing), and use of sterile packaged single-use manometer sets is necessary.
  - Vascular damage – distal vascular insufficiency may result directly from cannulation, or arise from subsequent thrombosis of the cannulated artery. This risk is increased by insufficient collateral circulation, which should always be checked for before cannulation. Emboli (air or thrombus) can cause distal vascular occlusion.

Sources of error in arterial pressure monitoring

- *Air bubbles* – as noted above, a recording system with a high resonant frequency and critical damping is preferable. Standard pressure transducers have a natural frequency in the region of 100 Hz, but the addition of the connecting tubing, tap and cannula markedly reduces this. The presence of air bubbles in the system also decreases the resonant frequency of the system and increases the damping.
- *Catheter wall compliance* – if compliant tubing is used to connect the cannula and transducer it will distend with the pulse wave, and like the presence of air will cause decreased resonant frequency and increased damping.
- *Blood clot* – if this forms within the cannula it will increase the flow resistance of the cannula and also the flow velocity of the saline. These factors will also tend to increase system damping and decrease resonant frequency.
- *Zero point* – the importance of choosing a zero reference point in order to minimise hydrostatic errors has

been described above. This effect can be reduced by periodic zeroing of the system.

Gas flow measurement

The measurement of gas flow and volumes is applied in clinical practice for the following applications:
- To test pulmonary function in patients
- To monitor gas flows in anaesthetic machines
- To monitor respiratory flows and tidal volumes in patient breathing circuits

Devices used in pulmonary function testing are described below.

Benedict Roth spirometer

This consists of a light bell which traps a closed volume of air over water. The subject breathes in and out of this trapped gas, causing the bell to rise and fall following the inspired and expired volumes. A sensor or pen coupled to the bell traces its movement, giving a spirometric trace from which gas flow rates and lung volumes can be derived (Figure 45.22). This device is relatively large in size and not portable.

Vitalograph

The vitalograph records expiratory flow rates and volumes by collecting expired gas from the subject in a bellows. A recording pen is coupled to the bellows, tracing an expired volume graph (Figure 45.23). This device is more portable than the Benedict Roth spirometer but only measures forced expiratory volumes and flows. The results obtained are also very dependent on subject technique.

Wright respirometer

This is another continuous volume recorder, designed specifically for clinical application. It operates by using the gas flow to drive a spinning vane, which is coupled by clockwork gears to the display dials. Total volumes up to 1000 litres can be recorded. Like the dry gas meter, its accuracy and reliability is dependent on the mechanical quality of its clockwork mechanism. It can only measure unidirectional flow but has the advantages of being small and portable, and requiring no power supply. Flow rates again can only be derived by averaging recorded volumes over time (Figure 45.24).

Dry gas meter

This machine is based on the gas meters used for measuring domestic gas consumption. It measures large volumes of gas by continually feeding the gas flow into a pair of reciprocating bellows. As each bellows fills alternately, its movement records an increase in volume by a clockwork counter and operates inlet and exhaust valves to direct the gas flow through the machine. In this way the flow of very large volumes (10^6 litres) of gas can be measured, compared to the several litres capacity of the closed-volume spirometers. However, average flow rates can only be estimated over time, and cannot be measured directly.

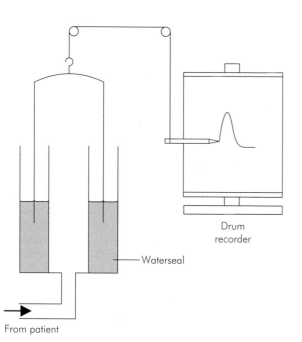

Figure 45.22 Benedict Roth spirometer

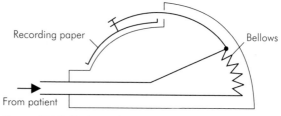

Figure 45.23 Vitalograph

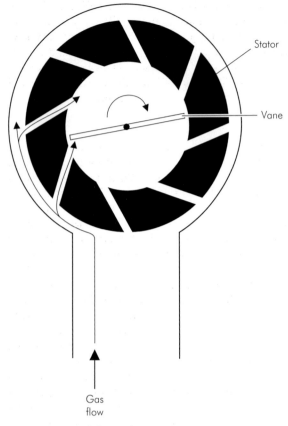

Figure 45.24 Wright respirometer

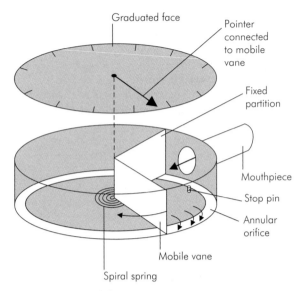

Figure 45.25 Peak flow meter

Electronic volume meter

In this device the spinning vane mechanism described above in the Wright respirometer has been adapted to give an electronic signal. One method uses fixed blades to create a spiral flow to drive the blades of the vane. The spinning blades interrupt a light signal from light-emitting diodes (LEDs), which is then picked up by photoelectric cells. These provide an electrical signal which can be processed and calibrated to give volume measurements. This device has the advantages of being free from the mechanical errors associated with clockwork mechanisms, and being able to measure volumes from bidirectional (inspiratory and expiratory) flow. It does, however, require a power supply, and a signal processing and display unit.

Peak flow meter

This device records the maximum expiratory flow of patients by using the expired gas to operate a shutter controlling a variable orifice through which the gas escapes to the atmosphere. The greater the expiratory flow, the larger the orifice opened up by the shutter. The displacement of the shutter is non-returnable and is recorded by a pointer which thus records the maximum expiratory flow reached (Figure 45.25).

Gas flow measurement in anaesthetic machines

Rotameter

Gas flows from an anaesthetic machine into a ventilator or patient circuit are most commonly measured using rotameters. The rotameter is a variable-orifice flow meter in which the gas flow to be measured is passed upwards through a vertically mounted glass (or plastic) tube. This tube has a tapering internal diameter, wider at the top and narrower at the bottom. Gas flow through the rotameter is controlled by a needle valve at the bottom (Figure 45.26).

A bobbin with a smaller diameter than the internal diameter of the rotameter tube acts as a pointer, and is moved up or down the tube by the force of the gas flow as it increases or decreases. The bobbin may vary in design, but the most common type is shaped like a spinning top, with spiral grooves cut in the sides causing it to spin in the gas flow. The spin reduces friction and sticking of the bobbin. With this type of bobbin, readings are taken from the top edge.

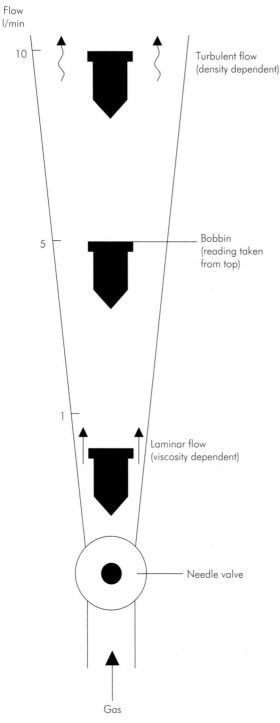

Flow
l/min

10

Turbulent flow
(density dependent)

5

Bobbin
(reading taken
from top)

1

Laminar flow
(viscosity dependent)

Needle valve

Gas

Figure 45.26 Rotameter

When the gas flow is steady the bobbin settles at a point where the force of the gas flow acting on it and passing round it equals the bobbin weight. At high flows the bobbin is near the top of the rotameter and the cross-section of the annular space around the bobbin is greater than at low flows, when the bobbin is near the bottom of the rotameter and the orifice cross-section is small.

Gas flow pattern in a rotameter

The pattern of gas flow through a rotameter is a mixture of turbulence and laminar flow, due to the flow conditions as the gas passes the bobbin. When the cross-sectional area open to flow is small (i.e. the bobbin is near the bottom of the rotameter), flow past the bobbin is like flow in a 'tube'. This is because the cross-sectional area open to flow is small, and a tube in this context is defined by having diameter < length (see *Flow through tubes* in Chapter 44). In this case flow is laminar and gas viscosity is the main determinant of flow. When the bobbin is near the top of the rotameter, at high flows, the annular cross-sectional area open to flow is large. Flow here is similar to that through an 'orifice', an orifice being defined by having diameter > length. In this case flow is turbulent and density becomes the most important gas property determining flow. The importance of the flow pattern is that because the viscosities and densities of gases can differ significantly (e.g. oxygen and helium have similar viscosities but their densities are 1.33 and 0.17 kg m^{-3}), a rotameter can only be calibrated accurately for a specific gas or mixture.

- *Advantages* – simple design and reliable, does not require power supply, no signal transmission path, conditioning unit or display to go wrong.
- *Disadvantages* – only calibrated for specific gas under standard pressure and temperature conditions. Actually part of the gas circuit, so failure may be hazardous, and sensitive to circuit changes downstream (see below).

Features of the rotameter block

Rotameters on an anaesthetic machine are arranged in an array, a different one for each gas, with the most distal gas (left-hand side – usually oxygen) entering the common flow first. The design of this array, or rotameter block, displays certain features for increased safety:

- If the first gas to enter the flow line is oxygen (Figure 45.27a), it can leak from the breakage of any subsequent rotameter, potentially giving rise to a

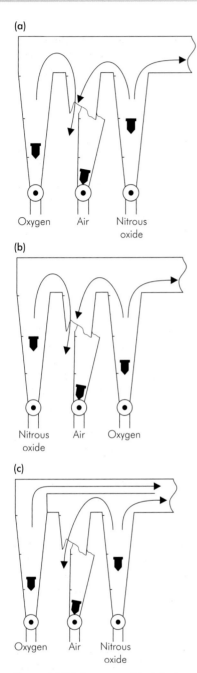

(a)

Oxygen   Air   Nitrous oxide

(b)

Nitrous oxide   Air   Oxygen

(c)

Oxygen   Air   Nitrous oxide

Figure 45.27 Rotameter block faults

hypoxic gas mixture. Thus the order of gases entering the flow line can increase the risk of hypoxia, and theoretically the safest position for oxygen would be last in order of entering the common flow

(Figure 45.27b). A change in the rotameter order would however bring its own risks, and internal channelling is therefore used to separate the individual gas flows. Thus even when the oxygen control knob is first in order, channelling can ensure that oxygen is the last gas to enter the flow line (Figure 45.27c).

- The oxygen control can be mechanically linked to other gases to prevent hypoxic mixtures being selected.
- Positioning vaporisers at the outlet of the rotameters can increase the pressure in the rotameters and thus affect their calibration, since the density of the gases would be altered.

Gas flow measurement in breathing circuits
Pneumotachograph

The pneumotachograph obtains a signal dependent on the gas flow by using a pneumotachograph head that is inserted into the breathing circuit, or which a patient can breathe through directly during pulmonary function testing. Common types of pneumotachograph heads are:

- **Fixed resistance** – The signal is a differential pressure signal produced by gases flowing through a fixed-flow resistance. These include the screen and Fleisch heads.
- **Hot wire** – The flow signal is produced by the gas flow cooling a heated resistance wire.
- **Pitot tube** – The flow signal is dependent on the pressure difference between dynamic and static pressures in the centre of the pneumotachograph head.

The flow signal is passed to a signal conditioning unit from which it can be analysed and displayed. Tidal volumes are calculated by integrating the flow signal over the duration of inspiration or expiration. Linearity of a pneumotachograph head signal is important in making calibration and calculation of volumes easier. Flow should be corrected for changes in gas mixture. Correction will include gas viscosity if flow is laminar, but gas density for turbulent flow. More detail for different devices is given below.

Screen pneumotachograph

This is the most commonly used design, and consists of a short connector with a gauze screen mounted across the middle, through which the gas flows (Figure 45.28a). The diameter of the head must be large enough to ensure laminar flow through the screen. The screen acts as a flow

(a) Screen

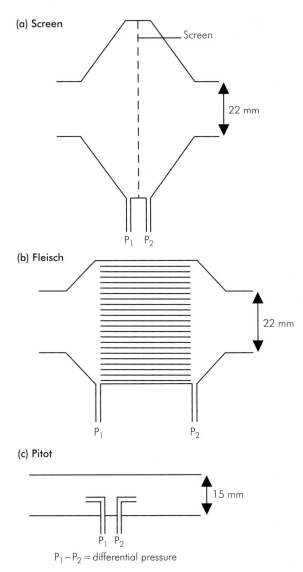

Screen

22 mm

P_1 P_2

(b) Fleisch

22 mm

P_1 P_2

(c) Pitot

15 mm

P_1 P_2

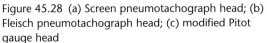

$P_1 - P_2 =$ differential pressure

Figure 45.28 (a) Screen pneumotachograph head; (b) Fleisch pneumotachograph head; (c) modified Pitot gauge head

resistance and produces a small pressure drop across it. This pressure drop is sampled by a pair of pressure ports, one on either side of the screen, which feed the differential pressure to a differential pressure transducer. The pressure transducer produces a small electrical signal for conditioning, analysis and display. This pneumotachograph head is linear over a wide range and of a convenient size, but turbulence may be produced at high flow rates.

Fleisch pneumotachograph
This pneumotachograph head passes the flow through an array of fine-bore ducts to ensure laminar flow over a wide range (Figure 45.28b). It is larger and bulkier than the screen head.

Hot-wire pneumotachograph
In this device two 'hot' wires are mounted at right angles to each other, across the lumen of the pneumotachograph head. The hot wires are resistive wires heated by a controlled current passing through them. The gas flow produces cooling of the wires which is dependent on the flow rate, which in turn varies their resistance, giving a small electric signal. Disadvantages are limited frequency response and the requirement for a stabilised power supply.

Modified Pitot tube pneumotachograph
This device is based on the Pitot tube which is used to measure local gas speed (as in an aircraft airspeed gauge). It consists of a connector with two small-diameter (1–2 mm) pressure sampling tubes mounted axially in the centre of the gas flow path, the open ends of these tubes acting as pressure sampling ports (Figure 45.28c). One sampling port faces downstream and one upstream. The downstream port measures the 'static' pressure. The upstream port gives a 'total' pressure reading, which is greater than the static pressure, since gas impacts on the port creating an additional pressure ('dynamic' pressure) due to its kinetic energy. The difference between the total pressure and static pressure port is measured by a differential pressure transducer and is dependent on the gas speed. The pneumotachograph is calibrated for gas flow but is non-linear, requiring linearisation in the signal processing unit. It has the advantage of being mechanically simple, small in size (and dead space) and cheap to produce. The flow through this head is turbulent.

Gas and vapour concentrations
In the past the analysis of gas concentrations in gas mixtures and blood samples relied on chemical methods. These were relatively slow, laborious and inaccurate compared to modern methods. They included:
- The Haldane apparatus – a volumetric technique based on gas absorption, used to measure component gases in a respiratory gas mixture. Oxygen was absorbed by passage through pyrogallol.

- The Van Slyke apparatus – a method for the measurement of blood gases. Haemoglobin was released from red cells by inducing rapid haemolysis with saponin. Carbon dioxide was displaced by lactic acid and oxygen displaced by potassium ferrocyanide, enabling volumetric measurements to be made.

These chemical methods have been largely superseded by gas analysers based on physical principles. These have improved accuracy, and can also provide continuous breath-to-breath measurement.

Gas analysers
All modern gas analysers generate electrical signals that are a real-time measure of the concentration of gas. The signals are small and require signal processing to improve accuracy and compensate for non-linearity.

Step response of gas analysers
Gas analysers, like many other instruments, suffer a finite delay before registering a change in sample composition. This time lag may be measured as:

- *The delay time* – the time from a stepped change in concentration/partial pressure at the sampling site, to detection of a 10% increase at the sample chamber. This is largely due to the time required for the sample to pass from the sampling orifice to the measurement chamber.
- *The rise time* – the time required for the display to rise from 10% to 90% of the stepped change in gas concentration/partial pressure at the sampling site.
- *The response time* – the time from the gas reaching the sample chamber to the analyser displaying 95% of the final measurement (Figure 45.29).

Types of gas analyser
Gas and vapour analysers can be usefully divided into *discrete analysers* (extremely accurate) and *continuous analysers* (accurate).

Discrete analysers
Discrete analysers are rarely used in clinical anaesthesia. An example of discrete analysis is provided by:

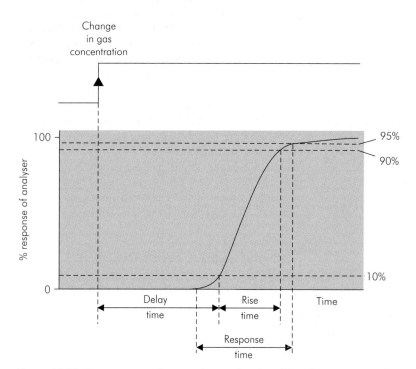

Figure 45.29 Step response of gas analyser – showing delay time, response time and rise time

Gas/liquid chromatography – in this method the unknown gas mixture is injected into a stream of 'carrier gas' (e.g. nitrogen) flowing through a column of liquid-coated particles, the 'stationary phase' (e.g. polyethylene glycol). As the gas mixture passes through the column the various component gases are slowed down according to their solubility in the stationary phase liquid, and thus appear separated out at the end of the column. On exit from the column the gases are assayed by a method such as infrared absorption or thermal conductivity detection, which yields a series of 'peaks' corresponding to the component gases. The gases are identified by comparison of the time lags of the different peaks with those for known gas samples, and their concentrations are given by the height of their peaks. This method is very accurate, very sensitive, but expensive, and is usually only used for research purposes.

Continuous analysers

Continuous analysers include:

- Mass spectrometers
- Infrared absorption
- Ultraviolet absorption
- Paramagnetism
- Thermal conductivity
- Polarography
- Galvanic fuel cells

Mass spectrometers

These instruments can separate complex mixtures of gases. The sample is continuously drawn into the apparatus through a narrow sampling tube. Some of the sample passes into an evacuated steel ionising chamber, where it is ionised by a beam of electrons. The resulting mixture of ions then diffuses through a slit in the chamber, and they are accelerated by a negatively charged plate. These charged ions are then separated to give a spectrum (Figure 45.30). There are two methods of separating the ions:

Magnetic sector – The ions, once accelerated, are deflected by a strong magnetic field, which separates out different particle streams according to mass and charge. Each of the deflected ion streams is then measured at a different detector plate. The number of gases that can be measured is determined by the number of detector plates (usually 4–6). As most ions have the same charge, separation mainly depends on molecular mass.

Quadrupole – This spectrometer, despite possessing only one detector, can measure up to eight different species of particle. The ions reach the detector through a passage formed by four steel rods, the quadrupole. These rods are energised by a radiofrequency signal, which enables them to selectively allow ions with a specific mass to pass through to the detector. The quadrupole signal can be varied to scan for ions of different masses, thus producing a sequential assay for different gases. The mass range is less than that of a magnetic sector spectrometer, and the use of a single shared detector makes it less accurate.

- *Advantages* – versatile, allowing measurement of a variety of component gases in a mixture, and has a rapid response time (< 0.1 s).

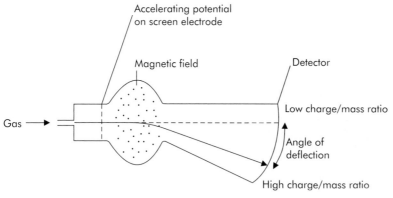

Figure 45.30 Mass spectrometer

• *Disadvantages* – complex equipment with high capital, installation and maintenance costs. The presence of water vapour can interfere with sample measurement and prolong the rise time. For this reason many mass spectrometers incorporate a correction for the presence of water vapour.

Infrared (IR) absorption (in capnographs)

This method is commonly used in capnographs. A molecule composed of two or more dissimilar atoms will absorb IR light. Absorption of wavelengths between 2.5 and 25 μm will cause covalent bonds to bend and vibrate, increasing the molecule's rotational speed. Different gas molecules absorb specific wavelengths of IR light (Figure 45.31). Thus by detecting increased absorption at particular frequencies gases can be identified and their concentrations determined. These instruments can be classified as:

• *Dispersive* – usually multiple gas analysers, where the radiation from the IR source is split and delivered to the sample sequentially: e.g. IR spectrophotometer.
• *Non-dispersive* – single gas analysers, where only one wavelength is used: e.g. the capnograph specifically used for carbon dioxide.

The most frequently used IR gas analyser is the IR spectrophotometer. Modern machines use specific LEDs to split the IR irradiation into different wavelengths. The sample chamber is transilluminated, and the absorption of IR radiation measured and compared with that of a reference chamber.

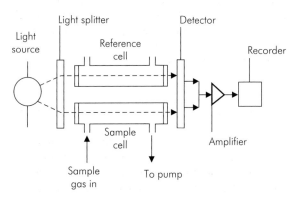

Figure 45.31 Infrared absorption gas analyser (capnograph)

• *Advantages* – this type of analyser is fast enough to follow breath-to-breath changes of CO_2, N_2O and volatile anaesthetics.
• *Disadvantages* – as the response time increases with molecular size (250 ms for CO_2, increasing to 750 ms for a volatile anaesthetic agent), rapid respiratory rates may decrease the accuracy of end-tidal/inspiratory volatile agent concentrations.

Ultraviolet (UV) absorption

Gases composed of similar atoms (O_2, H_2, N_2) will not absorb IR radiation, but will absorb UV light (as will halothane). These molecules all possess characteristic UV absorption spectra, absorbing light of very short wavelength. The only clinical analyser based on this method measures halothane, with a quoted accuracy of ± 0.2% over the range 0–5%.

• *Advantages* – acceptable accuracy.
• *Disadvantages* – the absorbed quanta are of sufficient energy to disrupt the molecule, producing toxic breakdown products, which cannot be returned to the breathing circuit unless passed through soda lime. The response time is slow (> 1 s).

Paramagnetism (in oxygen analysers)

This method is commonly used in oxygen analysers. Molecules can be either paramagnetic (attracted towards a magnetic field) or diamagnetic (repelled by a magnetic field). Paramagnetic molecules (e.g. oxygen) possess two unpaired electrons spinning in the same direction in the outer electron shell. The Pauling analyser uses the ability of oxygen to distort a non-homogeneous magnetic field as the basis to detect the presence of oxygen in a gas mixture. The analyser consists of a cell with a sealed glass dumbbell (containing nitrogen, a weakly diamagnetic gas) and a mirror, suspended by wires (but free to rotate) between the poles of a magnet. The paramagnetic effect of oxygen displaces the dumbbell, causing it and the mirror to rotate. The degree of rotation of both dumbbell and mirror is proportional to the concentration of oxygen present in the mixture. By reflecting a beam of light off the suspended mirror, the degree of rotation can be detected using a photocell. The resulting electrical signal, after processing, provides a measure of oxygen concentration. No other gases of clinical interest have this property (Figure 45.32).

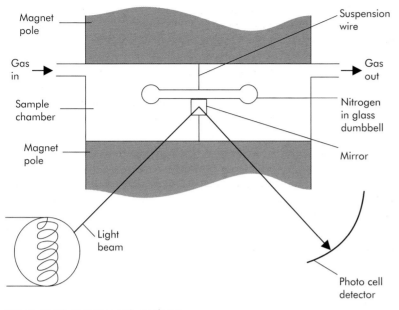

Figure 45.32 Paramagnetic analyser

Various modifications have been made to the basic design to compensate for external vibration, excessive gas flow rates, and pressurisation of the cell.
- *Advantages* – the commercial versions of this type of analyser are compact, relatively cheap, and remain unaffected by other common gases.
- *Disadvantages* – slow response times (5–20 s), mainly the result of large sample chambers.

Thermal conductivity
A gas with a high thermal conductivity will conduct heat more readily than one with a low conductivity (in comparison with air, CO_2 has 35% conductivity, whereas helium has 600%). This is the basis of instruments known as katherometers. When a gas is passed over a heated wire, the wire is cooled to a temperature which depends on the temperature of the gas, its flow rate, and the thermal conductivity of the gas.

The fall in wire temperature causes a decrease in electrical resistance. This fall in resistance is used to produce a small signal related to gas concentration, by connecting the wire as one arm of a Wheatstone bridge circuit. These analysers have been used mainly to measure CO_2 and helium concentrations, and have also found use in gas chromatography systems.

- *Advantages* – relatively simple and inexpensive technology.
- *Disadvantages* – slow response times (approximately 5 seconds) unless operated at low pressure (100 mmHg).

Electrochemical gas analysers
These instruments are based on an electrochemical reaction occurring between two electrodes in an electrolyte solution. The electrochemical reaction produces an electrolytic current passing between the electrodes whose magnitude is dependent on the partial pressure of dissolved gas molecules. There are two main devices, which are described in more detail under *Oxygen measurement* and *Carbon dioxide measurement*, below. These are the polarographic electrode and the fuel cell.

Other methods of gas analysis
Several other physical properties have been used as the basis for analysers:
- *Solubility* – this is the basis of the Drager Narkotest, which measures the effect of different concentrations of various volatile anaesthetic agents (cyclopropane, methoxyflurane, halothane, diethyl ether) on the length of four bands of silicon rubber. There is a linear relationship between the concentration of the volatile agent and the

The polarographic electrode

This consists of a pair of electrodes of specific materials (depending on the gas being measured) in an electrolyte solution. When a potential difference is applied across the electrodes, a current is produced between them through the electrolyte solution, which is dependent on the concentration of the gas in solution. In this device the redox potentials of the electrodes *oppose* the flow of current between the electrodes, and an externally applied potential difference is required to drive the reaction.

The fuel cell

This is effectively a primary cell (as in a battery), again consisting of two electrodes of specific materials in an electrolyte solution. In this device the redox potentials of the electrodes produce a potential difference which *generates* a current between the electrodes. Again the current in the solution is dependent on the dissolved gas concentration. This device drives the reaction itself, by the current it generates, but ultimately the reagents in the cell will be used up, and the reaction will cease. Hence the name 'fuel cell'.

measured length of the rubber bands. Measurements require correction for the presence of nitrous oxide.

- *Density* – this is the basis for the Waller chloroform balance. A sealed glass bulb filled with air is counter-balanced with a small weight in a gas-tight chamber. If a gas with a density greater than air is introduced into the chamber, there is an apparent decrease in the weight of the glass bulb. This reduction in weight is proportional to the difference in density between air and the vapour/air mixture, and can be used as the basis for calculating the amount of volatile present.
- *Refractive index* – The difference in the velocity of light passing through a vacuum and through a transparent substance/gas determines the refractive index of that substance. The measured delay in the passage of light through a gas is dependent on the number of molecules present. The Rayleigh Refractometer measures this transmission delay. If the refractive index of the gas is known, it is possible to calculate gas concentration.
- *Velocity of sound* – When a gas oscillates at a particular frequency, its structure will begin to resonate. The resonance depends on the velocity of sound in the gas

mixture, which is in turn a function of gas composition.
- *Raman light scattering* – When photons of light energy pass through a gas, a small fraction of them give up a portion of their energy to some of the gas molecules, raising their electron energy levels. This energy is then re-emitted at a longer wavelength characteristic of the gas as the excited molecules return to their original state.

Sources of error in gas and vapour measurements

Gas sampling errors can arise when sampling gases from a breathing circuit, due to:
- *Contamination* – gas samples can become contaminated with secretions, debris or water vapour.
- *Poor gas mixing* – significant concentration gradients may occur in a circuit and be sustained by laminar flow conditions, giving anomalous results.
- *Altered vapour pressure* – significant temperature gradients occur between inspired and expired gases, which can alter the vapour pressure in the sampled gas.
- *Altered pattern of flow at the sampling point* – excessive sampling rates can cause local flow and gas concentrations to change at the sampling point.
- *Variation in absolute pressure* – pressure may vary from point to point in a circuit, which can give rise to different results depending on the location of the sample site.

Instrument error – A major source of instrument sampling error is the 'ram-gas effect'. The flow velocity of gas as it enters the sampling port can alter sample composition. This effect can be reduced by using lower sampling rates, and ensuring that the sampling port is set at right angles to the main gas flow.

Patient error – Chronic lung disease can lead to increased non-homogeneity of the alveolar time constants throughout the lung. This results in a corresponding variation of alveolar gas composition between different lung units. Thus expiratory gas samples may not be representative of lung performance as a whole.

Oxygen measurement

Oxygen measurements in arterial blood can be made using various parameters including arterial partial pressure (PaO_2), arterial blood oxygen content (CaO_2) and haemoglobin oxygen saturation (SaO_2).

These parameters are all related to each other in the oxyhaemoglobin dissociation curve (ODC), which is a sigmoid-shaped curve describing the relationship between the oxygen saturation of blood and the partial pressure of oxygen in the blood (see *Gas exchange* in Chapter 17, and Figure 17.17).

Current measurement techniques can be applied either 'in vitro', i.e. remote from the patient using samples of gases or blood collected from the patient; or alternatively they can be applied directly to the patient, enabling 'in vivo' measurements to be made.

'In vitro' measurements of oxygen concentrations
Measurement in fresh gas mixtures
This can be done using the following methods, which have already been described in more detail above:

- Paramagnetic analyser – These instruments have slow response times owing to their large sample chambers, which limits their practical use.
- Mass spectrometer – Although versatile, with a rapid response, these instruments are too complex and expensive for widespread use.

Measurement in blood samples
This is almost universally done using electrochemical methods and forms the basis for both 'in vitro' and 'in vivo' techniques. The two most common techniques already mentioned above are the polarographic electrode and the galvanic fuel cell.

These devices are based on the electrochemical reduction of oxygen at a cathode, using electrons generated at the anode. For each molecule of O_2 reduced, four electrons move between the electrodes in an external circuit connecting the electrodes. This generates an electrical current which is dependent on the concentration of oxygen present in the sample. Application of Henry's law (the number of molecules in solution is proportional to the partial pressure) enables the partial pressure of oxygen to be calculated from the current measured.

Clark electrode (polarographic electrode)
The Clark electrode is used to measure the partial pressure of oxygen in arterial blood samples. This device is a system of two electrodes, a negative platinum cathode and a positive silver/silver chloride anode, which are immersed in an electrolyte solution (KCl). These are separated from the sample by a permeable membrane, which allows oxygen to filter from the sample through

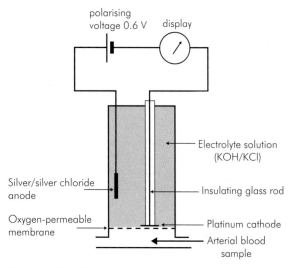

Figure 45.33 Clark electrode

into the electrolyte solution (Figure 45.33). The oxygen reacts with electrons at the cathode to produce OH^- ions, which migrate to the anode in the electrolyte solution. The reaction at the anode then produces electrons which flow through the external circuit to supply the redox reaction at the cathode. This small current in the external circuit can be measured by a galvanometer or digital readout, and is dependent on the oxygen in solution at the cathode. Therefore at equilibrium the current is a measure of the concentration of oxygen in the sample.

The Clark electrode

The redox potentials of the anode and cathode produce a small potential difference which *opposes* the flow of electrons to the cathode in the external circuit, because the silver anode is electropositive relative to the cathode (hydrogen).

Thus a small polarising voltage supply (0.6 V) is required to remove electrons from the anode and supply them to the cathode.

The redox reaction which occurs at the platinum *cathode* can be summarised as:

$$O_2 + 2H_2O + 4e^- \rightarrow 4(OH)^-$$

These OH^- ions produced at the cathode migrate to the silver/silver chloride *anode*, where electrons are produced by the oxidation of silver in the anode by Cl^-. This occurs as follows:

$$4Ag + 4Cl^- \rightarrow 4AgCl + 4e^-$$

The Cl$^-$ at the anode is provided by the displacement of Cl$^-$ from the KCl electrolyte solution by OH$^-$.

Initially the generated current increases with applied polarising voltage until it reaches a plateau, where no further increase occurs in spite of increasing the applied voltage. The plateau value is the point where the rate of oxygen reduction has become the limiting factor, and is proportional to the oxygen concentration in the sample.

The permeable membrane covering the electrodes serves to protect the cathode from protein deposition, which increases with applied voltage, reduces the available electrode surface area, and reduces the localised depletion of oxygen that can occur around the cathode. However, although this membrane prolongs electrode life it also increases response time of the electrode.

- *Advantages* – it is robust, and can be battery-powered, making it portable.
- *Disadvantages* – it has a limited lifespan, the silver anode of the silver/silver chloride electrode being eventually consumed by the current.

Galvanic fuel cell

This device is similar to the Clark electrode in that it is composed of two electrodes in an electrolyte solution (KOH). The electrodes are a lead anode and a gold mesh cathode (Figure 45.34). Oxygen is reduced by electrons at the cathode (the 'sensing' electrode), producing OH$^-$ ions which migrate to the anode. The redox reaction at the anode provides electrons at the cathode via the external circuit, producing a small current which is measured by a galvanometer or digital readout.

The fuel cell

In this device, *unlike the Clark electrode*, the redox potential difference between the cathode and anode *favours* the flow of current in the external circuit from anode to cathode, since the lead anode is electronegative compared to the cathode. Thus no external polarising voltage is required.

The reduction of oxygen at the cathode takes place as follows:

$$O_2 + 2H_2O + 4e^- \rightarrow 4OH^-$$

The OH$^-$ ions migrate to the anode under the influence of the redox potential difference between the electrodes.

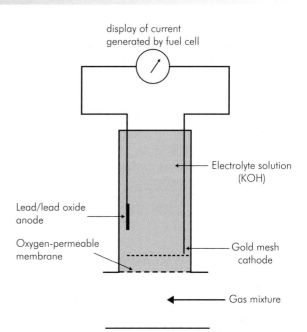

Figure 45.34 Galvanic fuel cell

At the anode electrons are produced by the oxidation of the lead anode:

$$2Pb + 4(OH)^- \rightarrow 2PbO + 2H_2O + 4e^-$$

This device is a primary cell which maintains itself by the consumption of the oxygen supplied by the sample. Theoretically its working life is only determined chemically by consumption of the lead anode.

- *Advantages* – compact, does not require a power supply, inexpensive and low maintenance.
- *Disadvantages* – relatively slow response time (approximately 30 s), too slow to measure breath-to-breath changes. Basic cells can be contaminated by N$_2$O, which reacts with the lead anode to produce nitrogen. Working lifespan of 6–12 months.

Sources of error with electrochemical methods

- *Blood gas factor* – the measured oxygen values are lower for blood than for gas samples. This is thought to reflect the delay caused by oxygen diffusion in blood, and the localised depletion of oxygen that occurs at the cathode; this is a consistent effect requiring mathematical correction.
- *Stability* – these systems utilise a two-point calibration (gas containing zero oxygen, and one containing a

fixed concentration); calibration drift occurs when protein and lipid deposits build up on the membrane or bubbles form in the electrolyte solution. To prevent this, a combination of regular electrode cleaning and quality control is necessary.

- *Interference* – erroneous effects can result from substances other than oxygen being reduced at the cathode (including N_2O). This can be avoided by specific membrane selection.
- *Temperature correction* – all modern blood gas analysers measure at 37 °C. If a patient has a temperature that differs from this by more than 2 °C, mathematical correction is necessary.

'In vivo' measurement of oxygen concentration
Intravascular oxygen electrodes
This is a bipolar variant of the Clark electrode in which both the anode and the cathode are mounted within a fine tube covered by an oxygen-permeable membrane. The whole assembly is small enough to pass through an 18G cannula. Response times vary between 5 and 60 seconds.

- *Advantages* – they provide a continuous measurement of arterial oxygen tension.
- *Disadvantages* – like its monopolar variant, the electrode is temperature-sensitive, and subject to calibration drift due to protein deposition. Access of oxygen to the cathode is flow-dependent, which can introduce error at low blood flow states (largely overcome by using a pulsed polarising current). Rapid response times are only achieved at the expense of poor accuracy at low flow rates.

Transcutaneous oxygen electrodes
These provide a measure of the oxygen that has diffused from capillaries in the dermis of the skin. The electrode comprises a ring-shaped anode, a central cathode, and electrolyte solution enclosed by an oxygen-permeable membrane. The electrode housing contains a heating element and a thermistor to allow temperature compensation. The whole assembly is held in direct contact with the skin by adhesive tape. Locally heating the skin increases capillary blood flow, improving the correlation between transcutaneous and arterial PO_2. Transcutaneous PO_2 increases with local temperature up to the point where tissue damage occurs, approximately 44–46 °C.

- *Advantages* – useful in neonatal monitoring, particularly in detecting hyperoxia. Response times are a function of diffusion distance, and vary from 10–15 seconds in infants to 45–60 seconds in adults.
- *Disadvantages* – excessive heating can increase the oxygen diffusion distance (oedema) and eventually lead to burns. Heating also increases skin metabolism, and causes the ODC to shift to the right. Essentially, transcutaneous PO_2 is a better index of skin oxygen delivery than PaO_2 (correlation between cutaneous and arterial PO_2 is best in infants); changes in cutaneous PO_2 lag behind changes in PaO_2.

Conjuctival oxygen tension electrode
The electrode consists of a ring cathode (gold or platinum), an anode (silver or silver/silver chloride) and a thermistor (for temperature compensation). These elements are covered by a membrane composed either of silicon oxide or polyethylene, and mounted on an ophthalmic former. This is placed under the eyelid in the conjuctival fornix (local anaesthesia is necessary for the awake patient), and held in place by the orbicularis oculi. Response times are similar to those obtained with transcutaneous electrodes.

- *Advantages* – this is an improvement over transcutaneous measurement, the shorter diffusion distance makes heating unnecessary, and correlation with arterial PO_2 is generally better.
- *Disadvantages* – the preparation and expense of these electrodes have limited their use.

Mass spectrometer
In addition to its in vitro application, the mass spectrometer can also be used as an in vivo analyser. In vivo, the mass spectrometer is in direct continuity with the patient via either an intravascular perforated metal catheter covered with a gas-permeable membrane or a transcutaneous oxygen electrode. The estimated response time varies between 3 and 50 seconds.

Optodes
This method differs from the others described, in that measurement does not depend on the consumption of oxygen. Oxygen will 'quench' the fluorescence of certain dyes. The magnitude of this 'quenching' effect is a function of oxygen concentration. This provides the basis for the technique, which uses an intravascular probe, composed of an optical fibre with a dye-coated tip, covered by

an oxygen-permeable membrane. Sequential illumination of the fibre causes the dye to fluoresce. The intensity of fluorescence depends on the concentration of oxygen present at the tip and is measured using a photomultiplier. The inclusion of a thermocouple allows for temperature compensation.

- *Advantages* – this method is independent of blood flow. Initial results suggest favourable stability and response times.
- *Disadvantages* – probes are expensive and subject to fibrin deposition. In addition, prolonged use may result in the deterioration of the dye, making measurements invalid.

Carbon dioxide measurement

Carbon dioxide (CO_2) is the metabolic end product of the aerobic oxidation of glucose. It is a soluble gas and is an important determinant of tissue pH. CO_2 is transported in the blood as carbamino-Hb compounds, as bicarbonate, or dissolved in solution.

The direct measurement of the partial pressure of CO_2 in arterial blood ($PaCO_2$) can provide information regarding pH, adequacy of ventilation and metabolic status.

The indirect measurement of end-tidal CO_2 reflects cardiac output and pulmonary blood flow, and can confirm correct endotracheal intubation.

The relationship between CO_2 and pH is described by the Henderson–Hasselbalch equation (see Chapter 16):

$$pH = pK_a + \log_{10} \frac{[HCO_3^-]}{[PaCO_2]}$$

An early method of measuring CO_2 levels indirectly was the Astrup technique, which used pH measurements to derive the PCO_2 level of a sample from a Siggard–Andersen diagram, by interpolation. This technique was time-consuming and inaccurate.

Modern techniques measure either arterial or end-tidal CO_2 ($ETCO_2$) levels. These can be applied 'in vitro', where the measurements are made on blood or gas samples remote from the subject, or 'in vivo', where the CO_2 measurement system is in direct continuity with the patient.

'In vitro' carbon dioxide measurement
The carbon dioxide electrode

This technique is used in blood gas analysers. It uses two electrodes, a glass pH electrode and a silver/silver chloride

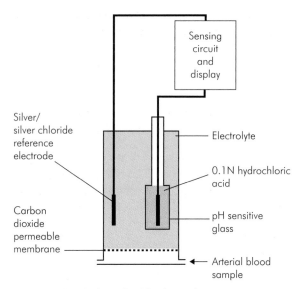

Figure 45.35 Carbon dioxide electrode

reference electrode, both maintained at 37 °C. The glass electrode is covered by a layer of cellophane or nylon mesh with a thin layer of sodium bicarbonate between the electrode and the covering. Both electrodes are enclosed within a membrane (Teflon or silicon rubber) which, while permeable to CO_2, is impermeable to blood cells, plasma and hydrogen ions (Figure 45.35). Using a two-point calibration system, buffers of known CO_2 concentration are used to establish the relationship between pH and CO_2. The system relies on the carbonic acid equilibrium:

$$H_2O + CO_2 \leftrightharpoons H_2CO_3 \leftrightharpoons H^+ + HCO_3^-$$

The diffusion of CO_2 across the membrane causes the equilibrium to shift to the right in accordance with the law of mass action. This generates hydrogen ions and causes a fall in pH which is proportional to the concentration of CO_2 (0.01 pH units for every 0.1 kPa change in CO_2).

- *Advantages* – generally regarded as accurate and stable.
- *Disadvantages* – response times are governed by the permeability properties of the membrane, and the rate of conversion of CO_2 into bicarbonate (the rate of reaction can be accelerated by inclusion of the enzyme carbonic anhydrase). Accuracy depends on membrane integrity, since it is vital to ensure that the only change in pH at the electrode results from the shift in the carbonic acid

equilibrium. This can be monitored by measurement of electrical resistance across the membrane.

'In vivo' measurement of carbon dioxide concentration

Transcutaneous electrodes

The measurement of transcutaneous CO_2 requires a modification of the basic CO_2 electrode. The electrode is part of a housing which also contains a heating element and thermistor (for temperature compensation). This is held in direct contact with the skin by adhesive tape. The skin is heated to a temperature of 42–44 °C. This increases capillary blood flow, CO_2 production in the skin, and CO_2 solubility. As described by Severinghaus, the measured transcutaneous CO_2 is usually greater than arterial CO_2 ($PaCO_2$):

$$\text{Transcutaneous } CO_2 = 1.33 \times PaCO_2 + 0.5 \text{ kPa}$$

- *Advantages* – gives a continuous measurement of carbon dioxide concentration in capillary blood.
- *Disadvantages* – as with the oxygen electrode, there is the risk of skin burns. Response times are slow, and the correlation between transcutaneous and arterial CO_2 is variable.

Intravascular probes

Miniaturised versions of the CO_2 electrode have been commercially produced that are small enough to be inserted through an arterial cannula.

- *Advantages* – give a continuous measurement of arterial carbon dioxide tension.
- *Disadvantages* – these are fragile, unstable, and subject to calibration drift.

Optodes

Similar to those used to measure oxygen 'in vivo', these measure CO_2 indirectly, by measuring the change in pH of a buffer, which in turn causes a change in the intensity of fluorescence of a pH-sensitive dye. The intravascular probe is composed of an optical fibre with a dye-coated tip covered by a thin layer of buffer. This is separated from the blood by a CO_2-permeable membrane. Any change in light intensity is proportional to the change in buffer pH, caused by the diffusion of CO_2 across the membrane. Changes in fluorescence are detected by a photomultiplier.

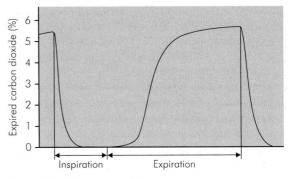

Figure 45.36 Capnograph trace

The capnograph: end-tidal CO_2 ($ETCO_2$)

In normal individuals, the $ETCO_2$ usually measures 0.5–0.8 kPa less than the arterial CO_2. The magnitude of this difference increases with respiratory disease, particularly where there is significant ventilation/perfusion mismatch. The capnograph provides a continuous display of repeated $ETCO_2$ estimations (Figure 45.36).

The majority of the commercial capnographs are based on infrared spectrophotometry, and can be classified as either *sidestream* or *mainstream* monitors according to their sampling system.

Sidestream capnograph

The most common type of capnograph is of the sidestream type. In this the sample gas is drawn from the main respiratory flow through a side port via a narrow tube to the sample cuvette (flow rates of 50–500 mL min^{-1}). Following CO_2 measurement, the gas is either returned to the expiratory limb of the breathing circuit (of particular relevance to low-flow anaesthesia) or scavenged.

- *Advantages* – these are generally more convenient than mainstream monitors; the patient attachment is less bulky, and more robust.
- *Disadvantages* – without elaborate water traps/filters to remove water vapour, the measured value of $ETCO_2$ would be invalid. A suction pump transfers the sample from the site of sampling to the measurement chamber; this sampling rate can in itself introduce error. The response time of these instruments tends to be longer than that of mainstream analysers.

Mainstream capnograph

In the mainstream capnograph, the measuring head inserts into the breathing or ventilator circuit so that it carries the main gas flow. The capnograph head acts as the sampling chamber, and is transilluminated by IR light through side windows.

- *Advantages* – the position of the probe makes removal of a sample of gas from the breathing circuit unnecessary. The system is far less complicated (no suction pump required); the errors due to gas sampling are eliminated. Response times are significantly less than with the sidestream type.
- *Disadvantages* – the probes are fragile, expensive, heavy, and require support (unsupported, they can cause the tracheal tube to kink); direct contact with the skin may cause a burn. The sensor window must remain clean to prevent inaccuracy and calibration problems.

Clinical uses of the capnograph trace

In anaesthesia the capnograph trace can provide immediate verification of successful tracheal intubation. However, in addition to this, both the shape of the capnogram and the value of the ETCO$_2$ measurement can reflect clinical changes (Figure 45.37).

Infrared absorption spectroscopy

This is the technology most widely used in monitoring end-tidal CO$_2$. The molecular structure of a more complex gas molecule such as carbon dioxide (compared to a simpler gas molecule such as oxygen) enables the gas to absorb infrared radiation. This is due to the specific mode of molecular oscillation excited at a characteristic frequency and wavelength. In the case of carbon dioxide this occurs at a wavelength of 4.3 µm in the infrared range.

pH measurement

Sorenson in 1909 defined pH as the log to the base 10 of the reciprocal of the hydrogen ion concentration [H$^+$].

$$pH = -\log_{10}[H^+]$$

Under normal conditions, buffer systems within the body (bicarbonate, phosphate, haemoglobin and protein) maintain the pH within a narrow range (7.38–7.42). The pH scale can be used as a clinical measure of acid–base status; this has both diagnostic and therapeutic value. The SI unit of pH is the hydrogen ion concentration expressed as nmol L^{-1}.

Indirect estimation of pH

Because of difficulty in measuring [H$^+$] directly, blood pH was estimated by derivation from the Henderson–Hasselbalch equation:

$$pH = pK_a + \log\frac{[HCO_3^-]}{H_2CO_3}$$

or

$$pH = pK_a + \log\frac{[HCO_3^-]}{\alpha PCO_2}$$

where pK$_a$ is the equilibrium constant for the dissociation of carbonic acid, and α is the solubility coefficient for carbon dioxide.

This method is inaccurate because the values of pK$_a$ and α vary with temperature.

Figure 45.37 Causes of changes in end-tidal CO$_2$ concentration

Change	Cause	Diagnosis
↓ ETCO$_2$	↑ Alveolar ventilation	↑ respiratory rate, ↑ tidal volume
	↓ CO$_2$ production	hypothermia
	↑ Dead space	pulmonary embolus, shock, hypotension
	Technical error	calibration error, air contamination, patient disconnection
↑ ETCO$_2$	↓ Alveolar ventilation	↓ respiratory rate, ↓ tidal volume
	↑ CO$_2$ production	sepsis, hyperpyrexia, thyrotoxicosis
	↑ inspired CO$_2$	rebreathing, CO$_2$ added to inspired gases, administration of NaHCO$_3$

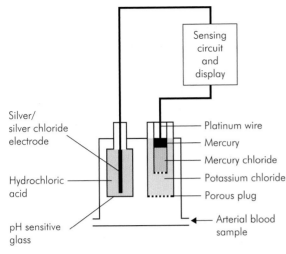

Figure 45.38 pH electrode

The pH electrode

Measurement of pH uses a system of two electrodes: one is the measuring electrode (silver/silver chloride in glass) while the other is a reference electrode (silver/silver chloride in reference solution, 0.1 mol L^{-1} KCl). Selectivity for H^+ is achieved by enclosing the measuring electrode in glass which is permeable to H^+ only (Figure 45.38).

The redox reaction at the measuring electrode is dependent on the H^+ activity in the sample, while the potential of the reference electrode remains constant. Together, the two electrodes form a galvanic cell in which the small current flowing through the external circuit is dependent on H^+ activity in the sample and can be measured with a galvanometer or digital display. The voltage differences by changes in sample pH are very small, in the order of tens of millivolts for each change of 1.0 in pH. Modern pH electrodes can be constructed as portable probes to test the pH of solutions using a pH meter. Since it is a galvanic cell, a pH electrode will have a finite life like other fuel cells.

Oximetry

Oximetry is a spectrophotometric technique (transillumination of a sample and measurement of absorbed radiation) that measures percentage haemoglobin saturation (SaO_2). In addition, it can also provide an indirect measure of oxygen tension and content, by use of the oxyhaemoglobin dissociation curve (ODC).

> **There are two forms of oximetry:**
>
> - Transmission (or absorbance) oximetry
> - Reflectance oximetry

Of the two techniques, transmission oximetry is the most commonly used for both 'in vitro' and 'in vivo' measurements.

Transmission oximetry

In transmission oximetry a section of perfused tissue (fingertip or earlobe) is transilluminated by infrared light. The absorption of the infrared illumination by the tissue layer is measured and is dependent on the concentrations of oxygenated (HbO_2) and deoxygenated (Hb) haemoglobin present.

Basic principles

The absorption of radiation by a layer of solution is determined by the Lambert–Beer law, which is discussed in more detail under *Light transmission and absorbance* in Chapter 44.

> **Lambert–Beer law**
>
> This relates the transmitted light to both molar concentration and thickness of the solution layer by expressing the absorbance as
>
> $$Absorbance = \varepsilon \, c \, d$$
>
> where ε = molar extinction coefficient, c = molar concentration, d = thickness.
>
> The Lambert–Beer law describes the absorption by HbO_2 and Hb individually, and algorithms are applied in order to calculate haemoglobin saturation.

Absorbance curves for HbO_2 and Hb

Absorbance can be plotted against wavelength to give curves for HbO_2 and Hb as shown in Figure 45.39. It can be seen that the absorbance of both compounds is high for shorter wavelengths (< 600 nm) of light, since they are both basically red in colour. However, at longer wavelengths in the red and infrared regions of the electromagnetic spectrum, the absorbance of HbO_2 is less than that of Hb. This gives HbO_2 a brighter red appearance

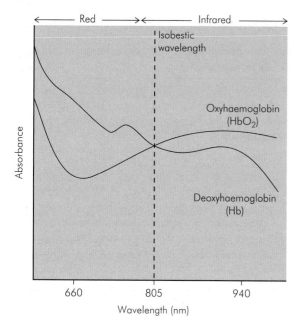

Figure 45.39 Absorbance curves for HbO$_2$ and Hb in oximetry

than Hb. At these longer wavelengths, the curves display secondary peaks in absorbance, one at 660 nm for oxyhaemoglobin (HbO$_2$) in the red region, and a different peak for deoxyhaemoglobin (Hb) at 940 nm in the infrared region.

Isobestic points – these are the two points at which the absorbances for HbO$_2$ and Hb are equal, i.e. they are the points at which the absorbance curves cross. They are dependent only on haemoglobin concentration. Some earlier oximeters corrected for haemoglobin concentration using the wavelength at the isobestic points.

Functional saturation

In order to determine haemoglobin saturation, monochromatic light at these two wavelengths must be used to transilluminate the sample. Measurement of the absorbances at these wavelengths enables the concentrations of HbO$_2$ and Hb to be calculated, and hence the haemoglobin saturation.

This saturation measurement is referred to as the 'functional saturation' because it is based only on the principal form of haemoglobin and ignores the presence of minor haemoglobin species such as

carboxyhaemoglobin (HbCO), methaemoglobin (HbMet), sulphaemoglobin (HbSul), and fetal haemoglobin (HbF). It is calculated as shown here:

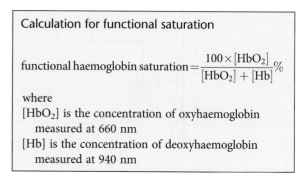

Calculation for functional saturation

$$\text{functional haemoglobin saturation} = \frac{100 \times [\text{HbO}_2]}{[\text{HbO}_2] + [\text{Hb}]}\%$$

where
[HbO$_2$] is the concentration of oxyhaemoglobin measured at 660 nm
[Hb] is the concentration of deoxyhaemoglobin measured at 940 nm

Fractional oxygen saturation

Most co-oximeters measure light absorbance at a minimum of four different wavelengths. This enables inclusion of the minor haemoglobin species in addition to the principal forms, oxyhaemoglobin and deoxyhaemoglobin. The more accurate 'fractional saturation' may then be calculated by:

Fractional haemoglobin saturation

$$= \frac{100 \times [\text{HbO}_2]}{[\text{HbO}_2] + [\text{Hb}] + [\text{HbCO}] + [\text{HbMet}]}\%$$

The two most commonly detected minor species of haemoglobin are HbMet and HbCO, which constitute < 1% and < 2% (in non-smokers) of the total of Hb concentration respectively. This means that under normal circumstances it is adequate to measure functional SaO$_2$.

Co-oximeter

This instrument requires haemolysis of the blood sample (by either chemical or physical means), prior to measurement of haemoglobin saturation. It is often incorporated into a blood gas machine.

- *Advantages* – light absorbance is measured at several different wavelengths, enabling fractional saturation to be estimated.
- *Disadvantages* – does not provide continuous saturation monitoring; moderately expensive capital cost and maintenance to obtain fractional saturation, which is not normally significantly different from functional saturation.

Pulse oximeter

> A **pulse oximeter** consists of a peripheral probe and a processing/display unit. The probe contains two light-emitting diodes (LEDs), which transilluminate the chosen tissue with monochromatic light at 'red' (660 nm), and 'infrared' (940 nm) wavelengths.
> A photodiode (PD) detects the transmitted light, converting it to an electrical signal. The functional haemoglobin saturation (SaO_2) is then calculated from the signal by the processing unit and displayed.

Sequential LED cycling – One LED emits red and the other infrared light, but the PD is unable to differentiate between wavelengths. To overcome this problem only one LED transilluminates at a time, the LEDs switching on and off alternately. The pulses in the PD signal are then identified in time to give separate values for red and infrared absorbances. Multiple pulses are used in each measurement cycle to minimise any motion artefact, and a specifc sequence is set up including a period of no transillumination. The time period when both LEDs are switched off is used to provide a correction for ambient light conditions.

The pulse oximeter signal

The transillumination signal of a pulse oximeter can be divided into two components:
- *The AC component* – This is a rapidly changing signal that corresponds to the light absorbed during the pulsatile portion of arterial blood flow.
- *The DC component* – This represents the light absorbed constantly by the resting volume of tissues and arterial blood.

The AC component constitutes a small proportion of the total signal, but is the major determinant of accuracy. It ranges from 1% to 5% of the DC component in a normal pulse wave. These signals are processed by the oximeter's own internal algorithms in order to calculate SaO_2.

Oximeters are calibrated using data previously obtained from human volunteer studies, in which saturations were recorded while the subjects breathed various inspired oxygen concentrations, including hypoxic levels. On ethical grounds, these studies were limited to minimum measured saturations of 80%. As a result, commercial oximeters are most accurate over the saturation range 80–100%. Any saturation values below this level are obtained by extrapolation, and suffer from increasing errors. Even within the normal range, the intrinsic error of some oximeters has been estimated to vary between 0% and 13%.

Increased response times in pulse oximeters

The response time is particularly important in pulse oximeters. Prolonged response time can be attributed to:
- *Instrumental delay* – This relates to the averaging time used to reduce movement artefact. Increasing the averaging time prolongs the response time.
- *Circulatory delay* – Response time is the time taken for changes in central saturation to reach the peripheral circulation. It varies according to probe site (approximately 10–15 seconds for an ear probe, and > 60 seconds for a finger probe). Both cold-induced vasoconstriction and venous engorgement can increase response times 2–3-fold.

Reflectance oximetry

This technique is used for continuous invasive measurement, i.e. monitoring mixed venous saturation with an oximetric pulmonary artery catheter (OPAC). Light of specific wavelength passes along a fibreoptic channel to the tip of the catheter, where it is reflected back up a second channel in the OPAC by the passing blood. The intensity of the reflected light is measured by a photodiode.
- *Advantages* – the detector (photodiode) can be remote from the sampling point.
- *Disadvantages* – the intensity of reflected light depends on the depth of penetration of the light into the blood, and on the concentration of Hb. The concentration–wavelength relationship is non-linear, and is affected by changes in pH, body temperature, haematocrit and cardiac output.

Sources of error in oximetry

These include:
- *Light-emitting diodes* – Each emits light over a narrow spectral range either side of the central or principal wavelength, i.e. 660 nm or 940 nm. This can vary up to ± 15 nm between LEDs of the same type, introducing an error in the measurement of absorbance and the calculation of SaO_2. Oximeters compensate for this using internal software.

- *Ambient light* – This can be minimised by using shielded probes, and sequential LED cycling (see above).
- *Low perfusion states* – The amplitude of the probe signal depends on tissue perfusion (decreased perfusion reduces signal amplitude). The oximeter attempts to compensate by amplifying the total signal (AC and DC components). This has the effect of making the signal-to-noise ratio worse. Under poor conditions the noise may become the predominant signal. When this occurs, the ratio of scaled signals for both 660 and 940 nm approaches unity, corresponding to a falsely displayed saturation of 85%. To prevent this happening, modern machines have signal-to-noise ratio limits, which if exceeded interrupt the display.
- *Motion artefact* – As mentioned, motion artefact can be reduced by increasing the signal averaging time, but only at the expense of response time. Alternatively, some oximeters employ sophisticated internal algorithms which help identify obviously spurious readings.
- *External dyes* – Methylene blue has the most dramatic effect: as concentration increases, SaO_2 values decrease. This reduces oximeter readings by up to 65% at a concentration of 2–5 mg kg^{-1} for 10–60 minutes. Some dark nail polishes can also interfere with oximetry.
- The effect of additional haemoglobin species on absorbance:
    - HbMet – light absorption is greater than both principal species at 940 nm, and simulates reduced Hb at 660 nm. At high saturations ($>$ 85%) the true value is underestimated; at low values ($<$ 85%) it is overestimated.
    - HbCO – has minimal absorption at 940 nm, but has a similar absorbance to HbO_2 at 660 nm; this results in overestimation of SaO_2.
    - HbF – essentially the same absorption spectra as adult haemoglobin and has no effect on oximetry.
    - HbS – has no reported effect on oximetry. It should be noted that in patients with sickle disease there is a shift in the ODC to the right. Thus, for any given PaO_2, the corresponding saturation is less than expected.
- *Anaemia* – There is a linear trend to underestimate SaO_2 as the concentration falls; at haemoglobin levels of 8 g 100 mL^{-1} this can be 10–15%. Polycythaemia has no effect. Accuracy is less at low saturation levels in anaemic patients.
- *Bilirubinaemia* – Does not appear to affect oximeters, though when severe it may result in elevated estimation of HbMet, and HbCO when using in vitro methods.
- *Diathermy* – The interference effect largely depends on the particular oximeter. This can be reduced by using suppression filters.
- *Probes* – Different probes have different performance characteristics. Using a different probe with the same oximeter without modification of the oximeter's internal algorithm can introduce error.

Neuromuscular monitoring

Neuromuscular monitoring is used in the following applications:

- Assessment of neuromuscular blockade during surgical anaesthesia in order to guide the use of muscle relaxants
- Identification of the type of neuromuscular blockade present (depolarising, non-depolarising, or type II block)
- Localising peripheral nerves during regional anaesthetic techniques

Methods of neuromuscular monitoring

The basic technique involves two stages: first the pulsed electrical stimulation of a peripheral motor nerve, and secondly the assessment of the muscular response.

Electrical stimulation of a peripheral nerve

Needle or surface electrodes are located over or close to a peripheral motor nerve. A standard electrical pulse stimulates the nerve, producing a measurable muscle twitch. It should be noted that muscle response is related to delivered current and not applied voltage.

The stimulator pulse – the electrical characteristics of the stimulator pulse are:

- A square-wave pulse with a uniform amplitude.
- A pulse current amplitude appropriate for the particular application: i.e. low amplitude for needle electrodes (0.5–5.0 mA), and higher amplitude for skin electrodes (10–40 mA).
- An optimal pulse length of 0.2 ms. This is a result of the compromise between current pulse amplitude and duration of current flow, since an excessive value of either increases the risk of neural damage.
- Various patterns of pulses, including single or trains of pulses at 1–2 Hz, and tetanic bursts at 50–100 Hz.

All currently used nerve stimulators are battery powered and are isolated electrically from all other objects. Skin electrodes are used for intraoperative neuromuscular monitoring and require relatively high current pulse amplitudes. This provides 'supramaximal' stimulation, which ensures maximum recruitment of muscle fibres, thus providing a baseline for a control twitch when using relaxants. Peripheral nerve location for local anaesthetic blocks is performed using needle electrodes, insulated except for the needle tips. These stimulate with much lower currents. Dual-function stimulators operate for both neuromuscular monitoring ('external' mode) and nerve location ('internal' mode).

Assessment of neuromuscular blockade

The assessment of muscular response to electrical stimulation provides the basis for neuromuscular monitoring during neuromuscular blockade. A variety of methods providing an indirect measure of contractile force have been employed. These include:

- Vision and touch
- Mechanomyography
- Accelomyography
- Electromyography

For effective clinical application of neuromuscular blockade monitoring, the method of assessment needs to combine accuracy with practical convenience.

Different muscle groups in neuromuscular blockade

When monitoring neuromuscular blockade, it is important to realise that different muscle groups demonstrate different sensitivities to muscle relaxants.
Some muscles reflect respiratory muscle response better than others.

Vision and touch

The muscle twitch that results from the electrical stimulation is assessed either by observation (i.e. either degree of contraction or a simple count of pulse when using 'train of four'), or by palpation.

- *Advantages* – this method is simple and convenient.
- *Disadvantages* – it is inaccurate, and provides only a gross assessment of muscle response.

Mechanomyography

In this method the muscle becomes a force-displacement transducer. A small preload is attached to the muscle to maintain isometric conditions. Electrical stimulation causes the muscle to contract against the preload, generating a tension that is proportional to the force of contraction. This 'generated' tension is converted to an electrical signal, which can then be measured. For access and convenience, adductor pollicis is the muscle normally used.

- *Advantages* – more accurate than 'vision and touch'.
- *Disadvantages* – the need for correct positioning of the transducer, selection of the preload, and immobilisation of the hand makes this method inconvenient and difficult to maintain.

Accelomyography

This method requires careful positioning of a joint, usually a digit, such that the distal end remains free hanging. Electrical stimulation of the appropriate motor nerve causes muscle contraction and movement of the digit. The measured acceleration of the distal part is directly proportional to the force of muscle contraction. By fixing a piezoelectric wafer to the distal part of the digit, it is possible to convert the measured acceleration into an electrical signal which can then be measured.

- *Advantages* – more objective than 'vision and touch'.
- *Disadvantages* – as with mechanomyography, there are problems with joint positioning, which make this technique inconvenient and inconsistent.

Electromyography

This measures muscle activity by recording the magnitude of the evoked compound action potentials from either skin or needle electrodes overlying a particular muscle (adductor pollicis or the hypothenar eminence is the most commonly used site). The active electrode is placed over the motor nerve, the indifferent electrode is placed over the tendon insertion.

- *Advantages* – avoids the mechanical problems of using and calibrating transducers attached to joints.
- *Disadvantages* – simple alteration in hand position can alter electrode geometry enough to change the measured response.

Despite offering improved objectivity and accuracy, the above techniques are more suited to use as research tools.

Currently, observation and palpation provide the basis for clinical neuromuscular monitoring.

Stimulation patterns in neuromuscular monitoring

Several patterns of current pulses for neuromuscular stimulation have been developed to improve sensitivity in the monitoring. These are designed to exaggerate specific characteristics of non-depolarising muscle blockade – for example:

Fade – decreased muscle twitch amplitude with repeat stimulation.

Post-tetanic facilitation – an increase in the response following tetanic stimulation due to increased mobilisation of acetylcholine (ACh). The various stimulation patterns include:

- Single twitch
- Train of four
- Tetanic stimulation
- Post-tetanic count
- Double burst

Single twitch

A supramaximal electrical stimulus is delivered at 1 Hz. At this frequency there is sufficient time for complete muscle fibre recovery between stimuli, avoiding any misinterpretation of twitch height arising from fade. The ratio of the measured twitch height after relaxant administration (T_1) to the control twitch height before relaxant (T_c) provides a measure of muscle relaxation. Normal muscle function corresponds to a T_1/T_c ratio of 1.0. This falls steadily to zero as receptor occupancy increases from 75% to 100%, reflecting ACh receptor occupancy at the neuromuscular junction.

- *Advantages* – useful for assessment of neuromuscular blockade with depolarising relaxants (suxamethonium chloride), where there is neither fade nor post-tetanic facilitation.
- *Disadvantages* – the usefulness of this pattern is limited by the narrow range of receptor occupancy detected (i.e. 25%) and the requirement for a means of measuring twitch height, e.g. mechanomyography.

Train of four (TOF)

This pattern consists of four identical stimuli delivered at 2 Hz. Non-depolarising muscle relaxants cause a reduction in height of the first twitch compared to a pre-

Figure 45.40 Acetylcholine receptor occupancy corresponding to number of TOF twitches detectable.

Detectable twitches	% Receptor blockade
4	< 75
3	75
2	80
1	90
0	100

relaxant supramaximal stimulus, and also a serial reduction in height of the four response twitches. There is a relationship between receptor occupancy and the number of visually detectable twitches (Figure 45.40).

The degree of neuromuscular blockade can be more objectively assessed by calculating the ratio of the fourth (T_4) and first (T_1) measured twitch heights (T_4/T_1). The consensus of opinion is that for adequate respiratory function, the T_4/T_1 ratio must be $> 70\%$.

- *Advantages* – more sensitive than the single twitch. Gives a quantitative result with simple visual assessment.
- *Disadvantages* – although more sensitive than the single twitch, TOF remains a basically innaccurate method. The fade of TOF pulses on administration of relaxant does not correlate with the reappearance of TOF pulses during recovery.

Tetanic stimulation

The extent of detectable fade following a tetanic stimulation depends on:

- The degree of muscle blockade
- The amplitude and duration of the tetanic burst

By increasing the amplitude of the tetanic burst, it is possible to detect fade at much lower levels of receptor occupancy. A tetanic burst of 50 Hz for 5 seconds produces a muscle response comparable to a maximal voluntary effort. The absence of fade following this stimulus can be interpreted as the return to full muscle power (Figure 45.41).

- *Advantages* – can be used to assess neuromuscular blockade at relatively low levels of receptor occupancy.
- *Disadvantages* – cannot quantify receptor occupancy from post-tetanic fade. It is an unpleasant sensation in

Normal neuromuscular junction

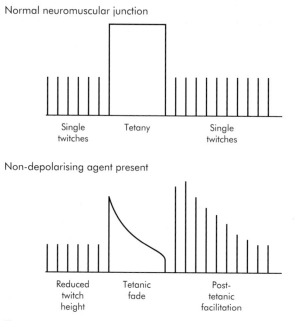

Figure 45.41 Tetanic stimulation and fade

Normal neuromuscular junction

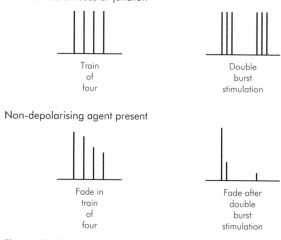

Figure 45.42 Double-burst stimulation

the conscious patient, and leaves an unpleasant sensory aftermath when applied to the unconscious patient.

Post-tetanic count (PTC)

This pattern is sometimes known as post-tetanic potentiation or facilitation. Intense muscle blockade can completely abolish the response to a train of four. Tetanic stimulation increases the mobilisation of ACh in the presynaptic membrane. Subsequent electrical stimulation uses twitches at 1-second intervals, releasing supranormal concentrations of ACh sufficient to overcome the effect of non-depolarising relaxants. The number of resultant twitches (the PTC) depends on the frequency of the tetanic burst, the amplitude and duration of the burst, and the degree of neuromuscular blockade present.

- *Advantages* – this method can produce a response at relatively high levels of receptor occupancy, and a PTC < 5 indicates profound neuromuscular blockade. A PTC > 15 is at least equivalent to two twitches of a TOF, and at this level, successful pharmacological reversal of the remaining muscle blockade is possible.
- *Disadvantages* – the mobilisation of ACh at the neuromuscular junction produced by the tetanic stimulus may last for some time. Therefore repetition

of two PTCs in quick succession (< 6 minutes apart) may lead to underestimation of the degree of neuromuscular blockade.

Double-burst stimulation (DBS)

This variant pattern was introduced to improve the manual assessment of fade. It consists of two tetanic bursts of 50 Hz. Each burst is composed of three tetanic twitches (at 20 ms intervals), the bursts being separated by 750 milliseconds. Muscle response is clinically detected as just two separate twitches (T_1 and T_2). The DBS ratio (T_2/T_1) is closely related to the TOF ratio (Figure 45.42).

- *Advantages* – easier to assess small degrees of residual neuromuscular blockade with DBS than with TOF.
- *Disadvantages* – Relies on the degree of fade between the first and second bursts. Best appreciated by palpation rather than visually. In TOF, twitches can be counted visually.

Depth of anaesthesia

Historical background

In 1845, Snow made the first documented attempt to assess anaesthetic depth, describing five levels of ether anaesthesia. During the First World War this was refined by Guedel, who developed the chart classification of ether anaesthesia based on lacrimation, pupil size and position, respiratory pattern, and peripheral movements. Advances in anaesthesia (in particular the introduction of curare soon after the Second World War) made previous classifications obsolete. As a consequence, a new system was developed based on the graded assessment of autonomic activity, which includes lacrimation, a parameter surviving from Guedel's chart classification.

> The ideal measuring system for assessing anaesthetic depth would:
>
> - Identify a universally acceptable indicator of conscious awareness
> - Translate this measurement into a convenient clinical scale
> - Eliminate the risk of conscious awareness
>
> To date no system fulfils any of these criteria.

Methods for the assessment of anaesthetic depth that are mainly of historical interest include the following:

- Tunstall's 'isolated arm' technique – this provided a gross visual indicator of inadequate anaesthesia by detecting movement in forearm muscles isolated from the effect of muscle relaxants by means of a tourniquet.
- Integrated clinical scores (e.g. Evans score)
- Lower oesophageal contractility
- Frontalis electromyogram

Integrated clinical scores

The most commonly quoted score is the Evans or PRST score. This scoring system was designed to assess the elements of autonomic activity: P (systolic blood pressure), R (heart rate), S (sweating) and T (tears). The scoring system is outlined in Figure 45.43.

PRST scores thus range from 0 to 8, but in practice the midpoint of the range is rarely exceeded, reflecting the redundancy within this scoring system.

- *Advantages* – simple, requiring no specialised equipment.
- *Disadvantages* – the parameters are not specific for the effects of anaesthesia. Values vary widely amongst individuals and can be significantly affected by various drugs and pre-existing disease states.

Figure 45.43 Evans PRST scoring for depth of anaesthesia

Parameter	Measurement	Score
P	< Control + 15	0
	< Control + 30	1
	> Control + 30	2
R	< Control + 15	0
	< Control + 30	1
	> Control + 30	2
S	Nil	0
	Skin moist to touch	1
	Visible beads of sweat	2
T	No excess tears, eye open	0
	Excess tears, eye open	1
	Tear overflow, eye closed	2

Lower oesophageal contractility

Monitoring oesophageal contractions has been used in the past to assess anaesthetic depth. There are two types of smooth muscle contraction described in the lower oesophagus:

Provoked lower oesophageal contractions – these result from sudden distention of the oesophagus, and are induced by the rapid inflation of a balloon catheter in the lower oesophagus.

Spontaneous lower oesophageal contractions – these arise spontaneously, and can be induced by emotion and stress in the awake individual.

Anaesthetic depth was related to an index dependent on the recordings of these contractions.

- *Advantages* – easy to interpret, can be used in the presence of muscle relaxants.
- *Disadvantages* – unproven relationship with anaesthetic depth.

Frontalis electromyogram (FEMG)

The frontalis muscle was chosen for this purpose because:

- It receives both visceral and somatic fibres from the facial nerve.

- It is less sensitive than other muscles to the effects of muscle relaxants.

The dual nerve supply means that this muscle can be influenced by autonomic activity. Using two surface electrodes, compound action potentials from this muscle are recorded.

- *Advantages* – non-invasive, convenient and easy to apply electrodes.
- *Disadvantages* – recording EEG signals poses technical problems because of low amplitude and interference. There is a wide inter-individual variability in measured FEMG values. Thus single FEMG values are of limited use as an assessment of anaesthetic depth.

Current methods of assessing anaesthetic depth: electrical activity of the brain

These methods remain in use currently and are considered to have a more reliable relationship with anaesthetic depth. They include:

- The electroencephalogram (EEG)
- Evoked responses – including auditory evoked responses (AER), brainstem auditory evoked responses (BAER) and visual evoked responses (VER)
- Bispectral index (BIS)

Electroencephalogram (EEG)

This method provides a continuous non-invasive assessment of cerebral activity. The generated electrical signal is the summated product of excitatory and inhibitory post-synaptic activity controlled and paced by subthalamic nuclei. To have any clinical use, these signals require extensive processing.

The EEG is a varying voltage signal, with amplitudes between 1 and 500 µV. For the purposes of interpretation, the frequency spectrum is divided into five bands (Figure 45.44).

If the EEG frequency spectrum for a patient undergoing deepening anaesthesia is plotted, sequential changes are noted. The EEG of an awake patient has a low amplitude and high frequency. Deepening anaesthesia causes a progressive increase in signal amplitude and reduces frequency. All volatile anaesthetics induce these sequential changes in the EEG signal.

Cerebral function analysing monitor (CFAM)

This device produces a continuous display of an analysed EEG signal from two symmetrical pairs of scalp electrodes. The display consists of two traces. One trace shows the

Figure 45.44 Frequency bands in the EEG signal

Band	Frequency range (Hz)	Psychological state
δ	< 3	Unconscious, non-REM sleep
θ	4–7	Trance, drifting, may be lateralised/focal
α	8–12	Conscious, relaxed, meditating
β	> 13	Alert, focused, mentally active
γ	40	Thinking, high level processing

mean amplitude of the EEG signals plotted in time, while the second trace shows the mean power in each frequency band (δ, θ, α and β).

Compressed spectral array

This system plots sequential segments of the EEG power spectrum, to give a three-dimensional picture of power amplitude vertically (y-axis), frequency horizontally (x-axis) and time (z-axis). This creates a 3D plot of 'peaks' and 'valleys' showing how the power spectrum of the EEG changes with the course of time (Figure 45.45).

- *Advantages* – EEG monitoring reflects cerebral electrical activity rather than peripheral muscular or autonomic function.
- *Disadvantages* – none of the methods are completely reliable predictors of depth of anaesthesia. At best they provide a trend of information that needs to be combined with clinical observation.

Depth of anaesthesia and the EEG

The EEG is a general indicator of cerebral perfusion and metabolic activity. Signal output can be depressed by hypoxia, hypotension, cerebral oedema and metabolic encephalopathy. Any change in the character of the EEG signal needs to be interpreted with this in mind, and cannot be entirely attributed to depth of anaesthesia. Interpretation is further complicated in that different anaesthetic agents have different effects on the EEG signal.

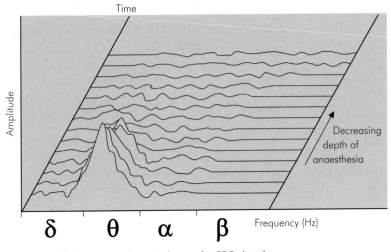

Figure 45.45 Compressed spectral array for EEG signals

Evoked responses

These signals are of very low amplitude (1–2 µV), compared to the EEG background trace (10–300 µV) and electrical noise due to neuromuscular activity. They are extracted from the background EEG and noise signal by computer averaging. The signals consist of a series of identifiable peaks and troughs, each with a time delay relative to the stimulus, which is referred to as the latency. The early signal (between 0 and 10 ms) is the 'brainstem response', based on its presumed origin. Signals between 10 and 100 ms are middle latency, and contain the early cortical response. Signals beyond this (100–1000 ms) represent the late cortical response arising mainly from the frontal cortex and association areas.

The signal latencies are increased, and the peaks and troughs are attenuated or even abolished, by anaesthesia, sedation and sleep. There is an increasing volume of data suggesting that the early cortical waves of the AER can detect dose-related changes in a range of general anaesthetic agents, respond to surgical stimulation, and correlate with the explicit and implicit memory of events during anaesthesia.

Brainstem auditory evoked responses (BAERs) – These are generated using an auditory stimulus and are sometimes referred to as auditory evoked responses (AERs). The signal has six distinguishable peaks (I–VI), the anatomical origin of which has caused much debate. It is suggested that the first is derived from the cochlear nerve, the second from the cochlear nucleus, the third from the superior olivary complex, the fourth and fifth from the inferior colliculus. BAERs are not affected significantly by intravenous anaesthetic agents, limiting their use in total intravenous anaesthesia.

Visual evoked response (VERs) – These signals arise from stimulation of the visual pathway by a pulsed flash of light. This modified flash test produces variable results, and as such is more suited to a qualitative rather than quantitative assessment. The signals represent a mainly cortical response.

Bispectral index (BIS) monitoring

BIS monitoring relies on the calculation of an index derived from the anaesthetised patient's EEG. It uses several parameters from the EEG, including time domain, frequency domain and frequency spectrum parameters. The details of the algorithms used to calculate the BIS index remain undisclosed by the developers of the original device.

The BIS index ranges from 0 to 100, where 0 is equivalent to an isoelectric (silent) EEG.

Acceptable levels for the BIS index during general anaesthesia are between 40 and 60.

As yet the reliability of this index in correlating with depth of anaesthesia and in avoiding awareness remains controversial.

Temperature measurement

Temperature measurement is an important part of clinical practice and has particular relevance to anaesthetic management. Anaesthesia impairs normal thermoregulation, causing a biphasic fall in body temperature that begins soon after induction. Extremes of body temperature (more commonly hypothermia) increase the risk of patient morbidity (see *Body temperature and thermoregulation* in Chapter 21). Body temperature is usually taken to be 37 °C or 98.6 °F.

Temperature scales
- Fahrenheit (1714) developed his temperature scale using the first mercury thermometer. The zero point was set using a mixture of sodium chloride and ice. According to this scale, ice melted at 32 °F, water boiled at 212 °F, and body temperature was assumed to be 100 °F.
- Celsius (1742) developed his scale with two fixed points, 0 °C for the melting point of ice and 100 °C for the boiling point of water.
- Kelvin (absolute temperature scale) uses two fixed points of absolute zero, 0 K (−273.15°C), and the triple point of water, which is 273.16 K (0.01 °C).

Conversion between temperature scales

Simple conversion between temperature scales can be made as follows:

$$°F = (°C \times 9/5) + 32$$
$$°C = (°F - 32) \times 5/9$$
$$K = (°C + 273)$$

Temperature measurement site
Small temperature gradients exist between different parts of the body in normal subjects. The ability of a measured value to reflect core temperature depends on the site chosen. This will also determine the response time, i.e. the speed with which a change in body temperature is registered.
- **Oesophagus** – The correct probe position is in the lower 25% of the oesophagus. When it is correctly placed, the measured values provide a good estimate of cerebral blood temperature. If placed above this level however, the probe may under-read due to the cooling effect of the inspired gases.
- **Nasopharynx** – The probe is positioned just behind the soft palate. Compared with the oesophageal probe, this provides a less accurate measure of core temperature.
- **Tympanic membrane** – Aural canal temperature provides an accurate measure of hypothalamic temperature. It has a short response time, and correlates well with the results obtained from an oesophageal probe.
- **Blood** – Blood temperature can be measured using the thermistor of a pulmonary flotation catheter. This method provides the best continuous measure of core temperature.
- **Rectal** – The recorded temperature is influenced by the heat generated by gut flora, the cooling effect of blood returning from the lower limbs, and the insulation of the temperature probe by faeces. The rectal temperature is normally 0.5–1% higher than core temperature, and compared with other sites the response time is slow.
- **Bladder** – More accurate than rectal temperature, the probe is usually part of an indwelling catheter. These probes are expensive, invasive, and slow to respond when the urine flow exceeds 270 mL h^{-1}.

Thermometers
These can be classified as:
- *Direct-reading thermometers* – the display and site of measurement are in direct contact.
- *Remote-reading thermometers* – the display is distant from the site of measurement.

The choice of thermometer is determined by the application, the clinical environment, the required accuracy, and whether a continuous display is needed. Clinical measurement of temperature may use:
- A mercury glass thermometer
- A chemical thermometer
- A resistance thermometer
- A thermistor
- A thermocouple

Environmental temperature measurement usually employs a dial thermometer.

Direct-reading thermometers
Liquid expansion thermometers
These consist of a glass bulb filled with either alcohol or mercury, which is connected to a narrow evacuated glass capillary tube. When warmed, the liquid expands, causing a column of liquid to rise up the capillary tube. The temperature corresponds to a point on a calibrated temperature scale measured by the height of the fluid column. If the cross-sectional area of the capillary tube is constant, then the relationship between expansion of the liquid and the column height will remain linear.
- *Advantages* – simple, and no power supply required.
- *Disadvantages* – poor visual display of temperature, slow response time, limited temperature range (requiring a low-reading thermometer for hypothermia), cannot be read remotely, easy breakage, unsuitable for insertion into cavities.

Chemical thermometers
These consist of a series of cells, each containing a mixture of chemicals, the colour of which is temperature-dependent. The particular chemical mixture is chosen to suit the required temperature range, and the colour change usually occurs within 30 seconds. The older single-use thermometers relied on a series of dye-containing crystals. The newer reusable thermometers use liquid crystal technology. In these, the solid crystals are colourless, and as they melt the realignment of the composite molecules produces the change in colour.
- *Advantages* – faster response time, no breakage problem, disposable.
- *Disadvantages* – despite the selection of suitable material, it is usually only possible to differentiate temperature intervals of approximately 0.5 °C.

Dial thermometers
These are of two types:
Bimetallic – a typical example consists of a flattened spiral spring made up of two dissimilar metals each with a different coefficient of expansion. One end of the spring is fixed, the other attached to a pointer. As the temperature increases the spring either winds or unwinds, causing the pointer to move across a temperature scale.
Pressure gauge type – this is based on the Bourdon pressure gauge, and consists of a hollow spiral metal tube. The tube forms a spring and terminates at one end in a temperature-sensing bulb. The bulb contains either volatile liquid or vapour which expands as the temperature increases, causing an increase in pressure within the tube. This results in an unwinding movement which is coupled to a pointer on a temperature scale.

- *Advantages* – relatively cheap and robust, providing a continuous easily readable measurement.
- *Disadvantages* – the accuracy of these thermometers is only ± 0.25 °C, and they are prone to calibration errors.

Remote-reading thermometers
Resistance thermometers
These devices are based on the change in electrical resistance of a coil of wire with temperature. This occurs according to the relationship

$$R_t = R_o \left(1 + at + bt^2\right)$$

where R_t is the resistance at temperature t °C, R_o is the resistance at 0 °C, and a and b are constants.

The change in resistance is detected using a Wheatstone bridge circuit and galvanometer. Platinum is most commonly used for this purpose because it resists corrosion and has a large temperature coefficient of resistance. This type of thermometer has the ability to measure very small changes in temperature, i.e. ± 0.0001 °C. Over the range 0–100 °C, the relationship between temperature and resistance is largely linear.
- *Advantages* – accuracy.
- *Disadvantages* – physical size of the coil, making it difficult to produce a small probe; fragile, slow response time.

Thermistors
Composed of the fused oxides of heavy metals (including of manganese, nickel, zinc, cobalt and iron), a thermistor is a semiconductor that possesses a negative temperature coefficient of resistance. The components are compressed into minute beads (ranging in diameter from 0.012 to 0.25 cm) with very small thermal capacities and rapid response times (as little as 0.2 seconds). A greater temperature coefficient makes thermistors more sensitive than wire resistance thermometers.

- *Advantages* – small size, rapid response time.
- *Disadvantages* – the relationship between resistance and temperature is non-linear and subject to wide variation. This requires signal conditioning and calibration. Thermistors from the same batch show wide variation in their electrical resistance, and as they age their electrical resistance changes. Thermistors exhibit hysteresis, and the relationship between resistance and temperature when heating up is different from that when cooling. To minimise these effects, commercial thermistors are batched and pre-aged.

Thermocouple

This is an electric circuit composed of two different metals, joined to form two separate identical junctions. If these junctions are maintained at different temperatures, an electromotive force (EMF) is generated that is proportional to the temperature difference between the two junctions and can be measured using a galvanometer. This is the 'Seebeck effect'.

The metals commonly used include copper-constantin (copper/nickel alloy), and platinum-rhodium.

- *Advantages* – the junctions may be very small and versatile. Low thermal capacity means rapid response times. Acceptable accuracy ($\pm$ 0.1 °C). All junctions made with the same metals behave identically. They are relatively cheap.
- *Disadvantages* – the voltage output per degree Celsius is small (approximately 50 mV) and requires signal amplification. The non-linear relationship between EMF and temperature requires signal processing.

Humidity measurement

Historically the measurement of humidity was an important contribution to the safe practice of anaesthesia. The combination of static electric sparks, and the use of flammable anaesthetic gases (e.g. ether) constituted a significant risk to the wellbeing of both patient and anaesthetist. One of the measures used to reduce static electricity, and hence the incidence of fires and explosions, was to maintain the relative humidity in the operating theatre above 50%. While this is no longer a major consideration in current practice, an understanding of humidity, with its influence on thermal balance and respiratory function, is important. Failure to adequately humidify respiratory gases by using a heat and moisture exchanger (HME) or circle circuit, can result in:

- Failure to maintain patient temperature
- Mucosal drying and decreased ciliary activity
- Increased viscosity of secretions

Definition of humidity

Humidity can be defined in two ways:

Absolute humidity – the mass of water vapour present in a given volume of gas at defined temperature and pressure (expressed as g H_2O m^{-3} of gas)

Relative humidity – the mass of water vapour present in a given volume of gas, expressed as a percentage of the mass of water vapour required to saturate the same volume of gas at identical temperature and pressure.

For further discussion of humidity and saturated vapour pressure see Chapter 44.

Measurement of humidity

Instruments used to measure humidity are called hygrometers, examples include:

Regnault's hygrometer (Figure 45.46) – Based on the cooling effect of evaporating ether on the temperature of a silver tube. When the temperature of the tube decreases to the 'dew point' small droplets of water condense on the outside. The temperature of the ether at the dew point corresponds to the absolute humidity of the surrounding air, and can be determined from tables.

Hair hygrometer – Hair protein is organised into β-pleated sheets. This biochemical structure elongates in the presence of moist heat. The increase in hair length

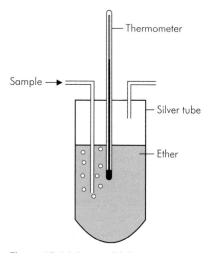

Figure 45.46 Regnault's hygrometer

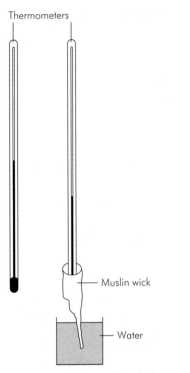

Figure 45.47 Wet and dry bulb thermometer

Thermometers

Muslin wick

Water

is proportional to the humidity of the surrounding air. If one end of the hair is fixed to a light lever the change in length can be amplified and measured. Once calibrated, the instrument can be used to measure relative humidity. The accuracy is poor, and the measured range limited to 15–85% relative humidity (though this is still adequate to measure humidity in the operating theatre).

Wet and dry bulb thermometers (Figure 45.47) – This method uses two mercury bulb thermometers, a 'dry' thermometer which is exposed to air, and a 'wet' thermometer which is surrounded by a wick that draws water from a small reservoir. The temperature of the wet thermometer depends on the rate of evaporation of water from the wick, and hence the humidity of the surrounding air. This temperature will always be lower than that recorded on the dry thermometer. The difference between the two recorded temperatures decreases as the humidity increases. Using specific tables, the relative humidity can be obtained from the measured temperature difference.

Humidity transducers – These measure a change in electrical current in response to a change in humidity. The electrical conductivity of certain substances varies depending on the amount of absorbed water. When such a substance is incorporated into a simple electrical circuit as either a resistor or a capacitor, any increase in the humidity results in a detectable change in either resistance or capacitance. This method provides a rapid, sensitive measure of humidity, and is often used in control systems for air-conditioning systems. These transducers display hysteresis.

Mass spectrometry – As used in the measurement of other gases, these instruments provide a rapid, accurate measurement of water content, which can be measured breath to breath.

Pain measurement

Pain is one of the most difficult physiological phenomena to quantify, but its impact on the individual patient, and its significance to health care in general, make assessment of pain an essential part of clinical practice.

Pain has been defined as follows by the International Association for the Study of Pain:

An unpleasant sensory and emotional experience associated with actual or potential tissue damage

Pain is thus multidimensional and has to be assessed using both objective and subjective methods of measurement.

Objective measurement is performed by an observer. In addition to assessment of the pain dimensions outlined in Figure 45.48, objective measurements also include measurements associated with the physical changes accompanying pain.

Subjective measurement consists of data that are self-reported by the patient.

Most of the methods of assessing pain dimensions are common to both patient and observer.

Dimensions characterising pain

Pain can be characterised by the dimensions summarised in Figure 45.48.

Figure 45.48 Dimensions characterising pain

Dimension	Parameter measured or described
Physical	Location
	Intensity and character
	Frequency and duration
Functional	Aggravating and relieving factors
	Disability, e.g. walking distance, self care
	Productivity, e.g. employment, recreation
Behavioural	Rubbing, grimacing, guarding, vocalisation
	Gait and posture
	Medication frequency and dosage
Affect	Degree of depression
Cognition	Degree of understanding

Acute and chronic pain

A further dimension defining the nature of a pain condition is the classification into acute pain or chronic pain.

Acute pain is pain occurring in the first few days following surgery or trauma.

Chronic pain is pain persisting beyond the acute period or associated with chronic disease.

These pain conditions differ in prognosis, management and outcome, but there does exist a 'grey' area between them, in cases where acute pain conditions evolve into chronic ones.

Physiological changes associated with pain

Physiological changes associated with both acute and chronic pain conditions. In acute pain, these signs are reflected by autonomic changes, which can be recorded and scored. They are particularly useful when assessing pain in unconscious or obtunded patients, but are not specifically associated with pain and are open to misinterpretation. They include those shown in Figure 45.49.

Single-dimension pain measurement

These methods apply to both acute and chronic pain situations and include:

Figure 45.49 Physical signs associated with pain

Pain	Signs
Acute pain	↑ Heart rate
	↑ Blood pressure
	↑ Respiratory rate
	↑ Lacrimation
	↑ Sweating
Chronic pain	Changes in limb size and muscle bulk
	Changes in skin temperature and sweating
	Localised swelling
	Muscle spasm

- **Use of body chart for pain location** – This is a simple diagram on which the patient or observer marks the areas corresponding to the pain.
- **Visual analogue scale** – This is a straight line drawn between two extremes, e.g. 'no pain' and 'worst pain imaginable'. The patient marks a point on this line to represent their current status. It can be used for various parameters such as pain, mood, pain relief, disability. The value is taken as the distance of the mark along the scale from the origin. The validity of these scales is questioned concerning their reproducibility and reliability. Current opinion is that visual analogue scales are reliable when used with the appropriate group of patients and under controlled circumstances. These scales are not suitable for very young children or visually impaired people, or in the immediate postoperative period.
- **Numerical ranking or pictoral ranking** – This is an alternative to using visual analogue scales, and may be more suitable for some groups of patients (e.g. children). These scales are marked by numbers or pictures to represent increasing or decreasing pain. The gradation is thus not continuous, but is limited to a finite number of choices. This may make the results more reproducible in some cases, and the method may be easier to use for patients, but a loss of sensitivity can result.
- **Word descriptor ranking** – In this method, assessment is dependent on a choice of a word descriptor from a list. The assessment is obtained by scoring for

each word to give a pain rating index (PRI). Alternatively, using free choice from non-scored word lists, the total number of words chosen (NWC) can be recorded. Multiple word descriptor lists can be used to produce multidimensional pain assessment. This method can be adapted for visually impaired patients.

Multidimensional pain measurement

These methods can be applied to produce a more complete assessment of a pain condition by combining assessment of multiple pain dimensions. They include:

- **McGill questionnaire** – This questionnaire was first decribed by Melzack in 1975. It consists of a body map and word descriptor sections for evaluating the intensity and other characteristics of pain. It is a relatively involved questionnaire taking around 20 minutes or more to complete, depending on patient skills. This limits its application, since it is not suitable for children, highly anxious patients or patients in the immediate postoperative period. It is commonly used in research.
- **Brief Pain Inventory** (BPI) – This questionnaire was originally developed by Cleeland in 1991 for the measurement of pain in cancer patients. It measures worst, least, average and current pain as well as interference effects of pain on relations with others, enjoyment of life, sleep, mood, walking and working. Over the years the BPI has been validated for many chronic pain conditions such as neuropathic pain, osteoarthritis and fibromyalgia. It is based on the measurement of 11 indices, using 10-point scales.
- **Memorial pain assessment card** – This is a collection of linear analogue scales for different pain dimensions such as intensity, pain relief or mood. It can also include a limited set of word descriptor lists.

Figure 45.50 Methods of pain assessment in children

Age (years)	Method
Infant	Observation – crying, motor withdrawal
1–3	Observation – crying, withdrawal, facial expression, lip smacking, aggressive behaviour
3–5	Pictorial ranking scales
	Colour-matching scales
5–12	Visual analogue scales
	Number ranking scales
> 12	Multidimensional scales

- **Pain observation chart** – This can be designed for patients to record a number of pain dimensions on a diary basis, e.g. pain intensity, pain relief and drug side effects in order to optimise drug regimes. Alternatively pain charts can be designed for observers or carers to record objective assessment data on a diary/timetable basis in order to optimise postoperative analgesia.
- **Beck depression inventory** – This provides a self-reported index of depression, which can be used to quantify changes in depression levels due to treatment of chronic pain conditions.

Assessment of pain in children

Pain assessment in children depends on the age and skills of the child, and is affected significantly by their interaction with their parents. Some of the methods used are summarised in Figure 45.50.

CHAPTER 46

Anaesthetic equipment

Ted Lin and Rajani Annamaneni

Medical gas pipeline services

The medical gas pipeline system (MGPS) provides wall gas and vacuum supplies in working areas such as operating theatres, resuscitation and recovery areas. The MGPS consists of the following:

- Oxygen (at 420 kPa)
- Nitrous oxide
- Medical air (at 420 and 700 kPa)
- Medical vacuum
- Scavenging vacuum

The gases and services are distributed by a medical pipeline network to specialised terminal outlets. Equipment can then be connected to these outlets by non-interchangeable flexible hosing.

Fundamentals of Anaesthesia, 4th edition, ed. Ted Lin, Tim Smith and Colin Pinnock. Published by Cambridge University Press. © Cambridge University Press 2017.

The MGPS distribution network consists of specially cleaned and degreased medical-quality copper pipes. These are colour-coded and installed to government-specified standards. Different areas of the network are isolated by special valves connected into the network by non-interchangeable screw-threaded (NIST) unions.

The pipeline terminal outlets consist of Schrader sockets that are clearly labelled and colour-coded for the service or gas. They are matched for a specific connecting flexible pipeline by a collar indexing system. Each flexible pipeline is colour-coded with unique terminal and equipment ends. The terminal end consists of an indexed Schrader probe that fits into its specific terminal socket. The other end of the hose is a non-interchangeable (NIST) union, which connects onto a piece of equipment. These design features of the hoses and terminal sockets ensure that the gases or services cannot be cross-connected to equipment.

Oxygen supply

Oxygen is stored centrally in a vacuum-insulated evaporator (VIE). This consists of an inner stainless-steel tank with an outer steel jacket. A vacuum is maintained between the tank and jacket for insulation.

The VIE has the following features:

- It contains liquid and gaseous oxygen with an inner temperature between –160 and –180 °C (lower than the critical temperature of oxygen, which is –118 °C, but higher than the boiling point at 1 atm, –183 °C).
- The pressure within the VIE is approximately 1100–1300 kPa, varying with oxygen demand.
- There is a main outlet at the top of the VIE, for oxygen withdrawal to supply the distribution pipeline.
- Liquid oxygen may also be withdrawn via a separate outlet and fed through a superheater, in order to 'top up' the supply line and maintain pressure during periods of high demand.
- A reserve supply, provided by a cylinder bank, is available in case of VIE failure.
- The VIE normally contains enough oxygen for 10 days' supply, while the reserves are adequate for 24 hours' use.

A schematic diagram of a VIE is shown in Figure 46.1.

Nitrous oxide supply

Nitrous oxide is supplied from a central bank of gas cylinders, which contain a mixture of liquid and gas (critical temperature of nitrous oxide is 36.5 °C). These are connected to the distribution pipeline network by a control panel, which regulates the gas pressure. The control may also provide local heating in order to avoid condensation and freezing due to the cooling caused by the evaporation of the liquid nitrous oxide. A reserve bank of cylinders is also provided.

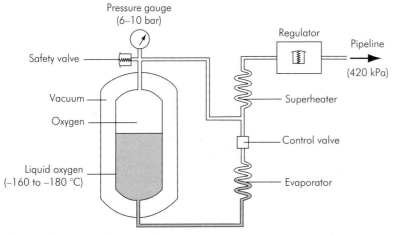

Figure 46.1 Vacuum-insulated evaporator

Medical compressed air

Compressed air for medical use must be much purer than its industrial equivalent. It is generated by compressors and will contain oil mist as well as water vapour. In a hospital two types of supply are required, a low-pressure supply (420 kPa) for anaesthetic machines and ventilators, and a higher-pressure supply (700 kPa) to provide power for surgical equipment. The pipeline network may be supplied either by a bank of air cylinders or by a local compressor system. If a local compressor is used care must be taken to ensure the purity of the compressed air produced.

Medical vacuum

Medical vacuum is required for suction, and BS4957 specifications suggest a vacuum level of 53 kPa (400 mmHg). Medical vacuum is also required for scavenging of anaesthetic gases, but it is not recommended that the same vacuum supply is used for both purposes because:

- Suction requires relatively low flow rates but high levels of vacuum, which if applied inadvertently to a patient's airway would be harmful.
- Scavenging requires low vacuum levels with high flow rates. The high flow rates used to remove waste anaesthetic gases could reduce suction levels during surgery.
- Waste anaesthetic gases contain volatile vapours which may be absorbed by lubricants and ultimately cause system failure.

Suction vacuum systems incorporate bacterial filtration and drainage to dispose of aspirated body fluids.

Gas cylinders

Gases and vapours are supplied from cylinders in the absence or failure of piped gas supplies. The cylinders are made of molybdenum steel, which is stronger than carbon steel. This enables cylinders to be made with thinner walls and therefore lighter in weight. They are used to supply the gases and vapours shown in Figure 46.2.

Cylinder identification

Cylinders are identified visually by a symbol and colour coding, as listed in Figure 46.3. They also have markings on them and labels giving information about their contents.

Cylinder markings/labels

- Tare weight of cylinder
- Hydraulic test pressure of cylinder
- Identity of gas (symbol)
- Density of gas
- Serial number of cylinder
- Owner of cylinder and manufacturer of gases

Pin index system (PIS)

Gas cylinders are also identified mechanically by a pin indexing system, which conforms to both British Standard (BS) and equivalent International Organization for Standardization (ISO) specifications. This system prevents the wrong cylinder from being connected to an anaesthetic machine.

Figure 46.2 Gases and vapours supplied in cylinders

Content	Gas/vapour	Cylinder pressure kPa (psi)	Boiling point at 1 atm (°C)	Critical temperature (°C)
Oxygen	gas	13,700 (1980)	– 183	– 118
Nitrous oxide	vapour	4400 (640)	– 89	36.5
Entonox	gas and vapour	13,700 (1980)	gas separation at – 6 °C	
Air	gas	13,700 (1980)		
Carbon dioxide	vapour	5000 (723)	– 78.5	31
Helium	gas	13,700 (1980)	– 269	– 268

Figure 46.3 Colour coding of gas cylinders (British and ISO standards)

Substance	Gas/vapour	Symbol	Colour coding	
			Cylinder	Shoulder
Oxygen	gas	O_2	black	white
Nitrous oxide	vapour	N_2O	blue	blue
Entonox	gas and vapour	N_2O/O_2	blue	white/blue
Air	gas	AIR	black	white/black
Carbon dioxide	vapour	CO_2	grey	grey
Helium	gas	He	brown	brown

The pin index system is designed into the outlet valve block of the cylinder, and is illustrated in Figure 46.4. The cylinder valve block face matches up to the inlet port of the anaesthetic machine. This face contains the gas outlet from the cylinder, which is made gas-tight by a metal and rubber ring seal, the Bodok seal. Beneath the outlet are six possible positions for indexing holes. Pins on the anaesthetic machine inlet fit into these holes. If the positions of these pins do not match the index holes on the valve block outlet, the cylinder cannot be fitted to that particular inlet on the anaesthetic machine. Figure 46.4 shows PIS positions for some of the gases commonly used, and details of the cylinder head arrangement.

Cylinder testing

Cylinders are hydraulically tested every 5 years using water under high pressure. Water or water vapour remaining in a cylinder may represent a hazard because it may condense and freeze (affecting the operation of the outlet valve) if the cylinder empties rapidly. Random cylinders from a batch may be destructively tested by the manufacturers using water under pressure.

Cylinders are inspected by the manufacturer endoscopically for cracks and defects on their inner surfaces, and they can also be tested ultrasonically.

Estimation of cylinder contents

The contents of a cylinder, for both gases and vapours, are estimated by weighing the cylinder and subtracting the weight of the empty cylinder or tare weight, which is recorded on the cylinder itself.

Cylinder sizes can be identified by a letter (BOC coding) according to internal volume (water capacity). A reserve oxygen cylinder on an anaesthetic machine may be an 'E' cylinder, with a water capacity of 4.7 litres. A tall standing cylinder with a side spindle pin index valve may be a 'J' cylinder, with a water capacity of 47 litres.

Gases

In the case of gases, such as oxygen and air, cylinders are initially filled to a given pressure (13,700 kPa = 137 bar). Since gases are not liquefied in the cylinder (temperature < critical temperature), the cylinder contents can also be estimated by the cylinder pressure. This gradually decreases as the cylinder empties. The mass of gas present is directly proportional to the pressure according to the universal gas law, and the volume of the contents available at atmospheric pressure can be estimated using Boyle's law.

What are the contents of a full 'E' cylinder at atmospheric pressure (1.0 bar)?

An 'E' cylinder has a water capacity of 4.7 litres ($V1$) and is filled to a pressure of 137 bar ($P1$). Its contents ($V2$) at atmospheric pressure ($P2 = 1.0$ bar) are given by Boyle's law:

$$P2.V2 = P1.V1$$
$$\begin{aligned} V2 &= P1.V1/P2 \\ &= 4.7 \times 137 \\ &= 643.9 \text{ litres} \end{aligned}$$

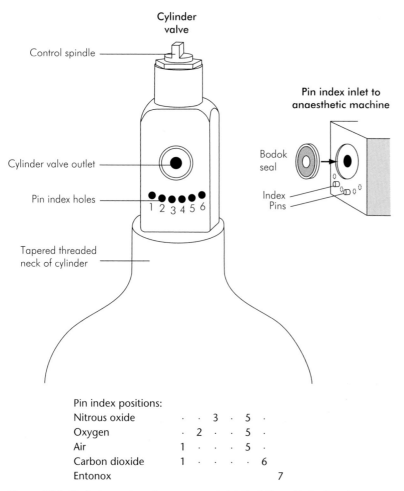

Pin index positions:

Nitrous oxide	.	. 3	.	5	.
Oxygen	.	2 .	.	5	.
Air	1	. .	.	5	.
Carbon dioxide	1	. .	.	. 6	
Entonox					7

Figure 46.4 Pin index system for gases, and detail of the cylinder head

Vapours

In the case of vapours (such as nitrous oxide or carbon dioxide) the contents of the cylinders are a mixture of gas and liquid. The cylinders are initially filled to a given *filling ratio*. The filling ratio is defined as the weight of the substance contained divided by the weight of a volume of water equal to the internal volume of the cylinder. This ratio is set at 0.75, since if the cylinders are overfilled there is a risk of rupture with increases in ambient temperature.

Cylinder pressure, in the case of vapour content only, varies if the temperature changes. This can occur when the cylinder is emptied rapidly, due to absorption of latent

> **With vapours the cylinder pressure cannot be used to estimate cylinder contents**, because it does not vary as the cylinder empties. This is because the cylinder pressure is maintained at saturated vapour pressure (SVP) while liquid is present. The cylinder pressure only falls when the cylinder is nearly empty and all of the liquid contents have evaporated.

heat of vaporisation causing cooling of the contents. Under these circumstances the cylinder pressure will decrease with cooling but will be restored as the cylinder warms up again (Figure 46.5).

(a) Slow emptying of cylinder

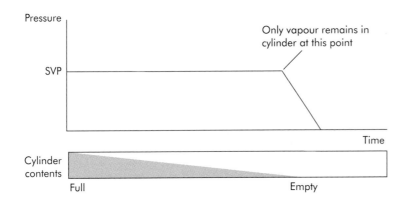

(b) Rapid emptying of cylinder

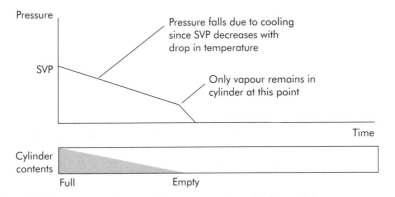

Figure 46.5 Pressure and temperature changes in a cylinder containing vapour

Pressure regulators

The high pressure inside gas cylinders is reduced by a pressure regulator before connection to equipment such as an anaesthetic machine. An example of a single-stage regulator which might be used to reduce oxygen cylinder pressure from 13,700 kPa to 420 kPa is shown in Figure 46.6. Cylinder pressure (P) is reduced to the supply pressure (p) as oxygen passes through the small inlet valve (area = a) into the control chamber. The pressure in the control chamber (p) is controlled by a compression spring acting on a diaphragm (area = A) which is coupled mechanically to the inlet valve. The supply pressure is thus controlled by the force (F) in the spring. This can be expressed by the following equation:

$$F = \text{Force acting on conical valve}$$
$$+ \text{Force acting on diaphragm}$$
$$= Pa + pA$$

It is assumed that the force in the spring remains constant, i.e. the range of movement in the spring is small compared to its total length. Then any change in the supply or cylinder pressures will cause a compensating change as the diaphragm moves and varies the effective area of the inlet valve. In the above equation, if F is constant, a decrease in pA (drop in supply pressure due to increased demand) causes an increase in Pa (increased flow from cylinder). Alternatively if Pa decreases (due to cylinder pressure falling as it empties), pA will increase (increased flow from cylinder).

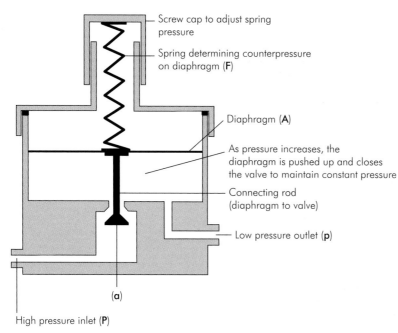

Screw cap to adjust spring pressure

Spring determining counterpressure on diaphragm (**F**)

Diaphragm (**A**)

As pressure increases, the diaphragm is pushed up and closes the valve to maintain constant pressure

Connecting rod (diaphragm to valve)

Low pressure outlet (**p**)

(**a**)

High pressure inlet (**P**)

Figure 46.6 Single-stage pressure regulator

> **The pressure regulator** reduces the cylinder pressure from 137 bar in an O_2 cylinder, or 44 bar in an N_2O cylinder, to a lower supply pressure of approximately 4 bar (400 kPa). It also compensates for changes in demand or cylinder pressure. The sensitivity of this control depends on the ratio of the area of the control-chamber diaphragm to the area of the conical valve, which is usually 200:1.

Anaesthetic machines
Surgical anaesthesia is usually provided through a continuous-flow anaesthetic machine which consists of the following components:
- Metal framework and pipeline circuitry
- Medical gas pipeline service connections
- Connections for gas cylinders and pressure gauges for cylinder contents
- Safety mechanisms
- Back bar including vaporiser connections
- Common gas outlet and auxiliary gas outlets
- Vaporisers

- Rotameters (see *Gas flow measurement in anaesthetic machines* in Chapter 45)
- Scavenging circuitry
- Suction circuitry

The basic arrangement of these components is illustrated in Figure 46.7. Modern machines often incorporate electronic monitoring, safety features and a mechanical ventilator.

Metal framework and pipeline circuitry
The metal framework of the anaesthetic machine is usually made of stainless steel and is electrically earthed via antistatic wheels, which reduce risks of electric shock, interference with rotameters, and fire or explosion of inflammable agents. The frame incorporates pipeline circuitry with both fixed and detachable joints. The pipes are usually brass or copper with brazed fixed joints. More recently nylon pipes have been introduced. Detachable joints are screw-threaded and sealed with a compressible washer, O-ring seal or polytetrafluoroethylene (PTFE) tape. Different diameter pipes are used for each gas to prevent cross-connection.

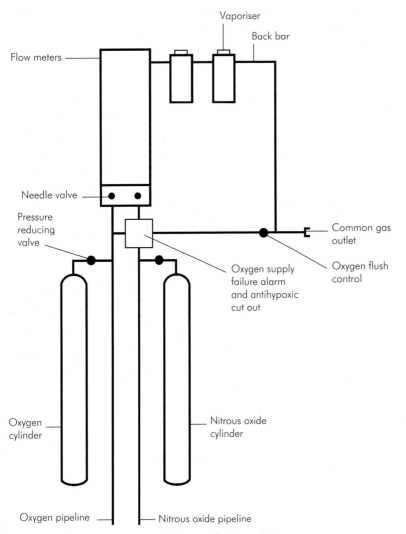

Vaporiser

Back bar

Flow meters

Needle valve

Pressure
reducing
valve

Oxygen supply
failure alarm
and antihypoxic
cut out

Common gas
outlet

Oxygen flush
control

Oxygen
cylinder

Nitrous oxide
cylinder

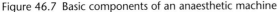

Oxygen pipeline

Nitrous oxide pipeline

Figure 46.7 Basic components of an anaesthetic machine

Medical gas pipeline service (MGPS) connections

Non-interchangeable screw-threaded (NIST) connections are used for MGPS supplies. Flexible colour-coded hoses are used to connect to gas-specific wall terminals. The machine end of these hoses is a male NIST.

NIST connectors are made gas-specific by:

- A non-interchangeable threaded nut
- A specific diameter shoulder with O-ring seal
- A specific diameter forward shaft

The machine MGPS connections are the female counterparts of the above hose connectors. They also incorporate metal gauze filters and one-way non-return valves to prevent retrograde leakage.

Pin index system (PIS) connections for gas cylinders

The PIS connections for the cylinder gas supplies consist of a gas inlet with the male counterpart of the PIS, i.e. pins corresponding to the indexing holes on the cylinder valve block. A yoke with an arrangement secured by a screw fitting holds the cylinder valve block in place. The cylinder inlets also incorporate metal gauze filters and one-way non-return valves to prevent retrograde leakage. Retrograde leakage through gas inlets, if great enough, has been known to alter the gas mixture delivered to the patient, and can lead to the delivery of a hypoxic mixture. The PIS connection is made gas-tight by a metal and rubber ring seal in the cylinder valve block (Bodok seal). Pin index positions have been described in Figure 46.4.

Safety mechanisms

Several safety mechanisms are incorporated into the design of an anaesthetic machine. These include:

- **Secondary pressure regulators** – Smooth out gas pressure fluctuations within the anaesthetic machine, which occur due to changes in pipeline pressure or variations in demand from the machine. Such fluctuations in machine pressure can cause inaccuracies in the fresh gas mixture, or disturb the performance of rotameters and oxygen monitors. Secondary pressure regulators are set to pressures below the anticipated pressure fluctuations and are designed to maintain working pressures within 10% over a wide range of flow rates, from hundreds of millilitres to tens of litres.
- **Oxygen failure warning device** – Monitoring of the delivered fresh gas oxygen concentration is mandatory, but the anaesthetic machine also has a built-in oxygen failure device. This is mounted upstream of the rotameter block and is designed according to BS4272 specifications, which include:
  o Audible alarm > 60 dB at a distance of 1 metre from the machine, for 7 seconds or more
  o Activation when the oxygen supply falls to 200 kPa
  o Power supply derived from the oxygen supply pressure
  o Alarm that cannot be switched off or reset until the oxygen supply is restored
  o Alarm coupled to a gas cutoff valve that cuts off anaesthetic gases and opens the machine pipeline circuitry to air
  An early oxygen failure warning device was the Ritchie whistle (1960), and many modern devices are similar in principle. Figure 46.8 shows how such a device works.
- **Oxygen bypass circuit** – Bypasses the rotameter block and back bar to provide an emergency oxygen flow of at least 30 litres per minute to the common gas outlet. The control is usually a push-button situated near the common gas outlet, which is recessed to prevent accidental operation, and which cannot be locked, to prevent barotrauma to the patient.

Back bar

The back bar is the horizontal part of the anaesthetic machine circuit between the rotameter block and the common gas outlet. It is downstream of the rotameter block and feeds fresh gas mixture to the common gas outlet. Vaporisers are mounted on the back bar, enabling volatile agents to be added to the fresh gases. The pressure in the back bar is approximately 1 kPa at the outlet end, and may be 7–10 kPa at the rotameter end, depending on:

- Total gas flow
- Circuit connection to common gas outlet
- Vaporisers used and their settings

Total occlusion of the common gas outlet produces pressures of approximately 30 kPa in the back bar. The maximum pressure that can be produced in the back bar is limited by a 'blow off' or pressure relief valve at the outlet end (threshold set to 30–40 kPa). This protects the rotameter block and vaporisers from overpressure damage, and to a very limited degree protects the patient from barotrauma.

Vaporiser connections

The system for connecting vaporisers to the anaesthetic machine back bar is designed with specific features.

Vaporiser connections to the back bar

- Prevent gas leakage from the back bar with or without a vaporiser in place
- Prevent volatile agent leakage into the back-bar circuit
- Allow convenient installation and removal of vaporisers
- Have a safety interlock mechanism to prevent use of more than one volatile agent simultaneously

---

Figure 46.9 illustrates some of these design features. The potential hazards caused by poor design or usage of the vaporiser connection system include:

- Leakage of gas, causing inadequate fresh gas mixtures or pressures to be delivered to the patient
- Leakage of volatile agent into the fresh gas flow

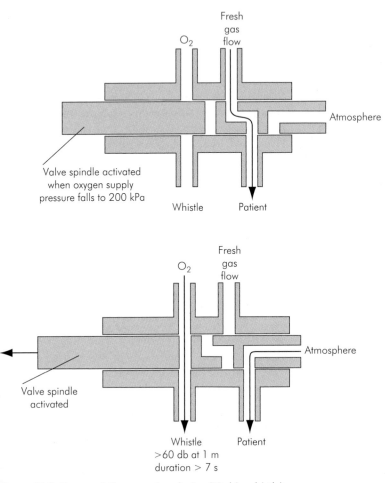

Figure 46.8 Oxygen failure warning device (Ritchie whistle)

- Damage or injury caused by difficulty in attaching or detaching vaporisers
- Contamination of downstream vaporisers by upstream volatile agent, when no safety interlock mechanism is present
- Contamination of soda lime in the breathing circuit by trichloroethylene (no longer used in the UK), which produces a neurotoxin

In early machines, where more than one vaporiser could be switched on at a time, a more volatile agent (e.g. halothane), if placed upstream, could be absorbed by a less volatile agent (e.g. trichloroethylene). This could lead to the release of a maximal concentration (determined by the saturated vapour pressure) of the absorbed agent on subsequent use of the downstream vaporiser. In modern machines with a good safety interlock mechanism, the sequence of vaporisers on the back bar presents no significant hazard.

Gas outlets

The common gas outlet is a 22 mm male (external) and 15 mm female (internal) tapered outlet which supplies fresh gas mixture to the patient breathing circuit or a mechanical ventilator. It may be mounted on a swivel (Cardiff swivel) for increased convenience. It can withstand bending moments of up to 10 Nm (equivalent approximately to 40–50 kg weight hanging from the outlet). It may be threaded to prevent accidental disconnection.

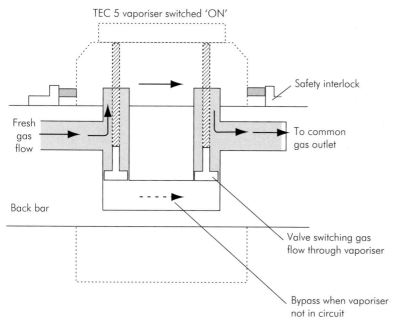

Figure 46.9 Vaporiser back-bar connections

The auxiliary gas outlets are Schrader oxygen or air sockets, which can be used to power devices such as a ventilator or a Venturi injector.

Anaesthetic machine maintenance

Servicing of machines should follow the manufacturer's guidelines. Typically servicing is performed at 3- to 6-month intervals. Each machine should have an attached log-book to record commissioning date, servicing dates, faults, repairs and modifications.

Anaesthetic machine checklist

The anaesthetic machine should be checked by the anaesthetist before each operating session. A checklist is published by the Association of Anaesthetists of Great Britain and Ireland (2012), designed to be attached to each machine (Figure 46.10).

Vaporisers

The design of a vaporiser is determined by the clinical application and the volatile agent being used. Choice of a vaporiser for use in the absence of compressed gas supplies will differ from that where piped supplies are available, while a vaporiser suitable for use with desflurane will be very different from one for use with isoflurane.

Functions of a vaporiser
• To produce vaporisation of the volatile anaesthetic agent
• To mix the vapour with the fresh gas flow to the patient
• To control the mixture so that a given concentration of volatile agent is delivered to the patient, in spite of varying gas flow rates and ambient temperature conditions

The important properties of volatile agents when considering vaporiser design are saturated vapour pressure (SVP), boiling point (BP) and minimum alveolar concentration (MAC). These are shown for some commonly used agents in Figure 46.11.

Two different types of vaporiser are considered here, **variable bypass** and **measured flow**.

Variable bypass vaporiser

In this vaporiser the fresh gas flow to the patient circuit is split into two streams by a flow-splitting valve. One stream bypasses the vaporising chamber and is free

Checklist for Anaesthetic Equipment 2012
AAGBI Safety Guideline

Checks at the start of every operating session
Do not use this equipment unless you have been trained

Check self-inflating bag available

Perform manufacturer's (automatic) machine check

Power supply	• Plugged in • Switched on • Back-up battery charged
Gas supplies and suction	• Gas and vacuum pipelines – 'tug test' • Cylinders filled and turned off • Flowmeters working (if applicable) • Hypoxic guard working • Oxygen flush working • Suction clean and working
Breathing system	• Whole system patent and leak free using 'two-bag' test • Vaporisers – fitted correctly, filled, leak free, plugged in (if necessary) • Soda lime - colour checked • Alternative systems (Bain, T-piece) – checked • Correct gas outlet selected
Ventilator	• Working and configured correctly
Scavenging	• Working and configured correctly
Monitors	• Working and configured correctly • Alarms limits and volumes set
Airway equipment	• Full range required, working, with spares

RECORD THIS CHECK IN THE PATIENT RECORD

Don't Forget!	• Self-inflating bag • Common gas outlet • Difficult airway equipment • Resuscitation equipment • TIVA and/or other infusion equipment

This guideline is not a standard of medical care. The ultimate judgement with regard to a particular clinical procedure or treatment plan must be made by the clinician in the light of the clinical data presented and the diagnostic and treatment options available.

© The Association of Anaesthetists of Great Britain & Ireland 2012

Figure 46.10 Association of Anaesthetists of Great Britain and Ireland: checklist for anaesthetic equipment 2012. Reproduced from *Anaesthesia* 2012; **66**: 660–8, with permission from AAGBI.

CHECKS BEFORE EACH CASE

Breathing system	Whole system patent and leak free using 'two-bag' test Vaporisers – fitted correctly, filled, leak free, plugged in (if necessary) Alternative systems (Bain, T-piece) – checked Correct gas outlet selected
Ventilator	Working and configured correctly
Airway equipment	Full range required, working, with spares
Suction	Clean and working

THE TWO-BAG TEST

A two-bag test should be performed after the breathing system, vaporisers and ventilator have been checked individually

i. Attach the patient end of the breathing system (including angle piece and filter) to a test lung or bag.

ii. Set the fresh gas flow to 5 l.min⁻¹ and ventilate manually. Check the whole breathing system is patent and the unidirectional valves are moving. Check the function of the APL valve by squeezing both bags.

iii. Turn on the ventilator to ventilate the test lung. Turn off the fresh gas flow, or reduce to a minimum. Open and close each vaporiser in turn. There should be no loss of volume in the system.

Figure 46.10 (*cont.*)

from volatile agent. The other stream passes through the chamber and becomes saturated with vapour. This second stream then rejoins the bypass flow to give the required concentration of vapour in the fresh gas flow to the patient (Figure 46.12). The final vapour concentration is controlled by using the flow-splitting valve to vary the fraction of the gas flow passing through the vaporising chamber. Accuracy is therefore dependent on the flow-splitting valve maintaining a

Figure 46.11 Properties of some commonly used volatile agents

Volatile agent	SVP (kPa) at 20 °C	BP (°C) at 100 kPa	MAC
Isoflurane	31.5	48	1.15
Sevoflurane	21.3	58	2
Desflurane	88.5	23	6

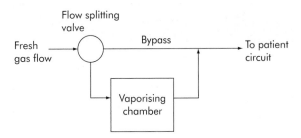

Figure 46.12 Principles of a variable bypass vaporiser

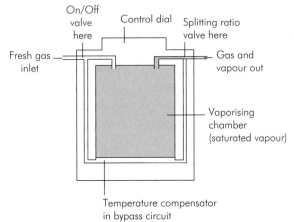

Figure 46.14 Basic design of a plenum vaporiser

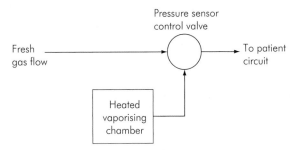

Figure 46.13 Principles of measured flow vaporiser

In the plenum vaporiser the inspired gases are at higher than atmospheric pressure by 1–8 kPa, and pressurise the vaporiser chamber. Pressurisation increases the density of the carrier gas in the chamber, thus ensuring better mixing with the vapour at low flows.

When the vaporiser chamber is at atmospheric pressure, carrier gas density is less than vapour density, and at low flow rates gas will tend to pass across the top of the chamber without mixing.

The plenum vaporiser is the most commonly used type in hospital practice. Plenum vaporisers have a relatively high flow resistance (approximately 0.4 kPa per litre per minute of flow) and are therefore unsuitable for placing 'in line' in a spontaneously breathing circuit.

constant *flow-splitting ratio* over the range of flow rates used. There are two main types of variable bypass vaporiser, described below: **plenum vaporisers** and **draw-over vaporisers**.

Measured flow vaporiser

This vaporiser has a chamber in which the volatile agent is heated by an electrical element to produce pure vapour under pressure. The pressure produced in the chamber is equal to the SVP of the volatile agent at the preset temperature. The vaporiser then controls the addition of the pressurised vapour to the fresh gas flow using a pressure sensor-controlled valve, to maintain a given volatile percentage in the patient's inspired gases. This type of device is used for desflurane (Figure 46.13).

Plenum variable bypass vaporisers

Examples – Blease Datum, Drager Vapor, Ohmeda TEC 5

A plenum vaporiser during spontaneous ventilation

In order to develop a peak inspiratory flow rate of 30 litres per minute through this vaporiser, a patient would need to develop a peak inspiratory pressure of $30 \times 0.4 = 12$ kPa (> 120 cmH$_2$O), compared with a normal inspiratory pressure of < 2 kPa. Effectively the plenum vaporiser acts as a flow restrictor, and for a spontaneously breathing patient a *circuit with a reservoir bag is needed* to supply the peak inspiratory flow rates. Figure 46.14 illustrates the design of a simple plenum vaporiser.

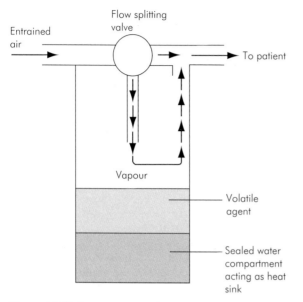

Figure 46.15 Draw-over vaporiser

Flow-splitting ratio

The performance of variable bypass vaporisers depends on the flow-splitting ratio, which is the ratio of the bypass flow to the gas flow through the chamber.

Calculation of flow-splitting ratio from gas flows

If total gas flow through the anaesthetic machine back bar is 5 litres per minute, and flow through the vaporiser is 0.2 litres per minute, what is the flow-splitting ratio?

Vaporiser chamber flow $= 0.2$
Bypass flow $= 5.0 - 0.2 = 4.8$
Flow splitting ratio $= 4.8/0.2 = 24$

Draw-over variable bypass vaporisers

Examples – Epstein, Goldman, Macintosh, Oxford (EMO), Oxford Miniature

In the draw-over vaporiser the inspiratory gases are at atmospheric pressure and are drawn through the vaporiser chamber by the inspiratory efforts of the patient. The vaporiser and flow-splitting valve must therefore have low resistance. This type of vaporiser has the advantage that atmospheric air can be used as the carrier gas (supplemented by cylinder oxygen if required).

Calculation of flow-splitting ratio to produce a final concentration of 1% isoflurane

First find the concentration of vapour in an isoflurane vaporiser chamber at 20 °C (SVP for isoflurane at 20 °C = 31.5 kPa; assume ambient pressure in the vaporiser chamber to be 105 kPa).

Saturated vapour concentration in the vaporiser chamber is given by the ratio

$$\frac{SVP}{\text{pressure in vaporiser chamber}} \times 100\% = \frac{31.5}{105} \times 100\%$$
$$= 30\%$$

Final concentration
$$= \frac{\text{concentration in vaporiser chamber}}{(\text{flow splitting ratio} + 1)}$$

Flow splitting ratio
$$= \frac{\text{concentration in vaporiser chamber}}{\text{final concentration}} - 1$$
$$= 30 - 1$$

Therefore a flow-splitting ratio of 29 is required, i.e. 1/30 (3.3%) of the total flow must pass through the chamber.

The more potent the volatile agent, the greater the dilution of the vapour required, and the greater the flow-splitting ratio.

However, accuracy is poor in this type of vaporiser since flow rates vary considerably through the vaporiser with the respiratory cycle. The ability of the flow-splitting valve to maintain a constant splitting ratio becomes poor over the wide range of flows. At low flow rates the resistance of the flow-splitting valve will become relatively more significant and gases will tend to bypass the vaporiser, causing a fall in volatile concentrations. At high flow rates there will be increased dilution of the vapour in the vaporiser chamber, and again concentrations will tend to be reduced. Figure 46.15 shows a simple draw-over vaporiser.

Measured flow vaporisers

Example – Ohmeda TEC 6 Desflurane vaporiser

The measured flow vaporisers produce a separate independent flow of vapour or saturated carrier gas. This flow is then metered into the patient's fresh gas flow to produce

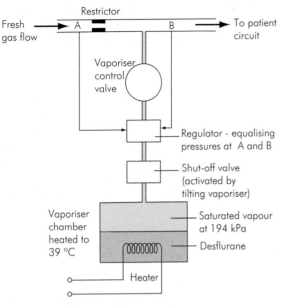

Figure 46.16 Measured flow vaporiser

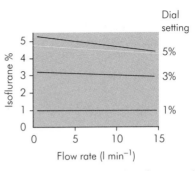

Figure 46.17 Concentration changes with flow in a plenum vaporiser

the required concentration of volatile agent (Figure 46.16). Thus no splitting of the fresh gas flow occurs.

Desflurane requires a measured flow vaporiser (TEC 6)

This is because the boiling point of desflurane at sea level is 23.6 °C, which is close to room temperature. In such a case, use of a plenum vaporiser with an intermittently boiling volatile agent would make its performance unpredictable. The desflurane vaporiser therefore heats the volatile agent to 39 °C to produce a chamber pressure of approximately 194 kPa.
A continuous flow of desflurane vapour from the chamber is then added to the fresh gas flow via the concentration control valve.

Features of a desflurane vaporiser include:
- Mains supply, with backup battery
- Three built-in heaters to boil the desflurane and to prevent condensation in different parts of the vaporiser
- A warm-up time of 10 minutes, during which the control dial is locked
- Electronic circuitry to indicate 'ready for use', to warn of low levels of desflurane or disconnection, and to switch off when tilted
- Supplies concentrations up to 18% (3 MAC)

Vaporiser performance

Vaporiser performance is dependent on the range of flow rates, the ambient conditions and the carrier gas mixture used, together with the design and maintenance of the vaporiser.

Flow rate

Flow rate of carrier gas passing through the vaporiser is important because as flow rate increases, an increasing amount of vapour is required to saturate the carrier gas. At higher flow rates the carrier gas in the vaporiser chamber may not become fully saturated, and thus the concentration of the volatile agent delivered to the patient tends to fall. Figure 46.17 shows how volatile agent concentration might vary with increasing flow rate in a plenum vaporiser. In addition, high flow rates will accentuate the temperature effects in the chamber (see below). Performance of a vaporiser will therefore be more consistent if variations in flow rates are minimised. A large surface area for vaporisation in the vaporiser chamber will be able to maintain saturation of the carrier gas over a wider range of flow rates.

Temperature

The concentration of vapour in the vaporiser chamber is dependent on the SVP of the volatile agent and the ambient pressure in the chamber. Temperature affects the performance of a vaporiser due to the variation of SVP with temperature. A main cause of temperature falling in the chamber is the absorption of latent heat as vaporisation occurs. This will become more marked at higher flow rates, when the rate of vaporisation is increased.

Compensation to correct for such fluctuations is achieved by adjusting the gas flow through the vaporiser chamber. Temperature compensation was performed manually in early vaporisers by altering the flow-splitting

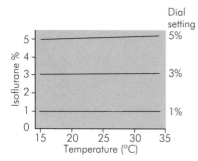

Figure 46.18 Concentration changes with temperature in a plenum vaporiser (TEC 4) at 5 L min^{-1} oxygen flow

valve according to the temperature in the vaporiser, or by using a simple automatic device, such as a bimetallic-strip-controlled flow valve. However, modern plenum vaporisers may incorporate electronically controlled flow valves, which are also integrated into the machine by a microprocessor. However, the basic principle of increasing the flow through the vaporiser chamber if the temperature in the chamber starts to fall remains the same.

Further compensation is obtained by increasing the thermal capacity of the vaporiser in order to smooth out temperature fluctuations. This was achieved in the EMO draw-over vaporiser by filling a compartment in the base of the vaporiser with water. Alternatively, in the later plenum vaporisers, a large heavy mass of copper is incorporated into the vaporiser body. This enhanced thermal capacity acts as a heat source in case of temperature falls, and a heat sink should ambient temperature rise, thus smoothing out the effects of temperature fluctuations. Figure 46.18 shows how vaporiser performance might vary with temperature in a typical modern vaporiser.

Atmospheric pressure

From the calculation example for plenum vaporisers given above (see *Flow-splitting ratio*), the concentration of volatile agent in the vaporiser chamber is dependent on the ratio

$$\frac{SVP}{\text{Pressure in the vaporiser chamber}}$$

The pressure in the vaporiser chamber is essentially atmospheric pressure, so if atmospheric pressure is increased the final volatile concentration delivered will be reduced. On the other hand, at altitude, where atmospheric pressure is reduced, the volatile concentration delivered is increased.

It should be noted that although the delivered concentration may increase at altitude, the partial pressure exerted by the volatile agent in the tissues will remain unchanged.

'Pumping effect'

This effect is produced by repetitive changes in circuit resistance at the common gas outlet. It can be produced when the outlet is periodically obstructed by assisting ventilation or attaching a minute volume divider ventilator (e.g. Manley) to the outlet. This results in alternating compression and release of the saturated gas in the vaporiser chamber, which in turn produces surges of volatile agent concentration in the patient circuit. Mechanisms to reduce this pumping effect include increasing the flow resistance of the vaporiser and insertion of a non-return valve at the outlet of the vaporiser.

Carrier gas composition

Increasing the nitrous oxide content of the carrier gas can produce a small reduction in the volatile concentration delivered. This is because the nitrous oxide reduces the viscosity and increases the density of the gas mixture, which decreases the gas flow through the vaporiser chamber owing to the flow-splitting valve characteristics. Nitrous oxide also has increased solubility in volatile agents, which can cause a further transient fall in volatile agent concentration when the nitrous oxide fraction is increased. This effect is not clinically significant.

Mechanical stability

Poor fitting of the vaporiser to the back bar can result in gas leaks, loss of back-bar pressure or tilting, which can allow leakage of volatile agent into the bypass circuit. Regular checking of vaporiser seating and improvements in vaporiser and back-bar design can minimise the risk of these problems.

Overfilling

Direct leakage of volatile agent into the patient circuit can also be caused by overfilling of the vaporiser, and this is potentially fatal. Care should be taken in filling and checking vaporisers.

Vaporiser maintenance

Vaporisers should be serviced annually, and calibration should also be checked regularly. Drainage and cleaning of vaporiser chambers (2-weekly intervals) can prevent the build-up of unwanted substances (such as thymol, a waxy stabilising agent used in halothane), which can reduce evaporation rates in the vaporiser chamber and cause moving parts to stick if they accumulate.

Design features of a vaporiser

The desirable features of a vaporiser depend to some extent on the specific application (portable or fixed, compressed gas supplies available or not), but some general specifications include:

- Large surface area for vaporisation in the vaporiser chamber
- Large heat sink
- Temperature compensation valve to control flow through the vaporiser
- Accurate flow-splitting valve
- Low flow resistance for draw-over vaporiser
- Stable mechanical mounting
- Safeguard against leakage into patient circuit
- Safety interlock device
- Clear liquid-level gauge
- Agent-specific filling port
- Easy emptying and cleaning

Breathing systems

Breathing system describes the equipment used to deliver fresh gases and volatile agents to a patient. The following general terms are used to describe breathing systems:

1. **Open system** – In its simplest form a breathing system may just be a method of augmenting room air, an open hose and a cupped hand, nasal cannulae delivering oxygen or a clear plastic oxygen mask. These are referred to as *open* breathing systems.
2. **Closed system** – This controls the gas mixture delivered to the patient, using a sealed mask and circuit. Closed systems can be divided into *rebreathing* and *non-rebreathing* systems.
   - *Rebreathing* is the inhalation of previously expired gases, including carbon dioxide and water vapour. Many of the breathing systems used in practice allow rebreathing, but are normally used with high enough fresh gas flow rates to prevent rebreathing. These types of system include the Bain and Magill circuits, and are described below in the Mapleson classification.
   - *Non-rebreathing* describes breathing systems in which rebreathing is prevented. This can be achieved by a non-rebreathing valve, a carbon dioxide absorber or high fresh gas flow rates in a rebreathing system.

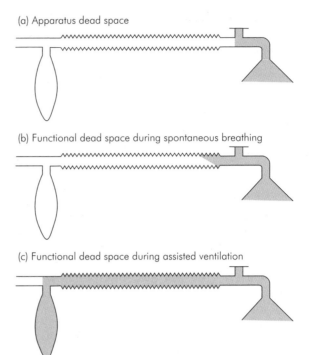

(a) Apparatus dead space

(b) Functional dead space during spontaneous breathing

(c) Functional dead space during assisted ventilation

Figure 46.19 Functional dead space within Magill circuit

Most practical **breathing systems** function as semi-closed and partially rebreathing systems. They are often capable of operating as non-rebreathing systems, depending on the magnitude of fresh gas flow (FGF) used.

Breathing system performance

Breathing systems may have to work in different environments, each of which may influence the design of the circuit. The optimum circuit for a given application will be a compromise between various features, which include:

- Low dead space. **Apparatus dead space** is the volume between the patient and the expiratory valve. **Functional dead space** extends to all of the volume contaminated with expired gases during each ventilatory cycle. It may be greater than apparatus dead space in an inefficient circuit, or less in other cases, where FGF flushes out expired gases before inspiration (Figure 46.19).

- Efficient operation in both spontaneously breathing (SV) patients and those requiring controlled/assisted ventilation (CV). Efficiency in this context is measured by minimum fresh gas flow (FGF) required to prevent rebreathing, expressed as a multiple of the patient's minute volume (MV). The Magill attachment requires an FGF > 0.7 MV to prevent rebreathing in a spontaneously breathing patient.
- Economical use of fresh gas supply and volatile agent. Economy of usage of anaesthetic gases is needed where supplies are restricted, or to minimise costs. In the operating theatre piped gas supplies are usually available. In other areas gas supplies may be limited, and occasionally pressurised supplies may not even be available. Environmental considerations and pollution are also a concern in the work environment.
- Physical size or weight. The weight and bulk of a circuit's components may be a factor discouraging its use, as the circuit may drag on endotracheal tubes or laryngeal masks, and displace them from a patient's airway. Factors such as apparatus dead space are likely to be in proportion to the size of the circuit's components. It is not always convenient to use breathing systems via an anaesthetic machine in resuscitation areas, and a simpler system such as the Waters circuit may be more practical.

Breathing system components

A breathing system may consist of all or some of the following components:
- Face mask
- Gas hoses and connectors
- Adjustable pressure-limiting (APL) expiratory valve (Figure 46.20)
- Reservoir bag (inflating or self-inflating)
- Carbon dioxide absorber
- A valve to switch between controlled (CV) and spontaneous (SV) ventilation modes
- One-way valves to prevent rebreathing

Masks and hoses

Masks and hoses are lightweight, disposable and transparent or semi-transparent. These features make the components easier to handle, cheaper and safer. Hoses come in three standard sizes: 22 mm diameter for adult breathing circuits, 15 mm diameter for paediatric breathing circuits and 30 mm diameter for scavenging circuits.

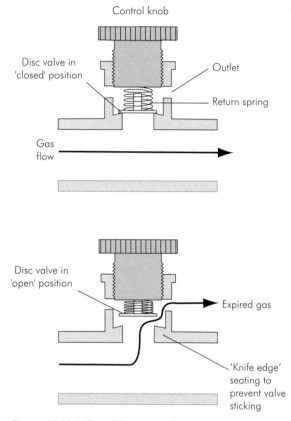

Figure 46.20 Adjustable pressure-limiting expiratory valve

Hose connectors

Standard male and female sizes to fit the hose diameters. They are also designed with standardised tapers to allow convenient but secure push-fitting between circuit components. 22 mm (15 mm for paediatric circuits) connections fit the breathing circuit hoses together and to valves, reservoir bags and masks. 15 mm connectors join the circuit to endotracheal tubes and laryngeal masks. Tapers are designed according to ISO and BS standards. Some connectors possess 22 mm external and 15 mm internal tapers to facilitate connection between the circuit hoses and an endotracheal tube or laryngeal mask.

Reservoir bags

Come in 0.5 litre, 2 litre and 4 litre sizes and are made of distensible synthetic material. The compliance of the bag is designed to be low enough to prevent development of harmful pressures if the system valves are accidentally closed.

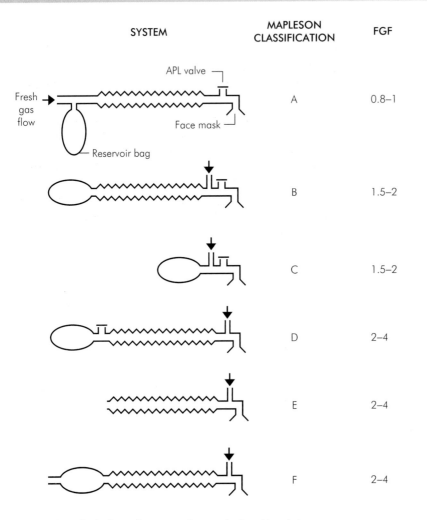

SYSTEM	MAPLESON CLASSIFICATION	FGF
	A	0.8–1
	B	1.5–2
	C	1.5–2
	D	2–4
	E	2–4
	F	2–4

FGF is the fresh gas flow required to avoid rebreathing during spontaneous ventilation quoted as multiples of minute volume

Figure 46.21 Mapleson classification system for breathing systems

Mapleson classification for breathing systems

This system classifies breathing systems according to the configuration of the following components:

- Reservoir bag
- Flexible hosing
- Adjustable pressure-limiting (APL) expiratory valve
- Face mask

The different configurations are described and illustrated in Figure 46.21.

Practical breathing systems

Various breathing systems have been developed empirically for different applications. Some systems consist of the basic components described in the Mapleson classification and therefore fit into the system described. Some examples are described in Figure 46.22.

Circle system

A typical circle system is shown in Figure 46.23. The system consists of a carbon dioxide absorber, a reservoir

Figure 46.22 Examples of commonly used circuits

Circuit	Mapleson	Comments
Magill	A	Good for SV. May be used for CV but requires twice MV. APL valve convenient near patient, but drags on endotracheal tube or mask.
Lack	A	Coaxial circuit delivering FGF via outer hose. Expiratory limb through inner hose with APL valve at anaesthetic machine. Disadvantages are high inspiratory resistance and large apparatus dead space. Also parallel twin-hose Lack circuit offers low flow resistances but more bulky.
Bain	D	Coaxial circuit. FGF delivered through inner hose. Suitable for SV or CV; less efficient for SV than Magill but more efficient for CV. Disadvantages of coaxial system are that cracks or disconnection in inner hose may go unnoticed.
Waters circuit	C	Practical circuit for resuscitation. Requires low-pressure oxygen supply. Low dead space. Suitable for SV or CV.
Ayre's T-piece	E	Suitable for paediatrics. The expiratory limb forms apparatus dead space but also acts as an inspiratory reservoir. This limb should be equal to the tidal volume to prevent dilution of inspired gases by entrained air. Requires 2–4 times MV to avoid rebreathing.
Jackson–Rees modification of Ayre's T-piece	F	Paediatric circuit. Open-ended reservoir modification of bag in expiratory limb.
Humphrey	ADE	Twin-hose system which switches between Mapleson A for SV and D/E for CV.

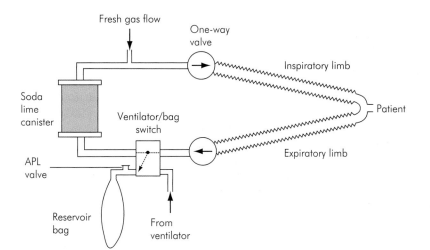

Figure 46.23 A typical circle system

bag, one-way valves to ensure unidirectional gas flow and hoses with a Y-piece to connect the patient into the circuit. The circle system can be used with a spontaneously breathing patient, or control/assist can be given manually using the reservoir bag.

The optimum configuration for the components has the FGF and reservoir bag located between the carbon dioxide absorber and the one-way inspiratory valve. This arrangement minimises the inspiratory resistance of the circuit.

Advantages of the circle system

- Low FGF rates can be used without causing rebreathing of expired carbon dioxide, resulting in economy of anaesthetic gas usage.
- Recirculation of volatile agent gives economy and low pollution rates.
- Low functional dead space, equal to the volume of the patient Y-piece, due to removal of carbon dioxide by the absorber.

Disadvantages of the circle system

- More components than simpler systems (such as Magill or Bain) create a bulky system requiring a separate mounting on the anaesthetic machine.
- One-way valves to ensure unidirectional flow increase flow resistances and are a potential source of problems such as sticking.
- Inspiratory and expiratory flow resistances are higher than in the case of the Magill or Bain systems. These higher flow resistances are dependent on FGF rates in the circle. Low FGF rates increase inspiratory resistance but decrease expiratory resistance. High FGF rates produce the opposite effect, decreasing inspiratory resistance and increasing expiratory resistance. Work of breathing is therefore lowest with high FGF rates. This effect is not significant in a fit adult, but can become important in frail patients or children.

Controlled ventilation (CV) with the circle system

CV can be applied using the circle system, by using a 'bag in the bottle' type of ventilator. This effectively acts as a 'bag squeezer', and the ventilator is connected into the circle system in place of the reservoir bag. In such a case the tidal volume delivered may depend on both the ventilator setting and the FGF. Modern circle systems

incorporate ventilators which monitor the delivered tidal volume and compensate for changes in FGF.

An alternative arrangement is the use of a servo-type ventilator which delivers 'driving' gas (oxygen) via the reservoir bag limb and allows expiration through the same limb. In such a configuration the driving gas must not 'contaminate' the patient circuit. This means FGF must be greater than MV, and the length of the reservoir limb tubing must have a volume greater than 1.5 times the tidal volume.

Use of volatile agents with the circle

When volatile agents are used with the circle the commonest configuration is with a plenum vaporiser located out of the circle (vaporiser outside circle, VOC). The FGF thus passes through the vaporiser first, and then into the circle system. In the past, draw-over vaporisers were used positioned within the circle system (vaporiser inside circle, VIC).

Both methods have disadvantages at low FGF. In summary:

- **VOC** – Expired gas dilutes the inspired gases and reduces inspired volatile concentrations, until equilibrium is reached, when end-tidal volatile concentrations equal inspired concentrations. Also the performance of many plenum vaporisers may be inaccurate at low flow rates.
- **VIC** – Inspired gases are recirculated through the vaporiser, resulting in continually increasing volatile concentrations, which may reach saturation levels.

Carbon dioxide absorption

Carbon dioxide absorption is used to prevent rebreathing, and is most commonly used in the circle system in combination with low FGF rates. A combination of chemical reactions is used to absorb carbon dioxide. First carbon dioxide is dissolved in water to form carbonic acid, and the carbonic acid then reacts with calcium hydroxide to form calcium carbonate and water:

$$CO_2 + H_2O = H_2CO_3 = H^+ + HCO_3^-$$
$$Ca(OH)_2 + H^+ + HCO_3^- = CaCO_3 + 2H_2O$$

This reaction is exothermic and produces water, providing a warm moist environment in the carbon dioxide absorber for the FGF to pass through. The pH of the reagents increases as the reaction proceeds, enabling an indicator to be used to show when the calcium hydroxide is exhausted.

Some practical points concerning the use of carbon dioxide absorbers are as follows:

- **FGF rates** – Use of carbon dioxide absorption with the circle system can reduce FGF rate to a few hundred millilitres per minute, once equilibrium has been reached. This FGF is required to replace absorbed oxygen (100–300 mL min^{-1}) and gases lost through leakage and the APL valve.
- **Calcium hydroxide preparation** – The most commonly used preparation is soda lime, which is a mixture of 80% $Ca(OH)_2$, 4% NaOH and 16% H_2O. The soda lime is in the form of granules, which are designed to be small enough to give low spaces between granules and thus high-efficiency absorption, but not so small as to provide excessive resistance to gas flow.
- **Soda lime** – The absorption capacity of soda lime is in the order of 25 litres of carbon dioxide per 100 g of soda lime. The colour change indicating exhaustion of the granules (commonly pink to white) may occur before full-capacity absorption due to surface reaction on the granules. This can lead to apparent regeneration of granules as the surface and core of the granule equilibrate when used soda lime is left standing. Soda lime dust is caustic and can cause morbidity if a soda lime canister is located too close to the patient's airway in the breathing system. This can occur in the to-and-fro configuration used with a Waters canister (Mapleson C) system. 'Channelling' may occur in soda lime canisters which are poorly packed. This is the formation of channels through the soda lime granules through which gases pass without adequate exposure to the soda lime, and it results in incomplete carbon dioxide absorption

Toxic products due to reaction between volatile agents and soda lime

Reactions between volatile agents and soda lime have been noted which can result in the production of toxic substances:

Carbon monoxide may be produced by volatiles containing $-CHF_2$ in their structure (isoflurane, desflurane, enflurane) when they pass through dessicated soda lime. This is an artificial situation, since soda lime absorbers normally have a high humidity content due to the water produced in the absorption reaction between carbon dioxide and soda lime (see above). However, animal studies have demonstrated clinically significant levels of inspired CO, and carboxyhaemoglobin can be produced when using dry soda lime.

Compound A – Soda lime can decompose sevoflurane to produce a number of compounds. One of these has been identified as being toxic, Compound A, a pentafluoroisopropenyl fluoromethyl ether. The concentrations of Compound A produced in normal clinical conditions (< 30 ppm) are only a fraction of the toxic levels (> 150 ppm).

A **neurotoxin (dichloroethylene)** can be produced by trichloroethylene (Trilene), an agent no longer in current use, when it is decomposed by soda lime.

Oxygen delivery systems

In the spontaneously breathing patient, various systems exist to provide enhanced fraction of inspired oxygen (F_IO_2) for the spontaneously breathing patient. These can be required in locations such as recovery areas, resuscitation areas, labour suites and ambulances. The types of device used include nasal cannulae, face masks and attachments for enhancing the F_IO_2 through laryngeal masks or endotracheal tubes.

Oxygen delivery systems may be described in terms of **variable** or **fixed performance**, and **low**, **medium** or **high dependency**. Figure 46.24 outlines some characteristics of commonly used devices.

Variable performance

This term refers to the F_IO_2 delivered by a particular system. In a variable-performance system (Figure 46.25) the F_IO_2 delivered is dependent on the oxygen flow rate. The range of flow rates used is usually between 2 and 15 litres per minute, and such devices are capable of producing F_IO_2 up to 0.8–0.9. Variable-performance systems require an inspiratory oxygen reservoir in order to achieve the higher F_IO_2 levels, and may be classified as being of 'no capacity' if they have no reservoir capacity (nasal cannulae), 'small capacity' in the case of face masks, and 'large capacity' when a reservoir bag is included. Non-return valves are also incorporated in order to restrict entrainment in face masks and to prevent rebreathing from reservoir bags.

Fixed performance

A fixed-performance device (Figure 46.26) delivers an F_IO_2 which is independent of the oxygen flow rate used. These systems are usually based on a Venturi jet that is fed by the

Figure 46.24 Oxygen delivery systems for spontaneously breathing patients

Device	Type	F_iO_2	Comments
Nasal cannulae	Variable, no capacity	0.21–0.3	Alternative for patients who cannot tolerate masks. Performance unpredictable, affected by nasal obstruction and mouth breathing.
Face mask	Variable, low capacity	0.21–0.5	Performance depends on entrainment through holes in mask and around mask. Enhanced by flap valves. Increases functional dead space.
Face mask with reservoir and non-rebreathing valve	Variable, large capacity	0.21–0.80	Provides high F_iO_2. Suitable for head-injury patient. Recommended by ATLS.
Venturi face mask	Fixed	0.24–0.60	Performance depends on colour-coded Venturi jets. F_iO_2 determined by jet size and entrainment ratio. Requires reservoir tubing between jet and face mask. Dependent on tidal volume.
Venturi T-piece	Fixed	0.24–0.60	Used for laryngeal masks or endotracheal tubes. F_iO_2 determined by jet size and entrainment ratio. Requires high flow rates and reservoir tubing in expiratory limb.

oxygen supply and entrains room air. They are often applied in patients with chronic respiratory disease in whom oxygen-dependent respiratory drive is suspected.

Low dependency
Describes systems used to increase F_iO_2 in patients breathing spontaneously at atmospheric pressure.

Medium dependency
Describes a system which supplies a degree of positive airway pressure to a spontaneously breathing patient (e.g. a continuous positive airway pressure (CPAP) system). These systems are used in high dependency areas or intensive care units.

The F_iO_2 delivered in variable-performance systems depends on:

- Oxygen flow rate
- Tidal volume
- Respiratory rate
- Capacity of the system
- Use of non-return valves

High dependency
Describes systems used to control the F_iO_2 in patients requiring mechanical ventilation.

Resuscitation breathing systems
Such systems are used during resuscitation, to apply artificial ventilation to patients who are not breathing spontaneously. They also allow the patient to breathe spontaneously through them. There are two commonly used systems, the Ambu system and the Laerdal system.

The basic components of these systems are:
- **Self-inflating bag** – This has a volume of approximately 1500 mL for an adult (500 mL for a child, 250 mL for an infant). The walls are reinforced to make the bag self-inflating. One end of the bag is the inlet for fresh gas, and this is sealed by a flap valve. This also possesses an inlet for oxygen supplementation. The other end of the bag is connected to the patient via a non-rebreathing valve (Figure 46.27).
- **Non-rebreathing valve** – There are several designs for this valve in common use. These include the Rubens valve, the Laerdal valve and different types of Ambu valve. These valves open the patient's airway to the bag during inspiration, and then during expiration close the connection to the bag and allow the patient's gases

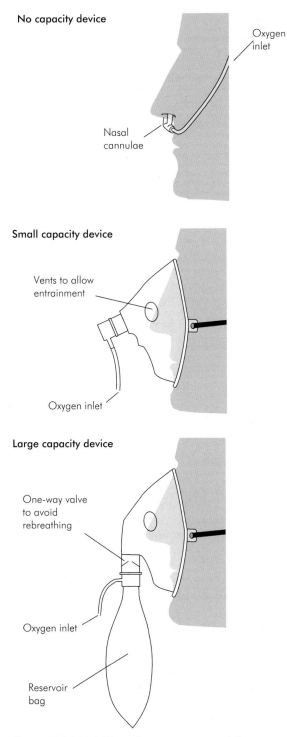

No capacity device

Oxygen inlet

Nasal cannulae

Small capacity device

Vents to allow entrainment

Oxygen inlet

Large capacity device

One-way valve to avoid rebreathing

Oxygen inlet

Reservoir bag

Figure 46.25 Variable-performance oxygen delivery systems

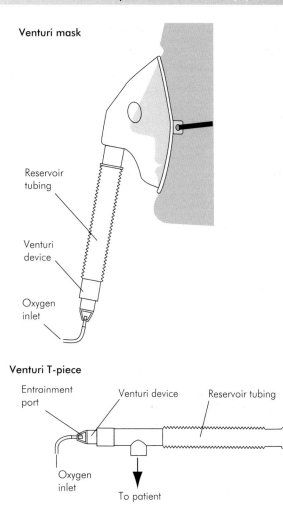

Venturi mask

Reservoir tubing

Venturi device

Oxygen inlet

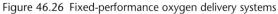

Venturi T-piece

Entrainment port

Venturi device

Reservoir tubing

Oxygen inlet

To patient

Figure 46.26 Fixed-performance oxygen delivery systems

to expire to the atmosphere. Figures 46.28 and 46.29 show examples of some non-rebreathing valves used in resuscitation systems. The Rubens valve possesses a spring-loaded bobbin which slides to open the patient's airway to the bag during inspiration (or inflation). During expiration the spring closes the airway to the bag and opens it to the atmosphere. High pressures in the bag can hold the bobbin in the inspiratory position. The Ambu valve Type E (Figure 46.29) uses 'mushroom' (labial flap) valves to produce the same reciprocal inspiratory and expiratory functions.

- **Oxygen reservoir bag** – This is fitted over the fresh gas inlet to the self-inflating bag and is inflated by the supplementary oxygen supply. It also possesses an inlet

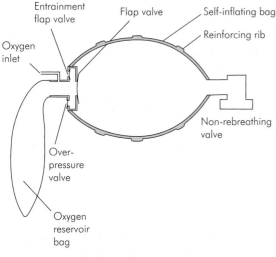

Figure 46.27 Self-inflating bag

INSPIRATION

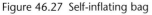

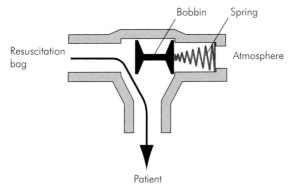

Figure 46.28 Rubens non-rebreathing valve

flap valve to allow entrainment from the atmosphere should the demand of the patient exceed its capacity. Without the reservoir bag the delivered F_IO_2 is limited to < 0.5. Using a reservoir bag can increase the F_IO_2 to 1.

INSPIRATION

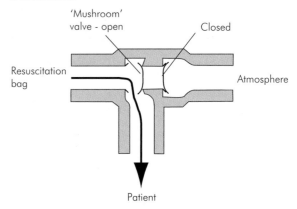

EXPIRATION

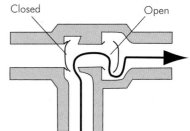

Figure 46.29 Ambu non-rebreathing valve

- **Oxygen supply** – This enters the bag or reservoir via narrow-bore tubing and a nipple connector. The flow rate used is between 2 and 15 litres per minute. The final inspired oxygen concentration delivered to the patient will depend on the oxygen flow rate, respiratory rate, tidal volume and whether a reservoir is used.

Endotracheal tubes

The endotracheal tube (ETT) is a plastic or rubber tube inserted into the trachea. It provides a definitive airway, allowing positive-pressure ventilation while preventing contamination of the lungs from the contents of the pharynx. The original tubes were made by Rowbotham and Magill in 1920 from rubber tubing of varying diameter and cut to the correct length by hand. Both oral and nasal tubes were designed, and these were connected to the breathing circuit by a metal adapter. Later developments included the cuff with pilot balloon, double-lumen

Figure 46.30 Original design features of LMA

Feature	Notes
Wide-bore tube	Lower resistance to spontaneous respiration
Large oval inflatable cuff	Overlies larynx. May obstruct if displaced. Partial inflation. May aid insertion. Does not prevent aspiration
Soft bars across distal lumen of tube	In earlier designs, to stop epiglottis from obstructing lumen of tube. Not used in later designs
Reusable/disposable	Original design was reusable (autoclavable up to 40 times). Later types are disposable

tubes for thoracic surgery, and anatomically shaped tubes such as the Oxford or RAE (Ring, Adair, Elwyn) tubes.

Red rubber produced inflammatory reactions at the site of contact and has been superseded by non-irritant transparent plastic. The tubes are often marked with the initials IT (implant tested) or Z79 (which refers to a room number related to the toxicity subcommittee of ANSI) to indicate compliance with the standards defined by the American National Standards Institute. The tube is marked with the internal and external diameters in millimetres, the length in centimetres, and usually also a radio-opaque line to aid visualisation on chest x-ray. High-volume cuffs when inflated are associated with a lower pressure on the tracheal mucosa and are appropriate for long operations or intensive care use. The pressure in the cuff can also increase as nitrous oxide diffuses through the thin plastic wall. While this can be prevented by filling the balloon with saline, some tubes have been designed with an oversize pilot balloon (Brandt pattern) or with a cuff filled with self-expanding foam and the connecting tube left open to the atmosphere. The requirements of ENT surgery have led to designs which minimise the obstruction to the surgeon's vision (microlaryngoscopy tubes), or which cannot be kinked (wire-reinforced tubes), and tubes resistant to ignition by the operating laser.

To describe an endotracheal tube, identify the following features:

- Single or double lumen
- Material
- Cuff and pilot balloon with self-sealing valve
- Bevel with or without eyes
- Special features

Laryngeal mask airway

First produced commercially in 1986 to the design of Dr Archie Brain, the laryngeal mask airway (LMA) offered an airway intermediate between the face mask and the tracheal tube, and represents one of the most significant advances in airway design. It consists of a wide tube terminating at one end in a 15 mm connection and at the other in an inflatable cuff that is placed over the laryngeal opening. When inflated, the cuff provides an airtight seal sufficient to permit gentle positive-pressure ventilation if the chest compliance is normal, although it does not protect the trachea from soiling by stomach contents and should not therefore be used if aspiration is a possibility. The LMA is produced in a range of sizes from #1 (neonate) to #5 for large adults. Some features of the original LMA are noted in Figure 46.30.

Further variations in laryngeal mask design have evolved. These include:

- Reinforced LMA for ENT or prone positioning
- ProSeal double-lumen LMA for passage of orogastric tube through second lumen
- Intubating LMA, allowing passage of fibreoptic bronchoscope or blind intubation
- iGel LMA, with gel-filled non-inflatable cuff

Scavenging systems

An appropriate scavenging system is mandatory in each anaesthetic room and operating theatre in order to avoid pollution by anaesthetic gases and agents. Although there are no studies proving side effects caused by chronic exposure to low levels of anaesthetic gases or vapours, the alleged side effects include:

- Increased incidence of spontaneous abortion.
- Vitamin B_{12} inactivation by nitrous oxide, with neurological sequelae.

- Increased incidence of female births.
- Reduced fertility in females exposed to nitrous oxide.
- Increased incidence of minor congenital abnormalities.
- Increased incidence of leukaemia and lymphoma in exposed females.
- Potential contribution to global warming effect of atmospheric pollutants. Although the contribution of nitrous oxide and volatile agents is estimated to be small in comparison to that of carbon dioxide, the cumulative effect over decades could become significant.

Recommended levels of pollutants

> ### COSHH and NIOSH
>
> Pollutants are covered by the Control of Substances Hazardous to Health (COSHH) Regulations in the UK, and in the USA the National Institute for Occupational Safety and Health (NIOSH) issues similar regulations. These control exposure levels to many pollutants, including anaesthetic agents.

Some of the recommended maximum levels of exposure (averaged over any 8-hour time period) are listed in Figure 46.31.

Types of scavenging system

Scavenging systems are designed to collect the waste gases and vapours from the anaesthetic machine and dispose of them, without affecting the breathing or ventilation of the patient, and without affecting the safe operation of the anaesthetic machine.

Figure 46.31 Anaesthetic pollutant levels (COSHH regulations)

Pollutant	Maximum level (ppm)
Nitrous oxide	100
Halothane	10
Enflurane	50
Isoflurane	50
Sevoflurane	20 (manufacturer's recommendation)

> **The different types of scavenging system** include:
> - Passive systems
> - Active systems
> - Absorber systems

All scavenging systems require a device for collecting the waste gas from the breathing system, ventilator or patient. To cope with wide fluctuations in gas flow (from 0 to 130 L min^{-1}) there needs to be a reservoir to collect waste gases. The patient may be protected either by positive and negative pressure relief valves or, in an active system, by an open-ended reservoir. The standard size of connections is 30 mm, to avoid wrong connections, and the risk of obstruction of the patient's expiratory pathway must be minimised. Figure 46.32 shows the design of scavenging systems.

Passive systems

Early scavenging systems were passive in that the patient's expiratory effort was required to propel waste gas down an additional length of tubing to the outside atmosphere. While the flow of gas could be assisted either by placing the end near the air-conditioning outlet or by terminating the roof vent with an extractor cowl, these systems were notably inefficient. Despite a maximal tubing resistance of 0.5 cmH$_2$O the increased resistance to expiration and the potential for complete obstruction represented a distinct hazard to the patient without measurably protecting theatre staff.

Active systems

Modern active scavenging is usually driven by a fan unit remote to the theatre unit which produces a sub-atmospheric pressure capable of large gas flows (75 L min^{-1}, peak flow 130 L min^{-1} per patient) in a piped distribution system. Distribution is terminated in each theatre, where it is connected to the reservoir collection system. The reservoir usually houses a visual flow indicator, which should be periodically checked to ensure the system is working. The system should operate within the pressures of −0.5 cmH$_2$O and +5 cmH$_2$O at 30 L min^{-1} flow.

Absorbers

Absorbers are usually based on activated charcoal and can, to a limited extent, absorb volatile agents (which may be released again by the use of heat).

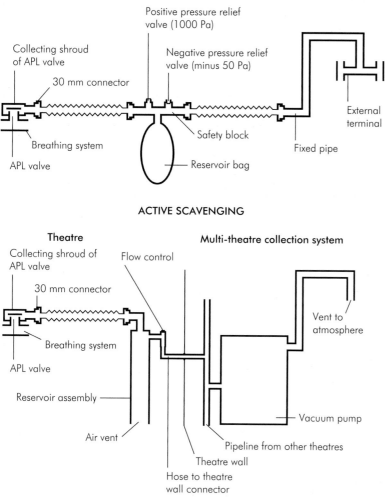

Figure 46.32 Scavenging systems

Mechanical ventilators

A mechanical ventilator is designed to automatically inflate the lungs when a patient is unable to breathe spontaneously. This is most commonly achieved by applying positive pressure to the patient's airway, as in intermittent positive-pressure ventilation (IPPV). Alternative techniques also include high-frequency methods such as high-frequency jet ventilation (HFJV), and the use of negative pressure applied to the patient's chest wall (cuirass).

Ideal characteristics of a ventilator

The ideal specifications for a ventilator will vary according to its clinical application. Clearly the requirements of a ventilator for the intensive care unit will be very different from those for a ventilator to be used in an ambulance. Usually clinical application will dictate the physical parameters of the ventilation cycle and the mechanics of the ventilator.

Within the limitations of its clinical application a ventilator should:

A ventilator can be described by different characteristics:

- **Ventilation cycle parameters** – This term refers to the parameters (pressure, flow rate) which are defined during the inspiratory and expiratory phases of each ventilation cycle. It also defines how the ventilator switches between inspiratory and expiratory phases. Detailed discussion is presented below under *Mapleson classification for ventilators*.
- **Mechanics** – The mechanism and power supply used to generate the ventilation cycle, e.g. minute volume divider, 'bag in the bottle'. These characteristics will often determine its physical size and power requirements.
- **Clinical features** – The features which determine its clinical field of application (operating theatre, ICU, neonatal unit). These include its ability to provide ancillary modes such as positive end-expiratory pressure (PEEP), continuous positive airway pressure (CPAP) and synchronised intermittent mandatory ventilation (SIMV).

- Provide appropriate ventilation modes for its particular application
- Have easy switching between automatic and manual functions
- Be simple and practical to use
- Be mechanically well designed and reliable
- Have appropriate, reliable and readily visible monitoring and alarms
- Be easy to clean and sterilise

Mapleson classification for ventilators

The Mapleson scheme classifies positive-pressure ventilators according to the different phases of the ventilation cycle:
- Inspiratory phase
- Cycling between inspiration and expiration (inspiratory cycling)
- Expiratory phase
- Cycling between expiration and inspiration (expiratory cycling, inspiratory triggering)

Inspiratory phase

During inspiration, either pressure or flow rate can be determined by the ventilator mechanism. Thus a ventilator can be described either as a **pressure generator** or as a **flow generator**. Flow generators and pressure generators are basically different in mechanical design.

A pressure generator must be capable of providing high flow rates at the preset inspiratory pressure, which means it must have a low internal impedance to flow. This means that variations in the mechanics of the respiratory system will affect the ventilator performance.

A flow generator delivers a preset flow rate irrespective of variations in lung compliance, so its internal impedance must be very high to attenuate the effect of variations in lung compliance on ventilator performance. The preset flow rate means that a flow generator can be used to deliver a fixed tidal volume and minute ventilation no matter how the mechanics of the respiratory system vary.

Some properties of pressure and flow generators are listed in Figure 46.33.

Inspiratory pressures and flow rates during mechanical ventilation

In a mechanically ventilated patient, inspiratory pressures and flow rates are affected by both lung compliance and the type of ventilator used.

Ventilator performance and reduced lung compliance

The differences between pressure and flow generators when ventilating patients with normal or reduced lung compliances can be illustrated by the pressure and flow curves during a ventilation cycle. The flow curve also gives information about the tidal volume, since volume is obtained from the area under the flow curve. The inspired tidal volume delivered is thus equal to the area under the flow curve during inspiration. Expired tidal volume is given by the area under the flow curve during expiration.

Figure 46.34 shows a **pressure generator** delivering constant inspiratory pressure. Flow rate increases to a peak during inspiration and then decreases exponentially

Figure 46.33 Comparison between pressure and flow generator ventilators

Property	Pressure generators	Flow generators
Inspiratory pressure	Inspiratory pressure and pattern (e.g. constant, sinusoidal, triangular) preset on ventilator	Inspiratory pressure will vary according to respiratory mechanics of patient. High inspiratory pressures may be produced with low lung compliance (e.g. acute respiratory distress syndrome)
Inspiratory flow rate	Inspiratory flow rate (and hence tidal volume) will vary according to respiratory mechanics of patient. High flow rates may be produced with high lung compliance (e.g. neonates)	Inspiratory flow rate and pattern (e.g. constant, ramp) preset on ventilator
Tidal volume	Tidal volume will vary according to lung compliance. Decreased lung compliance will reduce tidal volume	Preset tidal volume will be delivered at the expense of airway pressure, unless an inspiratory pressure limit is preset
Risk of barotrauma	Low risk	High risk unless pressure limit preset on ventilator
Risk of volutrauma (excessive tidal volumes)	High risk unless limit on tidal volume preset on ventilator	Low risk
Compensation for leakage	Some limited ability to compensate for small leaks in circuitry between ventilator and patient, since ventilator always acts to deliver preset inspiratory pressure	Any leakage from connecting circuit will be lost, as it is counted by ventilator as delivered flow (tidal volume)
Clinical application	Suitable for paediatrics or neonates because of low risk of barotrauma and ability to compensate for small leaks. Requires tidal volume limit. Safer for emphysematous lungs	Appropriate for ICU because of ability to deliver flow (tidal volume) with low lung compliance. Requires inspiratory pressure limitation to reduce risk of barotrauma

during expiration, which is passive. The areas (tidal volumes) under the inspiratory and expiratory parts of the flow curve are approximately equal. When lung compliance is reduced the peak inspiratory flow rate reached is lower and the inspiratory and expiratory tidal volumes are reduced.

Figure 46.35 shows a **flow generator** delivering constant flow during inspiration with a **preset tidal volume**. Inspiratory pressure initially rises rapidly to reach a peak, and then decreases exponentially during expiration. When lung compliance is reduced the ventilator still delivers the same constant inspired flow with the same duration (preset tidal volume), but peak

inspiratory pressure is increased. The lower the compliance (i.e. the stiffer the lungs), the greater the inspiratory pressures required to deliver the preset flow and tidal volume.

Figure 46.36 shows a **flow generator** delivering constant flow with **pressure limitation** and a **preset tidal volume**. With normal lung compliance the pressure limit is not exceeded and an inspiratory pressure curve like that in Figure 46.35 is produced. When reduced lung compliance is present the inspiratory pressures are increased. If the pressure exceeds the preset limit, inspiration is cut short and the tidal volume delivered is reduced below the preset value.

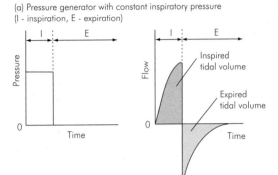

(a) Pressure generator with constant inspiratory pressure
(I - inspiration, E - expiration)

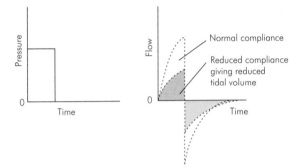

(b) Effect of reduced compliance in pressure generator

Figure 46.34 Inspiratory patterns from a pressure generator

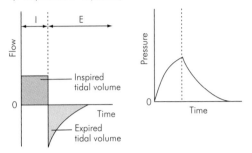

(a) Flow generator with preset tidal volume
(I - inspiration, E - expiration)

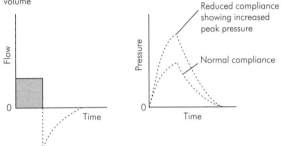

(b) Effect of reduced compliance on flow generator with preset tidal volume

Figure 46.35 Inspiratory patterns from a flow generator with preset tidal volume

Cycling between inspiration and expiration (inspiratory cycling)

The change between inspiration and expiration can be triggered by various parameters. This function is referred to as cycling, and it may be described as follows:

- Volume cycling – Inspiration stops and expiration begins when the preset tidal volume is delivered. An inspiratory pause may be used, which prolongs the inspiratory phase.
- Pressure cycling – Inspiration occurs up to a preset inspiratory pressure, at which expiration is then triggered.
- Time cycling – The inspiratory phase occurs for a fixed duration, which is preset, and at the end of this time expiration is triggered. This type of cycling will effectively preset tidal volume in a flow generator.

Expiratory phase

Expiration is normally passive, but during the expiratory phase positive pressure can be applied to give positive end-expiratory pressure (PEEP). This technique is usually applied in the intensive care unit to improve oxygenation and recruit lung volume in patients with certain lung pathologies such as acute respiratory distress syndrome (ARDS). Surgical anaesthesia in the operating theatre does not usually involve the use of PEEP.

Cycling between expiration and inspiration (expiratory cycling)

The change from expiration to inspiration usually occurs on a timed basis (i.e. expiratory time cycling) as determined by the preset ventilation frequency. For example, if a frequency of 12 breaths per minute is preset, then expiratory cycling will occur (i.e. inspiration will be triggered) every 5 seconds.

Alternatively, inspiration may be triggered by negative pressure changes or flow rates generated by the patient's own spontaneous inspiratory efforts. This approach is adopted in supported or assisted ventilation modes (e.g. SIMV) used to give ventilatory support to patients with some degree of spontaneous respiratory effort or who are being weaned from mechanical ventilation.

(a) Flow generator with preset tidal volume and pressure limitation

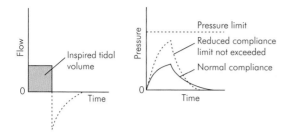

(b) Effect of reduced compliance on flow generator with pressure limitation causing reduction of tidal volume

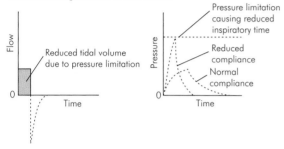

Figure 46.36 Inspiratory patterns from a flow generator with pressure limitation and preset tidal volume

Ventilator mechanics

The mechanical design of ventilators centres around the driving mechanism which delivers fresh gas to the patient. Secondary aspects such as the power supply, control mechanisms, monitoring and reliability are often equally important in determining the ventilator's clinical performance. Some examples of the different mechanical designs used for ventilators are summarised in Figure 46.37. A ventilator may have the advantages of simplicity and reliability, or may be very complex in design, in order to cope with more specialised clinical applications.

Clinical features of ventilators

Most ventilators can be used to ventilate normal lungs. For the more specialised clinical applications, for patients with respiratory pathology, or for weaning from mechanical ventilation, additional clinical features or ancillary modes may be required in a ventilator. Some examples of these modes are outlined in Figure 46.38.

Humidifiers

Humidity refers to the amount of water vapour present in a gas or the atmosphere. It is defined in two ways (see Chapter 44):

Absolute humidity (AH) is the mass of water vapour present in a given volume of air or gas (g m^{-3} or kg m^{-3}). This value will not vary with the temperature of the air.

Relative humidity (RH) is the ratio of the mass of water present in a given volume of air at a given temperature, to the mass of water required to saturate that given volume at the same temperature. RH is usually expressed as a percentage, and it will decrease as temperature increases. Fully saturated air at 20 °C contains 17 g m^{-3} while at 37 °C it contains 43 g m^{-3}.

It is important for us to control the humidity of medical gases and the atmosphere in order to decrease the risk of the following problems:

- Heat and moisture loss from the patient's respiratory tract
- Damage to the mucosa of the respiratory tract
- Corrosion or frost damage to gas pipes, cylinders and valves
- Discomfort and fatigue of operating theatre staff
- Accumulation of static electrical charges (risk of microshock) in the operating theatre

Humidifiers for medical gases

Ideally, inspired fresh gases should be supplied at body temperature with an RH of 100% (i.e. saturated). Inspiration of cool unhumidified gases by a patient can potentially lead to a loss of more than 10% (> 10 W) of basal metabolic energy requirements. In addition, the prolonged use of under-humidified gases in a ventilated patient can cause severe damage to the mucosa (inflammation, ulceration) and lungs (inspissation of secretions, micro-atelectasis).

Various mechanisms have been used to humidify inspired gases. The most commonly used types of humidifier are listed below.

Bottle humidifier

This method, often seen on wards, relies on passing or bubbling oxygen through a bottle containing water at room temperature. From the values for water content at room temperature and body temperature, it can be seen that this is at best only likely to achieve an RH of approximately 40% at body temperature. In practice, complete saturation of the gas is not even achieved at room temperature.

Figure 46.37 Ventilator mechanics

Ventilator	Mechanism	Comments
Minute volume divider	Driven by the fresh gas supply. The fresh gas flow passes into bellows, which divide it up into tidal volumes by filling repeatedly. The first bellows empty into second bellows, which deliver the tidal volume to the patient	Of historical interest (e.g. Manley MP3 ventilator). Simple reliable mechanism. No additional power supply required. Limited capability for patients with abnormal lungs. Workhorse ventilator for theatres and anaesthetic rooms
'Bag in bottle' or 'bag squeezer'	Fresh gas flow for the patient enters bellows (bag) mounted in a container (bottle). The ventilator compresses the bellows downwards, by pressurising the bottle during inspiration. The bag is then opened to an expiratory port during expiration. Different sizes of bellows used for adults and children. Modern versions microprocessor controlled	The patient circuit is isolated from the ventilator circuit. This means the ventilator is used as a servoventilator, to ventilate a patient through a separate breathing system such as a circle or Bain. Often incorporated into anaesthetic machines (e.g. Ohmeda 7800)
Microprocessor-controlled electronic ventilator	Usually employs a bellows mechanism driven mechanically (e.g. spring loaded). Sophisticated electronics and monitoring to provide accurate control and triggered modes of ventilation	Used for intensive care. Complex and software driven. Provides ancillary modes for difficult lung pathologies (ARDS, bullous lung disease) and weaning
High-frequency jet ventilator	Uses high-pressure MPGS supply (400 kPa) to inject into an endotracheal tube, tracheostomy tube, or other interface circuit, which connects to the patient's airway. The ventilator–patient interface is an important factor in determining performance	Used for intensive care and thoracic surgery. Does not require a sealed airway to ventilate patient. Increased risk of barotrauma and problems with humidification when applied for prolonged periods (e.g. Accutronic Monsoon Jet Ventilator)

Soda lime absorber in the circle breathing system

This device is primarily used to prevent rebreathing at low flow rates, by absorbing carbon dioxide. The reaction of the carbon dioxide with the soda lime results in the production of calcium carbonate, heat and water. As a result an RH of 60–70% can be produced in the inspired gases at body temperature.

Heat and moisture exchanger (HME)

These passive devices consist of a capsule containing a condensing filter (stainless-steel mesh), hygroscopic material (paper coated with calcium chloride) or hydrophobic material (ceramic fibres). The capsule is fitted with 22 mm and 15 mm ports so that it can be fitted in-line between the breathing circuit and the patient's airway (endotracheal tube or laryngeal mask). Expired gases, saturated with water vapour, pass through the capsule, causing water to be deposited and heat to be retained by the contained element. Condensation causes a further temperature rise (latent heat of evaporation), producing a warm, moist environment for the incoming cool dry inspired fresh gas flow to pass through. Effective operation of the HME relies on the humidity and temperature gradient between the capsule and the fresh gas flow, and can result in an RH of 60–70% at body temperature. The HME is made of low-thermal-conductivity plastic to preserve the temperature inside the capsule. It may also be combined with a port for end-tidal CO_2 monitoring and a bacterial/viral filter.

Disadvantages with the use of this device include increased dead space, increased flow resistance, water

Figure 46.38 Ancillary modes in ventilators

Mode	Description	Comments
Positive end-expiratory pressure (PEEP)	0–15 cmH$_2$O of positive airway pressure maintained during expiration	Applied to improve oxygenation, recruit lung volume and prevent micro-atelectasis
Continuous positive airway pressure (CPAP)	0–15 cmH$_2$O of positive airway pressure maintained during inspiration and expiration	Applied to assist patients' spontaneous breathing by improving oxygenation and reducing the work of breathing
Intermittent mandatory ventilation (IMV)	This mode supports patients who are breathing spontaneously, but inadequately. It supplies a minimum minute volume, as a preset number of mandatory breaths per minute. The patient breathes spontaneously between mandatory breaths	Applied to patients who are being weaned from mechanical ventilation. A disadvantage is that mandatory breaths may 'stack' on top of spontaneous breaths, giving high airway pressures
Synchronised intermittent mandatory ventilation (SIMV)	This form of IMV synchronises the mandatory breaths with the patient's spontaneous breathing	Avoids 'stacking' of mandatory breaths and spontaneous breaths
Pressure support (PS)	An 'assisted' mode in which the ventilator provides a mechanical breath when triggered by the patient's spontaneous effort. The ventilator is set to act as a pressure generator in this mode	Used as a supporting mode in spontaneously breathing patients being weaned from mechanical ventilation or with respiratory failure

accumulation in the filter and decreased efficiency with large tidal volumes.

Hot water bath

This consists of a thermostatically controlled water tank through which the inspired fresh gas flow is passed (Figure 46.39). Temperature is monitored at the airway by a thermistor which feeds back to control the water temperature. The water tank has a large surface area to ensure full saturation of the inspired gases. Performance depends on the fresh gas flow rate passing through the humidifier. 100% RH (full saturation) can be achieved by setting the water tank temperature higher than body temperature, to allow for cooling in the patient circuit.

Disadvantages with this method include risk of scalding and electric shock, risk of water and condensation passing into the patient's respiratory tract (so humidifier and water traps must be kept below level of patient), risk of infection due to colonisation of humidifier, and the need for a power supply.

Nebulisers

These devices produce a fine mist of water droplets in the inspired gases, and can be used to deliver drugs as well as humidification. The diameter of these droplets may range from less than 1 μm up to 20 μm, depending on the mechanism used to produce them. Droplets of less than 1 μm in diameter can reach the lower airways and alveoli, while larger particles of 5–10 μm tend to deposit in the trachea and pharynx. Since the water is in the form of droplets, there is no saturation limit to the amount of water contained by the inspiratory gases, and excessive quantities of water can be readily deposited in the trachea and larger airways, particularly with the smaller particles. Different mechanisms are used to nebulise solutions, including:

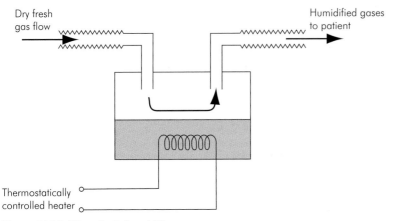

Figure 46.39 Water bath humidifier

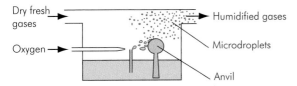

Figure 46.40 Gas jet nebuliser

- **Gas jet nebuliser** – This device is driven by a high-pressure gas jet passing across the top of a small tube fed by water from a reservoir (Figure 46.40). The negative pressure produced at the jet orifice entrains water from the tube, creating a spray, which is broken into finer droplets by impact on an anvil. This method produces a majority of droplets in the range 2–5 μm diameter.
- **Ultrasonic nebuliser** – This method uses an ultrasonic (1–3 MHz) transducer to break up a water feed dripping on to it. The resultant droplets are finer than those produced by the gas jet nebuliser, and are in the range 0.5–2 μm. This is the more effective technique for delivering nebulised drugs.

Disadvantages of nebulisers are that they are more complex devices than other techniques, can easily result in excessive delivery of water to the respiratory system, and have variable performance according to the droplet sizes produced.

Intravenous equipment
Historically, vascular pressures, especially the central venous pressure, were measured using a water column manometer and three-way tap. More information is obtained if the pressure changes can be converted to an electronic signal and processed by a monitor. The waveform can be displayed and stored as a trend, calculations are performed automatically, and staff are alerted when preset limits are exceeded. Transducers are incorporated into a modified giving set incorporating a sampling port and a flushing device that delivers 3 mL of fluid per hour to keep the catheter patent. A coloured stripe aids identification – red for arterial line, blue for central venous, yellow for pulmonary artery catheter. Disposable, integrated transducer giving sets are designed so that the compliance of the tubing and transducer are matched to transmit the pressure wave with minimal distortion (Figure 46.41). Earlier arrangements made with separate components were prone to either over- or under-damping of the waveform and hence inaccurate systolic or diastolic readings. The value for mean arterial pressure can usually be relied upon, since it is least distorted, and arguably should be charted instead of the more familiar systolic and diastolic values. Coincidentally, it is also the more accurate when measured by automated cuff methods.

Intravenous cannulae
These vary from the simple winged steel needle of the 'butterfly' pattern to the multi-lumen central venous catheter. The winged steel needle is now rarely used in the UK except for subcutaneous infusions. It has been superseded by the plastic cannula over needle pattern, which is associated with a much lower incidence of extravasation. Those made of translucent plastic are somewhat easier to place, but the smoothness and mechanical strength of

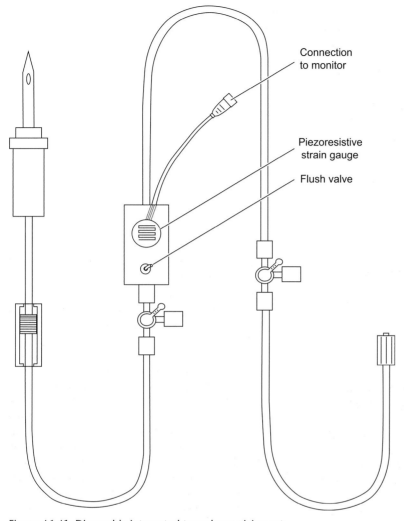

Connection
to monitor

Piezoresistive
strain gauge

Flush valve

Figure 46.41 Disposable integrated transducer giving set

the material are important considerations. Some needle types are made ultra-sharp with a double-angled bevel, and all include a flashback chamber to indicate successful venepuncture. Cannulae are colour-coded by the manufacturer to indicate the gauge. Some terminate with a Luer lock fitting whereas others also have an injection port. Other designs have resulted from attempts to reduce needlestick injuries.

Although central venous catheters can be placed by an over-the-needle approach, this limits the length of the combination to about 15 cm. A 'through-the-needle' method enables longer catheters to be placed, but then

larger-diameter catheters require even larger needles. A safer approach was pioneered by Seldinger, who used a fine-gauge needle to seek the central vein into which he inserted a thin guide wire. The track was then enlarged with a vein dilator passed over the wire, allowing the larger-diameter catheter to be similarly placed. Those intended for short-term monitoring or drug administration are sutured to the skin by the hub. This method of fixation is not appropriate for lines intended to be used over a period of weeks or months for chemotherapy or long-term parenteral nutrition. Instead, such lines are retained by having a cuff of fibrous material bonded to the line that becomes firmly anchored by the ingrowth of scar tissue after 2–3 weeks.

Intravenous giving sets

Giving sets consist of a clear plastic tube terminating at one end in a Luer lock adapter for the IV cannula and the other end in a spike for insertion into the bag of fluid. Manually controlled adult sets produce a drop size of 20 per millilitre, whereas paediatric sets are more easily regulated since the drop size is 60 per millilitre. While some automated drip controllers use standard giving sets, the majority require the use of the manufacturer's own disposables. Simple giving sets intended just for low-viscosity crystalloid administration deliver an acceptable flow rate through cheaper, narrow-gauge tubing. Blood is more viscous and is best given through wider tubing and a drip chamber that incorporates a 150 μm mesh filter. Most designs either terminate in a rubber end or have a dedicated injection port so that bolus doses of drugs can be given. Additional filters can be placed in-line to remove undesirable leucocytes and platelet aggregates from fresh blood. Crystalloid filters with an even finer mesh can retain microscopic particles of undissolved drugs, plastic, glass, rubber and bacteria as well as preventing air embolism. In theory, drugs too can be adsorbed onto these filters and the plastic of the giving sets, but this is only a problem with very potent drugs given in microgram doses.

Blood warmers

The earliest method of warming refrigerated blood was to use an extended giving set that was dipped into an electrically heated water bath. Later versions consisted of a modified giving set sandwiched between electrically heated dry plates. At slow flow rates, though the blood leaves the warmer at 37 °C it cools significantly before reaching the patient. The maximum flow rate of the dry plate type is limited even when using a pneumatic pressure bag. If the blood loss can be measured in litres per minute there are designs ('level 1' blood warmer) which will permit resuscitation at this rate. The conducting tubing is all large-bore, and obviously the intravenous cannula should be as large as possible too.

Regional anaesthesia equipment

Although standard intravenous needles can be used for regional anaesthesia, success rates can be improved by using needles specifically designed for the purpose. These have a shorter bevel, which, although more difficult to insert through the skin, affords a greater 'feel' as it penetrates the tissues, and this results in less trauma to the nerve. The needles come in a range of sizes, and some incorporate a short length of flexible plastic tubing so that movement of the tip is minimised during the injection of local anaesthetic. Other needles are electrically insulated for connection to a nerve stimulator. These are battery-powered devices that produce a small current at the tip of the advancing needle, which produces parasthesiae or motor stimulation when correctly placed.

Ultrasound needles

The use of ultrasound guidance when performing peripheral nerve blocks is becoming increasingly widespread in order to improve efficacy and reduce the incidence of complications. It is particularly recommended when blocks are performed in areas such as the head and neck, where there can be a risk of serious complications such as pneumothorax or intravascular injection.

Specialised needles have been developed for use in ultrasound-guided blocks, which have laser-etched shafts and tips in order to improve their ultrasound reflectivity. This enhances the visibility of the needles during scanning, thus reducing the likelihood of unwanted perforation of structures.

Spinal needles

These are needles modified to access the subarachnoid space. Adult needles are 10 cm long and are produced in a range of sizes and tip types. Needles of size 22 G to 29 G are used in anaesthesia, whereas the larger 18 G needle is only needed to obtain CSF if it is expected to be purulent in suspected meningitis. The needles incorporate an inner stylet that helps to stiffen the needle during its insertion and prevents the lumen from being occluded by a core of tissue. The hubs are made of translucent plastic so that the emerging CSF can be easily seen. Usually the plastic component of the needle is colour-coded to identify the needle gauge. While an incidence of headache is inevitable after dural puncture, it is related to the size of the hole or tear in the dura. This can be minimised by using a needle with an *atraumatic* tip such as the pencil-tipped Whitacre or Sprotte type, and by using the smallest possible gauge.

Epidural needles and catheters

A modified needle is used to place a catheter into the epidural space. The most widely used needle in the UK is the Tuohy (1945) needle. Adult needles are 10 cm long and marked at 1 cm intervals. They are either 16 or 18 G and come with a metal or plastic stylet. The hub has a Luer lock fitting to accept the *loss of resistance syringe* (glass or plastic) and is supplied with or without wings. The bevel has been rounded to a blunt Huber tip designed to give the maximum 'feel' when inserted through the ligaments and not be so sharp as to penetrate the more delicate dura. The angled tip helps direct the epidural catheter in the desired direction. While there are epidural catheters that are open-ended, the most widely used pattern in the UK has a blind end, with the local anaesthetic exiting by three small holes near the tip. This style is said to be less likely to enter a dural vein and should reduce the chances of intravascular injection of local anaesthetic. The catheter is marked in centimetres at the distal end to aid placement of the intended length in the epidural space. The proximal end is fitted to a Luer lock connector, and all injections should be given through a filter to remove particles of glass or bacteria.

The increasing popularity of the combined spinal and epidural (CSE) technique for obstetric analgesia has resulted in the introduction of kits containing modified epidural needles, catheters and matching spinal needles.

Infusions of drugs into the epidural space are best delivered from one of the purpose-designed pumps now available. Potential confusion with drip controllers is prevented, and the additional security features are an important safeguard so that patients or their relatives or unauthorised staff are prevented from altering the infusion rates.

Methods of sterilisation

There is a range of methods for cleaning equipment, from decontamination through disinfection to sterilisation:
- **Decontamination** – the physical removal of infected material by washing or scrubbing

Figure 46.42 Methods of disinfection and sterilisation

Disinfection
(1) Pasteurisation
• 20 minutes at 70 °C or
• 10 minutes at 80 °C or
• 5 minutes at 100 °C
(2) Chemical
• formaldehyde or
• 70% alcohol or
• 0.1–0.5% chlorhexidine or
• 2% gluteraldehyde or
• 10% hypochlorite solution or
• hydrogen peroxide or
• phenol
Sterilisation
(1) Dry heat
• 150 °C for 30 minutes
(2) Moist heat (steam under pressure: autoclaving)
• 30 minutes at 1 atmosphere 122 °C or
• 10 minutes at 1.5 atmospheres 126 °C or
• 3 minutes at 2 atmospheres 134 °C
(3) Ethylene oxide
(4) Gamma irradiation

- **Disinfection** – the killing of non-sporing organisms
- **Sterilisation** – the killing of all microorganisms including viruses, fungi and spores

Methods of disinfection and sterilisation are listed in Figure 46.42.

Index